MW01013089

The Sports Medicine Resource Manual

The Sports Medicine Resource Manual

Peter H. Seidenberg, MD, FAAFP
President and Co-Founder
King Medical Care, Inc.
Bloomsburg, Pennsylvania

Anthony I. Beutler, MD
Chief
Injury Prevention Research Laboratory
Assistant Professor
Department of Family Medicine
Uniformed Services University of the Health Sciences
Bethesda, Maryland

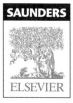

SAUNDERS

ELSEVIER

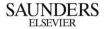

1600 John F. Kennedy Blvd.
Ste 1800
Philadelphia, PA 19103-2899

THE SPORTS MEDICINE RESOURCE MANUAL   ISBN: 978-1-4160-3197-0

Copyright © 2008 by Saunders, an imprint of Elsevier Inc.

All rights reserved. No part of this publication may be reproduced or transmitted in any form or by any means, electronic or mechanical, including photocopying, recording, or any information storage and retrieval system, without permission in writing from the publisher. Permissions may be sought directly from Elsevier's Rights Department: phone: (+1) 215 239 3804 (US) or (+44) 1865 843830 (UK); fax: (+44) 1865 853333; e-mail: healthpermissions@elsevier.com. You may also complete your request on-line via the Elsevier website at http://www.elsevier.com/permissions.

Notice

Knowledge and best practice in this field are constantly changing. As new research and experience broaden our knowledge, changes in practice, treatment, and drug therapy may become necessary or appropriate. Readers are advised to check the most current information provided (i) on procedures featured or (ii) by the manufacturer of each product to be administered to verify the recommended dose or formula, the method and duration of administration, and contraindications. It is the responsibility of the practitioner, relying on their own experience and knowledge of the patient, to make diagnoses, to determine dosages and the best treatment for each individual patient, and to take all appropriate safety precautions. To the fullest extent of the law, neither the Publisher nor the Editors assume any liability for any injury and/or damage to persons or property arising out of or related to any use of the material contained in this book.

The Publisher

Library of Congress Cataloging-in-Publication Data

Seidenberg, Peter H.
   The sports medicine resource manual / Peter H. Seidenberg, Anthony I. Beutler. — 1st ed.
      p. ; cm.
   Includes bibliographical references.
   ISBN 978-1-4160-3197-0
   1. Sports medicine. 2. Sports injuries. I. Beutler, Anthony I. II. Title.
   [DNLM: 1. Athletic Injuries—diagnosis. 2. Athletic Injuries—therapy. 3. Physician's Role. 4. Sports Medicine—methods. QT 261 S458s 2008]

RC1210.S43 2008
617.1'027—dc22

2007041856

Acquisitions Editor: Rolla Couchman
Developmental Editor: Pamela Hetherington
Publishing Services Manager: Joan Sinclair
Design Direction: Karen O'Keefe Owens

Printed in the United States of America

Last digit is the print number: 9 8 7 6 5 4 3 2 1

Working together to grow
libraries in developing countries

www.elsevier.com | www.bookaid.org | www.sabre.org

ELSEVIER   BOOK AID International   Sabre Foundation

Dedication

We would like to thank our many teachers—those wonderful men and women who cared and took time from their busy lives to explain complex things to simple minds.

This book is dedicated to our families—our parents; our children; but most of all to our patient and wonderful wives, Jen and Angie.

Contributors

MAJ Chad Asplund, MD
Sports Medicine Coordinator; Department of Family and Community Medicine; Eisenhower Army Medical Center; Fort Gordon, Georgia

Michael Barron, MD
Family Physician; Department of Family Medicine; Southern Illinois Healthcare Foundation; Belleville, Illinois

Anthony I. Beutler, MD
Chief; Injury Prevention Research Laboratory; Assistant Professor; Department of Family Medicine; Uniformed Services University of the Health Sciences; Bethesda, Maryland

Barry P. Boden, MD
Adjunct Associate Professor in Surgery; Department of Orthopaedic Surgery; F. Edward Herbert School of Medicine; Uniformed Services University of the Health Sciences; Bethesda, Maryland; Orthopaedic Surgeon; The Orthopaedic Center; Rockville, Maryland

Jimmy D. Bowen, MD, FAAPMR, CSCS
Assistant Professor; Departments of Surgery and Physical Medicine; Uniformed Services University of the Health Sciences; Bethesda, Maryland; Clinical Instructor; Southeast Missouri State University; Medical Director; Department of Sports Medicine; St. Francis Medical Center; Staff Psychiatrist; Orthopedic Associates of Southeast Missouri; Cape Girardeau, Missouri

Lori A. Boyajian-O'Neill, DO
Associate Professor and Chair; Department of Family Medicine; Kansas City University of Medicine and Biosciences; Kansas City, Missouri

Fred H. Brennan, Jr, DO, FAOASM, FAAFP
Director; National Capital Consortium Tri-Service Primary Care Sports Medicine Fellowship Program; Bethesda, Maryland; Assistant Team Physician; George Mason University; Fairfax, Virginia

Jorge Cabrera, MD, PhD
Resident; Department of Family Practice; Womack Army Medical Center; Fort Bragg, North Carolina

Gregg Calhoon, ATC
Athletic Trainer; Department of Physical Education; United States Naval Academy; Annapolis, Maryland

Michael Cannon, MD, MS
Assistant Professor; Department of Community and Family Medicine; Saint Louis University School of Medicine; St. Louis, Missouri

Dennis A. Cardone, DO
Children's Sports Center; Pediatric Orthopedics of South Florida; Fort Myers, Florida

Elizabeth J. Caschetta, MS, ATC
Certified Athletic Trainer; Illini Sports Medicine; Belleville, Illinois

Marc A. Childress, MD
Assistant Professor; Department of Family Medicine; Uniformed Services University of the Health Sciences; Bethesda, Maryland; Teaching Physician; Deparment of Family Medicine; Malcolm Grow Medical Center; Andrews Air Force Base, Maryland

Raymond D. Chronister, ATC
Assistant Athletic Trainer; Department of Physical Education; United States Naval Academy; Annapolis, Maryland

Greg Dammann, MD
Resident; Department of Orthopaedic Surgery; Tripler Army Medical Center; Honolulu, Hawaii

W. Scott Deitche, MD
Director of Sports Medicine; Family Medicine Residency Center; Carl R. Darnall Army Medical Center; Fort Hood, Texas

Patricia A. Deuster, PhD, MPH
Professor; Department of Military and Emergency Medicine; Uniformed Services University of the Health Sciences School of Medicine; Scientific Director; Consortium for Health and Human Performance; Bethesda, Maryland

LTC Kevin deWeber, MD, FAAFP
Director; Military Primary Care Sports Medicine Fellowship; Assistant Professor of Family Medicine; Uniformed Services University of the Health Sciences; Bethesda, Maryland

Pierre A. d'Hemecourt, MD
Director of Primary Care Sports Medicine; Division of Sports Medicine; Boston Children's Hospital; Harvard Medical School; Boston, Massachusetts; Team Physician; Department of Health Services; Boston College; Chestnut Hill, Massachusetts

David A. Djuric, MD
Resident; Department of Family Medicine; Dewitt Army Community Hospital; Fort Belvoir, Virginia

Timothy Dwyer, MD
Senior Medical Officer; Ray Hall Branch Medical Clinic; The Basic School; Quantico, Virginia

Adam J. Farber, MD
Chief Resident; Department of Orthopaedic Surgery; Johns Hopkins Hospital; Baltimore, Maryland

CPT David D. Farnsworth, MD
Resident; Saint Louis University Family Medicine Residency; Cardinal Glennon Children's Hospital; St. Louis, Missouri; Department of Family Medicine; St. Elizabeth's Hospital; Belleville, Illinois

Karl B. Fields, MD
Professor and Associate Chairman; Department of Family Medicine; University of North Carolina; Director; Family Practice Residency and Sports Medicine Fellowship; Moses H. Cone Health System; Greensboro, North Carolina

Scott D. Flinn, MD
Clinical Professor; University of California, San Diego; Force Surgeon; Commander Naval Surface Forces; United States Navy; San Diego, California

Bradley D. Fullerton, MD, FAAPMR
Physical Medicine and Rehabilitation Preceptor; University of Texas Medical Branch; Galveston, Texas; Consulting Physiatrist in Ultrasound Research; Human Engineering Research Laboratory; University of Pittsburgh; Pittsburgh, Pennsylvania; Medical Director of Spasticity Clinic; Dell Children's Hospital; Austin, Texas

CPT Richard Geshel, DO
Staff Physician; Department of Family Medicine; Reynolds Army Community Hospital; Fort Sill, Oklahoma

MAJ Rodney Gonzales, MD
Family Medicine Residency Program; Martin Army Community Hospital; Fort Benning, Georgia

Norman W. Gill III, PT, DSc, Cert MPT, OCS, FAAOMPT
Department of Orthopaedics and Rehabilitation; Walter Reed Army Medical Center; Washington, DC

Elise T. Gordon, MD
Physician; Department of Family Medicine/Sports Medicine; Naval Hospital of Pensacola; Pensacola, Florida

Lyndon B. Gross, MD, PhD
Assistant Professor; Department of Orthopedic Surgery; Saint Louis University; Active Provisional Staff; Department of Orthopedic Surgery; Des Peres Hospital; Active Provisional Staff; Department of Orthopedic Surgery; St. Joseph's Hospital; Courtesy Staff Physician; Department of Orthopedic Surgery; Missouri Baptist Medical Center; St. Louis, Missouri

Philip Ham, DO
Director; Board Certified Family Practice Physician; Department of Family Practice; United States Air Force; Cannon Air Force Base, New Mexico

Yuval Heled, PhD
Assistant Professor; Department of Military and Emergency Medicine; Uniformed Services University of the Health Sciences School of Medicine; Bethesda, Maryland; Researcher; Heller Institute of Medical Research; Sheba Medical Center; Tel Hashomer; Ramat Gan, Israel

MAJ Duane R. Hennion, MD
Department of Family Medicine; Uniformed Services University of the Health Sciences; Bethesda, Maryland

Thomas M. Howard, MD
Assistant Clinical Professor; Department of Family Medicine; Virginia Commonwealth University School of Medicine; Richmond, Virginia; Program Director; Virginia Commonwealth University; Fairfax Family Practice Sports Medicine Fellowship; Fairfax, Virginia

Allyson S. Howe, MD
Director of Sports Medicine; Department of Family Medicine; Malcolm Grow Medical Center; Andrews Air Force Base, Maryland

Wesley R. Ibazebo, MD
Resident; Department of Physical Medicine and Rehabilitation; University of North Carolina at Chapel Hill; Chapel Hill, North Carolina

MAJ Christopher G. Jarvis, MD, FAAFP
Senior Sports Medicine Fellow; Department of Family Medicine; Uniformed Services University of the Health Sciences; Bethesda, Maryland

Shawn F. Kane, MD
Family Physician; Primary Care Sports Medicine; Blanchfield Army Community Hospital; Fort Campbell, Kentucky

Brandon D. Larkin, MD
Primary Care Sports Medicine Fellow; Department of Community and Family Medicine; Saint Louis University; St. Louis, Missouri

LTC Jeff C. Leggitt, MD
LTS US Army

James D. Leiber, DO
Assistant Professor; Department of Family Medicine; Department of Osteopathic Principles and Practice; Lake Erie College of Osteopathic Medicine; Bradenton, Florida

Christopher J. Lettieri, MD
Associate Professor of Medicine; Department of Medicine; Uniformed Services University of the Health Sciences; Bethesda, Maryland; Medical Director; Sleep Disorders Clinic; Pulmonary, Critical Care, and Sleep Medicine; Walter Reed Army Medical Center; Washington, DC

Jeffrey L. Levy, DO
Director; Primary Care Sports Medicine; Family Medicine
Residency Clinic; Womack Army Medical Center; Fort Bragg,
North Carolina; Team Physician; Methodist College; Fayetteville,
North Carolina

MAJ Guy R. Majkowski, PT, DSc, OCS, FAAOMPT
Director of Rehabilitation Services; Malcolm Grow Medical
Center; Andrews Air Force Base, Maryland

Geof D. Manzo, MS, ATC
Approved Offsite Clinical Instructor; Athletic Training;
McKendree College; Lebanon, Illinois; Certified Athletic Trainer;
Illini Sports Medicine/Professional Therapy Services; St.
Elizabeth's Hospital; Belleville, Illinois; Head Athletic Trainer;
Gateway Grizzlies Independent Minor League Baseball Club;
Sauget, Illinois

Timothy J. Mazzola, MD
Team Physician (Former); US Air Force Academy; United States
Air Force Academy, Colorado; Chief; Pagosa Springs Sports
Medicine; Pagosa Springs, Colorado

Andrew T. McDonald, MD
Team Physician; Primary Care and Sports Medicine; Rose-
Hulman Institute of Technology; Sports Medicine Physician;
Bone & Joint Center; AP&S Clinic; Terre Haute, Indiana

MAJ Howard J. McGowan, MD
Assistant Professor; Department of Family Medicine; Uniformed
Services University of the Health Sciences; Bethesda, Maryland;
Teaching Physician; Department of Family Medicine; Malcolm
Grow Medical Center; Andrews Air Force Base, Maryland

MAJ Christopher D. Meyering, DO
Sports Medicine Fellow; Primary Care Sports Medicine; DeWitt
Army Community Hospital; Fort Belvoir, Virginia; Sports
Medicine Fellow; Tri-Service Primary Care Sports Medicine
Fellowship; Uniformed Services University of the Health
Sciences; Bethesda, Maryland

William A. Mitchell III, MD
Fellow; Primary Care Sports Medicine Fellowship; Saint Louis
University; St. Louis, Missouri; Fellow; Department of Family
and Community Medicine; St. Elizabeth's Hospital;
Belleville, Illinois

Ryan E. Modlinski, MD
Fellow; Primary Care Sports Medicine; Moses H. Cone Family
Medicine Residency; Greensboro, North Carolina

Sean T. Mullendore, MD
Adjunct Assistant Professor; Department of Family Medicine;
University of Nebraska Medical Center; Staff Family/Sports
Physician; 55 MDOS/SGOPR; Ehrling Bergquist USAF Clinic;
Offutt AFB; Omaha, Nebraska

Daniel L. Munton, MD
Staff Physician; Physical Medicine and Rehabilitation;
Department of Sports Medicine; Abilene Sports Medicine and
Orthopedics; Abilene, Texas

Melissa Nebzydoski, DO
Resident; Department of Family Medicine; Dewitt Army
Community Hospital; Fort Belvoir, Virginia

Jay E. Noffsinger, MD
Professor of Pediatrics; Saint Louis University School of
Medicine; Director of Medical Student Education; Pediatric
Sports Medicine; Cardinal Glennon Children's Medical Center;
St. Louis, Missouri

Rochelle M. Nolte, MD
Sports Medicine Physician; Aviation Medical Officer; US Coast
Guard; San Diego, California

Francis G. O'Connor, MD, MPH
Medical Director; Human Performance Lab; Military and
Emergency Medicine; Associate Professor of Family
Medicine; Department of Military and Emergency Medicine;
Uniformed Services University of the Health Sciences; Bethesda,
Maryland

CPT Jessica A. Pesce, MS, PT
Assistant Chief; Physical Therapy; Womack Army Medical
Center; Fort Bragg, North Carolina

James Phillips, MD
Captain; United States Army Medical Corps; Darmstadt Health
Clinic; Darmstadt, Germany

Nicholas A. Piantanida, MD
Assistant Professor; Department of Family Medicine; Uniformed
Services University of the Health Sciences; Bethesda, Maryland;
Director; Primary Care Sports Medicine; Primary Care
Department; Keller Army Community Hospital; West Point,
New York

Scott A. Playford, MD
Sports Medicine Physician; Camp Geiger Sports Medicine; Naval
Hospital Camp Lejeune; Jacksonville, North Carolina

MAJ Christopher M. Prior, DO, FAAFP
Assistant Professor; Department of Family Practice; Uniformed
Services University of the Health Sciences; Bethesda, Maryland;
Director of Sports Medicine; Family Medicine; Columbine
Medical Center; Family Physician; Department of Family
Practice; Littleton Adventist Hospital; Littleton, Colorado;
President; Rocky Mountain Sports Medicine Association; Castle
Rock, Colorado

Bernard Purcell, MS
Manager; Injury Prevention Research Laboratory; Department of
Family Medicine; Uniformed Services University of the Health
Sciences; Bethesda, Maryland

Scott W. Pyne, MD, FAAFP, FACSM
Assistant Professor; Department of Family Medicine; Uniformed
Services University of the Health Sciences; Bethesda, Maryland;
Director of Health Services; Chief of the Medical Staff; Team
Physician; United States Naval Academy; Naval Health Clinic
Annapolis; Annapolis, Maryland

Ahmed A. Radwan, MD
Family Medicine Attending/Sports Medicine Fellowship Staff
Physician; Family Medicine/Sports Medicine; Saint Louis
University; St. Louis, Missouri; Family Medicine Attending/
Sports Medicine Fellowship Staff Physician; Family Medicine/
Sports Medicine; St. Elizabeth's Hospital; Belleville, Illinois

LCDR Leslie H. Rassner, MD
Assistant Professor; Department of Family Medicine; Uniformed
Services University of the Health Sciences; Bethesda, Maryland;
Head; Division of Sports Medicine; Department of Orthopedics;
Residency Staff Physician; Department of Family Medicine;
Naval Hospital Camp Lejeune; Camp Lejeune, North Carolina

Jennifer Reed, MD, FAAPMR
Professor; Eastern Virginia Medical School; Norfolk, Virginia;
Attending Physician; Bone & Joint/Sports Medicine Institute;
Naval Medical Center; Portsmouth, Virginia

K. Dean Reeves, MD
Clinical Associate Professor; Physical Medicine and
Rehabilitation; University of Kansas Medical Center; Lawrence,
Kansas; Rehabilitation Medical Director; Meadowbrook
Rehabilitation Hospital; Gardner, Kansas

Peter H. Seidenberg, MD, FAAFP
President and Co-Founder; King Medical Care, Inc.;
Bloomsburg, Pennsylvania

Joel L. Shaw, MD
Assistant Professor; Department of Family Medicine; Uniformed
Services University of the Health Sciences; Bethesda, Maryland;
Assistant Fellowship Director; Tri-Service Primary Care Sports
Medicine Fellowship; Dewitt Army Community Hospital; Fort
Belvoir, Virginia

Mark A. Slabaugh, MD
Associate Professor; Department of Surgery; Uniformed Services
University of the Health Sciences; Bethesda, Maryland; Chief of
Orthopaedics; Department of Orthopaedics; Malcolm Grow
Medical Center; Andrews Air Force Base, Maryland

Mark B. Stephens, MD, MS
Associate Professor; Family Medicine; Uniformed Services
University of the Health Sciences; Bethesda, Maryland

Janiece N. Stewart, MD
Fellow; Primary Care Sports Medicine; Saint Louis University; St.
Louis, Missouri; Assistant Professor; Illini Sports Medicine; St.
Elizabeth's Hospital; Belleville, Illinois

Patrick St. Pierre, MD
Assistant Professor; Orthopaedic Surgery; Uniformed Services
University of the Health Sciences; Bethesda, Maryland;
Associate Director; Nirschl Orthopaedic Sports Medicine
Fellowship; Virginia Hospital Center; Arlington, Virginia

Timothy L. Switaj, MD
Resident; Department of Family Medicine; Dewitt Army
Community Hospital; Fort Belvoir, Virginia

Sean Thomas, MD
Family Medicine Residency Faculty; Womack Army Medical
Center; Fort Bragg, North Carolina

Stephen J. Titus, MD
Assistant Professor; Department of Family Medicine; Uniformed
Services University of the Health Sciences; Bethesda, Maryland;
Teaching Faculty; Family Medicine Residency; Malcolm Grow
Medical Center; Andrews Air Force Base, Maryland

Gaston Topol, MD
Team Physiatrist; Rosario Rugby Union; Rosario, Argentina

Brian K. Unwin, MD
Vice Chair for Education; Assistant Professor of Family Medicine
and Geriatrics; Department of Family Medicine; Uniformed
Services University of the Health Sciences School of Medicine;
Faculty Physician; National Naval Medical Center; Bethesda,
Maryland; Faculty Physician; Dewitt Army Community Hospital;
Fort Belvoir, Virginia; Faculty Physician; Walter Reed Army
Medical Center; Washington, DC

Charles W. Webb, DO, FAAFP
Assistant Professor; Department of Family Medicine; Oregon
Health and Science University; Portland, Oregon; Director;
Primary Care Sports Medicine; Department of Family Medicine;
Madigan Army Medical Center; Tacoma, Washington

John H. Wilckens, MD
Associate Professor; Orthopaedic Surgery; Johns Hopkins
University School of Medicine; Attending Orthopaedic Surgeon,
Chairman; Orthopaedic Surgery; Johns Hopkins Bayview
Medical Center; Team Physician; Baltimore Orioles; Baltimore,
Maryland; Orthopaedic Consultant; Naval Academy Athletic
Association; Annapolis, Maryland

Pamela M. Williams, MD
Assistant Professor; Department of Family Medicine; Uniformed
Services University of the Health Sciences; Bethesda, Maryland

Derek A. Woessner, MD
Staff Physician; Martin Army Community Hospital; Fort Benning,
Georgia

Nicole T. Yedlinsky, MD
Family Practice Physician; Department of Primary Care; Bayne-
Jones Army Community Hospital; Fort Polk, Louisiana

The views expressed in this textbook are those of the authors and should not be construed as official policy of the Department of the Air Force, the Department of the Army, the Department of the Navy, or the Department of Defense.

Foreword

Francis G. O'Connor, MD, MPH

"You find what you look for, and diagnose what you know."

—Dr. Jack Houston

The late Dr. Jack Houston, founder of the Houston Sports Medicine Clinic and educator of many of today's leaders in sports medicine, is credited with the above quote, which invites all clinicians to "think outside the box." As a clinical educator, I have invoked this quote for years in an attempt to inspire primary care sports medicine fellows and family medicine residents. My goal is to remind them that they are limited only by their own imagination and that, in many respects, they are their patients' most important risk factor.

Primary care sports medicine has been a discipline practiced by primary care providers for many years. In 1988, Tucker and O'Bryan published that the great majority of physicians who were field side on Friday night in New York state for high-school football games were family physicians.[1] Many of us with a little gray hair have fond memories of that first preparticipation examination in high school being performed in a busy gymnasium by the community family physician—the sports doc—who may well also have delivered us.

About the same time as Tucker and O'Bryan's study, a steady sentiment was growing in the primary care community that additional training (fellowship) in primary care sports medicine would be of great service to family physicians, internists, physical medicine and rehabilitation physicians, pediatricians, and emergency medicine physicians who were interested in gaining more expertise in this area. Sports medicine fellowships soon became quite popular and were sponsored throughout the country in academic family medicine departments, orthopedics departments, and private practice groups. The journal *The Physician and Sportsmedicine* became a must have, with its annual issue updating fellowships across the country.[2]

In April 1993, the first board examination in sports medicine, which was a certificate of added qualification, was offered to family physicians, internists, and pediatricians. At that time, a variety of fellowships were offered, there was no formal accreditation process, and physicians who could demonstrate practical experience were "grandfathered" into the board examination. In addition, there was a fair amount of anxiety among the growing number of primary care sports physicians because the discipline had not yet been clearly defined, and there were few if any core textbooks or published curricula.[3-5]

Since that time the field of primary care sports medicine has dramatically changed. Fellowships are now accredited by the Accreditation Council for Graduate Medical Education by strict criteria. An examinee who desires to sit for the Certificate of Added Qualifications examination must be a graduate of an accredited fellowship. Physiatrists will sit for the board examination in sports medicine for the first time in 2007.

Hundreds of graduates abound from many fine fellowships, and they have found excellent clinical opportunities as academic leaders and private-practice clinicians. The American Medical Society of Sports Medicine was founded in 1991, with the mission being to offer a forum that fosters a collegial relationship among dedicated, competent, primary care sports medicine physicians as they seek to improve their individual expertise and raise, with integrity, the general level of sports medicine practice.[6] In addition, the American College of Sports Medicine, which was founded in 1954, inaugurated its first family physician, William O. Roberts, MD, as College President in 2004.[7]

Accordingly, the written field has also changed. The discipline now has several leading journals, as well as clinical sections in other sports medicine journals. In addition to the journal literature, textbooks that were rare in 1993 abound as leaders and fellowship graduates have been quick to define the discipline. Books currently available for primary care sports medicine physicians range in scope, from definitive texts addressing defined areas to broad-based, evidence-based review texts to books devoted to exploring the idiosyncrasies of field-side coverage and monographs comprehensively detailing physical examination techniques. Missing in this picture, however, has been a definitive text that seeks to identify and describe in detail the core procedures that define the sports medicine practitioner, both in the office as well as at the field side.

Peter Seidenberg and Anthony Beutler, both of whom are fellowship-trained primary care sports medicine physicians and accomplished clinical educators and researchers, recognized this missing piece. They have identified the skill set, assembled a host of talented authors, and produced a textbook that defines the integrated cognitive and procedural approach necessary to succeed as a sports medicine clinician.

For those of us who have seen the birth and growth of the discipline of primary care sports medicine, we remember pivotal moments that helped to shape the specialty: board certification, accredited fellowships, the founding of the American Medical Society of Sports Medicine, the first family physician to lead the American College of Sports Medicine, and key advancements in sports medicine literature that have shaped our specialty. Just as a Strauss or Birrer text was instrumental for the first Certificate of Added Qualifications and a Mellion handbook was a necessary companion for all sports physicians attending a training room, I have no doubt that this Seidenberg/Beutler *Sports Medicine Resource Manual* will become a "must have" for every graduating family medicine resident and beginning sports medicine fellow as well as a cornerstone teaching text for their attending physicians.

Returning to Dr. Houston's quotation, Drs. Seidenberg and Beutler have been out-of-the-box thinkers, and they have truly edited a unique manuscript that will assume a fundamental position for sports medicine providers. I'm proud to have had a role in their education, and I'm sure that Dr. Houston would have admired their contribution to the field of sports medicine.

REFERENCES

1. Tucker JB, O'Bryan JJ, et al: Medical coverage of high school football in New York state. Phys Sportsmed 1988;16(9):120-128.
2. The Physician and Sportsmedicine home page (Web site). Available at www.physsportsmed.com. Accessed March 27, 2007.
3. Strauss RB: Sports Medicine, 2nd ed. Philadelphia, WB Saunders, 1991.

4. Birrer RB: Sports Medicine for the Primary Care Physician. Philadelphia, Appleton & Lange, 1984.

5. Mellion MB, Walsh WM, Shelton GL (eds): The Team Physician's Handbook. Philadelphia, Hanley & Belfus, 1990.

6. American Medical Society for Sports Medicine home page (Web site). Available at www.amssm.org. Accessed March 27, 2007.

7. American College of Sports Medicine home page (Web site). Available at www.acsm.org. Accessed March 27, 2007.

Preface

"You never know how big the field is, until you try and walk across it..."

When we sat down to design "the one sports medicine textbook" for graduating family medicine residents and all sports fellows, we really did not imagine creating something 650 pages long. Sports medicine seemed a relatively simple thing, just muscles and bones and people hurting themselves. But as we tried to compile a single text describing the philosophy, examinations, treatments, procedures, and special considerations inherent in our daily practice, we soon gained a firsthand appreciation for how big the field is and how long it takes to walk across it.

This is a unique text. It is largely written by primary care sports medicine physicians for primary care sports medicine physicians. The orthopedists, athletic trainers, physical therapists, and other professionals who we invited to participate were chosen because of their knowledge and also because of their proven track records in training primary care sports medicine professionals. The authors in this book are not only experts in their subject matter, but they also understand how to teach their subject matter to primary care physicians. They understand it because they do it every day. As editors, we express our sincere appreciation to these dedicated professionals who have poured their souls into these chapters.

The text is organized into sections that parallel the process of sports medicine diagnosis. The opening section contains the philosophy of sports medicine: the essential duties to consider before even stepping foot on a sideline or seeing athletes in a training room. Section 2 presents the history and physical exam: how to examine and diagnose the injured athlete. After proper examination, diagnosis and treatment are presented in Section 3. In this section we have provided the basics of casting, splinting, and fracture care, as well as the treatment of traditional soft-tissue injuries. Section 4 outlines rehabilitation and bracing: the art and science of augmenting and allowing the body to heal itself. An overview of the myriad procedures and special tests in sports medicine follows in Section 5. Finally, as an overarching capstone, the appendices outline the role of exercise in maintaining health and fitness in the pediatric, pregnant, and geriatric populations.

At the turn of the twenty-first century, evidence-based medicine is fast becoming a cliché. However, the need to assess the evidence that underlies treatment recommendations remains critical. It is essential to understand not only what the evidence shows, but also what it does not show or what it has not shown yet. The evidence base of sports medicine can perhaps best be described as "growing." Applying a mature evidence scale to the growing body of sports medicine evidence would result in having nearly all evidence rated a C or a 3. Rather than do that, we have tried to create a scale that allows for and distinguishes the small study sizes typical of the current sports medicine evidence base. This text uses the following evidence scale:

Level of evidence (LOE):
A—Double-blind study
B—Clinical trial more than 20 subjects
C—Clinical trial fewer than 20 subjects
D—Series 5 or more subjects
E—Anecdotal case reports

Other levels of evidence (meta-analysis, consensus opinion, etc.) are noted as such in the text.

The age of textbooks may be drawing to a close. With so many online sources boasting up-to-date treatment recommendations and the push to make all things digital, one might wonder how this book will compete. Long after leeches are no longer fashionable for treating patellofemoral pain (that is a joke, at least in 2007!), we hope that the well-worn pages of your *Sports Medicine Resource Manual* will still be a valuable physical examination review, a familiar procedure reference, and a trusted affirmation of sports medicine and team physician philosophy.

So, whether you are a family medicine doctor trying to review and learn more about musculoskeletal medicine or a sports medicine fellow preparing to dive into your fast-paced fellowship, we hope you find this book valuable. It was lots of fun to create, and it was written for you.

Peter H. Seidenberg, MD, FAAFP
Anthony I. Beutler, MD

Contents

SECTION 3:   FRACTURES AND SOFT-TISSUE INJURIES

SECTION 4:   REHABILITATION

SECTION 5:   SPECIAL TESTS AND PROCEDURES

APPENDICES

INDEX

SECTION 1

General Principles

CHAPTER 1

The Sideline Physician

John H. Wilckens, MD

KEY POINTS

- Although being well-read and technically competent are key qualifications, engendering trust is the most important attribute of an effective sideline physician, and participating in the team chemistry will build that trust.
- The effective sideline physician must also be able to communicate well: articulating and defining the issues to the athletes, the coaches, the training staff, and the parents will provide realistic expectations that everyone understands.
- The primary goals of the sideline physician are to manage emergencies on the playing field and to evaluate injured athletes for return to competition.
- Sideline physicians should anticipate the emergencies that are unique to each particular sport. Emergency response should be planned for and rehearsed to include athletic trainers, emergency medical services personnel, event support staff, and local hospital emergency department staff.
- Same-day return-to-play criteria should include the consideration of the safety of the injured athlete and the other competitors, the risks and consequences of reinjury, the effectiveness of playing hurt, and the consequences that may affect ultimate healing.

INTRODUCTION

Athletics (i.e., playing sports) represents an important part of our society **(Figure 1.1).** In its purest and simplest form, it gives participants an opportunity to compete with others and themselves and to develop cardiovascular fitness, strength, and agility, which are seen as positive factors for a productive and long life. It also teaches teamwork, encourages development of a work ethic, and prepares individuals for the hard knocks of life. However, participation in athletics also involves the risk of injury, which is greatest during actual competition, be it youth soccer or a professional sport. Because of this risk, the profession of sports medicine has evolved to make athletics as safe as possible. The ultimate sports medicine participation is as the sideline physician during games, when the risk of injury is the greatest.

The sideline is a daunting place in which to practice medicine **(Figure 1.2).** First, the sideline physician does not have the comforts and amenities of the "ivory tower" office, with its receptionists, nurses, ancillary technicians, and easily accessible diagnostic tests and imaging. Second, the sideline physician is expected to evaluate an injured athlete, make the correct diagnosis, treat the condition, and return the athlete to optimum performance, immediately if not sooner! Evaluation of the injured player often takes place without the privacy of an examination room or the option of undressing the patient: the sideline physician may have to examine, in front of 80,000 screaming spectators, an athlete who is dressed in a uniform and bulky protective equipment and who is out of breath and writhing in pain. After the diagnosis is made, the coaching staff, the fans, the athlete, and even the parents of the athlete expect the sideline physician to treat the condition and return the athlete to play. In the office, that evaluation and discussion about the return to play allows for dialog and education; there is no such luxury on the sideline.

To define the roles and responsibilities of the sideline physician, this chapter offers not evidence-based medicine, but "eminence-based" medicine, presenting the art of sideline "physicianship" gleaned from years of experience working with respected team physicians, trainers, and coaches. Technically speaking, the terms *team physician* and *sideline physician* incorporate different concepts. The team physician takes care of the day-to-day medical needs of the team and is responsible for preparticipation evaluations, training rooms, scheduling referrals for medical conditions, and return-to-play timelines. However, he or she may not be on the sideline because of conflicting commitments. The sideline physician is the medical expert who is "on the scene" during the game. The role of the sideline physician is best fulfilled by the team physician because of the inherent knowledge of the players and related personnel and because the physician has the trust and confidence of both. However, many times the sideline physician may not have any formal connection with the team, thus making the job of caring for injured players even more difficult. No matter how competent the physician, without those relationships, the job is harder. Because the team physician and the sideline physician are most often one and the same, the terms may be used interchangeably, assuming that relationship.

REQUIREMENTS AND RESPONSIBILITIES

As in clinical medicine and athletics, preparation is critical to the success of the sideline physician. In addition to having a broad

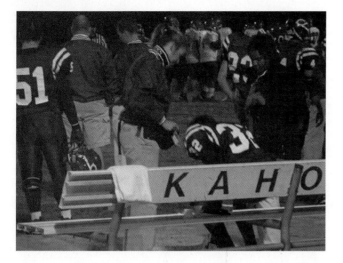

Figure 1.1   A physician *(right)* attends to an athlete with a dislocated finger.

knowledge of all aspects of sports medicine, the sideline physician needs to understand the specific sport within which he or she is working; to be familiar with the patterns of injuries and possible emergency conditions that are unique to that sport; and to develop a trusting, working relationship with all members of the team and its staff.

Sport-specific knowledge

Understanding the sport prepares the physician for the sideline. Previous participation in that sport by the physician is helpful for but not critical to understanding the sport. Each sport has a unique constellation of injuries, and the effective sideline physician will be familiar with them. Because the sideline physician is at the scene, he or she is in a unique position to witness the injury, which provides important information for the clinical examination. However, such information offers another advantage: it permits the sideline physician to make recommendations for rules modification in an attempt to make the sport safer. The most profound advances in sports medicine are not surgical techniques but rather

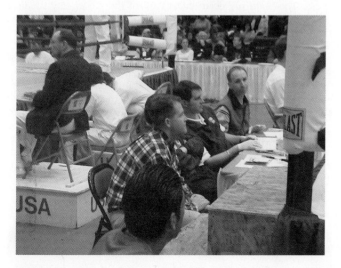

Figure 1.2   A ringside physician at the 2003 USA Boxing National Championships.

injury prevention. Injury surveillance is an important responsibility of the sideline physician.

Just as each sport has a unique constellation of injuries, it also has unique emergencies. The single most important responsibility of the sideline physician is to be able to identify and treat emergencies rapidly and appropriately. The knowledgeable sideline physician can anticipate and plan for such emergencies, and, more importantly, he or she can arrange for the rehearsal of such emergencies and the necessary responses. For example, the time to learn how to use a spine board or to discover that a player on an oversized backboard cannot be accommodated in a helicopter's patient bay is not on game day. To avoid such dangerous (and embarrassing) moments, it is essential to conduct planned drills for potential emergencies. Although it is critical to rehearse and assign responsibilities to the training staff on the field, such rehearsals also need to include local emergency medical technicians, event medical staff, and local emergency department personnel.

The sideline physician also needs to consider that the athletes are not the only individuals who are at risk for injury during a game. The officials represent a special group that is at risk for injury because—except for the home plate umpire in baseball—most wear no special protective equipment even though they are on the playing field. In addition, many are older and not as conditioned or as quick as the athletes they are regulating. There is also a risk of injury to the sideline participants, the coaching staff, the officiating staff, other players, injured players, photographers, media personnel, mascots, and of course to the most susceptible person: the one with his or her first sideline pass. The edges of the field of play can be a dangerous place because contact does not always end at the sideline. Of athletes crossing the perimeters of the playing field, 93% extend up to 12 feet past the boundaries, although approximately half (59%) travel less than 6 feet.[1] At the collegiate and professional levels, 10% of the out-of-bounds athletes travel more than 12 feet.[1] The athletes are wearing protective equipment, but the sideline personnel are not. Athletes are focused on the action, whereas sideline personnel may be distracted by taking pictures, talking on headsets, and so on. Although seasoned sideliners are usually cognizant of this extended potential injury zone, new sideline spectators and injured players may not be aware of the risks. The sideline physician can guide personnel away from a developing play. It is much easier to prevent an injury than to treat one.

Relationships

To be a good sideline physician, one has to be a good *team* physician. As such, one's effectiveness is based not only on medical and sports knowledge but also on relationships with the athletic trainers, the athletes, the coaching staff, the athletes' parents, and the team's administrative personnel. Those relationships are best built on trust, and trust develops from establishing the fact that the sideline physician is a team player who understands the mechanics, personalities, and needs of the team; who has the athletes' best interests at heart; who embraces and supports the mission and vision of the team; and who shares a common bond with the team. When it is clear that the team's and the athletes' interests are above those of the physician, then the coaches and other personnel will be more willing to accept and comply with the physician's decisions—not only the easy ones but also the difficult ones that may affect the outcome of the competition. Many times, building this relationship means going to the training room and the athletic field on a regular basis, not just to see injured athletes, but also to understand the sport and to participate in the team effort. Athletics is all about teamwork. A great technical surgeon or a compassionate, well-read physician does not always translate to an effective team physician. A physician's competence is, of course, respected, but he or she will not gain the team's confidence and trust until he or she demonstrates participation in and identification with the team. Participation in the team's chemistry will facilitate the building of that important trust. The purpose of the sideline physician in this scenario is the team's success rather than his or her practice marketability.

The most crucial relationship is the one with the athletic trainers, and the time invested in building that relationship is time well spent. These hardworking, talented providers are an important resource because they know the athletes and the coaches well. Not only during the game but also during practice and the surrounding time in the training room, they are the sideline physician's eyes and ears. A seasoned athletic trainer is a blessing: he or she can triage and manage the injured athletes effectively, and he or she can also represent the physician to the coaching staff, translating medical terminology into coaching terminology. Alternatively, a young, inexperienced athletic trainer also can be an opportunity: the physician will need to be more hands-on with regard to the medical management of the team, but the athletic trainer will be responsive and eager to learn.

Communication with the training staff is critical for the team physician, and rehearsing scenarios and practicing emergency protocols will identify opportunities to improve communication and thus the medical care provided. Much of the physician's direct involvement depends on the quality of and the trust in the training staff. If there are deficiencies in the training staff, they need to be addressed and improved. With young staff, the physician really has to take a hands-on role during the game. A seasoned and veteran staff may relieve the physician's anxiety somewhat, but effective communication still is required.

Team practice

Visits by the physician during team practice allow for visibility and the ability to meet with all members of the team without the distraction of actual playing conditions. Getting to know the athletes and coaches in this less stressful environment can provide important clues to each athlete's profile. For example, some athletes are very stoic, and only knowledge of that fact will permit the correct interpretation of a subtle finding as the indication of a substantial injury. Other athletes are "high maintenance" and require a lot of attention even with minor injuries. It is helpful to know this information before game day. Again, understanding the team is important. A team may have some positions that are deep in talent and for which the loss of one player is not critical to the team's success. Other athletes are "franchise players," and an injury that takes such a player out of the game can alter the whole team's structure, character, and chance of success. In addition, some athletes are impact players who can play at 80% capacity and still contribute, whereas other injured players who can function at 95% capacity (e.g., a quarterback with a finger injury or turf toe) will not be able to help the team at all. Such information is gleaned only after spending time with and developing a bond of trust with the team, the trainers, and the coaches. The importance of this bond of trust between the physician and the team cannot be overemphasized. It is built and earned, and it is the means of equipping and preparing the physician and the team for the difficult decisions that must be made on the sideline during competition.

Pregame considerations

To maximize effectiveness, it is critical that the physician command and control his or her schedule to allow adequate time to cover the sporting event properly. This coverage means that the physician must end clinics, office hours, and surgery schedules well in advance of game time; he or she must not be saddled with on-call responsibilities; and he or she must have a plan in place to direct his or her office staff, colleagues, midlevel providers, and

nurses to handle emergencies that may occur during the sporting event.

The sideline physician must arrive with or before the team because his or her responsibilities begin well before the opening whistle or the first pitch. If the physician is traveling with the team, arriving with the team is easy. For home events, arriving with the team is more difficult because of potential conflicts with family and practice priorities. Getting there before the team ensures timely arrival and less hassle with traffic, parking, and credentials. In addition, since the physician's last visit with the team, an athlete may have become ill, thus making playing status questionable; also there may be several "wait-and-see" injuries that need to be reevaluated. Arriving early can allow for early intervention, with improved chances for the athlete's participation in the game; it can also permit coaches to make last-minute adjustments to their game plan and roster.

In addition to caring for the "home" team, the sideline physician may also need to care for the visiting team, which may not have a traveling physician. This is a courteous and responsible gesture: seeing the visiting team, staff, and families also sets a precedent that may be reciprocated if the situation is reversed. If the visiting team has a physician, it is still appropriate for the home team's physician to meet him or her early before game time to review emergency protocols and the available medical facilities.

Arriving early also allows the physician to visit and meet with the stadium support staff, the referees, the umpires, and other event administrators, presenting another opportunity to establish or confirm the trust relationship. Not only is it a warm gesture, but doing so also provides an opportunity to review with the training staff emergency equipment, their location, and protocols. During the game, these individuals may require the physician's services, services that can be facilitated by previous acquaintance.

As a visiting team physician, it is important to search out the emergency medical services staff and home medical staff. Although the team may have played in a certain venue before, things can change that may have an impact on decisions on the field, such as radiology capability, the closest emergency department, and magnetic resonance imaging availability. The visiting sideline physician should become familiar with the local emergency protocols. It is wise to remember that the responsibility of being the team's physician is applicable not only to injured players during the game but also until that player reaches home, which may include a long aircraft ride.

Dealing with an ill athlete on game day requires the physician's early presence at the field. In brief, a low-grade fever can be treated with hydration and acetaminophen. If symptoms are limited to the upper respiratory tract, the player can be allowed to warm up. If he or she feels better, the athlete can be allowed to compete. If the athlete has general malaise, body aches, gastrointestinal symptoms, and fever, then more caution about playing should be exercised. Strenuous activity can make some viral illnesses more virulent and protracted.[2] It should be pointed out to the coach who insists on the sick player being available that there are serious drawbacks to this plan of action: (1) The illness is contagious and may inoculate other team members through shared water bottles, towels, and contact; (2) sick athletes are not as effective as well ones and have reduced strength, energy, and endurance; and (3) sick athletes are prone to making mistakes and incurring injury, thus increasing their downtime. This recommendation by the physician may be more palatable to the coaching staff if they have confidence and trust in that physician.

Always a subject of controversy is the role of precompetition injections, particularly cortisone and ketorolac (Toradol). These injectables have a use and should be included in the team physician's sideline medical bag, but their routine use before competition is challenged. Injury and pain are part of athletic competition: hence the role of the team physician. However, pain has some salvific value in that it helps identify and protect an injured body part. Eliminating that pain can lead to additional injury and delayed full recovery. Cortisone is an effective anti-inflammatory drug, but it can soften and weaken the soft tissues that it contacts. Ketorolac is an injectable nonsteroidal anti-inflammatory drug and a potent analgesic. In addition to potential injection-site problems, it may mask an injury, it can affect platelet function and bleeding, and it poses a small but identifiable risk to renal function.[3] This risk may be increased among athletes who are taking supplements.

Each team physician must make his or her own decision about the use of injectables before and during competition. The physician must carefully weigh the risks and benefits to the patient athletes, and he or she must make a decision that he or she can defend in court and sleep with at night. Some issues to consider are, for example, what happens if a pitcher requests and receives a pregame injection, the game is then cancelled, and he is scheduled to pitch the following day? Does he receive another injection? Is it safe? Also, if such an injection is offered to one player, is it then available to all on demand? Some physicians use pregame ketorolac for athletes without any symptoms, and other physicians refuse to use it at all. There are two situations in which this author would consider using a precompetition injection: an acromioclavicular separation and a hip pointer. These two conditions can be quite painful and limit one's ability to compete because of pain alone. Injecting the acromioclavicular joint or hip pointer with xylocaine/bupivacaine will allow an athlete to warm up without pain and see if he or she can play effectively.

In the absence of a definitive sports-wide ruling on this issue, the decision about the use of injectables before or during competition is the physician's personal preference. That decision should be made well in advance of game day, and it is important to communicate that decision clearly and specifically to athletes, coaches, and training staff. If the line is clearly drawn and communicated, the team may test it but will ultimately respect it. If the communication is not clear, then there may be an endless barrage of requests for injectable medication.

The physician should take an active role in the team's warm-ups so that he or she can watch and individually assess those athletes who are ill or injured. In addition to observing, the physician should not hesitate to communicate with the athlete or his or her position coach; this communication should be done not to interfere with the pregame preparation but rather to share awareness of the situation, which can build trust and confidence. In all communications with the training staff, athletes, and coaches, it is important to support the overall mission of the team. There will be risks with any decision; they should be communicated clearly, and the good coaches will understand. Just because it is safe for an injured or ill athlete to play does not mean that he or she will be effective or provide a good quality of play.

No sideline physician's preparation is complete without a thoughtfully stocked "sideline physician's bag." Recommendations are available regarding what kind of medication and equipment should be in such a bag,[4] but two practical points should be taken into consideration: (1) There is no reason to stock the bag with unfamiliar medication or equipment that the physician is unable to use, and (2) the bag needs to be well organized so that the physician can find a needed item quickly and so that he or she can also direct someone else to retrieve it while he or she is attending to an athlete (see Chapter 3 for specifics regarding the physician's bag).

Game-time position

The physician exists on the sideline for two main reasons: (1) to provide medical care in the event of an emergency, and (2) to assess an athlete's ability to return to competition after an injury.

The sideline physician should not let any other task interfere with these two priorities, and he or she should position himself or herself to be in full view of the entire playing field. Many injuries can occur away from the action, so the sideline physician should not just follow the ball. Pacing the sideline will allow one to assess players as they come off of the field. In addition, the sideline physician has a responsibility that requires great attention to detail, and he or she must not be distracted with the emotion, the drama, and the rush of competition.

MEDICAL CARE

These game-position concepts frame this author's philosophy about the participation of the sideline physician in the on-field evaluation of an injured athlete: The physician belongs on the sideline—not on the field—except for during certain specific circumstances (described later). Although this stance is controversial and may not represent what happens every weekend on television, the team physician has a limited role on the playing surface. The training staff are the first, and usually the only, responders; most calls for medical assistance on the playing field are not emergencies. The training staff should be trained to evaluate the injured athlete; the physician involved in this initial evaluation only complicates and delays the process (with a few notable exceptions, outlined later). A system that works nicely is to have the head athletic trainer and an assistant be the first responders. After the trainers are on the field, regardless of which team is involved, the sideline physician can take two to three steps onto the playing field to be in full view of the trainers on the field and to observe what is happening. The trainers will then signal if they need physician assistance. This process allows the physician to collect his or her thoughts and to anticipate the worst-case scenario on the field. Typically, during those first few seconds, the trainers will try to relieve the anxiety and agitation of the injured athlete and keep the athlete on the ground until a primary assessment can be obtained. Talking to the athlete assists with the assessment and focuses the athlete on reducing his or her agitation. Asking the athlete to move an injured extremity will provide substantial basic information.

On-field physician examinations

Each downed athlete does represent a possible medical emergency, and, for these notable exceptions (possible spine injury, lower extremity dislocation, fracture–dislocation, and unstable or open fracture), the physician should rush onto the field.

Spine injury/loss of consciousness

If there appears to have been a spine injury or a loss of consciousness, the physician is needed for the execution of the emergency protocol. Typically, an athlete with a spine injury lands face down, and a quick and systematic stabilized rollover is needed to assess the athlete. The physician should stabilize the neck and direct the spine management protocol as practiced. Any athlete who loses consciousness should be treated as having a spine injury until the athlete regains consciousness and a spine injury can be ruled out. It is critical in sports that require helmets and shoulder pads (e.g., gridiron football, lacrosse, hockey) that this equipment is left in place for the assessment and transportation of the potentially spine-injured athlete. Removing the helmet with the shoulder pads in place causes increased neck extension. In addition, the helmet typically has a snug fit, and it can help immobilize a sweaty head to the spine board. If an airway needs to be established, remove the facemask and leave the helmet on[5] (see Chapter 5 for a full discussion of emergency procedures).

Lower-extremity dislocation, fracture–dislocation, and unstable or open fracture

The physician needs to be on the field for the initial management of lower-extremity dislocation, fracture–dislocation, and unstable or open fracture, all of which may require a gentle reduction, immobilization, or both before transport off of the playing surface. The actual reduction of a displaced fracture, dislocation, or fracture–dislocation should be attempted only by personnel who are adequately trained to do so. A simple reduction by gentle exaggeration of the deformity, followed by in-line traction and correction of the deformity, can reduce most displaced fractures and dislocations; however, an improperly performed reduction can cause more injury. If the extremity becomes cyanotic and is pulseless, a reduction maneuver is indicated, regardless of physician experience. After he or she has been splinted, the athlete should be transported off the field by vehicle (i.e., by a modified golf cart ["gator"]); these athletes are usually big and sweaty, and there are possible adverse environmental conditions that make transport by stretcher difficult, painful, and dangerous.

Injury clock

Finally, if there is an injury clock (e.g., as in wrestling or lacrosse), immediate involvement of the sideline physician will save valuable time with regard to the assessment and the availability of the injured athlete.

Sideline events
Nonemergencies

For nonemergencies, the training staff's on-field examination of an injured knee, ankle, or shoulder will be repeated on the sideline under more favorable circumstances. No physician can effectively examine an injured athlete in full uniform on the playing field while under the observation of both teams, officiating staff, tens of thousands of fans (via the JumboTron [scoreboard]), and possibly a television audience (and lawyers). To do so is to create a flawed examination with little ultimate value. In addition, the patient is usually still in extreme pain and thus cannot cooperate with a thorough examination.

Emergencies

Fortunately, medical emergencies are very rare among young athletic individuals, but they do exist, and the sideline physician should think about each one in advance and develop a strategy for addressing the injury in accordance with sound medical judgment and the standard of care. Although specific emergencies are topics of other chapters, a short discussion is in order to frame them for the sideline physician.

The management of all emergencies, whether on the sideline or in the emergency department, starts with the ABCs: airway, breathing, and circulation.[6]

Respiratory distress/stridor When evaluating the downed athlete, an airway needs to be established. Again, unconscious athletes should be assumed to have a spine injury, and appropriate precautions should be taken with gentle in-line traction. A jaw thrust should establish an airway. Check for tobacco, chewing gum, and broken teeth, all of which represent potential obstructions to an airway. The mouthpiece should be removed. If an airway cannot be established, the physician must insist on the early activation of the emergency medical system. Helmets should be left in place, but faceguards should be removed.

Direct trauma to the laryngeal area (e.g., a direct blow to the larynx by a ball, puck, stick, or opponent) represents an acute airway emergency.[7] If an athlete is unable to talk and demonstrates respiratory distress, immediate plans should be formulated to establish a surgical airway.

Other causes of stridor and respiratory distress in the downed athlete include pneumothorax (patients usually can talk but are short of breath and tachypneic), tension pneumothorax (usually manifests as a more emergent shortness of breath and deviation of the trachea; usually treated with a thoracotomy on the side away from the deviation[8]), and posterior sternoclavicular dislocation (characterized by stridor, shortness of breath, or difficulty swallowing[9]). Loose bodies lodged in the airway can be displaced with a well-executed Heimlich maneuver. Respiratory distress can also occur as a result of acute anaphylaxis from medication, food, or an insect bite; injectable epinephrine should be immediately available.[10]

Cardiac arrest Cardiac arrest is rare during athletic competition. However, for those competitions involving patients who are more than 30 years old, cardiac disease is the most common cause of sudden death. Among younger patients, cardiac arrest may occur from a variety of causes, including congenital anomalies and structural, vascular, or conduction defects. Many attempts have been made to screen for these conditions. The most sensitive predictors seem to be a family history of sudden death and syncope with exercise. Athletes with either of these red flags require at a minimum that the family history be evaluated and an electrocardiogram and echocardiogram be obtained.[4] Drug abuse—specifically cocaine—can lead to cardiac irritability and sudden death. Another cause of cardiac arrest among young athletes is commotio cordis.[11] A young athlete typically is struck with a batted baseball, a thrown lacrosse ball, or a hockey puck to induce this condition. If an automated external defibrillator is available, these patients usually can be shocked and resuscitated. Without an automated external defibrillator, cardiopulmonary resuscitation should be initiated.

Neck pain The athlete with neck pain represents a particularly urgent sideline encounter. Many times the athlete is ambulatory, has mild neck pain, and is adamant about returning to play. If the athlete has pain, cervical muscle spasm, reduced range of motion, or neurologic findings, the discussion should not focus on return to play but rather on what type of immobilization, transportation, and imaging should be done urgently.[12]

Burners and stingers The burner or stinger (i.e., transient brachial plexopathy) represents another difficult decision for the sideline physician. A thorough neck and neurologic examination should be made. Any athlete with continuing symptoms should not be allowed to return to play. If symptoms clear completely during the game, consideration can be given to return to play. Athletes and concerned parties should understand that a recurrent stinger is very common. If the athlete has had a recurrent stinger, he or she can return to play that day only if symptoms have resolved, if he or she has had fewer than three previous stingers, and if those previous symptoms resolved in less than 24 hours.[13]

Bleeding Bleeding is common in athletics and may not represent an emergency. However, as a result of blood-borne pathogens (including the human immunodeficiency virus and hepatitis), most governing athletic authorities have specific guidelines for handling the bleeding athlete.[2] The sideline physician should be familiar with the recommendations set forth by the governing body of the event that is being covered. In general, the bleeding needs to be stopped and covered. Blood-soaked equipment and uniforms should be cleaned, covered, or changed to prevent possible blood-borne disease transmission. Although contracting a blood-borne disease under these conditions is a rare possibility, it represents an emotional issue.

Infectious diseases aside, actual bleeding becomes an important issue when it occurs near the face because it may interfere with the athlete's vision. The area around the orbit of the eye is vascular, and lacerations in this area may generate enough bleeding to make vision difficult. For example, in boxing, if an athlete cannot see, he or she cannot compete effectively or defend himself or herself adequately against the opponent.

Most bleeding responds to direct pressure. If there is urgency to returning the athlete to competition, a pressure dressing should be applied. As a rule, the physician should refrain from definitive wound closure on the sideline. Most wounds require irrigation and anatomic closure, which is difficult to achieve in this setting. After the competition, when conditions in the training room or the emergency department are more conducive to definitive treatment with appropriate lighting, irrigation, local anesthetic, sutures, and equipment, lacerations can be sutured. If appropriate conditions do not exist, the injured player should be referred to a place in which those conditions are met. For wound closure, the physician should use suture material that is of sufficient strength to withstand additional trauma but that is also small enough to effect a cosmetic closure. Although Dermabond represents technology with which to close most wounds effectively and cosmetically, its ability to withstand repeat trauma is unknown, and it is difficult to apply to the sweating athlete. The physician should become familiar with its storage and handling requirements because it will not work above a certain temperature.

Head injuries Head injuries are extremely difficult to examine and monitor, and they have been the cause of many shortened athletic careers, even professional ones. These injuries affect not only athletic competition but also employment, relationships, and activities of daily living. In addition, the brain is very sensitive to reinjury. To date, there is no sideline device with which to assess and definitively treat head injuries; the Standardized Assessment of Concussion (SAC) represents an early attempt at such a device.[14] However, to have worth with regard to validity, the test must be administered during the preseason, and the recorded score must be available on the sidelines. After a player is concussed, the SAC can give some insight into the brain injury. If the score is lower than baseline, it is clear evidence for keeping the athlete out of competition. Alternatively, a similar SAC score is only suggestive evidence, and it may underrepresent the injury. In this scenario, the physician's knowledge of the athlete will provide valuable information about his or her personality, responsiveness, and mood. The more unfamiliar the physician is with the athlete, the more conservative the assessment should be.

There are many criteria and classification systems for closed head injuries, and each has its own strengths and weaknesses. The sideline physician should become very familiar with one system and use it as a guide for treating closed head injuries. Decisions to play or to not play a concussed athlete should be articulated with a classification system that is appropriate for the physician's clinical acumen. The physician should refrain from modifying, mixing, and matching classification systems.

The real emergency that can occur when allowing concussed athletes to play is reinjury and the "second impact syndrome." This neurologic emergency has a 50% mortality rate[15] and appears to be more prevalent among young and adolescent athletes. The potential for autonomic deregulation can exist for up to 30 days after a closed head injury. In general, there are very few circumstances in which a concussed athlete should be allowed to return immediately to competition.[13,16,17]

Heat injury Heat injury represents a potential emergency **(Figure 1.3)**. Usually poor play from heat injury will force the athlete to the sideline long before the risk of heat stroke. Physicians should be sensitive to the temperature and humidity. Treatment begins the

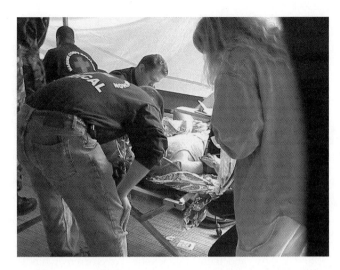

Figure 1.3 A medical team attending to a marathon participant who suffered exertional collapse.

night before with forced hydration and liberal use of salt. For heavy sweaters with a history of heat cramps, additional electrolyte solutions can be used precompetition. During competition, the liberal drinking of water and sports drinks should be encouraged. (Particular attention should be given to the officials to make sure that they are adequately hydrated.) If the athlete begins cramping, passive stretching will help break the spasm. However, after cramps start, the athlete is probably a couple of liters behind, and it will be difficult to catch up with oral hydration alone. Such athletes typically respond well to intravenous hydration (for healthy athletes, 1 or 2 L of normal saline), which is best done in the training room. Again, prevention is the best treatment: heavy sweaters should be identified, and fluids should be pushed.

RETURN-TO-PLAY DECISIONS

As discussed, on-field emergencies trigger protocols that just require execution. A broken bone or a torn anterior cruciate ligament represents a severe injury, but the decision about return to play is simple. In reality, the more minor the injury, the more consuming it is for the sideline physician because a decision must be made whether or not to return the athlete to competition.

General criteria

Same-day return-to-play criteria are extremely subjective, and they depend on the age and skill level of the athlete, the injury sustained, and the type of sport being played. Common sense represents an important element of this type of decision making, and the following thoughts should be taken into consideration **(Figure 1.4):**

1. Will clearance to play be safe for the injured athlete? Is the athlete at increased risk of injury because of his or her injury or illness? What are the risks of reinjury? What are the consequences of reinjury?

2. Will clearance to play be safe for the other competitors? Sometimes an athlete can return to competition with a splint, brace, or cast. Although doing so may protect the injured player and his or her body part, can it injure an opponent or teammate?

3. Can the athlete compete effectively? Many injuries can be treated and return to play can be safe, but the athlete is less

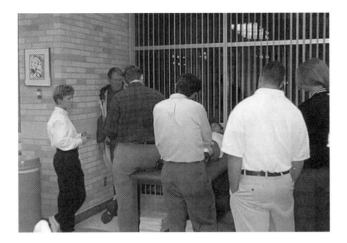

Figure 1.4   A sports medicine team gathers around an athlete to discuss the plan for safe and effective return to play.

effective. A sprained ankle may be adequately taped and braced and the athlete considered for return to play, but lost agility and speed inhibit the athlete's ability to perform. This situation may be obvious for skilled players, such as running backs, but particular concern should also be shown for those athletes whose speed and agility is not showcased, such as interior linemen. "Losing a half step" may not be so obvious on the sideline, but in the trenches, a loss of quickness in one player can put the whole backfield at increased risk.

4. Although the athlete can play safely while hurt, will continued play affect healing and his or her later ability to play effectively? For example, a pitcher with a high pitch count who is throwing well but with pain may win that game but pitch less effectively for the rest of the season.

In addition, athletes perform at high levels of skill. Subtle changes in their performance, such as lost velocity or accuracy in pitching, may signal fatigue, be a harbinger of an impending injury, or both.

The sideline physician should be aware of the context of the injury. He or she may need to inform the athletes, the coaches, and the parents about the risks and benefits of playing injured or ill. In addition, an injury that occurs at the beginning of the season may have a different solution than one that occurs during the last game of the season.

As a general working guideline, some basic principles can be applied to evaluating the injured athlete and determining the appropriateness of return to play. First, the injured part should have a functional (although not necessarily full) range of motion. Second, athletes should have protective strength. Again, an injured part may seem weaker because of the injury or as a result of pain. If the patient is allowed to return to play, the strength of the injured part should be adequate enough to function and to provide protection.

For lower-extremity injuries, a simple "hop test" will help with the decision making. After the evaluation of a strain or sprain is performed and the injury is treated, if the athlete expresses a desire to return to play, the sideline physician can ask him or her to hop or jump on the *uninjured* leg three times to provide an idea of the injured leg's preinjury ability. Next, the athlete should hop three times using both legs, and the physician should watch to see if the athlete favors the injured leg; this two-leg hop also will give the athlete some gradual confidence. Then, the athlete should hop on the injured leg. If the hop on the injured leg is adequate, the player can try to assume the playing position, attempt some jogging, and then make an effort to run. If these responses are acceptable, a sideline agility test is performed. If the physician is convinced that

the athlete is safe to play, then the decision to play rests with the position coach, who determines the athlete's effectiveness.

Some decisions regarding return to play are difficult. The injured athlete may be an impact player whose presence may be critical to the outcome of the competition. Again, decisions about athletes with major injuries are easy: they cannot return to play. However, with some injuries, the athlete can play, but he or she has limited effectiveness and may be exposed to a greater risk of reinjury. As best as he or she can, the sideline physician needs to spell out the risks, and preestablished trust will go a long way in this situation. Some injured players have significantly affected the outcome of a contest. However, how many more have not? How many never return to their previous level of play? A good litmus test for the sideline physician is to ask himself or herself if this athlete would be allowed to return to play if he or she were the physician's son or daughter.

Specific anatomic area
Ankle
Ankle injuries—particularly sprains—are very common sporting injuries. In fact, when evaluating the athlete, it may be difficult to determine whether the observed laxity is acute, chronic, or acute in the presence of a chronically unstable ankle. Swelling suggests acuteness. Although some ankle sprains can be braced or taped sufficiently to allow return to competition, it is the responsibility of the sideline physician to be sure that the athlete does not have an ankle fracture. In Canada, the Ottawa criteria[18] were developed to allow emergency department medical staff to triage ankle injuries and to eliminate the obtaining of unnecessary radiographs for ankle sprains without missing an ankle fracture. The Ottawa criterion for an ankle radiograph after acute injury is tenderness to palpation, specifically over the medial malleolus, the lateral malleolus, or the proximal fifth metatarsal. Tenderness over any of these regions suggests fracture and requires a radiograph. If there is no tenderness over these bony landmarks, even with substantial local soft-tissue swelling and generalized tenderness, radiography is not indicated.[19] Recently, at West Point, the Ottawa criteria were validated for use during the evaluation of athletic and training injuries.[20]

Some ankle sprains are "bad actors" and may require prolonged rehabilitation before the injured player can return to play; early return to play may delay eventual healing. Athletes with ankle sprains associated with a deltoid injury or a syndesmosis injury should not immediately return to play. If the ankle has medial swelling, tenderness just below the medial malleolus, or tenderness between the distal tibia and fibula (the syndesmosis), then the ankle should be iced initially and protected with immobilization and non–weight-bearing restrictions.

If an athlete sustains a minor ankle sprain and is not prophylactically braced or taped, he or she should be given an opportunity for taping, bracing, or both and evaluated for return to play. If the ankle is already taped or braced and the athlete wears a cleated shoe, the ankle and shoe can be "spatted" with tape over both the ankle and shoe to provide more stability. If the athlete is still symptomatic, the ankle may need to be retaped or braced before evaluation for return to play.

If the decision is made to not return the athlete with an ankle sprain to competition, the ankle should be iced and elevated. This early treatment may allow for quicker recovery from this injury.

Knee
Examining the knee on the field with the athlete in full gear is difficult. In addition, the athlete is typically still in too much pain for a proper examination. Transporting the patient to the sideline allows for a complete systematic evaluation of the injured and uninjured knee. From the history and mechanism of a knee injury, the sideline physician usually has a good idea of what may be injured.

It is best to examine the injured structure last. It hurts less that way, and the "bad news" comes last, thus keeping the athlete focused on the examination. The sideline examination represents a golden opportunity to obtain a sensitive examination. The first bout of pain from the injured structure(s) is gone, swelling has not occurred, and the adrenaline of the competition is still present. Most athletes will be comfortable with a complete examination. An hour later, the same examination would be more difficult.

If the knee is stable and no injury is identified by the sideline examination, the knee should be observed for a short period (10 to 15 minutes) for swelling. If no swelling occurs, the player can try to return to play.

Knee injuries are common and range from simple contusions to complete dislocations. The medial collateral ligament is commonly injured from a contact or an impact to the lateral aspect of the knee, which produces a valgus stress on that ligament. If on examination the athlete has medial collateral ligament laxity from a noncontact injury, the physician should suspect an associated anterior cruciate ligament injury. Isolated lateral collateral ligament injuries are rare; they are usually associated with a cruciate ligament injury. With lateral collateral ligament injuries, the physician should check for peroneal nerve function. The anterior cruciate ligament is commonly injured via a noncontact mechanism, with the athlete recalling a "pop." The Lachman test is the most sensitive test for this injury. In addition to eliciting the amount of translation, the quality of the end point can suggest an anterior cruciate ligament injury. The posterior cruciate ligament is most commonly injured from a direct blow to a flexed knee, and it is best evaluated with a posterior drawer test. Any one of these ligamentous injuries probably precludes return to competition that day. In addition to pain and swelling, the knee is unstable, even with bracing and taping, which precludes running, pivoting, or jumping.

Other acute knee injuries include a patellar dislocation, which usually occurs from a twisting maneuver with the knee straight. A dislocated patella usually self-reduces, but if it does not, the knee can be extended, and gentle lateral to medial pressure on the patella should reduce it easily.

Meniscal injuries can occur with a knee ligament injury or in isolation. Athletes describe the knee as being "tweaked" with a contact or noncontact mechanism. These injuries have delayed swelling.

Any of the above injuries precludes return to play. The knee should be packed in ice and immobilized, and the athlete should be transported to the training facility or the bench.

Shoulder

The three most common traumatic shoulder injuries are clavicle fracture, acromioclavicular joint separation, and shoulder dislocation. Athletes with these injuries can usually walk off of the field. Palpating the clavicle, the acromioclavicular joint, and the shoulder under the jersey and pads can help with the preliminary diagnosis, but the shoulder is best evaluated with the jersey and equipment off. Players with a clavicle fracture should be examined for possible pneumothorax and neurovascular injury. The injured arm should be placed in a sling, and ice should be applied to the fracture site.

Acromioclavicular joint separations have varying degrees of severity, but they are all painful. These injuries are also treated with ice and a sling. Most of these injuries preclude return to play, but under unusual circumstances, a grade I or II[21] acromioclavicular joint separation can be injected with an anesthetic and the prominence over the acromioclavicular joint can be padded for relief in an attempt to return the athlete to play.

The shoulder is the most commonly dislocated major joint. Athletes complain of having a "dead arm" and being unable to touch the opposite shoulder. These dislocations can be reduced with gentle traction and relaxation without medication, which is best done in the training facility or the locker room with the athlete's equipment off. Attempting to do this on the field or the bench is not recommended because patient relaxation is critical to a gentle reduction. Players with recurrent dislocations sometimes can self-reduce the dislocation. Pain and recurrent instability usually preclude return to play, and the shoulder should be treated with ice and a sling. Alternatively, patients with recurrent instability may have little pain; with taping, bracing, or both, an athlete with this condition can be considered for return to competition.

In general, fractures anywhere, from the ankles to the fingers, are painful, and they usually preclude return to play, except under the most unusual circumstances (e.g., an offensive lineman with a metacarpal fracture that has been treated with a playing cast). The injured extremity should be iced, immobilized, and elevated. Radiographs obtained early will provide indisputable documentation and allow the player, the coach, and the physician to make the appropriate adjustments to the game plans.

Abrasions should be cleaned and dressed immediately. With the emergence of community-acquired methicillin-resistant *Staphylococcus aureus*, this procedure becomes even more important.[22]

Muscle contusions and strains are very common. Hamstring and quadriceps strains are particularly annoying, and they can remove an athlete from play. A tight wrap might provide some relief and a hope of return to play, but continuing to play carries the risk of extending the muscle strain. Some physicians have advocated a local injection of an anesthetic with a corticosteroid to the area of the muscle injury after the competition; this protocol is associated with improved pain control, gait, and earlier return to play at a later time.[23]

Contused muscles should be stretched and, if possible, immobilized in that position overnight.[20] This procedure, which reduces swelling and tightness, returns athletes to play in days instead of weeks, and it is best done on the sideline before substantial pain and swelling commence. The timely application of ice and appropriate protected immobilization on the sideline (after the player accepts that he or she cannot return to play) may facilitate quicker rehabilitation and return to function and ability later on.

CONCLUSION

The first level of confidence that a team will have for the physician is in his or her technical ability. However, being a great diagnostician or an innovative surgeon will only get a foot in the door (or rather, on the sideline). Preparation is equally important to the sideline physician. An old Chinese proverb states, "The more you sweat during peacetime, the less you will bleed during war." This quote is appropriate not only for the athlete and the team but also for the sideline physician. With validated knowledge and consummate preparation, the sideline physician who involves himself or herself in the team chemistry will be elevated to a whole new level of confidence and respect. That respect will provide the leverage needed to represent and articulate the medical issues of the injured athlete and the vision and mission of the team; these concepts should be one and the same. When the lines between the two become blurry, the effective sideline physician can deliver a safe, thoughtful decision, no matter how unpopular.

REFERENCES

1. Garrick JG, Collins GS, Requa RK: Out of bounds in football: player exposure to probability of collision injury. J Safety Res 1977;9(1):34-38.
2. Wilckens JH, Glorioso JE Jr: Risk assessment and management of nonorthopaedic conditions. Section A. Viral disease. In DeLee JC, Drez D Jr, Miller MD (eds): DeLee & Drez's Orthopaedic Sports Medicine: Principles and Practice, 2nd ed. Philadelphia, WB Saunders, 2003, pp 251-263.

3. Lee A, Cooper MC, Craig JC, et al: Effects of nonsteroidal anti-inflammatory drugs on postoperative renal function in adults with normal renal function. Cochrane Database Syst Rev 2004;(2):CD002765.

4. Madden CC, Walsh WM, Mellion MB: The team physician: the preparticipation examination and on-field emergencies. In DeLee JC, Drez D Jr, Miller MD (eds): DeLee & Drez's Orthopaedic Sports Medicine: Principles and Practice, 2nd ed. Philadelphia, WB Saunders, 2003, pp 737-768.

5. Waninger KN, Richards JG, Pan WT, et al: An evaluation of head movement in backboard-immobilized helmeted football, lacrosse, and ice hockey players. Clin J Sport Med 2001;11(2):82-86.

6. American College of Surgeons Committee on Trauma: Advanced Trauma Life Support Program for Doctors, 6th ed. Chicago, American College of Surgeons, 1997.

7. Hanft K, Posternack C, Astor F, et al: Diagnosis and management of laryngeal trauma in sports. South Med J 1996;89(6):631-633.

8. Levy AS, Bassett F, Lintner S, et al: Pulmonary barotrauma: diagnosis in American football players. Three cases in three years. Am J Sports Med 1996;24(2):227-229.

9. Gove N, Ebraheim NA, Glass E: Posterior sternoclavicular dislocations: a review of management and complications. Am J Orthrop 2006;35(3):132-136.

10. Gomez JE: Sideline medical emergencies in the young athlete. Pediatr Ann 2002;31(1):50-58.

11. Link MS, Wang PJ, Maron BJ, et al: What is commotio cordis? Cardiol Rev 1999;7(5):265-269.

12. Haight RR, Shiple BJ: Sideline evaluation of neck pain. When is it time for transport? Phys Sportsmed 2001;29(3):45-62.

13. Shah S, Luftman JP, Vigil DV: Football: sideline management of injuries. Curr Sports Med Rep 2004;3(3):146-153.

14. McCrea M: Standardized mental status testing on the sideline after sport-related concussion. J Athl Train 2001;36(3):274-279.

15. Cantu RC: Second-impact syndrome. Clin Sports Med 1998;17(1):37-44.

16. Almquist J, Broshek D, Erlanger D: Assessment of mild head injuries. Athlet Ther Today 2001;6(1):13-17.

17. Kelly JP, Rosenberg JH: The development of guidelines for the management of concussion in sports. J Head Trauma Rehabil 1998;13(2):53-65.

18. Stiell IG, McKnight RD, Greenberg GH, et al: Implementation of the Ottawa ankle rules. JAMA 1994;271(11):827-832.

19. Derksen RJ, Bakker FC, Geervliet PC, et al: Diagnostic accuracy and reproducibility in the interpretation of Ottawa ankle and foot rules by specialized emergency nurses. Am J Emerg Med 2005;23(6):725-729.

20. Ryan JB, Wheeler JH, Hopkinson WJ, et al: Quadriceps contusions. West Point update. Am J Sports Med 1991;19(3):299-304.

21. Rockwood CA Jr, Williams GR Jr, Young DC: Disorders of the acromioclavicular joint. Rockwood CA Jr, Matsen FA III, Wirth MA, et al (eds): The Shoulder, 3rd ed. Philadelphia, WB Saunders, 2004, pp 521-595.

22. Rihn JA, Michaels MG, Harner CD: Community-acquired methicillin-resistant *Staphylococcus aureus*: an emerging problem in the athletic population. Am J Sports Med 2005;33(12):1924-1929.

23. Levine WN, Bergfeld JA, Tessendorf W, et al: Intramuscular corticosteroid injection for hamstring injuries. A 13-year experience in the National Football League. Am J Sports Med 2000;28(3):297-300.

The Preparticipation Evaluation

Jay E. Noffsinger, MD

KEY POINTS

- The primary objectives of the preparticipation physical evaluation (PPE) are to detect conditions that may be life-threatening or disabling or that may predispose an athlete to injury or illness.
- The secondary objectives of the PPE include determining general health and serving as an entry point into the health-care system for adolescents.
- The purpose of the PPE is to facilitate and encourage safe participation rather than to exclude athletes from participation.
- A comprehensive history will identify up to 75% of problems that affect athletes.
- Only after this history is supplemented by a careful physical examination can appropriate clearance decisions be made.

INTRODUCTION

Without question, the practice of primary care sports medicine has become more and more reliant on evidence-based medicine. This textbook will be filled with examples of evidence-based medicine. Unfortunately, recommendations regarding a comprehensive preparticipation physical evaluation have been primarily based on clinical observations and "expert opinions." Before 1992 there were virtually no national guidelines for a PPE for this very reason. That year representatives from many important organizations got together and published the first PPE monograph. The second edition came out in 1997, and the third was published in 2005.[1] Organizations sponsoring this monograph include the American Academy of Family Physicians, the American Academy of Pediatrics, the American College of Sports Medicine, the American Medical Society for Sports Medicine, the American Orthopaedic Society for Sports Medicine, and the American Osteopathic Academy of Sports Medicine. National endorsements have come from the National Athletic Trainers Association, the Sports Physical Therapy Section of the American Physical Therapy Association, and the Special Olympics Medical Committee. This impressive list of organizations is a testament to the importance and significance of the monograph. The work of the representatives of these organizations is ongoing, and future editions of their work will include more evidence-based medicine. Recommendations may ultimately change from guidelines to standards.

GOALS AND OBJECTIVES

The obvious primary objective of a well-done PPE is to detect conditions that may be life-threatening or disabling or that predispose an athlete to injury or illness. Unfortunately, cost analyses and other factors preclude the kind of evaluation that would be 100% sensitive and specific. For example, without an echocardiogram, most cases of hypertrophic cardiomyopathy will go undetected, even with a comprehensive history and physical. A final primary objective of a PPE is to meet legal and administrative requirements.

For most adolescents, this PPE will be the only health maintenance visit for the year. Of course, this is not ideal, but it is reality. Therefore, secondary objectives of this evaluation are to determine general heath, to serve as an entry point into the health-care system for adolescents, and to provide an opportunity for the discussion of health and lifestyle issues.

TIMING, SETTING, AND STRUCTURE

Although multiple health-care professionals may play a role in conducting the PPE, ultimate responsibility should be assigned to a physician who is a doctor of medicine or osteopathy. Different states have different regulations regarding the qualifications of practitioners. The optimal time to conduct the PPE is 6 weeks before the onset of preseason practice. This allows time to follow up on abnormalities that are discovered, but it is not so soon that new problems are likely to appear. With an estimated 7 to 8 million required PPEs occurring at the high-school level and probably an equal number at the middle-school and college levels, it may be impossible to have each evaluation performed within this timetable; however, the above principles should be considered. The monograph recommends a comprehensive PPE at entry to middle and high school, with yearly interim updates as directed by the history. The American Academy of Pediatrics recommends biannual evaluations with interval history updates. Unfortunately, state laws prevail, and most states require yearly evaluations. Other organizations that may have requirements include school districts, athletic conferences, and insurance companies.

No routine screening tests, including blood tests, are recommended currently. Rather, these tests are to be directed by findings on the PPE. Earlier recommendations included a urinalysis; this often resulted in a workup for the protein discovered and resulted in a diagnosis of benign orthostatic proteinuria after substantially alarming the athlete and parents while awaiting further tests.

Ideally, the preferred setting for the PPE is the primary care physician's office. This setting is optimal for privacy, lighting, proper instruments, familiarity with the patient (including immunization records), and ready access to appropriate referrals if necessary to follow up on identified problems. Certainly pursuing the secondary objectives of the PPE is better done in this setting. Problems include expense, availability to provide timely PPEs to all athletes, lack of direct contact with school officials (including coaches), and, unfortunately, a lack of expertise by many primary care physicians with regard to the ideal conduct of such an evaluation. A properly performed "station-method" PPE is an acceptable alternative. Stations may include vital signs, visual acuity assessment, fitness, flexibility, nutrition, and a physical examination that can be divided into as many stations as desired to meet the expertise of the examiners present. Advantages of this method include low expense, greater availability, likely appropriate expertise of the coordinated medical team (e.g., an orthopedist to do the musculoskeletal assessment and a cardiologist to listen to hearts), and on-site coordination with coaches and other school officials. The old "last-minute" locker-room method is now condemned.

THE PREPARTICIPATION PHYSICAL EVALUATION MEDICAL HISTORY

It is felt that a complete history will identify 75% of the problems that affect athletes. It is important that athletes and parents complete the history together because it has been found that if each completes the form separately, there is only a 39% correlation.[2] The PPE medical history form suggested by the monograph is included (Figure 2.1), and it incorporates all of the questions recommended by the American Heart Association[3] (revised in 1998).[4] Many states have adopted this form or use one that is very similar. Although readers of this text understand that they may be forced to use state forms that are not ideal, they are encouraged to develop their own supplementary history document to make sure that all appropriate history is obtained. Unfortunately, only about half of the United States even requires a medical history.[5,6] The most common cause of nontraumatic sudden death in athletes is definitely cardiac (80% to 95%), and this is followed distantly by heat illness and then asthma. Among patients who are less than 35 years of age, any cardiac problems are usually congenital; alternatively, among those who are 35 years of age and older, arteriosclerotic cardiovascular disease predominates. The best chance of detecting hypertrophic cardiomyopathy, which is the most common congenital heart defect that causes sudden death in the United States, is the history rather than the physical. The collapse of an athlete during (rather than after) competition or a positive family history demands a comprehensive cardiologic evaluation. Participation guidelines for athletes with cardiovascular problems are covered by the 36th Bethesda Conference, which was published in 2005.[7] It is known that 0.5% to 1% of all humans are born with a congenital heart defect. Approximately 1% of these defects are potentially life-threatening, and 10% of individuals with this condition will die as a result of the problem. It can be concluded that one of these ultimately fatal defects would be present for every 200,000 PPEs. If echocardiograms were required for all PPEs, it would cost nearly $250,000 to detect each fatal defect or at least $18,000 for a typical sports program.[8] Clearly, this is not financially feasible. In the United States, cardiologists do not recommend screening electrocardiograms because they will not rule out hypertrophic cardiomyopathy; instead, electrocardiograms often detect worrisome changes that ultimately turn out to be "athlete's heart," which is a known entity that consists of normal physiologic changes. In some countries (e.g., Italy) other heart conditions that can be detected by electrocardiograms (e.g., arrhythmogenic right ventricular dysplasia) predominate, which makes electrocardiography a sensible and inexpensive screen.

The heat-illness spectrum includes heat edema, heat cramps, heat syncope, heat exhaustion, and heatstroke. Heat-illness predisposition includes a history of problems in the heat as well as a pertinent family history, and these elements of the history should be pursued. I have seen heat stroke occur in twin male athletes competing in college cross-country during successive seasons. If a prior heat illness has ever included central nervous system dysfunction, heatstroke should be assumed. Recurrences may be associated with a mortality rate of as high as 10%. In cases of exertional heatstroke the athlete may still be sweating profusely. Only in cases of classical heatstroke is the skin dry. Other predisposing factors include dehydration, old or young age, inadequate acclimatization, poor aerobic fitness, large body size with excess body fat, febrile condition, overexertion, and certain medications and supplements. Inquiries regarding sickle cell trait status should be made, and strong consideration should be given to testing those whose status is unknown. Approximately 8% of blacks and a small percentage of whites carry this trait. Although it is normally benign, under extremes of strenuous activity (particularly in the heat and at altitude), rhabdomyolysis and sudden death have occurred.[9,10] Preventive measures are strongly advised, including adequate acclimatization, maintaining good hydration, avoiding diuretics, and avoiding all-out sprints or timed miles early during training. It is quite possible that the deaths of many black athletes that have been attributed to heat alone may actually be related to sickle cell trait. Most of these problems have occurred in the first 1 to 2 weeks of practice during the summer, so medical observers need to be particularly vigilant at these times.

Questions about asthma may point out very poor control and lead to recommendations that will lessen the probability of serious consequences. Many athletes have very poorly controlled asthma and abuse their "rescue" inhalers. Other athletes with a diagnosis of exercise-induced asthma may actually have other conditions, such as paradoxical vocal cord dysfunction. Alternatively, the incidence of exercise-induced asthma is often underestimated. A detailed allergy and asthma history questionnaire was developed by the Sports Medicine Committee of the American College of Asthma, Allergy & Immunology to assist with raising awareness of exercise-induced asthma.[11] Suspected cases can be confirmed by changes in peak expiratory flow rates from baseline to after exercise followed by a positive response to preventive medication, such as a short-acting β-agonist, 5 to 10 minutes before exercise.

It has been said that the most common injury in sports medicine is a recurrence of a prior injury. The identification of prior injuries by the taking of a history often confirms totally inadequate rehabilitation and certainly dictates a very careful musculoskeletal examination to look for persistent problems, such as poor flexibility, strength (including core strength), proprioception, or even residual pathologic laxity of a joint.

A history of concussions or repetitive "burners" demands a careful assessment of full recovery as well as checking for anatomic and other predispositions to recurrences that may be less benign than prior injuries. Isolated stingers are not considered to be serious, but severe or repeated injuries can lead to permanent motor or sensory sequelae. Radiologic investigation can exclude cervical spinal stenosis or degenerative disk disease.

Preparticipation Physical Evaluation

HISTORY FORM

DATE OF EXAM _____

Name _____ Sex _____ Age _____ Date of birth _____

Grade ____ School _____ Sport(s) _____

Address _____ Phone _____

Personal physician _____

In case of emergency, contact

Name _____ Relationship _____ Phone (H) _____ (W) _____

Explain "Yes" answers below.
Circle questions you don't know the answers to.

	Yes	No
1. Has a doctor ever denied or restricted your participation in sports for any reason?	☐	☐
2. Do you have an ongoing medical condition (like diabetes or asthma)?	☐	☐
3. Are you currently taking any prescription or nonprescription (over-the-counter) medicines or pills?	☐	☐
4. Do you have allergies to medicines, pollens, foods, or stinging insects?	☐	☐
5. Have you ever passed out or nearly passed out DURING exercise?	☐	☐
6. Have you ever passed out or nearly passed out AFTER exercise?	☐	☐
7. Have you ever had discomfort, pain, or pressure in your chest during exercise?	☐	☐
8. Does your heart race or skip beats during exercise?	☐	☐

9. Has a doctor ever told you that you have (check all that apply):

☐ High blood pressure ☐ A heart murmur
☐ High cholesterol ☐ A heart infection

	Yes	No
10. Has a doctor ever ordered a test for your heart? (for example, ECG, echocardiogram)	☐	☐
11. Has anyone in your family died for no apparent reason?	☐	☐
12. Does anyone in your family have a heart problem?	☐	☐
13. Has any family member or relative died of heart problems or of sudden death before age 50?	☐	☐
14. Does anyone in your family have Marfan syndrome?	☐	☐
15. Have you ever spent the night in a hospital?	☐	☐
16. Have you ever had surgery?	☐	☐
17. Have you ever had an injury, like a sprain, muscle or ligament tear, or tendinitis, that caused you to miss a practice or game? If yes, circle affected area below:	☐	☐
18. Have you had any broken or fractured bones or dislocated joints? If yes, circle below:	☐	☐
19. Have you had a bone or joint injury that required x-rays, MRI, CT, surgery, injections, rehabilitation, physical therapy, a brace, a cast, or crutches? If yes, circle below:	☐	☐

Head	Neck	Shoulder	Upper arm	Elbow	Forearm	Hand/ fingers	Chest
Upper back	Lower back	Hip	Thigh	Knee	Calf/shin	Ankle	Foot/toes

	Yes	No
20. Have you ever had a stress fracture?	☐	☐
21. Have you been told that you have or have you had an x-ray for atlantoaxial (neck) instability?	☐	☐
22. Do you regularly use a brace or assistive device?	☐	☐
23. Has a doctor ever told you that you have asthma or allergies?	☐	☐

	Yes	No
24. Do you cough, wheeze, or have difficulty breathing during or after exercise?	☐	☐
25. Is there anyone in your family who has asthma?	☐	☐
26. Have you ever used an inhaler or taken asthma medicine?	☐	☐
27. Were you born without or are you missing a kidney, an eye, a testicle, or any other organ?	☐	☐
28. Have you had infectious mononucleosis (mono) within the last month?	☐	☐
29. Do you have any rashes, pressure sores, or other skin problems?	☐	☐
30. Have you had a herpes skin infection?	☐	☐
31. Have you ever had a head injury or concussion?	☐	☐
32. Have you been hit in the head and been confused or lost your memory?	☐	☐
33. Have you ever had a seizure?	☐	☐
34. Do you have headaches with exercise?	☐	☐
35. Have you ever had numbness, tingling, or weakness in your arms or legs after being hit or falling?	☐	☐
36. Have you ever been unable to move your arms or legs after being hit or falling?	☐	☐
37. When exercising in the heat, do you have severe muscle cramps or become ill?	☐	☐
38. Has a doctor told you that you or someone in your family has sickle cell trait or sickle cell disease?	☐	☐
39. Have you had any problems with your eyes or vision?	☐	☐
40. Do you wear glasses or contact lenses?	☐	☐
41. Do you wear protective eyewear, such as goggles or a face shield?	☐	☐
42. Are you happy with your weight?	☐	☐
43. Are you trying to gain or lose weight?	☐	☐
44. Has anyone recommended you change your weight or eating habits?	☐	☐
45. Do you limit or carefully control what you eat?	☐	☐
46. Do you have any concerns that you would like to discuss with a doctor?	☐	☐

FEMALES ONLY

	Yes	No
47. Have you ever had a menstrual period?	☐	☐

48. How old were you when you had your first menstrual period? _____

49. How many periods have you had in the last 12 months? _____

Explain "Yes" answers here: _____
_____
_____
_____
_____
_____
_____
_____
_____

I hereby state that, to the best of my knowledge, my answers to the above questions are complete and correct.

Signature of athlete _____ Signature of parent/guardian _____ Date _____

Figure 2.1 Preparticipation physical evaluation: history form. (From the American Academy of Family Physicians, American Academy of Pediatrics, American College of Sports Medicine, et al: Preparticipation Physical Evaluation, 3rd ed. Minneapolis, The Physician and Sportsmedicine/McGraw-Hill, 2005.)

Preparticipation Physical Evaluation

PHYSICAL EXAMINATION FORM

Name _____ Date of birth _____

Height _____ Weight_____ % Body fat (optional) _____ Pulse_____ BP___/____ (___/___ , ___/___)

Vision R 20/ _____ L 20/ _____   Corrected: Y N   Pupils: Equal _____ Unequal _____

Follow-Up Questions on More Sensitive Issues	Yes	No
1. Do you feel stressed out or under a lot of pressure?	☐	☐
2. Do you ever feel so sad or hopeless that you stop doing some of your usual activities for more than a few days?	☐	☐
3. Do you feel safe?	☐	☐
4. Have you ever tried cigarette smoking, even 1 or 2 puffs? Do you currently smoke?	☐	☐
5. During the past 30 days, did you use chewing tobacco, snuff, or dip?	☐	☐
6. During the past 30 days, have you had at least 1 drink of alcohol?	☐	☐
7. Have you ever taken steroid pills or shots without a doctor's prescription?	☐	☐
8. Have you ever taken any supplements to help you gain or lose weight or improve your performance?	☐	☐
9. Questions from the Youth Risk Behavior Survey (http://www.cdc.gov/HealthyYouth/yrbs/index.htm) on guns, seatbelts, unprotected sex, domestic violence, drugs, etc.	☐	☐

Notes: _____
_____
_____

	NORMAL	ABNORMAL FINDINGS	INITIALS*
MEDICAL			
Appearance			
Eyes/ears/nose/throat			
Hearing			
Lymph nodes			
Heart			
Murmurs			
Pulses			
Lungs			
Abdomen			
Genitourinary (males only)†			
Skin			
MUSCULOSKELETAL			
Neck			
Back			
Shoulder/arm			
Elbow/forearm			
Wrist/hand/fingers			
Hip/thigh			
Knee			
Leg/ankle			
Foot/toes			

*Multiple-examiner set-up only.
†Having a third party present is recommended for the genitourinary examination.

Notes: _____
_____

Name of physician (print/type) _____ Date _____

Address _____ Phone _____

Signature of physician _____, MD or DO

Figure 2.2 Preparticipation physical evaluation: physical evaluation form. (From the American Academy of Family Physicians, American Academy of Pediatrics, American College of Sports Medicine, et al: Preparticipation Physical Evaluation, 3rd ed. Minneapolis, The Physician and Sportsmedicine/McGraw-Hill, 2005.)

For persistent symptoms, electrodiagnostic studies may be warranted. Prevention tools may include neck strengthening, equipment changes (including neck rolls), and reviewing tackling techniques. An athlete who reports bilateral or upper and lower extremity symptoms would never be diagnosed with a stinger, and a central cause is assumed. Transient quadriparesis should initially be handled as a catastrophic cervical spine injury. After fractures and ligamentous instability have been ruled out, further investigation is needed to exclude congenital or acquired predispositions. Even with a totally negative workup, return-to-play recommendations remain controversial and should include neurosurgical or neurologic consultation.

Although there is some debate about second impact syndrome, there is no question that someone who has experienced a concussion is 4 to 6 times is more likely to have a recurrence than someone who has not.[12,13] The term *second impact syndrome* was coined to describe massive cerebral edema with collapse and death after minor head trauma in an athlete who was still symptomatic from an earlier concussion. The theory is that autonomic dysfunction of the cerebral vessels resulted from the first injury and caused them to dilate significantly after the second impact, thus resulting in catastrophic cerebral edema. Although future studies are needed to settle the debate regarding second impact syndrome, described cases have occurred almost exclusively among very young athletes. There is also much debate regarding the classification of concussions and subsequent management decisions. International experts have recently reported their recommendations from the Second International Conference on Concussion in Sports,[14] and the American College of Sports Medicine also released a consensus statement regarding concussion and the team physician.[15] It is universally agreed that athletes should not be allowed to return to play until they are asymptomatic both at rest and with exertion; however, the problem is with determining what qualifies as asymptomatic. Recently developed computer-based programs to assess neuropsychological function as compared with baseline may become standard in the future as their validity is confirmed. Cumulative damage is another concern, including dementia pugilistica (punch-drunk syndrome).

THE PREPARTICIPATION PHYSICAL EVALUATION

The PPE form recommended by the monograph is included here **(Figure 2.2).** Note that it includes follow-up questions about more sensitive issues. The physical examination can be conducted without the parents present, and it is an ideal time to explore these issues. The presence of anisocoria is noted to prevent future misinterpretation as possibly resulting from a serious head injury. Best corrected vision should be 20/40 or better, otherwise clearance considerations include appropriate protection of the good eye in many sports. I have personally seen individuals with a BB injury, a bottle-rocket injury, and a congenital cataract, and I also worked with an athlete who underwent multiple eye surgeries after a retinal detachment. Each of these individuals had almost no vision in one of their eyes, and each had been inappropriately playing contact sports for years with no protection for their good eye. **Table 2.1** provides the categories of sports-related eye-injury risk to the unprotected players. Good athletic trainers may be consulted for help with designing custom protective eyewear for sports in which standards are not available, such as wrestling. **Table 2.2** outlines recommended eye protectors for selected sports. Although at one point I had trouble convincing a high-school football player about the importance of placing a visor in his helmet to protect his

Table 2.1 Categories of Sports-Related Eye-Injury Risk to the Unprotected Player

High Risk

SMALL, FAST PROJECTILES
Air rifle
BB gun
Paintball

HARD PROJECTILES, "STICKS," CLOSE CONTACT
Baseball/softball
Basketball
Cricket
Fencing
Hockey (field and ice)
Lacrosse (men's and women's)
Racquetball
Squash

INTENTIONAL INJURY
Boxing
Full-contact martial arts

MODERATE RISK
Badminton
Fishing
Football
Golf
Soccer
Tennis
Volleyball
Water polo

LOW RISK
Bicycling
Diving
Noncontact martial arts
Skiing (snow and water)
Swimming
Wrestling

EYE SAFE
Gymnastics
Track and field*

*Javelin and discus have a small but definite potential for injury. However, good field supervision can reduce the extremely low risk of injury to nearly negligible.
Adapted with permission from Vinger PF: Phys Sportsmed 2000;28(6):49-69.
In American Academy of Family Physicians, American Academy of Pediatrics, American College of Sports Medicine, et al: Preparticipation Physical Evaluation, 3rd ed. Minneapolis, The Physician and Sportsmedicine/McGraw-Hill, 2005.

good eye, it has recently become necessary to prove medical necessity for the wearing of a shaded visor because players now want them so that they can conceal the direction in which they are looking.

Height, weight, and body mass index determinations allow for the addressing of both obesity and possible eating disorders. A general musculoskeletal screening examination is mandatory, and a more comprehensive examination should be performed for areas in which prior injuries have occurred. At this time, the determination of the Tanner stage is not recommended; however, for those in the middle-school age group, I think it would at least be wise to consider. For example, in a

Table 2.2   Recommended Eye Protectors for Selected Sports

Sport	Minimal Eye Protector	Comment
Baseball/softball (youth batter and base runner)	ASTM standard F910	Face guard attached to helmet
Baseball/softball (fielder)	ASTM standard F803 for baseball	ASTM specifies age ranges
Basketball	ASTM standard F803 for basketball	ASTM specifies age ranges
Bicycling	Helmet plus street wear/fashion eyewear	
Boxing	None available; not permitted in the sport	Contraindicated for functionally one-eyed athletes
Fencing	Protector with neck bib	
Field hockey (men's and women's)	ASTM standard F803 for women's lacrosse (goalie: full face mask)	Protectors that pass for women's lacrosse also pass for field hockey
Football	Polycarbonate eye shield attached to helmet-mounted wire face mask	
Full-contact martial arts	None available; not permitted in the sport	Contraindicated for functionally one-eyed athletes
Ice hockey	ASTM standard F513 face mask on helmet (goaltenders: ASTM standard F1587)	HECC-certified or CSA-certified full face shield
Lacrosse (men's)	Face mask attached to lacrosse helmet	
Lacrosse (women's)	ASTM standard F803 for women's lacrosse	Should have option to wear helmet
Paintball	ASTM standard F1776 for paintball	
Racket sports (badminton, tennis, paddle tennis, handball, squash, and racquetball)	ASTM standard F803 for selected sport	
Soccer	ASTM standard F803 for selected sport	
Street hockey	ASTM standard F513 face mask on helmet	Must be HECC or CSA certified
Track and field	Street wear with polycarbonate lenses/fashion eyewear*	
Water polo/swimming	Swim goggles with polycarbonate lenses	
Wrestling	No standard available	Custom protective eyewear can be made

*Eyewear that passes ASTM standard F803 is safer than street wear eyewear for all sports activities with impact potential.
ASTM, American Society for Testing and Materials; CSA, Canadian Standards Association; HECC, Hockey Equipment Certification Council.
Adapted with permission from Vinger PF: Phys Sportsmed 2000;28(6):49-69. In American Academy of Family Physicians, American Academy of Pediatrics, American College of Sports Medicine, et al: Prepariticipation Physical Evaluation, 3rd ed. Minneapolis, The Physician and Sportsmedicine/McGraw-Hill, 2005.

sport like football, there is a huge difference between a Tanner-I, 210-pound overweight male and a Tanner-V athlete of the same age and weight who looks like a National Football League linebacker.

An example of a general musculoskeletal screening examination as outlined in the PPE monograph is included **(Figure 2.3)**. Unfortunately, this is one of the most common parts of the evaluation that is left out. This examination would be particularly amenable to the station method, and it could be performed by an athletic trainer, a physical therapist, or even an orthopedic surgeon.

Male testicular examination allows not only for the identification of problems but also for the discussion of the importance of periodic self-examination to assist with the early detection of testicular cancer, which is the most common malignancy found in young adult males.

The cardiovascular examination recommended by the American Heart Association includes checking pulses, determining blood pressure, looking for signs that are suggestive of Marfan's syndrome, and auscultating the heart in at least two different positions to look for dynamic changes that may suggest hypertrophic cardiomyopathy (e.g., increased intensity of a systolic murmur with the Valsalva maneuver). Marfan's syndrome is an autosomal-dominant connective tissue disease that manifests with characteristic phenotypic findings that include the following: kyphosis, high-arched palate, pectus excavatum, arachnodactyly, arm span that is greater than height, mitral valve prolapse, aortic insufficiency murmur, myopia, lenticular dislocation, a thumb sign, and a wrist sign. Screening for this disorder is recommended for men who are 6

feet tall or taller and women who are 5 feet and 10 inches tall or taller, who have two or more physical manifestations, or who have a family history of Marfan's syndrome. The importance of identifying Marfan's syndrome is because of the associated aortic root dilatation, which can progress to dissection and rupture with ensuing sudden death.[16] Blood-pressure measurement should be accomplished using the largest appropriate cuff. The regular adult cuff is too small for many large male athletes, and it results in a false elevation of the blood-pressure measurement. The finding of elevated blood pressure for age is probably the most common abnormality found during the PPE. If decreased pulses are found in the lower extremities, blood-pressure measurements should also be taken from the legs to rule out coarctation of the aorta. Blood-pressure measurements should be repeated on at least two separate occasions to ensure that the elevation is persistent. If elevated blood pressure is confirmed, investigation for end-organ damage should follow. **Table 2.3** outlines the classification of hypertension in children and adolescents, and **Table 2.4** covers the classification of hypertension in adults. Specific recommendations for participation for athletes with hypertension are found in the PPE monograph and the results of the 36th Bethesda Conference.[7] In general, aerobic or dynamic exercise is beneficial for hypertension, whereas high static activities may be contraindicated. It is only necessary to restrict activity while further evaluation is performed and blood-pressure control is achieved for adults with stage 2 hypertension or children with measurements that are above the 99th percentile (in whom end-organ damage is likely) or for those in whom a secondary cause is suspected.

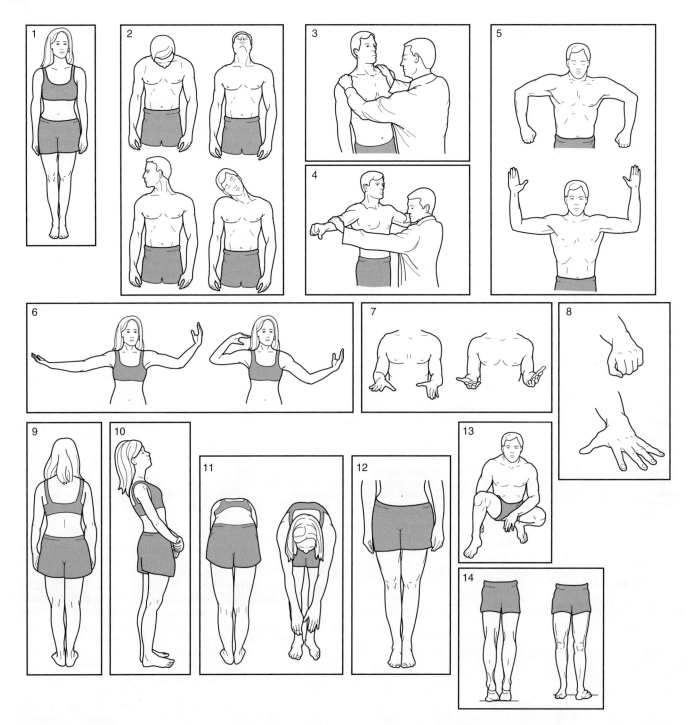

Figure 2.3 General musculoskeletal screening examination. (From the American Academy of Family Physicians, American Academy of Pediatrics, American College of Sports Medicine, et al: Preparticipation Physical Evaluation, 3rd ed. Minneapolis, The Physician and Sportsmedicine/McGraw-Hill, 2005.)

The neurologic examination should be much more comprehensive when the history reveals prior concussions or multiple "burners" or "stingers," as discussed previously.

DETERMINING CLEARANCE

Because the goal of the PPE is to facilitate and encourage safe participation rather than to exclude athletes from participation, it is fortunate that most large studies find an ultimate disqualification rate of less than 1%. Between 3.1% and 13.9% of athletes require

further evaluation before a final clearance determination can be made. One of the largest studies on this subject, which was performed by Magnes and colleagues,[17] looked at more than 10,000 athletes and resulted in a final disqualification rate of only 0.4% after an initial conditional referral rate of 10.2%. Reasons for a delay in the final clearance determination pending further investigation or referral included hypertension (38%), ophthalmologic reasons (12%), genitourinary reasons (10%), neurologic reasons (8%), infectious mononucleosis (4%), and musculoskeletal reasons (4%). The monograph-suggested clearance form is included **(Figure 2.4),** and clearance options include the following: (1) clearance without restriction; (2) clearance with recommendations for further evaluation or treatment; (3) no clearance for any sport; and (4) no clearance for certain sports. Decisions may be based in part on the classification of sports by contact **(Table 2.5)** and the classification of sports by strenuousness **(Table 2.6)**. These tables as well as the table regarding medical conditions and sports participation **(Table 2.7)** come from the American Academy of Pediatrics

Committee on Sports Medicine and Fitness. As with neuropsychologic testing after concussions, with further research, future editions of the monograph will hopefully have more standards and fewer "qualified yes" recommendations. When the station method is used to conduct this examination, the most experienced practitioners may be at the last station, where clearance determinations are

Table 2.3   Classification of Hypertension in Children and Adolescents

Blood Pressure Classification*	Systolic and Diastolic Blood Pressure Measurement[†]
Normal	< 90th percentile for age, sex, and height
High normal	90th-95th percentile for age, sex, and height
Hypertension	> 95th-99th percentile for age, sex, and height
Severe hypertension	> 99th percentile for age, sex, and height

*Charts for classification by age, sex, and height percentile can be found at http://www.nhlbi.nih.gov/guidelines/hypertension/child_tbl.htm.
[†]On repeated measurement.
Adapted from Update on the 1987 Task Force Report on High Blood Pressure in Children and Adolescents: Pediatrics 1996;98(1):649-658. In American Academy of Family Physicians, American Academy of Pediatrics, American College of Sports Medicine, et al: Preparticipation Physical Evaluation, 3rd ed. Minneapolis, The Physician and Sportsmedicine/McGraw-Hill, 2005.

Table 2.4   Classification of Hypertension in Adults

Blood Pressure Classification*	Systolic Blood Pressure (mm Hg)	Diastolic Blood Pressure (mm Hg)[†]
Normal	<120	and <80
Prehypertension	120-139	or 80-89
Stage 1 hypertension	140-159	or 90-99
Stage 2 hypertension	≥160	or ≥100

*Classification determined by highest systolic or diastolic blood pressure category.
[†]Based on the average of two or more properly measured, seated readings on each of two or more office visits.
Adapted from The Seventh Report of the Joint National Committee on Prevention, Detection, Evaluation, and Treatment of High Blood Pressure (JNC 7). Washington, DC, US Department of Health and Human Services, National Institutes of Health, National Heart, Lung, and Blood Institute, 2003. In American Academy of Family Physicians, American Academy of Pediatrics, American College of Sports Medicine, et al: Preparticipation Physical Evaluation, 3rd ed. Minneapolis, The Physician and Sportsmedicine/McGraw-Hill, 2005.

Preparticipation Physical Evaluation   **CLEARANCE FORM**

Name _____ **Sex** _____ **Age** _____ **Date of birth** _____

❑ **Cleared without restriction**
❑ **Cleared, with recommendations for further evaluation or treatment for:** _____

_____

_____

_____

❑ **Not cleared for** ❑ **All sports** ❑ **Certain sports:** _____ **Reason:** _____
Recommendations: _____

_____

EMERGENCY INFORMATION
Allergies _____
Other Information _____

IMMUNIZATIONS (eg, tetanus/diphtheria; measles, mumps, rubella; hepatitis A, B; influenza; poliomyelitis; pneumococcal; meningococcal; varicella)

❑ **Up to date (see attached documentation)** ❑ **Not up to date** Specify _____

Name of physician (print/type) _____ **Date** _____

Address _____ **Phone** _____

Signature of physician _____ **, MD or DO**

© 2004 American Academy of Family Physicians, American Academy of Pediatrics, American College of Sports Medicine, American Medical Society for Sports Medicine, American Orthopaedic Society for Sports Medicine, and American Osteopathic Academy of Sports Medicine.

Figure 2.4   Preparticipation physical evaluation: clearance form. (From the American Academy of Family Physicians, American Academy of Pediatrics, American College of Sports Medicine, et al: Preparticipation Physical Evaluation, 3rd ed. Minneapolis, The Physician and Sportsmedicine/McGraw-Hill, 2005.)

Table 2.5 Classification of Sports by Contact, High to Moderate Intensity

Contact or Collision	Limited Contact	Noncontact
Basketball	Baseball	Archery
Boxing*	Bicycling	Badminton
Diving	Cheerleading	Bodybuilding
Field hockey	Canoeing or kayaking (white water)	Bowling
Football, tackle		Canoeing or kayaking (flat water)
Ice hockey†	Fencing	Crew or rowing
Lacrosse	Field events (high jump, pole vault)	Curling
Martial arts	Floor hockey	Dancing (ballet, modern, jazz)§
Rodeo	Football, flag	
Rugby	Gymnastics	Field events (discus, javelin, shot put)
Ski jumping	Handball	
Soccer	Horseback riding	Golf
Team handball	Racquetball	Orienteering¶
Water polo	Skating (ice, in-line, roller)	Power lifting
Wrestling		Race walking
	Skiing (cross-country, downhill, water)	Riflery
		Rope jumping
	Skateboarding	Running
	Snowboarding‡	Sailing
	Softball	Scuba diving
	Squash	Swimming
	Ultimate Frisbee	Table tennis
	Volleyball	Tennis
	Windsurfing or surfing	Track
		Weight lifting

*Participation not recommended by the American Academy of Pediatrics.
†The American Academy of Pediatrics recommends limiting the amount of body checking allowed for hockey players who are 15 years old and younger to reduce injuries.
‡Snowboarding has been added since the previous statement was published.
§Dancing has been further classified into ballet, modern, and jazz since the previous monograph was published.
¶A race in which competitors use a map and compass to find their way through unfamiliar territory.
Reprinted with permission from American Academy of Pediatrics Committee on Sports Medicine and Fitness: Pediatrics 2001;107(5):1205-1209. In American Academy of Family Physicians, American Academy of Pediatrics, American College of Sports Medicine, et al: Preparticipation Physical Evaluation, 3rd ed. Minneapolis, The Physician and Sportsmedicine/McGraw-Hill, 2005.

Table 2.6 Classification of Sports by Strenuousness

High to Moderate Intensity		
High to Moderate Dynamic and Static Demands	High to Moderate Dynamic and Low Static Demands	High to Moderate Static and Low Dynamic Demands
Boxing*	Badminton	Archery
Crew or rowing	Baseball	Auto racing
Cross-country skiing	Basketball	Diving
Cycling	Field hockey	Horseback riding (jumping)
Downhill skiing	Lacrosse	
Fencing	Orienteering	Field events (throwing)
Football	Race walking	Gymnastics
Ice hockey	Racquetball	Karate or judo
Rugby	Soccer	Motorcycling
Running (sprint)	Squash	Rodeo
Speed skating	Swimming	Sailing
Water polo	Table tennis	Ski jumping
Wrestling	Tennis	Waterskiing
	Volleyball	Weight lifting

Low Intensity		
Low Dynamic and Low Static Demands		
Bowling		
Cricket		
Curling		
Golf		
Riflery		

*Participation not recommended by the American Academy of Pediatrics.
Reprinted with permission from American Academy of Pediatrics Committee on Sports Medicine and Fitness: Pediatrics 2001;107(5):1205-1209. In American Academy of Family Physicians, American Academy of Pediatrics, American College of Sports Medicine, et al: Preparticipation Physical Evaluation, 3rd ed. Minneapolis, The Physician and Sportsmedicine/McGraw-Hill, 2005.

made. Strict standards are indeed difficult, and there will always be room for case-by-case individual judgment. It is vital that all abnormalities that are described are followed up with the ultimate goal of maximal safe participation in physical activity and minimal disqualifications.

SPECIAL NEEDS

A new section in the third edition of the PPE monograph deals with athletes with special needs. A much more comprehensive work addressing PPE for Special Olympians will be published soon. Surely athletes with intellectual and special disabilities as well as other special needs deserve at least as comprehensive of an evaluation as mainstream athletes. Indeed, many of them have problems that will require a more complex investigation before clearance decisions can be made. Participation in sports for this population has innumerable benefits, including improved physical fitness, mood state, socialization, perceived health, discipline, self-confidence, self-esteem, personal satisfaction, and the satisfaction of being a part of a team. Many of the principles of the evaluation are the same as for mainstream athletes. The Special Olympics PPE is optimally performed by personal physicians, but it is often conducted using a station-method model called *Medfest*. A primary goal of PPE in this population, maybe even more than with "normal" athletes, is to identify events in which these athletes may safely participate with minimal risk, despite the presence of disability and chronic medical conditions. Because of potential impaired communication, the importance of a thorough physical evaluation is increased. Although a comprehensive discussion of special needs athletes is beyond the scope of this chapter, a few common conditions deserve mention. Visual and hearing problems are more common in this population and demand careful investigation. Obesity and sedentary lifestyle are also very prevalent, and they lend support to the further encouragement of athletic participation.

In 1983, Special Olympics Inc. disseminated its recommendation that every athlete with Down syndrome undergo a neurologic evaluation and a radiographic evaluation of the cervical spine.[18] These recommendations were based on the increased incidence of atlantoaxial instability among patients with this condition. Views include that of a lateral cervical spine in the straight, flexed, and extended positions. Movement of more than 5 mm of the atlantodens interval in cervical spine films with flexion and extension

Table 2.7 Medical Conditions and Sports Participation*

Condition	May Participate
Atlantoaxial instability (instability of the joint between cervical vertebrae 1 and 2) Explanation: Athlete needs evaluation to assess risk of spinal cord injury during sports participation.	**Qualified yes**
Bleeding disorder[†] Explanation: Athlete needs evaluation.	**Qualified yes**
Cardiovascular disease	
Carditis (inflammation of the heart) Explanation: Carditis may result in sudden death with exertion.	**No**
Hypertension (high blood pressure) Explanation: Those with significant essential (unexplained) hypertension should avoid weight and power lifting, bodybuilding, and strength training. Those with secondary hypertension (hypertension caused by a previously identified disease) or severe essential hypertension need evaluation. The National High Blood Pressure Education Working group defined significant and severe hypertension.	**Qualified yes**
Congenital heart disease (structural heart defects present at birth) Explanation: Those with mild forms may participate fully; those with moderate or severe forms or who have undergone surgery need evaluation. The 26th Bethesda Conference defined mild, moderate, and severe disease for common cardiac lesions.	**Qualified yes**
Dysrhythmia (irregular heart rhythm) Explanation: Those with symptoms (chest pain, syncope, dizziness, shortness of breath, or other symptoms of possible dysrhythmia) or evidence of mitral regurgitation (leaking) on physical examination need evaluation. All others may participate fully.	**Qualified yes**
Heart murmur Explanation: If the murmur is innocent (does not indicate heart disease), full participation is permitted. Otherwise, the athlete needs evaluation (see "Congenital heart disease," above, and mitral valve prolapse discussion in the text).	**Qualified yes**
Cerebral palsy[†] Explanation: Athlete needs evaluation.	**Qualified yes**
Diabetes mellitus Explanation: All sports can be played with proper attention to diet, blood glucose concentration, hydration, and insulin therapy. Blood glucose concentration should be monitored every 30 minutes during continuous exercise and 15 minutes after completion of exercise.	**Yes**
Diarrhea Explanation: Unless disease is mild, no participation is permitted, because diarrhea may increase the risk of dehydration and heat illness. See "Fever," below.	**Qualified no**
Eating disorders	
Anorexia nervosa, bulimia nervosa Explanation: Patients with these disorders need medical and psychiatric assessment before participation.	**Qualified yes**
Eyes	
Functionally 1-eyed athlete, loss of an eye, detached retina, previous eye surgery, or serious eye injury Explanation: A functionally 1-eyed athlete has a best-corrected visual acuity of less than 20/40 in the eye with worse acuity. These athletes would suffer significant disability if the better eye were seriously injured, as would those with loss of an eye. Some athletes who previously have undergone eye surgery or had a serious eye injury may have an increased risk of injury because of weakened eye tissue. Availability of eye guards approved by the American Society for Testing and Materials and other protective equipment may allow participation in most sports, but this must be judged on an individual basis.	**Qualified yes**
Fever Explanation: Fever can increase cardiopulmonary effort, reduce maximum exercise capacity, make heat illness more likely, and increase orthostatic hypertension during exercise. Fever may rarely accompany myocarditis or other infections that may make exercise dangerous.	**No**
Heat illness, history of Explanation: Because of the increased likelihood of recurrence, the athlete needs individual assessment to determine the presence of predisposing conditions and to arrange a prevention strategy.	**Qualified yes**
Hepatitis Explanation: Because of the apparent minimal risk to others, all sports may be played that the athlete's state of health allows. In all athletes, skin lesions should be covered properly, and athletic personnel should use universal precautions when handling blood or body fluids with visible blood.	**Yes**
Human immunodeficiency virus (HIV) infection Explanation: Because of the apparent minimal risk to others, all sports may be played that the athlete's state of health allows. In all athletes, skin lesions should be covered properly, and athletic personnel should use universal precautions when handling blood or body fluids with visible blood.	**Yes**

*This table is designed for use by medical and nonmedical personnel. "Needs evaluation" means that a physician with appropriate knowledge and experience should assess the safety of a given sport for an athlete with the listed medical condition. Unless otherwise noted, this is because of variability of the severity of the disease, the risk of injury for the specific sports, or both.
[†]Not discussed in the text of the monograph.

Continued

Table 2.7   Medical Conditions and Sports Participation—cont'd

Condition	May Participate
Kidney, absence of one	**Qualified yes**
Explanation: Athlete needs individual assessment for contact, collision, and limited-contact sports.	
Liver, enlarged	**Qualified yes**
Explanation: If the liver is acutely enlarged, participation should be avoided because of risk of rupture. If the liver is chronically enlarged, individual assessment is needed before collision, contact, or limited-contact sports are played.	
Malignant neoplasm[†]	**Qualified yes**
Explanation: Athlete needs individual assessment.	
Musculoskeletal disorders	**Qualified yes**
Explanation: Athlete needs individual assessment.	
Neurologic disorders	
History of serious head or spine trauma, severe or repeated concussions, or craniotomy	**Qualified yes**
Explanation: Athlete needs individual assessment for collision, contact, or limited-contact sports and also for noncontact sports if deficits in judgment or cognition are present. Research supports a conservative approach to management of concussion.	
Seizure disorder, well-controlled	**Yes**
Explanation: Risk of seizure during participation is minimal.	
Seizure disorder, poorly controlled	**Qualified yes**
Explanation: Athlete needs individual assessment for collision, contact, or limited-contact sports. The following noncontact sports should be avoided: archery, riflery, swimming, weight or power lifting, strength training, or sports involving heights. In these sports, occurrence of a seizure may pose a risk to self or others.	
Obesity	**Qualified yes**
Explanation: Because of the risk of heat illness, obese persons need careful acclimatization and hydration.	
Organ transplant recipient[†]	**Qualified yes**
Explanation: Athlete needs individual assessment.	
Ovary, absence of one	**Yes**
Explanation: Risk of severe injury to the remaining ovary is minimal.	
Respiratory conditions	
Pulmonary compromise, including cystic fibrosis	**Qualified yes**
Explanation: Athlete needs individual assessment, but generally, all sports may be played if oxygenation remains satisfactory during a graded exercise test. Patients with cystic fibrosis need acclimatization and good hydration to reduce the risk of heat illness.	
Asthma	**Yes**
Explanation: With proper medication and education, only athletes with the most severe asthma will need to modify their participation.	
Acute upper respiratory infection	**Qualified yes**
Explanation: Upper respiratory obstruction may affect pulmonary function. Athlete needs individual assessment for all but mild disease. See "Fever," on previous page.	
Sickle cell disease	**Qualified yes**
Explanation: Athlete needs individual assessment. In general, if status of the illness permits, all but high exertion, collision, and contact sports may be played. Overheating, dehydration, and chilling must be avoided.	
Sickle cell trait	**Yes**
Explanation: It is unlikely that persons with sickle cell trait have an increased risk of sudden death or other medical problems during athletic participation, except under the most extreme conditions of heat, humidity, and, possibly, increased altitude. These persons, like all athletes, should be carefully conditioned, acclimatized, and hydrated to reduce any possible risk.	
Skin disorders (boils, herpes simplex, impetigo, scabies, molluscum contagiosum)	**Qualified yes**
Explanation: While the patient is contagious, participation in gymnastics with mats; martial arts; wrestling; or other collision, contact, or limited-contact sports is not allowed.	
Spleen, enlarged	**Qualified yes**
Explanation: A patient with an acutely enlarged spleen should avoid all sports because of risk of rupture. A patient with a chronically enlarged spleen needs individual assessment before playing collision, contact, or limited-contact sports.	
Testicle, undescended or absence of one	**Yes**
Explanation: Certain sports may require a protective cup.	

Reprinted with permission from American Academy of Pediatrics Committee on Sports Medicine and Fitness: Pediatrics 2001;107(5):1205-1209. In American Academy of Family Physicians, American Academy of Pediatrics, American College of Sports Medicine, et al: Preparticipation Physical Evaluation, 3rd ed. Minneapolis, The Physician and Sportsmedicine/McGraw-Hill, 2005.

meets the radiographic criteria for atlantoaxial instability, which is reported at rates of 10% to 30% among patients with Down syndrome, and approximately 12% to 16% of these patients develop neurologic signs and symptoms. Obviously, most patients with radiographic abnormalities never develop problems. Conversely, patients with normal x-rays can later develop abnormalities. If problems are found, patients with atlantoaxial instability are restricted from events that put undue stress on the cervical spine. Clearly, carefully looking for symptoms is the most important consideration. Because patients with Down syndrome have a nearly 50% incidence of congenital heart defects, they should be carefully evaluated.

Seizures are also more common among patients with intellectual disabilities. If seizures are controlled by medication, restriction is not necessary. Special consideration should be given to the inherent dangers of a seizure occurring in certain settings (e.g. diving, open-water swimming, events occurring at heights, and equestrian sports). Reasonable seizure control and medication compliance are essential for all sports participation.

Autonomic dysreflexia is an acute, life-threatening syndrome of excessive, uncontrolled sympathetic output that can occur in athletes with spinal-cord injuries at or above the sixth thoracic level. This reflex can occur spontaneously, or it can be triggered by things such as bowel or bladder distension, infections, sunburn, ingrown toenails, and wearing tight garments; it may also be self-induced by an athlete in an attempt to improve performance (a practice known as *boosting*). Findings may include significant blood-pressure elevation, a pounding headache, bradycardia, flushing of the face, and sweating above the level of the spinal cord injury. Paraplegic athletes are also prone to premature osteoporosis, which increases the risk of occult fractures.[19] For a more comprehensive review of athletes with special needs, look for the monograph addressing PPE for Special Olympians, which will be coming out soon.

FUTURE DIRECTIONS

In the future, the medical community must work toward the acceptance of nationally standardized forms and the creation of databases to measure the effectiveness and validity of the PPE process. The appropriate place for neuropsychological testing after concussion is currently being studied; this is an example of how many recommendations will subsequently be more based on evidence. In many cases, very sports-specific evaluations may be appropriate. As an example, findings such as generalized ligamentous laxity may even result in recommendations for safer sports selection by young athletes. There is already a move toward the electronic handling of athletic health information, which has obvious potential advantages but also inherent dangers, such as security issues, cost, and the need to keep up with changing technologies. This change will be a part of the national trend to move toward electronic health records for everyone.

CONCLUSION

Although the PPE monograph may be far from perfect, it certainly represents the best effort at consensus that has been arrived at thus far by experts from multiple important national organizations. These groups will continue to meet periodically as new information becomes available, and this will result in new additions to the publication. Without question, this is a work in progress. A second monograph addressing athletes with special needs will be equally comprehensive and provide a valuable reference for practitioners who are involved in their care. There will always be room for case-by-case individual judgment regarding clearance and return-to-play decisions. Whenever abnormalities are found, it is critical that they be investigated expeditiously so that the ultimate restriction from sports participation is minimal; one only has to consider the national obesity epidemic to understand the significance of this recommendation. Without question, the true goal of the optimal PPE is the encouragement of maximal safe physical activity for all athletes and potential athletes.

REFERENCES

1. American Academy of Family Physicians, American Academy of Pediatrics, American College of Sports Medicine, et al: Preparticipation Physical Evaluation, 3rd ed. Minneapolis, The Physician and Sportsmedicine/McGraw-Hill, 2005.
2. Risser WL, Hoffman HM, Bellah GG Jr: Frequency of preparticipation sports examinations in secondary school athletes: are the University Interscholastic League guidelines appropriate? Tex Med 1985;81(7):35-39.
3. Maron BJ, Thompson PD, Puffer JC, et al: Cardiovascular preparticipation screening of competitive athletes: a statement for health professionals from the Sudden Death Committee (clinical cardiology) and Congenital Cardiac Defects Committee (cardiovascular disease in the young), American Heart Association. Circulation 1996;94:850-856.
4. Maron BJ, Thompson PD, Puffer JC, et al: Cardiovascular preparticipation screening of competitive athletes: addendum: an addendum to a statement for health professionals from the Sudden Death committee (Council on Clinical Cardiology) and the Congenital Cardiac Defects Committee (Council on Cardiovascular Disease in the Young). American Heart Association. Circulation 1998;97:2294.
5. American Academy of Family Physicians, American Academy of Pediatrics, American Medical Society for Sports Medicine, et al: Preparticipation Physical Evaluation. Minneapolis, McGraw-Hill, 1992.
6. Sullivan JA, Grana WA: Preparticipation Evaluation, The Pediatric Athlete, American Academy of Orthopaedic Surgeons Seminar. 1990, pp 53-61.
7. 36th Bethesda Conference: Recommendations for determining eligibility for competition in athletes with cardiovascular abnormalities. J Am Coll Cardiol 2005;45(8):1312-1375.
8. Epstein SE, Maron BJ: Sudden death and the competitive athlete: perspectives on preparticipation screening studies. J Am Coll Cardiol 1986;7:220-230.
9. Pretzlaff RK: Death of an adolescent athlete with sickle cell trait caused by exertional heat stroke. Pediatr Crit Care Med 2002;3(3):308-310.
10. Kark JA, Posey DM, Schumacher HR, et al: Sickle-cell trait as a risk factor for sudden death in physical training. N Engl J Med 1987;317(13):781-787.
11. American College of Allergy, Asthma and Immunology: Asthma Disease Management Resource Manual. Available at http://allergy.mcgs.edu/physicians/manual/manual.html. Accessed August 9, 2004.
12. Gerberich SG, Priest JD, Boen JR, et al: Concussion incidences and severity in secondary school varsity football players. Am J Public Health 1983;73:1370-1375.
13. Zemper E: Analysis of cerebral concussion frequency with the most commonly used models of football helmets. J Athletic Train 1994;29:44-50.
14. McCrory P, Johnston K, Meeuwisse W, et al: Summary and agreement statement of the 2nd International Conference on Concussion in Sport, Prague 2004. Br J Sports Med 2005;34(4):196-204.
15. Concussion (mild traumatic brain injury) and the team physician: a consensus statement. Med Sci Sports Exerc 2005;37(11):2012-2016.
16. Hosey RG, Armsey TD: Sudden cardiac death. Clin Sports Med 2003;22(1):51-66.
17. Magnes SA, Henderson JM, Hunter SC: What conditions limit sports participation? Experience with 10,540 athletes. Phys Sportsmed 1992;20(5):143-160.
18. Special Olympics International: Participation by individuals with Down syndrome who suffer from atlantoaxial dislocation condition. March 31, 1983.
19. Dec K, Sparrow K, McKeag DB: The physically-challenged athlete: medical issues and assessment. Sports Med 2000;29(4):245-258.

The Team Physician's Bag

Scott D. Flinn, MD, and Elise T. Gordon, MD

KEY POINTS

- Emergency resuscitation material should be carried on the physician's person in an easily accessible bag, like a fanny pack.
- Inventory of the physician's bag should be taken at the beginning of every season, and items should be replaced as they are used because it is important to maintaining the bag at its peak readiness.
- If the team is traveling, the physician must remind all team members to bring adequate personal supplies of their medicines, eyeglasses, contacts, and any other personal medical supplies that they routinely use.
- What to carry in the game bag depends on the sport covered, how many participants there are, the location of the event, the availability of other resources, the philosophy of the care to be rendered (triage alone or treatment), and the ability to carry the materials.
- It is important to know what medications you can give to athletes if they participate in a sport and/or organization that tests for banned substances.

INTRODUCTION

The team physician is an integral part of the medical team that provides care for athletes before, during, and after athletic events. Occasionally, the team physician is called on to cover the staff and the spectators as well. Whether covering a local field event, a mass participation event, or a team traveling to an international competition, the team physician's coverage bag should contain materials to address anything from routine medical problems to emergency field situations. Planning for the medical coverage of the event will help determine what specific items that the physician will carry.

In 2000, the American College of Sports Medicine in conjunction with the American Academy of Family Physicians, the American Academy of Orthopedic Surgeons, the American Medical Society of Sports Medicine, the American Orthopedic Society of Sports Medicine, and the American Osteopathic Academy of Sports Medicine published a team physician consensus statement that contained recommendations for event planning, including recommended medical supplies that are either available on-site at the venue or carried in the physician's coverage bag.[1] Other team physicians have provided similar recommendations.[2-6] The type of event, the sport, the location, the number of competitors, the expected available resources, and the usual weather at the competition site dictate variations in the range of required medical supplies.

THE GAME BAG

Choices for the physician's game bag come in many shapes, sizes, colors, and materials.[3,5,6] There are medical bags that are specifically designed for carrying event-coverage medical equipment. Some prefer a hard-shell case because it provides added protection for breakable materials. These can come with wheels for ease of portability, and they may be lockable. Alternatively, bags made of soft material are usually lighter and easier to carry with a shoulder strap or in a backpack configuration. Other options include fishing tackle boxes and luggage that has been modified to suit the event.

Competitive events may be located in interesting venues that require the gear to be hand carried some distance or up and down stairs. A padded shoulder strap, a backpack, or wheels make this easier. The bag should be large enough to carry the necessary gear but not so large as to be overly cumbersome to transport.

Regardless of the type of bag selected, the physician must be able to readily access supplemental emergency equipment that cannot be carried on the physician's person. This other gear should be quickly accessible. Movable dividers in the main compartment allow for flexibility with the placement of gear. Side and top pockets with clear panels and zippers or Velcro closures allow for secure, rapid access to small items, and they allow for the easy identification of contents. Others prefer labeled plastic bags or color-specific nylon bags for the storage of specific gear. The outside of the bag should be marked with colored markers, stickers, or embroidery to allow for the easy identification of the bag.

A fanny pack is helpful for carrying immediately available emergency equipment onto the field, mats, ice, or track. If one is going on a long trip, more than one bag may be necessary. International travel can make transporting some items difficult. If possible, ship some of the medical kit with the team supplies ahead of time and carry only the essentials.

Maintaining the items on an inventory list keeps the bag always at the ready. At least once a year, the contents of the bag should be reviewed to eliminate expired medications and to update the equipment and supplies. After an event during which items are used, the bag should be restocked before the next coverage. It is particularly important to review the inventory list before covering new types of events because special sport- or event-specific items may need to be added.

TRAVEL

Overnight and international travel involves a unique set of challenges.[7] For example, the destination may have limited supplies and medication. The team physician should be aware of any and all medical problems of the personnel who are traveling, and he or she should advise all traveling members to pack an adequate supply of their medications in their original containers with the prescription label. A spare pair of glasses and/or contacts should also be carried.

The Centers for Disease Control and Prevention Web site provides information about any required vaccines or travel health risks and whether a yellow card for proof of vaccination is needed for specific destinations.[8] The US Department of State Web site provides information that details any travel warnings.[9] Many destination countries will have limited medical resources.

During travel, the team physician may have to provide more services than are normally expected while at home. It is prudent to carry the fanny pack with travel and emergency supplies and medications for easy access during travel. The medicines that are most likely to be needed are those for traveler's diarrhea, cellulitis, dermatitis, and upper respiratory infections. An albuterol inhaler and some diphenhydramine would also be advisable. If air or sea travel is involved, motion sickness medications for those who are susceptible may be quite helpful.

THE EVENT

Covering any event takes forethought and planning. The physician should know whether he or she is covering a game, a tournament, or a mass-participation event. The number of personnel to be covered, including athletes and coaches, affects the quantity of material to take. Sometimes the physician will be responsible for providing care for spectators as well. It is also essential to know what equipment is available at the event site and what other medical assets are immediately available.[10-13] The response time and skill level of the local emergency response should be taken into account. Some sports have unique or frequent injuries, and the provider should be prepared to handle these (e.g., nosebleeds in wrestling).

If the physician is covering an unfamiliar sport or event, various resources can be used to ensure proper sideline preparedness. Discussing the medical coverage of the event with the local athletic trainer and with colleagues with experience can be especially valuable. Literature searches can provide data regarding sport-specific injury patterns; physicians should refer to the National College Athletic Association Injury Surveillance System.[14] Many sports medicine–related Web sites have links to consensus statements regarding preparation for mass-participation events, sideline preparedness, and game bag inventory.[1,10,15]

Because no list can be comprehensive and cover every contingency, the following are some guidelines for what to take in the game bag. Physicians have their personal preferences, which are developed with experience. Consideration as to how material will be transported and staged is important; one does not want to have to carry undue amounts of material over long distances. The physician should be prepared to carry the medical gear unless other arrangements have been made. Appropriate additions, deletions, and substitutions should be made as required or desired to tailor the physician coverage bag appropriately.

MEDICAL EMERGENCY GEAR

Although they are uncommon, medical emergencies should be handled promptly by the coverage physician and support personnel using basic life support skills with universal precautions.[11] Planning before the event should include determining what emergency gear is available at the venue, what emergency services are available and how to contact them, and the average response time. The basic emergency equipment should be carried on the physician's person in a small fanny pack or in a rapidly accessible container in the game bag that is kept within easy reach on top of the bag (also called a *blowout kit*).

Medical emergency equipment may be grouped into categories that are similar to life-support categories: airway, breathing, circulation, disability/drugs, and exposure. Recommended gear for emergencies is listed in **Table 3.1.** Not all of the material may be applicable to each situation, and the items should be adjusted accordingly. Some of the gear is large and should be supplied at the venue. The physician should carry a pocket mask or another means of delivering mouth-to-mouth resuscitation. If it will take a prolonged time for emergency crews to respond, consideration should be given to carrying a bag–valve–mask device. When covering a football event, it is necessary to have the ability to remove the mask to obtain airway access without removing the helmet. Items are readily available and include polyvinyl chloride pipe cutters and trainer's angels.[16] Screwdrivers seldom work because the screws are often rusted or stripped. If there is a potential for facial trauma that can compromise the airway and make mouth-to-mouth and bag–valve–mask support difficult or impossible, consideration should be given to being able to perform an emergent surgical airway. Because it is very unusual to have cardiac emergencies that need to be treated on the field other than ventricular fibrillation or pulseless ventricular tachycardia, an automatic external defibrillator is recommended to be on site, whereas the numerous cardiac medications associated with advanced cardiac life support are not recommended.

Diagnostic instruments

The basic diagnostic instruments are listed in **Table 3.2.** A glucometer is recommended when covering events in which diabetic athletes are participating. If the physician is taking fluorescein strips, he or she must remember to take an appropriate blue light. If heat casualties are a concern, a rectal thermometer should be available to determine accurate core temperatures.

Wound care

The equipment and supplies needed to treat various wounds are noted in **Table 3.3.** Controlling bleeding and cleaning gross blood from uniforms is necessary to remain in competition in most sports, so appropriate materials for this (e.g., peroxide) should be in the bag. In addition to the usual medical instruments, a multitool device such as a Leatherman or Gerber can have many uses in the field, including opening stuck chinstraps.

Orthopedic material

Sufficient materials to provide immediate care for orthopedic injuries should be in the game bag.[13] A suggested list is provided in **Table 3.4.** If there is a likelihood of a femoral shaft fracture, a Hare traction splint should be available.

Table 3.1 Emergency Equipment

General/Diagnostic
Communication: cell phone or radio with local emergency numbers

Paper and pen

Gloves

Stethoscope

Penlight

Multitool (e.g., Leatherman, Gerber)

At the Venue
Oxygen, tubing, and mask

Automatic external defibrillator

Backboard with cervical spine stabilization material

Crutches

Airway
Face shield/pocket mask

Oral airways (small, medium, and large)

Nasal airways (26, 28, and 30) with lube packet

Trainer's angels, polyvinyl chloride pipe cutter, screwdriver, or facemask extractor for football helmets

Intubation and/or cricothyrotomy materials if the need to establish a definitive airway is anticipated

Breathing
Pulse oximeter

Bag—valve—mask/ambubag if prolonged ventilation may be necessary

Suction

Vaseline gauze and/or Asherman chest seal if there is a risk for pneumothorax

Circulation
Intravenous infusion set

Roll of sterile gauze dressing

4×4 inch sterile gauzes pads

Tape: athletic self-adhesive wrap

Tourniquet if there is a risk for severe laceration (e.g., speed skating)

Disability and Drugs
Cervical collar

Glucose tablets

Albuterol inhaler

Epinephrine, 1:1000, 2-3 mL (e.g., EpiPen)

Diphenhydramine, injectable, 50 mg

Aspirin, 81 mg

Nitroglycerin, sublingual, 0.4 mg or spray

Exposure
Penlight/flashlight/headlamp

Trauma shears

Medications

This is often the most variable part of the bag.[7] In particular, cardiac conditions are rare in the athletic population. Ventricular fibrillation and pulseless ventricular tachycardia would be the most likely life-threatening situations to occur, and they may respond to the rapid administration of electricity by automatic external defibrillator. Otherwise, the physician will rarely encounter other cardiac conditions that can be addressed adequately in the field. Therefore, carrying additional cardiac medications and a full defibrillator that can provide a pacing capability is not recommended.

Table 3.2 Diagnostic Instruments

Stethoscope

Thermometer (rectal if heat casualties are anticipated)

Blood-pressure cuff

Oto-ophthalmoscope

Penlight

Fluorescein strips with blue-light ophthalmoscope

Reflex hammer

Vibrating fork

Eye chart

Goniometer

Headlamp (enables illumination while leaving hands free for rendering treatment)

Glucometer

Spare batteries

Pregnancy test

Peak flow meter

Table 3.3 Wound Care Supplies

Scissors: trauma, Iris

Hemostats

Forceps: tissue, splinter

Scalpels: #10 and #15

Stapler and staple remover

Steri-Strips: various sizes

Benzoin

Band-Aids: multiple sizes, including knuckle and four-wing bandages

Dermabond

Fingernail polish remover/acetone (for Super glue removal)

Alcohol swabs

Iodine swabs

Syringes: tuberculin, 3 mL, 5 mL, 10 mL

Needles: 18 gauge, 22 gauge, 25 gauge, 1.5 inches

Suture material: various sizes and types

Suture packs

Tape: athletic 0.5, 1, and 1.5 inch; Elastikon 2 and 3 inch; Coban 1 and 2 inch; Expandover

Bandages: Tegaderm; Telfa; blister bandages; Second Skin, 1 inch; Adaptik; Vaseline gauze

Nonstick bandages: 8×3 inch

4×4 inch: sterile and nonsterile

2×2 inch: sterile and nonsterile

Neosporin packets

Benzocaine sticks (Medco)

Styptic (Monsel's solution)

Dental rolls (for nosebleeds)

Alcare Plus or Hibiclens for potential methicillin-resistant *Staphylococcus aureus* (Steris: 1-800-548-4873)

Moleskin

Corn shaver

Cuticle cutter

Nail clippers

Sting Xtractor (TECNU Enterprises: 1-800-Itching)

Tube gauze and applicator

Lancets (for blister care)

Table 3.4   Splinting and Bracing Materials

Crutches
Sam splint or plaster
Orthoplast (especially if the facility has a hydrocollator to mold it)
Shoulder slings
Straight-leg immobilizer
Ankle brace
High-density foam (e.g., to cut donuts for acromioclavicular joint)
Ace bandages: 3, 4, and 6 inch
Triangular bandage and safety pins
Finger splints (put into small tackle box)
AlumaFoam and trauma shears to cut it
Thumb splint
Wrist splint
Neoprene knee sleeve
Hare traction splint

Table 3.5   Medications

Essential Medications
Diphenhydramine, oral and injectable
Epinephrine, 1:1000, 2 or 3 mL (e.g., EpiPen)
Glucose tablets
Albuterol inhaler
Medicine envelopes

Altitude Medications (for Travel to Areas over 10,000 Feet)
Diamox
Dexamethasone
Nifedipine

Antibiotics
Amoxicillin/clavanulate
Ciprofloxacin
Cephalexin
Erythromycin or clindamycin
Doxycycline
Trimethoprim—sulfamethoxazole (for methicillin-resistant *Staphylococcus aureus*)
Rocephin
Acyclovir or valacyclovir

Anti-inflammatory Drugs, Muscle Relaxants, and Pain Relievers
Ibuprofen
Indomethacin
Celebrex
Acetaminophen
Flexeril
Prednisone

Controlled Medications for Special Circumstances
Acetaminophen with codeine
Morphine
Naloxone

Antiallergy Drugs, Antihistamines, and Motion-Sickness Drugs
Meclizine
Diphenhydramine
Loratadine
Scopolamine patch

Cardiac Medications
See emergency section

Eyes, Ears, Nose, and Throat Drugs
Tobramycin ophthalmic drops
Ophthalmic anesthetic drops
Otic suspension or fluoroquinolone otic drops
Mydriatic agent
Eyewash
Artificial tears
Nasal steroid
Saline nose spray
Afrin
Pseudoephedrine
Cough syrup

Gastrointestinal Medications
Over-the-counter antacid
Proton-pump inhibitor
Antiemetic, injectable, oral, suppositories
Loperamide
Stool softener
Magnesium citrate or another laxative
Pepto-Bismol

Gynecologic Medications
Oral contraceptive pack
Fluconazole, 150 mg, or clotrimazole vaginal cream
Metronidazole or clindamycin vaginal cream
Sulfanilamide cream

Injectable Drugs
Lidocaine with or without epinephrine
Marcaine
Triamcinolone, 10 mg/mL and 40 mg/mL
1 ampule of 50% Dextrose solution
Tetanus immunization
EpiPen (or EpiPen Jr)
Diphenhydramine
Phenergan

Pulmonary Drugs
Albuterol inhaler
Inhaled steroid (for travel)
Spacer
Paper bag

Sleep-Inducing Medications
Ambien or Sonata

Topical/Dermatologic Drugs
Antifungal cream
Antibacterial ointment or cream
Mupirocin ointment (for methicillin-resistant *Staphylococcus aureus*)
Betadine
Medicated first aid spray
Hydrocortisone cream, varying strengths
Peroxide, another blood remover, or a 10% bleach solution
Zinc

Continued

Table 3.5   Medications—cont'd

Calamine/Caladryl

Lip balm

Head lice treatment

Urinary Medications

Pyridium, 200 mg

Table 3.6   Head, Eyes, Ears, Nose, and Throat Supplies

Nose packs

Fluorescein and otoscope or penlight with a blue light

Small mirror (for putting contact lenses in)

Small eye suction cup (for removing contact lenses from lid)

Contact case and saline eye flush

Eye protector (hard eye shell for protection in a case of suspected or confirmed globe trauma)

Eyeglass repair kit

Eyewash

Ear and eye medications (see Table 3.5)

Dental floss

Save-A-Tooth emergency dental kit (found in any drug store)

Dental wax/sugarless gum (for protection of braces)

Medications should be carried to address the usual routine and field issues. When traveling, the physician should carry antibiotics to cover routine illnesses like skin infections, upper respiratory congestion and infections, and gastrointestinal problems. Suggested medications to carry are listed in **Table 3.5.** Vaccinations should be performed as required before any travel, and proper documentation should be carried as needed.

Eye, ear, nose, and throat

Supplies to handle field care for eye, ear, nose, and throat issues are listed in **Table 3.6.** If an orbital globe rupture is suspected, pressure should not be applied to the eye, but a firm protective covering should be placed around the bony orbit to protect the globe contents.

Miscellaneous items

Other items that should be considered for the team bag are listed in **Table 3.7.** A knife and a multitool device may also be useful, depending on the location of the event.

Comfort items

Comfort items for the physician and the athletes are listed in **Table 3.8.** This list can be modified as needed to fit personal taste. Coaches seem to always have headaches, so appropriate over-the-counter medication may be handy.

Administrative supplies

A certain amount of reference material and paperwork may be necessary, depending on the event covered, and forms to document medical care may be required. Depending on the athletes and the medications involved, the US Anti-Doping Agency handbook may be particularly useful for covering a competition in

Table 3.7   Miscellaneous Equipment

Hand sanitizer

ToughSkin

Petroleum jelly

Skin lubricant

Icy Hot

Tissues

Zip-top bags

Biohazard bags

Tape Shark (for cutting tape)

Tape measure

Small sharps container

Examination gloves, regular and latex free

Sterile gloves, regular and latex free

Cotton-tipped applicators

Tongue depressors

Tiger Balm

Cooling balm

Shoelaces

Safety pins

Sewing kit

Salt/electrolyte replacement packets

Ice bags and wraps to hold them on

Lighter (use caution when boarding an airplane; the rules are constantly changing)

Ring cutter

Duct tape

Baby powder

Whistle

Velcro

Hot sauce (mix with water and drink to decongest nasal passages; can also eat wasabi)

Silly Putty or reaction ball (for occupational therapy)

---

which athletes may be drug tested.[17] See the list of suggested administrative supplies in **Table 3.9.**

Sport-specific supplies

Specific sports may have a particular problem that is frequently encountered. Some suggestions for supplies are listed in **Table 3.10.** For example, having enough supplies to cover numerous skin scrapes would be important when covering a game on artificial turf.

CONCLUSION

Covering events can be as logistically easy as volunteering at the local basketball game or as complex as a multination international tour. Planning for the event enables the physician to provide an adequate first response to field emergencies. The materials to be carried in the game bag are dependent on a number of factors, including physician experience and preference. A rather thorough set of recommended equipment and supplies has been presented for the physician to use to tailor the game bag to best meet the coverage needs for a specific event. In this day of evidence-based medicine, the items in the team physician's coverage bag remain the product of expert opinion, consensus, experience, and personal choice.

Table 3.8   Comfort Items

Sunscreen/aloe

Over-the-counter headache and pain medications (e.g., acetaminophen, ibuprofen)

Over-the-counter antacid

Hard candy

Towel

Wipes, bleach wipes

Emery board

Disposable razor

Playing cards

Lock

Earplugs

Space blanket

Back plaster

Poncho

Eye black

Alarm clock

Arch supports

Insect repellent

Massage cream/baby lotion/hand lotion

Tampons/sanitary napkins

For International Travel

Small packets of tissues (may need to use as toilet paper in remote areas)

Electric transformers

Table 3.9   Administrative Supplies

Patient care documentation form

Notebook

Concussion assessment form

Prescription pad

Pens

Permanent markers

Head-injury assessment form

References (e.g., Sanford Guide,* EMS Field Guide, 5-Minute Sports Medicine Consult[†]; may also be available for personal digital assistant)

US Anti-Doping Agency Guide[‡]

Business cards or phone numbers for local specialists (e.g., dentist, orthopedist, neurosurgeon)

*Sanford Guide to Antimicrobila. Available at www.sanfordguide.com.
[†]Bracker MD (ed): 5-Minute Sports Medicine Consult. Philadelphia, Lippincott Williams & Wilkins, 2001.
[‡]US Anti-Doping Agency: USADA 2007 guide to prohibited substances and prohibited methods of doping (Web site): Available at www.usantidoping.org/files/active/what/usada_guide.pdf. Accessed April 10, 2007.

Table 3.10   Sport-Specific Supplies and Concerns

Skiing

Hat

Mittens

Ski tool

Warm Weather

Salt packets

Rectal thermometer

Basketball

Eye injuries

Crew

Skin issues

Cycling

Acromioclavicular separations

Clavicle fractures

Road rash

Football

Helmet-removal tool (screwdriver, pliers, football facemask removal tool; many versions can be found online)

Spare mouth guards

Ice Hockey

Lacerations

Dental injuries (have a dental kit and phone numbers for referral)

Mass-Participation Event

Blister care

Hyponatremia (salt packets)

Heat and/or cold injuries

Running

Blister care

Chafing

Swimming

Chafing (petroleum jelly)

Eye irritation (Visine, Vasocon-A)

Tampons

Rugby

See Wrestlers/boxers

Special Populations

PEDIATRIC ATHLETES

Suspensions and chewable medications

SPECIAL OLYMPICS ATHLETES

Lorazepam or diazepam for seizures

DISABLED ATHLETES

Hand blisters

Thermoregulation issues

Autonomic dysreflexia

Syncope

FEMALE ATHLETES

Sanitary napkins and tampons

Naproxen and Motrin

Vaginal infections (for Candida and bacterial vaginitis)

WRESTLERS/BOXERS

Nasal hemopack

Cotton nose packs (dental pledgets or junior tampons will do in a pinch)

Vaseline

Gauze

Drysol or styptic (these athletes are too sweaty to keep Steri-Strips in place)

REFERENCES

1. Herring SA (chair): Team physician consensus statement. Med Sci Sports Exerc 2000;32(4):877-878.
2. Ray RL, Feld FX: The team physician's medical bag. Clin Sports Med 1989;1(8): 139-146.
3. Cabasso A: The athletic team physician's medical bag. N J Med 1991;88(9):625-626.
4. Stricker PR: The sports medicine kit: basics of the bag. Ped Ann 2002;31(1):14-16.
5. Yan CB, Rubin AL: Equipment and supplies for sports and event medicine. Curr Sports Med Rep 2005;4(3):131-136.
6. Buettner CM: Sports pharmacology: the team physician's bag. Clin Sports Med 1998;17(2):365-373.
7. Brown DW: Medical issues associated with international competition. Guidelines for the traveling physician. Clin Sports Med 1998;17(4):739-754.
8. Center for Disease Control and Prevention home page (Web site): Available at www.cdc.gov. Accessed April 10, 2007.
9. US Department of State home page (Web site): Available at travel.state.gov. Accessed April 10, 2007.
10. Herring SA (chair), Bergfeld J, Boyd J, et al: Sideline preparedness for the team physician: a consensus statement (Web site): Available at www.acsm.org/AM/ Template.cfm?Section=Clinicians1&Template=/CM/ContentDisplay.cfm&ContentID= 1620. Accessed April 10, 2007.
11. Gomez JE: Sideline medical emergencies in the young athlete. Pediatr Ann 2002;31(1):52-57.
12. Hutchison M, Tansey J: Sideline management of fractures. Curr Sports Med Rep 2003;2(3):125-135.
13. Roberts WO: Mass-participation events. In Lillegard WS, Butcher JD, Rucker KS (eds): Handbook of Sports Medicine, 2nd ed. Boston, Butterworth-Heinemann, 1999, pp 27.
14. National Collegiate Athletic Association Injury Surveillance System home page (Web site): Available at www.ncaa.org/iss. Accessed April 10, 2007.
15. Herring SA, Bergfeld JA, Boyajian-O'Neill LA: Mass participation event management for the team physician: a consensus statement. Med Sci Sports Exerc 2004;36(11):2004-2008.
16. Roberts WO: Helmet removal in head and neck trauma, The Physician and Sportsmedicine (serial online): Available at www.physsportsmed.com. Accessed December 20, 2005.
17. US Anti-Doping Agency: USADA 2007 guide to prohibited substances and prohibited methods of doping (Web site): Available at www.usantidoping.org/files/active/what/ usada_guide.pdf.

CHAPTER 4

Mass-Participation Event Coverage

Scott W. Pyne, MD, FAAFP, FACSM

KEY POINTS

- Advanced planning and preparation are essential to the successful medical management of mass-participation events.
- Medical leadership should follow clear lines of communication and must interact with event leadership with mutual respect and shared common goals.
- The establishment of the level of medical care provided and a contingency plan for the disposition of more severe conditions requires cooperation, communication, and coordination with numerous supporting organizations.
- Injury prevention, medical condition identification, and specific treatment plan education of participants and event and medical support staff is recommended both before and during an event.
- Documentation and summarization after an event are helpful for the planning of future events.

INTRODUCTION

The medical coverage of mass-participation events presents a unique, exciting, and challenging opportunity to literally bring medical care to the masses. Although sports doctors are adept at treating athletes individually, additional skills and advanced planning are required to provide optimal care in these diverse settings. Mass-participation events, which are those in which many people participate simultaneously, are generally spread out over several miles, many distinct sites, and variable terrain. They may include single-discipline or multiple-discipline events with competition for individuals or teams. Advanced planning and preparation are critical to successfully accommodate the medical needs of the event participants.[1-4] As the leader of the medical team, the medical director's main goal is to implement strategies to prevent serious injury and illness.[5] This is accomplished through the numerous responsibilities of planning, communicating, and organizing in addition to caring for injured athletes. An awareness of the rules of the event is essential for providing care within the framework of the competition.[6] The needs of the athletes who are competing must be considered well before the event, with specific consideration given to the type of event, the number of participants, any course peculiarities,

and environmental predictions; all of these are guiding principles when determining the medical assets required.

EPIDEMIOLOGY

To best understand the requirements of a given event, it is helpful to review epidemiologic data regarding like events. Injury rates have been well documented in the medical literature: running (< 21 km), 1% to 5%; triathlon (51 km), 2% to 5%; Nordic skiing (55 km), 5%; cycling (variable distances), 5%; youth wrestling, 12.7%; ice-skating marathon, 14.3%; running (42 km), 1% to 20%; triathlon (225 km), 15% to 30%; and, wilderness multisport endurance event, 70%.[7-11]

Team sports injury rates are often expressed as frequency per 1000 player hours. Documented rugby tournament injury rates are interesting in that they vary from 32 to 97.9 injuries per 1000 player game hours.[12-16] A 10-year experience of USA CUP soccer injuries revealed an overall decrease in injury rates from 19.87 in 1988 to 9.89 in 1997.[17] Team-sport tournament coverage has the additional medical challenges of physical contact in combination with endurance and recovery requirements between multiple competitions.[6,18] The disparity of injury-rate data may also be explained by differing definitions of injury, different inclusion criteria, and variable athlete experience levels.

Increased distance and environmental temperature during endurance events have been shown to increase injury rates.[19-21] Similar data have not yet been demonstrated for team sports, except with regard to the incidence of heat injury.[17]

The experience of previous years is very helpful during the medial planning process for subsequent years' events; this stresses the importance of a reliable injury data tracking system. Similar events in similar elements can also be considered during the initial planning and preparation stages of new events.

Injury type and distribution data are also useful when planning for medical supplies and staffing expertise. Fortunately, the risk for morbidity and mortality in mass-participation events is quite small.[22]

MEDICAL DIRECTOR

As a key advisor to the event director, the medical director must lead the medical team and ensure that the event is conducted with the safety of the competitors being of utmost importance.

Often this is lower on the list of the competing priorities that face event organizers, who must balance sponsor, financial, and community concerns. Mutual respect, common goals, and direct lines of communication between the event directors and the medical directors are essential to the smooth conduct of mass-participation events. It is strongly suggested that a written agreement outlining the mutual responsibilities of the medical team and of the organizing body be agreed upon during the initial planning phases of the event.[1]

In extreme conditions, the medical director may advise that the event be cancelled, modified, or rescheduled. It is best that these possibilities and contingency plans be discussed with event management and that action plans be prepared and published before the day of the event. It is helpful to have clearly delineated criteria to use to make these decisions. Wet-bulb globe thermometers, wind-chill calculations, and lightning warning systems are all objective evaluation tools that can be used on site and frequently reassessed.[1]

It is advisable to assess the course for any potential trouble spots or hazards and to take steps that are designed to mitigate injury. The start and the finish are common sites of medical concern. The start area should be on a large, level surface that is devoid of obstacles, allowing the athletes to more easily accommodate the surge that invariably occurs as an event begins. The finish area should also be large enough to prevent the athletes from bunching up and being forced to stand in one place, thereby risking postexercise hypotension and collapse.[19,23] It should have necessary facilities and resources to allow the athletes to properly cool down, warm up, and recover after the event, and it should also offer easy access to medical treatment areas.

Likewise, fields of play and rest areas should be reviewed for team sports. Playing areas should be free of hazards, and the playing surface should be in good condition. The medical director should evaluate the availability of shade, access to water, bathroom facilities, and warming areas specific to the event.

Biking, swimming, and skiing events carry additional risk elements,[24] such as water safety and trauma potential associated with high speeds and hard surfaces. Water temperature and sea conditions; road conditions; transition, acceleration, and deceleration areas; and protective equipment must be carefully scrutinized.

The medical director is often responsible for recruiting, training, and supplying the medical support staff as well as ensuring their safety and comfort. Shelter from the elements, efficient transportation to and from the medical care site, the provision of bathroom facilities, and a generous feeding plan often go a long way toward ensuring support staff during subsequent years.

MEDICAL PHILOSOPHY

The medical philosophy defines the level of medical care that will be available at the event and to whom it will be provided. Risk assessment incorporates the multiple variables considered during the conduct of the event and the likelihood of injury on the basis of that risk. By defining risk, strategies to prevent and treat injury can better be developed.[25] This assessment should be reviewed and agreed upon by the medical director and the event director during the early event-planning stages. The risk level may differ among the aid stations throughout the course, with the most robust resources usually being provided at the finish area. Differences may also exist that are based on the number and demographics of the participants and on resource availability.

A decision must be made regarding how spectators requiring medical assessment and care will be addressed. Spectators are still exposed to the same elements as the athletes, and they share common injury and illness risks (albeit to a lesser extent). A level of responsibility for the provision of their medical needs

exists for event management, and this often falls to the medical team. Several reviews of mass-gathering medical care and coverage have been published to aid in the assessment of need requirements for this population.[26-30]

Coordination with the local emergency medical service (EMS) and emergency departments and hospitals is absolutely required. It is unlikely and unreasonable to expect all event medical stations to have access to the same level of care as these fixed facilities. Although the medical team should address patient safety and the conservation of assets, it should also include a decision mechanism regarding when and where to transport injured athletes. Many diagnoses may be appropriately evaluated and dispositioned from a more robust medical aid station rather than involving EMS and hospital assets, which are more appropriately reserved for cases with higher levels of acuity.

Fortunately, EMS organizations can often assist with patient distribution through their dispatch systems; this ensures that patients are transported to facilities with available access and a necessary level of care to meet their needs. The medical director should be well versed in both local and state EMS laws regarding the initiation of patient contact and the on-site physician responsibilities and limitations when dealing with these EMS units. Pre-event collaboration among clinicians is an opportune time to review facility capabilities and common event-specific injuries and illnesses that may otherwise be infrequently encountered in the hospital setting.

Mobile medical assets in the form of bike, canoe/kayak, all-terrain vehicle teams, and ambulance EMS units provide an excellent means of accessing injured competitors throughout the course[31] **(Figure 4.1)**. Their ability to easily move to injured participants allows for earlier evaluation and the initiation of definitive care.

Medical documentation with patient identification should be performed for all contacts, especially those requiring transportation to higher levels of care. Remember that written patient assessment should remain confidential. These documents should be maintained for reassessment after the event.

It is essential to provide basic life support and first aid[1] **(Figure 4.2)**. Access to external automated defibrillators has been shown to improve survival in cases of out-of-hospital cardiac arrest.[32] The use of and type of intravenous fluids and the availability of oxygen, medications, and advanced cardiac and trauma life support equipment are areas that require clarification. A decision must be made regarding the provision of medication on the event course and in the medical aid stations. For longer events,

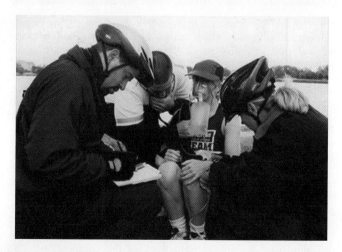

Figure 4.1 Mobile medical assets in the form of bike, canoe/kayak, all-terrain vehicle teams, and ambulance emergency medical service units provide an excellent means of accessing injured competitors throughout the course.

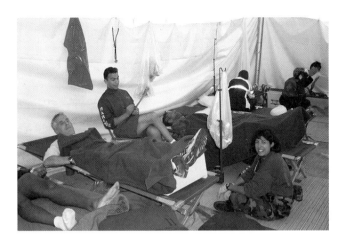

Figure 4.2 The use and type of intravenous fluids and the availability of oxygen, medications, and advanced cardiac and trauma life support equipment are areas that require clarification. Decisions must be made regarding the provision of medication on the event course and in the medical aid stations.

it is not uncommon for athletes to carry and take their own medication during the event. This must be anticipated to best treat the competitor and to prevent overprescribing. Urgent or emergency medications such as aspirin, epinephrine (auto-injector), albuterol (metered-dose inhaler), glucose, and advanced cardiac life support medications should be considered with regard to the time required to access definitive medical care. All medications should be tightly controlled by the medical team, and their use should be clearly documented.

Medical aid stations may or may not have basic laboratory capabilities. The ability to assess an athlete's blood glucose and sodium levels will assist with rapid evaluation and allow for the appropriate treatment of a collapsed athlete.[33] Handheld glucose and electrolyte monitors are readily available, and they have become part of the standard medical kit for many endurance events.[34]

MEDICAL CHAIN OF COMMAND

The importance of identifying an individual to serve as the medical director deserves discussion. Their responsibilities include planning, event-day medical decision making, and medical troubleshooting. The medical support staff, the event director, and the media all benefit from having individuals who are clearly identified by specific roles (rather than a general medical committee) to answer questions and to provide leadership regarding medical issues.

It is also recommended that each aid station have an assigned medical leader who is well versed in the event's medical philosophy and plan. This medical leader can organize the support staff; coordinate the medical care that is provided locally; familiarize those on the medical team who are unable to assemble before the event with the plans for the event; and update members with less knowledge about the event's medical philosophy.

MEDICAL AID STATION STAFFING

The appropriate staffing of medical treatment areas with both medical and nonmedical staff is important for the safe conduct of the medical aid station. The composition and number of this staff will vary, depending on the location and the nature of the

event. The number makeup can be best derived from previous experience, through comparison with similar events in similar conditions, or by using risk-assessment analysis. A helpful guide from the American College of Sports Medicine[2] for distance running events is to provide the following medical personnel per 1000 runners: 1 to 2 physicians; 4 to 6 podiatrists; 1 to 4 emergency medical technicians; 2 to 4 nurses; 3 to 6 physical therapists; 3 to 6 athletic trainers; and 1 to 3 assistants. Approximately 75% of these personnel should be stationed at the finish area. Nonmedical staff can assist with the transport of injured athletes, documentation, medical tracking, and the provision of information within the medical aid station and to the event staff.

After the event, it is most important to elicit feedback from both medical and nonmedical staff. This often identifies areas that had not been considered during the initial planning and execution phases of the event, and it demonstrates to the staff the value of their participation and critique. A written after-action report as a follow-up to these comments is highly recommended because it allows for the documentation of areas of concern, the development of solutions, and the preparation for subsequent events.

COMMUNICATION PLAN

It is vital that event medical support sites have the ability to communicate with each other, with EMS assets, with local hospitals, with the event director, and with competing athletes before, during, and after the competition. This becomes increasingly important when vast distances and terrain are covered by the event.

Various communication networks have been used that have included cellular phones, computer networks, ham radio networks, handheld radios, flag systems, and large signs. These systems should be tested well before the event, and a secondary system and a backup plan should be established in case there is a failure of the primary means of communication. Cellular phone and radio reception are especially problematic in remote settings, and they may vary with terrain features and weather conditions.

A communication plan outlining how EMS will be requested and dispatched and when various members of the medical and event team need to be contacted will increase the efficiency of the medical care provided. Often a medical command center with the medical director, an EMS dispatcher, and a communications coordinator is established near the medical aid station with the highest volume of patients.

The event information plan also requires a functional and timely communication system. This plan often involves a separate information area. The medical team must establish a protocol for sharing information regarding the status of injured and medically transported participants while maintaining patient privacy. Aid stations should have a patient-tracking mechanism that includes intake, disposition, and discharge information that is communicated to the information center for dissemination according to the event plan. One common indication for a predefined system is when worried family members and friends who are unable to link up with competitors present to the medical aid stations requesting information. An information area that is separate from the medical aid station allows for the accurate provision of information according to the event plan while minimizing the disruption of the efficiency of medical aid station functioning.

FINANCE AND LOGISTICS PLANNING

The conduct of mass-participation events both requires and has the potential to generate money. Medical directors must ensure that the safety of the participants and the support staff is not compromised by decisions to increase revenue for the event. The medical director must be involved in any plans that may have medical implications. He or she must be a core member of most preplanning activities.

Exacting care should be taken when reviewing the financial aspects of event medical coverage because insufficient funds should not result in insufficient medical care. Calculating the costs of medical supplies, transportation, and personnel compensation must be performed and agreed upon early in the event-planning process. The groups that are responsible for payment should be identified and the funds verified. Supply lists should be generated, and agreements regarding procurement and payment should be made in writing. Additionally, all contracted medical staff should have signed agreements.

Accurate course maps are useful to both competitors and event staff. It is best that maps be to scale and that aid, fluid, and feed stations and prominent landmarks be identified. Terrain maps are especially useful for long-distance wilderness endurance events. Maps should be liberally distributed and available at all medical aid stations.

The spacing of medical aid stations throughout the course is determined by many variables **(Figure 4.3)**. The course must be previewed, and the location of medical aid stations should be established on the basis of anticipated need, appropriate location, and course-specific considerations.[35] Medical aid stations must be easily identifiable to both competitors and EMS units. Large inflatable balloons, flags, and placards with a red cross on a white background are universally recognizable. Uniforms, shirts, vests, or identification badges are just a few ways to make the medical staff clearly and distinctly identifiable to all.

The logistics of staging, setup, security, and the movement of supplies and personnel before, during, and after the event generally falls to event management. As part of the pre-event preparation, the medical team must be confident in the plan to deliver temporary facilities, cots, chairs, and medical supplies to the medical aid station sites. The ability to resupply aid stations during the event must be balanced with the considerations of availability and ease of movement to and from these areas during the event. It is generally preferred to have all supplies on site before the start of the event.

The medical team should also advise the event coordinators about fluid and food composition, availability, and distribution throughout the event to optimize competitor safety.[1] The increased availability of fluid stations may result in an increased risk of exercise-associated hyponatremia in slower runners.[36]

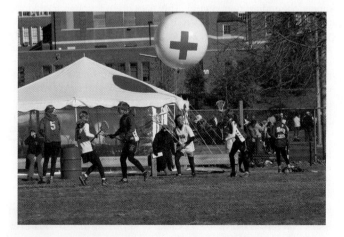

Figure 4.3 Medical aid stations must be easily identifiable to competitors and emergency medical service units. Large inflatable balloons, flags, and placards with a red cross on a white background are universally recognizable.

TRANSPORTATION PLAN

The transportation of people, supplies, and injured competitors requires planning and coordination on multiple levels, and the plan must be carefully scrutinized. Medical evacuation routes must be established to avoid conflict with the event in progress and to ensure the most efficient means of transport. This includes access from the event site to the medical aid stations and EMS access from the event or medical aid station to a higher level of medical care. These routes should remain clear of obstructions and crowds, and they should be prominently identified. If the event risk assessment identifies the possibility of patient injury requiring transportation via helicopter, landing sites should be predetermined and clearly marked.

Medical team members must be able to arrive at their assigned location in advance of the start of the event. The time required to set up and organize the aid station, assign roles, and provide on-site medical education should be accounted for accordingly. The medical team must also have a means to depart the aid station and dispense with any equipment and supplies when the event concludes. The staff may make use of personal or public transportation; in some settings, the transportation plan will be included as part of the overall event plan.

It is not unusual for participants to decide that a medical treatment area is a good place to end their participation in the event. If this decision is realized in the middle of the course, a plan for the removal of these athletes must be implemented. Many events have a "sweep" vehicle that follows the last competitors and that can transport these participants to the finish area. Other transport arrangements may be available, depending on the nature of the event, but the need for them and arrangements for their use must be anticipated before the event.

MEDICAL TRAINING

Participant training

Competitors should be given medical information before the event. This is most easily provided with the event information, and it can be coordinated through the event director. Additions to event Web sites, handouts to accompany the event pick-up packet, and information posters displayed in common areas before and during the event are several effective examples.

Common medical conditions and their prevention, the location of medical aid stations on the course, and available services at these areas assist the participants with their planning and preparation for a safe event. Medical presentations to the athletes and interest groups are often well received, and they may be coordinated through local or national athletic groups or as part of pre-event meetings.

Race-day information regarding weather conditions and health warnings has been used with success at numerous events.[35] This provides the participants and coaches with information that can be useful when planning their level of participation and for determining specific changes in their pre-event preparation.

Medical staff training

It is common for the medical support for mass-participation events to be gathered from diverse backgrounds and experience levels. Most of these individuals are better versed in medical care within a clinical or hospital facility than in the field environment. The medical plan, philosophy, chain of command, and level of care provided must be reviewed with the medical staff. It is helpful (although not always practical) to provide an education session before the day of the event. Group training allows for the introduction of key members of the medical and event team, and it allows for the review of overall plans and strategies for the safe conduct of the event. Questions from within a larger group are often quite helpful for each individual. Providing triage and treatment guidelines specific for the event in writing is very useful, and it is also helpful to provide administration information about the course, parking, proximity to water, food and facility stations, and communication and transportation plans. Computer Web sites, Listservs, and e-mails are other means of disseminating this information.

TRIAGE AND TREATMENT GUIDELINES

The majority of the medical conditions presenting at a given event can be predicted well in advance by a review of previous events and numerous examples in the medical and event literature. Preparing, training, and practicing for these conditions are important for the evaluation, treatment, and disposition of injured participants.

The initial evaluation of an athlete in the medical aid station should focus on the severity of the injury.[19] Fortunately, most complaints are nonsevere in nature, and these patients can be quickly treated and released. Common presenting conditions include sprains, strains, aches, pains, and dermatologic conditions.

Severe medical conditions include cardiac events, hypothermia, hyperthermia, hyponatremia, near drowning, and head and neck trauma. These should be quickly differentiated from nonsevere conditions by the evaluation of mental status, rectal temperature,[37] blood pressure, and pulse. Serum glucose and sodium levels may also aid in the diagnosis. Depending on the medical care plan of the event, some of these severe conditions may be treated at the medical aid station or transported via EMS to the most appropriate medical treatment facility.

Medical conditions such as exercise-associated collapse, heatstroke, chest pain, and hyponatremia can further be triaged and separated from musculoskeletal and dermatologic conditions in the treatment area **(Figure 4.4)**. This separation of care allows for the assignment and preparation of support staff in the area of care in which they are most experienced. It also allows those patients with more severe conditions to be treated in an area with readily available access to medical testing, injury-specific supplies, and close monitoring.

The establishment of a medical holding area has proven successful.[38] This area is reserved for athletes who are waiting for transportation for nonsevere conditions or for those who are not prepared to leave the medical area but who do not require further care. This group is continuously observed and encouraged to make their way back to the after-event areas.

Medical treatment guidelines have been used successfully in these settings. The guidelines should consider standards of medical care, the event's medical philosophy, the available level of care, and decision points regarding continued on-site treatment or transportation to higher levels of medical care.

One of the most anxiety-producing occurrences during the medical coverage of mass-participation events is the collapsed athlete. Fortunately, the majority of cases of exercise-associated collapse are the result of predictable physiologic events associated with exertion, and they respond rapidly to positioning with the head down and the legs and pelvis elevated.[19] These athletes generally have a normal mental status.

Individuals with altered mental status should be rapidly evaluated with a rectal temperature for hyperthermia or hypothermia. A patient with a persistent altered mental status and with a relatively normal rectal temperature should be treated as suspected of having hyponatremia until proven otherwise.[19] On-site sodium assessment allows for rapid diagnosis and the initiation of treatment.[39] Hyperthermic individuals should be rapidly cooled on site, preferably with ice water immersion[19,24]; hypothermic patients should be warmed.

MEDICAL–LEGAL

An additional responsibility of the medical director is the assurance of medical staff liability coverage. Unfortunately, general event insurance packages usually exclude medical coverage.[40] Options for medical liability coverage should be discussed with legal representation in advance of the event and include individual or group policies. Good Samaritan laws for the state and country of the medical care should be considered, and medical licensure laws should also be addressed if practicing out of state or country.

EMS laws and regulations vary from state to state, and it is advisable that the medical director have a working understanding of them to ensure compliance.

CONCLUSION

The medical management of mass-participation events is a gratifying experience that offers clinicians unique opportunities. Thorough medical planning and preparation are absolute requirements for the successful conducting of these events. By following established medical plans and treatment guidelines and by remembering limitations with a focus on competitor and staff safety, event medical care results in a fulfilling experience for everyone involved.

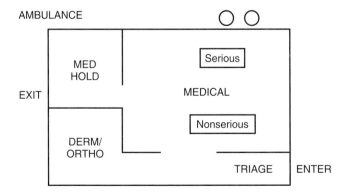

Figure 4.4 Patients with medical conditions such as exercise-associated collapse, heatstroke, chest pain, and hyponatremia can be further triaged and separated from patients with musculoskeletal and dermatologic conditions in the treatment area.

REFERENCES

1. American College of Sports Medicine: Mass participation event management for the team physician: a consensus statement. Med Sci Sports Exerc 2004;36(11):2004-2008.
2. American College of Sports Medicine: Position statement on heat and cold illness during distance running. Med Sci Sports Exerc 1996;28(12):i-x.
3. Kleiner DM, Glickman SE: Considerations for the athletic trainer in planning medical coverage for short distance road races. J Ath Train 1994;29:145-147.
4. Anderson JC, Courson RW, Kleiner DM, McLoda TA: National Athletic Trainer's Association position statement: emergency planning in athletics. J Ath Train 2002;37(1):99-104.
5. Jaworski CA: Medical concerns of marathons. Curr Sports Med Rep 2005;4(3):137-143.
6. Bugbee S, Knopp WD: Medical coverage of tennis events. Curr Sports Med Rep 2006;5(3):131-134.

7. Roberts WO: Exercise-associated collapse in endurance events. A classification system. Phys Sportsmed 1989;17:49-57.

8. Jones BH, Roberts WO: Medical management of endurance events: incidence, prevention and care of casualties. In Cantu C, Micheli LJ (eds): ACSM's Guidelines for the Team Physician. Philadelphia, Lea & Febiger, 1991, pp 255-286.

9. Borland ML, Rogers IR: Injury and illness in a wilderness multisport endurance event. Wilderness Environ Med 1997;8(2):82-88.

10. Zijlstra JA: Medical consequences of the 15th eleven-cities skating marathon. Ned Tijdschr Geneeskd 1998;142(7):331-335.

11. Lorish TR, Rizzo TD Jr, Ilstrup DM, Scott SG: Injuries in adolescent and preadolescent boys at two large wrestling tournaments. Am J Sports Med 1992;20(2):199-202.

12. Bathgate A, Best J, Craig G, et al: A prospective study of injuries to elite Australian rugby union players. Br J Sports Med 2002;36:265-269.

13. McIntosh AS, Best J, Orchard J, et al. Rugby union injury surveillance study: report on seasons 2000-2002. Sydney, Australia: University of New South Wales Press; 2004.

14. Jakoet I, Noakes TD: A high rate of injury during the 1995 Rugby World Cup. S Afr Med J 1998;88(1):45-47.

15. Best J: Injuries During the 2001 Under 21 Rugby Championship, Report to International Rugby Board Medical Advisory Committee, June, 2001.

16. Best JP, McIntosh AS, Savage TN: Rugby World Cup 2003 injury surveillance project. Br J Sports Med 2005;39:812-817.

17. Elias SR: 10-year trend in USA Cup soccer injuries: 1988-1997. Med Sci Sports Exerc 2001;33(3):359-367.

18. Feehan M, Walter AE: Precompetition injury and subsequent tournament performance in full-contact taekwondo. Br J Sports Med 1995;29(4):258-262.

19. Holtzhausen LM, Noakes TD: Collapsed ultraendurance athlete: proposed mechanisms and an approach to management. Clin J Sports Med 1997;7(4):292-301.

20. Hiller WD, O'Toole ML, Fortess EE, et al: Medical and physiological considerations in triathlons. Am J Sports Med 1987;15(2):164-168.

21. Crouse B, Beattie K: Marathon medical services: strategies to reduce runner morbidity. Med Sci Sports Exerc 1995;28(9):1093-1096.

22. Maron BJ, Poliac LC, Roberts WO: Risk for sudden cardiac death associated with marathon running. J Am Coll Cardiol 1996;28:428-431.

23. Holtzhausen LM, Noakes TD: The prevalence and significance of post exercise (postural) hypotension in ultramarathon runners. Med Sci Sports Exerc 1995;27(12):1595-1601.

24. Mayers LB, Noakes TD: A guideline to treating ironman triathletes at the finish line. Phys Sportsmed 2000;28(8):33-50.

25. Bahr R, Holme I: Risk factors for sports injuries—a methodological approach. Br J Sports Med 2003;37:384-392.

26. Ma OJ, Millward L, Schwab RA: EMS medical coverage at PGA tour events. Prehosp Emerg Care 2002;6(1):11-14.

27. Baker WM, Simone BM, Niemann JT, Daly A: Special event medical care: the 1984 Los Angeles Summer Olympic experience. Ann Emerg Med 1986;15(2):185-190.

28. Parrillo SJ: Medical care at mass gatherings: considerations for physician involvement. Prehospital Disaster Med 1995;10(4):273-275.

29. Perron AD, Brady WJ, Custalow CB, Johnson DM: Association of heat index and patient volume at a mass gathering event. Prehosp Emerg Care 2005;9(1):49-52.

30. Delaney JS, Drummond R: Mass casualties and triage at a sporting event. Br J Sports Med 2002;36:85-88.

31. Laird RH: Medical care at ultraendurance triathlons. Med Sci Sports Exerc 1989;21(5):S222-S225.

32. Nichol G, Stiell IG, Laupacis A, et al: A cumulative meta-analysis of the effectiveness of defibrillator-capable emergency medical services for victims of out-of-hospital cardiac arrest. Ann Emerg Med 1999;34(4 Pt 1):517-525.

33. Davis DP, Videen JS, Marino A, et al: Exercise associated hyponatremia in marathon runners: a two-year experience. J Emerg Med 2001;21(1):47-57.

34. Speedy DB, Noakes TD, Holtzhausen LM: Exercise-associated collapse. Phys Sportsmed 2003;31(3):23-29.

35. Cianca JC, Roberts WO, Horn D: Distance running: organization of the medical team. In O'Connor FG, Wilder RP (eds): Textbook of Running Medicine. New York: McGraw-Hill; 2001, pp 489-503.

36. Hew TD, Chorley JN, Cianca JC, et al: The incidence, risk factors, and clinical manifestations of hyponatremia in marathon runners. Clin J Sports Med 2003;13:14-17.

37. Roberts WO: Assessing core temperature in collapsed athletes: what's the best method? Phys Sportsmed 2000;28(9):71-76.

38. O'Connor FG, Pyne SW, Brennan FH: Exercise-associated collapse: an algorithmic approach to race day management. Part I of II. Am J Med Sports 2003;5:212-217, 229.

39. Hew-Butler T, Almond C, Ayrus JC, et al, and the Exercise-Associated Hyponatremia (EAH) Consensus Panel: Consensus statement of the 1st International Exercise-Associated Hyponatremia Consensus Development Conference, Cape Town, South Africa, 2005. Clin J Sport Med 2005;15:208-213.

40. Dooley JW: Professional liability coverage (medical malpractice). Road Race Manage 1999;October:3.

CHAPTER 5

Emergency Planning for Athletic Events

Scott D. Flinn, MD, and Timothy Dwyer, MD

KEY POINTS

- There are three phases in the development and execution of the emergency medical plan: the planning phase, the event phase, and the review phase.
- When scheduling any athletic event, both environmental conditions and community impact must be considered.
- A "wave start" is an option for larger events in which the amount of space at the starting area may be inadequate for all of the competitors at once.
- The medical staff should receive training before the event that addresses the overall medical strategy and intervention level, medical record documentation, communication methods, the disqualification of participants, the medical protocols to be used, and the chain of command.
- The term exercise-associated collapse is used to describe athletes who are unable to stand or walk unaided as a result of light-headedness, faintness, dizziness, or syncope. Treatment protocols should address immediate actions for the common causes of exercise-associated collapse, including cardiac arrest, exertional heat illness, hypothermia, and exertional hyponatremia.

INTRODUCTION

As the scope and frequency of various athletic events broadens, so does the role of the medical director. Developing a comprehensive and appropriate plan for emergency medical coverage for athletic events—whether game-day coverage for single or multiple venues or a mass-participation event—requires much forethought. With the use of proper planning techniques and resources, the medical director, working in concert with the event organizer, can develop a comprehensive medical plan that is focused on the safety of the event participants. A clearly delineated agreement between the event-organizing body and the medical director should define

the medical care and administrative responsibilities for the development of a cohesive functional emergency medical plan.

The primary function of the medical plan is to prevent serious injury or illness to competitors that may result in permanent disability or death. Additional consideration should be given to the safety of all staff and spectators. For the scope of this discussion, we will concentrate primarily on the planning and management for the medical care of the competitors who are participating in athletic events.

There are three phases in the development and execution of the emergency medical plan: the planning phase, the event phase, and the review phase.[1] As the planning process is started, any review material from previous events is highly valuable to leverage the successes and prevent the repetition of errors from earlier events.

Considerations during the development of the emergency medical plan include event scheduling, reviewing the course or venue, determining the medical strategy to be employed, making decisions about competitor-specific items, establishing the logistical requirements, and training personnel, including elucidating any specific protocols to be used.[1-4]

SCHEDULING

When scheduling any athletic event, both environmental conditions and community impact must be considered. For events in which heat injuries are a potential, starting events earlier in the day may limit heat casualties. Likewise, events in colder conditions should be planned to start later in the day and finish during daylight, thus enabling the last finisher to be off of the course before the onset of darkness and dropping temperatures.[2-6]

When planning the event, the medical director and event organizers should consider the establishment of a formal event-cancellation policy for extreme circumstances.[2] This policy should include specific reasons for event cancellation or postponement (e.g., extreme heat or cold, lightning). If undue heat risk or other factors may cause the cancellation or postponement of an event, a policy should include a clear description of the process to inform competitors and event staff members and to refund or credit event fees, as applicable.

Various data may be used to aid in the decision making regarding whether an event should be cancelled or postponed as a result of heat, including the heat index and the Wet Bulb Globe

The authors would like to acknowledge Ms. Lynne Johnson for all of her hard work on this chapter.

Table 5.1   Wet Bulb Globe Temperature and Heat Risk

Wet Bulb Globe Temperature	Level of Risk	Comments
<65°F or <18°C	Low	Risk low but still exists on the basis of individual risk factors
65°F-73°F or 18°C-23°C	Moderate	Risk level increases as event progresses through the day
73°F-82°F or 23°C-28°C	High	All competitors should be aware of injury potential; individuals at risk should not compete
>82°F or >28°C	Hazardous	Consider rescheduling or delaying the event until safer conditions prevail; if the event proceeds, take added precautions to reduce risk factors

Formula: Wet bulb globe temperature = 0.7 (wet bulb) + 0.2 (dry bulb) + 0.1 (globe).
Adapted from Armstrong LE, Epstein Y, Greenleaf JE, et al: Med Sci Sports Exerc 1996;28(10):139-148; Seto CK, Way D, O'Connor N: Clin Sports Med 2005;24(3):695-718.

Temperature Index. The National Weather Service has created a heat index chart (available at http://www.crh.noaa.gov/pub/heat.php) that combines humidity and temperature measurements to construct a scale that describes the relative heat and the risk of heat illness. A more specific means for determining heat risk was developed at the Marine Corps Recruit Depot in Parris Island, South Carolina: the Wet Bulb Globe Temperature Index (available at http://www.usariem.army.mil/heatill/appendc.htm). It is considered the standard for measuring heat stress, and it is used by the US Armed Forces to anticipate troop heat exposure. The measurement takes into account the ambient temperature, the radiant heat, and the humidity to calculate a risk score. This score can then be charted and the category of risk of heat-related illness assessed. Wet bulb globe thermometers are available commercially. The American College of Sports Medicine has published standards regarding the heat risk for participating in athletic events on the basis of the Wet Bulb Globe Temperature Index; these are shown in **Table 5.1**.[3,7]

When considering the impact of an event on the local community, other scheduled events and local capabilities must be taken into account. The availability and capability of local emergency departments, 911 services, ambulances, and air evacuation should be considered during the scheduling of the event.[1,2]

COURSE REVIEW

The event or competition venue requires careful preview and evaluation. Single or multiple venues may be involved. For mass-participation events, particular attention must be paid to the event start area. In particular, adequate room should be available for all participants to start the event without danger of trampling. A "wave start" is an option for larger events in which the amount of space at the starting area may be inadequate for all of the competitors at once. Varying skill levels and ages of competitors can be used when planning a wave start. Other sport-specific issues of starting area safety, such as avoiding downhill starts in cross-country skiing, should be considered.[6] Hazards of the event course itself may include road conditions, altitude changes, currents, reduced visibility because of hills or trees, overlapping or looping courses, and multisport transition zones. Additionally, traffic and crowd control and emergency vehicle access need to be taken into consideration.[2-6]

Aid stations and shelters should be strategically positioned based on the type of event, the number of participants, the skill level of the participants, and the accessibility of emergency transport. Ideally, stations should be spaced approximately every 15 to 20 minutes along the event course. Aid stations should provide adequate protection from the elements for both the event participants and the medical personnel. The extent of protection should vary with expected climate and weather conditions.[1-3,6]

The finish area should provide for ease of competitor flow, for the appropriate triage and treatment of competitors who require medical intervention, and for easy access to emergency transport. The proper routing of participants who do not require medical care is essential for an effective and efficient medical response at the finish line.

MEDICAL STRATEGY

In concert with race organizers, the medical director develops the medical strategy for treating injured participants. The primary consideration is what level of care will be offered. This depends on a number of factors, including the size of the event, the available resources, and the talent of the medical team. Provisions for basic first aid and basic life support are usually the baseline. Decisions must then be made whether further care will be rendered on site or whether the participant should be transported to another medical facility. Medical team members should be trained for triage, appropriate intervention, and either transport, disqualification, or return to play, as appropriate.[1-4] The medical director should also provide the team with casualty estimates and specific treatment protocols. Specifically, an exercise-associated collapse protocol and an adverse event protocol are crucial parts of the medical strategy.[8,9] Depending on the strategy employed, medical team members should have the equipment and supplies available to accomplish the mission.

Competitor-specific interventions

Before the event, certain competitor-specific safety-related issues must be considered. First is whether or not participants need a preparticipation medical clearance and need to sign a medical waiver.[1,2] Ensuring the fitness and appropriate health of competitors can prove to be a difficult task. The use of the precompetition medical examination supplemented by blood and urine testing may be appropriate, and it may be required by sponsoring agencies for certain high-risk venues and levels of competition. Although liability is highly unlikely unless there is gross negligence, the consideration of a medical waiver for participants should involve legal counsel. Bib coding with medical information may be used for the identification of high-risk competitors or of those with concerning medical conditions. A policy for the involvement and inclusion of disabled competitors and any special provisions should be developed and reviewed as appropriate for the specific nature of the athletic event. The medical disqualification of participants should be reviewed and stated clearly to all competitors and event staff members.[1-5] The identification of medical team members should be clearly explained to all competitors and support staff. Signs, tents, name tags, shirts, hats, and jackets are typically used with good success.

Competitors should be informed about what type of hydration and feeding (if any) will be provided along the course. Specific gear or equipment may be required, optional, or restricted for the competitors. For example, wet suits and bicycle helmets might be

Table 5.2   San Diego County Recommendations for Support Staff Based on Event Size

Anticipated Crowd Size	Knowledge of 911 Access and CPR	Basic First Aid Stations	First Aid Stations Including Nurse	First Aid Stations Including Physicians	BLS Ambulances	ALS Ambulances	Mobile Teams
Less than 2500	*	*	†				
2500-15,000	*		*	†	*	†	
15,000-50,000	*			*	*	*	*
Over 50,000	*			*	*	*	*

*Required resource; multiple such resources should be considered depending on the boundaries of the event or the size of the crowd.
†Recommended resource; intended to ensure the safety of participants.

Basic First Aid Station	First Aid Station Including Nurse	First Aid Station Including Physician
The basic first-aid station is staffed by a person who is trained and certified to render first aid and cardiopulmonary resuscitation. The basic first-aid station should contain three items: (1) a plan for accessing 911; (2) someone trained in cardiopulmonary resuscitation; and (3) a basic first-aid kit that contains compresses, ice packs, bandages, and antiseptic.	The first-aid station that includes a nurse has the same elements as the basic first-aid station plus a registered nurse with an appropriate license. The registered nurse's medical service skills should include (but not be limited to) triage and basic airway management.	The first-aid station that includes a physician has the same elements as the basic first-aid station plus staffing by an appropriately licensed medical physician, and it may include advanced cardiac life support medications and defibrillator capabilities.

Adapted from The City of San Diego Office of Special Events: Planning the medical services for your special event (Web site): Available at www.sandiego.gov/specialevents/pdf/medical.pdf. Accessed April 13, 2007.

required for a triathlon, whereas headphones or earplugs may be restricted. Nontherapeutic braces or hard casts may be restricted in some sports. For warm-weather events, information regarding the use of sunscreen and the prevention of heat illness and hyponatremia should be included in information packets, with particular attention paid to fluid- and salt-intake recommendations.[2,3,7,10-13]

Logistics

Medical logistics for the race include determining the number and type of medical personnel, the location and supply of aid stations, and the communication and transportation requirements. The estimation of the required support is usually based on the casualty estimates. Casualty estimates will vary on the basis of the number of competitors, the number of spectators, the level and extent of competition, and environmental factors. For example, a weekly high school football game will have far different requirements than an iron-man triathlon. Historic injury rates and knowledgeable local personnel are excellent sources of casualty estimates.

Consideration must be given to the number of trauma casualties versus the number of medical casualties. High-speed events have a higher incidence of traumatic injuries, whereas events involving extremes of distance and of environmental conditions produce a greater number of medical casualties. In marathons, an estimated 5% to 10% of competitors will require some medical intervention.[12] Triathlons usually have 2% to 5% of competitors seeking medical assistance, whereas 15% to 35% of iron-man competitors require assistance.[14] Finally, one should consider the age range of the participants because extremes of age may require special equipment sizes and/or medications.

Aid stations

The location and function of the course aid stations will vary, depending on length of the course, their position along the course, and the extent of care being provided. In addition to the basic aid stations along the route, there should be one or more major aid stations at the start/finish and in the more remote areas

along the event route.[2,3] These major aid stations should be staffed and equipped to provide more care than other aid stations along the route because more patients will likely be seen.

Special considerations may affect the location and supply of recommended medical resources. These include the time of the event (night versus day); the number of active participants and spectators; alcohol availability and anticipated use; the demographics of crowd; the location of the event and different event components; the weather and the time of year; the length of the event; and problems that have been encountered with the event in the past.[1-6,12-14]

The number and type of personnel available to staff aid stations are important. The skill level required depends on the level of care to be offered, whereas the number of staff is determined by the casualty estimate.[2] Consultation with the local authorities and the municipal office of special events may help determine the number and type of personnel needed for aid stations. For example, the City of San Diego Office of Special Events requires and recommends various services based on the size of the crowd and the type of event.[15] See **Table 5.2** for recommendations.

Aid stations should be built and supplied to provide adequate protection, comfort, and access for both competitors and race staff. Tents, chairs, tables, cots, litters, and backboards should be placed on the basis of casualty estimates. Lights, generators, heating/cooling equipment, and blankets provide improved visibility and comfort. Sinks, hand-washing stations, toilets, and trash facilities enable good hygiene.

An adequate supply of fluids and food may be provided for the competitors. A good estimate for fluid supply is 200 to 300 mL per competitor per 10 to 20 minutes of competition, with more available at the start and the finish areas.[2,3,5]

Medical supplies

The extent of medical supplies required for each venue or aid station will vary depending on expected casualties and the level of training of the staff. General supplies include first-aid supplies and basic resuscitation equipment. Recommended medical supply and equipment lists for the major medical aid stations are shown in **Table 5.3.** This is not intended to be an exhaustive list, and these recommendations should be tailored to the expected needs of each event.[1-3] Supplies should include items such as first-aid supplies for blister care, oral rehydration fluids, ice for heat casualties and sprains, heating supplies (if it is a cold-weather event), and basic cardiopulmonary resuscitation gear.

Different events and medical strategies require the tailoring of medical supplies. If more invasive measures are to be offered, intravenous fluids, advanced cardiac life support equipment and medications, and advanced trauma life support equipment may be required. If children are participants, appropriate pediatric sizes should be available. Medications may include oxygen, subcutaneous epinephrine, and diazepam. If heat casualties are a consideration, a means of cooling (e.g., an ice-water bath in a small plastic pool) should be considered as one of the simplest, most-effective means of cooling in the field.[3,16-18]

Medical-record materials should be provided for recording patient contacts. Additionally, aid stations should be provided with appropriate sharps and biohazard containers, with their method for disposal clearly stated.

Communications

A reliable system of communication is crucial for a successful emergency medical plan. The primary and backup communication systems should be tested before the event. Communications should be coordinated with the local emergency medical services, police systems, and office of special events, as applicable. This is particularly important for radios because specific types of radios and frequencies must be used, depending on the location and terrain. Furthermore, other events may be occurring simultaneously within the emergency service area.

In addition to having adequate systems, personnel must be trained regarding how and when to use the system. It should be clearly stated when communication with the medical director for information about severely injured participants is appropriate. Furthermore, it should be clearly delineated who can order emergency transportation and under what conditions. At large events with multiple aid stations, it is especially important that personnel use good radio discipline so that idle chatter does not interfere with necessary discussions.

Outside communications are also an issue. Injured athletes may need to contact family members. Often, designating a particular rendezvous site is helpful. Media interactions can also be sources of conflict. Delineation of who should speak to the press regarding any patient care is a Health Insurance Portability and Accountability Act concern in addition to a potentially problematic issue.[2] This responsibility should be clearly spelled out, and it usually resides with the medical director.

Transportation

Traffic control and parking issues should be included in the overall event planning. Access routes for emergency transport vehicles should be established and clearly marked for whatever transport vehicle is to be used, whether it is an ambulance, a helicopter, a snowmobile, or a safety boat. The presence of other traffic along the route and the use of sweep vehicles at the end of the event should be included in the planning process.

Personnel

Estimates for the both number and type of personnel for the aid stations at games or mass-participation events are based on casualty estimates, past experience, and the available literature. The management of medical personnel and equipment and the

Table 5.3 Medical Supply Recommendations

Medical Supplies
Gloves
Airway kit
Pocket mask
Rectal thermometers
Blood-pressure cuff
Stethoscope
Penlight, oto-opthalmoscope
Oxygen and delivery system
Intravenous fluids and administration kits; tourniquet
Medications: aspirin, albuterol inhaler, epinephrine (1:1000 for subcutaneous administration), diphenhydramine (injectable and oral), diazepam, glucagon, and magnesium sulfate
Glucose monitor
Sodium monitor
Oxygen saturation monitor
Cricothyrotomy kit (as indicated)
Automatic or manual external defibrillator (as indicated)
Advance cardiac life support drugs (as indicated)
Intubation equipment (as indicated)
Musculoskeletal Supplies
Trauma shears
Tape cutters
Ice; immersion tubs
Plastic bags
Splints/slings/braces/crutches
Athletic tape
Blister-care products
Elastic bandages
Suture materials/wound-care supplies
Other Supplies
Patient record form; pens
Communications; phone numbers
Shelter
Stretchers/cots
Chairs
Tables
Blankets/towels
Security fencing
Heating/cooling equipment for shelter
Generator or electricity source
Lights
Sharps containers
Contaminated waste disposal container
Portable sink/waterless hand cleaner
Toilet
Backboards; semirigid neck collars

The physician's game bag may contain many of these articles, although perhaps not in the quantity necessary to service multiple venues or a mass-participation event. Adapted from Herring SA, Bergfeld J, Boyd J, et al: Med Sci Sports Exerc 2001;33(5):846-849; Herring SA, Bergfeld J, Boyajian-O' Neill LA, et al: Med Sci Sports Exerc 2004;36(11):2004-2008; Armstrong LE, Epstein Y, Greenleaf JE, et al: Med Sci Sports Exerc 1996;28(10):139-148; Daniels JM: Phys Sportsmed 2005;33:12.

development of and adherence to treatment protocols fall under the realm of the medical director. The overall medical care for the event must be a coordinated effort between the aid-station captains and the event's medical director. In addition, the protection of the medical staff is a key responsibility of the medical staff leadership. Preparations must be made to establish a clearly delineated chain of command, appropriate uniforms, adequate shelter, traffic control, and security fencing.[1-3,19]

The medical staff should receive training before the event that includes the overall medical strategy and intervention level, medical-record documentation, communication methods, disqualification of participants, medical protocols to be used, and the chain of command. Protocols for universal precautions, sharps disposal, and medical treatment must be established and disseminated. These treatment protocols should be designed to remain within the training and certification level of the respective provider while meeting the expected incidence of casualties and casualty estimates. Furthermore, the issues of medical responsibility and legal liability must be carefully delineated with the event organizers and appropriately clarified with the entire medical staff.

Treatment protocols

The basis for each protocol should follow the medical strategy regarding treatment at the aid station or transfer. Although it is not possible to plan for every adverse event or patient presentation, each aid station should be provided with written protocols including lists of common problems that have been seen during similar events and their expected interventions. In addition, protocols for emergency transport must include minimal preliminary evaluation, specific indications for transport, and directions regarding who may call for transport. For example, anyone can call for transport for a suspected myocardial infarction.

A triage protocol provides the initial evaluation that will direct the medical team with regard to further treatment protocols and the need for emergency transport. Basic attention to the airway with cervical spine precautions, breathing, circulation, disability, and exposure is paramount. Protocols should specify what vital signs will be determined (including a core temperature) and whether basic blood chemistries will be obtained. The protocol should then direct further evaluation or transfer as needed.

Specific protocols that should be prepared include common musculoskeletal injuries, basic cardiopulmonary resuscitation, and event-specific situations. Determinations should be regarding whether or not intravenous fluid administration will be given for non–life-threatening illnesses and under what parameters. Additional protocols should be developed as indicated, including automatic external defibrillator usage, advanced cardiac life support, advanced trauma life support, exercise-associated collapse, hyperthermia/hypothermia, and hyponatremia. When developing treatment protocols, they need to be kept simple and concise.

Exercise-associated collapse can be seen in athletes of all ages. The term *exercise-associated collapse* is used to describe athletes who are unable to stand or walk unaided as a result of light-headedness, faintness, dizziness, or syncope.[8,9] Although syncope is generally benign, exercise-related syncope may signal the possibility of sudden death. The cause of the collapse is not always apparent on initial evaluation. Life-threatening neurologic, cardiac, and metabolic causes must be considered and appropriate management provided. A careful triage should direct subsequent care in an appropriate direction. The limited capabilities of the medical aid stations and the benefits of immediate transfer must be considered when caring for these athletes. Athletes who collapse before the end of the event should be handled as medical emergencies. **Table 5.4** lists some of the causes of collapse that should be considered.[8,9] The protocol should address immediate actions for the common causes of exercise-associated collapse,

Table 5.4 Exercise-Associated Collapse Causes

Trauma
Cardiac contusion
Head trauma
Neurologic
Neurocardiogenic syncope
Seizure
Cardiac
Myocardial infarction
Supraventricular tachyarrhythmias
Hypertrophic cardiomyopathy
Myocarditis/pericarditis
Valvular heart disease
Prolonged QT syndrome
Coronary artery anomalies
Metabolic
Exertional heat illness
Heatstroke
Hypothermia
Exertional hyponatremia

Adapted from O'Connor FG, Oriscello RG, Levine BD: Am Fam Physician 1999;60(7):2001-2008; O'Connor FG et al: The American Journal of Medicine and Sports 2003;5(3):212-217.

including cardiac arrest, exertional heat illness, hypothermia, and exertional hyponatremia.

Neurocardiogenic syncope is the most common cause of syncope in young adults. It is a result of the high levels of resting vagal tone and orthostatic intolerance after exercise, which results in sudden reflex vasodilation and/or bradycardia. These athletes collapse after completing the competition, and prevention includes continuing participant movement after the finish line. These athletes should be encouraged to consult their private physician to rule out any significant pathologic causes for their syncope before further competition.[8]

Exertional heat illness protocols should address actions for all levels of heat illness that may be encountered during an event. Heat-related illness comprises a spectrum of disorders that ranges from minor illness such as sunburn and heat cramps to severe forms such as heat stroke. These illnesses continue to be significant problems, particularly among competitive athletes and most commonly during the summer months. Heatstroke is the third most common cause of death among high school athletes, and it is responsible for at least 240 deaths per year in the United States alone.[7] There are multiple risk factors associated with heat-related illnesses. Of these risk factors, those that can be readily influenced by the medical plan include the appropriate prescreening of competitors; proper education and awareness of heat illness among the competitors; appropriate access to shade, sunscreen, and fluids; the prevention and treatment of dehydration or overhydration; and the proper planning and design of an emergency plan for the early recognition and treatment of heat-related illness.[2,3,7]

Sunburn can be a significant problem of summertime and tropical competitions. All athletes should be reminded to maintain a liberal application of a sunscreen throughout the competition. Heat cramps can occur in the larger musculature as a result of fluid and electrolyte depletion; "salty sweaters" may be at a higher risk for this condition. Treatment involves rest, cooling, stretching, and massage. In addition, oral rehydration with an electrolyte solution (i.e., a sports drink), salty pretzels, or salt packets may be part of the prevention and treatment protocol.[10-13]

Heatstroke should be treated as a medical emergency because the associated morbidity and mortality are related to both the degree of temperature elevation and the duration of exposure. The protocols should reflect the urgency of proper evaluation and treatment. A common misconception that should be pointed out in the protocol is the fact that many heat-exhaustion and heatstroke patients are still sweating profusely. Important considerations include core-temperature measurement techniques and cooling methods. The practice of intravenous hydration at the event site has been the subject of extensive discussion in the sports medicine community. Intravenous hydration should be carefully and thoroughly discussed with the medical staff and the event organizers during the planning of the event.

Athletic activity outdoors in cold environments is accompanied by a risk for cold injury. Activities performed in cold environments include skiing and hiking; those involving water immersion, such as swimming, diving, and windsurfing; and those involving prolonged activity, such as running and biking. Hypothermia occurs when the body loses more heat than it generates, and the body's core temperature drops to below 95°F or 35°C.[3] Most often, hypothermia occurs when inexperienced athletes find themselves in situations in which unpredictable changes in weather exhaust their resources, and the core body temperature drops drastically. Protocols should include the proper determination of core temperature; the removal of cold, wet clothing; the protection of the athlete from further heat loss; the prevention of arrhythmias; and field measures to be used for rewarming. The risk of a subsequent drop in body temperature caused by the return of cold peripheral blood into the circulation can be minimized by using passive rewarming techniques until the patient can be transported to a more stable environment.[3,5]

Hyponatremia occurs when serum sodium levels drop from the normal range to less than 130 mEq/L.[10] This can lead to significant intracellular swelling and the altering of central nervous system function. A hyponatremia protocol is important in the correct setting because symptoms can progress with cerebral and pulmonary edema and lead to seizure, coma, and cardiopulmonary arrest.[10,20] The protocol should reflect whether a mechanism for measuring actual serum sodium levels will be available. The prevention of hyponatremia is facilitated by providing contestants with proper hydration recommendations that are based on the American College of Sports Medicine consensus statement regarding hydration and physical activity.[13] Additionally, the use or restriction of fluid should specifically be addressed. Urgent transfer to the nearest medical facility is indicated for all patients with physical findings of severe or progressing hyponatremia.

CONCLUSION

Developing an emergency medical plan for events is a challenging task. Ensuring the provision of adequate medical evaluation and treatment is the fundamental base of the medical plan. A thorough review of the successes and failures of previous events and input from previous staff can help with the shaping of the plan. The plan should specifically address the scheduling of the event, the course layout, the medical strategy, competitor issues, logistics, and treatment protocols. Important considerations include environmental conditions, casualty estimates, and sport-specific issues. The medical team should be trained to provide safe and appropriate care. Participants should know what to expect and how to minimize the risk of injury. A well-designed emergency plan is an essential component of a successful competitive athletic event.

REFERENCES

1. Sideline preparedness for the team physician: a consensus statement. Med Sci Sports Exerc 2001;33(5):846-849.
2. American College of Sports Medicine: Mass participation event management for the team physician: a consensus statement. Med Sci Sports Exerc 2004;36(11): 2004-2008.
3. Armstrong LE, Epstein Y, Greenleaf JE, et al: American College of Sports Medicine position stand. Heat 1996;28(10):139-148.
4. Andersen J, Courson RW, Kleiner DM, McLoda TA: National Athletic Trainer's Association Position Statement: Emergency Planning in Athletics. J Athl Train 2002;37(1):99-104.
5. Castellani JW, Young AJ, Ducharme MB, et al, and the American College of Sports Medicine: American College of Sports Medicine position stand: prevention of cold injuries during exercise. Med Sci Sports Exerc 2006;38(11):2012-2029.
6. Roberts WO: Mass participation events. In Lillegard WA, Butcher JD, Rucker KS (eds): Handbook of Sports Medicine, 2nd ed. Boston, Butterworth-Heinemann Publications, 1998, pp 27-45.
7. Seto CK, Way D, O'Connor N: Environmental illness in athletes. Clin Sports Med 2005;24(3):695-718.
8. O'Connor FG, Oriscello RG, Levine BD: Exercise-related syncope in the young athlete: reassurance, restriction or referral?. Am Fam Physician 1999;60(7): 2001-2008.
9. O'Connor FG, et al: Exercise-associated collapse: an algorithmic approach to race day management. Am J Med Sports 2003;5(3):212-217.
10. Speedy DB, Noakes TD, Schneider C: Exercise-associated hyponatremia: a review. Emerg Med (Fremantle) 2001;13(1):17-27.
11. Noakes T and the International Marathon Medical Directors' Association: Fluid replacement during marathon running. Clin J Sports Med 2003;13(5):309-318.
12. Sanchez LD, Corwell B, Berkoff D: Medical problems of marathon runners. Am J Emerg Med 2006;24(5):608-615.
13. Casa DJ, Clarkson PM, Roberts WO: American College of Sports Medicine roundtable on hydration and physical activity: consensus statements. Curr Sports Med Rep 2005;4(3):115-127.
14. Dallam GM, Jonas S, Miller TK: Medical considerations in triathlon competition: recommendations for triathlon organisers, competitors and coaches. Sports Med 2005;35(2):143-161.
15. The City of San Diego Office of Special Events: Planning the medical services for your special event (Web site): Available at www.sandiego.gov/specialevents/pdf/medical.pdf. Accessed April 13, 2007.
16. Hadad E, Rav-Acha M, Heled Y, et al: Heat stroke: a review of cooling methods. Sports Med 2004;34:501-511.
17. Glazer JL: Management of heatstroke and heat exhaustion. Am Fam Physician 2005;71(11):2133-2140.
18. Armstrong LE, Crago AE, Adams R, et al: Whole-body cooling of hyperthermic runners: comparison of two field therapies. Am J Emerg Med 1996;14:355-358.
19. Daniels JM: Optimizing the sideline medical bag: preparing for school and community sports events. Phys Sportsmed 2005;33:12.
20. Flinn SD, Sherer, R: Seizure after exercise in the heat—recognizing life-threatening hyponatremia. Phys Sportsmed 2000;28(9):61-67.

Physical Examination

CHAPTER 6

Victim or Culprit: A Pathoanatomic Approach to the Correct Diagnosis

Anthony I. Beutler, MD

KEY POINTS

- Overuse injuries, the most common injuries in athletes, usually require more sophisticated diagnosis and treatment than the traditional rest, ice, nonsteroidal anti-inflammatory drugs (NSAIDs), and gradual return to play.
- In the system of victims and culprits, *victims* are the structures being injured; *culprits* are the forces, tissues, or objects causing the victims' injuries.
- A proper understanding of the kinetic chain is essential to a complete search for hidden culprits that underlie the patient's injuries.
- Optimal treatment regimens should focus on eradicating the culprit that is causing the injury, rather than simply focusing on treating the victim.
- Understanding the concept of victims and culprits can assist in the proper diagnosis, full rehabilitation, and safe return to play for injured athletes.

INTRODUCTION

Injury is a part of sports participation, and it is a common but potentially devastating event in the life of an athlete. Sports medicine physicians seek to prevent injuries and to quickly return injured athletes to sports participation. In the case of many acute injuries, this is relatively simple and easily done. The broken radius is detected on x-ray, reduced, and then immobilized with plaster. After 6 weeks, the cast is removed, gradual rehabilitation is started, and the athlete is gradually progressed until he or she is ready to return to the field of play. However, many subacute or overuse injuries do not predictably respond to rest, ice, compression, elevation, and a little time away from sport. Too often athletes patiently take NSAIDs, rub ice on the affected part, maybe do a few stretches, and then try to return to activity only to find that the pain recurs with more intensity and at a lower level of activity than before.

Being trapped in the overuse injury cycle is incredibly exasperating for an athlete, and it is often frustrating for the physician who is treating that athlete. Why does plantar fasciitis persist despite rest, ice, and time away from running? Why does subacromial shoulder pain continually crescendo even when the patient is completely resting the arm? Will a patient with chronic Achilles tendinitis ever be able to run again?

These are common questions for sports medicine providers and their patients with overuse injuries. Although not as glamorous or as likely to make the evening edition of SportsCenter as more violent, acute events, overuse injuries are the most common injuries that occur in athletes.[1,2] Learning to correctly diagnose and effectively treat these injuries is an essential skill for the musculoskeletal provider. Many frameworks exist for conceptualizing the process of injury and injury treatment. Chapters 33 and 34 discuss a few of these frameworks. Additionally, the concept of "victims and culprits" is very useful for conceptualizing and ensuring the adequate treatment of overuse injuries.[3]

VICTIMS AND CULPRITS? WHAT IS THIS, CSI: MUSCULOSKELETAL?

Just like in the movies, all injuries involve trauma. In all trauma situations, there is a victim (the thing that gets hurt) and a culprit (the thing that does the hurting). In acute injuries, this can be fairly straightforward. If a soccer goalie collides with the goalpost and breaks an arm, the victim is the arm, and the culprit is the goalpost. However, in overuse injuries, the situation is more complex. A 42-year-old runner complains of heel pain that is worse with the first steps in the morning. The pain has progressively increased for the past 3 months until she can no longer run with a normal stride. What's the diagnosis? What are the victim and culprit in this scenario?

In the movies, identifying the victim is easy: the victim is the one lying in a pool of blood with a chalk police line drawn around him. So it is with the musculoskeletal system. Physicians are typically well trained in "victim identification," and most physicians would agree that the plantar fascia is the victim in the 42-year-old runner presented previously. However, great detectives don't make the big bucks for correctly identifying the victim. The real question is, "Whodunit?" Who or what culprit has injured this runner's plantar fascia? These steps of identifying the victim and discovering the culprit are essential elements of a complete pathoanatomic diagnosis.

IDENTIFYING THE VICTIM

A thorough history is the key to successful diagnosis or "victim identification," because it allows for correct syndrome recognition. A successful musculoskeletal provider will soon recognize how a meniscal tear *sounds* different from patellofemoral pain during the history. Understanding injury mechanisms and common symptomatology allows the physician to arrive at a working diagnosis and a relatively narrow differential diagnosis before even beginning the physical examination. Diagnoses should be confirmed rather than completely determined by physical examination and imaging. The physician should begin the history by asking the athlete questions that identify the transition that may have contributed to the overuse. When did the injury first occur? Did you recently purchase new shoes or a new racquet? Have you changed training locations or your training regimen?

After taking a history and performing a physical examination and appropriate imaging, a pathoanatomic diagnosis should be reached: you should be able to clearly identify the victim. Vague diagnoses, such as runner's knee and shin splints, do not clearly identify the anatomic dysfunction and should be avoided. Diagnoses such as patellar tendinopathy and chronic exertional compartment syndrome more clearly identify the painful, presenting structure. However, even these diagnoses are limited because they may not accurately describe the pathologic process of the injury, and they offer no insight into associated dysfunctions that occur along the rest of the kinetic chain.

Despite the inconsistencies between diagnostic terms and the underlying pathology they describe, most physicians are reasonably adept at victim identification. They can correctly identify the region and often even the specific structure that has been injured. (If they cannot, then reading the next several chapters about examination should help them tremendously!) But as previously discussed, identifying the victim is typically the easy part of the crime scene investigation; discovering the culprit is a more advanced and difficult task.

DISCOVERING THE CULPRIT: WHODUNIT?

In acute traumatic injury, the culprit is typically easy to apprehend. The patient was fine and functioning well until he or she was

struck by a baseball, was tackled by a defender, or landed awkwardly from a jump. However, in cases of overuse injury, the onset of symptoms may be more subtle, and the precise circumstances surrounding the injury may be less clear cut. Overuse injuries might be the result of cumulative trauma **(Figure 6.1)**, or they might result from an acute event that would not have caused injury if it were not for a background of chronic dysfunction. Determining the cause(s) of injury or the culprit(s) who injured the victim is complex because, for most victims, there are many potential culprits. In addition, overuse injuries occur over time, thus allowing the victim to be exposed to many suspected culprits. Figuring out who did what, when, where, and how is a challenge for even the most experienced clinician.

Potential culprits in overuse injuries are typically grouped into extrinsic and intrinsic groups **(Table 6.1)**. Intrinsic factors are biomechanical abnormalities that are unique to a particular athlete. An example of an intrinsic risk factor is high foot arches, which have been demonstrated in military recruits to predispose an individual to a greater risk of musculoskeletal overuse injury than low arches or "flat feet."[4] Extrinsic factors that commonly contribute to overload include poor technique, improper equipment, and improper changes in the duration or frequency of activity. These improper changes in activity or "training errors" are the most common cause of overuse injuries in recreational athletes. Vulnerability to extrinsic overload is also dependent on the intrinsic risk factors of an individual athlete.

When attempting to identify the culprit of a specific injury, the entire extremity and kinetic chain need to be thoroughly examined. A runner who presents with running-related anterior knee pain requires a detailed examination of the knee as well as an examination of the entire lower extremity and pelvis. Leg-length discrepancies, sacral rotations, hamstring inflexibility, forefoot pronation, and gluteal weakness are only a few of the many potential culprits in this case. The tennis player with elbow pain almost routinely demonstrates weakness in the rotator cuff. Indeed, the tennis player, the baseball pitcher, or any athlete who performs overhead actions who presents with upper-extremity pain needs an examination that includes the lower extremity as well as the trunk because all of these are involved in upper-extremity motion in sports. The assessment of core strength should be included for both upper- and lower-extremity athletes (e.g., pelvic bridge assessment, single-leg squat test, and single-leg Trendelenburg examination for gluteal weakness). This awareness of and ability to search

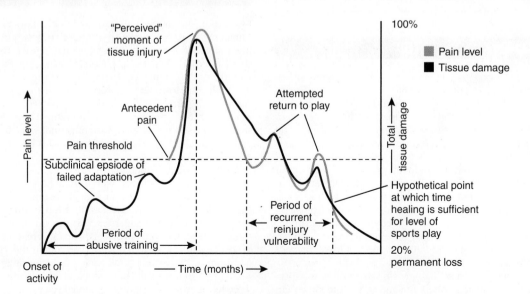

Figure 6.1 Pain and tissue-damage timeline in overuse injuries. (Redrawn from Leadbetter WB: Clin Sports Med 1992;11[3]:533-578.)

Table 6.1 Risk Factors That Contribute to Overuse Injuries

Intrinsic	Extrinsic
Malalignment	Training errors
Muscle imbalance	Equipment
Inflexibility	Environment
Muscle weakness	Technique
Instability	Sports-imposed deficiencies

for culprits along the entire kinetic chain is what separates the novice practitioner from the expert musculoskeletal diagnostician.

Throwing is a classic example of the concept of the kinetic chain, and it illustrates just how wide ranging the search for culprits can be. Chronic throwing overuse can cause a disparity of muscular balance between the internal and external rotators of the shoulder. The external rotators, which are continually required to eccentrically decelerate the arm, are subject to overuse fatigue, which subsequently produces strength and flexibility deficits. However, although this simple construct is useful when beginning to think about the shoulder, it vastly underestimates the sophisticated coordination of the throwing action.

Throwing is a complex process that begins in the legs and that involves force transfer through the hips, trunk, scapula, shoulder, elbow, and wrist. Kibler and colleagues describe this system of force production and transfer as "the kinetic chain."[5] According to this model, the production of throwing forces begins in the legs and trunk with the shoulder and elbow contributing relatively little to normal throwing force. Rather, the joints of the upper extremity serve to fine tune the tremendous forces of throwing, delivering the forces with optimal timing for accurate performance and ensuring the proper arm position for injury prevention. Biomechanical studies support the validity of the kinetic chain model, consistently showing that more than 50% of throwing forces originate in the legs and trunk.[6] Therefore, examination of the throwing athlete with shoulder or elbow pain must also include examination of the scapula, back, and lower extremities because injury, weakness, or anatomic abnormality of these more "proximal" portions of the kinetic chain may result in injury to the shoulder or elbow.

Overuse injury in throwers typically occurs as the athletes attempt to make up for lost force production in the trunk by increasing arm velocity. Alternatively, the abnormal trunk forces may propel the arm into positions of biomechanical disadvantage, thus allowing the large forces of the trunk to directly injure the susceptible connective tissue of the malaligned shoulder and elbow. Hence, biomechanical changes along any portion of the throwing kinetic chain may have a role in the pathogenesis of the commonly diagnosed rotator cuff tendinopathy in an overhead athlete. More importantly for our purposes, tracing the kinetic chain of an injured structure (victim) will often identify the offending culprit.

WHAT'S THE BIG DEAL ABOUT IDENTIFYING THE CULPRIT? CAN'T WE JUST TREAT THE VICTIM?

Too often patients with musculoskeletal complaints are given vague diagnoses and equally vague rehabilitation plans. Patients who are told that they have tendinitis that should improve with rest and 2 weeks of NSAID therapy have usually been imprecisely diagnosed and inadequately treated. Some patients may indeed return to their activities without difficulty after the prescribed 2 weeks despite this inadequacy, but most will not.

Improving the specificity and accuracy of the diagnosis will help. Instead of tendinitis, a more specific diagnosis for the patient would be patellar tendinitis. However, a more precise diagnosis will yield no benefit if the prescribed therapy remains the vague: the patient's outcome will remain unchanged. Patients will likely try to return to their sport after 2 weeks only to find that things are no better and may indeed be worse now that they have been deconditioned by weeks of rest.

Returning to the crime scene analogy, the patient's lack of improvement should not surprise us. By prescribing NSAIDs and rest, we have effectively resuscitated and bandaged our victim (the patellar tendon). However, we have not identified and apprehended the offending culprit. Hence, if we allow the victim to resume normal activities while the culprit is still at large, we should not be surprised to find the same victim stabbed again by the very same culprit in the very same place. It is foolish indeed to allow the victim (the patellar tendon) to return to sports activity before the culprit (a tight quadriceps muscle) is identified and before both the victim and the culprit have been thoroughly rehabilitated.

PUTTING IT ALL TOGETHER: WHEN I KNOW THE VICTIM, HOW DO I FIND THE CULPRIT?

Victim identification

Let's return to our 42-year-old runner with heel pain that is worse with the first steps that she takes in the morning. On the basis of that history alone, we can surmise that this patient probably has plantar fascial pain. Sure enough, when we press on the medial calcaneal tubercle, our patient winces with pain. So, to follow the model **(Box 6.1),** the victim in our case is the plantar fascia.

Box 6.1: A 42-Year-Old Runner with Heel Pain

Victim
Plantar fascia

Culprit
Tight heel cords

Mechanism
Tight heel cords cause heel off to occur earlier during the stance phase and before the midfoot has returned to a supinated (locked) position. Heel off while the midfoot is pronated (unlocked) leads to excess strain on the plantar fascia.

Common Treatments
Victim-based treatments:
- Nonsteroidal anti-inflammatory drugs (noninflammatory, despite the "-itis")
- Heel cups/heel pads
- Ice massage
- Steroid injection

Culprit-based treatments:
- Gastrocnemius/soleus stretching
- Intrinsic foot-muscle strengthening
- Night splints
- Orthotics

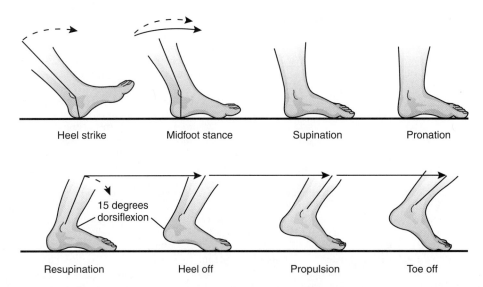

Figure 6.2 Normal gait cycle. In the usual gait cycle with normal gastrocnemius/soleus flexibility, heel off occurs at approximately 10 to 15 degrees of ankle dorsiflexion, after midfoot supination, pronation, and resupination have occurred. This allows the supinated midfoot to engage the bony lock of Chopart's joint before heel off and propulsion occur.

Discovering the culprit

As we review possible culprits, we discover that the patient is an experienced runner who regularly changes her shoes and who has not changed her running style or pace recently. She did have her gallbladder removed earlier this year, and she reports that her heel pain started a few weeks after she returned to running after the surgery. On physical examination, she has normal arches, normal bony alignment, and no leg-length discrepancy. Strength in all muscle groups and in the core musculature tests normal, but she has a maximum of 0 degrees of passive dorsiflexion in both ankles when her knees are fully extended. Thus, we will propose that the culprit responsible for injuring this patient's plantar fascia is gastrocnemius/soleus tightness or tight heel cords (see Box 6.1).

Understanding the kinetic chain and the mechanism of injury

How can tight heel cords result in plantar fascial pain? The answer requires an understanding of the normal gait cycle **(Figure 6.2).** In normal walking and usual jogging, heel strike occurs on the lateral aspect of the heel, and this is followed closely by midfoot stance. The midfoot is initially supinated, but pronation rapidly occurs to assist with shock absorption and cushioning. After this, the midfoot then resupinates. All of this is performed "on the clock" of ankle dorsiflexion. Figure 6.2 illustrates how each of these proceeding steps occurs while ankle dorsiflexion progresses. At the point of an individual's maximal ankle dorsiflexion, the Achilles tendon will drag the calcaneus off the ground, thereby initiating the "heel off" portion of the gait. However, it is

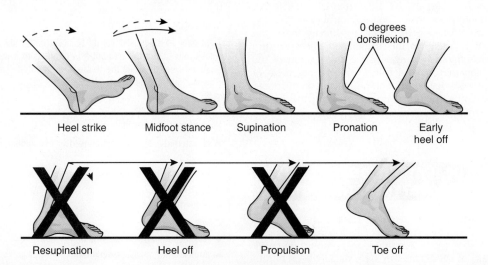

Figure 6.3 Abnormal gait cycle caused by tight heel cords. With gastrocnemius/soleus tightness, heel off occurs before resupination is complete. This results in an unlocked Chopart's joint, and it causes the forces of propulsion to be absorbed along the soft tissues of the foot (including the plantar fascia) rather than along the usual bony structures.

biomechanically *essential* that the midfoot resupinate before the Achilles tendon causes heel off to occur. The midfoot (specifically Chopart's joint) engages a bony lock when it is in the supinated position. This bony lock allows the foot to function as a stiff lever during the propulsive, heel-off phase of the gait cycle. However, if heel off occurs while the midfoot is still pronated and Chopart's joint is unlocked, the force of propulsion cannot be transmitted along the midfoot bones and thus must be absorbed by the plantar fascia, the intrinsic muscles, and the other soft-tissue structures of the foot.

In patients with tight heel cords (such as our runner with 0 degrees of dorsiflexion), heel strike, midfoot stance, initial supination, and pronation occur normally. However, as depicted in **Figure 6.3,** the patient's tight heel cords result in early heel off. Because this early heel off occurs before resupination is complete and before Chopart's joint can engage the bony lock that is essential to normal gait mechanics, the propulsive force of running and walking overloads the plantar fascia and thus can result in plantar fascial pain. Hence, tight heel cords are indeed the culprits that cause injury to the victimized plantar fascia in this case.

Choosing the correct treatment

The most common treatments for plantar fascia pain include NSAIDs, heel cups/pads, ice massage, and steroid injections. However, by applying our model of victims and culprits, it becomes clear that each of these treatments is designed to bandage up the victim rather than deal with the offending culprit. Our patient can take buckets of NSAIDs, use the best heel cups available, religiously practice ice massage, and receive perfectly placed steroid injections, but she will continue to have pain as long as her abnormal gait mechanics continue to stress her plantar fascia.

The secret to successfully "curing" this patient's plantar fascia pain comes from addressing the culprit (see Box 6.1). Gastrocnemius and soleus stretching will allow for greater dorsiflexion, which will permit the complete resupination of the midfoot before heel off. Intrinsic foot-muscle strengthening will allow for more active, soft-tissue shock absorption, and it will offload the overworked plantar fascia. Night splints may also be beneficial for increasing maximum ankle dorsiflexion. Only after both the victim and the culprit have been successfully rehabilitated can the patient expect to return to sport without an increased risk of reinjury.

CONCLUSION

The model of victims and culprits is, after all, only a model, with all of the associated inherent fallibilities and limitations. However, the model of victims and culprits does provide a useful framework for thinking about the diagnosis, the treatment, and even the prevention of many injuries. Although there are no comprehensive lists of every conceivable victim and associated culprits, **Table 6.2** gives a few examples of well-known overuse victims and culprits and their commonly associated treatments. These lists are decidedly incomplete, but they are intended to guide your thinking and organize your learning as you read the upcoming chapters. As sports medicine physicians, we cannot simply accept repeated injury as being a necessary part of athletics and physical activity. Hopefully the victim-and-culprit model will assist you with looking beyond the obvious, immediate injury and lead you to focus instead on how to avoid the cycle of reinjury or even perhaps on how to prevent the initial injury from occurring.

Table 6.2   Common Overuse Victims, Culprits, and Treatments

Diagnosis	Victim	Victim-Based Treatment	Common Culprits	Culprit-Based Treatment
Plantar fasciitis	Plantar fascia	NSAIDs	Tight heel cords	Gastrocnemius/soleus stretching
		Heel cups/heel pads		Night splints
		Ice massage	Training error	Decrease mileage by 50%, then increase
		Steroid injection		no more than 10% per week
			Muscular weakness	Intrinsic foot-muscle strengthening
			Overpronation	Orthotics
			Improper/worn-out shoes	Shoe prescription after foot and gait analysis
Patellofemoral (anterior) knee pain	Patellofemoral joint	NSAIDs Rest	Muscular (quadriceps or gluteal) weakness	Tailored physical therapy to strengthen muscles
			Poor flexibility (quadriceps, hamstrings, gastrocnemius)	Stretching prescription
			Poor alignment	Orthotics for pes planus
				Patellar taping/bracing for patellar malalignment
Patellar tendinitis	Patellar tendon	NSAIDs Patellar strap	Quadriceps/hip flexor tightness	Stretching prescription
			Quadriceps weakness	Tailored physical therapy to strengthen muscles
				Eccentric quadriceps-strengthening program
Trochanteric bursitis	Trochanteric bursa	NSAIDs Steroid injection	Tensor fascia lata or gluteal weakness (especially gluteus medius)	Tailored physical therapy to strengthen muscles
Subacromial pain	Rotator cuff/ subacromial bursa	NSAIDs Steroid injection	Rotator cuff weakness	Tailored physical therapy to strengthen the rotator cuff
			Subacromial spurring	Subacromial decompression
			Scapular dyskinesis	Scapular retraining

NSAIDs, nonsteroidal anti-inflammatory drugs.

REFERENCES

1. Baquie P, Brukner P: Injuries presenting to an Australian sports medicine centre: a 12-month study. Clin J Sport Med 1997;7(1):28-31.
2. Brukner P, Bennell K: Overuse injuries: where to now? Br J Sports Med 1997;31(1):2.
3. Macintyre JG, Lloyd-Smith DR: Overuse running injuries. In Renstrom PA (ed): Sports Injuries—Basic Principles of Prevention and Care. Boston, Blackwell Scientific Publications, 1993, pp 139-160.
4. Cowan DN, Jones BH, Frykman PN, et al: Lower limb morphology and risk of overuse injury among male infantry trainees. Med Sci Sports Exerc 1996;28(8):945-952.
5. Kibler WB, Chandler TJ, Pace BK: Principles of rehabilitation after chronic tendon injuries. Clin Sports Med 1992;11(3):661-671.
6. Kibler WB: What makes the ball go and what happens when it doesn't. Presentation at American College of Sports Medicine Annual Meeting, St. Louis, May 2002.

CHAPTER 7

Physical Examination of the Wrist and Hand

William A. Mitchell III, MD, and Ahmed A. Radwan, MD

KEY POINTS

- Most sports require the use of both wrists and hands, and all sports require the use of these body parts in either transient or complementary roles.
- The common diagnosis of a "sprain" and the pressure to continue playing often compels the athlete back onto the field or court without proper treatment. Improper diagnosis and treatment, however, may lead to chronic pain or dysfunction in the wrist and hand.
- Simple screening tests like range of motion, strength, and palpation can highlight potential abnormalities; special tests of the wrist and hand allow the practitioner to carefully examine these specific areas of concern. It is important to remember that, although a positive test may strongly suggest a particular diagnosis, a negative test does not rule one out.

INTRODUCTION

Appropriately functioning wrists and hands are essential to sports participation. The very essence of athletics involves the skillful use of one's body, and the wrists and hands are common focuses of this skill. Most sports require the use of both wrists and hands, with the possible exceptions of distance running, some soccer positions, and certain one-handed sports. However, it may be argued that these sports also require the use of the wrist and hand, if only in a transient or complementary role.

The incidence of wrist and hand injury varies with the study population, but it ranges from 3% to 25% of all athletic injuries.[1] Those physicians who work in a referral setting (especially those who treat elite or professional athletes) should expect to see a greater percentage of fractures, whereas those on the sidelines or in the training room will see more soft-tissue injuries.

The sideline physician has a distinct advantage in the evaluation of injuries to the wrist and hand. He or she has access to facts that may significantly aid the early diagnosis and treatment of these injuries, including the mechanism of injury, the force of the impact, and the relative stoicism of the patient in question.[1] Such information can contribute considerably to the accuracy of a diagnosis.

Because of their detailed anatomy and complex motions and functions, the wrist and hand are sometimes considered enigmatic.[1,2] This can especially be true when a practitioner sees injuries to these members only rarely. Such mystery commonly leads to the diagnosis of a "sprain," and the pressure to continue playing compels the athlete back onto the field or court without proper treatment.[2] Improper diagnosis and treatment, however, may lead to chronic pain or dysfunction in the wrist and hand, possibly bringing an early end to an athletic career. Thus, the injunction to us as medical professionals to push our capabilities to their limits—but to know those limits well and to refer quickly when we have reached them—is doubly true with wrist and hand injuries.

Considering the importance of the wrist and hand in sports, the frequency of injury, and the consequences of delay in diagnosis and treatment, the value of competency with these structures becomes clear. All practitioners caring for athletes would do well to strive to understand the complex anatomy and physiology of the wrist and hand, the unique demands placed on these structures by different sports, and the physical examination techniques recommended by the medical literature.

ANATOMY

The wrist is composed of two transverse rows of carpal bones, with only the scaphoid crossing the midcarpal joint[1] **(Figure 7.1).** The placement of the scaphoid prevents the distal row from displacing under compressive loads, which would allow for the collapse of the midcarpal joint.[2] This location also places the scaphoid at significantly greater risk for injury than the remaining carpal bones.

The pisiform is considered by some authors to be sesamoidal rather than a true carpal bone. One reason for this is that no tendons originate on or insert into the carpal bones except the pisiform, which is found at the junction of the flexor carpi ulnaris and the abductor digiti minimi tendons. Because of this, wrist motion is always passive.[2] The tendons responsible for this motion are the extensor carpi radialis longus and brevis, the extensor carpi ulnaris, the flexor carpi radialis, the flexor carpi ulnaris, and the palmaris longus **(Figures 7.2 and 7.3).**

The joints of the wrist include the distal radioulnar joint, the radiocarpal joint, the intercarpal joints, the midcarpal joint, and the

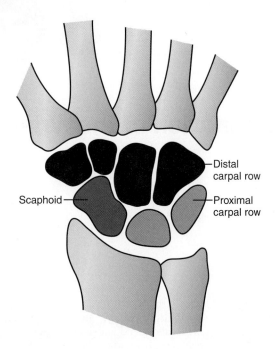

Figure 7.1 The carpal bones are aligned in two transverse rows, with the scaphoid crossing the midcarpal joint. (From DeLee JC, Drez D, Miller MD: DeLee and Drez's Orthopaedic Sports Medicine, 2nd ed. Philadelphia, Saunders Elsevier, 2003, p 1337.)

carpometacarpal joints **(Figure 7.4).** The radius articulates with the scaphoid and lunate bones; this joint bears 60% of an axial load applied to the wrist.[3] The lunate and triquetrum articulate not with the ulna but rather with the triangular fibrocartilage complex (TFCC).

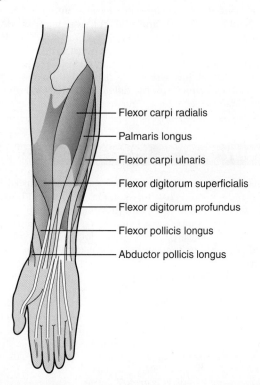

Figure 7.2 The wrist flexors. (From Jenkins DB: Hollinshead's Functional Anatomy of the Limbs and Back, 7th ed. Philadelphia, WB Saunders, 1998, p 160.)

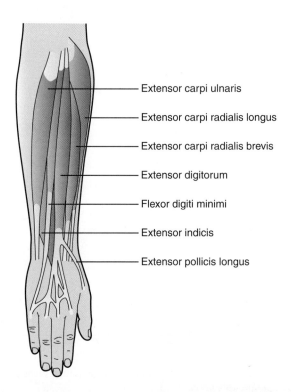

Figure 7.3 The wrist extensors. (From Jenkins DB: Hollinshead's Functional Anatomy of the Limbs and Back, 7th ed. Philadelphia, WB Saunders, 1998, p 160.)

Wrist stability is maintained by the intracapsular ligamentous anatomy, with the stronger ligaments on the volar aspect **(Figure 7.5).** One of the most important is the scapholunate ligament, which contributes significantly to wrist stability and is commonly injured.[1]

The anatomy of the hand is intricate, and an exhaustive description is beyond the scope of this text. However, an understanding of the bony structures, the musculotendinous articulations, the neurovascular bundles, and the compartmental anatomy is essential when caring for athletes.

The hand is composed of 21 bones distal to the carpus, including the metacarpals, the phalanges, and the two sesamoids of the thumb[4] **(Figure 7.6).** Each metacarpal has a base proximally and a head distally, with a body interposed. The phalanges have a similar construction; each finger has three phalanges, and the thumb has two.

The joints of the hand include the carpometacarpal joints, the metacarpophalangeal (MCP) joints, and the interphalangeal (IP) joints. Each finger has a proximal interphalangeal joint (PIP) and a distal interphalangeal joint (DIP); the thumb has only one IP joint. The second and third metacarpals articulate with one another and with the distal carpals such that they are nearly immobile. The fourth and fifth metacarpals, however, are considerably more mobile (although not as mobile as the thumb),[3] and this allows for increased grip strength. The collateral ligaments at the MCP joints allow for considerable sideways movement with the fingers in extension. During flexion, however, they become tight, and this restricts such side-to-side mobility. The IP joints are hinge joints, allowing only for flexion and extension. Both the MCP and IP joints have thick palmar ligaments on the volar surface that prevent hyperextension.[4]

The extrinsic muscles of the hand originate in the forearm and elbow. The flexor tendons of the fingers include the flexor digitorum superficialis and the flexor digitorum profundus. These travel in a fibro-osseous tunnel between the metacarpals and the

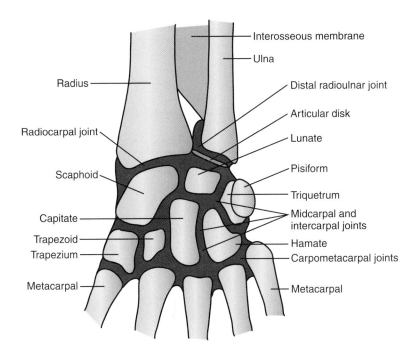

Figure 7.4 The bones and joints of the wrist. (From Jenkins DB: Hollinshead's Functional Anatomy of the Limbs and Back, 7th ed. Philadelphia, WB Saunders, 1998, p 166.)

DIP joints, and they insert onto the base of the middle and distal phalanges, respectively **(Figure 7.7)**. The extensor tendons of the fingers pass over the dorsum of the wrist in six separate compartments.[4] They include the extensor digitorum communis, the extensor indicis proprius, and the extensor digiti minimi. The latter two are accessory extensors of the index and little fingers, respectively.[5]

The intrinsic muscles of the hand include the thenar, hypothenar, lumbrical, and interosseous groups. The thenar muscles control the abduction and opposition of the thumb, whereas the flexion and extension of the thumb are controlled by forearm muscles. The interosseous and lumbrical groups flex the MCP joints and help extend the IP joints. They also abduct and adduct the fingers[6] **(Figure 7.8)**.

The median nerve is the motor supply to the thenar muscles and the two radial lumbricals. It also provides sensory innervation to the palmar aspect of the first three digits and the radial half of the ring finger. The ulnar nerve provides motor control for the remaining intrinsic hand muscles and sensation for the fifth digit and the ulnar half of the ring finger. The radial nerve provides sensory innervation to the dorsum of the hand[6] **(Table 7.1 and Figure 7.9)**.

RANGE OF MOTION

Active

Many authors recommend beginning with a simple screening examination for active range of motion, such as having the patient move the wrists in all four cardinal directions or having him or her extend the fingers with the palms down, supinate, and then slowly flex the digits into a fist. Any abnormality noticed on this screening may then be more carefully examined.[2]

Active pronation and supination of the forearm and wrist from neutral position are both 85 to 90 degrees **(Table 7.2)**. There are marked differences between individuals, however, and the affected arm should always be compared with the unaffected arm to determine what is normal for the individual. Radial deviation is about 15 degrees, whereas ulnar deviation is 30 to 45 degrees. The wrist can flex 80 to 90 degrees and extend 70 to 90 degrees.[3]

Flexion of the fingers will decrease with concomitant flexion of the wrist. With the wrist in neutral, the MCP joints will flex 85 to 90 degrees, the PIP joints 100 to 115 degrees, and the DIP joints 80 to 90 degrees. Finger extension also occurs at the MCP joints (30 to

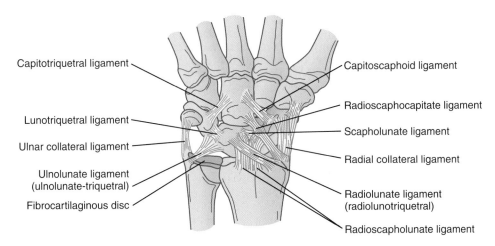

Figure 7.5 Volar ligaments of the wrist. (From Magee DJ: Orthopaedic Physical Assessment, 4th ed. St. Louis, Saunders Elsevier, 2006, p 357.)

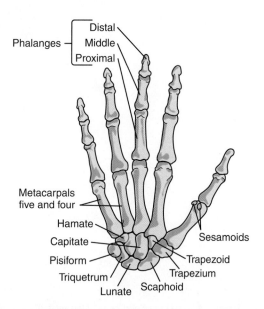

Figure 7.6 Bones of the wrist and hand, palmar view. (From Jenkins DB: Hollinshead's Functional Anatomy of the Limbs and Back, 7th ed. Philadelphia, WB Saunders, 1998, p 164.)

45 degrees) and the DIP joints (20 degrees).[3] The PIP joints have 0 degrees of extension, which makes them prone to dorsal dislocation.

Unlike the fingers, the thumb is also able to flex at its carpometacarpal joint (45 to 50 degrees). Otherwise, the flexion mechanism is similar to the fingers at the MCP joint (50 to 55 degrees) and the IP joint (80 to 90 degrees). Thumb extension occurs solely at the IP joint (0 to 5 degrees). Abduction of the thumb reaches 60 to 70 degrees, whereas adduction is normally 30 degrees. Of note is that the flexion and extension of the thumb occur in a plane that is parallel with the palm. Abduction and adduction occur perpendicular to this plane.[3]

Passive

If there is limitation of the active ranges of motion, the examiner should proceed with a passive range examination. The passive movements are the same as the active and essentially have the same extremes.[3]

STRENGTH TESTING

Strength testing should be performed with the patient seated and the elbows flexed to 90 degrees. With the following strength tests, the examiner should not be able to easily overcome a normal patient's strength. For a complete list of the names, actions, and innervation of the muscles being tested, see **Table 7.3**.

To test the wrist extensors, the patient sits with the forearm pronated and makes a fist. The examiner supports the forearm and asks the patient to extend the wrist. The examiner then presses downward on the dorsum of the hand, attempting to overcome the patient's strength. To isolate the extensor carpi ulnaris, the patient may extend the wrist while holding the fist in ulnar deviation. Similarly, extending the wrist held in radial deviation will isolate the extensor carpi radialis longus and brevis[5] **(Figure 7.10)**.

The finger extensors are usually tested together because the tethering of the extensor tendons makes it difficult to hold the middle and ring fingers in extension while the other fingers are flexed. With the hand pronated and supported by the

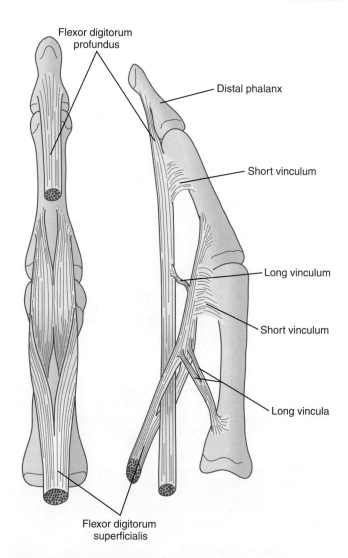

Figure 7.7 The digital flexor tendons, palmar and lateral views. (From Jenkins DB: Hollinshead's Functional Anatomy of the Limbs and Back, 7th ed. Philadelphia, WB Saunders, 1998, p 172.)

examiner, the patient extends and adducts the four fingers. The patient holds this position as the examiner attempts to passively flex the fingers. Each finger joint may also be tested individually by supporting the finger proximal to that joint and having the patient extend against resistance.

The wrist flexors are tested with the forearm supinated. The patient makes a fist and flexes the wrist. Supporting the patient's forearm with one hand, the examiner attempts to extend the wrist with the other hand. Placing the patient's fist in ulnar deviation will isolate the flexor carpi ulnaris, whereas radial deviation will isolate the flexor carpi radialis.[5]

Finger flexor strength may be tested together by the examiner hooking his or her fingers under the patient's. The patient makes a tight fist, and the examiner attempts to extend the patient's fingers **(Figure 7.11)**. The examiner should be able to overcome the patient only with difficulty. For a complete examination, the fingers should also be tested individually. To test the flexor digitorum profundus, the examiner stabilizes the PIP in extension, and the patient flexes the DIP. Normal flexion is 45 degrees in this position **(Figure 7.12)**. The flexor digitorum superficialis is tested by having the patient flex each finger one at a time while the others are held in full extension **(Figure 7.13)**. The MCP and the PIP should flex in all of the fingers when they are tested this way. The DIP of the

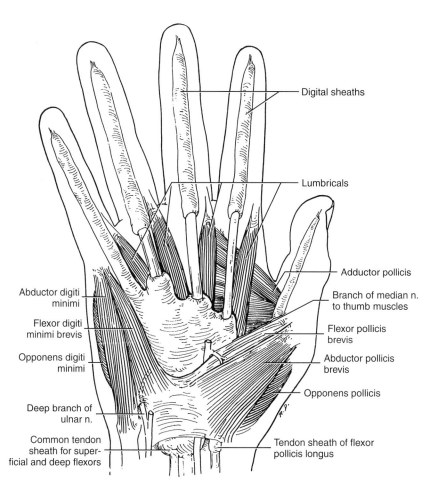

Digital sheaths

Lumbricals

Adductor pollicis

Branch of median n.
to thumb muscles

Flexor pollicis
brevis

Abductor pollicis
brevis

Opponens pollicis

Tendon sheath of flexor
pollicis longus

Abductor digiti
minimi

Flexor digiti
minimi brevis

Opponens digiti
minimi

Deep branch of
ulnar n.

Common tendon
sheath for super-
ficial and deep flexors

Figure 7.8 The intrinsic muscles of the hand.
(The included figure identifies the thenar and
hypothenar groups.) (From Jenkins DB:
Hollinshead's Functional Anatomy of the Limbs
and Back, 7th ed. Philadelphia, WB Saunders,
1998, p 171.)

Table 7.1   Motor Nerve Functions at the Wrist

Nerve	Muscle Innervated	Test for Function
Radial	Extensor carpi radialis, brevis, and ulnaris	Resist wrist extension*
	Extensor pollicis brevis/longus	Push against extended thumb
	Abductor pollicis longus	Push against abducted thumb
	Extensor digitorum communis	Wrist neutral; extend MCP with flexed PIP (prevents use of intrinsics)
	Extensor indicis	
	Extensor digiti minimi	
Median	Flexor digitorum superficialis	Hold all fingers in extension (isolates superficialis); patient flexes isolated PIP
	Flexor pollicis longus	Patient holds flexed thumb against hypothenar eminence; examiner attempts to pull it away
	Abductor pollicis longus	Patient abducts thumb against resistance
	Opponens pollicis	Patient apposes small finger and thumb; examiner attempts to separate them
	Flexor pollicis brevis, lateral portion	Patient makes O with thumb and index finger; examiner pulls them apart*
	Radial two lumbricals	
Ulnar	Flexor digitorum profundus (ulnar two digits)	Stabilize MCP and PIP in extension; patient actively flexes DIP
	Dorsal interossei (DAB: dorsal abducts)	Patient fans extended fingers; examiner forces each pair together*
	Palmar interossei (PAD: palmar adducts)	Patient holds extended fingers together; examiner attempts to force them apart
	Adductor pollicis	Patient adducts thumb against resistance
	Opponens digiti minimi	Test as for opponens pollicis (described previously)
	Flexor pollicis brevis, medial portion	
	Abductor digiti minimi	Patient attempts to abduct small finger against examiner's resistance (most specific for ulnar nerve)
	Flexor carpi ulnaris	

*Most commonly used screening test.
MCP, metacarpophalangeal (joint); PIP, proximal interphalangeal (joint); DIP, distal interphalangeal (joint).
From Lillegard WA, Butcher JD, Rucker KS: Handbook of Sports Medicine: A Symptom-Oriented Approach, 2nd ed. Boston, Butterworth-Heinemann, 1999, p 161.

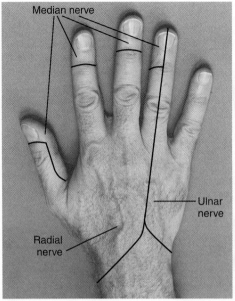
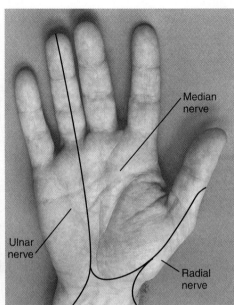

Figure 7.9 The dermatomes of the hand. (From Reider B: The Orthopedic Physical Examination, 2nd ed. Philadelphia, WB Saunders, 2005, p 145.)

A B

index finger should flex as well because its flexor digitorum profundus tendon is not tethered to the others, thus allowing the DIP to flex even while the other fingers are held in extension.[5]

The muscles that enact the radial and ulnar deviation of the wrist have been previously discussed (see Table 7.3). The strength of these actions may be tested by having the patient deviate the wrist radially and then resist the examiner's effort to force it into ulnar deviation. The opposite would test the strength of the ulnar deviators.[5]

Table 7.2 Active Movements of the Forearm, Wrist, and Hand

Pronation of the forearm (85 to 90 degrees)

Supination of the forearm (85 to 90 degrees)

Wrist abduction or radial deviation (15 degrees)

Wrist adduction or ulnar deviation (30 to 45 degrees)

Wrist flexion (80 to 90 degrees)

Wrist extension (70 to 90 degrees)

Finger flexion (MCP, 85 to 90 degrees; PIP, 100 to 115 degrees; DIP, 80 to 90 degrees)

Finger extension (MCP, 30 to 45 degrees; PIP, 0 degrees; DIP, 20 degrees)

Finger abduction (20 to 30 degrees)

Finger adduction (0 degrees)

Thumb flexion (CMC, 45 to 50 degrees; MCP, 50 to 55 degrees; IP, 85 to 90 degrees)

Thumb extension (MCP, 0 degrees; IP, 0 to 5 degrees)

Thumb abduction (60 to 70 degrees)

Thumb adduction (30 degrees)

Opposition of little finger to thumb (tip to tip)

Combined movements (if necessary)

Repetitive movements (if necessary)

Sustained positions (if necessary)

MCP, metacarpophalangeal; PIP, proximal interphalangeal; DIP, distal interphalangeal; CMC, carpometacarpal; IP, interphalangeal.
From Magee DJ: Orthopaedic Physical Assessment, 4th ed. St. Louis, Saunders Elsevier, 2006, p 373.

Finger abduction strength is tested by having the patient fully abduct the fingers and then resist as the examiner forces them into adduction with his or her own fingers while supporting the forearm with the other hand **(Figure 7.14)**. Adduction may be tested by having the patient hold the fingers adducted against one another and resist the examiner's attempt to separate the fingers. These actions may also be tested by placing the patient's hand on a table with the fingers comfortably separated. This allows the examiner to test the strength of each finger individually.[5]

The movement of the thumb is similar to that of the fingers, with the notable exception of opposability. Extension of the thumb can be tested by having the patient extend the thumb as if hitchhiking. The examiner should apply force dorsally to the proximal phalanx, which will test the extensor pollicis longus and brevis together. He or she should then should stabilize the proximal phalanx and apply a similar force to the distal phalanx; this will test the extensor pollicis longus in isolation[5] **(Figure 7.15)**.

Thumb flexion may be tested by having the patient flex the thumb across the palm. The examiner may then attempt to extend the thumb against resistance. MCP flexion is controlled by the flexor pollicis longus and brevis together, whereas the flexor pollicis longus alone controls IP flexion[5] **(Figure 7.16)**.

Thumb abduction can be described as palmar or radial. Palmar abduction is controlled by the abductor pollicis brevis, and it is tested by having the patient abduct the thumb perpendicularly away from the plane of the palm. The examiner attempts to force the thumb back toward the palm **(Figure 7.17)**. Radial abduction is powered by the abductor pollicis longus, and it may be tested with the hand flat on a table. The thumb is abducted in a plane that is parallel to the palm; the examiner attempts to push the thumb back toward the palm.[5]

Thumb adduction, which is similar to abduction, occurs in planes that are both parallel and perpendicular to the palm. Both are primarily controlled by the adductor pollicis. A patient's strength may be tested using Froment's test (described later) or by placing the examiner's finger in the patient's palm and having the patient hold the examiner's finger in place with the thumb. The examiner then attempts to bring the thumb into abduction against resistance[5] **(Figure 7.18)**.

Opposition of the thumb relies on the cooperation of the opponens pollicis with the abductor pollicis brevis. While the first

Table 7.3   Muscles of the Forearm, Wrist, and Hand

Action	Muscles Acting	Nerve Supply	Never Root Devation
Supination of forearm	1. Supinator	Posterior interosscous (radial)	C5-C6
	2. Biceps brachii	Musculocutaneous	C5-C6
Pronation of forearm	1. Pronator quadratus	Anterior interosscous (median)	C8, T1
	2. Pronator teres	Median	C6-C7
	3. Flexor carpi radialis	Median	C6-C7
Extension of wrist	1. Extensor carpi radialis longus	Radial	C6-C7
	2. Extensor carpi radialis brevis	Posterior interosscous (radial)	C7-C8
	3. Extensor carpi ulnaris	Posterior interosscous (radial)	C7-C8
Flexion of wrist	1. Flexor carpi radialis	Median	C6-C7
	2. Flexor carpi ulnaris	Ulnar	C7-C8
Ulnar deviation of wrist	1. Flexor carpi ulnaris	Ulnar	C7-C8
	2. Extensor carpi ulnaris	Posterior interosscous (radial)	C7-C8
Radial deviation of wrist	1. Flexor carpi radialis	Median	C6-C7
	2. Extensor carpi radialis longus	Radial	C6-C7
	3. Abductor pollicis longus	Posterior interosscous (radial)	C7-C8
	4. Extensor pollicis brevis	Posterior interosscous (radial)	C7-C8
Extension of fingers	1. Extensor digitorum communis	Posterior interosscous (radial)	C7-C8
	2. Extensor indiees (second finger)	Posterior interosscous (radial)	C7-C8
	3. Extensor digiti minimi (little finger)	Posterior interosscous (radial)	C7-C8
Flexion of fingers	1. Flexor digitorum profundus	Anterior interosscous (median)	C8, T1
	2. Flexor digitorum superficialis	Anterior interosscous (median): lateral two	C8, T1
	3. Lumbricals	digits	C8, T1
	4. Interossei	Ulnar: medial two digits	C7-C8, T1
	5. Flexor digiti minimi (little finger)	Median	C8, T1
		First and second; median; third and fourth:	C8, T1
		ulnar (deep terminal branch)	C8, T1
		Ulnar (deep terminal branch)	
		Ulnar (deep terminal branch)	
Abduction of fingers (with fingers extended)	1. Dorsal interossei	Ulnar (deep terminal branch)	C8, T1
	2. Abductor digiti minimi (little finger)	Ulnar (deep terminal branch)	C8, T1
Adduction of fingers (with fingers extended)	1. Palmar interossei	Ulnar (deep terminal branch)	C8, T1
Extension of thumb	1. Extensor pollicis longus	Posterior interosseous (radial)	C7-C8
	2. Extensor pollicis brevis	Posterior interosseous (radial)	C7-C8
	3. Abductor pollicis longus	Posterior interosseous (radial)	C7-C8
Flexion of thumb	1. Flexor pollicis brevis	Superficial head: median (lateral terminal	C8, T1
	2. Flexor pollicis longus	branch)	C8, T1
	3. Opponens pollicis	Deep head: ulnar	C8, T1
		Anterior interosseous (median)	C8, T1
		Median (lateral terminal branch)	
Abduction of thumb	1. Abductor pollicis longus	Posterior interosseous (radial)	C7-C8
	2. Abductor pollicis brevis	Median (lateral terminal branch)	C8, T1
Abduction of thumb	1. Adductor pollicis	Ulnar (deep terminal branch)	C8, T1
Opposition of thumb and little finger	1. Opponens pollicis	Median (lateral terminal branch)	C8, T1
	2. Flexor pollicis brevis	Superficial head: median (lateral terminal	C8, T1
	3. Abductor pollicis brevis	branch)	C8, T1
	4. Opponens digiti minimi	Median (lateral terminal branch)	C8, T1
		Ulnar (deep terminal branch)	

From Magee DJ: Orthopaedic Physical Assessment, 4th ed. St. Louis, Saunders Elsevier, 2006, p 377.

rotates the thumb to face the other fingers, the second brings the thumb away from the palm. The strength of this function is tested by having the patient touch the tips of the thumb and little finger and inspecting the hand carefully to ensure that the distal phalanges form a reasonably continuous line with one another. A significant angle between the two indicates that the thumb lacks appropriate rotation; the abductors may be working alone. Strength is tested as follows: with the hand appropriately positioned, the examiner hooks his or her index fingers around the thumb and little fingers palmarly and attempts to separate the two[5] **(Figure 7.19).**

PALPATION

Dorsal wrist

Palpation of the dorsal wrist should begin at the radial tubercle **(Figures 7.20 and 7.21).** Just distal to the bony radial tubercle,

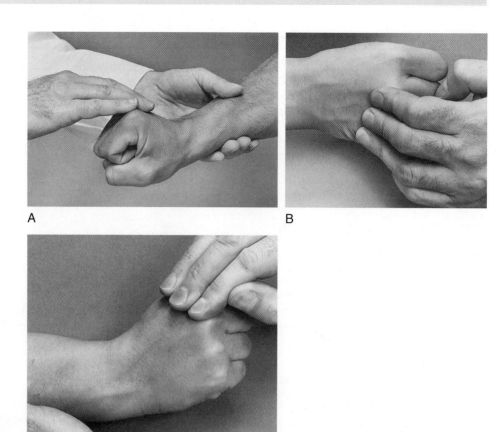

A

B

Figure 7.10 *A*, Assessing wrist extensor strength. *B*, Assessing the strength of the extensor carpi ulnaris. *C*, Assessing the strength of the extensor radialis longus and brevis. (From Reider B: The Orthopedic Physical Examination, 2nd ed. Philadelphia, WB Saunders, 2005, p 138.)

C

the examiner will find the abductor pollicis longus and the extensor pollicis brevis. These tendons form the volar border of the anatomic snuffbox and lie in the first dorsal compartment of the wrist. The floor of the anatomic snuffbox itself is formed by the waist of the scaphoid bone. Tenderness in this location is concerning for a scaphoid fracture, especially in a patient whose history involves falling on an outstretched hand. Immediately distal to the snuffbox

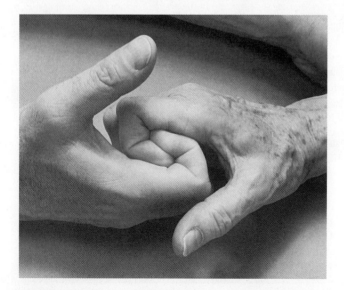

Figure 7.11 Assessing overall finger flexor strength. (From Reider B: The Orthopedic Physical Examination, 2nd ed. Philadelphia, WB Saunders, 2005, p 140.)

floor, the examiner will find the pulsating dorsal branch of the radial artery and, beyond this, the bony prominence of the trapezium.[5]

The dorsal border of the anatomic snuffbox is formed by the extensor pollicis longus, which comprises the third dorsal compartment. Passing just beneath this tendon are the extensor carpi radialis longus and brevis, thus forming the second dorsal compartment. These are most easily felt with the wrist extended against resistance. Near the intersection of these tendons, the examiner will palpate Lister's tubercle, which is approximately 2 cm in the ulnar direction from the radial styloid.[5] Palpating distal to Lister's tubercle will reveal the distal edge of the radius followed by the scapholunate ligament. From this point, the scaphoid extends radially and the lunate ulnarly.

The wrist's fourth dorsal compartment contains the extensor digitorum communis, which can easily be felt over the midline of the wrist dorsally as the patient actively extends his or her fingers. Palpating 1 cm further in the ulnar direction reveals the extensor digiti minimi (quinti). This tendon, which acts as the sole extensor for the small finger, occupies the fifth dorsal compartment of the wrist and lies directly over the distal radioulnar joint.[5]

The head of the ulna is represented by a 1-cm protrusion on the ulnar aspect of the dorsal wrist. It is the most prominent landmark in this area, and it is easily visible on most people. Palpating along the head radially will reveal the indentation of the distal radioulnar joint. Palpating along the ulnar border, in turn, leads to the ulnar styloid. This protuberance anchors the TFCC, which connects the ulnar styloid to the distal radius. The TFCC may be directly palpated by starting at the ulnar head and moving distally until the examiner's fingertip falls into a small depression. Tenderness to palpation at this site strongly suggests a TFCC injury.[5]

The sixth and last dorsal compartment of the wrist houses the extensor carpi ulnaris, which travels through a groove on the ulnar side of the ulnar head before inserting at the base of the fifth

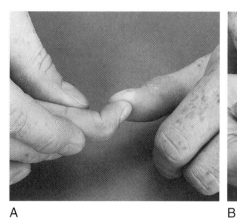
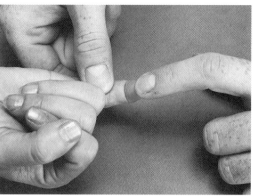

A   B

Figure 7.12 Assessing function of the flexor digitorum profundus. *A,* In the index finger. *B,* In the little finger. (From Reider B: The Orthopedic Physical Examination, 2nd ed. Philadelphia, WB Saunders, 2005, p 140.)

metacarpal. It is easily felt as the patient deviates the wrist ulnarly and extends against resistance. This tendon can subluxate if the restraining sheath tears. The examiner can reproduce this subluxation by taking the patient's wrist from pronation with slight extension into supination with slight flexion in one smooth motion.[5]

Moving distally from the TFCC, the examiner will feel another indentation that represents the lunotriquetral ligament. Just distal to this is the triquetrum itself, and this is followed by the hamate and finally the carpometacarpal joints, where the hamate articulates with the fourth and fifth metacarpals.[5]

Dorsal hand

For the palpation of the dorsal hand, the examiner should begin with the metacarpals. Each can be palpated from its base to its head for tenderness, crepitus, or swelling, which may indicate an underlying fracture. The phalanges should be palpated in much the same way. Particular attention should be paid to areas of obvious swelling, discoloration, or deformity.

At its head, each metacarpal articulates with a phalanx. Each of the MCP joints should be examined for collateral ligament injury by palpating both the radial and ulnar sides. Injury to the ulnar collateral ligament of the thumb is particularly common.[5] Pain over the joint dorsally may indicate an intra-articular fracture, osteoarthritis, or rheumatoid arthritis and should be differentiated from pain adjacent to the extensor tendon.[5] This tendon can be felt by having the patient hyperextend the MCPs. Pain in this area may signify injury to the restraining hood of the extensor mechanism, which could lead to the chronic subluxation of the tendon into the space between the metacarpal heads.

If one of the proximal interphalangeal joints is swollen, palpating carefully around the joint may reveal the area of greatest tenderness and thus, possibly injured structures. The most important structure dorsally is the insertion of the central slip of the extensor digitorum communis tendon at the base of the middle phalanx. Injury to

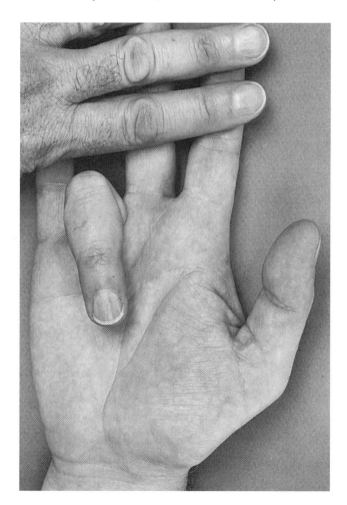

Figure 7.13 Assessing function of the flexor digitorum superficialis in the ring finger. (From Reider B: The Orthopedic Physical Examination, 2nd ed. Philadelphia, WB Saunders, 2005, p 140.)

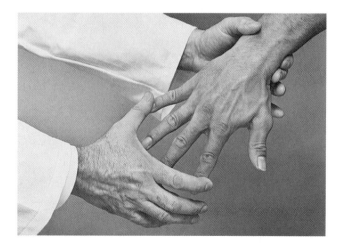

Figure 7.14 Assessing finger abduction strength. (From Reider B: The Orthopedic Physical Examination, 2nd ed. Philadelphia, WB Saunders, 2005, p 141.)

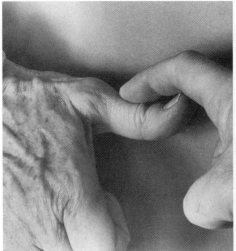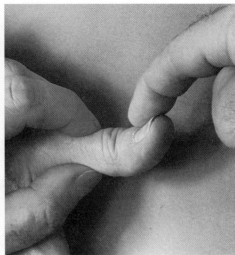

Figure 7.15 *A,* Assessing thumb extensor strength. *B,* Assessing extensor pollicis longus strength in isolation. (From Reider B: The Orthopedic Physical Examination, 2nd ed. Philadelphia, WB Saunders, 2005, p 143.)

A

B

this structure can lead to a boutonniere deformity without proper management.[5] Tenderness on the radial or ulnar aspects may indicate injury to the corresponding collateral ligament. Such a finding warrants the testing of collateral ligament integrity (described later). On the palmar aspect, the joint capsule thickens to form the volar plate. Pain at this site, as with any of the others, may indicate a periarticular fracture; radiographs are always warranted.[2]

The examiner may approach the distal interphalangeal joint in a similar fashion. At the base of distal phalanx, the extensor digitorum communis tendon (or the extensor pollicis longus tendon, in the case of the thumb) inserts dorsally. Pain at this site may indicate tendon injury or avulsion that can lead to a mallet-finger deformity.[5] The patient will be unable to extend the DIP against resistance. Pain over the radial or ulnar aspect of the joint is suspicious for injury to the corresponding collateral ligament. Pain located volarly raises the question of volar-plate injury.

Volar wrist

Similar to the dorsal wrist examination, this examination begins with the first dorsal compartment tendons, which form the volar border of the anatomic snuffbox. Immediately ulnar to these tendons, the examiner will feel the pulsations of the radial artery **(Figure 7.22)**. Moving distally just past the distal flexion crease of the wrist will locate the firm tubercle of the scaphoid. Continuing in a distal and slightly radial direction will lead the

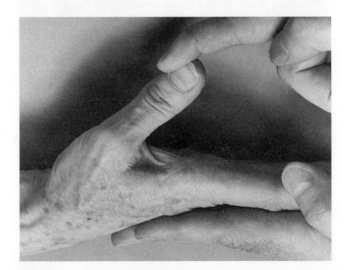

Figure 7.16 Assessing thumb flexion strength. (From Reider B: The Orthopedic Physical Examination, 2nd ed. Philadelphia, WB Saunders, 2005, p 143.)

Figure 7.17 Assessing the strength of the abductor pollicis brevis (palmar abduction) in isolation. (From Reider B: The Orthopedic Physical Examination, 2nd ed. Philadelphia, WB Saunders, 2005, p 143.)

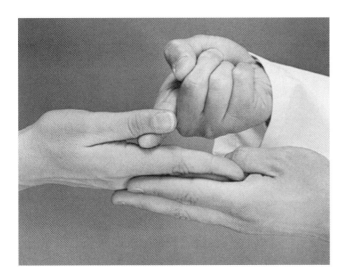

Figure 7.18 Assessing the strength of the adductor pollicis (palmar adduction). (From Reider B: The Orthopedic Physical Examination, 2nd ed. Philadelphia, WB Saunders, 2005, p 144.)

examiner to the trapezium and then to the basilar joint, which is the carpometacarpal joint of the thumb.

Returning to the radial artery and then palpating ulnarly will lead immediately to the flexor carpi radialis tendon, which inserts at the base of the second metacarpal. Continuing in an ulnar direction will next reveal the palmaris longus tendon, which is absent in 20% of the general population.[5] This tendon is most prominent when the wrist is slightly flexed and the tips of the thumb and little fingers are pinched **(Figure 7.23).**

Between the flexor carpi radialis and the palmaris longus is a depression overlying the median nerve. Percussion in this area may reproduce symptoms of median nerve compression in the carpal tunnel, which is known as *carpal tunnel syndrome.*[5] Immediately ulnar to the palmaris longus tendon are the flexor digitorum superficialis and profundus tendons. These cannot be seen in a patient with a palmaris longus, but they may be felt gliding under the examiner's fingers as the patient opens and closes his or her fist.[5]

Continuing in an ulnar direction, the examiner will come to the ulnar artery, which, unlike its radial counterpart, requires moderately firm palpation to feel. The artery lies just radial to the flexor carpi ulnaris tendon. This serves as a good landmark because the tendon is thick, and it becomes quite firm when the patient deviates the wrist ulnarly and flexes against resistance.[5] Following this tendon distally, the examiner will feel it insert onto the ovoid pisiform bone at the base of the hypothenar eminence.

From the pisiform, the examiner should palpate distally and toward the patient's index finger. Approximately 1 cm along this line, the examiner will find a small bony prominence that corresponds with the hook of the hamate bone **(Figure 7.24).** The fascial structure that the examiner has just traced is the pisohamate ligament, which forms the roof of the ulnar tunnel (Guyon's canal). This is a common site of ulnar nerve impingement.[5]

Volar hand

The palpation of the bones and joints for suspected pathology has been covered in the dorsal hand examination. As previously mentioned, particular attention should be paid to areas of obvious swelling, discoloration, or deformity.

The compartmental design of the volar hand makes it prone to closed-space infections.[5] Such infections will cause swelling, erythema, and pain that seem out of proportion to the examination.

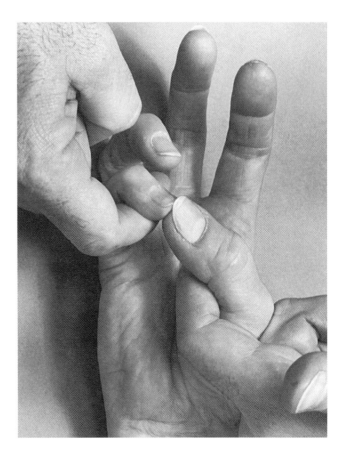

Figure 7.19 Assessing opposition strength. (From Reider B: The Orthopedic Physical Examination, 2nd ed. Philadelphia, WB Saunders, 2005, p 145.)

Palpation should be very gentle initially. See **Table 7.4** for possible closed-space infections. These diagnoses require urgent consultation with a surgeon for incision and drainage.

A common finding in the hand of middle-aged and older athletes is the nodular swelling associated with trigger finger. These nodules are usually felt at the transverse flexion crease of the palm or at the proximal flexion crease of the thumb.[5] The patient flexes the finger in question as the examiner palpates the associated A-1 pulley. The patient then extends the finger, which will cause a snap as the nodule slides through the A-1 pulley **(Figure 7.25).**

SPECIAL TESTS

Special tests of the wrist and hand can add valuable information to the physical examination. It is important to remember that, although a positive test may strongly suggest a particular diagnosis, a negative test does not rule one out.

Ligaments
Ligamentous instability test for the fingers[3]

The examiner stabilizes the finger to be tested proximal to the joint in question and then grasps the finger distally to apply a varus and valgus force while keeping the joint in 30 degrees of flexion. The results are compared with those of the unaffected hand. Generally, no laxity should be found. Pain alone indicates a grade 1 sprain of the corresponding collateral ligament. Pain with 20 to 30 degrees of laxity indicates a partial tear or a grade 2 sprain. Greater than 30 degrees of laxity indicates a grade 3 sprain, which is a complete tear.

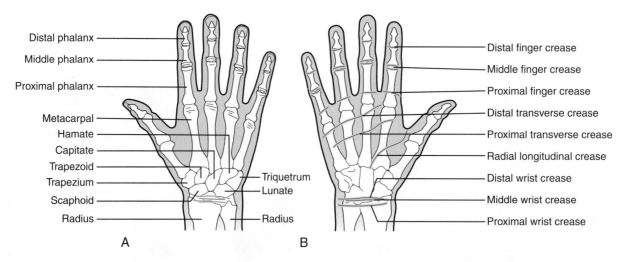

Distal phalanx
Middle phalanx
Proximal phalanx
Metacarpal
Hamate
Capitate
Trapezoid
Trapezium
Scaphoid
Radius

Triquetrum
Lunate
Radius

A

B

Distal finger crease
Middle finger crease
Proximal finger crease
Distal transverse crease
Proximal transverse crease
Radial longitudinal crease
Distal wrist crease
Middle wrist crease
Proximal wrist crease

Figure 7.20 Bony landmarks and skin creases of the wrist and hand. (From Tubiana: The hand. In Magee DJ [ed]: Orthopaedic Physical Assessment, 4th ed. St. Louis, Saunders Elsevier, 2006, p 411.)

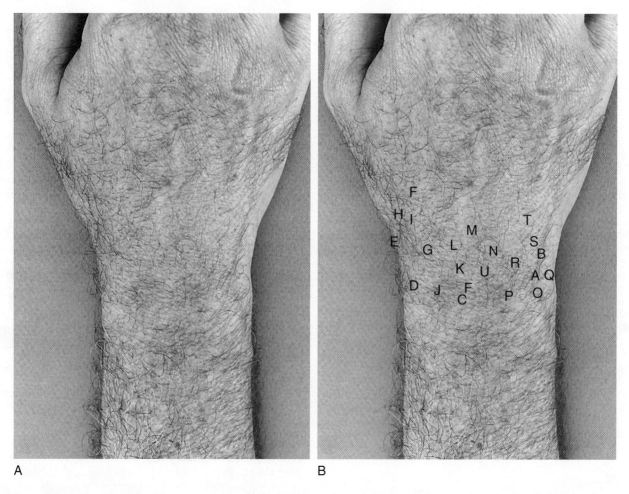

A

B

Figure 7.21 Dorsal view of the wrist. A, Triangular fibrocartilage complex. B, Extensor carpi ulnaris tendon. C, Lister's tubercle. D, Radial styloid. E, Abductor pollicis longus and extensor pollicis brevis tendons. F, Extensor pollicis longus. G, Scaphoid. H, Trapezium. I, Scaphotrapeziotrapezoid joint. J, Extensor radialis longus and brevis tendons. K, Scapholunate ligament. L, Scapholunate capitate joint. M, Head of the capitate. N, Extensor digitorum communis tendons. O, Ulnar head. P, Distal radioulnar joint. Q, Ulnar styloid. R, Lunotriquetral ligament. S, Triquetrum. T, Hamate. U, Lunate. (From Reider B: The Orthopedic Physical Examination, 2nd ed. Philadelphia, WB Saunders, 2005, p 107.)

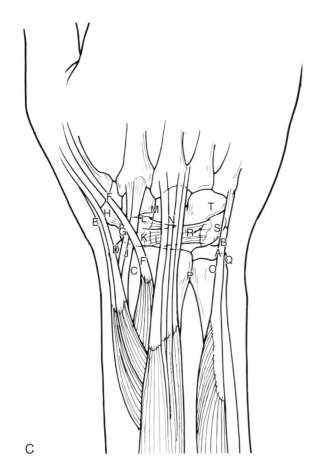

C

Figure 7.21 Continued.

Skier's thumb test[3,5]

The examiner takes the thumb into extension and then applies a valgus stress to the MCP joint, which will stress the ulnar collateral ligament and the accessory collateral ligament. Repeating the test with the MCP at 20 to 30 degrees of flexion will isolate the ulnar collateral ligament. Normal laxity of the ulnar collateral ligament is about 15 degrees. Laxity up to 35 degrees indicates a partial tear; more than 35 degrees of laxity represents a complete tear.

Finger extension (shuck) test[3]

The examiner holds the patient's wrist in flexion. With the fingers extended, the patient attempts to extend the wrist against resistance **(Figure 7.26).** Pain in the wrist indicates midcarpal instability, scaphoid instability, inflammation, or Kienbock's disease (osteonecrosis of the lunate).

Murphy's sign[3]

When making a fist, the head of the patient's third metacarpal will normally extend distally beyond that of the second and fourth metacarpals. If they are instead even, the sign is considered positive for lunate dislocation.

Capitate apprehension test[3]

The examiner stabilizes the patient's forearm and, with the other hand, holds the capitate **(Figure 7.27).** An anterior–posterior force is applied to the capitate. Apprehension, pain, or reproduction of symptoms indicates a positive test.

Piano keys test[3]

This will test the integrity of the distal radioulnar joint. The examiner stabilizes the distal radius and, with the other hand, attempts to displace the distal ulna dorsally and ventrally **(Figure 7.28).** Pain or laxity as compared with the opposite hand indicates a positive test. This test has been used to investigate the presence of TFCC injury. In patients with a complete peripheral TFCC tear, the piano keys test has a sensitivity of 59% and specificity of 96%[7] (LOE: B).

Supination lift test[3]

This test helps detect injury to the TFCC. The patient holds the forearm in full supination and applies an upward directed force against resistance **(Figure 7.29).** Pain over the ulnar aspect of the wrist or weakness with this test indicates a dorsal TFCC tear. Forced ulnar deviation may increase the patient's symptoms.

Axial load test[3]

While stabilizing the wrist, the examiner holds one of the digits and applies an axial load. Localized pain may indicate a fracture of the associated metacarpal or carpal bones. This test may also be positive with joint arthrosis.

Midcarpal pivot shift test[8]

This tests midcarpal instability. With the patient's forearm supinated, the examiner takes the wrist into full ulnar deviation and applies an axial load. The examiner then passively pronates the forearm. A painful click indicates a positive test.

Grind test[3]

This test is similar to the axial load test described previously. The examiner rotates the digit while applying axial compression. Localized pain indicates degenerative joint disease or other arthropathy. This test applies to any joint of the wrist or hand.

Linscheid test

There are two tests by this name that have been described in the literature. The first identifies lunotriquetral instability. The examiner applies a radially directed force over the ulnar border of the triquetrum. This compresses the lunotriquetral joint, and pain indicates lunotriquetral instability.[9] The other Linscheid test is for the instability of the second and third carpometacarpal joints. The examiner supports the metacarpal shafts with one hand and with the other applies a dorsally or palmarly directed force over the metacarpal heads. Localized pain over the carpometacarpal joints indicates a positive test for carpometacarpal instability[3,10,11] **(Figure 7.30).**

Muscles and tendons

The most common injury to a muscle or tendon is a strain. Resisting the activity of the injured structure will recreate the patient's pain, and direct palpation of the structure usually will as well. Because this is true with any muscle or tendon in the body, it is not considered a special test. The following tests are considered special in that they have gained acceptance for testing specific structures.

Table 7.4 Closed-Space Infections of the Hand

Location	Associated Infection
Volar fingertip	Felon
Volar finger	Infectious flexor tendonitis
Middle and distal palm	Midpalmar space infection
Thenar eminence	Thenar space infection

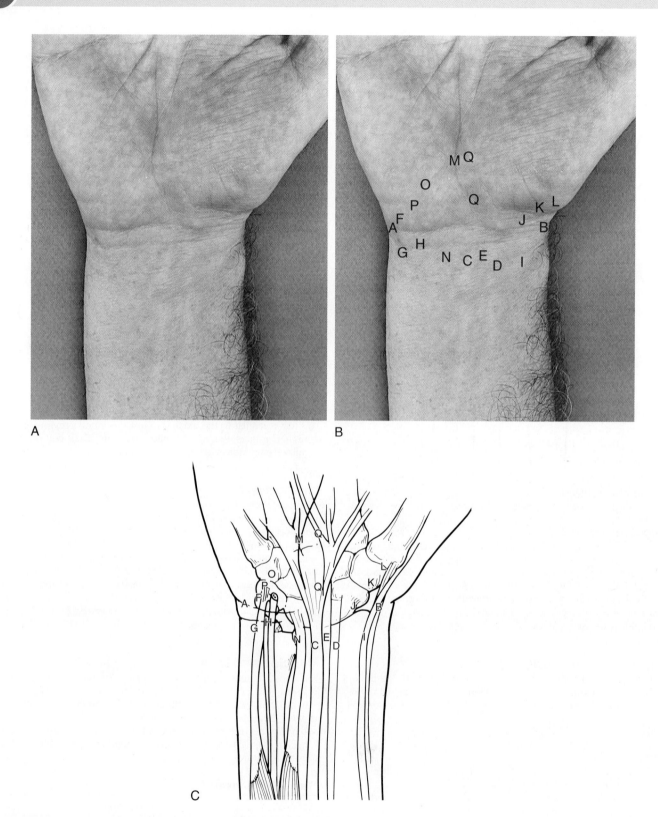

Figure 7.22 Palmar view of the wrist. *A*, Distal flexion crease. *B*, Abductor pollicis longus. *C*, Palmaris longus. *D*, Flexor carpi radialis. *E*, Median nerve. *F*, Pisiform. *G*, Flexor carpi ulnaris. *H*, Ulnar artery and nerve. *I*, Radial artery. *J*, Scaphoid tubercle. *K*, Trapezium. *L*, Basilar joint. *M*, Longitudinal interthenar crease. *N*, Flexor digitorum tendons. *O*, Hook of the hamate. *P*, Guyon's canal. *Q*, Proximal and distal margins of the transverse carpal ligament. (From Reider B: The Orthopedic Physical Examination, 2nd ed. Philadelphia, WB Saunders, 2005, p 115.)

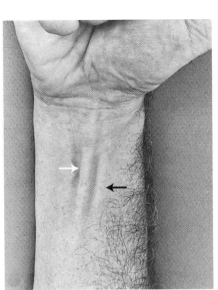

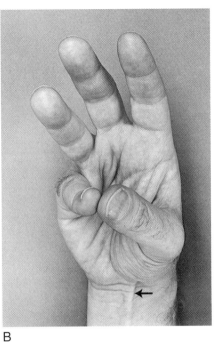

A

B

Figure 7.23 *A*, Prominence of the flexor carpi radialis *(solid arrow)* and the palmaris longus *(open arrow)* increased by active wrist flexion. *B*, Demonstration of the palmaris longus tendon by pinching. (From Reider B: The Orthopedic Physical Examination, 2nd ed. Philadelphia, WB Saunders, 2005, p 116.)

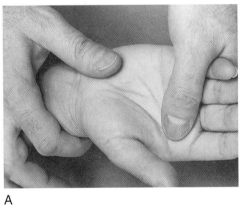

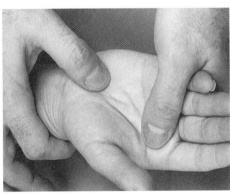

A

B

Figure 7.24 *A* and *B*, Palpation of the hook of the hamate. (From Reider B: The Orthopedic Physical Examination, 2nd ed. Philadelphia, WB Saunders, 2005, p 137.)

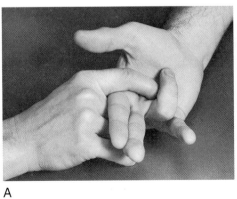

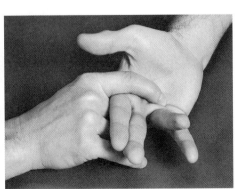

A

B

Figure 7.25 *A* and *B*, Palpation for trigger finger of the ring finger. (From Reider B: The Orthopedic Physical Examination, 2nd ed. Philadelphia, WB Saunders, 2005, p 136.)

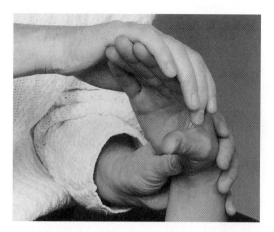

Figure 7.26 Finger extension (shuck) test. (From Magee DJ: Orthopaedic Physical Assessment, 4th ed. St. Louis, Saunders Elsevier, 2006, p 394.)

Finkelstein's test[3,12]

This test is used to detect de Quervain's or Hoffmann's disease, which is a paratenonitis of the thumb.[13] The patient makes a fist with the thumb inside the fingers **(Figure 7.31)**; the examiner then deviates the wrist ulnarly. Reproduction of the patient's symptoms (specifically pain over the extensor pollicis brevis and the abductor pollicis longus) is considered a positive test. Because this maneuver may cause pain in normal individuals, the affected thumb should be compared with the unaffected thumb.

Sweater finger sign[3]

The patient makes a fist, and the distal phalanges are observed lying in the palm. If one of the distal phalanges fails to flex, then the insertion of the flexor digitorum profundus tendon has failed either through rupture or avulsion **(Figure 7.32).** The ring finger is most often injured.

Extensor hood rupture

This test was first described by Elson.[14] The patient flexes the involved finger to 90 degrees at the PIP joint (classically over the edge of a table). As the examiner holds the middle phalanx in position, the patient extends the finger. An absence of extension force at the PIP joint coupled with fixed extension at the DIP joint comprises a positive test for central extensor hood rupture.

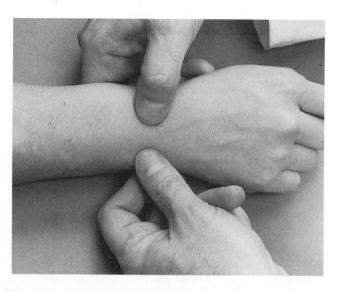

Figure 7.28 Piano keys test. (From Reider B: The Orthopedic Physical Examination, 2nd ed. Philadelphia, WB Saunders, 2005, p 153.)

Boyes' test[14,15]

This is another test for central extensor hood rupture. The PIP joint is held passively in extension, and the patient attempts to flex the DIP. An inability to flex the DIP indicates hood rupture. Unfortunately, this test only becomes positive when the extensor hood has retracted and adhered to surrounding structures. This is a late finding, and because these injuries benefit from early repair, the test by Elson that was previously described is considered superior.

Bunnel–Littler (Finochietto–Bunnell) test[3]

This test examines the structures surrounding the PIP joint, and it is also known as the intrinsic-plus test. The patient is passive during

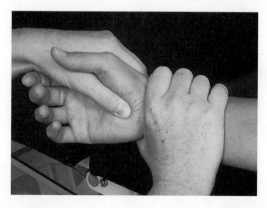

Figure 7.27 Capitate displacement test. The examiner's thumb is positioned over the capitate to displace it posteriorly. (From Magee DJ: Orthopaedic Physical Assessment, 4th ed. St. Louis, Saunders Elsevier, 2006, p 394.)

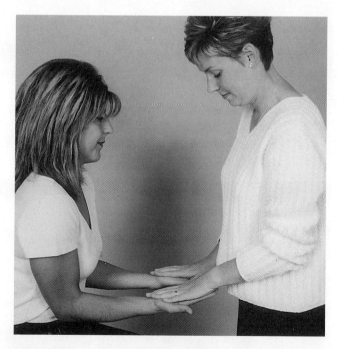

Figure 7.29 Supination lift test. (From Magee DJ: Orthopaedic Physical Assessment, 4th ed. St. Louis, Saunders Elsevier, 2006, p 395.)

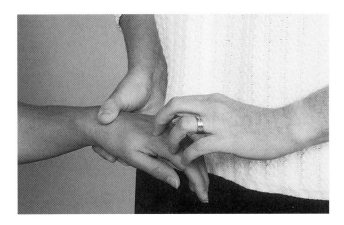

Figure 7.30 Linscheid test. (From Magee DJ: Orthopaedic Physical Assessment, 4th ed. St. Louis, Saunders Elsevier, 2006, p 395.)

this test. The examiner holds the MCP joint in extension and then attempts to flex the PIP joint. An inability to do this indicates either inflexible intrinsic muscles or a PIP joint capsule contracture. The test is then repeated with the MCP joint slightly flexed. Successful flexion implicates inflexible intrinsic muscles for the previous findings; continuing rigidity indicates joint capsule contracture.[16]

Froment's test[5]

This test evaluates the strength of a patient's key pinch, which is enacted by the adductor pollicis. To perform the test, the patient makes tight fists with both hands and places them against each other. The patient then uses the thumbs to hold an index card against the radial aspect of the index fingers. Normally the patient can resist the withdrawal of the card while keeping the PIP joints extended. If the adductor pollicis is weak, however, the patient will usually attempt to compensate by firing the flexor pollicis longus. This will result in flexion at the PIP on the affected hand, which is known as *Froment's sign.*

Subluxation of the extensor carpi ulnaris

The extensor carpi ulnaris tendon lies in the sixth dorsal compartment of the wrist. If the ulnar septum of this compartment is ruptured, the tendon will be free to subluxate in supination and then reduce in pronation. To complete the test, the patient may actively pronate and supinate the forearm while the examiner palpates the extensor carpi ulnaris at the wrist[1] (see Figure 7.21). Alternatively, the examiner may passively pronate and supinate the patient's forearm.[5] A painful snap is considered a positive test.

Intersection syndrome

This syndrome is characterized by pain over the dorsal wrist where the extensor pollicis brevis and the abductor pollicis longus cross the wrist extensors. It is an overuse syndrome that is common among athletes with repetitive stresses on the wrist (e.g., weightlifters, rowers, canoeists).[1] Clinical examination will reveal tenderness

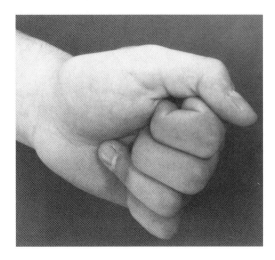

Figure 7.32 Sweater finger sign. Rupture of the flexor digitorum profundus tendon of the ring finger. (From Magee DJ: Orthopaedic Physical Assessment, 4th ed. St. Louis, Saunders Elsevier, 2006, p 396.)

to palpation over the dorsoradial wrist located 6 cm proximal to Lister's tubercle.[17] The test is positive if palpation reveals crepitus with or without an audible squeak.[1]

Nerves and reflexes
Median nerve entrapment

The following tests are for carpal tunnel syndrome, which is characterized by pain or paresthesias in the distribution of the median nerve (see Figure 7.9). This is the most common nerve entrapment in the hand.[5] Techniques for performing the tests have been compiled from various authors who have used the tests in clinical trials; otherwise, they have been compiled from expert opinion.

Phalen's test[3,5,18-33] For this test, the patient holds the wrist in 90 degrees flexion for 60 seconds. The dorsal aspects of the hands may be apposed or the hand hung over a table edge. The test is positive if the patient's symptoms are reproduced **(Figure 7.33A)**. In clinical trials, sensitivity ranges from 34% to 88% and specificity ranges from 40% to 100% (LOE: B).

Reverse Phalen's test[3,5] This test is similar to Phalen's test except that the wrists are held in 90 degrees extension for 60 seconds. The palmar aspects of the hands may be apposed (see Figure 7.33B). The test is positive if the patient's symptoms are reproduced.

Tinel's test[3,5,18-20,22-33] Tinel's test is performed with the patient's elbow flexed comfortably and the forearm supinated. The wrist is in a neutral position. The examiner taps with the index and middle fingers or a reflex hammer over the median nerve at the wrist and repeats this four to six times **(Figure 7.34).**

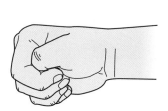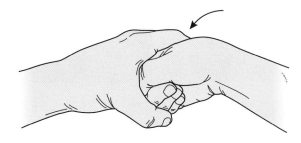

Figure 7.31 Finkelstein test. (From Magee DJ: Orthopaedic Physical Assessment, 4th ed. St. Louis, Saunders Elsevier, 2006, p 396.)

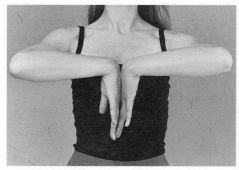
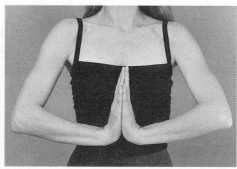

Figure 7.33 *A*, Phalen's test. *B*, Reverse Phalen's test. (From Reider B: The Orthopedic Physical Examination, 2nd ed. Philadelphia, WB Saunders, 2005, p 148.)

A

B

The test is positive if the patient reports pain or paresthesias in the distribution of the median nerve (see Figure 7.9). In clinical trials, Tinel's sign has a sensitivity of between 23% and 74%; specificity ranges from 77% to 100% (LOE: B). Tinel's test can also be used over other common sites of nerve entrapment to reproduce a patient's symptoms **(Figure 7.35).**

Carpal compression test[18,20,21,24,28-32]
To perform this test, the patient sits with the elbow flexed comfortably and the forearm pronated. The examiner applies pressure over the median nerve just distal to the distal flexion crease (see Figure 7.22). Most of the studies examining this test have used 30 seconds of compression, although some have used 5 seconds[28] and some have used 60 seconds.[29] The test is considered positive for carpal tunnel syndrome if pain, paresthesias, or numbness is reproduced in the median nerve distribution (see Figure 7.9). According to clinical trials, the carpal compression test has a sensitivity of between 28% and 89% and a specificity of between 30% and 95% (LOE: B).

Ulnar nerve entrapment
Ulnar nerve compression test[5] Compression of the ulnar nerve is the (distant) second most common nerve entrapment after carpal tunnel syndrome. The site of entrapment is usually Guyon's canal, which is formed by the pisohamate ligament that connects the pisiform with the hook of the hamate. To perform the test, the examiner compresses the ulnar nerve just radial to the pisiform bone on the volar aspect of the wrist **(Figure 7.36);** compression is held for 60 seconds. The test is positive if it produces pain or paresthesias in the distribution of the ulnar nerve (see Figure 7.9). This condition is common in cyclists and has been referred to as "handlebar palsy."[22]

Upper motor neuron lesion
Hoffman's sign This test will indicate the presence of an upper motor neuron lesion; it is considered the upper extremity equivalent of the Babinski's test.[3] The examiner holds the patient's middle finger and flicks the distal phalanx briskly. The test is positive if the thumb IP joint on the same hand flexes. Because upper motor neuron lesions will affect the upper and lower extremities, a positive test should prompt the examiner to also check for Babinski's sign and clonus in the feet.

Bones
Scaphoid fractures
Scaphoid fracture test[18] For this test, the examiner deviates the patient's wrist ulnarly while the forearm is pronated. Pain in the anatomic snuffbox indicates a positive test. One clinical trial showed a sensitivity of 100% and a specificity of 34%[34] (LOE: B).

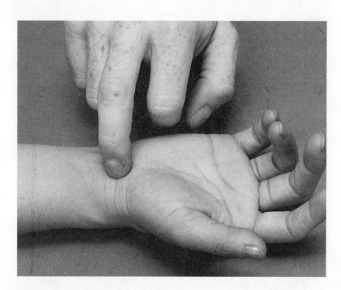

Figure 7.34 Tinel's test over the median nerve. (From Reider B: The Orthopedic Physical Examination, 2nd ed. Philadelphia, WB Saunders, 2005, p 147.)

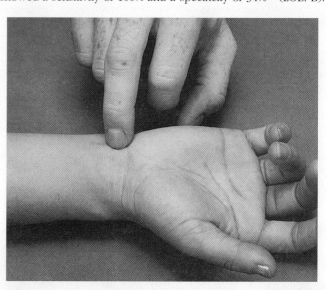

Figure 7.35 Tinel's test over the ulnar nerve at the wrist. (From Reider B: The Orthopedic Physical Examination, 2nd ed. Philadelphia, WB Saunders, 2005, p 148.)

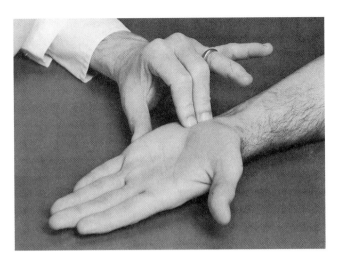

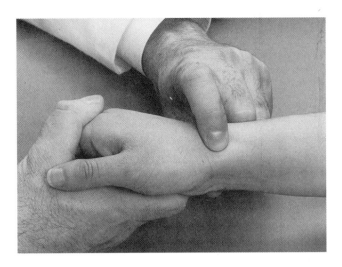

Figure 7.36 Ulnar nerve compression test at the wrist. (From Reider B: The Orthopedic Physical Examination, 2nd ed. Philadelphia, WB Saunders, 2005, p 148.)

Figure 7.37 Palpation of the scaphoid. (From Reider B: The Orthopedic Physical Examination, 2nd ed. Philadelphia, WB Saunders, 2005.)

Anatomic snuffbox tenderness The examiner exerts pressure over the anatomic snuffbox **(Figure 7.37).** The test is positive if pain is elicited in the radial wrist. Clinical trials showed a sensitivity of 100% and specificity of 29% to 98%.[35,36] Specificity improves markedly when the patient has a mechanism of injury that is suggestive of scaphoid fracture[18] (LOE: B).

Scaphoid tubercle tenderness The examiner applies pressure over the patient's scaphoid tubercle. The test is positive if pain is elicited. One clinical trial showed sensitivity of 83% and a specificity of 51%[18,35] (LOE: B).

Scaphoid compression test (axial load test) The examiner holds the patient's thumb and applies axial pressure through the first metacarpal and onto the scaphoid. The test is positive if pain is elicited in the radial wrist. Clinical trials showed a sensitivity of 100% and a specificity of 80% to 98%.[35,36] Again, specificity improves when the patient has a mechanism of injury that is suggestive of scaphoid fracture[18] (LOE: B). This test can also be performed on other digits to detect fractures of the metacarpals or associated carpal bones.

Resisted supination test The examiner holds the patient's hand in a handshake position. The patient supinates the forearm while the examiner resists. The test is positive if pain is elicited in the radial wrist. One clinic trial found this test to have a sensitivity of 100% and a specificity of 98% for patients with a mechanism that was suggestive of scaphoid fracture[18,36] (LOE: B).

Carpal instability

Watson test (scaphoid shift test)[3,17,18,37-39] The examiner holds the patient's wrist in full ulnar deviation and slight extension; the distal pole of the scaphoid is stabilized with the other hand **(Figure 7.38).** The examiner takes the wrist passively into radial deviation and slight flexion. An unstable scaphoid will sublux over the dorsal rim of the radius, causing pain and a characteristic "clunk" with relocation. The test is also considered positive for scaphoid instability if there is significant pain with the maneuver or if the patient's symptoms are reproduced. Clinical trials have shown the sensitivity of Watson's test to be from 64% to 69%; specificity ranges from 44% to 66% (LOE: B).

Lunotriquetral ballottement (Reagan's) test[1,3,18] The examiner stabilizes the patient's lunate bone with the thumb and index finger of one hand. The other hand mobilizes the pisotriquetral complex in a palmar direction that is followed by a dorsal direction **(Figure 7.39).** The test is positive for lunotriquetral instability if the patient's symptoms are reproduced or if excessive laxity is noted. One clinical trial showed this test to have a sensitivity of 64% and a specificity of 44%[40] (LOE: B).

Lunotriquetral shear test[3] This test will also determine the integrity of the lunotriquetral ligament. The examiner stabilizes the patient's wrist by placing his or her thumb in the patient's palm and his or her fingers over the lunate dorsally **(Figure 7.40).** An anterior–posterior directed force applied to the pisotriquetral joint will place a shearing force on the lunotriquetral joint. Pain, laxity, or crepitus indicates a positive test.

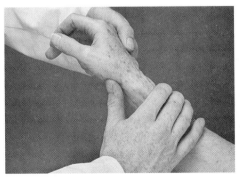

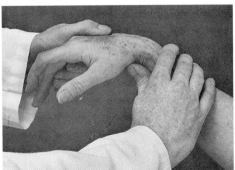

A

B

Figure 7.38 *A* and *B,* Scaphoid shift test. (From Reider B: The Orthopedic Physical Examination, 2nd ed. Philadelphia, WB Saunders, 2005, p 152.)

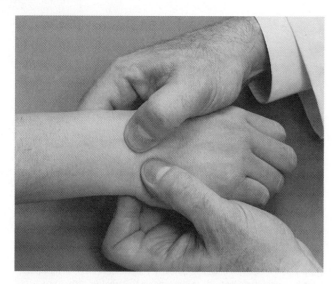

Figure 7.39 Lunotriquetral ballottement (Reagan's) test. (From Reider B: The Orthopedic Physical Examination, 2nd ed. Philadelphia, WB Saunders, 2005, p 152.)

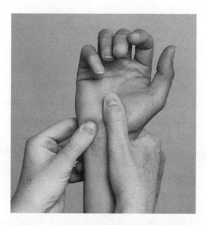

Figure 7.40 Lunotriquetral shear test. (From Magee DJ: Orthopaedic Physical Assessment, 4th ed. St. Louis, Saunders Elsevier, 2006, p 393.)

Ulnomeniscotriquetral dorsal glide[18,40] The patient is seated with the forearm resting on a table in a pronated position. The examiner places his or her thumb over the head of the ulna, and the index finger of the same hand then presses up on the pisotriquetral complex volarly. The examiner's thumb and finger are squeezed together. If this reproduces the patient's pain or if significant laxity is noted, then the test is positive for ulnomeniscotriquetral complex instability. The sensitivity of the test is 66%, and the specificity is 64% (LOE: B).

REFERENCES

1. DeLee JC, Drez D, Miller MD: DeLee and Drez's Orthopaedic Sports Medicine, 2nd ed. Philadelphia, Saunders Elsevier, 2003.
2. Lillegard WA, Butcher JD, Rucker KS: Handbook of Sports Medicine: A Symptom-Oriented Approach, 2nd ed. Boston, Butterworth-Heinemann, 1999.
3. Magee DJ: Orthopaedic Physical Assessment, 4th ed. St. Louis, Saunders Elsevier, 2006.
4. Jenkins DB: Hollinshead's Functional Anatomy of the Limbs and Back, 7th ed. Philadelphia, WB Saunders, 1998.
5. Reider B: The Orthopedic Physical Examination, 2nd ed. Philadelphia, WB Saunders, 2005.
6. Anderson BC: Evaluation of the patient with hand pain, UpToDate (online database): www.uptodate.com. Accessed September 24, 2006.
7. Lindau T, Adlercreutz C, Aspenberg P: Peripheral tears of the triangular fibrocartilage complex cause distal radioulnar joint instability after distal radial fractures. J Hand Surg 2000;25:(3):464-468.
8. Lichtman DM, Schneider JR, Swofford AR, et al: Ulnar midcarpal instability: clinical and laboratory analysis. J Hand Surg 1981;6:515-523.
9. Berdia S, Shin AY. Carpal ligament instability, eMedicine (online database): www.emedicine.com/orthoped/topic380.htm. Accessed October 5, 2006.
10. Beckenbaugh RD: Accurate evaluation and management of the painful wrist following injury. Orthop Clin North Am 1984;15:289-306.
11. Skervin T: Clinical examination of the wrist. J Hand Surg 1996;9:96-107.
12. Finkelstein H: Stenosing tendovaginitis at the radial styloid process. J Bone Joint Surg 1930;12:509-540.
13. Johnstone AJ: Tennis elbow and upper limb tendinopathies. Sports Med Arthro Rev 2000;8:69-79.
14. Elson RA: Rupture of the central slip of the extensor hood of the finger: a test for early diagnosis. J Bone Joint Surg Br 1986;68:229-231.
15. Boyes J: Bunnell's Surgery of the Hand. Philadelphia, JB Lippincott, 1970.
16. Hoppenfeld S: Physical Examination of the Spine and Extremities. New York, Appleton-Century-Crofts, 1976.
17. Dobyns JH, Sim FH, Linscheid RL: Sports stress syndromes of the hand and wrist. Am J Sports Med 1978;6:236-254.
18. Cleland J: Orthopaedic Clinical Examination: An Evidence-Based Approach for Physical Therapists. Carlstadt, Icon Learning Systems, 2005.
19. Ahn DS: Hand elevation: a new test for carpal tunnel syndrome. Ann Plast Surg 2001;46:120-124.
20. Durkan JA: A new diagnostic test for carpal tunnel syndrome. J Bone Joint Surg Am 1991;73:535-538.
21. Fertl E, Wober C, Zeitlhofer J: The serial use of two provocative tests in the clinical diagnosis of carpal tunnel syndrome. Acta Neurol Scand 1998;98:328-332.
22. Gellman H, Gelberman RH, Tan AM, et al: Carpal tunnel syndrome: An evaluation of the provocative diagnostic tests. J Bone Joint Surg Am 1986;68:735-737.
23. Gonzalez del Pino J, Delgado-Martinez AD, Gonzalez I, et al: Value of the carpal compression test in the diagnosis of carpal tunnel syndrome. J Hand Surg Br 1997;22:38-41.
24. Gunnarsson LG, Amilon A, Hellstrand P, et al: The diagnosis of carpal tunnel syndrome: Sensitivity and specificity of some clinical and electrophysiological tests. J Hand Surg Br 1997;22:34-37.
25. Hansen PA, Micklesen P, Robinson LR: Clinical utility of the flick maneuver in diagnosing carpal tunnel syndrome. Am J Phys Med Rehabil 2004;83:363-367.
26. Heller L, Ring H, Costeff PH: Evaluation of Tinel's and Phalen's sign in diagnosis of the carpal tunnel syndrome. Eur Neurol 1986;25:40-42.
27. Katz J, Larson M, Sabra A, et al: The carpal tunnel syndrome: diagnostic utility of the history and physical examination findings. Ann Intern Med 1990;112:321-327.
28. Kuhlman KA, Hennessey WJ: Sensitivity and specificity of carpal tunnel syndrome signs. Am J Phys Med Rehabil 1997;76:451-457.
29. Mondelli M, Passero S, Gianinni F: Provocative tests in different stages of carpal tunnel syndrome. Clin Neurol Neurosurg 2001;103:178-183.
30. Szabo RM, Slater RR Jr, Farver TB, et al: The value of diagnostic testing in carpal tunnel syndrome. J Hand Surg Am 1999;24:704-714.
31. Tetro AM, Evanoff BA, Hollstien SB, et al: A new provocative test for carpal tunnel syndrome: Assessment of wrist flexion and nerve compression. J Bone Joint Surg Br 1998;80:493-498.
32. Wainner RS, Fritz JM, Irgang JJ, et al: Development of a clinical prediction rule for the diagnosis of carpal tunnel syndrome. Arch Phys Med Rehabil 2005;86:609-618.
33. Williams TM, Mackinnon SE, Novak CB, et al: Verification of the pressure provocative test in carpal tunnel syndrome. Ann Plast Surg 1992;29:8-11.
34. Powell JM, Lloyd GJ, Rintoul RF: New clinical test for fracture of the scaphoid. Can J Surg 1988;31:237-238.
35. Grover R: Clinical assessment of scaphoid injuries and the detection of fractures. J Hand Surg Br 1996;21:341-343.
36. Waeckerle JF: A prospective study identifying the sensitivity of radiographic findings and the efficacy of clinical findings in carpal navicular fractures. Ann Emerg Med 1987;16:733-737.
37. Burton RI, Eaton RG: Common hand injuries in the athlete. Orthop Clin North Am 1975;4:309-338.
38. Taliesnik J: Carpal instability. J Bone Joint Surg Am 1988;70:1262-1268.
39. Watson HK, Ashmead D, Makhlouf MV: Examination of the scaphoid. J Hand Surg Am 1988;13:657-660.
40. LaStayo P, Howell J: Clinical provocative tests used in evaluating wrist pain: a descriptive study. J Hand Ther 1995;8:10-17.

CHAPTER 8

Physical Examination of the Elbow

Thomas M. Howard, MD; Joel L. Shaw, MD; and James Phillips, MD

KEY POINTS

- Because the muscles that originate in the elbow act in wrist motion, when evaluating elbow injuries, it is essential to also test wrist strength and range of motion.
- Lateral epicondylitis is diagnosed by examining wrist extensors, whereas medial epicondylitis is diagnosed by examining wrist flexors.
- Tinel's sign, the elbow flexion test, Wartenberg's sign, and Froment's sign are useful for the diagnosis of an ulnar nerve injury.
- The pronator teres syndrome test and the pinch grip test are useful for the diagnosis of a median nerve injury.
- The posterolateral rotatory instability test is used to identify the most common type of elbow instability.

INTRODUCTION

The increasing involvement in organized sports has resulted in an increase in sports-related injuries, including elbow injuries. Because of its location as the axis of the central joint of the upper extremity, the elbow is prone to both traumatic and overuse injuries.

Multiple types of elbow injuries occur in athletes, most often as a result of chronic repetitive forces, elbow overload, poor technique, or improper equipment. About 20% of overuse injuries in the young athlete involve the elbow.[1] In one study of young baseball pitchers over a 1-year period, the incidence of elbow injuries requiring treatment was 40%.[2] Bony and ligamentous injuries also occur in the elbow, usually in accordance with overuse, but these can be caused by direct trauma. This chapter will focus on the examination of the elbow and on differentiating among the possible injuries of this joint.

ANATOMY

The elbow joint is formed by three articulations that provide static and functional stability to allow for flexion, extension, supination, and pronation. Normal elbow motion is from approximately 0 to 135 degrees of flexion and about 90 degrees of pronation and supination.[3]

The bony anatomy includes the two condyles of the humerus, the trochlea and the capitellum, which articulate with the proximal ends of the radius and ulna. The trochlea (or medial condyle) is grooved, and it articulates with the semilunar notch of the ulna to form the humeroulnar joint. This articulation forms a modified hinge that allows for flexion, extension, and stability. The capitellum (or spherical-shaped lateral condyle) articulates with the radial head to form a combination hinge-and-pivot joint called the *humeroradial joint.* This joint allows for flexion, extension, and axial rotation. Finally, the radial head articulates with the lesser sigmoid notch of the ulna to form the radioulnar joint, which also provides axial rotation.[4]

As a result of the relative instability of the osseous articulations at the elbow, the ligaments are required to provide about 50% of elbow stability. The medial collateral ligament complex, which is the stronger of the collateral ligaments, is formed by anterior, posterior, and transverse ligaments. The anterior ligament provides about 70% of valgus stability and remains tight throughout the entire range of elbow flexion, thus providing the majority of this ligament's stability.[5,6] The posterior ligament only becomes tight past 90 degrees of flexion, thus providing minimal stability; the transverse ligament does not appear to provide any stability.

The lateral collateral ligament complex provides both rotational and varus elbow stability. This complex originates at the lateral epicondyle and inserts along the annular ligament. There are four ligaments that form this complex. The annular ligament, which surrounds the head of the radius, stabilizes it in the radial notch. The radial collateral ligament provides the majority of varus stability, remaining tight throughout flexion and extension; the lateral ulnar collateral ligament provides inferior rotatory stability. The accessory lateral collateral ligament assists the annular ligament with stabilizing the radial head during varus stress.[7]

There are four major muscle activities that are controlled by separate muscle groups that pass through the elbow joint. Flexion is performed by the biceps brachii, brachioradialis, and brachialis muscles. Extension is controlled by the triceps and anconeus muscles. Supination is controlled by the supinator and biceps brachii muscles. Pronation involves the pronator quadratus, pronator teres, and flexor carpi radialis muscles. Additionally, the flexor pronator muscles of the wrist originate from the medial epicondyle, and the wrist extensors originate from the lateral epicondyle.[8]

HISTORY

The first step is to determine from the patient whether the injury occurred traumatically or gradually over time. An understanding of the recreational and occupational activities of the patient may help determine the mode of the patient's elbow injury. Characteristics of the patient's pain, including timing, duration, intensity, location, character, frequency, and eliciting or relieving factors will help direct the diagnosis. The relationship of the pain to activity will help determine the severity of the injury. Finally, the physician needs to look for loss of function or symptoms that are suggestive of nerve damage or compression.

PHYSICAL EXAMINATION

After the differential diagnosis **(Table 8.1)** is narrowed down by the history, the definitive diagnosis is often determined by the physical examination. The initial examination involves the inspection of the elbow to look for bruising, atrophy, or swelling. Next, the patient should attempt to move through the range of motion to determine any loss in muscle function.

The palpation of several areas is essential. Posterior palpation should include the olecranon, the olecranon bursa, and the triceps. The palpation of both the medial and lateral epicondyle may suggest fracture, apophysitis, or epicondylitis. When testing for inflammation or injury of the extensor tendons of the wrist (especially the extensor carpi radialis tendon in cases of tennis elbow), resisted extension of the wrist will elicit pain at the lateral epicondyle.

Similarly, resisted flexion of the wrist will elicit discomfort at the medial epicondyle in patients with inflammation of the flexor tendons of the wrist.

Examination for the ligamentous stability of the medial and lateral collateral ligaments should be performed. Valgus stress applied to the elbow in both full extension and in several positions of flexion will determine the stability of the medial collateral ligament. Varus stress applied to the elbow will determine any damage to the lateral collateral ligament. Lastly, a neurovascular examination should be performed. This type of examination will be described in further detail throughout the rest of this chapter.

Range of motion

The elbow joint benefits from a wide range of motion. A limited range of motion would prevent important activities of daily living and, obviously, athletic activity. The range of motion in the elbow involves the following movements: elbow flexion, elbow extension, forearm supination, and forearm pronation. Flexion and extension are mainly produced at the humeroulnar and humeroradial joints. The radioulnar articulations proximally and distally are involved in supination and pronation. Range-of-motion testing can be accomplished with the patient either standing or sitting, and it should initially be tested actively.

Flexion

The patient should be asked to flex his or her elbow in an attempt to touch the hand to the shoulder. During this testing, the elbow should remain directly at the patient's side. Adequate range of motion should result in the patient being able to touch his or her anterior shoulder, and it can be measured to at least 135 degrees. This motion may be limited by anterior muscle mass.

Extension

The triceps, as will be discussed more in the strength section, controls extension. Extension is usually limited by the contact of the olecranon against the olecranon fossa. The patient should be instructed to straighten his or her elbow as far as possible, keeping the elbow directly at the side again. In most cases, a male will be able to extend to 0 degrees, although this may be limited by a tight biceps tendon. Most females will at least make it to 0 degrees, and they may even have 5 degrees of recurvatum.

Flexion and extension can be tested in a continuous motion. The left and right sides should be tested at the same time to determine any asymmetry.

Supination

The amount of supination is affected by the ability of the radius to rotate around the ulna and by any limitations at either the distal (wrist) or proximal (elbow) articulations.

Have the patient flex the elbow to 90 degrees and hold the elbow directly against the side. Start with the hand facing palm down in front of the patient. Next, have the patient attempt to rotate the forearm and palm up, remembering to keep the elbow against the side. Most patients should be able to rotate the forearm until the palm is facing up. Keeping the elbow against the patient's side prevents the patient from using shoulder adduction and flexion to assist with supination.

Pronation

Just like supination, pronation can be limited by abnormalities either proximally or distally that prevent the smooth rotation of the radius around the ulna. The patient will have his or her arm in the same position to test both pronation and supination.

Table 8.1   Differential Diagnosis of Elbow Injuries by Anatomic Area

Traumatic Injuries		
Medial	*Lateral*	*Posterior*
Medial epicondylar fracture	Lateral epicondylar fracture	Elbow dislocation
Supracondylar fracture	Capitellum fracture	Olecranon fracture
	Radial head fracture	
	Radial head subluxation	

Overuse Injuries			
Medial	*Lateral*	*Posterior*	*Anterior*
Medial epicondylitis	Lateral epicondylitis	Olecranon bursitis	Forearm splints
Ulnar collateral ligament sprain	Radial tunnel syndrome	Olecranon impingement	Median nerve compression syndrome
Osteochondritis dissecans	Posterior interosseous nerve syndrome	Triceps tendinitis	Pronator syndrome
Ulnar nerve entrapment			Biceps tendinitis

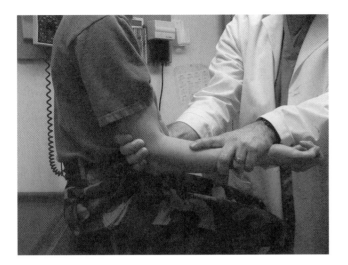

Figure 8.1 Elbow strength testing: flexion.

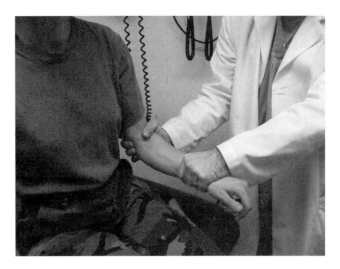

Figure 8.3 Elbow strength testing: supination.

Pronation involves starting in a position of full supination (palm facing up) and rotating to full pronation (palm facing down to the ground). Again, the patient must keep the elbow directly at the side and at 90 degrees of flexion to prevent any assistance from shoulder motion. Any asymmetry between the sides represents a pathologic limitation in motion.

As in flexion–extension, supination and pronation represent a common arc of motion. For this reason, they should be tested as a single, continuous test. Both arms should again be tested simultaneously to note any asymmetry in motion.

If a patient is unable to perform any motions with active testing, then the provider should proceed to passive motion testing. For the passive testing of flexion–extension, have the patient again hold his or her elbow at 90 degrees directly against his or her side. At this point, the provider should cup the olecranon in his or her hand and hold the elbow directly against the patient's side. With the other hand holding the arm just above the wrist, the provider will attempt to move the elbow through a normal range of motion in flexion and extension. The physician will be feeling for any limitation of motion related to an anatomic block or splinting related to pain. After determining the passive range of motion, the provider will have the patient attempt an active range

of motion again to compare passive and active limitations in motion.

For the passive testing of supination and pronation, the arm should be held in the same stable starting position. This time, stability will be provided by the physician holding the patient's hand as if shaking hands. The physician should use a firm enough grip to control the motion of the forearm. Slowly supinate and pronate the forearm to determine any limitation of motion and to measure the full range of motion. Feel for a sudden firm block or a slow stretch. This should again be compared with the patient's active range of motion.

Strength testing

The most common way to test the elbow musculature is through isometric and resisted motion. Studies have shown that flexion is most powerful between 90 and 110 degrees of flexion and with the forearm in a position of supination. Flexion power decreases to 75% at 45 and 135 degrees of flexion.[9] Other studies have shown that, in general, with isometric testing, men are twice as strong as women at the elbow joint, extension is 60% as strong as flexion, and pronation is 85% as strong as supination.[10] The movements that should be tested include elbow flexion, extension, supination, and pronation and wrist flexion and extension. For resisted isometric testing, the patient should be seated, with the provider standing in front of the patient.

For elbow strength testing, the provider should use one hand to stabilize the patient's elbow at the side by cupping the olecranon. For each motion, while the provider is pushing in one direction, the patient will push in the opposite direction. For example, to test flexion, the provider will attempt to move the elbow into extension while the patient resists by attempting to flex the elbow. This procedure will be used to test flexion, extension, supination, and pronation, as seen in **Figures 8.1 through 8.4**.

While examining the elbow, the provider should also test wrist flexion and extension because the muscles that control these motions originate from the elbow joint and act over both the elbow and the wrist. To test wrist strength, the provider should stabilize the forearm with one hand. The forearm should be positioned in pronation during the strength testing of the wrist. With the other hand, the provider will resist extension or flexion of the wrist, depending on the motion being tested **(Figures 8.5 and 8.6).**

Weakness on muscle testing of the elbow can indicate multiple potential injuries. If the patient has weakness with pain, the most likely diagnoses include tendinosis, a muscle tear, or a traumatic

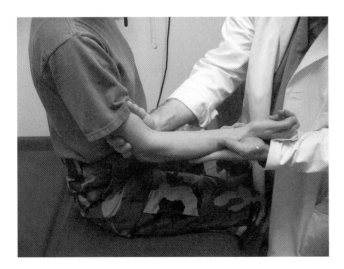

Figure 8.2 Elbow strength testing: extension.

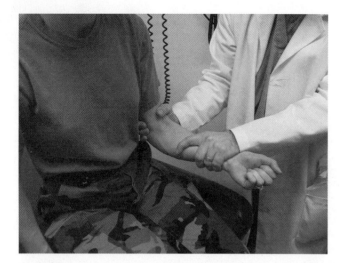

Figure 8.4 Elbow strength testing: pronation.

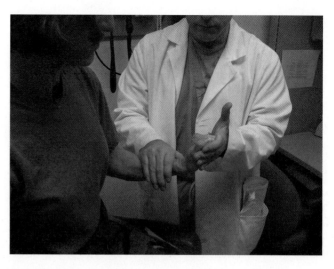

Figure 8.6 Elbow strength testing: wrist flexion.

injury such as a fracture. If the patient has weakness without pain, possible injuries include a severe strain of the muscle tissue or a neurologic injury. The distribution of muscle weakness and subsequent sensory testing can differentiate the location of neurologic injury (see Table 8.1). Sensation around the elbow and forearm is distributed anatomically as follows[3]:

C5: Lateral arm as a result of the axillary nerve
C6: Lateral forearm as a result of the musculocutaneous nerve
C8: Medial forearm as a result of the antebrachial cutaneous nerve
T1: Medial arm as a result of the brachial cutaneous nerve.

Along with strength testing, the provider should test associated reflexes at or involving the elbow. The common reflexes tested around the elbow include the biceps (C5-C6), the brachioradialis (C5-C6), and the triceps (C7-C8). This examination should be done in accordance with sensory testing, including the dermatomes and the cutaneous distribution around the elbow.

Palpation

Palpation should be accomplished with the patient as relaxed as possible, whether seated or in the supine position. This examination

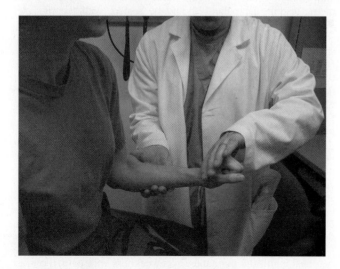

Figure 8.5 Elbow strength testing: wrist extension.

can start at the anterior aspect but should include all areas of the elbow, as discussed later.

Anterior aspect

The cubital fossa is the first area palpated anteriorly. Its boundaries include the pronator teres muscle medially, the brachioradialis muscle laterally, and a line superiorly connecting each epicondyle. Palpable structures within this fossa include the biceps tendon and the brachial artery. The brachial artery is significant as a result of the risk of injury with traumatic injuries such as fractures or dislocations. Injury to this artery can lead to compartment syndrome or Volkmann's ischemic contracture. Although they are not palpable, the median and musculocutaneous nerves also pass through this fossa. It is also possible to palpate the coronoid process of the ulna and the head of the radius through this fossa. Finally, the biceps and brachialis muscles may be palpated for abnormalities.

Medial aspect

The first and most obvious structure to palpate medially is the medial epicondyle. This structure is where the wrist flexor and forearm pronator muscles originate. The muscle bellies and their origins at the epicondyle should be palpated. Tenderness here suggests the presence of medial epicondylitis or golfer's elbow. The medial (ulnar) collateral ligament may be palpated as it originates from the medial epicondyle and extends to both the coronoid process (medial margin) and the olecranon process.

Posterior to the medial epicondyle, the provider will palpate the cubital tunnel, within which the ulnar nerve passes. Palpation here may cause a sensation that is consistent with compression of the ulnar nerve.

Lateral aspect

The first structure to palpate laterally is the lateral epicondyle. This provides the origin of the wrist extensor muscles. The provider again should palpate the muscle bellies along with their insertion at the lateral epicondyle. Tenderness at the origin of the common extensor tendon indicates potential lateral epicondylitis or tennis elbow. On palpation, the provider will notice that the extensor carpi radialis longus muscle inserts above the epicondyle along a ridge that extends to the humeral shaft. The provider should also be able to palpate the brachioradialis and supinator muscles laterally. The lateral (radial) collateral ligament can be palpated as a cord extending from the lateral epicondyle to the annular ligament and the lateral ulna. During the supination and pronation of the

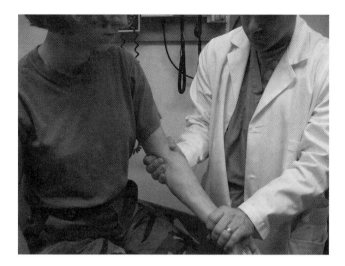

Figure 8.7 Varus testing of the lateral collateral ligament.

forearm, the physician should be able to feel the radial head and the annular ligament as they rotate.

Posterior aspect

The posterior aspect of the elbow is best palpated with the patient's elbow flexed at 90 degrees. The olecranon process becomes prominent distally at 90 degrees of flexion. At this point, if the skin is grabbed, the olecranon bursa will be palpated. The physician should be able to note any thickness of synovium or loose bodies that may put the patient at risk for developing olecranon bursitis in the future. Finally, the provider should palpate along the triceps tendon and the muscle belly of the triceps to note any abnormalities. To identify the distal triceps tendon, with the patient's elbow flexed at 90 degrees, the provider may palpate the tendon body within the olecranon fossa directly proximal to the olecranon process.

Special tests

Musculoskeletal literature has a paucity of studies evaluating the sensitivity and specificity of the following special tests. Until further research is conducted, the level of evidence for the majority of the tests described here is based on expert opinion rather than randomized studies.

Ligamentous tests

Ligamentous instability test This testing is used to identify varus (lateral or radial) and valgus (medial or ulnar) instability in the elbow. To stabilize the patient's arm, the examiner secures one hand at the patient's elbow and the other hand just above the patient's wrist. Each ligament is tested with the patient's forearm flexed at 20 to 30 degrees to unlock the olecranon from the fossa. To test the lateral collateral ligament (varus instability), the examiner exerts a varus or adduction force to the distal forearm while stabilizing the elbow and palpating the radial ligament **(Figure 8.7).** In a normal elbow, the provider will feel the ligament tense during this stress. Although several successive attempts are made, any change in pain or range of motion should be noted. Excessive laxity or a soft end point during this testing would indicate a positive test and joint instability.

For valgus (ulnar collateral ligament) testing, the patient's elbow and forearm should be placed in the same position. To test the medial collateral ligament (valgus instability), the examiner exerts a valgus or abduction force to the distal forearm while stabilizing the elbow and palpating the ulnar ligament **(Figure 8.8).** A positive test

again is signified by a change in pain or range of motion, excessive laxity, or a soft end point.

Milking maneuver The milking maneuver is a sensitive test for damage to the medial collateral ligament. To perform this test, have the patient place his or her forearm in supination with the shoulder extended and the elbow flexed to 90 degrees. The physician should then pull on the patient's thumb. With damage to the medial collateral ligament, the patient will report localized pain in the medial elbow and a sensation of apprehension and instability with this valgus tension. In a recent article,[11] a modification of this maneuver was described. In this maneuver, the provider stands next to the patient on the side of the elbow injury. The patient will then flex the shoulder to 90 degrees and supinate the forearm with the thumb pointed toward the provider. While grasping the thumb, the provider will provide valgus stress to the forearm while moving the elbow throughout its full range of motion. While performing this maneuver, the provider can palpate the areas of tenderness on the medial elbow. The possible advantages of this modification include testing the elbow through its full range of motion and the ability to identify at what point in the range of motion the stress and pain occurs.

Posterolateral rotatory apprehension test (posterolateral pivot–shift test) This test assesses the laxity of the ulnar insertion of the lateral collateral ligament. If present, this instability allows the humeroulnar joint to sublux, with secondary dislocation of the humeroradial joint. The ulna will displace on the humerus such that the ulna supinates or laterally rotates away from the trochlea. This is the most common type of instability within the elbow. During this test, the patient lies supine with the affected arm held overhead and with the shoulder rotated externally. The examiner grasps both the patient's wrist and the extended elbow. While standing at the head of the table, the physician provides a mild supination force at the wrist **(Figure 8.9).** Next, the physician will slowly flex the elbow while applying valgus and axial compression forces. A patient with posterolateral instability will become apprehensive with a sensation that the elbow will dislocate posterolaterally at approximately 20 to 30 degrees. If the examiner is able to continue flexing the elbow, at 40 to 70 degrees, there will be a sudden reduction of the joint that may be both palpated and seen[12] (LOE: E). Actual dislocation and reduction are usually only achieved in an unconscious or sedated patient.

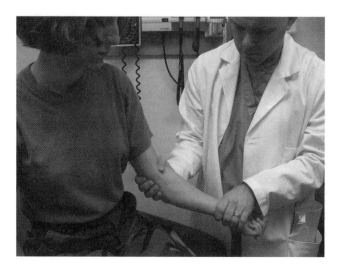

Figure 8.8 Valgus testing of the ulnar collateral ligament.

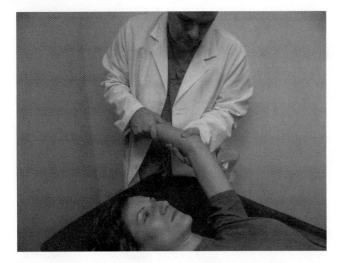

Figure 8.9 Posterolateral rotatory apprehension test.

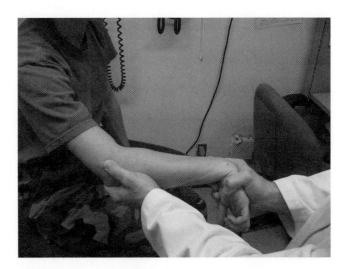

Figure 8.11 Lateral epicondylitis test, type 2.

Tests for epicondylitis

Lateral epicondylitis test, type 1 The provider should stabilize the patient's elbow with the thumb resting against the patient's lateral epicondyle. With the other hand, the provider should hold the patient's fist in an effort to resist motion **(Figure 8.10).** Direct the patient to form a fist, and then pronate the forearm. While resisting the patient's motion, have the patient deviate the wrist radially and extend the wrist. The test is considered positive if this resisted motion causes pain at the location of the lateral epicondyle as palpated by the examiner's thumb.[13]

Lateral epicondylitis test, type 2 As opposed to test type 1, this test is performed with the patient acting passively. The examiner should again position his or her hand along the patient's elbow with the thumb resting on the lateral epicondyle. The patient's forearm should then be passively pronated while the wrist is simultaneously flexed and the elbow is extended **(Figure 8.11).** Pain over the lateral epicondyle during this maneuver is considered a positive test. This test can potentially stress the radial nerve in patients with radial nerve compression, thus confusing the

diagnosis of lateral epicondylitis with radial nerve compression. Further diagnostic testing may be required to differentiate between these diagnoses.

Lateral epicondylitis test, type 3 The provider should have the patient position the elbow in a resting position of flexion. The provider will position his or her finger along the distal portion of the patient's long finger **(Figure 8.12).** In this position, the examiner should resist extension of the long finger distal to the proximal interphalangeal joint. This will specifically resist the action of the extensor digitorum muscle and tendon. A positive test is again signified by pain over the lateral epicondyle.

Medial epicondylitis test The examiner will position his or her hand supporting the elbow and with the thumb resting against the medial epicondyle. With the other hand, the provider should passively supinate the forearm while extending both the wrist and the elbow **(Figure 8.13).** This will stretch the origin of the flexor tendon complex at the medial epicondyle. Pain at the medial epicondyle indicates a positive test.

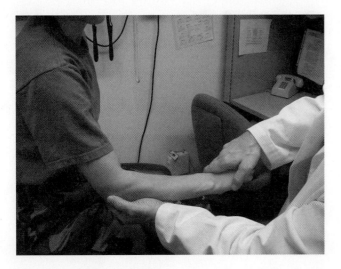

Figure 8.10 Lateral epicondylitis test, type 1.

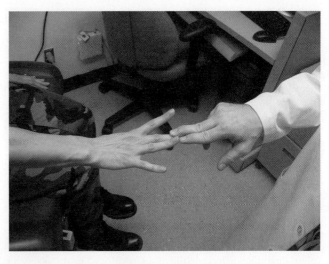

Figure 8.12 Lateral epicondylitis test, type 3.

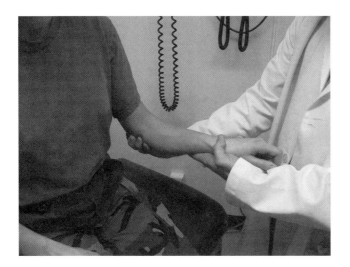

Figure 8.13   Medial epicondylitis test.

Tests for neurologic dysfunction[14]

Tinel's sign This test can be performed either on the ulnar or the radial side. For the ulnar nerve, the provider will tap in the ulnar groove between the olecranon process and the medial epicondyle. A positive test is signified by a tingling sensation in the medial forearm to the hypothenar area of the hand in the distribution of the ulnar nerve distal to the point of compression. To test the radial nerve, the provider should tap distal and anterior to the lateral epicondyle. If the test is positive, the patient will note a tingling sensation along the course of the radial nerve from the lateral forearm to the thenar eminence and radial digits.

Elbow flexion test For this test, the patient holds his or her elbow in maximal flexion with extension of the wrist and shoulder abduction for 3 to 5 minutes.[15] Patients with ulnar nerve compression may develop a tingling sensation or paresthesias in the distribution of the ulnar nerve into the forearm and hand.

Wartenberg's sign The term *Wartenberg's sign* refers to weakness of fifth finger abduction. The seated patient should rest his or her hands on the table, and then the provider will passively spread the patient's fingers apart. When asked to bring the fingers

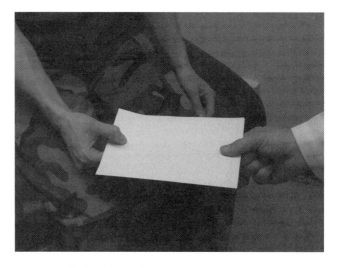

Figure 8.15   Positive Froment's sign.

together again, the patient with ulnar nerve entrapment will not be able to squeeze the little finger together with the rest of the hand.[16]

Froment's sign Froment's sign signifies weakness of the dorsal interosseous and adductor pollicis muscles in patients with ulnar nerve compression. The provider should ask the patient to pinch a piece of paper between the first and second metacarpals **(Figure 8.14)**. If the above muscles are weak, then the patient will not be able to hold the paper with the first and second metatarsals held together. Instead, the patient will flex the thumb with the flexor pollicis longus to hold the paper securely **(Figure 8.15)**.

Pronator teres syndrome test The provider will have the patient flex the elbow to 90 degrees. While the provider resists, the patient attempts to pronate and extend the elbow. A patient with compression of the median nerve by the pronator teres will develop tingling or paresthesias into the forearm and hand along the distribution of the median nerve.

Pinch grip test This test may also be referred to as the *"O" sign* or the *"OK" sign*. Patients with anterior interosseous nerve entrapment (a branch of the median nerve) will have difficulty pinching

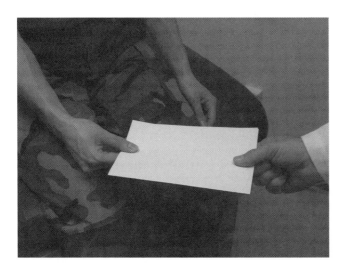

Figure 8.14   Negative Froment's sign.

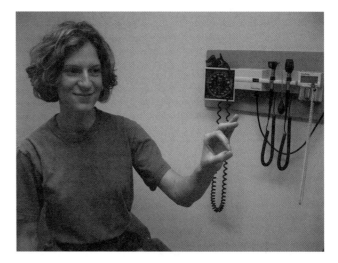

Figure 8.16   Negative pinch grip test.

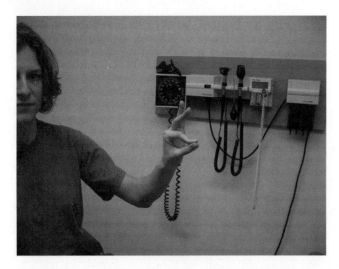

Figure 8.17 Positive pinch grip test significant for anterior interosseous nerve entrapment.

the tips of the index finger and the thumb together[17] **(Figure 8.16).** When asked to hold the tips of these digits together, the patient will not be able to keep them together against resistance. They may instead hold the distal phalanges flat against each other to hold the pinch **(Figure 8.17).** This will not be associated with any sensory deficit.

REFERENCES

1. Jobe FW, Nuber G: Throwing injuries of the elbow. Clin Sports Med 1986;5:(4):621-636.
2. Lyman SL, Fleisig GS, Osinski ED, et al: Incidence and determinants of arm injury in youth baseball pitchers: a pilot study (abstract). Med Sci Sports Exerc 1998;30:S4.
3. Hoppenfeld S, Hutton R: Physical Examination of the Spine and Extremities. Upper Saddle River, NJ, Prentice Hall, 1976, pp 35-57.
4. Lee MJ, Rosenwasser MP: Elbow trauma and reconstruction: chronic elbow instability. Orthop Clin North Am 1999;30:81-89.
5. Wilder RP, Guidi E: Anatomy and examination of the elbow. J Back Musculoskel Rehabil 1994;4:7-16.
6. Jackson MD, McKeag DB: Anatomy and biomechanics of the elbow and forearm. In Sallis RE, Massimino F (eds): Essentials of Sports Medicine. St. Louis, Mosby, 1997, pp 294-306.
7. O'Connor FG, Olivierre CO, Nirschl RP: Elbow and forearm injuries. In Lillegard WA, Butcher JD, Rucker KS (eds): Handbook of Sports Medicine: A Symptom-Oriented Approach, 2nd ed. Boston, Butterworth-Heinemann, 1999, pp 141-157.
8. Chumbley EM, O'Connor FG, Nirschl RP: Evaluation of overuse elbow injuries. Am Fam Physician 2000;61:691-700.
9. Kapandji AI: The Physiology of the Joints, Volume 1: Upper Limb. New York, Churchill Livingstone, 1970.
10. Askew LJ, An KN, Morrey BF, Chao EY: Isometric elbow strength in normal individuals. Clin Orthop 1987;222:261-266.
11. Callaway GH, Field LD, Deng XH, et al: Biomechanical evaluation of the medial collateral ligament of the elbow. J Bone Joint Surg Am 1997;79:(8):1223-1231.
12. O'Driscoll SW, Bell DF, Morrey BF: Posterolateral rotatory instability of the elbow. J Bone Joint Surg 1991;73:440-446.
13. Magee DJ: Orthopedic Physical Assessment, 4th ed. Philadelphia, WB Saunders, 2002, pp 321-353.
14. Vennix MJ, Wertsch JJ: Entrapment neuropathies about the elbow. J Back Musculoskel Rehabil 1994;4:31-43.
15. Buehler MJ, Thayer DT: The elbow flexion test: a clinical test for the cubital tunnel syndrome. Clin Orthop 1988;233:213-216.
16. Regan WD, Morrey BF: The physical examination of the elbow. In Morrey BF (ed): The Elbow and Its Disorders. Philadelphia, WB Saunders, 1993.
17. Bigg-Wither G, Kelly P: Diagnostic imaging in musculoskeletal physiotherapy. In Refshauge K, Gass E (eds): Musculoskeletal Physiotherapy: Clinical Science and Practice. Oxford, Butterworth-Heinemann, 1995.

CHAPTER 9

Physical Examination of the Shoulder

Sean T. Mullendore, MD

KEY POINTS

- Shoulder pain is a very common musculoskeletal complaint in primary care populations.
- Almost half of patients who present for the evaluation of shoulder pain will still have pain 1 year later.
- Neer's and Hawkins' impingement tests should be performed in a passive fashion
- Neck examination should always be included when evaluating shoulder pain in patients who are more than 35 years of age to rule out cervical radiculopathy.
- A focused shoulder examination should be systematic yet tailored to the most likely causes of symptoms on the basis of the clinical presentation.

INTRODUCTION

The shoulder joint (joints, actually) affords the largest range of motion (ROM) of any joint in the body with a relatively simple objective: placing the hand in the ideal position to accomplish fine motor tasks. Sounds simple, right? Unfortunately, the shoulder's "simple" task requires the interplay of three separate joints, one articulation, and more than a dozen muscles, many of which must function synergistically for proper shoulder motion and function. Not surprisingly, this complex interaction among muscles, ligaments, and joints allows ample opportunity for pathoanatomic problems that present as shoulder pain.

Physicians who practice primary care and musculoskeletal medicine will attest that shoulder pain is a common presenting complaint. The shoulder is the third most common site of musculoskeletal pain in the general population, after the back and the knee.[1] Surprisingly, only one third of shoulder pain is associated with an injury.[2] The annual incidence of shoulder pain in a general population ranges from 0.9% in patients between 31 and 35 years of age to 2.5% in patients between 42 and 46 years of age to 1.6% for those between 70 and 74 years of age.[3] Although the incidence of shoulder pain may not seem too taxing, its point prevalence in the general population ranged from 7% to 27% among adults less than 70 years of age to 13.2% to 26% for those more than 70 years of age, with a lifetime prevalence ranging from 7% to 67%.[3] Placing an even greater burden on medical systems than the sheer number of patients with shoulder pain is the finding that, after 12 months, only 60% of patients show complete recovery from their pain symptoms.[4]

ANATOMY

The shoulder joint, as mentioned previously, is actually composed of three separate synovial joints (glenohumeral, acromioclavicular, and sternoclavicular) and one articulation between the scapula and the posterosuperior thorax. Movement through a functional range at each of these interfaces is facilitated by any number of up to 16 muscles while being constrained by both static (i.e., ligaments) and dynamic (i.e., muscles and tendons) structures along the way. Let's look at the anatomy of the shoulder joint complex more closely from the inside out.

Bones/joints

The bones of the shoulder joint complex are shown in **Figure 9.1.** The scapula serves as the base of the shoulder joint complex and provides points of attachment for several muscles and ligaments as well as for the glenoid labrum. The humeral head joins the lower arm and, more importantly, the hand to the scapula at the glenohumeral joint through its articulation with the glenoid fossa. Because the articular surface area of the humeral head is approximately two to three times that of the glenoid fossa, only a fraction of the humeral head is in contact with the glenoid at any given time. This articular surface discrepancy contributes to the inherent instability of the glenohumeral joint, which is the most frequently dislocated major joint in the body. Fortunately, the glenoid's fibrocartilaginous labrum decreases the likelihood of glenohumeral dislocation by increasing the depth of the glenoid fossa and serving as a chock block, both of which decrease the translation of the humeral head on the glenoid. The acromioclavicular joint (ACJ) connects the acromion of the scapula to the clavicle, which serves as a strut to support the entire shoulder complex. The final connection between the bones of the shoulder and the axial skeleton is the sternoclavicular joint.

Ligaments

There are several ligaments in the shoulder that, if altered through trauma or degenerative changes, can contribute to the symptomatic instability of the glenohumeral joint or to painful

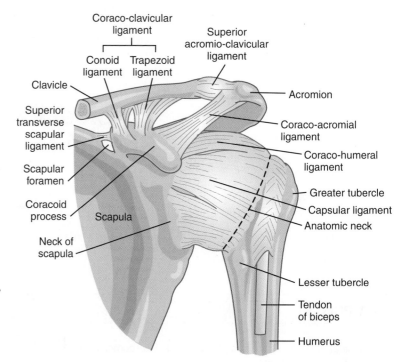

Figure 9.1 Bones, joints, and ligaments of the shoulder complex, anterior view. (Redrawn from Kuhn JE: The scapulothoracic articulation: anatomy, biomechanics, pathology and management. In Iannotti JP, Williams GR Jr [eds]: Disorders of the Shoulder: Diagnosis and Management. Philadelphia, Lippincott Williams & Wilkins, 1999, pp 817-845.)

rotator cuff disorders. The glenohumeral ligaments are actually thickenings of the joint capsule that form discrete superior, middle, and inferior ligaments. These serve as the primary static restraints of anterior glenohumeral translation and, to a lesser degree, of inferior glenohumeral translation.[5]

There are also ligaments that arise from the acromion that serve to stabilize the glenohumeral joint and the ACJ (see Figure 9.1). The coracohumeral ligament is an inferior stabilizer with the arm in adduction.[6] The coracoacromial ligament makes up part of the "roof" of the shoulder and, if it is thickened as a result of trauma or degenerative change, it can contribute to rotator cuff disorders like subacromial impingement.

Muscles/tendons

As already mentioned, there are more than a dozen muscles that have actions on the shoulder joint complex. To perform a seemingly simple movement like raising your hand, it takes several muscles working synergistically both at the glenohumeral and scapulothoracic articulations to produce a fluid, unobstructed motion. This concerted motion begins with the proper positioning of the scapula, which is facilitated by the scapular stabilizing muscles. The trapezius, rhomboids, and levator scapulae all elevate the scapula, while the first two muscles also retract the scapula toward the thoracic spinous processes. The serratus anterior serves to fix the scapula onto the thoracic rib cage as well as to produce scapular protraction and upward rotation. These muscles also serve to rotate the angles of the scapula either up or down.

The rotator cuff complex is perhaps the most frequently symptomatic soft-tissue structure in the shoulder. It consists of a group of four muscles that assist in the various glenohumeral movements while at the same time keeping the humeral head seated in the glenoid fossa. A common acronym for these muscles is *SITS* (supraspinatus, infraspinatus, teres minor, and subscapularis) **(Figure 9.2).** The supraspinatus extends from the supraspinatus fossa of the scapula to the greater tuberosity of the humerus. This muscle stabilizes the glenohumeral joint by compression while initiating elevation in the scapular plane. The infraspinatus and

the teres minor have respective points of origin from the infraspinatus fossa and the medial border of the scapula, and both insert on the greater tuberosity of the humerus. Each of these muscles resists posterior and superior glenohumeral translation and produces external rotation of the humerus. The subscapularis originates from the subscapular fossa and sends its tendon across the anterior aspect of the glenohumeral joint to insert over the intertubercular groove of the humerus. The subscapularis stabilizes the glenohumeral joint against anterior and inferior translation, and it is a strong internal rotator of the humerus.

The non–rotator-cuff scapulohumeral and thoracohumeral muscles, which I prefer to call "beach muscles," include the deltoid, the biceps, the triceps, the latissimus dorsi, and the pectoralis major. These muscles are responsible for most of the heavy lifting that is done with the upper extremity, and they get the most attention in the weight room. However, without adequately functioning rotator cuff and/or scapular stabilizing muscles, even the seemingly "strongest" individual may develop shoulder pain from subacromial impingement or other rotator cuff disorders as a result of pathologic shoulder biomechanics. These disorders will be discussed in more detail in Chapter 22.

RANGE OF MOTION

Shoulder range of motion (ROM) testing should be done actively, and, if it is abnormal, testing should be repeated passively. Limitations of both active and passive ROM may suggest adhesive capsulitis and/or glenohumeral arthritis, whereas a rotator cuff disorder usually limits only active ROM. The most commonly tested movements at the shoulder are external and internal rotation as well as elevation in the plane of the scapula (lying 20 to 30 degrees anterior to the frontal plane), which is a combination of forward flexion and abduction **(Figure 9.3).** The elevation of the arm is produced by a synchronized combination of glenohumeral and scapulothoracic motion in approximately a 2-to-1 ratio, and this is often referred to as *scapulohumeral rhythm.* By contrast, external/internal rotation occurs almost exclusively at the glenohumeral joint. ROM testing can be done with the patient in various positions

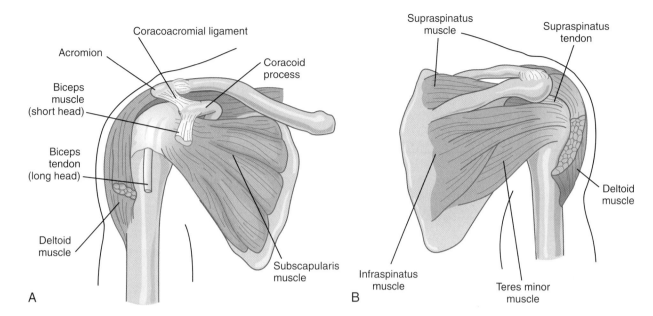

Figure 9.2   Anatomy of the shoulder and rotator cuff, showing anterior (*A*) and posterior (*B*) views.

(i.e., supine, seated, or standing), and it can measure pure movements in individual planes or more functional movements in combinations of planes (i.e., the "scratch" test). The reproducibility of ROM measurements between examiners (i.e., interrater reliability) is notoriously low; however, the intrarater reliability of ROM measurements is high, regardless of whether the patient is examined in the seated or supine position (LOE: D).[7,8]

Pure range of motion

A "normal" ROM will vary among patients, but most individuals can forward flex to 180 degrees, extend to 40 degrees, abduct to 120 degrees (with the palms down) or 180 degrees (with the palms up), and adduct to 45 degrees. The degrees of external and, to a lesser degree, internal rotation are dependent on the location of the arm when it is tested. With the arm at the side, a patient can externally rotate 40 to 50 degrees and internally rotate approximately 55 degrees. With the arm abducted 90 degrees, most subjects can externally rotate up to 80 to 100 degrees.

Functional range of motion

It may also useful to determine a functional ROM using the Apley "scratch" tests. To determine the amounts of combined internal rotation and adduction, the patient is asked to reach behind his or her back and touch the highest point toward the inferior angle of the opposite scapula **(Figure 9.4).** Combined external rotation and abduction is determined by having the patient reach behind his or her neck and trying to touch the superior angle of the opposite scapula (see Figure 9.4). Measurements are recorded by the thoracic spinous process level reached. These measurements are useful for determining a patient's ability or inability to perform activities of daily living, such as combing the hair or fastening a bra.

STRENGTH TESTING

As mentioned previously, there are more than a dozen muscles that have actions across the shoulder complex, many of which act synergistically to produce movements. This makes it nearly impossible to isolate individual muscles on physical examination;

however, it is possible to selectively examine several of the muscles that are most commonly affected by disorders of the shoulder (e.g., supraspinatus). The strength of the affected extremity should always be compared with the contralateral (and hopefully asymptomatic) side and graded on a standard 0-to-5 scale. The muscles most commonly tested are the rotator cuff or the *SITS* complex because these are the muscles that are most often affected by disorders of the shoulder complex. Other muscles may be tested indirectly through the visualization of active ROM (e.g., scapular stabilizer weakness may produce asynchronous scapulohumeral rhythm on shoulder abduction). Let's look at strength testing for each rotator cuff component, one by one.

Supraspinatus

The main function of the supraspinatus is to initiate elevation in the plane of the scapula. To isolate this muscle from the deltoid, testing should be performed with the arm elevated 80 to 90 degrees while it is positioned 20 to 30 degrees anterior to the frontal plane. Traditionally, the supraspinatus is tested with the arm internally rotated approximately 45 degrees (i.e., the "empty can" position); however, this position can provoke pain from impingement, which may confound muscle strength testing. Kelly and colleagues[9] showed that performing the test with the arm externally rotated 45 degrees (i.e., the "full can" position) most effectively isolated the supraspinatus muscle from other synergist muscles while decreasing the chance of provoking shoulder impingement (LOE: D). This test is shown in **Figure 9.5.**

Infraspinatus/teres minor

The infraspinatus and teres minor function together to externally rotate the humerus. Strength testing of these muscles can be done with the arm in varying amounts of elevation in a scapular plane and/or rotation from a neutral position (i.e., 0 degrees of external rotation). Kelly and colleagues[9] found that the best position from which to test the strength of these muscles is with the arm at 0 degrees of scapular elevation and 45 degrees of internal humeral rotation **(Figure 9.6).** This position provides for minimal activation/assistance from the posterior deltoid and supraspinatus muscles (LOE: D).

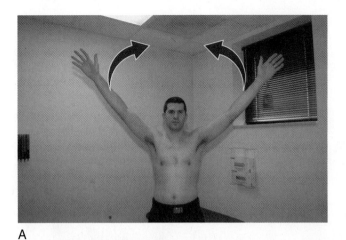

A

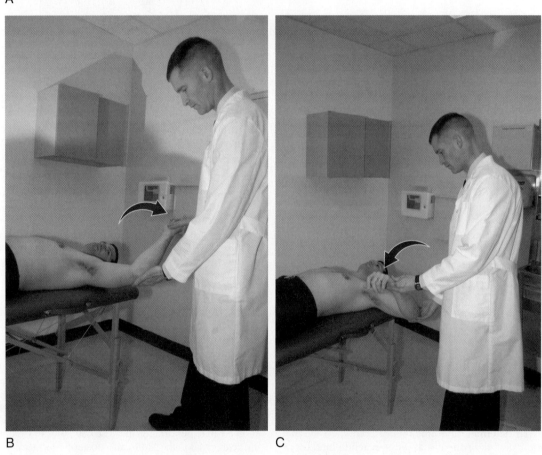

B   C

Figure 9.3 Shoulder movements. *A*, Elevation in the plane of the scapula, which lies 20 to 30 degrees anterior to a frontal plane. External rotation (*B*) and internal rotation (*C*) measured at 90 degrees of humeral abduction.

Subscapularis

The subscapularis muscle internally rotates the humerus. To test the strength of this rotator-cuff component, the subscapularis must first be isolated from the other internal rotators, namely the pectoralis major, teres major, and latissimus dorsi muscles. The most effective way to test the subscapularis in isolation is with the "lift-off test," which was first described by Gerber and Krushell[10] (LOE: C). The test is performed by having the patient internally rotate, extend, and adduct the arm to place the dorsum of the hand over the mid-lumbar spine. The patient is then asked to lift the hand off of his or her back against the examiner's

resistance **(Figure 9.7).** As with the maneuvers described previously, Kelly and colleagues[9] found the lift-off test against resistance to be the most effective way of isolating the subscapularis muscle from the other internal rotators of the humerus (LOE: D).

PALPATION

After inspecting the shoulder girdle and the surrounding anatomy for obvious deformity or atrophy, the shoulder complex should be palpated. Starting and finishing positions are not as important as

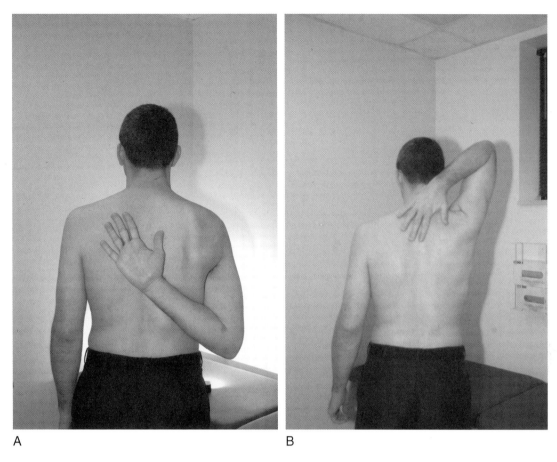

A   B

Figure 9.4   Apley "scratch" tests. The Apley scratch tests are measures of functional range of motion combining either internal rotation and adduction (*A*) or external rotation and abduction (*B*).

using a consistent and systematic approach to palpation. I prefer to begin palpation over the sternoclavicular joint and to proceed laterally along the clavicle to the ACJ. Any warmth, redness, or tenderness to palpation should be noted. In one study, ACJ tenderness on examination had a sensitivity of 96% for predicting ACJ-related shoulder pain; however, the corresponding negative predictive value was only 71%, perhaps as a result of the high

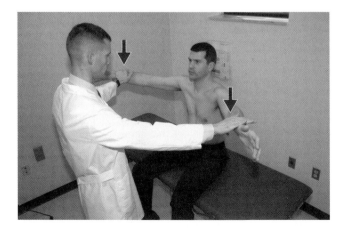

Figure 9.5   Supraspinatus strength testing. With the arm elevated 80 to 90 degrees in the plane of the scapula and externally rotated (i.e., the "full can" position), the subject resists the examiner's attempts to push the arm downward.

prevalence of some degree of ACJ pathology in subjects with shoulder pain[11] (LOE: B). Tenderness or crepitus over the acromion of the scapula may suggest fracture or a symptomatic accessory ossification center (os acromiale). The remainder of the scapula (the spine, superior and inferior angles) should be palpated for bony tenderness, as should the thoracic and cervical spinous processes. Posteriorly, the scapular stabilizers (i.e., the rhomboids, the trapezius, and the levator scapula) should be palpated for areas of tenderness or spasm. The subacromial bursa and rotator-cuff tendons can also be palpated for tenderness. To facilitate this examination, the examiner places the fingers of one hand anterior to the anterior margin of the acromion, between the anterior and medial portions of the deltoid muscle. The other hand is used to passively bring the subject's arm into extension, and this is followed by gentle internal and external rotation. This maneuver brings the rotator cuff tendons beneath the examiner's fingers anterior to the acromion. Experienced examiners may actually be able to appreciate a tear or "rent" in the rotator-cuff tendon complex. This "rent test," when performed properly, was shown in one study to have a diagnostic accuracy of 96% for predicting rotator-cuff tears at arthroscopy[12] (LOE: B).

SPECIAL TESTS

Because the shoulder complex is composed of multiple joints that are acted on by more than a dozen muscles working synergistically, it is often difficult for an examiner to determine the specific location of a patient's shoulder pain by history, inspection, palpation,

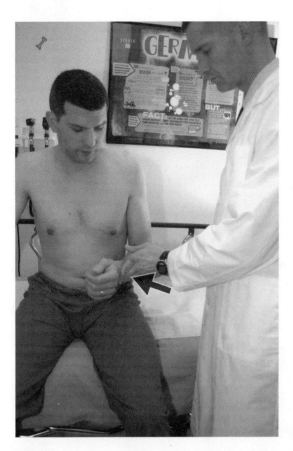

Figure 9.6 External rotation strength testing. With the arm at 0 degrees of elevation and approximately 45 degrees of internal humeral rotation, the subject resists the examiner's attempts to internally rotate the arm.

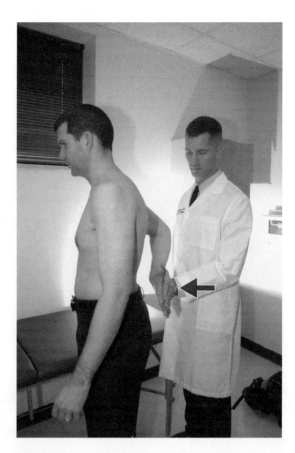

Figure 9.7 Subscapularis strength testing. The subject is asked to place the dorsum of the hand on the mid-lumbar region of the back and then to lift the hand off of the back against the examiner's resistance.

ROM, and strength testing alone. As a result, numerous special tests have been developed to pinpoint the pathoanatomic source of shoulder pain. For example, there have been more than a dozen special tests described and validated for glenoid labrum tears alone. The next section will describe some of the most common special tests for shoulder examination and the levels of evidence for each of them.

Impingement syndrome tests

Tests for impingement syndrome use various techniques to pinch or impinge soft-tissue structures (e.g., rotator-cuff tendons, bursae) between bones or ligaments. Most impingement tests have decent levels of sensitivity but low specificity because pain can originate either from the soft-tissue structure being impinged or the bony or ligamentous structure applying the impinging force. Below are some examples of impingement syndrome tests.

Neer's impingement sign

The technique for Neer's impingement sign is shown in **Figure 9.8.** The test was originally described as involving the patient being seated and the examiner standing. The examiner prevents scapular rotation by securing the patient's scapula with one hand and then raising the arm in forced forward elevation. This causes the greater tuberosity of the humerus to impinge against the acromion of the scapula, and the test is considered positive if pain is elicited. Because pain can also be provoked in patients with other shoulder conditions (e.g., glenohumeral or acromioclavicular

arthritis or frozen shoulder), it may be useful to inject a volume of 1% lidocaine into the subacromial space and to then repeat the test after 20 to 30 minutes. Pain from subacromial impingement should be significantly (i.e., 50% or greater) improved, whereas pain from other causes may not be relieved.

Regarding the sensitivity and specificity of this test, one study showed a sensitivity of 75% for bursitis and 88% for rotator cuff abnormalities, with respective specificities of only 48% and 51%.[13] This corresponded with positive predictive values (PPVs) of 36% and 40% and negative predictive values (NPVs) of 83% and 89%, respectively (LOE: B).

Hawkins' test

The impingement test described by Hawkins and Kennedy was originally published in 1980,[14] and it is shown in **Figure 9.9.** This test, like the Neer's impingement sign, is a passive maneuver. The examiner forward flexes the subject's humerus to 90 degrees and then forcibly internally rotates the shoulder. This maneuver drives the greater tuberosity of the humerus further under the coracoacromial ligament, which usually impinges the rotator cuff and/or biceps tendon in the process. Pain with this maneuver is a positive test.

An analysis by MacDonald and colleagues[13] examined the sensitivity, specificity, and predictive values of the Hawkins' test as compared with findings on shoulder arthroscopy. The test yielded a sensitivity of 92% for bursitis and 88% for rotator-cuff abnormalities, with specificities of 44% and 43%, respectively. The corresponding PPVs were 39% and 37%, and the NPVs were 93.1% and 90% (LOE: B).

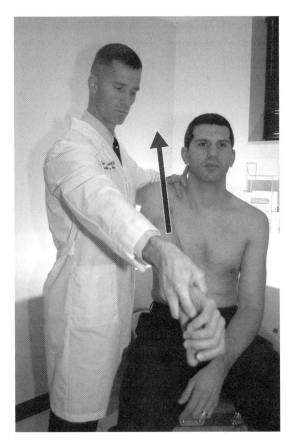

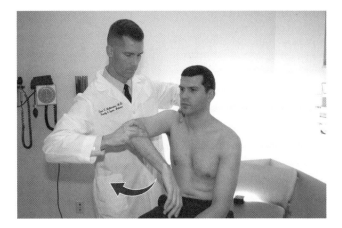

Figure 9.9 Hawkins' impingement sign. While securing the shoulder girdle with one hand, the examiner forward flexes the subject's arm to 90 degrees and then forcibly internally rotates the humerus. If the greater tuberosity of the humerus impinges against the coracoacromial ligament and produces pain, the test is positive.

supinate his or her forearm against the examiner's resistance. If the patient has pain localized to the bicipital groove, the test is positive, and this suggests biceps tendon pathology. The evidence basis for Yergason's sign is scant at best, and many clinicians do not find it very useful in narrowing down a pathoanatomic cause of shoulder pain.

Rotator-cuff integrity tests

The following tests are used to determine the integrity of the rotator-cuff tendon(s). Because the disruption of any of the rotator-cuff tendons can cause symptoms that mimic those of subacromial impingement, instability, glenoid labrum tear, or adhesive capsulitis, tests of rotator-cuff integrity should be included in all shoulder examinations.

Lift-off test

The lift-off test was mentioned previously in the section about strength testing, and it is shown in Figure 9.7. If the subject is unable lift the dorsum of his or her hand off of the back, this is considered a pathologic lift-off test, and it is suggestive of subscapularis rupture. Hertel and colleagues[17] evaluated this test and found a sensitivity and specificity for subscapularis rupture of 62% and 100%, respectively, with a corresponding PPV of 100% and an NPV of 69% (LOE: B).

Empty can test

The empty can test, which is also known as *Jobe's test* or the *supraspinatus test*, is used to test the integrity of the supraspinatus muscle. The subject is asked to elevate the arm 90 degrees in the plane of the scapula while maintaining maximum internal rotation of the shoulder (i.e., as if emptying a can of soda). The examiner then applies a downward force on the subject's arm. If the supraspinatus portion of the rotator cuff is torn, weakness will be appreciated by the patient either not being able to maintain the "empty can" position or by having the arm fall away with the slightest force from the examiner.

In one study by Itoi and colleagues,[18] the sensitivity and specificity of the empty can test using weakness (not pain) as the determining factor for a positive test were 77% and 68%, respectively. The corresponding PPV and NPV were 44% and 90% (LOE: B).

Figure 9.8 Neer's impingement sign. While securing the shoulder girdle with one hand, the examiner internally rotates and then forward flexes the subject's arm. If the greater tuberosity of the humerus impinges against the acromion of the scapula and produces pain, the test is positive.

Biceps tendinopathy tests

The long head of the biceps tendon travels through the bicipital groove in the proximal humerus before crossing the superior aspect of the glenohumeral joint and finally inserting on the superior glenoid labrum. There can be inflammation or degeneration of the long head of the biceps tendon anywhere from its myotendinous origin to its insertion. Below are two special tests for biceps tendon pathology.

Speed's test

Speed's test is performed by having the patient forward flex the arm against resistance with the elbow extended and the forearm supinated. The test is positive if pain is localized in the bicipital groove, and this suggests pathology of the biceps tendon or the biceps/labrum complex. In one prospective study of 45 patients undergoing shoulder arthroscopy, Speed's test yielded a specificity of 13.8% and a sensitivity of 90% for biceps tendon inflammation and/or superior labrum lesions[15] (LOE: B). With a PPV of 23% and an NPV of 83%, it was noted by this study's authors that Speed's test is often "positive with a various number of other pathological shoulder problems."

Yergason's sign

Also known as the "supination sign," this test was initially described in a case report by Yergason in 1931[16] (LOE: E). This test is performed by flexing the patient's elbow to 90 degrees with the forearm pronated and then asking the patient to actively

Drop sign

The drop sign is one of several "lag signs," and it is specific for the evaluation of the integrity of the infraspinatus tendon. To perform this test, the examiner holds the patient's affected arm in 90 degrees of forward flexion in the scapular plane at nearly complete humeral external rotation, with the elbow flexed to 90 degrees. The patient is asked to maintain this position, and the examiner releases the patient's wrist while still supporting the patient's elbow. The test is considered positive if a lag or "drop" toward internal rotation of more than 5 degrees occurs.

Hertel and colleagues[17] found that the sensitivity and specificity of this test for diagnosing tears of the infraspinatus were 21% and 100%, respectively. These corresponded with a PPV of 100% and an NPV of 32% (LOE: B).

Acromioclavicular joint tests

The ACJ tests are all designed to create shear force across the joint and to cause pain if a pathologic condition exists. Pain from the ACJ will most commonly be located on the top of the shoulder near the ACJ; however, Gerber and colleagues[19] found that, after injecting the ACJ of volunteers with saline, pain radiated to the trapezius in 80% of subjects (LOE: C). Some of the more common tests for ACJ pain are discussed here.

Active compression test

The active compression test was originally described by O'Brien and colleagues in 1998.[20] This test is performed by having the patient forward flex their arm to 90 degrees and then adduct it to 10 to 15 degrees. The patient is then asked to resist a downward directed force by the examiner first with the hand pronated and then with the hand supinated. The test, which is shown in **Figure 9.10,** is considered positive if pain that is localized to the ACJ during the first maneuver is reduced or eliminated during the second maneuver. In their original article, O'Brien and colleagues[20] found the test to be 100% sensitive and 97% specific for ACJ-related pain (LOE: B). However, Chronopoulos and colleagues[21] found the active compression test to be only 41% sensitive and 95% specific, with an overall accuracy of 92% (LOE: B).

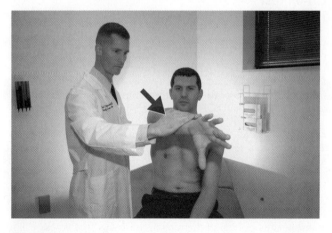

Figure 9.10 O'Brien's active compression test. The patient is asked to forward flex the arm to 90 degrees and then to adduct to 10 to 15 degrees. The subject is then asked to resist a downward force by the examiner, first with the hand pronated and then with the hand supinated. The test is considered positive if pain is elicited during the first maneuver and then reduced or eliminated during the second maneuver. Pain that localizes to the top of the shoulder suggests an acromioclavicular joint cause, whereas pain that localizes deep inside the shoulder joint suggests glenoid labrum pathology.

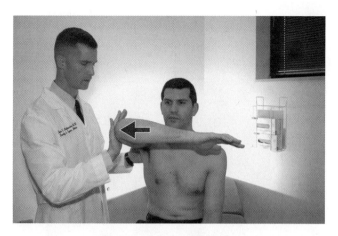

Figure 9.11 Acromioclavicular resisted extension test. The subject forward flexes the arm to 90 degrees, with the elbow flexed to 90 degrees. The subject then resists the examiner's attempts to adduct the arm. The test is positive if pain localizes over the top of the shoulder.

Acromioclavicular resisted extension test

The active compression resisted extension test was originally described by Jacob and Sallay in 1997.[22] This test is performed by having the patient forward flex his or her arm to 90 degrees with the elbow flexed to 90 degrees and then resisting the examiner's attempts to adduct the arm **(Figure 9.11).** In the study by Chronopoulos and colleagues,[21] the sensitivity of this test was 72%, with a specificity of 85% (LOE: B). In the same study, if the patient had both a positive active compression resisted extension test and a positive active compression test, the sensitivity improved to 81%, and the specificity was 89% (LOE: B).

Glenoid labrum tests

As mentioned previously, the glenoid labrum is a fibrocartilage structure that serves to enhance the stability of the glenohumeral joint as well as to be a point of attachment for the long head of the biceps tendon. When torn, the labrum can cause symptoms of pain, instability, locking, and catching. The most common location of labrum tears is the superior labrum anterior and posterior, at the origin of the long head of the biceps tendon. Below are some special tests for superior labrum anterior and posterior lesions.

Crank test

The crank test was first described by Liu and colleagues in 1996.[23] The test is performed with the patient in the upright or supine position, with the arm elevated to 160 degrees in the scapular plane. The examiner applies a joint load along the axis of the humerus and then internally and externally rotates the humerus **(Figure 9.12).** Pain during the maneuver with or without a click or reproduction of the patient's symptoms is considered a positive test. The sensitivity of the test was found to be 90%, with a specificity of 85% for labrum tear. The corresponding PPV was 95%, with an NPV of 85% (LOE: B).

Active compression test

The active compression test initially validated by O'Brien and colleagues[20] was described in the preceding section (see Figure 9.10); in addition, it is also very useful for the identification of labrum tears. The difference between a positive test for ACJ pathology versus that for a labrum tear was the location of the pain: it was on top of the shoulder for ACJ abnormality and pain, whereas painful clicking "inside" the shoulder was present for a labrum tear. In their study group of 318 patients, O'Brien and colleagues yielded a

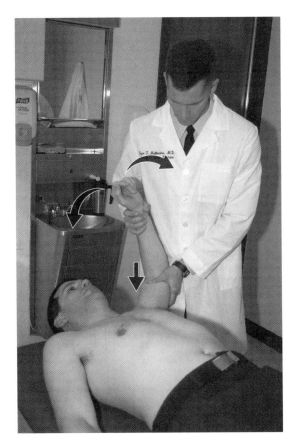

Figure 9.12 Crank test. After elevating the subject's arm approximately 160 degrees in the scapular plane, the examiner then internally and externally rotates the humerus while applying an axial load. Pain during this maneuver means that the test is positive.

sensitivity of 100% and a specificity of 99% for labrum tears confirmed at surgery (LOE: B).

Instability tests

Glenohumeral instability most commonly occurs in the anterior direction after traumatic glenohumeral dislocation or subluxation.

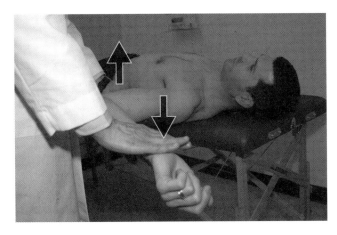

Figure 9.13 Apprehension test. The examiner abducts the subject's arm to 90 degrees with the elbow flexed 90 degrees and then maximally externally rotates the humerus while applying an anteriorly directed force on the proximal humerus. The test is positive if the subject feels a sense of apprehension that the shoulder is about to subluxate or dislocate.

Less frequently, instability occurs in posterior and/or inferior directions. Tests for glenohumeral instability are often divided into provocation/relief tests (i.e., tests causing/relieving pain or discomfort) and laxity tests (i.e., tests measuring the amount of glenohumeral translation).

Provocation/relief tests

Apprehension test In the apprehension test, the subject's arm is placed in the position of vulnerability for anterior glenohumeral luxation in an attempt to reproduce symptoms of anterior instability. With the subject either sitting or standing, the examiner abducts the subject's arm to 90 degrees with the elbow flexed 90 degrees. The subject's arm is then maximally externally rotated while an anteriorly directed force is applied on the proximal humerus **(Figure 9.13)**. The test is positive if the subject has pain anteriorly or a sense of apprehension that the shoulder is about to sublux or dislocate. In a meta-analysis of studies of this test, Luime and colleagues[24] found sensitivities and specificities ranging from 54% to 88% and from 44% to 100%, respectively (LOE: B).

Relocation test The relocation test is performed after a positive apprehension test, and it is shown in **Figure 9.14.** The subject's arm is brought out of maximal external rotation to a point at which the symptoms are relieved. A posteriorly directed force is then applied to the proximal humerus while the humerus is again maximally externally rotated. The test is considered positive if the subject felt a relief of the sense of apprehension produced during the apprehension test. In their meta-analysis, Luime and colleagues[24] found this test to have a sensitivity and specificity ranging from 30% to 85% and 58% to 100%, respectively (LOE: B).

Anterior release or surprise test The anterior release or surprise test is performed from the position of the relocation test, and it is shown in **Figure 9.15.** If the subject has a positive relocation test, the examiner's hand is quickly removed from the proximal humerus, and the subject's response is recorded. If the subject has a sudden return of the symptoms of the apprehension test, the anterior release test is considered positive. Luime and colleagues[24] found the sensitivity and specificity of the surprise

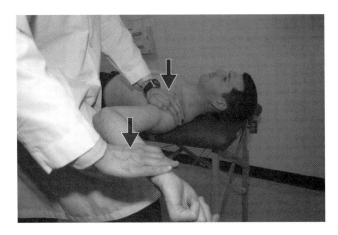

Figure 9.14 Relocation test. While the subject is still in the position for the apprehension test, the subject's arm is brought out of maximal external rotation to a point at which the symptoms of apprehension are resolved. A posteriorly directed force is then applied to the proximal humerus while the examiner again maximally externally rotates the humerus. A positive test results when the subject experiences relief from the previous sensation of apprehension.

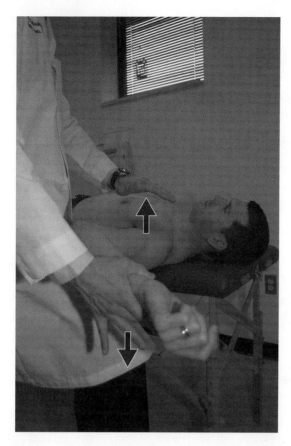

Figure 9.15 Anterior release test. This test is performed after a positive relocation test. The examiner's hand is quickly removed from the proximal humerus, and the subject's response is recorded. A positive test results when the subject has a sudden return of anterior apprehension symptoms (i.e., the feeling that the shoulder is about to subluxate or dislocate).

test to be 85% to 92% and 87% to 89%, respectively (LOE: B). If subjects had positive responses to all three of the instability tests described previously, the PPV was 94%, and the NPV was 72%[25] (LOE: B).

Laxity tests

Load-and-shift test The load-and-shift test is performed most effectively with the patient supine and with the scapula placed on the edge of the examination table. The patient's arm is placed in approximately 20 degrees of abduction, 20 degrees of forward flexion, and neutral rotation. The examiner then grasps the patient's arm above the elbow and "loads" the humeral head into the glenoid. The examiner's other hand is then placed on the patient's proximal humerus, and the humeral head is translated in anterior and posterior directions. The amount of laxity is graded as 0 (little to no movement), 1 (the humeral head rides up onto the glenoid rim), 2 (the humeral head can be dislocated but spontaneously relocates), or 3 (the humeral head is dislocated and cannot be relocated). Unfortunately, with positive likelihood ratios ranging from 1.7 to 2.5 and negative likelihood ratios from 0.59 to 0.99, the load-and-shift test is not very predictive of glenohumeral instability when it is performed on patients in the outpatient setting[26] (LOE: B). However, when it is performed with the patient under anesthesia, the positive and negative likelihood ratios improve to 13 and 0.02, respectively[27] (LOE: B).

Sulcus sign The sulcus sign tests for inferior glenohumeral instability. With the patient sitting or standing, the examiner grasps the patient's arm and pulls inferiorly. The test is positive if a dimple or sulcus appears beneath the acromion as the humeral head is translated inferiorly. There are several grading systems for the sulcus sign that rely on the measurement of the sulcus in centimeters. Tzannes and Murrell[28] found a sulcus sign of 2 cm or more to have a specificity of 97% for multidirectional instability; however, the corresponding sensitivity was only 28% (LOE: D). T'Jonk and colleagues[26] also found the sulcus sign to be ineffective for ruling out instability, with a negative likelihood ratio of 0.78 (LOE: B).

REFERENCES

1. Urwin M, Symmons D, Allison T, et al: Estimating the burden of musculoskeletal disorders in the community: the comparative prevalence of symptoms at different anatomical site, and the relation to social deprivation. Ann Rheum Dis 1998;57(11):649-655.
2. Wofford JL, Mansfield RJ, Watkins RS: Patient characteristics and clinical management of patients with shoulder pain in U.S. primary care settings: secondary data analysis of the National Ambulatory Mediacal Care Survey. BMC Musculoskelet Disord 2005;6(1):4.
3. Luime JJ, Koes BW, Hendriksen IJM, et al: Prevalence and incidence of shoulder pain in the general population: a systematic review. Scand J Rheumatol 2004;33(2):73-81.
4. van der Windt DA, Koes BW, Boeke AJ, et al: Shoulder disorders in the general practice: prognostic indicators of outcome. Br J Gen Pract 1996;46(410):519-523.
5. Doukas WC, Speer KP: Anatomy, pathophysiology, and biomechanics of shoulder instability. Orthop Clin North Am 2001;32(3):381-391, vii.
6. Halder AM, Itoi E, An KN: Anatomy and biomechanics of the shoulder. Orthop Clin North Am 2000;31(2):159-176.
7. Terwee CB, de Winter AF, Scholten RJ, et al: Interobserver reproducibility of the visual estimation of range of motion of the shoulder. Arch Phys Med Rehabil 2005;86(7):1356-1361.
8. Sabari JS, Maltzev I, Lubarsky D, et al: Goniometric assessment of shoulder range of motion: comparison of testing in supine and sitting positions. Arch Phys Med Rehabil 1998;79(6):647-651.
9. Kelly BT, Kadrmas WR, Speer KP: The manual muscle examination for rotator cuff strength. An electromyographic investigation. Am J Sports Med 1996;24(5):581-588.
10. Gerber C, Krushell RJ: Isolated rupture of the tendon of the subscapularis muscle. Clinical features in 16 cases. J Bone Joint Surg Br 1991;73(3):389-394.
11. Walton J, Mahajan S, Paxinos A, et al: Diagnostic values of tests for acromioclavicular joint pain. J Bone Joint Surg Am 2004;86-A(4):807-812.
12. Wolf EM, Agrawal V: Transdeltoid palpation (the rent test) in the diagnosis of rotator cuff tears. J Shoulder Elbow Surg 2001;10(5):470-473.
13. MacDonald PB, Clark P, Sutherland K: An analysis of the diagnostic accuracy of the Hawkins and Neer subacromial impingement signs. J Shoulder Elbow Surg 2000;9(4):299-301.
14. Hawkins RJ, Kennedy JC: Impingement syndrome in athletes. Am J Sports Med 1980;8:151-158.
15. Bennett WF: Specificity of the Speed's test: arthroscopic technique for evaluating the biceps tendon at the level of the bicipital groove. Arthroscopy 1998;14(8):789-796.
16. Yergason RM: Supination sign. J Bone Joint Surg 1931;13:160.
17. Hertel R, Ballmer FT, Lambert SM, et al: Lag signs in the diagnosis of rotator cuff rupture. J Shoulder Elbow Surg 1996;5(4):307-313.
18. Itoi E, Kido T, Sano A, et al: Which is more useful, the "full can test" or the "empty can test," in detecting the torn supraspinatus tendon? Am J Sports Med 1999;27(1):65-68.
19. Gerber C, Galantay RV, Hersche O: The pattern of pain produced by irritation of the acromioclavicular joint and the subacromial space. J Shoulder Elbow Surg 1998;7(4):352-355.
20. O'Brien SJ, Pagnani MJ, Fealy S, et al: The active compression test: a new and effective test for diagnosing labral tears and acromioclavicular joint abnormality. Am J Sports Med 1998;26(5):610-613.
21. Chronopoulos E, Kim TK, Park HB, et al: Diagnostic value of physical tests for isolated chronic acromioclavicular lesions. Am J Sports Med 2004;32(3):655-661.
22. Jacob AK, Sallay PI: Therapeutic efficacy of corticosteroid injections in the acromioclavicular joint. Biomed Sci Instrum 1997;34:380-385.

23. Liu SH, Henry MH, Nuccion S, et al: Diagnosis of glenoid labral tears. A comparison between magnetic resonance imagine and clinical examination. Am J Sports Med 1996;24(2):149-154.

24. Luime JJ, Verhagen AP, Miedema HS, et al: Does this patient have instability of the shoulder or a labrum lesion? JAMA 2004;292(16):1989-1999.

25. Lo IK, Nonweiler B, Woolfrey M, et al: An evaluation of the apprehension, relocation, and surprise tests for anterior shoulder instability. Am J Sports Med 2004;32(2):301-307.

26. T'Jonk L, Staes F, Smet L, Lysens R: The relationship between clinical shoulder tests and the findings in arthroscopic examination. Geneeskunde Sport 2001;34:15-24.

27. Cofield RH, Nessler JP, Weinstabl R: Diagnosis of shoulder instability by examination under anesthesia. Clin Orthop 1993;291:45-53.

28. Tzannes A, Murrell GA: Clinical examination of the unstable shoulder. Sports Med 2002;32(7):447-457.

Physical Examination of the Cervical and Thoracic Spine

Derek A. Woessner, MD, and Charles W. Webb, DO, FAAFP

KEY POINTS

· Neck and back pain are common and costly clinical problems.
· When evaluating for cervical spine injuries with radiographic studies, the clinician must ensure that the cervicothoracic junction is seen (C7-T1).
· When considering cervical fractures and dislocations, the most important concept is stability.
· The routine cervical series of x-rays consists of five views: the odontoid view, the lateral view, the posterior-anterior (PA) view, and two oblique views.
· In the thoracic spine, a significant amount of force is needed to cause a fracture.

INTRODUCTION

Neck and upper back pain are common clinical problems that are encountered by the primary care physician. Approximately 70% of all individuals will experience neck pain at some point in their lives.[1] In addition to being a common problem, neck and upper back pain can be very disabling. This type of pain is similar to low back pain in that the cause is poorly understood. Upper back and neck pain have become increasingly important as the costs of health care become a primary focus of attention. Neck and spinal disorders can account for approximately $25 billion in health-care costs annually. The primary focus of this chapter is to arm the sports medicine physician with the physical examination practices necessary to limit the costs of evaluating patients with these problems and to help the provider make the pathoanatomic diagnosis necessary to treat and rehabilitate the patient back to his or her preinjury state.

CERVICAL SPINE

Anatomy

The anatomy of the cervical spine is made up of seven vertebrae **(Figure 10.1).** The first two vertebrae, C-1 and C-2, differ considerably from C-3 through C-7. Anatomically, C-1 (which is also referred to as *the atlas*) articulates with the occiput of the skull

above and with C-2 (the axis) below. This atlanto-occipital joint primarily allows for flexion and extension. The axis, or C-2, is comprised of the odontoid process (also referred as *the dens*), and it articulates with the posterior aspect of the anterior arch of C-1.[2] This articulation, which is called the *atlantoaxial joint*, is stabilized by the transverse ligament, and it primarily provides rotation.[2]

Vertebrae C-3 through C-7 are all very similar, and they function as an interdependent group. These vertebrae allow for varying degrees of flexion, extension, lateral bending, and rotation. Specifically, flexion is focused at C-5 and C-6, and extension is focused on C-6 and C-7; therefore, degenerative changes and spine injuries commonly occur at these levels. Intervertebral disks are found between each pair of vertebral bodies between C-2 and C-7.

Next, there are eight pairs of cervical spinal nerves that exit through the intervertebral foramina bilaterally. The spinal nerve is named for the vertebra above which it exits.[3] For example, the C-5 nerve root exits above the C-5 vertebra; therefore, a herniated disk at the C4-5 level involves the C-5 nerve root.[3] The C-8 spinal nerve is the exception because this nerve exits between the C-7 and T-1 vertebrae.[3]

The facet joints, which are true synovial joints, are located in the posterior aspect of the cervical vertebrae. These joints are subject to degenerative changes that, on cervical extension as well as with lateral bending and rotation, may produce pain. Hypertrophy of these joints may affect the surrounding anatomic structures, including the spinal cord, the nerve roots, and the exiting spinal nerves.

For the clinician, the muscles of the neck may be divided into three major groups: anterior (flexion), posterior (extension), and lateral (lateral bending).[2] The muscles responsible for flexion are the sternocleidomastoid, the longus colli, and the longus capitis. The muscles involved in extension include the splenius, the semispinalis capitis, the semispinalis cervicis, the iliocostalis cervicis, the longissimus capitis, the longissimus cervicis, the trapezius, and the interspinales. Lastly, the muscles responsible for lateral bending are the sternocleidomastoid, the scalene muscles, the splenius, the longissimus capitis, the longissimus cervicis, the levator scapulae, and the longus colli.

History

Excluding cases of significant trauma, which require imaging studies to exclude fracture or instability, a detailed history and

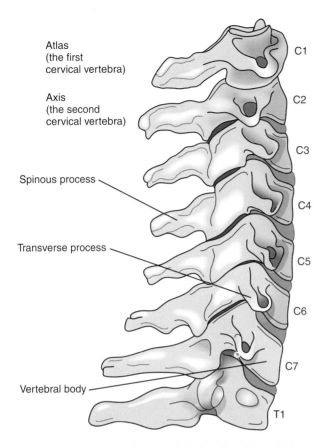

Atlas
(the first
cervical vertebra)

Axis
(the second
cervical vertebra)

Spinous process

Transverse process

Vertebral body

C1
C2
C3
C4
C5
C6
C7
T1

Figure 10.1 Bony anatomy of the cervical spine. (From The Hughston Clinic: Spine, Hughston Health Alert [serial online]: Available at www.hughston.com/hha/spine.jpg. Accessed April 23, 2007.)

physical examination can be enough to diagnose most clinically significant conditions involving the neck. As with any other medical examination, the history starts with the patient's age and the duration, frequency, and other characteristics of the symptoms. The patient's age helps with distinguishing different potential causes of the pain. For example, patients do not usually present with arthritis of the cervical spine until after the age of 60 years, with 85% of those patients with spondylosis presenting at 65 years of age or more.

With regard to pain duration and frequency, symptoms that resolve within a few days to a couple of weeks are usually the result of muscle strains. Ligamentous injury may take as long as 8 weeks for resolution, and disc injuries with radicular symptoms may take 12 to 24 weeks for recovery. Pain symptoms beyond the 6-month mark often indicate a degenerative process.

Symptom severity and mechanism of injury are other key parts of the history. If the cause was a motor vehicle accident, what was the speed of travel and the direction of the collision? If it was a sports-related injury, was it an axial blow from the front, the back, or one of the sides? This information will give the investigator clues as to the potential severity of injury. Traumatic, stretching, or overuse injuries help distinguish a thoracic outlet-type injury from a sprain/strain injury pattern.

In addition, as part of the history, the clinician needs to determine whether the pain experienced by the patient is localized or radiating. Often, pain that localizes is associated with muscle strains, ligament sprains, and degenerative processes. By contrast, pain that radiates into the upper limbs frequently indicates nerve involvement. The nature of the pain is crucial because tingling or a pins-and-needles sensation represents a neurologic injury, potentially of the nerve root **(Table 10.1).**

Range of motion

First, observe the patient's posture and general movements (i.e., rigid, guarded, general stiffness, or loose and free). From the front and the back of the patient, observe the overall muscle tone as well as the muscle bulk, comparing left and right side, and observe for muscle atrophy. Next, observe the soft tissue. Note the color of the patient's skin, and look for any swelling over the cervical spine. Finally, with the patient in the standing as well as the sitting position, observe the posture of the head, neck, thoracic spine, and upper limbs. To initiate proper medical care, the clinician must determine whether the patient's pain is localized to any of the following areas:

- The joints
- The muscles
- The neural structures
- Any combination of the above

Although some authors note the difficulty of accurately measuring cervical spine mobility as a result of the dearth of landmarks as well as of the depth of the soft tissue, clinicians rely on subjective observations.[4] In the clinical setting, qualitative and quantitative observations are evaluated for active and passive neck movements (e.g., flexion, extension, lateral bending, and lateral rotation).

Flexion/extension

Instruct the patient to touch the chin to the chest and then to look up at the ceiling. The normal range of motion for flexion is 80 to 90 degrees (two finger widths between the chin and the chest).[5] The normal range of motion for extension is limited to 70 degrees (this corresponds with the plane of the nose and forehead approaching a horizontal orientation).[5] The sternocleidomastoid muscles are the primary flexors; the paravertebral extensor and trapezius are the primary extensors.[5]

Lateral bending

Instruct the patient to touch the ear to the ipsilateral shoulder without raising the shoulder. The normal range of lateral bending is approximately 20 to 45 degrees; the primary lateral benders are the scaleni anterior, medial, and posterior.[5]

Lateral rotation

Instruct the patient to twist the chin toward the right and left. The normal range of rotation is 60 to 80 degrees; the sternocleidomastoid muscles are the primary rotators.[6] With passive range of motion, the patient is in the supine position, and the examiner passively tests flexion, extension, lateral bending, and lateral rotation. Document the following for each component of the passive and active ranges of motion: range of movement, pain, and quality of movement (i.e., clicking, resistance, or muscle spasms). Patients who are suspected of having acute cervical injury should not undergo passive range-of-motion testing until the possibility of fracture has been ruled out.

Flexion/extension

The examiner places his or her hands on either side of the patient's head and bends the head forward. As with active flexion, a normal examination is when the patient's chin is pushed forward to the chest. With normal extension, the examiner will be able to lift the patient's head backward so that the patient is able to see the ceiling directly above.[5]

Table 10.1   Differential Diagnosis of Neurologic Disorders of the Cervical Spine and Upper Limb

Cervical Radiculopathy (Nerve Root Lesion)	Cervical Myelopathy	Brachial Plexus Lesion (Plexopathy)	Burner (Transient Brachial Plexus Lesion)	Peripheral Nerve (Upper Limb)
Aim pain in dermatome distribution	Hand numbness, head pain, hoarseness, vertigo, tinnitus, deafness	Pain more localized to shoulder and neck (sometimes face)	Temporary pain in dermatome	No pain
Pain increased by extension and rotation or side flexion	Extension, rotation and side flexion may all cause pain	Pain on compression of brachial plexus	Pain on compression or stretch of brachial plexus	No pain early; if contracture occurs (late), pain on stretching
Pain may be relieved by putting hand on head (C5,6)	Arm positions have no effect on pain	Arm positions have no effect on pain*	Arm positions have no effect on pain*	Arm positions have no effect on pain*
Sensation (dermatome) affected	Sensation affected, abnormal pattern	Sensation (dermatome) affected	Sensation (dermatome) affected	Peripheral nerve sensation affected
Gait not affected	Wide-based gait drop attacks, ataxia; proprioception affected	Gait not affected	Gait not affected	Gait not affected
Altered hand function	Loss of hand function	Loss of arm function	Loss of function temporary	Loss of function of muscles supplied by nerve
Bowel and bladder not affected	Possible loss of bowel and bladder control	Bowel and bladder not affected	Bowel and bladder not affected	Bowel and bladder not affected
Weakness in myotome but no spasticity	Spastic paresis (especially in lower limb early, upper limb affected later)	Weakness in myotome	Temporary weakness in myotome	Weakness of muscles supplied by nerve
DTR[†] hypoactive	Lower limb DTR hyperactive	DTR hypoactive	DTR not affected	DTR may be decreased
Negative pathologic reflex	Upper limb DTR hyperactive Positive pathologic reflex	Negative pathologic reflex	Negative pathologic reflex	Negative pathologic reflex
Negative superficial reflex	Decreased superficial reflex	Negative superficial reflex	Negative superficial reflex	Negative superficial reflex
Gait not affected	Gait affected	Gait not affected	Gait not affected	Gait not affected
Atrophy (late sign), hard to detect early	Atrophy	Atrophy	Atrophy possible	Atrophy (not usually with neuropraxia)

*Except in neurotension test positions.
[†]Deep tendon reflexes (DTR).
From Magee DJ: Orthopedic Physical Assessment, 4th ed. Philadelphia, WB Saunders, 2002, p 129, Table 3-3.

Lateral bending

From the neutral position, the examiner bends the patient's head laterally toward the shoulder; the normal range of lateral bending is approximately 20 to 45 degrees.[5]

Lateral rotation

Again, from the neutral position, the examiner turns the patient's head in a side-to-side manner (i.e., the "no" motion) **(Figure 10.2)**. In a patient with normal lateral rotation, the head may be turned such that the patient's chin is virtually in line with the shoulders.[5]

Strength testing

To evaluate for strength and nerve root involvement, several maneuvers may be employed **(Table 10.2)**. To evaluate C-5 and C-6 nerve roots, use the following:

- Arm abduction (to test the deltoid muscle)
- Arm external rotation (to test the infraspinatus muscle)
- Elbow flexion (to test the biceps muscle)
- Wrist extension (to test the extensor carpi radialis)

Elbow extension evaluates the triceps muscle (which primarily assesses C-7, with some C-6 and C-8 involvement). Thumb extension

and ulnar deviation of the wrist are the movements of the C-8 nerve root. Lastly, by abducting the fingers, the T-1 nerve root may be assessed.[3]

Palpation

During the assessment of flexion and extension, the spinous processes and the interspinous ligaments from C-2 through T-1 can be palpated. The C-2 spinous process is palpated on the midline below the occiput. With slight flexion and extension of the cervical spine, the C3, C4, and C5 spinous processes may be palpated. Because C-4 has the shortest spinous process and is level with the angle of the jaw, the transverse process is more readily palpated. Both the spinous and transverse processes of C-6 are easily palpated. The C-7 and T-1 spinous processes are readily accessible and may be confused with one another. When the patient extends his or her neck, the examiner palpates what is thought to be the spinous process of C-7. If C-7 is being palpated, anterior movement will be noted. If T1 is being palpated, a minimal amount of movement is noted. To palpate the facet articulations, the examiner moves approximately 2 cm to either side of the spinous process. Next, the examiner should palpate the surrounding muscles and soft tissues of the neck and shoulder girdle. Specifically, the upper trapezius and paraspinal

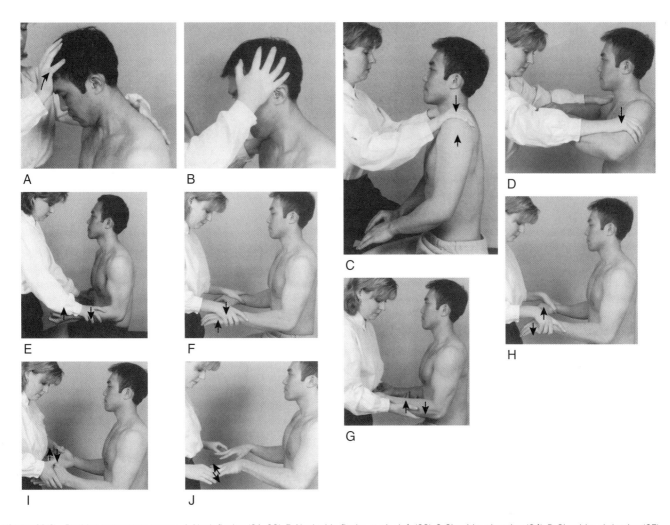

Figure 10.2 Position to test myotomes. *A*, Neck flexion (C1, C2). *B*, Neck side flexion to the left (C3). *C*, Shoulder elevation (C4). *D*, Shoulder abduction (C5). *E*, Elbow flexion (C6). *F*, Wrist extension (C6). *G*, Elbow extension (C7). *H*, Wrist flexion (C7). *I*, Thumb extension (C8). *J*, Finger abduction (T1). (From Magee DJ: *Orthopedic Physical Assessment*, 4th ed. Philadelphia, WB Saunders, 2002, pp 142-143.)

muscles should be palpated for spasms, trigger points, and deformities.

Special tests
Hoffman's sign
Hoffman's sign tests for upper motor neuron lesions above lower cervical spinal cord levels. When flicking the tip of the middle finger with the hand in a relaxed neutral position, the examiner will note a positive finding with the flexion of the thumb and index finger together in a pincer motion **(Figure 10.3).**

Spurling's sign
Spurling's sign involves pain radiating to the upper extremities after applying gentle, firm pressure to the patient's head with the head rotated and extended **(Figure 10.4).** This is often used to diagnose radicular pain syndrome. The sensitivity of Spurling's sign is 0.30 to 0.50, with a specificity of 0.74 to 0.93[7,8] (LOE: D).

Table 10.2 Cervical Nerve Root Testing

Nerve Root	Reflex	Myotome	Sensation	Nerve
C5	Biceps	Shoulder abduction	Lateral deltoid	Axillary
C6	Brachioradialis	Elbow flexion and/or wrist extension	First web space	Musculocutaneous
C7	Triceps	Elbow extension and/or wrist extension	Dorsal middle finger	
C8	N/A	Thumb extension and/or ulnar deviation	Ring finger	Medial antibrachial cutaneous
T1	N/A		Axilla	Medial brachial cutaneous

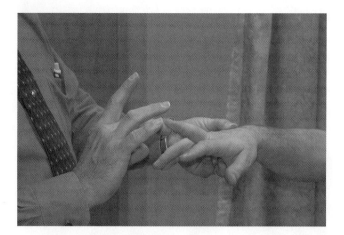

Figure 10.3 Hoffman's sign. The patient's hand is in a relaxed, neutral position, and the examiner flicks the middle finger. If this causes pinching of the thumb and middle finger, it is considered a positive test for an upper motor neuron lesion.

Abduction relief sign (Bakody's sign)

When disc protrusion is suspected as the cause of radicular pain, Bakody's sign is performed by having the patient place the hand of the affected upper extremity on the head. Arm abduction reduces symptoms by taking stretching pressures off of the affected nerve root. In a case series by Viikari-Juntura and colleagues,[9] this maneuver was discovered to have a sensitivity of 0.31 to 0.42 and a specificity of 1.0 (LOE: D) **(Figure 10.5).**

Bikele's sign

Bikele's sign occurs when a sitting patient is asked to raise the involved arm laterally into a horizontal, slightly backward position and to flex the elbow while laterally flexing the neck to the opposite side. If these motions reproduce radicular symptoms, then nerve-root inflammation is likely. The patient then actively extends the elbow. If this causes the radicular symptoms, then the stretching of the brachial plexus is instead the likely culprit **(Figures 10.6 and 10.7).**

Lhermitte's sign

Lhermitte's sign demonstrates a spinal or cervical myelopathy. With the patient sitting on the table, the examiner simultaneously

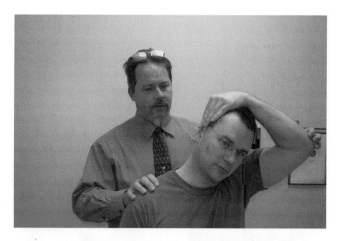

Figure 10.5 Disc protrusion causing radicular pain can be tested with the abduction relief sign. The patient places the hand of the affected upper extremity on his or her head. With arm abduction, symptoms are reduced by taking stretching pressures off of the affected nerve root.

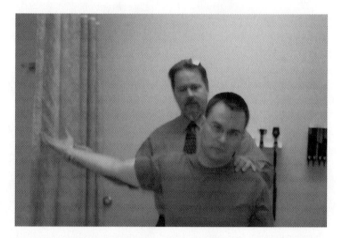

Figure 10.6 Bikele's sign tests for nerve root inflammation. The sitting patient is asked to raise the involved arm laterally to a horizontal, slightly backward position.

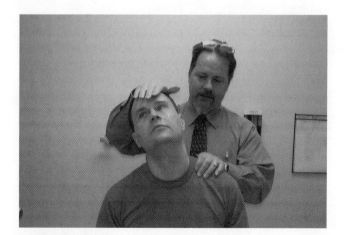

Figure 10.4 For Spurling's sign, the examiner applies gentle, firm pressure to patient's head with the head rotated and extended. Pain radiating to the upper extremity indicates radiculopathy.

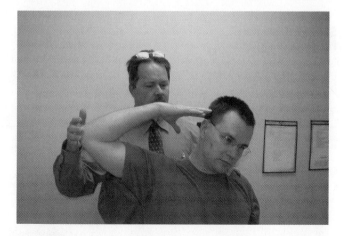

Figure 10.7 In the second part of Bikele's sign, the patient is asked to flex the elbow while laterally flexing the neck to the opposite side. Active extension of the elbow, which causes the brachial plexus to stretch, produces resistance and increased cervicothoracic radicular pain.

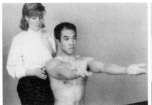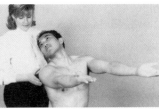

Figure 10.10 Hautant's test identifies insufficient blood flow through one or both vertebral arteries. The test is positive when the patient's hand pronates and/or shoulder flexion is difficult to maintain. (From Magee DJ: Orthopedic Physical Assessment, 4th ed. Philadelphia, WB Saunders, 2002, p 155.)

The patient is then instructed to rotate and extend the neck and head to one side and to close the eyes. This position is held for 15 to 30 seconds. A positive test is noted when the patient's hand(s) pronate and/or shoulder flexion is difficult to maintain **(Figure 10.10)**.

Sharp–Purser test

The Sharp–Purser test evaluates the sagittal stability of the atlantoaxial segment. The patient is asked to flex the head and relate to the examiner any signs or symptoms that this might evoke **(Figure 10.11)**. With the head semiflexed, the patient's forehead is supported by the examiner's palm. The index finger of the examiner's other hand is placed on the spinous process of the axis. Posteriorly directed pressure is applied to the forehead. If cardinal symptoms are provoked or the examiner palpates a sliding of the head in relation to the axis, the tentative assumption is made that they are caused by atlantoaxial instability. In patients with rheumatoid arthritis patients, this test was found to have a sensitivity of 0.69 and a specificity of 0.96[10] (LOE: D).

Radiographic testing

Cervical spine injuries are common for those participating in athletic events, from the "weekend warrior" to the well-conditioned athlete (10% of the 10,000 cervical spine injuries that occur annually in the United States are in individuals participating in athletic activities).[6] However, although the cervical injuries that result from participation in sports usually are self-limited, there still exist rare but catastrophic cervical spine injuries (e.g., quadriplegia). Therefore, guidelines have been created to assist medical providers with determining risk stratification for athletes after

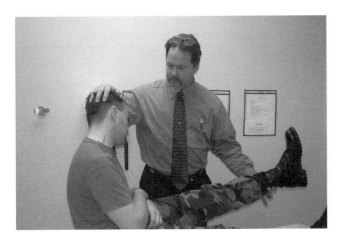

Figure 10.8 Lhermitte's sign indicates irritation of the spinal dura mater by a protruding cervical disc, a tumor, a fracture, or multiple sclerosis. With the patient seated, flexing of the patient's neck and hips simultaneously with the patient's knees extended may produce sharp pain that radiates down the spine and into the upper or lower extremities.

passively hyperflexes the patient's cervical spine and then flexes one of the patient's hips. If sharp pain is elicited down the spine or into the extremities, a myelopathy may be present. Testing for Lhermitte's sign is indicated when irritation of the spinal dura mater by a protruding cervical disc, a tumor, a fracture, or multiple sclerosis is considered in the differential diagnosis **(Figure 10.8)**.

Soto–Hall test

The Soto–Hall test is employed when a fracture of a vertebra is suspected. The patient is placed in a supine position without a pillow. One of the examiner's hands is placed on the patient's sternum, and mild pressure is exerted to prevent flexion at either the lumbar or the thoracic regions of the spine. The examiner's other hand is placed under the patient's occiput, and the head is slowly flexed toward the chest. Flexion of the head and neck toward the chest produces a pull on the posterior spinal ligaments from above. A positive result is recorded when acute, localized pain is experienced by the patient **(Figure 10.9)**.

Hautant's test

Hautant's test is performed to identify insufficient blood flow through one or both vertebral arteries. The seated patient elevates both upper extremities in the anterior plane with the shoulders flexed to 90 degrees, the elbows extended, and the hands supinated.

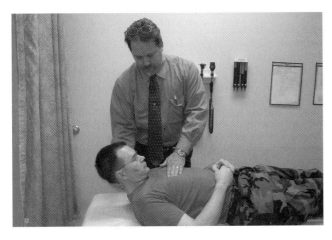

Figure 10.9 The Soto–Hall test.

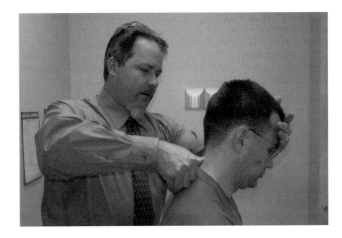

Figure 10.11 In the Sharp–Purser test, the sagittal stability of the atlantoaxial segment is assessed. The patient is asked to flex the head and relate to the examiner any signs or symptoms that this might evoke.

Table 10.3   Cervical Spine Injuries with No Contraindications for Sports Participation

Spina bifida occulta

Type 2 Klippel—Feil anomaly with no evidence of spinal instability

Developmental stenosis of the spinal canal (i.e., a canal—vertebral body ratio of less than 0.8)

A healed intervertebral disc bulge

Asymptomatic cervical disc herniations treated conservatively in the past

A stable, one-level, anterior or posterior fusion at C-3 or below (only if the individual is neurologically normal, is free of pain, and has a normal range of cervical motion)

Table 10.5   Cervical Spine Injuries with Absolute Contraindications for Sports Participation

Odontoid agenesis, hypoplasia, or os odontoideum; atlanto-occipital fusion

Type 1 Klippel—Feil mass fusion

Developmental canal stenosis with ligamentous instability, cervical cord neuropraxia with signs or symptoms lasting more than 36 hours, or multiple episodes of cervical cord neuropraxia

Atlantoaxial instability or atlantoaxial rotatory fixation

Spear-tackler's spine

Ligamentous laxity (more than 3.5 mm of anteroposterior displacement or 11 degrees of rotation)

Intervertebral disc herniation with neurologic signs or symptoms, pain, or limitations of cervical range of motion

Anterior or posterior fusion of more than three levels

cervical spine injuries[6] **(Tables 10.3, 10.4, and 10.5).** In addition, although abnormalities are often seen in asymptomatic patients, the confirmation of an intraspinal process requires radiographic imaging. The routine cervical series of x-rays consists of five views: the odontoid view, the lateral view, the PA view, and two oblique views.[3] Although the choice of test varies with the clinical features of the patient **(Tables 10.6 and 10.7),** the following general guidelines may be considered.

Odontoid views are appropriate in patients with acute trauma. With this view, the examiner is looking for an atlantoaxial articulation injury. **(Figure 10.12).** Specifically, the examiner is evaluating for a fracture of the dens, the body of C-2, and C-1:C-2 dislocation. The lateral view will allow the clinician to evaluate vertebral alignment, and it may be used to screen for osteoarthritis (facet and paravertebral joints), disk-space narrowing (osteoarthritis or radiculopathy), or bony pathology (compression fracture) **(Figure 10.13).** Oblique views are primarily used to determine the extent of foraminal encroachment. When the oblique views do not disclose narrowing of the foramina and there is high clinical suspicion, computed tomography scanning or magnetic resonance imaging should be obtained to evaluate for a herniated disk. Finally, computed tomography scanning or magnetic resonance imaging is indicated with the presence of objective neurologic impairment (weakness and/or reflex loss), persistent symptoms despite conservative care, evidence of cervical myelopathy, or plain films that are negative but physical findings that are suspicious for fracture.

THORACIC SPINE

Anatomy

The thoracic spine consists of twelve vertebral bodies, each of which articulates with the ribs. The first four thoracic segments, which are at the cephalic end of the spine, are similar to the lower cervical segments. Although the middle four vertebral bodies have thoracic

Table 10.4   Cervical Spine Injuries with Relative Contraindications for Sports Participation

No clear evidence of an increase in the risk for serious injury, but sequelae may include recurrent injury or temporary noncatastrophic injury (The player, the coach, and the parents must understand that there is some risk and agree to assume it.)

Developmental canal stenosis with one episode of cervical cord neuropraxia, the presence of intervertebral disc disease, or evidence of cord compression

Ligamentous sprain with mild laxity (less than 3.5 mm of anteroposterior displacement and 11 degrees of rotation)

Healed intervertebral disc herniation

Stable anterior or posterior fusion of two levels (if the individual is neurologically normal, is asymptomatic, and has full, painless cervical motion)

appearance, the last four have more of a lumbar configuration. From T-1 to T-12, the thoracic segments increase in size. The thoracic spine has a convex shape posteriorly, which is described as *kyphosis*. At C-7 and T-1 (the cervicothoracic juncture), the mobile cervical spine is linked to the less-mobile thoracic spine.

The first thing to note from the back, sides, and front of the patient is any obvious abnormality (observe the patient standing as well as sitting). Next, examine the skin for scars, sinuses, or color change and the soft tissues for swelling or warmth. Extending from the base of the occiput to T-12, the examiner will find the trapezius muscle. Next, located between the spinous processes of the upper thoracic spine and the medial border of the scapula, are the scapulae and the rhomboideus minor and major. Located in the middle to lower thoracic spine is the latissimus dorsi (a large superficial muscle that extends into the lumbar region). Finally, observe the erector spinae muscles (comprised of the spinalis, longissimus, and iliocostalis muscles) on either side of the spine. Specifically, note any spasm that may cause abnormal spinal curvature.

Range of motion

Although movements in the thoracic spine are relatively limited as compared with those of the cervical spine, flexion, extension, lateral bending (side bending), and lateral rotation can still be evaluated during passive and active range of motion. The main movements of the thoracic spine are as follows.

Flexion/extension

Instruct the patient to stand with the knees and the feet together. The patient should gently bend first forward and then backward. Normal forward flexion is between 20 to 45 degrees, and normal extension is between 25 to 45 degrees. An alternative method of assessing the degree of forward flexion is to measure (with the patient in the standing position) the length of the spine from the C-7 spinous process to the T-12 spinous process.[5] The patient bends forward, and the spine is measured again (from the C-7 spinous process to the T-12 spinous process); a 2.7-cm difference in the tape measure length is considered normal.[5]

While flexing and extending the patient's head, the examiner may palpate over and between the spinous processes of the lower cervical spine and the upper thoracic spine. (C-5 to T-3).[5] During this maneuver, the examiner notes any movement between the spinous processes.

Lateral flexion (side bending)

Instruct the patient to bend first to one side and then to the other. Ensure that the arms are kept close to the body as the patient attempts to touch the lateral side of the knee with the outstretched fingers (first on one side and then on the other side). Bending should be lateral rather than forward.

Table 10.6   Cervical-Spine—Specific Testing

Name	Indication	Test	Finding	Figure
Hoffman's sign	To test for an upper motor neuron lesion above lower cervical spinal cord levels	Flick the tip of the patient's middle finger with the hand in a relaxed, neutral position.	A positive finding is flexion of the thumb and index finger together in a pincer motion.	10.3
Spurling's sign	To diagnose radicular pain syndrome	Apply gentle, firm pressure to the patient's head with the head rotated and extended.	Pain radiating to the upper extremity indicates radiculopathy.	10.4
Abduction relief sign	To test for a disc protrusion causing radicular pain	The patient places the hand of the affected upper extremity on the head.	Arm abduction reduces symptoms by taking stretching tension off of the affected nerve root.	10.5
Bikele's sign	To test for nerve root inflammation	A sitting patient is asked to raise the involved arm laterally to a horizontal, slightly backward position and to flex the elbow while laterally flexing the neck to the opposite side.	Active extension of the elbow, which causes the brachial plexus to stretch, produces resistance and increased cervicothoracic radicular pain.	10.6 and 10.7
Lhermitte's sign	To test for irritation of the spinal dura mater by a protruding cervical disc, a tumor, a fracture, or multiple sclerosis	With the patient seated, the patient's neck and hips are flexed simultaneously with the patient's knees extended.	This may produce sharp pain that radiates down the spine and into the upper or lower extremities.	10.8
Soto—Hall test	To test for a fracture of a vertebra	The patient is placed supine without pillows. One hand of the examiner is placed on the sternum of the patient, and mild pressure is exerted to prevent flexion at either the lumbar or the thoracic regions of the spine. The other hand of the examiner is placed under the patient's occiput, and the head is slowly flexed toward the chest. Flexion of the head and neck toward the chest produces a pull on the posterior spinal ligaments from above.	Acute local pain is experienced by the patient.	10.9
Hautant's test	To identify insufficient blood flow through one or both vertebral arteries	The seated patient elevates both upper extremities in the anterior plane with the shoulders flexed by 90 degrees, the elbows extended, and the hands supinated. The patient is then instructed to rotate and extend the neck and head to one side and to close the eyes. This position is held for 15 to 30 seconds.	The test is positive when the patient's hand pronates and/or shoulder flexion is difficult to maintain.	10.10
Sharp—Purser test	To test sagittal stability of the atlantoaxial segment	The patient is asked to flex the head and to relate to the examiner any signs or symptoms that this might evoke.	If cardinal symptoms are provoked, the tentative assumption is made that they are caused by excessive translation of the atlas.	10.11
Thoracic outlet syndrome	To test for symptoms that are consistent with this syndrome	For the elevated arm stress test, the patient sits with the arms abducted 90 degrees from the thorax and the elbows flexed 90 degrees.	Patients with thoracic outlet syndrome cannot continue this test for 3 minutes because of the reproduction of symptoms.	10.14

Normal side flexion is between 20 to 40 degrees. Alternatively, the examiner can use a tape measure to determine the distance from the patient's fingertips to the floor (comparing the left and right sides).[5]

As the patient is flexing laterally and rotating, the examiner positions the middle finger over the spinous process and the index finger as well as ring finger on either side of the spinous process (i.e., the index finger and the ring finger are located between the spinous process of the vertebra being examined and the two abutting vertebra).[5] With this maneuver, the examiner notes any abnormal movement (e.g., hypermobility versus hypomobility) of C-5 to T-3.[5]

Rotation

Instruct the patient to cross the arms in front of the body and then to rotate to the right and left. Normal rotation for the thoracic spine is 35 to 50 degrees.[5]

Forward flexion/extension/lateral flexion/rotation (T-3 to T-11)

With the patient seated with the fingers intertwined behind the neck and the elbows together, the examiner positions one hand and arm around the patient's elbow and palpates over and

Table 10.7   Cervical Spine Indications for Diagnostic Testing

Indication	Diagnostic Test
Initial evaluation of patients with cervical disorders	Anteroposterior, lateral, odontoid, and oblique views
Cervical trauma	Cross-table lateral plain radiograph (must visualize C7-T1 disc space); "trauma" series of anteroposterior, open mouth odontoid, oblique, and controlled flexion and extension lateral views
Assessing stability of spine (nontrauma situation)/screening for abnormalities	Anteroposterior, flexion, neutral, and extension lateral radiographs
Presence of severe degenerative changes, severe end plate osteophytes	Computed tomography myelogram
Bony abnormalities of the cervical spine	Computed tomography scan with bone window settings
Persistent neurologic symptoms, cervical radicular syndromes	Computed tomography myelogram or magnetic resonance imaging
Suspected neurophysiologic impairment of the peripheral nerves, nerve roots, and spinal cord; conflicting diagnoses	Electrodiagnostic test (e.g., nerve conduction studies or electromyography)
Inability to visualize lower cervical spine	Swimmer's view or computed tomography scan

between the spinous processes.[5] To forward flex and extend the spine, the examiner lifts and lowers the patient's elbows.[5] Finally, with the same hand and arm position, the examiner can laterally flex and rotate the patient. Throughout these movements, the examiner is noting any abnormal movement (e.g., hypermobility versus hypomobility).[5]

Palpation

The vertebral spinous processes and interspinal ligaments should be carefully palpated for tenderness, gaps, and step offs, and they should also be percussed gently. Percussion allows the clinician to determine the location, size, and density of the underlying vertebral body. In addition, the muscles on each side of the spine should be palpated for spasm, trigger points, and defects. Finally, the spine should be palpated for any swelling.

Special tests

Because the thoracic spine is stabilized by the anterior and posterior ligaments, the costotransverse ligaments, and articulation with the spine and manubrium, a significant amount of force is needed to cause a fracture.[11] In addition, because there is little rotation in the thoracic spine as a result of rib support, most injuries occur in flexion and axial loading. Because thoracic spine injuries are difficult to detect on chest radiographs, dedicated thoracic spine radiographs should be obtained. Three types of fractures occur in the thoracic spine:

1. Wedge compression: This involves the anterior two thirds of the vertebral body, and it is considered stable.
2. Sagittal slice: This consists of an anterior fracture/dislocation with compression of the vertebral body below. This is unstable, and it is frequently associated with neurologic damage.
3. Posterior dislocation: This is a high-energy, unstable injury.

Physiologic wedging and Scheuermann's disease may mimic vertebral fractures in the thoracic spine. Physiologic wedging

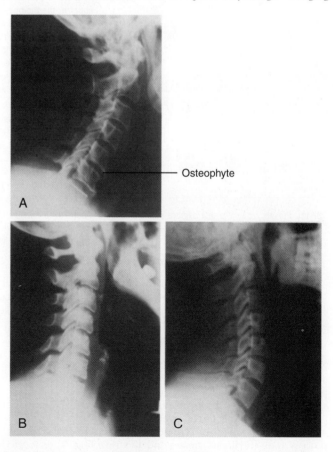

Figure 10.13   Lateral radiograph of the cervical spine. *A,* A normal curve showing osteophytic lipping. *B,* The cervical spine in flexion. *C,* The cervical spine in extension. (From Magee DJ: Orthopedic Physical Assessment, 4th ed. Philadelphia, WB Saunders, 2002, p 171.)

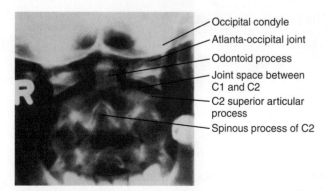

Figure 10.12   A through-the-mouth radiograph. (From Magee DJ: Orthopedic Physical Assessment, 4th ed. Philadelphia, WB Saunders, 2002, p 173.)

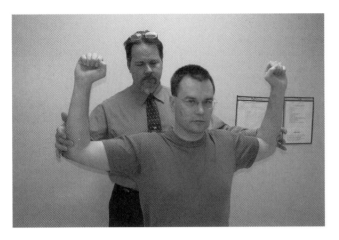

Figure 10.14 The Roos test.

occurs in the lower thoracic spine between T-8 and T-12. Scheuermann's disease involves the abnormal growth of cartilage with a weakening of the vertebral end plates. Currently, computed tomography scanning is the most effective method for examining the extent of the bony injury in the spine, and magnetic resonance imaging is the imaging modality of choice for patients with a neurologic deficit.

Kyphosis represents spinal deformity with anteroposterior angulation, and scoliosis represents lateral displacement or curvature of the spine. However, both of these may cause severe rib distortion. The severity of these two conditions is defined by the measurement of the Cobb angle of curvature, which is formed by the limbs of the convex primary curvature. The Cobb angle is defined by the relationship between two lines that are drawn parallel to the top and bottom of the vertebral bodies at the beginning and end of the curve. A scoliotic curve exists when this angle measures at least 10 degrees. Curves are considered significant they are if greater than 25 to 30 degrees; curves in excess of 45

to 50 degrees are considered severe, and they often require more aggressive treatment.

The term *thoracic outlet syndrome* refers to the symptoms that are associated with the compression of the blood vessels and nerves, which pass from the neck and thorax to the arm in the space between the rib cage and the clavicle. Patients may experience pain in the shoulder, arm, or hand. In addition, patients may develop paresthesias, loss of dexterity, cold intolerance, and headache. The elevated arm stress test or Roos' test may be used to evaluate for thoracic outlet syndrome **(Figure 10.14).** To perform this test, the patient sits with the arms abducted 90 degrees from the thorax and the elbows flexed 90 degrees (see Table 10.7). The patient then opens and closes the hands for 3 minutes. Patients with thoracic outlet syndrome cannot continue this for 3 minutes because of the reproduction of symptoms. Next, Adson's test is used to test for the impingement of vascular structures at the thoracic outlet. **(Figure 10.15).** During this test, the patient's arm is gradually elevated in an abduction arc while the examiner's fingers are held on the patient's radial pulse. As the arm is externally rotated and extended, the patient rotates and extends the head toward the arm being tested. The syndrome is often seen in patients who engage in repetitive motions that place the shoulder at the extreme of abduction and external rotation (e.g., athletes who participate in sports such as swimming, water polo, baseball, and tennis).

REFERENCES

1. Cook C, Brismee J, Sizer P: Identifiers suggestive of clinical spine instability: a Delphi study of physical therapists. Phys Ther 2005;85:895-906.
2. Al-Khateeb H, Oussedik S: The management and treatment of cervical spine injuries. Hosp Med 2005;66:389-395.
3. Levy H: Cervical pain syndromes: primary care diagnosis. Compr Ther 2000; 26(2):82-88.
4. Antonaci F, Ghirmai S, Bono G, Nappi G: Current methods for cervical spine movement evaluation. Clin Exp Rheumatol 2000;Mar-Apr:S45-S52.
5. Magee DJ: Orthopedic Physical Assessment, 4th ed. Philadelphia, WB Saunders, 2002.
6. Vaccaro A, Watkins B, Albert T, et al: Cervical spine injuries in athletes: current return-to-play criteria. Orthopedics 2001;24:699-703.
7. Tong H, Haig A, Yamakawa K: The Spurling test and cervical radiculopathy. Spine 2002;27:156-159.
8. Wainner R, Fritz J, Irrgang J, et al: Reliability and diagnostic accuracy of the clinical examination and patient self-report measures for cervical radiculopathy. Spine 2003;28:52-62.
9. Viikari-Juntura E, Porras M, Lassonen E: Validity of clinical tests in the diagnosis of root compression in cervical disc disease. Spine 1989;14:253-257.
10. Uitvlugt G, Indenbaum S: Clinical assessment of atlantoaxial instability using the Sharp-Purser test. Arthritis Rheum 1988;31:918-922.
11. Shapiro S, Abel T, Rodgers R: Traumatic thoracic spinal fracture dislocation with minimal or no cord injury. J Neurosurg 2002;96:333-337.

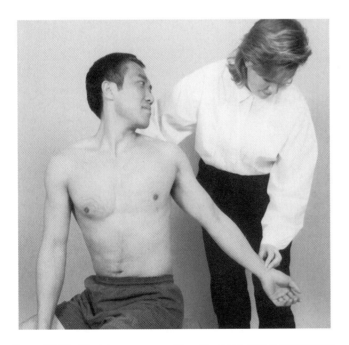

Figure 10.15 The Adson maneuver. (From Magee DJ: Orthopedic Physical Assessment, 4th ed. Philadelphia, WB Saunders, 2002, p 288.)

Physical Examination of the Lumbar Spine

Philip Ham, DO, and James D. Leiber, DO

KEY POINTS

- Low back pain is extremely common.
- The most consistent predictor of back injury is a history of back injury.
- Musculoligamentous sprains and strains are the most common causes of low back pain.
- Alarm symptoms can predict a life-threatening situation.
- The most important test is the straight leg raise.

INTRODUCTION

Low back pain (LBP) is an extremely common condition with major economic significance.[1] It is second only to the common cold as a cause for primary office visits, with an incidence at 5% annually.[2] Approximately 80% of the general population will have LBP at least once during their lifetime. It occurs in roughly 25% of the working population each year, and 14% of adults experience LBP that lasts for more than 2 weeks each year.[1] It is the fifth leading reason for medical office visits in the United States, and it is the leading cause of work-related disability. Direct medical costs as a result of LBP exceed $25 billion per year.[2] Approximately 75% of workers' compensation payments go to patients with LBP.[3,4]

LBP occurs most frequently in patients who are between 20 and 40 years of age, but it is more severe among older patients. High-risk jobs for this condition include miscellaneous labor, garbage collection, warehouse work, and nursing: basically, any job with extensive lifting, twisting, bending, or reaching. Studies show no strong association between LBP and sex, height, weight, or physical fitness.[1]

Participation in some leisure sports and attaining a good level of physical and aerobic fitness may be protective against LBP. In athletes, regardless of the sport, musculoligamentous sprains and strains are the most common cause of LBP.[5] However, skeletally immature athletes are also at a greater risk for occult fractures, spondylolysis, spondylolisthesis, scoliosis, tumors, and infections.[6] Younger athletes who participate in sports that require repetitive hyperextension maneuvers such as gymnastics, diving, figure skating, wrestling, and football may be at higher risk for the development of spondylolysis.[7,8]

Acute to chronic low back pain

Prognostic factors to help identify the subgroup of patients that is more likely to transition from acute to chronic LBP have been investigated. Some genetic information regarding predisposition to the development of lumbar disc disease is emerging, but much more study is required before it becomes clinically useful.[9] A systematic review of psychological risk factors for the development of chronic back pain showed a clear link with the transition from acute to chronic pain disability. Psychosocial variables generally have a greater impact than biomedical or biomechanical factors on back pain disability. Specific attitudes, cognitive styles, and fear-avoidance beliefs all have strong evidence for predicting this transition[10] (LOE: B). However, this has not been investigated fully in athletes. In addition, it is difficult to extrapolate from general workforce data in this regard because athletes may actually have a disincentive to report their pain as a result of the risk of losing playing time, monetary compensation, or scholarship opportunities.[8,11] One study found no relationship of psychosocial factors (limited to satisfaction with coach or teammates) to the onset of LBP[12] (LOE: B).

Risks

The preparticipation evaluation is used to identify athletes who are at risk of injury. Ideally, after these individuals have been identified, appropriate interventions can be made to decrease the likelihood of injury. The most consistent predictor of back injury appears to be a history of low back injury. Greene and colleagues[13] performed a prospective cohort study of 679 varsity athletes who were surveyed at a 1-year follow-up period; of these, 6.8% sustained a low back injury, and there was no difference in incidence between athletes involved in contact sports and those involved in noncontact sports. Of these athletes, those with a history of low back injury were three times more likely to sustain such an injury[13] (LOE: B).

Many other potential risk factors have been investigated. For example, smoking during adolescence seems to be a risk factor for the development of LBP.[14] However, a large population-based study of adolescent and adult monozygotic twins showed that the relationship was probably not causal[14] (LOE: B).

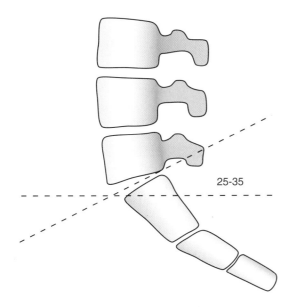

Figure 11.1 Ferguson's angle.

ANATOMY

A working knowledge of the lower back anatomy and biomechanics is a valuable tool when investigating LBP. There are five lumbar vertebrae that are distinguishable by their quadrangular spinous processes. They form a lordotic angle called *Ferguson's angle* **(Figure 11.1),** which averages 41 to 43 degrees. Their main motion is flexion and extension, along with minimal side bending. The large cross-sectional area of the lumbar vertebrae is built to sustain longitudinal loads **(Figure 11.2).** Nerve roots in the lumbar spine exit the inter-vertebral foramen below the corresponding segment but above the intervertebral disc, which is important when disc herniation is being considered **(Figure 11.3).** The first vertebra is named L1, and subsequent vertebrae follow in order. An individual vertebral unit consists of two vertebrae that sandwich a disk; the first vertebra names the unit. An important landmark to consider is the L4-L5 intervertebral disk, which is at the level of the iliac crest. As an example, the L4 vertebral unit would consist of L4, the intervertebral disk, and L5, and this can be further divided coronally into three elements (anterior, middle, and posterior). This anatomic division can be helpful when addressing the cause of a patient's back pain.[15]

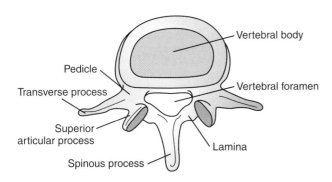

Figure 11.2 Lumbar vertebrae.

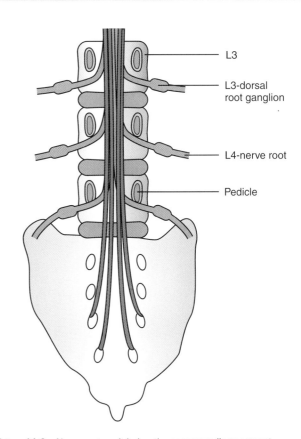

Figure 11.3 Nerve roots exit below the corresponding segment.

Vertebral anterior element

The major component of the anterior element is the vertebral body, which is wider transversely than it is in the anteroposterior dimension **(Figure 11.4).** It is also higher in the front than in the back, which creates a posterior facing wedge that helps maintain lumbar lordosis. The vertebral body is supported anteriorly by the anterior longitudinal ligament, which prevents hyperextension. It is further supported posteriorly by the posterior longitudinal ligament, which helps prevent hyperflexion (along with other ligaments and fascial attachments).[16] The intervertebral disk is composed of a central nucleus pulposus that consists of a colloidal gel that is approximately 80% water.[15] It is surrounded by the annulus fibrosus, which is a fibrous capsule that contains fibers that are arranged obliquely and that alternate in opposite directions for each layer, thus offering resistance to torsional stresses.[16] Because it is thinner posteriorly than anteriorly (most pronounced at L5-S1), disks preferentially herniate in this direction.[1] This disk will lose water within a few minutes when a compressive load is applied, but the water is typically restored when the load is removed. Therefore, with aging, the disk's capacity as a shock absorber is reduced as it loses resilience to return to its full height.[15]

The anterior element can be the source of pain from compression fractures of the vertebral body, disk herniations that result in pressure on the thecal sac, annulus fibrosus tears, infection (e.g., osteomyelitis or diskitis), or vascular causes (e.g., abdominal aneurysms).[15-17]

Vertebral middle element

The middle element consists of the spinal canal, the meninges, the spinal cord, and the nerves. These elements can be the source of pain in a variety of conditions, including compression of the spinal cord or nerve roots intrinsically from intradural tumors or

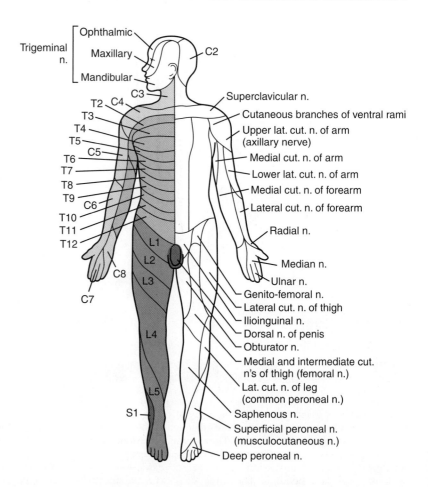

Figure 11.4 Anterior dermatomes. (Drawing by Jennifer Ham, OD.)

extrinsically from metastatic tumors, meningeal infections, herniated disks, osteophytic bone spurs, or spinal canal stenosis. Visceral disease may be referred to the spine via viscerosomatic reflexes.[15]

Vertebral posterior element

The posterior element consists of the spinous process, the transverse process, the lamina, the pedicles, the ligaments, the joint capsules, and the facet joints **(Figure 11.5).** Posterior muscular attachments occur primarily to these elements. It is in this region that the cause of most back pain is found.

Pain can occur in this region as a result of fractures (e.g., spondylolysis), spondylolisthesis, facet arthropathy that results in nerve root impingement, disk herniations, acute strains or sprains, chronic repetitive microtrauma that results in trigger points or myofascial pain syndromes, and somatic dysfunctions.[18,19] If one considers more superficial structures as part of the posterior element, then fibrofatty nodules, which are also known as *back mice,* may be the source of a patient's LBP; these likely result from chronic abnormal movement patterns.[15] In addition, herpes zoster can cause pain in the lumbar region that mimics LBP before or during rash development as well as in the form of a postherpetic neuralgia.[20]

Facets

The five lumbar vertebrae are controlled by the facet joints, which allow for minimal rotation. Injury, degeneration, or trauma to the facets may lead to spondylosis (the degeneration of the joints), spondylolysis (a defect in the par interarticularis), or spondylolisthesis (the forward displacement of one vertebrae over the other).[21]

Intervertebral disks

Intervertebral disks act as shock absorbers between vertebrae, and they separate vertebrae, thus allowing for functional movement between each and a space for the nerve roots to venture out of the spinal cord through the intervertebral foramina.[21] Disk degeneration (i.e., degenerative disk disease) and a loss of hydrophilic support results in the transfer of weight bearing and rotational loads to the facet joints; this may produce facet joint inflammation, arthropathy, and a degeneration cascade in the lumbar spine.[22] Disk pressure is maximally reduced by standing in a natural lordotic posture. Increased disk pressure can result in herniations of the nucleus pulposus (typically posterolaterally) into the vertebral body.

Lower extremities

The lumbar spine is supported by the lower extremities. Therefore, poor conditioning of the lower extremities places an athlete at greater risk for low back injury. An example would be fatigue of the lower extremities, which can lead to improper body mechanics such as keeping the knees straight and bending at the waist while trying to lift an object from the floor.[2]

Lumbar segmental mechanics

The alignment of the facets of the lumbar vertebrae in L1-L5 allows for a normal amount of sagittal plane (flexion/extension) and coronal plane (lateral side bending) movement at each vertebral level but minimal horizontal plane (rotation) movement, with the exception of L5-S1 junction, which permits a greater degree of rotation. The orientation of the facets results in both neutral and

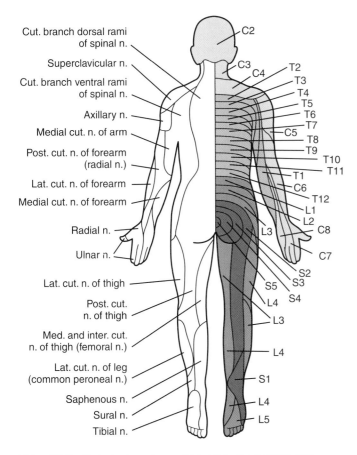

Cut. branch dorsal rami of spinal n.
Superclavicular n.
Cut. branch ventral rami of spinal n.
Axillary n.
Medial cut. n. of arm
Post. cut. n. of forearm (radial n.)
Lat. cut. n. of forearm
Medial cut. n. of forearm
Radial n.
Ulnar n.
Lat. cut. n. of thigh
Post. cut. n. of thigh
Med. and inter. cut. n. of thigh (femoral n.)
Lat. cut. n. of leg (common peroneal n.)
Saphenous n.
Sural n.
Tibial n.

Figure 11.5 Posterior dermatomes. (Drawing by Jennifer Ham, OD.)

non-neutral mechanics. When the spine is in a neutral position, side bending and rotation of the vertebrae should occur to opposite sides. However, in the non-neutral position, whether flexed or extended, the side-bending and rotation components occur to the same side.

With this basic understanding and practiced palpatory skills, specific assessments can be made to identify lumbar facets that are either remaining closed inappropriately or that are unable to fully close as expected. A segment that is dysfunctional in its movement is associated with a variety of identified neural reflexes, depending on the location, acuity, or chronicity of the problem. In the lumbar spine, sympathetic nerves associated with the nerve root can play a part in somatic–visceral, visceral–somatic, or somatic–somatic reflexes.[23] A cascade of biomechanical compensation and adaptation can ensue as time passes without correction of the segmental dysfunction.

HISTORY

The history is the most important part of the initial examination. Alarm symptoms known as *red flags* can be easily identified, and these may signify possible serious illnesses (infection or malignancy) that require urgent intervention.[1] Fever, malaise, and the inability to establish a position of comfort suggest conditions such as diskitis, osteomyelitis, or malignancy. Bowel or bladder dysfunction, saddle anesthesia, and progressive neurologic deficits may indicate cauda equina syndrome or nerve root compression and the need for emergency lumbar decompression.[2] Unremitting pain that is incompletely relieved by lying down or that is constant at night may indicate neoplasm or infection. It is also important to

watch for immunosuppression, intravenous drug use, and urinary tract or other infections.[1]

Pain quality, location, radiation, and exacerbating or relieving factors should be considered. Pain characterization and the determination of the presence or absence of sciatica are second only to the red flags in historical importance.[1] As outlined previously, an anatomic division of the vertebrae into anterior, middle, and posterior elements can be helpful for organizing a strong differential diagnosis.

Malignancy

In one study, 13 of 1975 patients who presented with LBP had an underlying malignancy.[9] Historical clues that suggest underlying malignancy (incidence in LBP, 0.7%) include the following: 50 years of age or older (positive likelihood ratio [+LR], 2.7; negative likelihood ratio [−LR], 0.32); history of previous cancer (+LR, 14.7; −LR, 0.70); unexplained weight loss (+LR, 2.7; -LR, 0.90); failure to improve after 1 month of therapy (+LR, 3.0; −LR, 0.77); no relief with bed rest (+LR, 1.7; −LR, 0.21); and duration of pain of 1 month or more (+LR, 2.6; −LR, 0.62) (LOE: B). Laboratory evaluation can be initiated with a complete blood count, erythrocyte sedimentation rate, urinalysis, and any other laboratory tests that are clinically indicated. Radiography, bone scanning, computed tomography scanning, or magnetic resonance imaging may help confirm or rule out one's clinical suspicion. If evidence of serious disease is uncovered, appropriate consultation is warranted (LOE: B).[24]

Spinal infection

Spinal infections (incidence, 0.01%) are suggested by the following red flags: fever (sensitivity, 0.27 to 0.83; specificity, 0.98) and spine tenderness (sensitivity, 0.86; specificity, 0.60). Other clues may be recent bacterial infection, intravenous drug use, and immunosuppression. Evaluation can proceed as outlined previously for suspicion of underlying cancer (LOE: B).[24-26]

Neurologic causes

Nerve root pain, peripheral nerve pain, and discogenic pain present differently. Nerve root pain is typical sharp and shooting; it is often increased by coughing, straining, standing, or sitting, and it is usually relieved by lying down, although only briefly. Peripheral nerve or lumbosacral plexus pain tends to be burning, like a "pins-and-needles," asleep, or numb quality. Discogenic pain is worsened with lumbar flexion.[1]

More than 95% of disc herniations affect the L4-5 or L5-S1 interspace.[27,28] Remember, a herniated disc in the lumbar vertebrae will affect the nerve root of the vertebrae below. For example, a disc herniation at L4-L5 will affect the S1 nerve root (see Figure 11.1). Classic features of disc herniation are sharp, burning, or aching pain in the buttock and paresthesias that radiate in a radicular pattern. A history of persistent leg numbness or weakness further increases the likelihood of neurologic involvement. If the athlete endorses dermatome-specific radicular symptoms that radiate below the knee, then disc herniation is highly likely (sensitivity, 0.95; specificity, 0.88) (LOE: B).[25,29]

Other causes of radicular pain include neoplasm, entrapment neuropathy, myofascial pain syndromes, trochanteric bursitis, endometriosis, diabetic radiculoneuropathy, shingles, the entrapment of the sciatic nerve by the piriformis muscle, and spinal stenosis.[1]

The hallmark of spinal stenosis is neurogenic claudication with symptoms of pain radiating down the buttock, thigh, and lower legs that is improved with lumbar spine flexion because forward flexion opens the foramina.[30] The possibility of spinal stenosis should be considered in athletes who are more than 65 years of age (+LR, 2.5; −LR, 0.33) if the pain endorses neurogenic claudication (sensitivity, 0.60; specificity, N/A), worsens with lumbar extension, and improves when the patient is seated (+LR, 3.1; −LR, 0.58). A wide-based gait noted on observation has a +LR of 14.3. Magnetic resonance imaging or computed tomography scanning can effectively confirm or rule out central stenosis[25,26] (LOE: B).

Bone injury

Thoracolumbar fractures typically present as back pain with segmental radiation in the distribution of the contiguous nerve roots. Sitting often aggravates the pain, and muscle spasm may disturb sleep. Other contributing factors are a history of trauma, corticosteroid use, osteoporosis, and an age of more than 70 years.[1] Compression fractures (incidence, 0.3%) should also be considered in the following groups of patients: those 50 years of age and older (+LR, 2.2, 5.5; −LR, 0.26, 0.81), those with a history of recent trauma (+LR, 2.0; −LR, 0.82), those with long-term corticosteroid use (+LR, 12.0; −LR, 0.94), and those with a history of osteoporosis[26] (LOE: B). Other bony causes of LBP include spondylosis, spondylolysis, and spondylolisthesis. Lumbar spine injuries are discussed further in Chapter 24.

Sprains and strains

Simple sprains and strains will typically present as a nonspecific dull ache in the low back, buttock, or posterior lateral thigh, sometimes with radiation. This pain will typically be worsened with prolonged standing or sitting.[1]

Myofascial pain

Myofascial LBP and fibromyalgia may present as diffuse LBP of gradual onset that worsens after sitting or resting, that is aggravated by cold, and that is relieved by warmth and movement. There is often stiffness and limited range of motion as well as a sensation of tightness in the back. Bilateral leg pain and paresthesia may occur. Tenderness is present within the affected muscle and soft tissues and often within the sacroiliac joint.

Rheumatoid

In a young athletic population, seronegative spondyloarthropathies (e.g., ankylosing spondylitis, Reiter's syndrome, psoriatic arthritis; incidence, 0.3%) should be considered. Patients characteristically have an onset of symptoms before the age of 40 years (+LR, 1.0; −LR, 0.0); they have an insidious onset of pain that lasts for more than 3 months (+LR, 1.5; −LR, 0.54), and they complain of morning back stiffness (+LR, 1.6; −LR, 0.61) that improves with movement and exercise. Radiographic evidence of sacroiliitis is often seen, as is an elevated sedimentation rate and C-reactive protein (LOE: B).[17,23]

PHYSICAL EXAMINATION

Inspection

A screening assessment can begin with simply observing the athlete in a standing position for posture and landmark asymmetries. Posture is best noted from the lateral perspective. Observe for an overall leaning (forward or backward) of the stance. This can begin to provide clues that may help focus further testing. For example, a relatively forward-bent posture may suggest a bilateral psoas muscle spasm or the protection of a painful area that worsens with extension (as in spondylolysis). Increased lumbar

lordosis (anterior pelvic tilt) may indicate a relative increase in hip flexor (iliopsoas and rectus femoris) to hip extensor (gluteus maximus and hamstring) strength and a weak abdominal musculature, whereas excessively tight hamstrings may cause a posterior pelvic tilt and a relatively decreased lumbar lordosis. Posteriorly, bilateral landmarks that are often used to determine symmetry are the mastoid process, the acromioclavicular joint, the inferior angle of the scapula, iliac crest heights, posterior iliac spines (PSISs), ischial tuberosities, and femoral heads. Observe for evidence of asymmetric muscular bulk and tone.

Observe for body type and gait alterations. Anteriorly, the head should be straight on the shoulders, with the nose in line with the manubrium, the sternum, and the umbilicus. The shoulders and clavicle should be even, although the dominant shoulder is typically lower. Iliac crest heights should be level; if they are not, there may be a leg-length discrepancy caused by altered bone length, a pronated foot, or a rotated pelvis. The anterior superior iliac spines should be level with the patellae, and the lower limbs should face straight ahead. The medial and lateral malleoli should be level.[21]

Viewing the patient from the side, the earlobes should be in line with the tip of the shoulder and the iliac crest. The lumbar spine should have a normal curve, without hyperlordosis or kyphosis. Posteriorly, the curvature of the spine should be free of scoliosis, and the PSISs should be level.[21]

Observe the skin for tufts of hair that are indicative of spina bifida occulta and for café-au-lait spots that are indicative of neurofibromatosis or collagen vascular disease.

Range of motion

Very little movement takes place in the lumbar spine because of the size of the vertebrae, the tightness of the ligaments, and the shape of the facets. What movement there is mostly takes place between L4-L5 and L5-S1.[21] Lumbar range of motion values may be helpful for getting an overall sense of flexibility and for determining change during rehabilitation programs. Range of motion should be assessed in the sagittal (flexion/extension), coronal (lateral side bending), and horizontal (rotation) planes. Although the spine flexibility of persons with LBP does not correlate with disability, reduced spinal mobility seems to be a negative predictor for successful rehabilitation. Be on the lookout for possible causes of decreased range of motion, such as pain, stiffness, and spasm.[15,17,31,32]

Lumbar forward flexibility can be determined with the use of the fingertip-to-floor test **(Table 11.1).** Have the athlete bend forward as far as possible while maintaining the knees, arms, and fingers in full extension. If the athlete bends at the knees while flexing, watch for tight hamstrings and nerve root symptoms. Normal forward flexion is between 40 and 60 degrees, normal extension is between 20 and 35 degrees, and normal side flexion is between 15 and 20 degrees. Pain while side flexing to the affected side could indicate an intra-articular lesion. Disc herniation commonly presents as increased pain with radiation down the affected side while forward or side flexing. Have the athlete combine extension and rotation. If this increases the pain, facet syndrome may be present.

Table 11.1 Average Range of Motion with Fingertip-to-Floor Test in the Healthy Adult Spine

Lumbar forward flexion	55.4 degrees
Lumbar extension	23.1 degrees
Lumbar lateral flexion	22.2 degrees
Lumbar rotation	13.6 degrees

From Alvarez DJ, Rockwell PG: Am Fam Physician 2002;65(4):653-660.

Table 11.2 Muscle Strength and Its Level of Nerve Root Innervation

Hip adduction	L1 and L2
Hip flexion	L2 and L3
Hip extension	S1 and S2
Knee flexion	L5 and S1
Knee extension	L3 and L4
Ankle dorsiflexion	L4
Plantar flexion	S1
Ankle inversion	L5
Ankle eversion	S1
Toe flexion	S1
Toe extension	L5

From Magee DJ: The lumbar spine. In Orthopedic Physical Assessment, 3rd ed. Philadelphia, WB Saunders, 1997.

Neurologic testing

A lower-extremity neurologic examination is an essential component of the lumbar spine evaluation. This examination should include the patella, the medial hamstring, the Achilles reflexes, a sensory examination, and motor testing.

Both sides should be compared, and the dermatomes of L1 through the first sacral dermatome (S1) can be tested by determining the patient's appreciation of a pinprick (or of a light touch, although this is less sensitive). Hoppenfeld[33] described a pattern that is relatively easy to remember. The anterior thigh is divided equally, with three lines going from superolateral to inferomedial, and the third line crosses the patella. The L1, L2, and L3 dermatomes are represented in these three regions when going from superior to inferior, respectively. A line drawn from the patella to the medial aspect of the big toe divides the L4 and L5 dermatomes. L4 is on the medial aspect of this line, and L5 is located lateral to this line. S1 is located on the lateralmost part of the foot.[15]

A single nerve root lesion usually causes only mild hypalgesia because there is a wide overlap of root distributions. Thus, the examiner may be unable to detect a sensory deficit. The great toe may be more specific for detecting L5 sensation. The lateral malleolus and the posterolateral foot may be more reliable for testing S1 sensation. Sensitivity and specificity are 0.50 each.[1]

After the sensory examination, motor testing is performed **(Tables 11.2 and 11.3).** Challenging the patient's maximal strength in both extremities can test the gross integrity of the motor nerves of the lumbar plexus. A simple method is to test the strength to resistance in flexion and extension at the hip, knee, ankle, and big toe as well as to test eversion and inversion at the ankle. The following

Table 11.3 Tendon Reflexes and Their Level of Nerve Root Innervation

Patellar	L3-L4
Medial hamstring	L5-S1
Lateral hamstring	S1-S2
Posterior tibial	L4-L5
Achilles	S1-S2

From Lehrich JR, Katz JN, Sheon RP: Approach to the diagnosis and evaluation of low back pain in adults, UpToDate Version 12.2 (online database): Available at www.uptodate.com. Accessed April 25, 2007; Magee DJ: The lumbar spine. In Orthopedic Physical Assessment, 3rd ed. Philadelphia, WB Saunders, 1997.

spinal nerves are tested with the muscle is in its actively shortened position: hip adduction (L1 and L2), hip flexion (L2 and L3), and hip extension (S1 and S2); knee flexion (L5 and S1) and extension (L3 and L4); ankle dorsiflexion (L4), plantar flexion (S1), inversion (L5), and eversion (S1); and toe flexion (S1) and extension (L5). Deep tendon reflexes can be used to test L4 (patella), L5 (medial hamstring), and S1 (Achilles).[15,34] The impingement of L3 or L4 is associated with a depressed knee jerk, whereas the impingement of S1 is associated with a depressed ankle jerk (sensitivity, 0.5; specificity, 0.6).[1]

PALPATION

Palpation and articular motion testing

Palpating for tissue texture abnormalities and assessing individual segment motion restrictions in the lumbar, thoracic, and cervical spines as well as in the pelvis, sacrum, and ribs allows the clinician to target treatment with the goal of restoring normal joint motion throughout the integrated spinal unit. Please see Chapter 34 for further review of this important skill.

Palpation of the paraspinal muscles may reveal tenderness or tissue texture changes that are indicative of muscle spasms or trigger points. Palpating the spinous processes may reveal tenderness that is indicative of subluxation or even fracture. A spinous process step deformity may indicate spondylolisthesis, and muscle tenderness may be caused by nerve root irritation (calf, S1; anterior tibial muscles, L5; quadriceps, L4).[1]

Palpation and trigger points

Trigger points are focal, discrete, hyperirritable spots that are located in taut bands of skeletal muscle. They are ubiquitous in the population, they can be found in nearly any muscle, and, by some accounts, they are responsible for the majority of chronic pain syndromes. It has been reported that the most commonly overlooked causes of myogenic LBP are trigger points in the quadratus lumborum. Other common myofascial trigger points occur in the following areas: the piriformis, the iliopsoas, the erector spinae, the rotatores, the multifidi, and the gluteus maximus, medius, and minimus muscles. Trigger points are detected when a suspicious muscle is palpated perpendicularly along the long axis of the muscle using the fingertips or, in some instances, a pincer grasp. Classic findings are the "jump sign," a wincing or voluntary withdrawal response by the patient, and a local twitch of the taut band. Patterns of referred pain can project peripherally and centrally, or they may be primarily localized. Mechanical and systemic perpetuating factors may include the following: lack of exercise, postural strains, muscle chilling, psychological stress, vitamin D deficiency, leg-length discrepancy, muscle overload, and a prolonged shortened position of a muscle (e.g., a long car ride with the hip maintained in external rotation that results in a sustained shortened piriformis muscle).[15,35,36]

SPECIAL TESTS

Seated flexion test (Figure 11.6)

This test evaluates for somatic dysfunction of the sacrum by assessing sacroiliac motion. The patient is in a seated position. The physician should hook his or her thumbs under the PSIS. The patient should slowly flex forward and attempt to touch his or her toes. The PSIS on the left and the right should start out at equal levels and remain equal throughout flexion. If one side moves and the other side does not, somatic dysfunction of the sacrum is on the side of the superior PSIS.

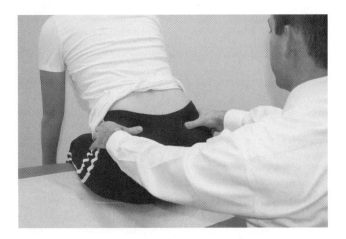

Figure 11.6 Seated flexion test/sacroiliac joint evaluation.

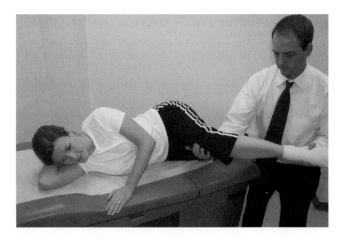

Figure 11.8 Modified straight leg raise test.

Standing flexion test

This test evaluates for somatic dysfunction of the pelvis by assessing iliosacral motion. With the patient standing, the physician should hook his or her thumbs under the PSIS. The patient should slowly flex forward and attempt to touch his or her toes. If one side moves and the other side does not, somatic dysfunction of the pelvis (more specifically in the innominate) is on the side of the superior PSIS. A sacral dysfunction would show a discrepancy during standing flexion, whereas a pelvic dysfunction would be evident by a discrepancy during seated flexion.

Straight leg raise test or Lasègue's test

The straight leg raise test is used to assess for the impingement of a nerve root from a herniated disc or from a space-occupying lesion by stretching that root. The patient should be in a supine position. The physician flexes the patient's hip with the patient's knee extended until the patient complains of pain or tightness in the back or the back of the leg. At this point, the physician brings the leg back down until the patient feels no pain. The physician should then dorsiflex the foot (Bragard's test); the neck may also be flexed (Soto–Hall test) **(Figure 11.7).** A positive test elicits pain in the leg, buttock, or back at 60 degrees or less of leg elevation. The pain is typically worsened by dorsiflexion of the ankle or neck flexion, and it is relieved with flexion of the knee and hip. A positive straight leg raise test usually indicates S1 or L5 root irritation. Sensitivity is about 91%, and specificity is 26%. Pain

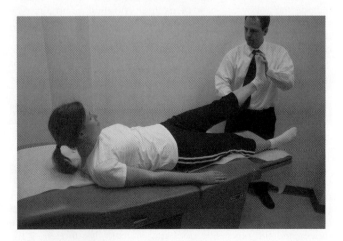

Figure 11.7 Straight leg raise test with Soto–Hall test.

that does not increase with dorsiflexion or neck flexion may indicate a lesion in the lumbosacral, sacroiliac, or hamstring area. Pain on the opposite side could indicate a large spac-occupying lesion.[1,17,37]

Modified straight leg raise test (Figure 11.8)

The patient is in a lateral recumbent position with the unaffected side down. The hip and knee are flexed at 90 degrees, and the knee is then slowly extended. Pain, resistance, or a reproduction of symptoms is a positive test.[21]

Reverse straight leg raise test (Figure 11.9)

This test looks for L3 or L4 root irritation. With the patient in the prone position, each thigh is extended one at a time at the hip joint. Pain over the involved nerve root may be reproduced, regardless of which leg is posteriorly raised.[1,38]

Crossed straight leg raise test

This test is much less sensitive (0.25), but it is also much more specific (0.90 to 0.97) for lumbar disc herniation. The patient should be in a prone position. Increased sciatica on raising the opposite leg with the knee extended is a positive test. This test predicts poor response to conservative therapy. Patients who have a positive crossed straight leg raise test may have a normal myelogram; however, 90% of these patients will be found to have a herniated disc.[1,28]

Prone knee bending test

With the patient in the prone position, the physician flexes the patient's knee as far as possible so that the patient's heel rests against the buttock for 45 to 60 seconds. Pain in the lumbar area, buttock, or posterior thigh may indicate an L2 or L3 nerve root lesion. Pain in the anterior thigh indicates tight quadriceps or femoral nerve tightness.[21]

Kernig–Brudzinski test (Figure 11.10)

This test is used to evaluate for meningeal irritation, dural irritation, or nerve root involvement. Place the patient in the supine position, and then place the patient's hands behind his or her head. Flex the patient's head to the chest, and flex the patient's hip with the leg extended until pain is felt. At this point, flex the knee. If the pain resolves, the test is positive.[21]

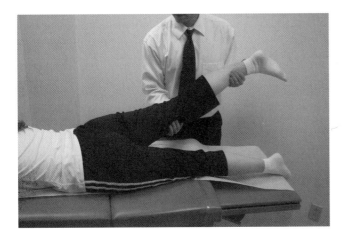

Figure 11.9   Reverse straight leg raise test.

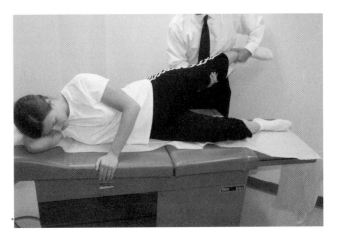

Figure 11.11   Femoral nerve traction test.

Femoral nerve traction test (Figure 11.11)

The patient should be in the lateral recumbent position with the unaffected side down. The unaffected limb should be flexed slightly at the hip and knee, the patient's back should be straight rather than hyperextended, and the head should be flexed. Take the patient's affected limb, and extend the knee while gently extending the hip approximately 15 degrees; this stretches the femoral nerve. Pain radiating down the anterior thigh is a positive test.[21]

Single-leg hyperextension test (stork test) (Figure 11.12)

Spondylolysis should be considered in athletes who are involved in hyperextension activities and who have pain on provocative clinical tests. Have the patient stand on one leg. The patient's lower back should be extended; this stresses the posterior elements, and pain will be greatest on the weight-bearing side, which is on the same side as the spondylolysis. However, it is important to remember that these fractures may be on both sides.[7,16]

Hopping test

Sacral stress fractures may be seen in long-distance runners who have focal sacral pain with a reproduction of the pain during the "hopping test."[7,17] The patient should stand and then hop on the affected leg.

Adam's forward bend test

This test helps screen for scoliosis. With the patient sitting or standing, have the patient bend over at the waist, and examine him or her from behind and from the side, horizontally along the contour of the back. If a rib hump is observed, this suggests a scoliosis curvature of at least 10 degrees, and it should prompt further evaluation with an x-ray.

Quadratus lumborum (Figure 11.13)

With the patient in the lateral recumbent position, have him or her flex the leg that is not to be tested. The tested leg is straight and slightly posterior to the trunk. While stabilizing the twelfth rib, the leg is abducted first to relax the quadratus lumborum, and then the leg is allowed to drop toward the floor for length testing.

Signs of the buttock

With the patient in the supine position, repeat the straight leg raise test. If there is unilateral restriction, flex the knee. If hip flexion increases, the problem is in the hamstrings or the lumbar spine. If hip flexion is still restricted, the examination is positive, and there is likely pathology in the buttock, such as bursitis, a tumor, or an abscess.[21]

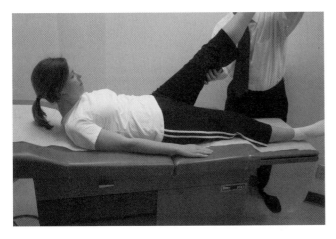

Figure 11.10   Kernig–Brudzinski test.

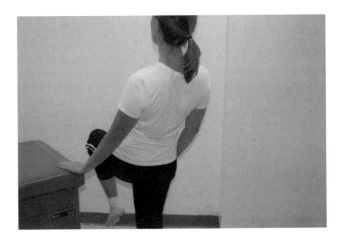

Figure 11.12   Single-leg hyperextension test.

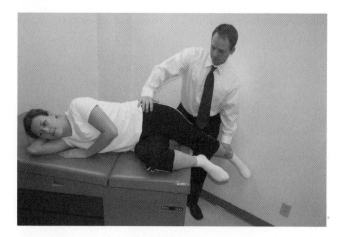

Figure 11.13 Quadratus lumborum range of motion testing.

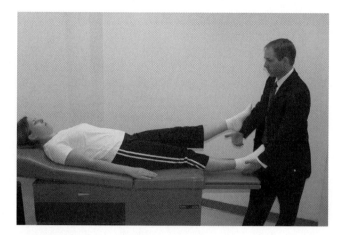

Figure 11.14 Hoover's test.

Bowstring test (cram test)

This test is used to evaluate for sciatic nerve tension. With the patient in the supine position, repeat the straight leg raise test. While maintaining the patient's thigh in the same position, the physician flexes the patient's knee to 20 degrees to reduce the symptoms. Thumb pressure is applied to the popliteal area to reestablish the painful radicular symptoms. If the radicular symptoms are reproduced, then the test is positive.[21]

Flip sign

This test helps distinguish between sciatic pain and lower lumbar spine pain. With the patient seated, have him or her extend the knees. Lay the patient supine, and perform the straight leg raise test. If both tests cause pain in the sciatic nerve distribution, the cause is likely to be sciatic. If only one test is positive, then the lumbar spine is likely the culprit.[21]

Babinski's test

This test is used to evaluate for an upper motor neuron lesion. With the patient sitting, the physician slides a fingernail down the plantar surface of the patient's foot. This should make the big toe flex. If the big toe extends and the other toes abduct, then the test is positive.[21]

Oppenheim's test

This test also tests for an upper motor neuron lesion. The physician slides a fingernail along the crest of the patient's tibia and then evaluates again for a positive Babinski sign.[21] This test is used to test for spinal thecal compression.

Naffziger's test

With the patient in the supine position, the physician gently compresses the jugular veins for 10 seconds. As the patient's face flushes, the patient is asked to cough. If coughing causes pain in the low back, then the spina theca is being compressed, which leads to increased intrathecal pressure. Increased lumbar spine pain with the Valsalva maneuver would indicate the same findings.[21]

Tests for malingering

Inconsistencies in the examinations may be signs of malingering. The next two tests may be helpful for determining whether this is an issue.

Axial loading

With the patient sitting or standing, press down on the top of the patient's head, or rotate the patient's body at the hips or shoulders. These movements should not bring about LBP.[1]

Hoover's test (Figure 11.14)

With the patient in the supine position, the physician places one hand under each calcaneous, with the patient's legs relaxed on the table. The patient should be asked to lift one leg off of the table with the knees straight. The physician should feel pressure under the patient's opposite heel. If no pressure is felt or if the patient does not lift the affected leg, the test is positive. Compare both sides.[21]

Hip special tests

The following special tests of the hip and pelvis should also be included in the low back evaluation: leg-length evaluation, flexion, abduction, and external rotation (FABER)/Patrick's test, Ober's test, Ely test, Thomas' test, and Trendelenburg's test. See Chapter 12 for information about how to perform these maneuvers.

REFERENCES

1. Lehrich JR, Katz JN, Sheon RP: Approach to the diagnosis and evaluation of low back pain in adults, UpToDate Version 12.2 (online database): Available at: www.uptodate.com. Accessed April 25, 2007.
2. Drezner JA, Herring SA: Low-back pain: essential muscle fatigue can cause reflex muscle spasm and pain. Clin Sports Med 1995;14(1):241-265.
3. Klein BP, Jensen RC, Sanderson LM: Assessment of workers' compensation claims for back strains/sprains. J Occup Med 1984;26(6):443-448.
4. Hart LG, Deyo RA, Cherkin DC: Physician office visits for low back pain. Frequency, clinical evaluation, and treatment patterns from a US National Survey. Spine 1995;20(1):11-19.
5. Eismont FJ, Kitchel SH: Thoracolumbar spine in the adult. In DeLee JC, Drez D Jr, Miller MD (eds): DeLee & Drez's Orthopaedic Sports Medicine: Principles and Practice, 2nd ed. Philadelphia, WB Saunders, 2003, pp 1525-1575.
6. Trombino LJ: Back pain in the young athlete. In Lillegard WA, Burcher JD, Rucker KS (eds): Handbook of Sports Medicine, A Symptom-Oriented Approach, 2nd ed. Boston, Butterworth Heinemann, 1999, pp 207-218.
7. Bono CM: Low-back pain in athletes. J Bone Joint Surg Am 2004;86-A(2):382-396.
8. Trainor TJ, Trainor MA: Etiology of low back pain in athletes. Curr Sports Med Rep 2004;3(1):41-46.
9. Sjolie AN, Ljunggren AE: The significance of high lumbar mobility and low lumbar strength for current and future LBP in adolescents. Spine 2001;26:2629-2636.
10. Linton SJ: A review of psychological risk factors in back and neck pain. Spine 2000;25(9):1148-1156.
11. Standaert CJ, Herring SA, Pratt TW: Rehabilitation of the athlete with low back pain. Curr Sports Med Rep 2004;3(1):35-40.
12. Herring SA: Predictors of low back injuries in varsity athletes. Clin J Sport Med 2002;12(4):261.

13. Greene HS, Cholewicki J, Galloway MT, et al: A history of low back injury is a risk factor for recurrent back injuries in varsity athletes. Am J Sports Med 2001;29(6): 795-800.

14. Leboeuf-Yde C, Kyvik KO, Bruun NH: Low back pain and lifestyle. Part I: Smoking. Information from a population-based sample of 29,424 twins. Spine 1998;23(20):2207-2213.

15. Curtis P, Gibbons G, Price J: Fibro-fatty nodules and low back pain. The back mouse masquerade. J Fam Pract 2000;49(4):345-348.

16. Taylor GW: Back pain and injuries in the athlete. In Lillegard WA, Burcher JD, Rucker KS (eds): Handbook of Sports Medicine, A Symptom-Oriented Approach, 2nd ed. Boston, Butterworth Heinemann, 1999, pp 195-206.

17. Drezner JA, Herring SA: Managing low-back pain. Steps to optimize function and hasten return to activity. Phys Sportsmed 2001;29(8):37-43.

18. Barr KP, Griggs M, Cadby T: Lumbar stabilization: core concepts and current literature, part 1. Spine 2005;84(6):473-480.

19. Cholewicki J, Panjabi MM, Khachatryan A: Stabilizing function of trunk flexor-extensor muscles around a neutral spine posture. Spine 1997;22:2207-2212.

20. Shapiro M: Herpes zoster related lumbar radiculopathy. Orthopedics 1996;19(11):976-977.

21. Magee DJ: The lumbar spine. In Magee DJ (ed): Orthopedic Physical Assessment. 3rd ed. Philadelphia, WB Saunders, 1997, pp 362-433.

22. Weinstein SM, Herring SA, Cole A: Rehabilitation of the patient with spinal pain. In DeLisa JA, Gans BM, Bockenek WL (eds): Rehabilitation Medicine: Principles and Practice, 3rd ed. Philadelphia, Lippincott-Raven, 1998.

23. White AA, Panjabi MM: Clinical Biomechanics of the Spine. Philadelphia, JB Lippincott, 1978.

24. Humphreys SC, Eck JC, Hodges SD: Neuroimaging in low back pain. Am Fam Physician 2002;65(11):2299-2306.

25. Harwood MI, Smith BJ: Low back pain: a primary care approach. Clin Fam Pract 2005;7(2):279-303.

26. Jarvik JG, Deyo RA: Diagnostic evaluation of low back pain with emphasis on imaging. Ann Intern Med 2002;137:586-597.

27. Liang M, Komaroff AL: Roentgenograms in primary care patients with acute low back pain: a cost-effectiveness analysis. Arch Intern Med 1982;142(6):1108-1112.

28. Hudgins WR: The crossed straight leg raising test. N Engl J Med 1977;297(20):1127.

29. Beattie PF, Meyers SP, Stratford P, et al: Associations between patient report of symptoms and anatomic impairment visible on lumbar magnetic resonance imaging. Spine 2000;25(7):819-828.

30. Deyo R, Tsui-Wu Y: Descriptive epidemiology of low-back pain and its related medical care in the United States. Spine 1987;12:264-268.

31. Perret C, Poiraudeau S, Fermanian J, et al: Validity, reliability, and responsiveness of the fingertip-to-floor test. Arch Phys Med Rehabil 2001;82(11):1566-1570.

32. McGill SM: Low back exercises: evidence for improving exercise regimens. Phys Ther 1998;78(7):754-765.

33. Hoppenfeld S, Hutton R: Orthopaedic Neurology: A Diagnostic Guide to Neurologic Levels. Philadelphia, Lippincott Williams & Wilkins, 1997.

34. Richardson CA, Snijders CJ, Hides JA, et al: The relation between the transversus abdominis muscles, sacroiliac joint mechanics, and low back pain. Spine 2002;27(4):399-405.

35. Alvarez DJ, Rockwell PG: Trigger points: diagnosis and management. Am Fam Physician 2002;65(4):653-660.

36. Simons DG: Myofascial pain syndrome due to trigger points. In Goodgold J (ed): Rehabilitation Medicine. St. Louis, Mosby, 1988.

37. Deville WL, van der Windt DA, Dzaferagic A, et al: The test of Lasègue: systematic review of the accuracy in diagnosing herniated discs. Spine 2000;25(9):1140-1147.

38. Deyo RA, Rainvelle J, Kent DL: What can the history and physical examination tell us about low back pain? JAMA 1992;268(6):760-765.

Physical Examination of the Hip and Pelvis

Peter H. Seidenberg, MD, FAAFP, and Marc A. Childress, MD

KEY POINTS

- Hip pain can originate from the hip joint, the groin, the surrounding musculature, the sacroiliac joints, the lumbar spine, the abdomen, or the pelvis, which makes this area a "black box" in sports medicine.
- A thorough history and physical can demystify the hip and provide an accurate diagnosis.
- A leg-length evaluation should be included in the hip and pelvis examination.
- Sacroiliac examination techniques include the flexion, abduction, and external rotation test; the supine-to-sit test; the standing flexion test; and Gillet's and Gaenslen's tests.
- The scour or quadrant test is the hip equivalent of McMurray's test for the knee.

INTRODUCTION

Hip and pelvis injuries are commonly seen in sports medicine, particularly among certain groups of athletes, such as dancers, runners, and soccer players.[1] These sports tend to involve a higher degree of force and extremes of movement across the hip, which may predispose the athlete to injury. Among adults who present to primary care physicians with musculoskeletal complaints, approximately 5% to 6% involve the hip. In the pediatric population, this percentage increases to 10% to 24%.[1]

Hip pain is viewed by many as the "black box" of sports medicine. The complexity of the joint itself, coupled with the variety of fashions in which injury or dysfunction can emerge, illustrates the need to begin with a very broad differential diagnosis that includes a wide range of both musculoskeletal and nonmusculoskeletal causes **(Table 12.1).** The ability to conduct a systematic evaluation of the hip and pelvis arms the physician with the tools required to tackle this intimidating area.

ANATOMY

The hip joint has a ball-and-socket configuration that results in an exceptional degree of stability while allowing for significant movement within three separate planes: frontal, sagittal, and transverse. Despite this degree of mobility, the partially spherical articulation between the femoral head and the acetabulum is required to distribute a large amount of pressure during activities of daily living. In fact, it has been calculated that walking and running can transmit up to three to five times the force of the patient's body weight through the hip joint.[2]

The bony joint results from the articulation between the head of the femur and the acetabulum. The acetabulum is derived from portions of three separate bones of the pelvis: the ilium, the ischium, and the pubis. These are often referred to as the *innominate bones*, and they collectively make up the "hip bone." The articular surface of the acetabulum is covered by a layer of cartilage that becomes more prominent at the periphery, which results in the thickened rim or labrum. The labrum also deepens the acetabulum, thus providing additional support to the femoral head. The joint's stability is further augmented by three ligaments that surround the joint capsule and a small ligamentum teres that attaches directly to the femoral head.[3] The innominate bones articulate anteriorly at the symphysis pubis, whereas the posterior portion of the pelvic girdle is completed by the sacrum and the coccyx.

The muscular structure of the joint includes the gluteal region, the lower lumbar area, and many muscles that originate in the pelvis and the lower back but that insert distally on the lower extremity **(Figures 12.1 and 12.2).** For examination purposes, most of these muscles can be grouped by their functional similarities. Flexors, extensors, abductors, adductors, and muscles that control internal and external rotation will all be discussed in more detail.

HISTORY

Patients and physicians may be tempted to focus on only the joint proper as the cause of hip or groin pain; however, pain can originate from many potential sources. Although the articulation of the hip takes place between the head of the femur and the acetabulum, one must also maintain an awareness of the nearby bony and soft-tissue anatomy of the region, including the low back and the pelvis. In the light of the large differential diagnosis (see Table 12.1), it is important during the evaluation to obtain a broad history and to perform a thorough examination before presuming a diagnosis.

Table 12.1 Differential Diagnosis of Hip Pain

Hip/Pelvis	Thigh
Stress fracture of the femoral neck	Muscle strains
	Adductor longus
Pubic ramus fracture	Rectus femoris
Osteitis pubis	Iliopsoas
Legg–Calvé–Perthes disease	Sartorius
	Gracilis
Slipped capital femoral epiphysis	Femoral hernia
	Lymphadenopathy
Avulsion fracture about the pelvis	**Abdomen**
	Lower abdominal wall
Snapping hip	Strain of the rectus abdominis
Acetabular labral tear	Inguinal hernia
Bursitis (iliopectineal, trochanteric)	Ilioinguinal nerve entrapment
	Sports hernia (hockey player's syndrome)
Avascular necrosis	Abdominal organ conditions
Osteoarthritis	Abdominal aortic aneurysm
Synovitis or capsulitis	Appendicitis
Low Back	Diverticulitis
Sacroiliitis	Inflammatory bowel disease
Sacroiliac dysfunction	Pelvic inflammatory disease
Sciatica	Sexually transmitted diseases
Nerve root impingement	Ovarian cyst
Degenerative disc disease	Ectopic pregnancy
Lumbosacral strain	

Adapted from Seidenberg PH, Childress MA: J Musculoskel Med 2005;22(7):337-344.

Similar to other musculoskeletal complaints, the differential diagnosis for hip pain varies dramatically with the age of the patient. As such, it is extremely important to assess both the chronologic and physiologic age of the patient. Apophyseal avulsion fractures occur more commonly among children, adolescents, and young adults in whom the growth plates have not yet closed **(Figure 12.3).** However, the likelihood of these injuries decreases significantly after the patient reaches skeletal maturity.[4] **Table 12.2** lists the apophyseal sites of the hip and the pelvis and the usual age ranges for appearance and fusion. In an older patient, the same mechanism of injury is less likely to produce a bony avulsion; rather, it is more likely to cause injury to the musculotendinous junction.

Other hip disorders, such as slipped capital epiphysis and transient synovitis, occur in children of specific age ranges.[5,6] Thus, the differential diagnosis for pediatric hip and groin complaints changes for different patients, depending on their age. Despite this variability, the evaluation of any patient with hip complaints can be performed systematically with a detailed history and examination.

Symptoms should always be qualified with the array of location, onset, duration, alleviating/aggravating factors, and characterization. Is the pain sharp, dull, burning, or tingling? Is there numbness or weakness? Is there any sense of clicking or snapping? Complaints of "snapping" are common to the hip, and they deserve closer attention to determine the perceived location, the provoking activities, and so on. Has the hip ever "locked?" Does the joint feel restricted? Is there any swelling, bruising, or pain in focal areas?

As with all joint complaints, the examiner must attempt to determine if the injury is acute, chronic, or acute on chronic in nature. Questions about the sport and position that the patient plays, the training regimen, the diet, and the equipment can be extremely

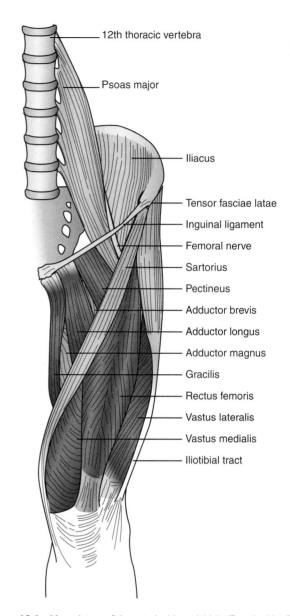

Figure 12.1 Musculature of the anterior hip and thigh. (From Jenkins DB [ed]: Hollinshead's Functional Anatomy of the Limbs and Back, 7th ed. Philadelphia, PA, WB Saunders, 1998, p 257.)

helpful when attempting to clarify the diagnosis in terms of both the victims and the culprits (see Chapter 7) involved in the injury. When did the pain begin? How long has it lasted? Has the pain changed? Has it improved or worsened? If the complaint is easily linked to an acute injury, then understanding the mechanism is imperative. Was the pain noted immediately, such as when a soccer player kicked the ball only to simultaneously meet the foot of an opposing player? Alternatively, did the pain start gradually and increase as the preseason training regimen intensified? Does the pain occur at a certain point during training? Has the marathon runner only noticed pain at mile 3 when she runs on the left side of the street?

The presence of radiating symptoms can be helpful for the diagnosis because the hip area is an obvious hub for nerves to the lower extremities and groin. Pain is the most common presenting complaint, and a clear description of the total distribution of discomfort should be sought. This can include descriptions of large affected areas (e.g., the distribution seen with sciatic nerve impingement)

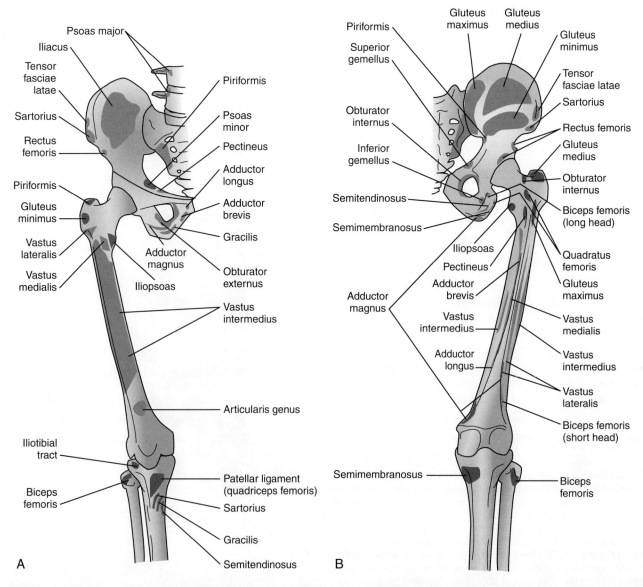

Figure 12.2 *A,* Anterior view of the origins and insertions of the hip and pelvis musculature. *B,* Posterior view of the origins and insertions of the hip and pelvis musculature. (From Jenkins DB [ed]: Hollinshead's Functional Anatomy of the Limbs and Back, 7th ed. Philadelphia, PA, WB Saunders, 1998, pp 259 and 275.)

as well as of small regions (e.g., entrapment of the less considered ilioinguinal nerve). For athletes in whom nerve impingement is suspected, it is important to ask about both weakness and numbness because the two may present independent of one another. In cases in which the complaint is predominantly functional (i.e., quadriceps weakness → femoral nerve, adductor weakness → obturator nerve, and so on), further inquiry is warranted. Areas of focus should include the middle and lower back, the hip, the pelvis, the groin (including the genitalia), the legs, and the feet.[7]

It is critical to know about any previous or concurrent injuries to the back or the lower extremities. Knowledge of the kinetic chain allows the clinician to see how changes in the gait cycle (relative muscular weakness) and attempts to compensate for pain or discomfort in other areas can easily affect the hip joint and its related structures. For this reason, injuries to both the ipsilateral and contralateral leg, knee, lower leg, ankle, or foot can be important.[8]

In the absence of acute trauma, close attention should be paid to constitutional symptoms such as fever, chills, or nausea, which could correlate with an infectious process in the abdominal or

pelvic region. For example, pain in the hip may prove to be a manifestation of appendicitis, pelvic inflammatory disease, or diverticulitis. Likewise, in the pediatric population, fever may suggest transient synovitis of the hip or, worse, a septic joint. A history of weight loss in the face of hip pain can be particularly alarming because the hip and pelvis are common locations for metastatic bony lesions.[9] Medical and medication histories are equally important. For example, if a patient presenting with new-onset hip pain was recently treated with steroids for an unrelated pulmonary issue, then the concern for avascular necrosis of the femoral head would be increased. Likewise, a patient with known osteoporosis would raise a higher suspicion for fracture of the femoral neck.

PHYSICAL EXAMINATION

The evaluation of hip complaints can often begin far before the formal history and physical as the clinician observes the patient walking to the examination room. Issues such as gait, posture, and

Table 12.2 Apophyses of the Hip and Pelvis

Apophysis	Appears	Fuses	Muscle Group
Ischial	12-15	19-25	Hamstrings
ASIS	12-15	16-18	Sartorius
AIIS	12-15	16-18	Rectus femoris
Iliac crest	12-15	15-17	Abdominals
Lesser trochanter	8-12	16-18	Iliopsoas
Greater trochanter	2-5	16-18	Gluteus maximus

Adapted from Anderson SJ: Curr Probl Pediatr Adolesc Health Care 2005;35(4):110-164; Paletta GA Jr, Andrish JT: Clin Sports Med 1995;14:591-628.

obvious deformity can offer quick clues as to the root of a complaint. A visual inspection can help identify muscular atrophy, pelvic obliquity (e.g., leg-length discrepancy, weak supporting musculature, or contractures), and significant scoliotic or lordotic curves.[10] For example, an excessive lordotic curve could be a patient's attempt to maintain balance in the face of flexion contractures of one or both hips.

Range of motion

This facet of the examination should be performed during every evaluation of the hip. The parameters for each movement are fairly well defined **(Table 12.3),** and they can be easily and quickly assessed in the clinical setting. In the supine position, the examiner can test flexion, abduction, adduction, and internal and external rotation. Flexion is best performed with the knees flexed as well so that the full range of hip joint motion will not be limited by hamstring tightness. Abduction and adduction **(Figures 12.4 and 12.5)** are tested by having the patient lay with the legs together and then moving one leg at a time. The degree of movement should be documented at the first sign that the pelvis is beginning to shift.

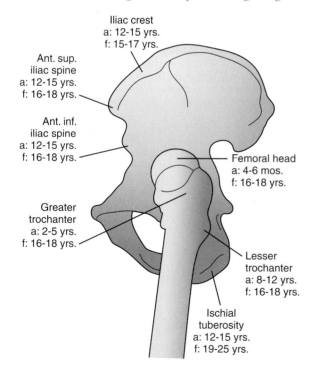

Figure 12.3 Secondary centers of ossification of the hip and pelvis. *a,* Average age of appearance; *f,* average age of fusion. (Redrawn with permission from Paletta GA Jr, Andrish JT: Clin Sports Med 1995;14:591-628.)

For this reason, it is critical that, before either examination, the pelvis should be level and stabilized by the hand of the examiner. Internal and external rotation can be assessed easily in this position by simply turning the foot of each extended leg **(Figure 12.6A and B).** This can also be tested by flexing the patient's knees to 90 degrees and rotating the lower leg around the vertical axis of the femur. If done in this fashion, it is important to remember that, when the lower leg is outwardly rotated, it is the internal rotation of the hip that is being assessed; likewise, with inward rotation of the lower leg, the external rotation of the hip is tested (see Figure 12.6C). Hip extension is best tested with the patient in the prone position. The patient flexes the knee of the leg that is to be examined; the examiner then lifts this leg with one hand while using the other to stabilize the pelvis **(Figure 12.7).**

Palpation

Palpation includes the musculature and the tendon origin and insertion sites both on the pelvis and more distally on the lower extremity, the bursae, the apophyses, the sacroiliac joints, and the pubic symphysis. Careful attention should be paid to any snapping or clicking sensations while guiding the patient through range of motion and special testing. For this reason, it is recommended that whichever hand is not guiding the patient through the desired motions be placed over the hip joint that is being assessed. This can also provide the patient with an added sense of stability because some of the tests can create some slightly precarious positions. Snapping or clicking may be from a relatively benign overlap of a tendon and a bony prominence, or it might be a sign of an intra-articular lesion, such as a loose body.[11] Chapter 30 discusses the causes of a snapping hip in more detail.

Neurologic testing

The neuromuscular examination is an integral part of the evaluation of hip and pelvis complaints. As was discussed previously, the hip and pelvis are foci for nerves that innervate the groin and the lower extremities. For this reason, even in cases in which nerve involvement is not immediately suspected, a basic assessment should still be performed to ensure that a lack of optimal neurologic or muscular function is not the cause or the effect of other hip pathology. Reflex and sensory testing of the distal extremities should be completed, especially in athletes who present with weakness or suspected nerve involvement. Next, strength testing of the cardinal muscle groups is performed, including the flexors (iliopsoas, rectus femoris), the extensors (gluteus maximus, hamstrings), the abductors (gluteus medius and minimus), and the adductors (adductor longus, adductor brevis, adductor magnus, pectineus, gracilis). Flexion strength can be tested by having the patient sit on an examination table with the lower legs hanging over the side (i.e., the knees bent to 90 degrees). The examiner should place a hand over the patient's thigh near the knee and

Table 12.3 Normal Parameters for Hip Range of Motion

Motion	Flexion	Extension	Abduction	Adduction	Internal Rotation	External Rotation
Range in degrees	110-120	0-15	30-50	30	30-40	40-60

Adapted from Seidenberg PH, Childress MA: J Musculoskel Med 2005;22(5):246-254.

instruct the patient to raise the leg off of the table against the examiner's hand. Extension can be evaluated by instructing the patient to assume a prone position and then to lift (extend) the leg off of the surface behind him or her against resistance placed just above the knee as well. Both adduction and abduction can be assessed by having the patient fully extend his or her legs in the supine position. From this position, resistance can be placed outside the malleoli as the patient attempts to separate the legs (abduction) and then along the medial malleoli as the legs are brought back together (adduction). To isolate more subtle deficits in abduction and adduction, it has been found to be helpful to perform the test with the patient lying in a lateral position with the hips in a neutral position and the knees fully extended. The patient then abducts the top leg approximately 30 degrees and resists the examiner's efforts to abduct and then adduct the leg.

SPECIAL TESTS

The examination components described previously can provide a good basis for further evaluation. On the basis of the findings of the history, observation, palpation, and range-of-motion testing, one can often accumulate a number of clues to the diagnosis. The following tests are designed to help the examiner with narrowing down the differential diagnosis. Although there is certainly crossover with regard to the specificity of each examination, patterns of positive and negative findings on these tests are very helpful for identifying particular disorders.

Trendelenburg's sign (Figure 12.8)

Trendelenburg's sign is used to evaluate for gluteus minimus weakness or, less commonly, hip joint instability. This examination involves asking the patient to stand comfortably on both feet and then to stand on one foot without using additional support. In a normal hip, the non—weight-bearing side will be slightly raised or parallel with the weight-bearing side, whereas a positive test results when the pelvis on the opposite side drops. When the body weight is transferred to the single leg, the hip abductors (including the gluteus medius) contract to keep the body in line. Both the weakness of the abductors and the instability of the hip (as a result of the significant increase in the amount of tension on the bony structures) could result in an inability to maintain this abduction, and this would allow the contralateral hip to fall.[12] If the only way that the patient is able to keep the pelvis level is by lateral flexion of the torso, it is considered a compensated positive test (see Figure 12.8C).

The Flexion, ABduction, and External Rotation test

The flexion, abduction, and external rotation (FABER) test is also known as *Patrick's test* or *Jansen's test*, and it is used to better isolate pathology to the hip joint or the sacroiliac joint or to isolate spasm to the iliopsoas muscle. This test is performed on a supine patient who has both legs fully extended and relaxed. The leg on the affected side is flexed, abducted, and externally rotated so that the foot rests on the unaffected leg, around the knee **(Figure 12.9).** The examiner applies gentle downward pressure on the knee of the test leg. With a positive test, the patient will be unable to complete this movement as a result of pain or limitation of mobility (remember to fully assess the range of motion for each individual movement separately as well; if there are known limitations in any of the movements alone, the test can be less specific).[13,14] Broadhurt and Bond[14] found patient pain at the sacroiliac joint while performing the maneuver to have a sensitivity of 0.77 and a specificity of 1.0 for sacroiliac dysfunction (LOE: A).

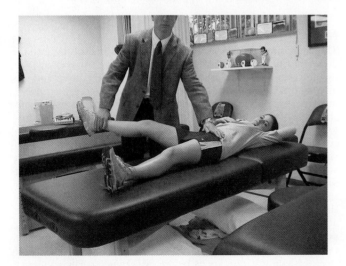

Figure 12.4 Abduction.

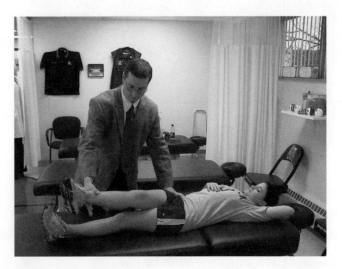

Figure 12.5 Adduction.

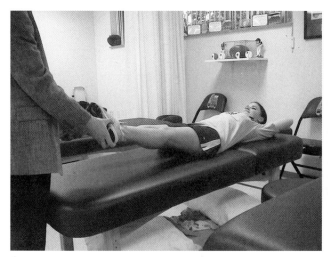

A

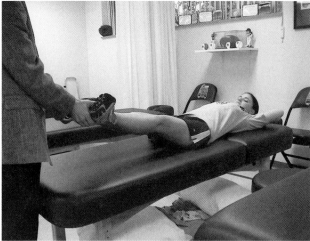

B

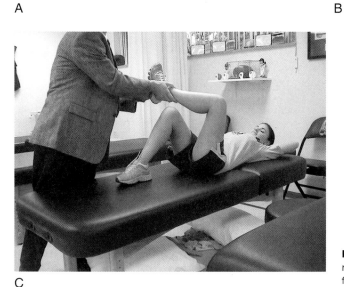

C

Figure 12.6 *A*, Hip internal rotation with the knees extended. *B*, Hip external rotation with the knees extended. *C*, Hip external rotation with the hip and knee in flexion.

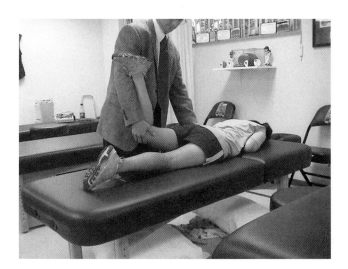

Figure 12.7 Extension.

Ober's test (Figure 12.10)

Ober's test is used to evaluate the trochanteric bursae and the tensor fasciae latae, which is contiguous with the iliotibial band. The patient should be instructed to lie on his or her side, with the affected leg up. The hips and knees should each be flexed to 90 degrees. The top hip should be brought passively into further flexion by the examiner and then guided into abduction and extension until the thigh is in line with the trunk. The leg should then be allowed to adduct passively into a neutral position. A positive test will result in the leg remaining in relative abduction, whereas, with a negative test, the subject may even be able to rest his or her knee on the table without discomfort.[15] Inability to adduct may result from excessive tightness in the tensor fasciae latae and the iliotibial band. The provocation of focal pain at the area overlying the greater trochanter suggests trochanteric bursitis. Ober's test and its modifications have been found to have an intra-examiner reliability of 0.91 and an inter-examiner reliability of 0.73 to 0.91[16,17] (LOE: D).

Thomas' test

To test the flexibility of the hip flexors, specifically the iliopsoas, the Thomas' test[10] is used. The patient lies supine and flexes one hip, pulling one knee to the chest. If a hip flexion contracture is present, the contralateral straight leg will rise off of the table.

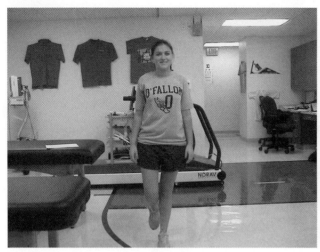

A

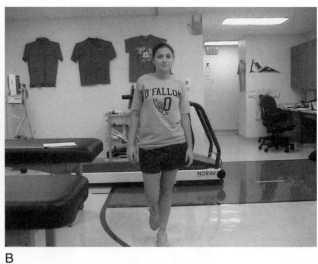

B

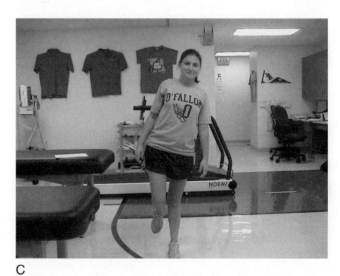

C

Figure 12.8 *A*, Negative Trendelenburg's sign. *B*, Positive Trendelenburg's sign. *C*, Positive compensated Trendelenburg's sign.

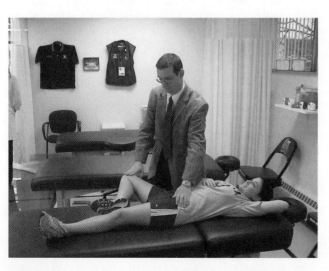

Figure 12.9 The flexion, abduction, and external rotation test.

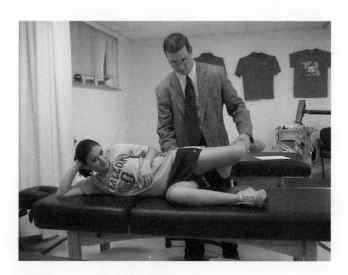

Figure 12.10 Positive Ober's test.

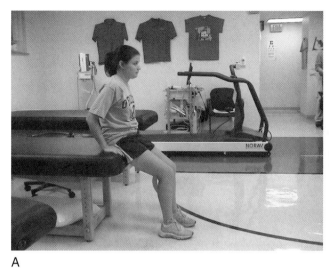

A

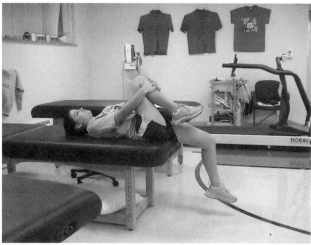

B

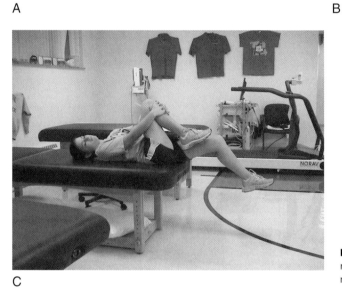

C

Figure 12.11   *A*, Starting position for modified Thomas' test. *B*, A negative modified Thomas' test. *C*, A modified Thomas' test that is positive for iliopsoas and rectus femoris contracture.

The modified Thomas' test **(Figure 12.11)** may be preferred. With this variation, the patient sits at the end of the examination table with the knees flexed to 90 degrees. Next, one knee is pulled tight to the chest. The patient is instructed to lie down while maintaining the knee against the chest. If a hip flexion contracture is present, the contralateral leg will rise off of the table. If a rectus femoris contracture is present, the contralateral knee will extend.

Piriformis test

The piriformis test[18] involves the patient again being on his or her side, with the upper leg flexed to 60 degrees. With one hand stabilizing the patient at the ipsilateral shoulder, the other hand is used to press down on the flexed leg at the knee **(Figure 12.12).** This maneuver is also called the FAIR test (flexion, adduction, and internal rotation).[19] Because the sciatic nerve can bisect, run above, or run below the piriformis muscle, spasm or tightness of the piriformis is theoretically capable of impinging the sciatic nerve and producing pain in the sciatic distribution. If the patient describes the classical "shooting" pain during the examination, the test is considered positive. However, because the maneuver creates pressure at the hip joint, pain can be elicited from other causes. As such, it is important to clarify the location of the pain that is provoked by the test. For patients with electrodiagnostically

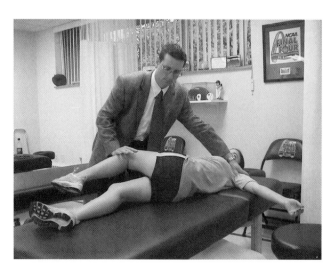

Figure 12.12   Piriformis test.

confirmed sciatic nerve impingement at the piriformis muscle, Fishman and Zybert[20] found this test to have a sensitivity of 0.88 and a specificity of 0.83 (LOE: B).

Log roll test

By passively internally and externally rotating the fully extended leg of a supine patient, the log roll test[21] can help evaluate the possibility of an acetabular injury or a femoral neck fracture. This test can be done easily, and it requires little effort on behalf of the patient or the examiner. In cases in which significant injury is suspected, this test can offer a rough assessment of the bony integrity before further examination is pursued so that appropriate caution may be taken.

The Stinchfield test

The Stinchfield test is also performed with the patient in a supine position. This involves the patient fully extending both the hips and the knees and then flexing the affected hip to approximately 20 degrees. The patient should be instructed to hold this position as the examiner places downward pressure on the distal end of the affected leg **(Figure 12.13)**. Pain elicited with this test at the anterior hip or groin suggests a fracture of the femoral neck, acetabular injury, or osteoarthritis.[22]

The Ely test (Figure 12.14)

The Ely test can be used to assess tightness of the rectus femoris muscle. The patient should lie prone with both legs fully extended. The examiner passively flexes the knee to the end of its range of motion, and the ipsilateral hip is observed to see if it lifts off of the examination table. If hip flexion does occur, the test is considered positive for rectus femoris contracture. Care should be taken to avoid any rotation of the hip or extension of the hip joint because this can elicit pain from other pathologies and diminish the value of the examination.[10]

The straight leg raise test

The straight leg raise test can be used to help differentiate pathology of the hip from that of the buttock. With the patient lying supine, the examiner passively raises (flexes) the leg in question with the knee fully extended. If there is pain present and flexion is limited, then the knee should be flexed and further flexion of the

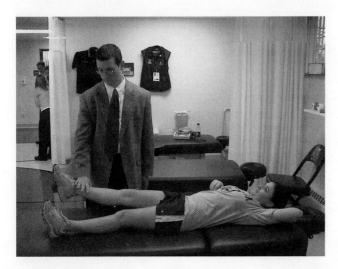

Figure 12.13 Stinchfield test.

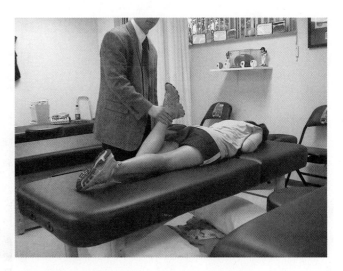

Figure 12.14 Ely test.

hip attempted. If hip flexion is unchanged after flexing the knee, this suggests that the pathology may be in the buttock rather than the hip. This would include diagnoses such as an abscess or ischial bursitis. Radiating pain distally on the flexed side can indicate sciatic nerve compression, although this may be less specific in many cases[23] (LOE: D).

Leg-length assessment

Leg-length is an important part of a hip pain evaluation,[24] because a leg-length abnormality may be the cause or the effect of the athlete's hip pain. Although there is debate in the musculoskeletal literature regarding the value of physical examination alone to diagnosis anatomic leg-length inequality,[25] the ability to detect the presence of a functional leg-length discrepancy will enable the examiner to complete a more thorough evaluation of the athlete's kinetic chain. A few of the most clinically practical techniques will be discussed here. In a standing patient, it is critical to ensure that the patient is standing with his or her feet comfortably apart (typically 6 to 8 inches) and not favoring one leg over the other, which would result in asymmetric abduction and adduction. The measurement of each side can be taken from the anterior superior iliac spine (ASIS) to either the medial or lateral malleolus, as long as both sides are measured to the same point.[10] The weaknesses of this method of measurement include the difficulty with ensuring a perfectly flat pelvis (because most patients who present with a hip complaint will preferentially shift weight away from the affected hip) and the possibility of interference in straight-line measurements by differing amounts of muscle mass or fat tissue. Also, when the measurement spans the entire length of the hip, the leg, and the lower leg, it is impossible to isolate any areas of focal discrepancy.

The Weber–Barstow maneuver

As an alternative for both patient comfort and technical reliability, the Weber–Barstow maneuver[10] may be used. This involves having the patient lie on his or her back with both knees and hips flexed. With the feet close together, the patient resets the pelvis by lifting it slightly off of the table and then gently lowering it back onto the table **(Figure 12.15A)**. By maintaining the malleoli at equal points, the patient can be examined at the knees to judge any length discrepancy. Although a discrepancy is more overt if one knee rises above the other, it is also helpful to inspect at the knees from the side and to look for any anterior or posterior displacement of the knees in relation to one another. The examiner

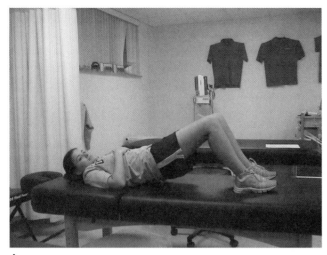 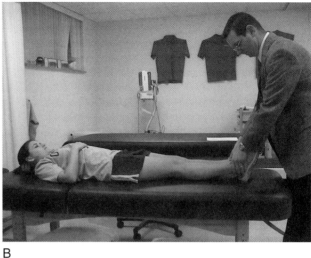

A   B

Figure 12.15 *A*, Resetting the pelvis for leg-length evaluation. *B*, Measuring position for Weber–Barstow maneuver.

then passively extends the knees, places his or her thumbs under the medial malleoli, and compares the positions of the thumbs (see Figure 12.15*B*). Differing thumb levels equate with possible leg-length inequality. The authors also find it helpful to compare thumb placement below the inferior poles of each patellae and below the anterior superior iliac spines.

Prone knee flexion test

As a follow up to the Weber–Barstow maneuver when leg-length inequality is suspected, the authors then do a prone knee flexion test.[10] This test is performed with the patient prone and the knees flexed to 90 degrees. The clinician's thumbs are placed transversely over the soles of the feet just distal to the calcaneus, and the heights of the thumbs are compared. If one side is lower, then that tibia is likely shortened **(Figure 12.16).**

Supine-to-sit test (long sitting test)

To assist with differentiating a true leg-length discrepancy from a functional one, the supine-to-sit test (long sitting test) is used. The patient lies supine with the legs straight, and the medial malleoli are lined up by the examiner. The patient is then asked to sit up

while keeping the legs straight in front of them. The examiner watches the medial malleoli to see if one leg moves more proximally than the other **(Figure 12.17);** this finding suggests that the pain is caused by pelvic dysfunction or malrotation.

Standing flexion test

Another method of evaluating pelvic dysfunction is the standing flexion test.[26] With the patient standing, the examiner palpates the posterior superior iliac spine. The patient is asked to maximally bend forward. If one posterior superior iliac spine moves more cranially, it is considered positive for ipsilateral sacroiliac joint hypomobility. Studies have found this test's inter-examiner reliability to be 0.32 to 0.68[27-31] (LOE: D).

Gillet's test

Gillet's test[32] also examines for sacroiliac dysfunction. The patient stands with the feet approximately 12 inches apart, and the examiner's thumbs are placed on the posterior superior iliac spines. The patient stands on one leg while pulling the opposite knee to the chest. The test is then repeated with the opposite leg **(Figure 12.18).** The test is positive if the posterior superior iliac

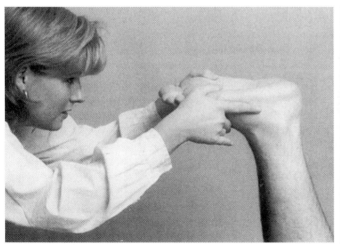 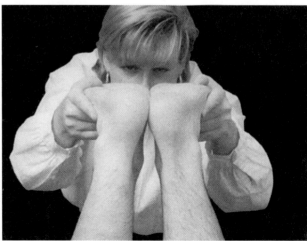

Figure 12.16 Prone knee flexion test. (From Magee DJ: Orthopedic Physical Assessment, 4th ed. Philadelphia, WB Saunders, 1997, p 630.)

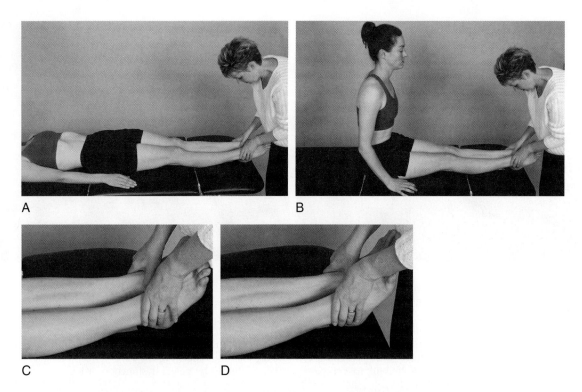

Figure 12.17   Long sitting test. (From Magee DJ: Orthopedic Physical Assessment, 4th ed. Philadelphia, WB Saunders, 1997, p 590.)

spine on the side of the flexed hip moves minimally or up; the ipsilateral sacroiliac joint is then considered hypomobile. Dreyfuss and colleagues[31] found this test to have a sensitivity of 0.43 and a specificity of 0.68 (LOE: B).

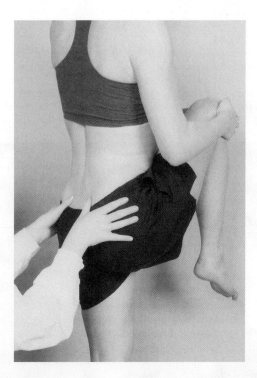

Figure 12.18   Gillet's test. (From Magee DJ: Orthopedic Physical Assessment, 4th ed. Philadelphia, WB Saunders, 1997, p 587.)

Gaenslen's test

Gaenslen's test[26,32] is also used to evaluate for sacroiliac disorders. The patient lies supine with both knees pulled up to the chest. The patient is positioned such that the test leg is able to be extended beyond the edge of the table. Pressure may be applied to the flexed leg while the extended one is stabilized **(Figure 12.19)**. Pain at the sacroiliac joint is considered a positive result. The sensitivity in studies has ranged from 0.21 to 0.71, with specificities between 0.26 and 0.72[31,32] (LOE: B).

Craig's test

Craig's test[34] can be used to estimate the degree of femoral anteversion. Femoral anteversion is the amount of forward projection

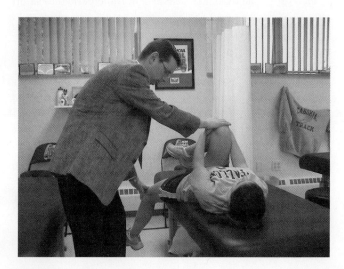

Figure 12.19   Gaenslen's test.

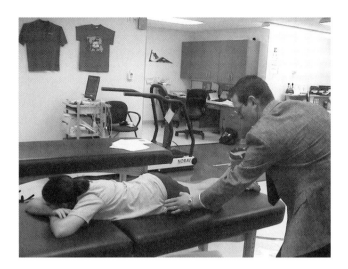

Figure 12.20   Craig's test.

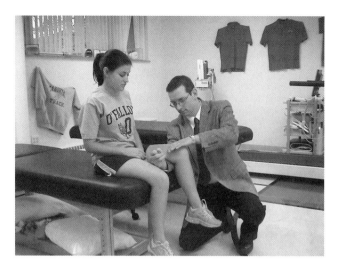

Figure 12.22   Fulcrum test for femoral stress fracture.

of the femoral neck. This is a normal finding, with average angles of between 8 and 15 degrees in adults and values closer to 30 to 40 degrees in infants. In excessive cases, which are usually seen in a pediatric population, patients can encounter additional difficulties. Although it is markedly less common, retroversion may also be problematic. The examination is performed on a supine patient with the pelvis on a flat and firm surface. The knee of the side in question should be flexed to 90 degrees, and the examiner should palpate the posterior aspect of the greater trochanter. Contact with the trochanter is maintained as the leg is rotated internally and externally, feeling for the point at which the trochanter becomes parallel with the examination surface. At this point, the degree of anteversion can be approximated by the angle of the leg from the vertical position **(Figure 12.20).**

Pathology of the pubic symphysis can produce groin pain, and, in athletes, osteitis pubis is a possible cause. By using passive abduction as well as resisted adduction of the hip,[35] the examiner can help distinguish this condition from a wide variety of disorders that could result in pain in the midline area of the groin. The examination is performed by having the patient lie on his or her side with both knees and hips flexed to 90 degrees. The patient may passively abduct both legs, or he or she may be instructed to

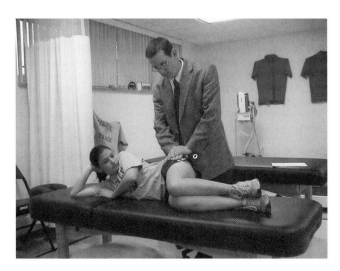

Figure 12.21   Lateral pelvic compression test.

adduct against the resistance of the examiner. Pain at the pubic symphysis with these movements is considered a positive test.

Lateral pelvic compression test

Additionally, the lateral pelvic compression test can be performed with the patient in the same starting position (hips and knees flexed to 90 degrees). The examiner then places direct downward pressure over the greater trochanter **(Figure 12.21).** A positive test will result in localized pain to the midline directly over the pubic bone.[21] As was discussed previously, cases of hip and groin pain require the physician to maintain a wide differential diagnosis that reaches far beyond musculoskeletal sources. Osteitis pubis serves as a good reminder of this warning because there are a number of concerning conditions that can produce pain in the pubic region, such as urinary tract infections, abdominal pathologies, sexually transmitted diseases, and other pelvic conditions.

Scour or quadrant test

The scour or quadrant test is a passive maneuver that is performed with the patient supine. The examiner axial loads, flexes, and adducts the hip to the end of its range of motion; in other words, the knee will be pointing at the patient's opposite shoulder. The hip is then taken into abduction in an arc-like motion. A positive test is any catching, pain, or apprehension with the maneuver; this is suggestive of labral pathology or loose bodies within the hip joint.[10] This test is for the hip what McMurray's test is for the knee.

Fulcrum test

The fulcrum test is used when there is a suspicion of a stress fracture of the femoral shaft. The patient sits with the knees flexed over the edge of the examination table with the feet not touching the ground. The examiner's forearm is placed under the thigh to be tested to act as a fulcrum. The fulcrum arm is moved from proximal to distal as the other hand applies downward pressure onto the ipsilateral flexed knee **(Figure 12.22).** If a stress fracture is present, the patient will experience sharp pain or apprehension during this test.[10]

REFERENCES

1.   Scopp M: The assessment of athletic hip injury. Clin Sports Med 2001;20(4): 647-659.

2. Hurwitz DE, Foucher KC, Andriacchi TP: A new parametric approach for modeling hip forces during gait. J Biomech 2003;36(1):113-119.
3. Jenkins DB: The bony pelvis, femur, and hip joint. In Jenkins DB (ed): Hollinshead's Functional Anatomy of the Limbs and Back. Philadelphia, WB Saunders, 1998, pp 239-248.
4. Seidenberg PH, Childress MA: Managing hip tendon and nerve injuries in athletes. J Musculoskel Med 2005;22(7):337-344.
5. Metzmaker JN, Pappas AM: Avulsion fractures in the pelvis. Am J Sports Med 1985;13(5):349-358.
6. Anderson SJ: Sports injuries. Curr Probl Pediatr Adolesc Health Care 2005;35(4):110-164.
7. Paletta GA Jr, Andrish JT: Injuries about the hip and pelvis in the young athlete. Clin Sports Med 1995;14:591-628.
8. Vijlbrief AS, Bruijnzeels MA, vand der Wouden JC, van Suijelkom-Smit LW: Incidence and management of transient synovitis of the hip: a study in Dutch general practice. Brit J Gen Pract 1992;42(363):426-428.
9. Tolat V, Carty H, Klenerman L, Hart CA: Evidence for a viral aetiology of transient synovitis of the hip. J Bone Joint Surg Br 1993;75(6):973-974.
10. Geraci MC Jr, Brown W: Evidence-based treatment of hip and pelvic injuries in runners. Phys Med Rehabil Clin N Am 2005;16(3):711-747.
11. Hage WD, Aboulafia AJ, Aboulafia DM: Orthopedic management of metastatic disease: incidence, location, and diagnostic evaluation of metastatic bone disease. OrtChop Clin North Am 2000;31(4):515-528.
12. Magee DJ: Hip. In Magee DJ (ed): Orthopedic Physical Assessment, 3rd ed. Philadelphia, WB Saunders, 1997.
13. Seidenberg PH, Childress MA: Evaluating hip pain in athletes. J Musculoskel Med 2005;22(5):246-254.
14. Allen WC, Cope R: Coxa saltans: the snapping hip syndrome. J Am Acad Orthop Surg 1995;3:303-308.
15. Hardcastle P, Nade S: The significance of the Trendelenburg test. J Bone Joint Surg Br 1985;67(5):741-746.
16. Ross MD, Nordeen MH, Barido M: Test-retest reliability of Patrick's hip range of motion test in healthy college-aged men. J Strength Cond Res 2003;17(1):156-161.
17. Broadhurst N, Bond M: Pain provocation tests for the assessment of sacroiliac dysfunction. J Spinal Disord 1998;11:341-345.
18. Gajdosik RL, Sandler MM, Marr HL: Influence of knee positions and gender on the Ober test for length of the iliotibial band. Clin Biomech (Bristol, Avon) 2003;18(1):77-79.
19. Reese N, Bandy W: Use of an inclinometer to measure flexibility of the iliotibial band using the Ober test and Modified Ober test: difference in magnitude and reliability of measurements. J Orthop Sports Phys Ther 2003;33:326-330.
20. Melchione WE, Sullivan M: Reliability of measurements obtained by use of an instrument designed to indirectly measure iliotibial band length. J Orthop Sports Phys Ther 1993;18:511-515.
21. Rodrigue T, Hardy RW: Diagnosis and treatment of piriformis syndrome. Neurosurg Clin N Am 2001;12(2):311-319.
22. Fishman L, Dombi G, Michaelson C, et al: Piriformis syndrome: diagnosis, treatment and outcome—a 10-year study. Arch Phys Med Rehabil 2002;83:295-301.
23. Fishman L, Zybert P: Electrophysiologic evidence of piriformis syndrome. Arch Phys Med Rehabil 1992;73:359-364.
24. McGrory BJ: Stinchfield resisted hip flexion test. Hosp Physician 1999;35(9):41-42.
25. Vroomen PC, de Krom MC, Wilmink JT, et al: Diagnostic value of history and physical examination in patients suspected of lumbosacral nerve root compression. J Neurol Neurosurg Psychiatry 2002;72(5):630-634.
26. Brady RJ, Dean JB, Skinner TM, Gross MT: Limb length inequality: clinical implications for assessment and intervention. J Orthop Sports Phys Ther 2003;33(5):221-234.
27. Rhodes DW, Mansfield ER, Bishop PA, Smith JF: The validity of the prone leg check as an estimate of standing leg length inequality measured by X-ray. J Manipulative Physiol Ther 1995;18(6):343-346.
28. Magee DJ: Pelvis. In Orthopedic Physical Assessment, 3rd ed. Philadelphia, WB Saunders, 1997.
29. Cleland J: Sacroiliac region. In Cleland J (ed): Orthopaedic Clinical Examination: An Evidence-Based Approach for Physical Therapists. New Jersey, Icon Learning Systems, 2005.
30. Riddle D, Freburger J: Evaluation of the presence of sacroiliac joint dysfunction using a combination of tests: a multicenter intertester reliability study. Phys Ther 2002;82:772-781.
31. Touissaint R, Gawlik C, Rehder U, Ruther W: Sacroiliac dysfunction in construction workers. J Manipulative Physiol Ther 1999;22:134-139.
32. Touissaint R, Gawlik C, Rehder U, Ruther W: Sacroiliac joint diagnosis in the Hamburg Construction Workers study. J Manipulative Physiol Ther 1999;22:139-143.
33. Vincent-Smith B, Gibbons P: Inter-examiner and intra-examiner reliability of the standing flexion test. Man Ther 1999;4:87-93.
34. Dreyfuss P, Michaelen M, Pauza K, et al: The value of the medical history and physical examination in diagnosing sacroiliac joint pain. Spine 1996;21:2594-2602.
35. van der Wuff P, Hagmeijer R, Meyne W: Clinical tests of the sacroiliac joint. Man Ther 2000;5:30-36.
36. Ryder CT, Crane L: Measuring femoral anteversion; the problem and a method. J Bone Joint Surg Am 1953;35-A(2):321-328.
37. Nuccion S, Hunter D, Finerman G, Hip and pelvis: In DeLee JC, Drez D Jr, Miller MD (eds): DeLee & Drez's Orthopaedic Sports Medicine: Principles and Practice, 2nd ed. Philadelphia, WB Saunders, 2003.

CHAPTER 13

Physical Examination of the Knee

Nicholas A. Piantanida, MD, and Nicole T. Yedlinsky, MD

KEY POINTS

- The astute clinician must have a precise understanding of the epidemiology and mechanism of sports knee injuries to obtain an accurate and complete history and physical examination.
- The number of patients presenting with knee pain is on the rise in the primary care setting as a result of increased activity levels among all age groups and the rising prevalence of obesity.
- The knee is a complex structure, but it is inherently stable, and it has limited vulnerabilities.
- The history will often give pertinent clues that will help guide and focus the knee examination. However, certain maneuvers should always be included in the examination.
- Evidence-based medicine narrows a diverse differential diagnosis by coupling individual examination maneuvers with a specific diagnosis.

INTRODUCTION

Musculoskeletal conditions that affect an athlete's knee and that ultimately impair athletic performance can present in various ways. An astute clinician must understand the patterns of disease and/or the mechanisms of injury that present as knee disorders. The knee examination should transition from a careful history to a meticulous physical examination. This chapter describes an approach to the knee examination that unites elements of critical thinking regarding the presenting symptoms or the mechanism of injury with the evidenced-based functional and manual examination of the knee.

EPIDEMIOLOGY

In the primary care setting, approximately 1 in every 20 visits are the result of knee pain.[1,2] Activity levels have increased at both ends of the age spectrum, from the growing number of children participating in organized sports to the baby boomer generation holding onto exercise regimens.[3,4] Special attention is warranted during the assessment of the pediatric athlete with knee pain because mechanical stress across the knee can injure the epiphyseal growth plate or create a traction apophysitis, such as is seen in cases of Osgood–Schlatter disease. The rising prevalence of obesity in the general population raises the necessity of managing knee osteoarthritis at even younger ages, and it creates new challenges in the management of chronic knee pain.

Acute knee pain accounts for more than 1 million emergency department visits and more than 1.9 million primary care outpatient visits annually.[5] Children and adolescent injuries reported by Arendt and Dick[6] indicate that knee injuries account for 15% to 50% of all sports injuries and that girls are at higher risk than boys. Data from the National Collegiate Athletic Association establish a knee injury rate of more than one injury for every 10 female athletes per year[7] for approximately 13,000 knee injuries each year. An estimated 28,000 knee injuries are statistically possible among the 2.8 million female athletes annually at the high school level because high school female athletes incur knee injuries at a rate that is one tenth that of collegiate athletes.[8] In terms of season-ending knee injuries, Chandy and Grana[8] showed that, as compared with high school male athletes, female athletes have an incidence that is 4.6 times higher (LOE: D).

ANATOMY

The knee is a complex structure that largely comprises soft tissue, with the distal femur articulating with the proximal tibia. It is a movable synovial hinge joint with limited vulnerabilities, and it is inherently stable as a result of its musculoskeletal geometry. Its structure permits flexion and extension in one axis for the most part, but it also allows for a minimal amount of medial femoral rotation with full extension. The ligamentous structures and associated musculature provide more stability than do the intrinsic compartmental shapes formed by its articular surfaces[9] **(Figure 13.1).**

The static stabilizers of the knee include the bones, the menisci, the ligaments, the capsule, and the articular cartilage. The patella is the body's largest sesamoid bone, and it is encapsulated superiorly by attachments with the quadriceps tendon and inferiorly by the patellar tendon. The patella forms a gliding articulation with the patellofemoral groove, and it is anchored distally at the tibial tubercle by the patellar tendon (see Figure 13.1). There exists asymptomatic ossification anomalies that produce a bipartite or tripartite patella in 1% to 4% of patients,[10] and these are often incidentally noted on radiographic examination. The distal femur comprises the trochlea and the medial and lateral condyles. Much of these

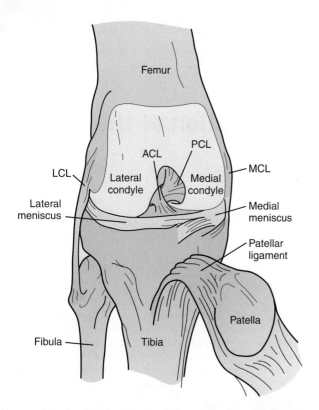

Figure 13.1 Anterior knee anatomy. ACL, anterior cruciate ligament; LCL, lateral collateral ligament; MCL, medial collateral ligament; PCL, posterior cruciate ligament. (From Brown JR, Trojian TH: Prim Care 2004;31:925-956.)

surfaces, as well as the underside of the patella and the proximal tibia, are lined by a hyaline-rich articular cartilage. Many types of collagen are present in articular cartilage. Type 2 collagen makes up 90% to 95% of the collagen fibers.

Between the weight-bearing surfaces of the femur and the tibia reside the crescent-shaped shock-absorbing menisci **(Figure 13.2)**. Meniscal tissue comprises primarily type 1 cartilage, and its

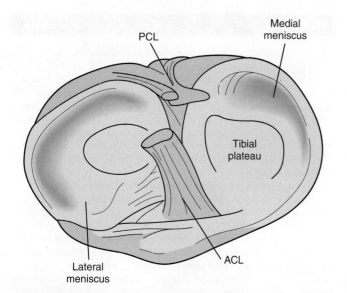

Figure 13.2 Tibial view. ACL, anterior cruciate ligament; PCL, posterior cruciate ligament. (From Brown JR, Trojian TH: Prim Care 2004;31:925-956.)

consistency is half as stiff as that of articular cartilage. The medial meniscus is fibrously integrated with the medial collateral ligament (MCL), which makes either vulnerable in the setting of injury to one structure. For comparison, the lateral meniscus covers 20% more tibial surface area, it is more circular in shape, and it is more loosely attached, translating 9 to 11 mm on the tibia when the knee is flexed. A discoid meniscus is a well-described anatomic variant (more commonly of the lateral meniscus), with an estimated incidence in the general population of 3% to 5%; it is one of the causes of "snapping knee syndrome."[11] The ligaments of Humphrey and Wrisberg are accessory meniscofemoral ligaments that originate from the medial segment of the lateral meniscus, with the former inserting anterior to the posterior cruciate ligament (PCL) and the latter inserting posterior to the PCL. An anterior transverse intermeniscal ligament joins the menisci anteriorly.

The cruciate complex establishes anterior–posterior ligamentous stability. The anterior cruciate ligament (ACL) provides restraint on the tibia from gliding anterior to the femur. The PCL provides restraint on the tibia traversing posterior to the femur.[12] When the knee is in full extension, the ACL serves as a secondary restraint to internal rotation of the tibia. The ACL originates from the lateral femoral condyle and is often described as two bands (anteromedial and posterolateral, named for their insertion sites on the medial tibia). The PCL originates from the lateral border of the medial femoral condyle, and it inserts in the PCL facet or fovea. The PCL's cross-sectional area is approximately 50% greater than that of the ACL at the femur and 20% greater at the tibia (LOE: C).[13] The PCL restrains external tibial rotation and also limits hyperextension of the knee. As a result of its close anatomic proximity to the posterolateral corner, the PCL acts as a secondary stabilizer of posterior tibial translation. Furthermore, 60% of significant PCL injuries are associated with a posterolateral corner disruption.[12]

Tensile stress creating varus (medially directed) forces to the knee are countered by the components of the posterior lateral corner. The posterolateral corner comprises two overlapping layers: superficial and deep. The iliotibial band (ITBand) and the biceps femoris tendon construct the superficial layer. The deep layer is more complex, and it includes contributions from the lateral collateral ligament (LCL), the capsular structures (the mid third lateral capsular ligament, the fabellofibular ligament, and the posterior arcuate ligament), and the popliteus muscle complex, which includes the popliteofibular ligament **(Figure 13.3)**. The LCL is the primary static restraint of the lateral knee. The LCL is taut at full extension, and it becomes lax after 30 degrees of flexion. The soft tissues along the lateral knee receive major contributions from the lateral retinaculum and the ITBand. The ITBand originates from the iliac crest and inserts on Gerdy's tubercle on the anterolateral aspect of the tibia. The ITBand contributes to lateral knee stabilization only at full extension. With cyclic knee flexion, the ITBand moves posteriorly, and the bicep femoris assumes dominant dynamic stabilization of the lateral knee.[14] Furthermore, in the overuse injured athlete, this posterior ITBand migration creates traction stress maximally at 30 degrees of knee flexion, which corresponds with the foot strike phase in the running gait. This pain is distributed from Gerdy's tubercle to the ITBand bursa that rests over the lateral femoral condyle.[15]

Tensile stresses creating valgus (laterally directed) forces to the knee are countered by static stabilizers that include the MCL and the posterior oblique ligament. The MCL is anatomically divided into several layers, with the superficial layer (extending 10 cm) coalescing with the deep layer to form secure attachments to meniscofemoral and meniscotibial surfaces. The posterior oblique ligament has attachments to the medial meniscus and the medial tibial joint line. The pes anserinus tendons (sartorius, gracilis, semitendinosus), the vastus medialis, and the semimembranosus muscle serve as dynamic constraints[14] **(Figure 13.4)**. The dynamic stabilization occurs only when the muscles are activated. Pope and

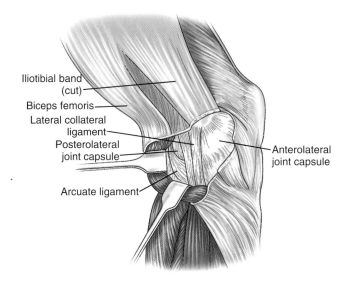

Figure 13.3 labels: Iliotibial band (cut); Biceps femoris; Lateral collateral ligament; Posterolateral joint capsule; Arcuate ligament; Anterolateral joint capsule

Figure 13.3 Lateral knee. The iliotibial band and superficial fascial layers are removed, exposing the lateral collateral ligament and the arcuate ligament. (From Insall JN, Scott WN: Surgery of the Knee, 3rd ed. Philadelphia, WB Saunders, 2000.)

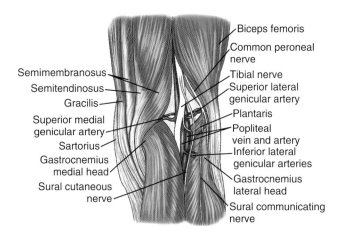

Figure 13.5 labels: Semimembranosus; Semitendinosus; Gracilis; Superior medial genicular artery; Sartorius; Gastrocnemius medial head; Sural cutaneous nerve; Biceps femoris; Common peroneal nerve; Tibial nerve; Superior lateral genicular artery; Plantaris; Popliteal vein and artery; Inferior lateral genicular arteries; Gastrocnemius lateral head; Sural communicating nerve

Figure 13.5 Posterior knee. (From Insall JN, Scott WN: Surgery of the Knee, 3rd ed. Philadelphia, WB Saunders, 2000.)

colleagues[16] found that, after a valgus stress is applied, the pain reflex arc is too slow to activate the dynamic stabilizers (LOE: B).

The dynamic stabilizers of the knee influence the patellofemoral joint significantly during the first 20 degrees of knee flexion, when the knee is most vulnerable. After 20 degrees of flexion, the bony and other static architecture is increasingly responsible for patellar control. The medial patellar stability is passively generated by the muscular attachment of the medial quadriceps: the vastus medialis. The vastus medialis is functionally divided into two parts: the vastus medialis obliquus and the vastus medialis longus. The vastus medialis obliquus is active during knee extension solely to position the patella centered in the trochlea of the femur. The vastus medialis longus, the rectus femoris, and the vastus lateralis function in concert to provide an anterolateral vector force while executing knee extension.[17]

The major flexors of the knee reside in the posterior thigh and include the long and short heads of the biceps femoris, the semitendinosus, the semimembranosus, and the adductor magnus **(Figure 13.5).** Posterior knee pain can arise from acute tendon strain or chronic injury resulting in tendinosis of any of the musculotendinous structures in or about the popliteal fossa. Ganglion cysts in the presence of tendon injury or a Baker cyst (popliteal

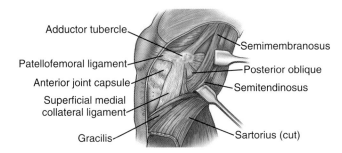

Figure 13.4 labels: Adductor tubercle; Patellofemoral ligament; Anterior joint capsule; Superficial medial collateral ligament; Gracilis; Semimembranosus; Posterior oblique; Semitendinosus; Sartorius (cut)

Figure 13.4 Medial knee. The sartorius is retracted to expose the superficial medial collateral ligament and the anterior joint capsule. (From Insall JN, Scott WN: Surgery of the Knee, 3rd ed. Philadelphia, WB Saunders, 2000.)

synovial cyst) may also contribute to the pain. Some of the more commonly injured structures posterolaterally include the lateral head of the gastrocnemius, the biceps femoris, and the popliteus tendons. Posteromedially, injuries to the semitendinosus and semimembranosus tendons are more common. Although they are unusual occurrences, strains or ruptures of the plantaris or the medial head of the gastrocnemius muscle may also cause posterior knee pain.[18]

The popliteus muscle group courses medially from the lateral femoral condyle to insert along portions of the medial tibia and the fibular head. Electromyographic studies show that the popliteus muscle serves as the primary internal rotator of the tibia and that, during initial flexion from an extended position, it will "unlock" the knee (LOE: C).[19] The popliteus assists the quadriceps and the PCL with maintaining normal tibial and femoral orientation. Hence, downhill running or rapid deceleration activities put a fatiguing stress on these groups.[20]

The posterior knee also contains the major neurovascular structures. The tibial nerve (L4-S3) and the common peroneal nerve (L4-S2) both branch from the sciatic nerve in the proximal popliteal fossa. Tibial nerve compression by popliteal cysts or by hemorrhage associated with popliteal muscle rupture has been reported.[21] Mastaglia[22] described six surgically proven cases of tibial nerve entrapment by the tendinous arch of the origin of the soleus muscle. The common peroneal nerve courses anterolaterally and winds around the fibular head to enter the peroneal or (fibular) tunnel. Within the tunnel, the nerve runs deep to the tendinous origin of the peroneus longus muscle and rests against the surface of the fibular neck. Common peroneal nerve compression can occur as the peroneus longus muscle contracts during plantar flexion or inversion of the foot to compress the nerve against the fibular neck. Peroneal nerve compression can occur at rest with cross-legged sitting or prolonged squatting, with activities that involve repetitive inversion or pronation of the foot (e.g., running), and in occupations that involve repetitive use of a pedal.[23]

The main vascular supply to the knee comes from branches of the popliteal artery. The genicular branches supply the articular capsule and the ligaments of the knee. They form a network of anastomoses, and they are named as follows: lateral superior and inferior, medial superior and inferior, and middle genicular arteries. The middle genicular artery directly pierces the posterior articular capsule to supply the ACL and the PCL.[12] Popliteal artery entrapment syndrome, which is an uncommon condition (primarily of young men), results from exertional compression of the popliteal artery and the medial head of the gastrocnemius

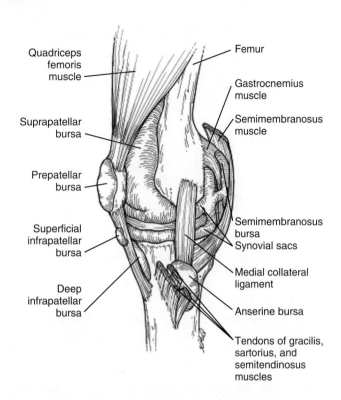

Quadriceps femoris muscle

Suprapatellar bursa

Prepatellar bursa

Superficial infrapatellar bursa

Deep infrapatellar bursa

Femur

Gastrocnemius muscle

Semimembranosus muscle

Semimembranosus bursa
Synovial sacs

Medial collateral ligament

Anserine bursa

Tendons of gracilis, sartorius, and semitendinosus muscles

Figure 13.6 Knee bursa. (From CanaleTS: Campbell's Operative Orthopaedics, 10th ed. Philadelphia Mosby, 2003).

muscle or adjacent musculotendinous structures. Exertional compression of the popliteal artery may occur during dynamic plantar flexion or passive dorsiflexion and cause intermittent claudication, an uncommon condition that is known as *popliteal artery entrapment syndrome.*[24]

Other soft tissues of the knee that cause disorders include the many bursa that lubricate and cushion bony–tendinous surfaces and the soft-tissue plicae that extend from either pole or lateral/medial margin of the patella.[25] Several of the bursa are depicted in **Figure 13.6** and include the prepatellar bursa, the pes anserinus bursa, and the infrapatellar bursa. Additionally, Hoffa's fat pad below the infrapatellar bursa can serve as a source of pain from impingement on extension. Hoffa's fat pad impingement can be confused with synovial proliferation syndromes such as pigmented villonodular synovitis.[26]

HISTORY

A careful history focuses the differential diagnosis and forms the substance that a meticulous knee examination strives to further develop or reproduce. The history should contribute to the assessment of the knee examination in ways that draw attention to the patient's description of the knee pain or injury. Other matters of age, skeletal maturity, prior injury/surgery, occupation, typical physical activity, and gender are excellent core reference points when assessing injury risk. For example, 80% to 90% of meniscal injuries in childhood and adolescence occur during sporting activities.[27]

As with all injuries, significant diagnostic importance exists with describing the mechanism of injury within the context of the anatomy. Specifically, the patient should describe the exact anatomic position of the leg at the time of injury. Traumatic menisci injuries, for example, occur in the setting of shearing forces that are created when the patient plants a foot and twists or pivots on the leg.

Secondary forces may contribute to the injury; these include external impact from a blow or other contact and stress in the form of an unanticipated movement such as the lateral football tackle that result in sprain or rupture of the MCL. The weight-bearing status at the time of injury and intentional or unanticipated rotational forces on the knee may injure specific structures. For example, 70% of ACL injuries are noncontact injuries and typically involve an unintentional sudden deceleration, hyperextension, or twist.[12] PCL injuries, by contrast, occur either in the setting of forced hyperflexion and a steady posterior compression of the proximal tibia or a traumatic hyperextension injury that also involves the posterior capsule.[28] In every case, the patient's recollection of the immediate events causing the injury starts with the mechanism.

The onset of knee pain may be acute or insidious; its location may be described as anterior, posterior, medial, or lateral. The severity of pain at the time of injury may be quantified on a pain scale (0 to 10) as well as by the degree of disability. An inability to continue play or to bear weight represents a greater degree of immediate disability. In every case, the examiner must delineate the formation of two distinct injury patterns. In one group, there exists a specific traumatic event that can be correlated with the onset of symptoms and a change in the functional level. For example, occult bone bruising or osteochondral lesions have been reported[29] in up to 80% of patients who rupture their ACLs. This group of athletes will have immediate impairment and potentially higher pain scores. In a second group, there is an insidious onset of symptoms and often a slow gradual worsening of functional limitations. In this second group, there exists a history of repetitive microtrauma that follows periods of exercise with underrecovery, where underrecovery is defined as inadequate time between exercise periods for tissues to adapt or rebuild. Symptoms are worse with activity and improve with rest. In both groups, aggravating and alleviating factors may be elicited from the history.[30]

Mechanical symptoms include any sound or sensation of popping or tearing. Mechanical symptoms might present at the time of injury or in association with the time course of the repetitive activity, such as 5 minutes into a run. ACL and PCL injuries are often accompanied by a "pop" sensation. True locking of the knee may present as a history of an inability to extend the knee that requires manual reduction; it may also be evident on examination as a persistent degree of flexion despite attempts to passively extend. The term *pseudolocking* refers to moments when the knee catches but manual reduction is not required. True locking is associated with bucket-handle meniscal tears. Patients with meniscal tears presenting subacutely will often report locking episodes and increased pain with squatting or walking down stairs. Clicking in association with flexion and extension is associated with numerous knee pathologies, including meniscal injury, plicae, an osteochondral defect, or degenerative disease.[14]

Instability or giving way of the knee may result from anatomic instability, or it may be the result of the inhibition of quadriceps function occurring as a reflex against painful stimuli or activity. Patellar instability may occur when patients with normal anatomy are exposed to direct high-energy forces. However, Sallay and colleagues[31] report that patellar instability occurs more commonly when patients with abnormal anatomy are exposed to indirect forces (LOE: B). These items of anatomic abnormalities include vastus medialis hypoplasia, increased medial retinaculum laxity, increased lateral retinaculum tightness, dysplastic patella, abnormal sulcus angle, patella alta, lateralization of the tibial tuberosity, a high Q angle, excess pronation, femoral anteversion, and general ligamentous laxity.

Swelling or ecchymosis of the knee that is relatively immediate (within 2 to 4 hours of the time of injury) likely represents hemarthrosis. This may signify injury to a relatively vascular structure such as the ACL, the MCL, the LCL, the extensor mechanism, or the juxtacapsular (outer third) meniscus, or it may mean patellar dislocation. Immediate swelling may also result from a tibial plateau fracture or another fracture. Swelling that is delayed in onset usually stems from synovial reaction or from injury to relatively avascular ligamentous and/or cartilaginous structures. However, significant swelling may not occur in the face of severe injury in the presence of a capsular tear. Recurrent knee effusion after activity is indicative of meniscal injury, particularly in the older athlete or in the patient with a previous ACL tear who has a degenerative injury to the meniscus.[27]

The tibial, common peroneal, and cutaneous nerves of the knee may be injured by direct trauma (crush or transection), traction, mechanical or functional compression, or repetitive local friction. A history of nerve injury or entrapment should identify symptoms of nerve conduction interruption that result in impairment of function (e.g., weakness, paralysis, and muscle atrophy when motor nerves are interrupted); subjective sensations of pain and paresthesia (e.g., numbness, tingling, burning, or crawling sensation); and objective findings of analgesia and anesthesia when sensory nerves are compromised. Almost any peripheral nerve in the body can be compressed, but nerve-signal interruption tends to occur at certain sites at which the area around the nerve is more constrained, such as fibrous or fibro-osseous tunnels. Compression injury can be acute, chronic, or intermittent.[23]

When knee pain is nontraumatic and/or chronic in nature, the history must focus on systemic diseases. A knee that is red, swollen, warm, and painful suggests an inflammatory process (Table 13.1), and the examiner needs to consider a diagnosis of septic arthritis. Further questions should include an inquiry of constitutional symptoms such as fever or chills and a brief dialog about recent sexual activity. The knee is not exempt from benign or malignant neoplasms. Additional appropriate review of symptoms includes unexplained weight loss, night sweats, or night pain.

Finally, the pertinent history should also include a description of any previous trauma or injury, sports and work histories, history of intervention and rehabilitation for prior injuries, and pertinent medical history (see Table 13.1). In every case, a careful history will advance the examiner's diagnostic accuracy, which he or she must then incorporate into the physical examination.

Table 13.1   Knee History Flow Sheet

Injury/trauma
  Mechanism
  Pain characteristics (location and severity)
  Disability (weight bearing, activity limiting)
  Time course of disease or swelling (acute or insidious)
Prior treatment
  Medications
Physical therapy/rehabilitation
Surgical history
Work history
Sports history
Medical history and differential diagnosis for inflammatory knee disorders
  Bursitis
  Crystal-induced synovitis (gout)
  Osteoarthritis
  Seronegative spondyloarthropathies (Reiter's syndrome, rheumatoid arthritis, inflammatory bowel disease, systemic lupus erythematosus, psoriasis, septic arthritis, rheumatic fever, Lyme disease)
Family history
  Pigmented villonodular synovitis
  Rheumatoid arthritis
  Systemic lupus erythematosus

Table 13.2   Knee Examination Flow Sheet

Inspection
Gait observation
Standing static examination
Range of motion
  Active and passive
  Palpation
Patellar assessment
  Knee effusion
  Retinacular tightness
  Patellar compression
  Plicae
Ligamentous stability
  Medial collateral ligament
  Lateral collateral ligament
  Anterior cruciate ligament
  Posterior cruciate ligament
Special tests
  Menisci
  Iliotibial band
  Flexibility
Neurovascular examination
Referred pain
Kinetic chain

PHYSICAL EXAMINATION

The examination is guided and narrowed by the history. Certain examination maneuvers should be performed on all patients because they form the basis for further maneuvers and they help the examiner to assess for the extent of injury suspected from the history. Knees with acute injuries and those with a single finding are significantly easier to diagnose on the basis of the clinical examination alone.[32] Without exception, the examiner must ensure that the patient is adequately exposed from the waist down; a gown or drape may be used, if needed. The examination sequence encompasses inspection, range of motion, palpation, patellar assessment, ligamentous stability, special tests, and assessment of the kinetic chain for associated factors and referred pain (Table 13.2).

Inspection

Inspection of the knee begins with the initial observation of the patient's gait when he or she enters the examination site. Ideally, this should involve at least 15 feet of ambulation. The examiner documents abnormalities of movement (e.g., shuffle, ataxia, or painful limp) and notes dynamic motion from the hips to the feet. These points of reference will assist with the identification of abnormal hip motion, excessive genu varus or valgus, ankle deformity, or foot overpronation. With the patient in the standing position, observe him or her for any visible static malalignment to include excessive knee varus or valgus and unusual patellar position (e.g., squinting with medial displacement). The skin is inspected for erythema, ecchymosis, and scars from previous injury or operative management. Any obvious asymmetry of landmarks and musculature is noted. The popliteal fossa is inspected from a posterior and lateral position for asymmetry and for discrepancy in the degree of the standing popliteal angle.

Range of motion

With the patient in a seated position, the knees are evaluated for active range of motion, and they are further evaluated for passive

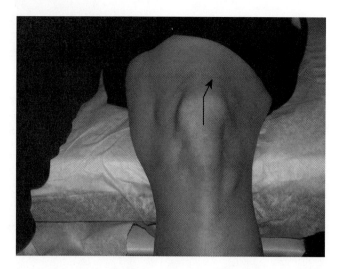

Figure 13.7 Lateral tracking or J-shift. (*Arrow* denotes lateral translation at full extension.)

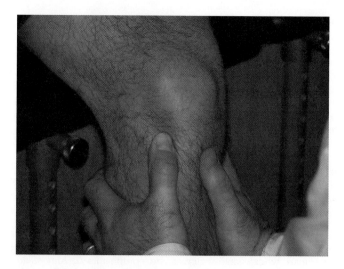

Figure 13.8 Palpation of the knee.

range of motion when there is a reduction in the active range. The normal range of knee flexion is 130 to 150 degrees; knee extension is normally 0 to −10 degrees. During flexion and extension of the knee, the examiner should evaluate for crepitus. Patellar tracking is observed in flexion and extension for evidence of maltracking, such as a lateral glide or a J-shift as the knee reaches full extension **(Figure 13.7).** Comparison of each of the above should always be made with the contralateral knee.

Palpation

The knee is palpated with the patient in the seated position for point tenderness to anterior, lateral, medial, and posterior structures **(Figure 13.8).** Point tenderness can accurately determine the location of a lesion 78% of the time (LOE-D).[14] The affected knee is also assessed for elevated temperature because infectious arthritis will commonly present as acute joint pain with erythema and warmth.

Patellar assessment
Brush, stroke, or bulge test

With the patient in the supine position, the knee is palpated to evaluate for an effusion and to apply manual tests of manual knee stability. Large knee effusions will often obliterate the normal recesses lateral and medial to the patella. They also will result in the knee assuming a resting position of 15 to 25 degrees of flexion, which maximally allows the synovial cavity to hold fluid. The presence of a small knee effusion is best assessed by a brush, stroke, or bulge test. The examiner commences by milking the synovial fluid proximally from the medial side of the patella and into the suprapatellar pouch. With the opposite hand, the examiner strokes distally from the suprapatellar pouch down the lateral patella. The examiner may be able to feel a fluid wave by tapping the index finger just below the lateral distal border of the patella and feeling for the impulse on the medial side. Normally, the knee contains approximately 1 to 7 mL of synovial fluid. This test shows as little as 4 to 8 mL of additional fluid within the knee.[33]

Patellar tilt and glide tests

The examiner may assess retinacular tightness in at least two ways. The examiner performs the lateral patellar tilt test by applying the forefingers to the lateral edge of the patella and creating a vector

force upward while the thumbs compress the medial edge **(Figure 13.9).** An abnormal test occurs if the lateral aspect of the patella fails to rise at least to a level that is horizontal to the table; this is indicative of a tight retinaculum. Medial and lateral patellar glide tests are also used to assess retinacular tightness. The examiner performs each test separately by applying both thumbs to push the patellar edge first medially and then laterally. The examiner notes the degree of translation when applying minimal translational force. Tightness of the lateral retinaculum is indicated by the inability to translate the patella medially more than one fourth of its width (2 cm). Hypermobility of the patella is indicated when the examiner is able to translate the patella medially or laterally by three fourths of its width or more (6 cm). The patellar apprehension test indicates recurrent subluxation if the patient feels instability with lateral patellar pressure. It is performed in the same fashion as the lateral patellar glide test.

Patellar compression or grind test (Clarke's sign)
(Figure 13.10)

The patellar compression or grind test (Clarke's sign) suggests the presence of patellofemoral dysfunction. The examiner performs the patellar compression test by placing the web of the hand over either the proximal or distal pole of the patella. The patient

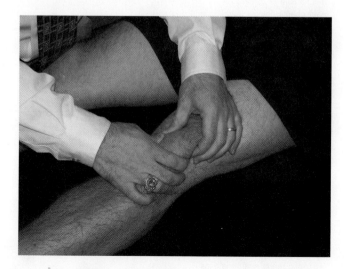

Figure 13.9 Patellar tilt test.

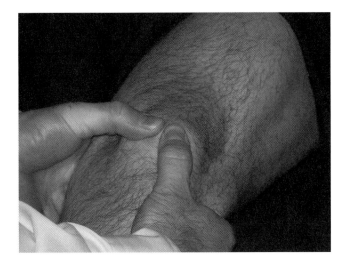

Figure 13.10 Patellar compression or grind test.

Table 13.3 Muscle Test Grading

Grade	Value	Movement
5	Normal	Full range of movement against gravity with maximal resistance (100%)
4	Good	Full range of movement against gravity with moderate resistance (75%)
3 +	Fair +	Full range of movement against gravity with mild resistance
3	Fair	Full range of movement against gravity (no resistance applied; 50%)
2	Poor	Full range of movement with gravity eliminated (25%)
1	Trace	Evidence of minimal contractility but no joint movement
0	Zero	No contraction palpated

is asked to contract the quadriceps muscles while the examiner pushes down on the patella directly. A negative test produces no pain. If this action produces pain and the patient cannot hold the contraction, then the test is considered positive. Ideally, this test is performed with a slight 15-degree to 20-degree knee flexion so that the patella is anatomically set in the trochlear groove.

In the knee, *plicae* are embryologic tissue folds that are occasionally a source of strain or that form a nidus for the growth of inflammatory tissue. On examination, plicae are palpable along the medial/lateral retinaculum and in the infrapatellar region. Some plicae are symptomatic and are tender fibrous bands that "snap" or "pop" over the femoral condyle as the knee is passively flexed and extended. These can mimic meniscal tears, but they are superficial.

Vastus medialis obliquus isometric strength test
(Figure 13.11)
The assessment of patellar and knee function is completed with quadriceps, hamstring, and hip muscle strength testing. While the patient remains in the supine position, each of these muscle groups should be tested. See **Table 13.3** for muscle test grading. To assess anterior knee pain, the examiner should isolate the vastus medialis obliquus by rotating the foot laterally while the

knee is extended. The patient is asked to perform an isometric quadriceps muscle contraction while the examiner applies downward resistance on the anterior tibia, and a comparison should be made with the opposite side. Pain with this quadriceps test may be the most specific physical examination finding in patients who have patellofemoral pain syndrome, with a specificity of 96% and a sensitivity of 40% (LOE: D).[25]

Q-angle test
The Q-angle, or the patellofemoral angle, is the angle between the quadriceps muscles and the patellar tendon. Both the hip and foot must be placed in neutral positions. Applying the goniometer to a midpoint on the patella, the examiner measures the angle formed from lines created from the tibial tubercle and the anterior superior iliac spines. Normal Q-angle measurements are 14 to 16 degrees and 16 to 18 degrees for males and females, respectively. Femoral neck anteversion and external tibial torsion increase the Q-angle. Femoral neck retroversion and internal tibial torsion decrease the Q-angle.

Ligamentous stability
Medial collateral ligament
Valgus stress test (Figure 13.12) The MCL is evaluated for injury and laxity via palpation, passive range of motion, and the valgus stress test. The patient will have tenderness to palpation

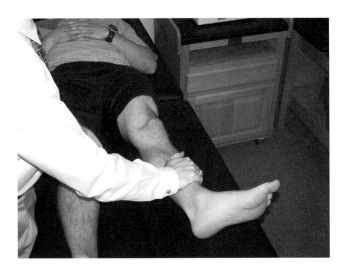

Figure 13.11 Vastus medialis obliquus isometric strength test.

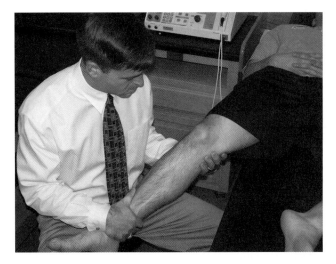

Figure 13.12 Valgus stress test.

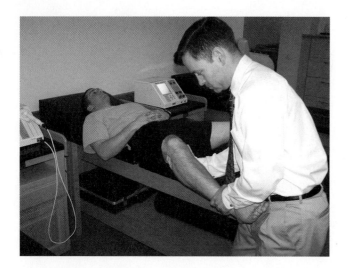

Figure 13.13 Varus stress test.

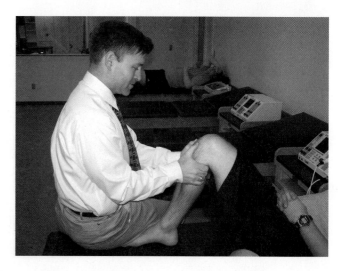

Figure 13.14 Anterior drawer test.

along the course of the MCL. Pain may be elicited with passive range of motion when flexing to more than 90 degrees and with hyperextension. To perform the valgus stress test, the examiner first stabilizes the joint with one hand palpating the knee along the medial joint line and the entire length of the MCL. The examiner evaluates the degree of laxity by holding the ankle with the other hand and applying a valgus force to the knee while keeping the ankle in a neutral position. The examiner performs the same maneuver at 0 and 30 degrees of knee flexion; the flexed position reduces static stabilization by the PCL and suggests PCL compromise if increased laxity exists at 0 degrees.

MCL injuries are graded on a scale of 1 to 3. A grade 1 injury is a stretch injury to the ligament without dissociation (0-mm to 5-mm opening), a grade 2 injury is a partial ligamentous disruption (6-mm to 10-mm opening), and a grade 3 injury is complete MCL disruption (> 10-mm opening).

Lateral collateral ligament
Varus stress test (Figure 13.13) Injury to the LCL is less common than that of the MCL, because the lateral stabilizing complex is less anatomically vulnerable than the MCL. Therefore, it is commonly associated with significant injury to other static knee stabilizers, such as the ACL, the PCL, and the arcuate ligament complex, of which it is a component.[10] The LCL is evaluated for injury in a similar manner to the way the MCL is and via the varus stress test. The patient notes tenderness along the course of the LCL. The varus stress test is performed in a similar manner to the valgus test for the MCL. The examiner repeats the test at 0 degrees and 30 degrees of knee flexion to disengage PCL contributions to the stability. The examiner stabilizes and palpates the joint with one hand while evaluating LCL laxity by holding the ankle with the other hand and applying a varus force to the knee.[14] LCL injuries are graded on a scale of 1 through 3 (as the MCL injuries are).

The anterior drawer test used to evaluate the ACL may demonstrate a grade 3 LCL injury. The patient is assessed with the knee flexed to 90 degrees and with the tibia placed in internal rotation. An anteriorly directed drawer force is then applied to the proximal tibia; the lateral tibia rotates anteriorly with a grade 3 LCL tear.[33]

Anterior cruciate ligament
Anterior drawer test (Figure 13.14) The integrity of the ACL is assessed with the anterior drawer test, Lachman's test, and the pivot shift test. The anterior drawer test is performed with the patient supine and the injured knee flexed to 90 degrees. The examiner stabilizes the foot in a neutral position and, with the thumbs placed at the tibial tubercle, applies an anterior force to the proximal tibia (see Figure 13.14). If the ACL is torn, the tibia will subluxate anteriorly from the neutral starting position. The anterior drawer test has a sensitivity of 48% and a specificity of 87% (LOE: D).[1]

Lachman's test (Figure 13.15) Lachman's test is the single best test for assessing the integrity of the ACL, with a sensitivity of 87% and a specificity of 93% (LOE: D).[1] The patient is again supine, with the injured knee flexed 20 to 30 degrees. The examiner uses one hand to stabilize the distal femur while the other hand grasps the proximal tibia. An anterior force is applied to the proximal tibia in an attempt to sublux the tibia. The modified Lachman's test incorporates the examiner's knee below the patient's posterior thigh to serve as the anchor. The test is positive if there is excessive anterior translation of the proximal tibia (at least 3 mm greater than the uninjured side) and a lack of a firm end point. Grading of ACL laxity is described as 1 through 3, as for the MCL.

Pivot shift test The pivot shift test to check for ACL tear requires good relaxation, and, therefore, it is best performed on the sideline before swelling and stiffness occur in the injured patient. It is performed with the patient supine and the knee fully extended. The foot and tibia are internally rotated, and a mild valgus stress is applied while the knee is gently flexed. At approximately 30 degrees, the tibia tends to subluxate anteriorly if the ACL is torn. The tibia will reduce on return to neutral. The sensitivity and specificity of the pivot shift test are 61% and 97%, respectively.[1] The pivot shift test has the highest positive predictive value of the three ACL tests (LOE: D).[12]

Posterior cruciate ligament
Posterior drawer test Patients with PCL injuries will more often present with vague symptoms or disability, and they are not as likely to describe an acute event. Inspection may reveal tibia vara, external rotation, and genu recurvatum as compared with the uninjured knee. Tenderness to palpation of the posterolateral knee and a joint effusion are often present with PCL injuries. Injury to the PCL may be noted on examination via stability testing by the posterior drawer test. The posterior drawer test is conducted with the patient in the supine position. The knee is

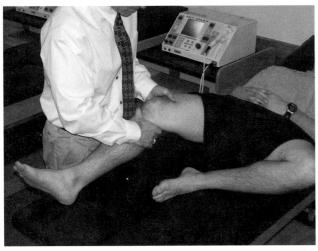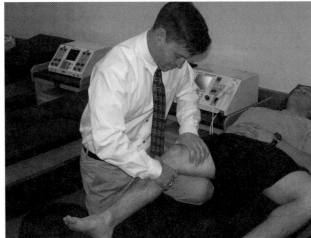

A   B

Figure 13.15 *A*, Lachman's test. *B*, Modified Lachman's test.

flexed to 90 degrees, with the foot stabilized on the table. Force is applied to the anterior tibial plateau in a posterior direction, and the degree of laxity is noted. PCL injury is graded as 1 through 3 (as for the MCL). The posterior drawer test is the most sensitive (90%) and specific (99%) test for the diagnosis of PCL injuries (LOE: D).[12]

Posterior sag or gravity sign The posterior sag or gravity sign is evaluated with the patient supine and with both knees and hips flexed to 90 degrees. The examiner holds the patient's legs and inspects them from a lateral direction to look for posterior tibial translation in the affected knee. The sensitivity of this finding is 79%, and the specificity is 100% (LOE: D).[12]

The varus and valgus stress tests as described for the evaluation of the MCL and LCL may be positive for PCL injury; this is most notable when the tests are performed in the setting of a concomitant collateral ligament injury.

Dial test (Figure 13.16) The dial test is used to assess posterolateral knee instability. Veltri[34] and Warren describe this test with the patient in the supine position, the foot/tibia passively drawn over

the side of the table, and the femur stabilized on the table. The examiner passively rotates the tibia laterally on the femur first at 30 degrees of knee flexion and then at 90 degrees of knee flexion. A comparison is made with the uninjured side. Compare the injured side with the uninjured side. If the affected tibia rotates more at 30 degrees, an isolated posterolateral injury is more likely. If the involved tibia rotates more at 90 degrees, injury to the PCL is likely.

Menisci

Meniscal injury produces a small effusion and joint line tenderness. The four specifically studied methods to detect meniscal injuries are McMurray's test, the joint line tenderness sign, the Apley compression test, and the "bounce home" test.

McMurray's test (Figure 13.17)

McMurray's test is performed with the patient supine and relaxed. The examiner grasps the patient's heel with one hand and the joint line of the knee with the other hand. The knee is flexed maximally, with external tibial rotation (medial meniscus) or internal tibial rotation (lateral meniscus). The knee

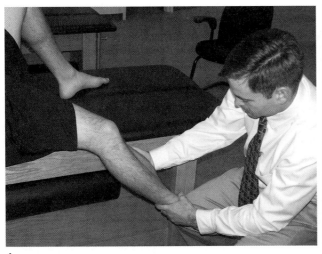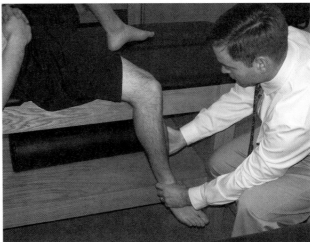

A   B

Figure 13.16 Dial Test at 30 degrees *(A)* and 90 degrees *(B)*.

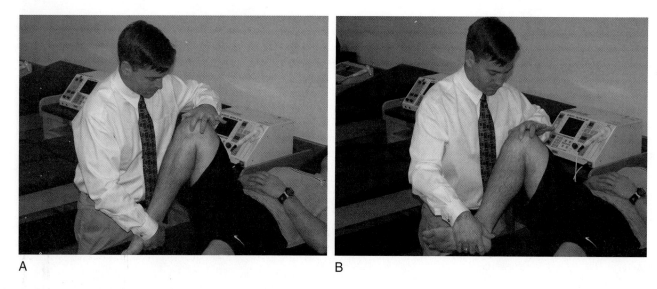

A   B

Figure 13.17   McMurray's test of the lateral meniscus *(A)* and the medial meniscus *(B)*.

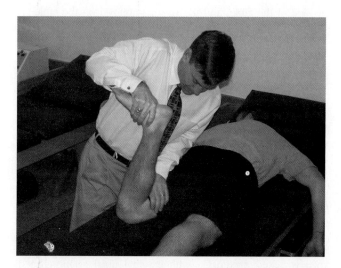

Figure 13.18   The Apley compression test (medial meniscus).

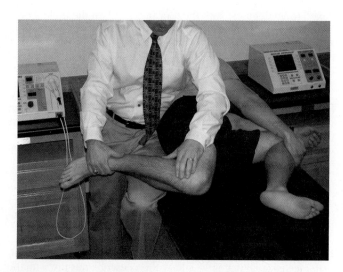

Figure 13.20   Ober's test.

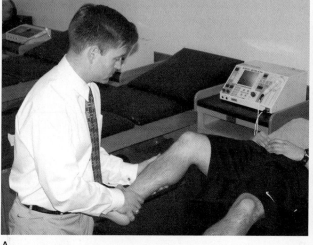

A   B

Figure 13.19   The start *(A)* and finish *(B)* of the "bounce home" test.

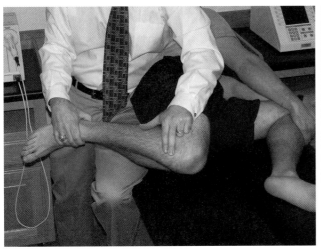 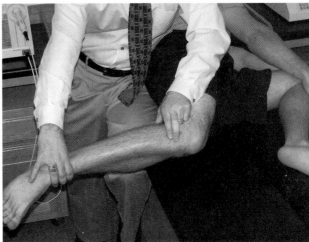

A B

Figure 13.21 The modified Noble test in flexion *(A)* and extension *(B)*.

is brought to full extension while maintaining rotation. A positive test produces a pop or click. Pain in a reproducible portion of the range of motion is described as part of McMurray's test. McMurray's test is specific (97%) but not very sensitive (52%) (LOE: D).[1]

Joint line tenderness sign

To check for joint line tenderness, the knee is first flexed to 90 degrees, with the patient supine. Joint line tenderness can also be assessed with the patient's knee hanging over the edge of the examining table, with a slight downward distracting force applied to the ankle. The joint line between the femur and the tibial condyles is palpated medially and laterally. The presence of pain on palpation is a positive finding. In contrast with McMurray's test, the joint line tenderness sign is sensitive (76%) but not very specific (29%) (LOE: D).[1]

Apley compression test (Figure 13.18)

The Apley compression test is performed with the patient in a prone position. The knee is flexed to 90 degrees, and a downward axial load is applied to the tibia while internally and externally rotating the tibia. A painful pop over the medial joint line is positive for a medial meniscal injury; a painful pop over the lateral joint line is positive for a lateral meniscal injury. The sensitivity of the Apley test ranges from 16% to 58%, and the specificity ranges from 80% to 82% (LOE: D).[9]

"Bounce home" or spring test (Figure 13.19)

The "bounce home" or spring test is performed with the patient supine and the heel cupped in the examiner's hand. The knee is allowed to passively extend from 30 degrees of flexion while the examiner supports the lower extremity. The test is positive if the knee does not reach full extension or if it has a springy end feel. Pain with this maneuver suggests meniscal injury.

Iliotibial band
Ober's test (Figure 13.20)

Patients with ITBand syndrome will often have tenderness to palpation of the lateral knee approximately 2 cm above the joint line, which will frequently worsen when the patient is standing and when the knee is flexed to 30 degrees. Ober's test is used to assess the flexibility of the ITBand. It is performed with the patient in the lateral decubitus position on the untested leg, with

the hip at the 90-degree position. The examiner stands behind the patient and grasps the top leg. The knee is flexed 90 degrees, and the hip is abducted and extended. The limb is allowed to passively adduct by gravity. Normal is considered to be when the knee drops level to or below the level of the examination table. This maneuver may replicate the lateral knee pain of ITBand syndrome.[34,35]

Noble compression test (Figure 13.21)

The Noble compression test is performed to demonstrate ITBand friction syndrome. The examiner positions the patient in the supine position with the hip flexed and proceeds to flex the knee 90 degrees while applying thumb pressure over the lateral femoral epicondyle. While the pressure is maintained, the knee is passively extended. A positive test is when the patient reports pain at approximately 30 degrees of knee flexion.[15] A variation of the Noble compression test that may be more helpful is performed with the patient in the lateral decubitus position on the untested leg (as for Ober's test). The examiner applies manual pressure at Gerdy's tubercle on the anterolateral aspect of the tibia while passively flexing and extending the knee. Again, pain symptoms are often most prominent when the knee is flexed to approximately 30 degrees.

Flexibility
Thomas' test (Figure 13.22)

Flexibility of the major muscle groups of the lower extremities should be assessed, particularly in the setting of an overuse injury of the knee. Thomas' test is used to assess quadriceps flexibility and hip flexion contracture. It is performed by having the patient lie supine with one hip and knee flexed and held against the chest. The contralateral leg is allowed to hang off the end of the examination table. If a hip flexion contracture is present, then the leg will not remain flush with the table. The angle formed between the involved leg and the examination table equals the number of degrees of flexion contracture present.[15]

Popliteal angle (Figure 13.23)

Hamstring flexibility is determined with the patient lying supine and the hip held at 90 degrees of flexion. The patient is asked to actively extend the knee, and a measurement is made of the popliteal angle using a goniometer. The normal range is less than 10 degrees short of full extension.[25]

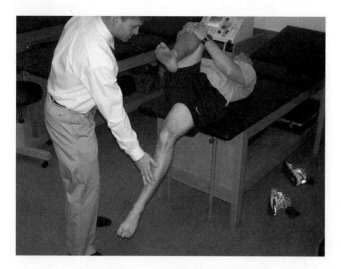

Figure 13.22 Thomas' test.

The flexibility of the ITBand is assessed using Ober's test, as described previously. Flexibility of the gastrocnemius–soleus complex should be assessed because decreased dorsiflexion of the ankle will often contribute to patellofemoral pain syndrome.

Neurovascular examination

The nerves that arise from the lumbar (L2-L5) and sacral (S2) spinal roots provide sensation to the skin over the knee and the surrounding areas. Decreased sensation of any of these dermatomes should prompt the examiner to search for proximal neuropathy. Posterolateral knee injuries will cause a common peroneal nerve injury in 15% of patients.[12] The examiner should assess for any sensory changes and examine the strength of ankle dorsiflexion and great toe extension.

Deep tendon reflexes of the lower extremities should be assessed at the patellar and Achilles tendons. The patellar reflex is mediated predominately through the L4 nerve root, although L2 and L3 also contribute. The reflex is tested by having the patient sit on the edge of the examination table with the legs hanging free. The patellar tendon is located and tapped at the level of the knee joint, and the reaction is compared with that of the opposite side. The medial hamstring reflex is mediated by the

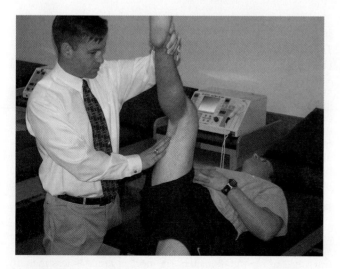

Figure 13.23 Popliteal angle.

L5 nerve root, with a contribution from S1. It is elicited by having the patient lie supine with the hip slightly flexed, externally rotated, and abducted. The examiner's index finger is placed over the medial hamstring tendon of the ipsilateral knee and struck with a reflex hammer.[33] The Achilles reflex is mediated primarily by the S1 nerve root, although S2 is also involved. It is tested by briskly tapping the Achilles tendon with the ankle and knee at 90 degrees of flexion. The neurologic examination should be completed by checking Babinski's reflex to rule out an upper motor neuron lesion.

Arterial pulses should be palpated at the popliteal, posterior tibialis, and dorsalis pedis arteries to document distal perfusion. This is particularly important in the setting of traumatic injury to the lower extremity and in knees that are dislocated or that have injuries to multiple ligaments. In combined ACL/PCL injuries, 14% of patients will have an associated vascular injury.[12]

Referred pain

Knee pain can arise from the knee itself, or it may be referred from conditions of the hip, the ankle, or the lower back. The nerves that provide sensation to the knee come from the lower back, and they also provide sensation to the hip, leg, and ankle. Pathologic conditions of the hip in pediatric patients (particularly slipped capital femoral epiphysis) commonly present as poorly localized knee pain. Other conditions that may present as knee pain include femoral neck fracture, avascular necrosis of the hip, and lumbar disc herniation.

The kinetic chain

Patients who present with knee pain, particularly in the absence of an acute knee injury, need to have a biomechanical evaluation of the lower extremity kinetic chain because malalignment can lead to dysfunction and pain. Inspection of the knee with the patient standing straight may reveal genu varum ("bowed legs"), genu valgum ("knock knees"), or genu recurvatum. The examiner should examine the patient for leg-length discrepancy, pes planus, and/or foot pronation. Excessive medial deviation of the knee beyond the second toe during a one- or two-legged squat indicates weakness of the hip abductors and external rotators.[15] Hip pathology can be detected by testing internal and external rotation in single planes; this is then followed by combined movements such as the flexion, abduction, and external rotation test and by passive movement of the hip quadrant (flexion, adduction, and internal rotation). Patients should be asked about any previous injuries because these may often result in kinetic chain dysfunction, particularly when rehabilitation has been inadequate.

REFERENCES

1. Jackson JL, O'Malley PG, Kroenke K: Evaluation of acute knee pain in primary care. Ann Intern Med 2003;139:575-588.
2. Kroenke K, Jackson JL: Outcome in general medical patients presenting with common symptoms: a prospective study with a 2-week and a 3-week follow-up. Fam Pract 1998;15:398-403.
3. National Center for Health Statistics: News release: Aging boomers drive up doctor visits (Web site): Available at www.cdc.gov/od/oc/media/pressrel/r030811.htm. Accessed June 15, 2004.
4. Adirim TA, Cheng TL: Overview of injuries in the young athlete. Sports Med 2003;33:75-81.
5. McCaig LF: National Hospital Ambulatory Medical Care Survey: 1992 emergency department survey. Adv Data 1994;Mar 2(245):1-12.
6. Arendt E, Dick R: Knee injury patterns among men and women in collegiate basketball and soccer: NCAA data and review of the literature. Am J Sports Med 1995;23:694-701.
7. Hutchinson MR, Ireland ML: Knee injuries in female athletes. Sports Med 1995;19:287-302.

8. Chandy T, Grana W: Secondary school athletic injury in boys and girls: a three-year comparison. Phys Sportsmed 1985;13:21-26.
9. Allen JE, Taylor KS: Physical examination of the knee. Prim Care 2004;31:887-907.
10. Bach BR: Acute knee injuries: when to refer. Phys Sportsmed 1997;25(5):45-52.
11. Kocher MS, Klingele K, Rassman SO: Meniscal disorders: normal, discoid and cysts. Orthop Clin North Am 2003;34(3):329-340.
12. Brown JR, Trojian TH: Anterior and posterior cruciate ligament injuries. Prim Care 2004;31:925-956.
13. Harner CD, Xerogeanes JW, Livesay GA: The human posterior cruciate ligament complex: an interdisciplinary study: ligament morphology and biomechanical evaluation. Am J Sports Med 1995;23:736-745.
14. Quarles JD, Hosely RG: Medial and lateral meniscus injuries: prognosis and treatment. Prim Care 2004;31:957-975.
15. Fredericson M, Guillet M, DeBenedictis L: Quick solutions for ITBand syndrome. Phys Sportsmed 2000;28(2):52-68.
16. Pope MH, Johnson RJ, Brown DW, Tighe C: The role of the musculature in injuries to the medial collateral ligament. J Bone Joint Surg Am 1979;61(3):398-402.
17. Malone T, Davies G, Walsh M: Muscular control of the patella. Clin Sports Med 2002;21:349-362.
18. Muche JA: Posterior knee pain and its causes. Phys Sportsmed 2004;32(3):23-30.
19. Basmajian JV, Lovejoy JF Jr: Functions of the popliteus muscle in man: a multifactorial electromyographic study. J Bone Joint Surg Am 1971;53(3):557-562.
20. Petsche TS, Selesnick FH: Popliteus tendonitis: tips for diagnosis and management. Phys Sportsmed 2002;30(8):27-31.
21. Sansone V, Sosio C, da Gama Malcher M, de Ponti A: Two cases of tibial nerve compression caused by uncommon popliteal cysts. Arthroscopy 2002;18:(2):E8.
22. Mastaglia FL: Tibial nerve entrapment in the popliteal fossa. Muscle Nerve 2000;23(12):1883-1886.
23. Hochman MG, Zilberfarb JL: Nerves in a pinch: imaging of nerve compression syndromes. Radiol Clin North Am 2004;42(1):221-245.
24. Adams MT, Wixon CL: Popliteal artery entrapment syndrome. J Am Coll Surg 2003;196(1):152-153.
25. LaBella C: Patellofemoral pain syndrome: evaluation and treatment. Prim Care 2004;31:977-1003.
26. Ofluoglu O: Pigmented villonodular synovitis. Orthop Clin North Am 2006;37:23-33.
27. Greis PE, Bardana DD, Holstrom MC, Burks RT: Meniscal injury: I. Basic science and evaluation. J Am Acad Orthop Surg 2002;10:168-176.
28. Margheritini F, Rihn J, Musahi V, et al: Posterior cruciate ligament injuries in the athlete. Sports Med 2002;32(6):393-408.
29. Birk GT, DeLee JC: Osteochondral injuries. Clinical findings. Clin Sports Med 2001;20(2):279-286.
30. Bruce EJ, Hamby T, Jones DG: Sports-related osteochondral injuries: clinical presentation, diagnosis, and treatment. Prim Care 2005;32:253-276.
31. Sallay PI, Poggi J, Speer KP, et al: Acute dislocation of the patella. A correlative pathoanatomic study. Am J Sports Med 1996;24:52-60.
32. Oberlander MA, Shalvoy RM, Hughston JC: The accuracy of the clinical knee examination documented by arthroscopy. A prospective study. Am J Sports Med 1993;21(6):773-778.
33. Magee DJ. Orthopedic Physical Assessment, 4th ed. Philadelphia, WB Saunders, 2002.
34. Veltri DM, Warren RF: Posteriolateral instability of the knee. J Bone Joint Surg Am 1994;76:460-472.
35. Khaund R, Flynn SH: Iliotibial band syndrome: a common source of knee pain. Am Fam Physician 2005;71(8):27-35.

Physical Examination of the Foot and Ankle

Karl B. Fields, MD; Wesley R. Ibazebo, MD; and Ryan E. Modlinski, MD

KEY POINTS

- Anatomy, biomechanics, and gait are key components of the examination of the foot and ankle.
- Structural changes in the foot reflect functional stress, and they can often be identified on visual inspection.
- Specific foot structures indicate a higher risk for sports injury (e.g., cavus feet and highly pronated feet).
- Certain areas of the foot are at high risk for poor outcomes and merit cautious examination after injury (e.g., the navicular and Lisfranc's joint).

INTRODUCTION

Clinical examination of the foot and ankle requires the assessment of the complex anatomy, biomechanics, and gait of the individual patient. Static evaluation alone misses critical factors that might interfere with the ability of the patient to stand, run, and jump. In addition to standard examination techniques, visual clues often suggest the correct diagnosis of many injuries. Integrating the findings from observation, physical testing, and gait assessment with an understanding of basic biomechanics is the cornerstone of the correct diagnosis of ankle and foot injuries.

FUNCTIONAL ANATOMY OF THE FOOT AND ANKLE

The foot functions as the body's only consistent contact point with the ground. A complex part of the human body in form and function, the foot has 26 major bones: 7 tarsals, 5 metatarsals, and 14 phalanges. Anatomists divide the foot into three distinct regions: (1) the hindfoot, which consists of the calcaneus and the talus; (2) the midfoot, which has the cuneiforms, the navicular, and the cuboid; and (3) the forefoot, which has the metatarsals and phalanges.

The hindfoot incorporates the tibiofibular joint, the talocrural (true ankle) joint, and the subtalar joint. Together, these structures function to help support the body's weight and the impact forces that occur during walking, running, jumping, and standing. As such, the talus and the calcaneus are strong, thick bones that tolerate impressive forces and form a stable attachment site for heavily burdened structures such as the Achilles tendon and the plantar fascia.

Midfoot bones provide the core of the foot arches. The navicular lends stability to the medial longitudinal arch, the cuboid provides the same for the lateral longitudinal arch, and the cuneiforms in the middle of the foot give shape to the transverse arch. The articulation of the hindfoot and the midfoot create the transverse tarsal joint, which is also known as *Chopart's joint*. This joint is a combination of the calcaneocuboid and talonavicular joints, and rotation around the Chopart's joint complex gives the foot its ability to adapt to uneven surfaces. The midfoot also serves as an attachment point for the tendons that facilitate inversion and eversion.

The forefoot begins at the tarsometatarsal joint, which is also known as *Lisfranc's joint*. Movement at this joint involves active flexion and extension, which are the keys to effective push off for running and jumping. For this motion to be effective, the long thin bones of the metatarsals and phalanges must function as levers to generate greater force.

The bones of the foot form two primary arches: (1) the longitudinal arch, which runs from the calcaneus to the distal ends of the metatarsals; and (2) the transverse arch, which extends horizontally across the foot and consists of the cuboid, the cuneiforms, and the metatarsals. The longitudinal arch is further divided into a medial part, which includes the calcaneus, the talus, the navicular, three cuneiforms, and three medial metatarsals, and a lateral part, which is formed by the calcaneus, the cuboid, and the fourth and fifth metatarsals. Ideally, the arches work like a spring for energy dissipation. The medial arch is thicker than the lateral arch to prevent hyperpronation during ambulation. During weight bearing, the arches compress to absorb and distribute the load. Ligaments like the plantar calcaneonavicular ligament (the spring ligament) and the short and long plantar ligaments assist with this force distribution. The integrity of the arches and their ability to absorb loads is maintained by the tight-fitting articulations between the bones of the foot, the action of the intrinsic foot musculature, and the strength of the plantar ligaments and plantar fascia.[1] The configuration of the arches and of Chopart's joint allow the foot the mobility necessary to adjust to landing on uneven ground surfaces and the rigidity to prepare for push off.

The anatomic structure of the plantar fascia helps create the solid platform that is necessary for propulsion. This aponeurosis originates at the medial border of the calcaneus and attaches distally to the capsule of the proximal phalanges. The plantar fascia also crosses Chopart's and Lisfranc's joints, and it serves as a passive restraint in addition to stabilizing the longitudinal arch. In biomechanical texts, the plantar fascia is likened to a Spanish windlass. Dugan and Bhat describe extension occurring at the metatarsophalangeal joint before toe off, with the plantar fascia tightening and pulling the calcaneal and metatarsal heads together.[2] This movement increases the height of the longitudinal arch, and it forces Chopart's joint into a flexed position that creates a solid structural support. The plantar fascia also serves as a trigger for the gastrocnemius–soleus complex. The stretch of the aponeurosis sends electrical stimulation to the complex, thus enabling it to fire.

The ankle or talocrural joint is a hinge joint that consists of the tibia, the fibula, and the talus. Superiorly, the anterior and posterior inferior tibiofibular ligaments and the interosseous membrane hold the tibia and fibula together. These structures collectively are known as the *syndesmosis*, and they stabilize the tibia and fibula to form the mortise, in which the talus sits. The tibia and fibula provide bony stability to the ankle joint as they extend down over the talus and form the medial and lateral malleoli.[3] The longer lateral malleolus provides greater bony stabilization, and it is supported by three relatively thin collateral ligaments: the anterior talofibular, the lateral calcaneofibular, and the posterior talofibular. The medial malleolus provides less bony restraint to injury, but it has the broad-based deltoid ligament attached and fanning down over the medial aspect of the rear foot to form a rigid structure that resists excessive eversion or subluxation. The ankle joint has a true synovial capsule.

The axis of rotation around any joint is perpendicular to the plane of motion. The ankle lies predominantly in the frontal and transverse planes, and, therefore, motion occurs in the sagittal plane. This, along with the bony structure, limits movement at the true ankle joint to predominantly plantarflexion and dorsiflexion. The average range of motion at the ankle joint is 45 degrees, with up to 20 degrees of dorsiflexion and 25 to 35 degrees of plantarflexion.[4] Inman[5] describes differences in dorsiflexion in the open versus the closed kinetic chain of the ankle as it relates to the rotation of the tibia. In the open kinetic chain, the tibia rotates externally, whereas, in the closed kinetic chain, the tibia rotates internally.

The subtalar joint lies between the talus and the calcaneus, and it is composed of three articular facets: anterior, middle, and posterior. These separate articulations function as a single joint and allow for the complex triplanar motions of pronation and supination. This composite motion is triplanar because it does not lie in any one of the three cardinal planes. Dugan and Bhat[2] liken the subtalar joint to an oblique hinge because of its unique configuration. The subtalar axis averages 23 degrees (with a range of 4 to 47 degrees) from the sagittal plane, and 41 degrees (with a range of 21 to 69 degrees) from horizontal.[6] Mann[6] defined supination in an open kinetic chain as plantarflexion, adduction, and inversion, and he defined pronation in the open kinetic chain as abduction, dorsiflexion, and eversion. In a closed kinetic chain, however, pronation changes as abduction results in the internal rotation of the tibia and the talus. With the foot planted, attempted dorsiflexion causes talar head plantarflexion and calcaneal eversion.[6]

The transverse tarsal axis (Chopart's joint) is a transitional area between the hindfoot and the midfoot. Motion at the joint consists of two axes that allow for pronation and supination. The longitudinal axis is inclined 15 degrees from the ground and rotated 9 degrees medially from sagittal plane, and it provides eversion/inversion and abduction/adduction. The oblique axis is inclined 52 degrees from the ground and rotated 57 degrees medially from the sagittal plane, and it provides plantarflexion/dorsiflexion.[7] With hindfoot eversion, the axes become parallel and allow for pronation and increased motion within this two-joint complex. With hindfoot inversion, supination occurs, and the axes converge, which causes the joint complex to lock into rigid configuration.[8] When examining ambulation, this mechanism defines why pronation creates a flexible foot for shock absorption, whereas supination creates a rigid lever for propulsion.

The tarsometatarsal joints (Lisfranc's joint) can be divided into five rays. The first ray is composed of the medial cuneiform and the first metatarsal. Motion at this joint is primarily a combination of dorsiflexion/inversion/adduction and plantarflexion/eversion/abduction.[9] The second ray contains the intermediate cuneiform and the second metatarsal, which is recessed and firmly placed into the base of the first and third metatarsal–cuneiform joints. Lisfranc's ligament locks this joint firmly into this recess to form the keystone for the longitudinal axis of the foot. This orientation subjects the bone to increased stress as a result of the inherent stability as the foot progresses through the stance phase.[9] The lateral cuneiform and the third and fourth metatarsals make up the third and fourth rays, with motion that is limited to plantarflexion/dorsiflexion.[9] The fifth ray allows for some pronation and supination as the fifth metatarsal rotates about the cuboid.

The metatarsal break is created by the metatarsophalangeal joints that extend about an oblique axis from the head of the second metatarsal to the head of the fifth metatarsal. Motion at this joint is predominantly flexion/extension.[9] The break averages 62 degrees from the long axis of the foot, and it helps with leg external rotation and foot supination during propulsion.[6]

WALKING GAIT

Walking gait incorporates a stance phase and a swing phase. The stance phase composes 62% of the cycle, and it is the weight-bearing portion.[6] The stance phase is subdivided into heel strike, midstance, and toe off. During heel strike, the tibia internally rotates, and the triple joint complex (subtalar, talonavicular, and calcaneocuboid) moves into an everted position. The cuboid follows the calcaneus, abducts the forefoot, and flattens out the medial longitudinal arch. Anterior compartment muscles contract eccentrically, thus providing control and cushioning as the foot approaches midstance to allow for smooth forefoot contact after heel strike.[10] At midstance, the weight centers over the middle of the foot at the second metatarsal. The motion of the body's center of gravity as it moves forward over the foot causes the tibia to externally rotate as the ankle dorsiflexes. The triple joint complex supinates, locking the joint into a slight varus position, and this creates a rigid lever of the medial longitudinal arch for push off.[1] Functionally, the foot must be flexible on ground contact and rigid for propulsion. Flexibility on contact provides shock absorption and accommodates footstrike on uneven terrain. Rigidity helps transfer the force that is generated by lower leg muscle action to the ground.

RUNNING GAIT

Running, like walking, is a series of pronations and supinations, but it is distinguished by an increased velocity. This means that there is decreased time in the stance phase and the presence of a phase in which the runner is airborne called the *float phase*.[2]

Studies comparing runners and walkers suggest that the stance phase decreases from approximately 62% of the gait cycle time in walking to 31% in running and 22% in sprinting.[11] The increased muscular force required to generate an airborne phase and the greater impact of landing that necessitates increased shock absorption both contribute to higher injury rates in runners. Just as in walking, the stance phase of running is divided into three phases: landing, midstance, and push off. Approximately half of stance phase occurs with the foot pronated to allow force absorption, whereas, during the second half of the phase, the foot supinates to allow for propulsion.[2]

At initial contact, most runners land with a lateral heel strike and with the foot in a slightly supinated position. At this point, the leg is in a functional varus of 8 to 14 degrees, and the calcaneus is inverted approximately 4 degrees.[12] The pelvis rotates anteriorly 40 degrees to maintain the center of gravity over the landing leg. The quadriceps extend the knee, and the hamstrings aid in stabilization at initial ground contact.[13] After first contact, the foot pronates at the subtalar and midtarsal joints, becoming flexible to absorb impact. This movement causes a mitered hinge effect during which pronation is accompanied by hindfoot eversion and tibial internal rotation.[2] The axes of Chopart's joint become parallel, which allows for increased mobility and a foot that can accommodate uneven surfaces. This mechanism is vitally important because the force generated at heel strike is 1.5 to 5 times body weight, and this force may be generated 800 to 2000 times a mile, depending on speed and stride length.[13]

At midstance, the ankle dorsiflexors flatten the foot eccentrically on the ground. Maximum pronation occurs when the body's center of gravity passes anterior to the base of support. This point marks the end of the absorptive component of stance phase.[2] At this stage, the hip and knee align vertically with the ankle, and the hip displaces laterally about an inch to maintain the center of gravity.[13]

With push off, the hip rapidly extends using the gluteus maximus and the hamstrings while the foot begins supination at the subtalar joint. The opposite limb swings forward, and pelvic rotation results in an external rotation of the tibia of the push-off leg, which in turn causes inversion at the calcaneus and supination.[13] This supination causes convergence of the triple joint axes, which provides a "locked" midfoot that can serve as a rigid lever for propulsion.[2] This motion requires complex biomechanical interactions. In addition to the external rotation of the tibia, the metatarsal break contributes to supination as extension occurs at the first metatarsophalangeal joint. This extension also leads to the tightening of the plantar fascia, which provides stability to the midfoot by pulling the other soft-tissue structures of the foot taut. Lastly, the intrinsic foot muscles that cross the transverse tarsal joint serve to stabilize the joint as well.[2]

After the foot leaves the ground, the leg enters the swing phase. The first portion of the phase is acceleration. During this part, the hip flexors lift the leg and hip off of the ground. The knee flexes to 65 degrees, and the ankle dorsiflexors fire to ensure that the foot clears the ground.[13] At the middle part of the phase, the hip rotates anteriorly using the opposite hip as a fulcrum. During deceleration, the leg prepares for the next heel strike by having the hamstrings contract, which slows the swing. The peroneals also fire, thus stabilizing the ankle for a coordinated landing.[13] Clinical examination of gait includes the observation of walking. Evaluation determines if the stance is even from side to side, if the pelvis and shoulder appear level during ambulation, and if there is excessive pronation or supination during either heel strike or toe off. Barefoot gait allows for the better interpretation of findings, but ambulation with shoes also suggests whether the degree of pronation or supination is partially corrected by footwear.

Observation of the running gait takes experience and careful analysis of the entire kinetic chain. Although the degree of pronation or supination is often a key finding, a number of changes occur with foot strike. For example, foot strike with asymmetric external rotation ("toeing out") of the foot may relate to a contracture of hip rotator muscles. Weakness of the gluteus medius muscle, which helps with the abduction of the hip during stance phase, can lead to genu valgus or to a rapid horizontal shift of the patella. Significant genu valgus may also relate to excess pronation at the rear or mid foot. Thus, the observation of the running gait triggers the careful evaluation of anatomic changes and muscular testing that may correlate with the observed abnormality. Abnormal gait may appear as the runner runs toward the observer by differences in foot strike position, knee lift, hip flexion, or arm swing. As the runner runs away from the examiner, the back swing should appear symmetric and extend straight behind the runner. Rotation at any level may affect this. Trendelenburg's position or a dropped shoulder may suggest leg-length inequality. A review of Chapter 43, Gait Analysis, will further assist the reader with the performance of the gait evaluation.

STATIC EXAMINATION OF THE ANKLE

Inspection of the ankle notes swelling, bruising, or any obvious anatomic deformity by comparing the injured ankle to the uninvolved ankle. Both passive and active range of motion should be assessed. Strength testing against resistance, repetitive motions, and stance may all help identify subtle weakness. Neurovascular examination may identify causes of specific weaknesses or referred pain. The palpation of the ankle focuses on direct bony tenderness that may indicate a fracture. Anatomic areas with higher fracture risk include the base of the fifth metatarsal, the navicular, the medial malleolus, and the posterior edge and tip of the lateral malleolus. (See the Ottawa ankle rules for the practical application of this type of examination.)

Specific tests of the ankle for injury and instability of the anterior talofibular ligament include the anterior drawer test **(Figure 14.1).** Using one hand, stabilize the distal tibia and the fibula. Then, with the other hand, grasp the heel, keeping the foot in slight plantar flexion of 10 to 20 degrees, and try to move the foot forward. Translating the foot 3 mm or more forward or a difference between the injured and uninjured ankles that exceeds 0.5 mm is considered a positive test. Van Dijk and colleagues[14] found the anterior ankle drawer test to have a 71% sensitivity and a 33% specificity for anterior talofibular ligament rupture when

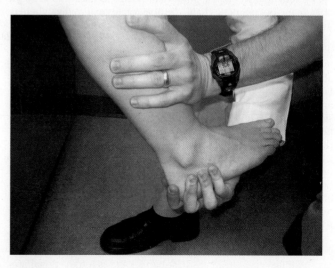

Figure 14.1 Anterior drawer test. (Used with permission by Dr. Karl B. Fields.)

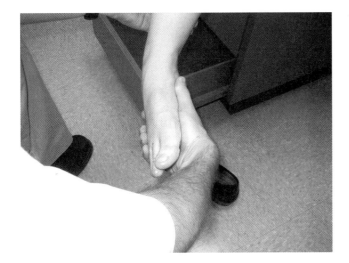

Figure 14.2   Talar tilt test. (Used with permission by Dr. Karl B. Fields.)

performed less than 48 hours after the inversion injury. This increased to a 96% sensitivity and an 84% specificity when repeated 5 days after the injury (LOE: D).[14]

The talar tilt test enables one to assess calcaneofibular ligament stability **(Figure 14.2)**. Again, stabilize the tibia and fibula with one hand. Grasp the heel with the foot in a neutral position, and invert the ankle with the other hand. Note the amount or degree of inversion of the injured ankle as compared with the other foot. Normal talar tilt ranges from 3 to 23 degrees, and anything greater than 23 degrees or a difference between the ankles of 5% to 10% is considered a positive test for calcaneonavicular instability.

Other specific examination techniques focus on specific conditions. Dorsiflexion tests look for evidence of anterior impingement. Plantarflexion stress tests may point to posterior impingement by os trigone, posterior talar process spurring, or other conditions. Thompson's test (a calf squeeze that results in plantar flexion) tests for Achilles integrity (96% sensitivity[15]; LOE: D) **(Figure 14.3)**. Kleiger's test (dorsiflexion and eversion) tests for syndesmosis injury, and it may also reproduce peroneal tendon subluxation.

STATIC EXAMINATION OF THE FOOT

Visual inspection first notes the overall shape of the foot. The normal foot has an overall "dome" shape as a result of the dominant medial longitudinal arch. The longitudinal arch of the foot can be further subdivided into the medial and lateral components.[16] The medial arch is composed of the calcaneus, the talus, the navicular, the medial cuneiforms, and three metatarsals.[16] The height of the arch should be measured from the base of the navicular to the ground with the patient in the standing position.[16] Abnormalities can include an excessively high arch (pes cavus) **(Figure 14.4)** or an excessively low arch (pes planus). A measurement of the navicular arch height of more than 3.12 cm is associated with an increased risk of injury.[17] The lateral longitudinal arch is much flatter, and it is composed of the calcaneus, the cuboid, and the lateral two metatarsals.[16] Attention must be paid during the examination of the arch during load bearing. The transverse arch is formed by the cuboid, the cuneiforms, and the bases of the metatarsals.[16] It is supported by the tendon of the peroneus longus as it crosses the plantar surface obliquely from the lateral foot to the base of the first metatarsal.[16] Breakdown of the transverse arch may lead to a widened forefoot. The normal ratio of the width of the forefoot to that of the hindfoot should be approximately 1.4 or 1.6 to 1. Wider

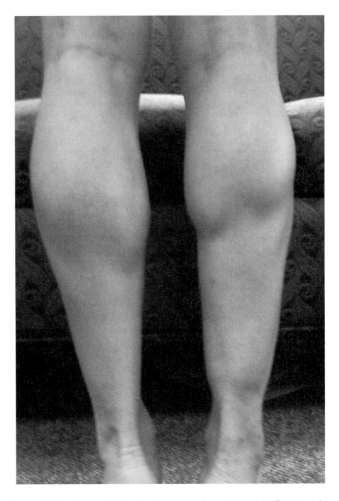

Figure 14.3   Partial right Achilles tendon rupture with nodule. Thompson's test would not show normal plantar flexion on calf squeeze. (Used with permission by Dr. Karl B. Fields.)

forefeet are seen in those individuals with a cavus foot who predominately bear weight on the forefoot.

Pes planus or "flatfoot" occurs from an inherited insufficient longitudinal arch, or it can develop from the breakdown of the longitudinal arch as a result of shifts in bony alignment from ligamentous breakdown or the collapse of support after rupture of the posterior tibialis tendon **(Figure 14.5)**. The foot often demonstrates calcaneal valgus **(Figure 14.6)** in combination with forefoot abduction and midfoot pronation. One sign of excess forefoot abduction is the "too many toes" sign. Looking from the rear, the examiner should not see more than two lateral toes unless the forefoot is excessively abducted. With a rigid flatfoot, when the patient stands on tiptoe, the longitudinal arch will not reappear. This is differentiated from the flexible flatfoot with which the arch is reestablished in non–weight-bearing positions or when the individual stands on his or her toes. This condition is mostly the result of posterior tibialis tendon contraction.

The term *forefoot* refers to the region of the foot from the base of the metatarsals to the tip of the phalanges. The prime function of the forefoot is push off, which requires long thin bones to function as a lever. This thinness promotes easier breakdown, including stress fractures, joint breakdown, and ligamentous strains. General inspection of the forefoot should assess for gross abnormalities of the skin, particularly thick callusing under the second metatarsal head, which is called *Morton's callus* **(Figure 14.7)**. Splaying of the toes often indicates metatarsal capsular

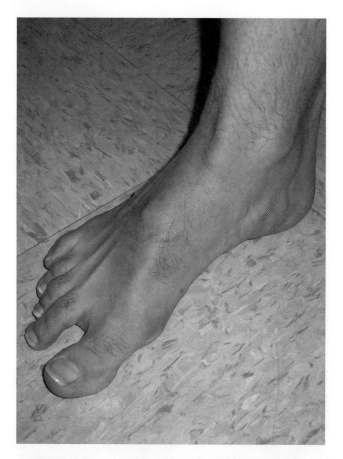

Figure 14.4 Cavus foot. (Used with permission by Dr. Karl B. Fields.)

breakdown, with the metatarsal head dropping through the plantar surface and leading to the rotation and separation of the toes. Palpation often reveals a dropped metatarsal head in the second, third, or fourth metatarsal that is indicative of transverse arch breakdown. Typically, only the first and fifth metatarsal heads make ground contact. Palpation that reveals hypermobile metatarsal heads may indicate a weakening of the intermetatarsal ligaments and precede transverse arch breakdown. Palpation of the metatarsal

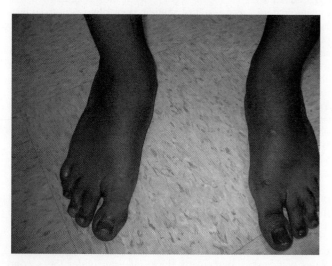

Figure 14.5 Pes planus with first ray dominance. (Used with permission by Dr. Karl B. Fields.)

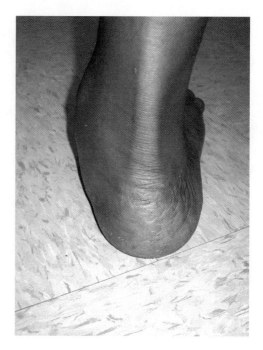

Figure 14.6 Calcaneal valgus with "too-many-toes" sign. (Used with permission by Dr. Karl B. Fields.)

shafts for direct tenderness or under the first metatarsophalangeal joint for sesamoid injury may be found in stress fractures.

An abnormal range of motion of the forefoot may suggest limitation elsewhere in the foot. The majority of forefoot abduction and adduction actually takes place in the junction of the hindfoot and midfoot at the talonavicular and calcaneocuboid joints. To examine these motions, stabilize the calcaneus with one hand, and move the forefoot both medially and laterally.[18] Normal values include

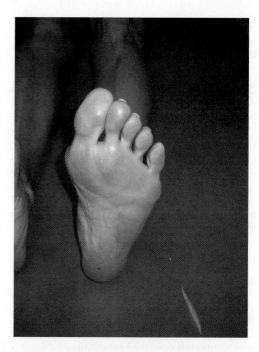

Figure 14.7 Morton's callus over second metatarsophalangeal (note also the fifth metatarsophalangeal callus.) (Used with permission by Dr. Karl B. Fields.)

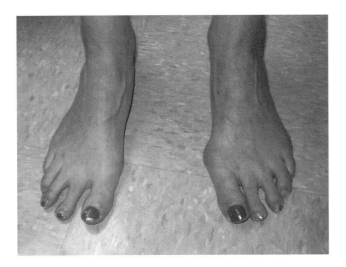

Figure 14.8 Bunion formation on the left in a runner with transverse arch breakdown bilaterally. (Used with permission by Dr. Karl B. Fields.)

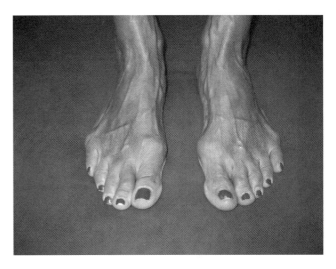

Figure 14.9 Bilateral bunionette with a prominent fifth metatarsophalangeal, a deviation of the fifth toe toward the fourth, and external rotation of the fifth toe. (Used with permission by Dr. Karl B. Fields.)

20 degrees of medial deviation and 10 degrees of lateral deviation.[18] The motion is assessed mainly by feel, and it is often difficult to measure accurately.

The examination and palpation of the bony structures of the forefoot should include the evaluation of each of the metatarsals and their associated phalanges. The examination should begin with the great toe because it plays an important role in the overall lever function and push off of the forefoot during the gait phase. After inspection is performed, the first test should be of the range of motion of the great toe. If any type of lateral deviation of the first metatarsal is present, range of motion should be tested in the reduced position. Given its importance as a lever, the first metatarsophalangeal joint must have good range of motion and joint stability. Normal range of motion includes 45 degrees of flexion and 30 to 90 degrees of extension. Less than 20 degrees of flexion and/or 30 degrees of extension limit function significantly. This decreased range of motion is referred to as *hallux rigidus*. Ideally, to obtain speed or power in jumping, 65 degrees of extension is optimal. Patients with hallux rigidus may demonstrate various compensatory measures to shift the force to the more flexible lateral four toes.

Hallux valgus change at the great toe occurs with the subluxation of the proximal phalanx at the metatarsophalangeal joint toward the second toe, which often displaces the second digit superiorly. The first metatarsal may migrate in the opposite direction, and the sesamoids often shift to the interspace between the first and second metatarsals.[16] This deformity may result in excess wear and friction over the medial metatarsophalangeal joint, which can result in a bursa or bunion[16] **(Figure 14.8).** Excess callus formation under the second or third toe indicates transition of the lever action laterally. When measuring the angle of hallux valgus, measure the angle formed between a line bisecting the shaft of the first metatarsal and a line bisecting the shaft of the first proximal phalanx. An angle of more than 15 degrees is considered pathologic for hallux valgus.

The evaluation of the other toes can reveal significant deformities. Claw toe is characterized by extension at the metatarsophalangeal joint and flexion at the proximal interphalangeal joint (and occasionally the distal interphalangeal joint). Significant claw toes arise from peripheral neuropathies, conditions such as Charcot-Marie-Tooth disease, and other neurologic disorders that lead to the weakness of extensor and intrinsic muscles or to changes in sensory input to the foot. Hammer-toe deformity is characterized by extension at the metatarsophalangeal joint and flexion at the

proximal interphalangeal joint when the toe is flat on the ground. This deformity arises from plantar displacement of the metatarsal head through the capsule, and it occurs with significant transverse arch breakdown that is possibly affected by poorly fitted shoes or trauma. The evaluation of the toes should also look for the presence of a prominent second toe. An elongated second ray is referred to as *Morton's foot*, and it is often associated with hyperpronation. When the fifth metatarsophalangeal breaks down, the metatarsal head becomes prominent, the phalanx deviates medially, and the toe externally rotates. This is called a *bunionette*, and it may appear similar in pathology to a bunion deformity **(Figure 14.9).**

Additional forefoot examination focuses on transverse arch breakdown. This leads to a variety of conditions, including metatarsalgia and Morton's neuroma. The "splayed-toe" sign indicates a plantar displacement of the metatarsal head and a stretch injury to the intermetatarsal ligaments **(Figure 14.10).** The pain of Morton's neuroma may be demonstrated by the palpation of the soft tissue

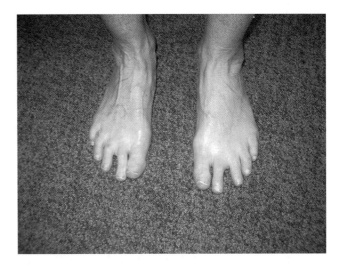

Figure 14.10 Bilateral "splayed-toe" sign between the second and third digits. On palpation and examination, this individual demonstrated subluxation of the second metatarsal heads and early hammer toe formation of the right second and third toes. (Used with permission by Dr. Karl B. Fields.)

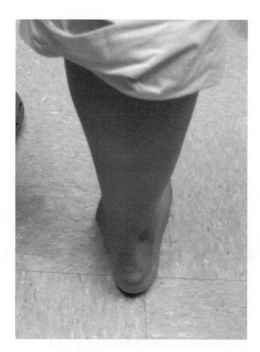

Figure 14.11 Haglund's deformity. (Used with permission by Dr. Karl B. Fields.)

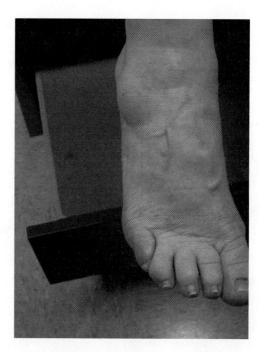

Figure 14.12 Sinus tarsi syndrome with marked puffiness anterior to the lateral malleolus. (Used with permission by Dr. Karl B. Fields.)

between the metatarsal heads using a web-space compression test.[19] Squeeze the metatarsal heads together using one hand, and then compress the web space between the thumb and the index finger of the opposite hand. Similarly, running a quarter in the dorsal web space between two metatarsals may also trigger severe pain in individuals with a Morton's neuroma.

Midfoot examination assesses tenderness, mobility, and the position of key bones, particularly the navicular and the cuboid. Tenderness over the medial arch and particularly over the navicular prominence requires specific diagnosis because navicular stress fractures rarely heal without non–weight-bearing treatment. Tenderness at the anterior ankle proximal to the tibialis anterior tendon may actually represent a proximal pole navicular stress fracture, and this location is labeled the "N spot." Failure to complete a "hop test" (i.e., the inability to hop 10 times on one foot) may indicate a stress fracture in an individual with an area of bony tenderness. Another condition presenting as medial arch pain may be an inflamed accessory navicular. These can be quite prominent, and they are easily visible on examination. Tenderness on the lateral foot more commonly occurs at the base of the fifth metatarsal, and this also requires diagnostic assessment to differentiate apophysitis, tendonitis, avulsion fractures, Jones fractures, and diaphyseal fractures. Palpation of the cuboid should test for hypermobility, which may be a sign of possible cuboid subluxation. Other key landmarks include the base of the second metatarsal, which is locked into a recess between the base of the first and third metatarsals. Tenderness here may represent injury to Lisfranc's ligament or along the entire Lisfranc's joint, which separates the midfoot and the forefoot. Valgus stress of the forefoot while stabilizing the midfoot also creates pain in a patient with this injury.

Rear foot examination includes the assessment of the attachment of the Achilles tendon. An excessive prominence at this location may represent *Haglund's deformity*, which is a traction exostosis from the posterior calcaneus **(Figure 14.11)**. The attachment of the plantar fascia, particularly to the medial border of the calcaneus, is the most common location of pain in plantar fasciitis. The calcaneal squeeze test, in which the examiner cups and compresses the calcaneus, helps differentiate stress fracture from

plantar fasciitis; this also elicits pain in patients with Sever's disease. Just below the medial malleolus lies the tarsal tunnel. Tenderness in this location should be further assessed with a Tinel's test and a heel raise. Tarsal tunnel syndrome may lead to a positive Tinel's test, whereas the heel will not shift into varus on heel raise if there is a tear of the posterior tibialis tendon. On the lateral rear foot, the sinus tarsi is the soft-tissue hollow between the calcaneocuboid joint and the tip of the fibula **(Figure 14.12)**. Swelling of the sinus tarsi may indicate excess pronation and impingement in this location. Palpation of the posterior clear space behind the calcaneus and proximal to the Achilles tendon may help identify retrocalcaneal bursitis, os trigone, or posterior talar process injuries.

REFERENCES

1. Van Boerum DH, Sangeorzan BJ: Biomechanics and pathophysiology of flat foot. Foot Ankle Clin N Am 2003;8:419-430.
2. Dugan SA, Bhat KP: Biomechanics and analysis of running gait. Phys Med Rehabil Clin N Am 2005;16:603-621.
3. Mahaffey D, Hilts M, Fields KB: Ankle and foot injuries in sports. Clin Fam Pract 1999;1:233-250.
4. Sammarco J: Biomechanics of the foot. In Frankle VH (ed): Basic Biomechanics of Skeletal Systems. Philadelphia, Lea & Febiger, 1980, pp 193-200.
5. Inman VT: The Joints of the Ankle. Baltimore, Williams & Wilkins, 1981.
6. Mann RA: Biomechanics of running. In Mack RP (ed): American Academy of Orthopaedic Surgeons Symposium on the Foot and Leg in Running Sports. St. Louis, Mosby, 1982, pp 1-29.
7. Manter JT: Movements of the subtalar and transverse tarsal joints. Anat Rec 1941;80:397-410.
8. Elftmann H: The transverse tarsal joint and its control. Clin Orthop Relat Res 1960;16:41-45.
9. Chan CW, Rudins A: Foot biomechanics during walking and running. Mayo Clin Proc 1994;69:448-461.
10. Inman VT, Ralston HJ, Todd F: Human Walking. Baltimore, Williams & Wilkins, 1981.
11. Mann RA, Hagy J: Biomechanics of walking, running, and sprinting. Am J Sports Med 1980;8:345-350.
12. Cavanagh PR: The shoe-ground interface in running. In Mack PR (ed): American Academy of Orthopaedic Surgeons Symposium on the Foot and Leg in Running Sports. St Louis, Mosby, 1982, pp 30-44.

13. Fields KB, Bloom OJ, Priebe D, Foreman B: Basic biomechanics of the lower extremity. Prim Care Clin Office Pract 2005;32:245-251.
14. van Dijk CN, Mol BW, Lim LS, et al: Diagnosis of ligament rupture of the ankle joint. Physical examination, arthrography, stress radiography and sonography compared in 160 patients after inversion trauma. Acta Orthop Scand 1996;67:566-570.
15. Maffulli N: The clinical diagnosis of subcutaneous tears of the Achilles tendon. Am J Sports Med 2004;26:266-270.
16. Moore KL, Dalley A: Clinically Oriented Anatomy, 4th ed. Philadelphia, Lippincott Williams & Wilkins, 1999.
17. Cowan D, Jones BH, Robinson JR: Foot morphologic characteristics and risk of exercise-related injury. Arch Fam Med 1993;2(7):773-777.
18. Garfinkel D, Rothenberger L: Foot problems in athletes. J Fam Pract 1984;19(2):239-250.
19. Wu K: Morton neuroma and metatarsalgia. Curr Opin Rheumatol 2000;12(2):131-142.

OTHER READINGS

Barr KP, Harrast MA: Evidence-based treatment of foot and ankle injuries in runners. Phys Med Rehabil Clin N Am 2005;16:779-799.
Coris EE, Lombardo JA: Tarsal navicular stress fractures. Am Fam Phys 2003;67(1):85-92.

Deland JT, Morris GD, Sung IH: Biomechanics of the ankle joint: a perspective on total ankle replacement. Foot Ankle Clin N Am 2000;5:747-759.
Gross MT: Lower quarter screening for skeletal malalignment-suggestions for orthotics and shoewear. J Orthop Sports Phys Ther 1995;21:389-405.
Hintermann B: Biomechanics of the unstable ankle joint and clinical implications. Med Sci Sports Exerc 1999;31:S459-S469.
Kannus VPA: Evaluation of abnormal biomechanics of the foot and ankle in athletes. Br J Sp Med 1992;26:83-89.
Ledoux WR, Sangeorzan BJ: Clinical biomechanics of the peritalar joint. Foot Ankle Clin N Am 2004;9:663-683.
Nigg BM: The role of impact forces and foot pronation: a new paradigm. Clin J Sport Med 2001;11:2-9.
Viitasolo J, Kvist M: Some biomechanical aspects of the foot and ankle in athletes with and without shin splints. Am J Sports Med 1983;11:125-130.
Wilder RP, Sethi S: Athletic foot and ankle injuries. Clin Sports Med 2004;23:55-81.

SECTION 3

Fractures and Soft-Tissue Injuries

CHAPTER 15

General Principles of Fracture Management

MAJ Howard J. McGowan, MD

KEY POINTS

- Pain, tenderness, loss of function, and refusal to perform certain actions are concerning for a potential fracture.
- Immobilization of the injured body part is key until more definitive care can be rendered.
- Describing fractures using a systematic and standardized method is essential.
- Along with functional and cosmetic concerns, the ultimate goal of fracture management is to return patients to their desired activities as soon as safely possible.

INTRODUCTION

Fractures are likely encountered by physicians who practice sports medicine and who cover athletic events. Often the primary care provider is the first responder to an athlete who has sustained a fracture on the playing field. Evaluating, acutely managing, describing, and following fractures through their course of healing are essential tools for the primary care sports medicine provider.

FRACTURE EVALUATION

When evaluating a patient with a musculoskeletal injury, the provider should take note of certain signs that should alert him or her to the possibility of a fracture. Pain and tenderness with an accompanying loss of function and refusal to perform certain actions are concerning for a potential fracture. Any deformity or swelling evident over the site of the injury also makes a fracture more likely. Abnormal motion or crepitus can be a sign of a bony injury as well. Although the x-ray can provide definitive proof of a fracture, this modality may not be readily available. A thorough clinical examination with an appropriately high index of suspicion for a fracture (especially in the presence of any of the above signs) can help a provider render safe care to an injured participant.

Marx describes 10 general principles to consider when evaluating patients with orthopedic injuries, including fractures[1]:

1. Most orthopedic injuries can be predicted by knowing the chief complaint, the age of the patient, the mechanism of injury, and an estimate of the amount of energy delivered.

2. A careful history and physical examination predict x-ray findings with a high degree of accuracy.
3. If a fracture is suspected clinically but x-ray films appear negative, the patient should be managed with immobilization as though a fracture were present.
4. Criteria for adequate radiographic studies exist; inadequate studies should not be accepted.
5. X-ray studies should be performed before attempting most reductions, except when a delay would be potentially harmful to the patient or in some field situations.
6. Neurovascular competence should be checked and recorded after all reductions.
7. Patients must be checked for the ability to ambulate safely before discharge from the emergency department, and they should not be discharged unless this can be established.
8. Patients should receive explicit aftercare instructions before leaving the emergency department. These instructions should cover such areas as monitoring for signs of neurovascular compromise or increasing compartment pressure, cast care, weight bearing, crutch use, and an explicit plan and timing for follow-up.
9. For a patient with multiple traumas, noncritical orthopedic injuries should be diagnosed and treated only after other, more-threatening injuries have been addressed.
10. All orthopedic injuries should be described precisely and according to established conventions.

With these 10 principles in mind, a few key points should be mentioned:

- Treating a participant for a fracture despite negative x-rays, as stated in the third principle, is not only prudent but advisable. If a fracture is suspected on the basis of a thorough history and physical and the initial radiograph is negative, then the provider should consider obtaining additional views or comparison views that could prove helpful for confirming the presence of a fracture.[2] Some injuries, such as a fracture of the scaphoid bone, often have negative x-ray findings initially. Treating such patients for a fracture with appropriate immobilization is advisable until follow-up x-rays or more definitive imaging can be done.
- As mentioned in the fourth principle, criteria exist for adequate radiographic studies. It should be stressed that at least two views (usually an anterior–posterior and a lateral) are a must for most orthopedic injuries. In addition, x-ray imaging should

be considered for the joints proximal and distal to the fracture site. Finally, if a patient presents to the training room or clinic with a splint or cast in place from an outside provider or emergency department, it is not unreasonable to check x-ray studies before removing the splint or cast.

- Regarding the fifth principle, in addition to checking x-ray studies before reductions, x-ray studies should also be performed *after* all reductions as well as after all splinting and casting.
- In addition to checking neurovascular competence after all reductions, as laid out in the sixth principle, it is important to check neurovascular competence at the time of the injury as well as after any splinting or casting. Vascular competence can be assessed by checking for pulses, capillary refill, and signs of pallor distal to the fracture site. Neurologic competence is assessed by checking for and documenting the presence of any sensory deficits distal to the site of the fracture.

Following these 10 principles and caveats will ensure that patients presenting for fracture management are treated appropriately and safely and that they are given the best chance for recovery.

EMERGENCY MANAGEMENT

When a fracture is suspected on the playing field, the first step is to immobilize the injured body part until the patient can be transported for more definitive care. Splinting the injured body part helps to protect against further injury, to relieve pain, and to decrease the chance of a fat embolism or shock, and it facilitates the transport of the patient. A variety of materials are available to fabricate a splint (see Chapter 16), but anything rigid may be used, if needed. As noted previously there are signs that should alert the clinician to the possibility of a fracture, and, as laid out in Marx's principles, a careful history and physical can predict x-ray findings with a high degree of accuracy. Splinting a suspected fracture should therefore not be delayed while awaiting transport or x-ray. A common axiom is to splint the injured body part as it lies. This generally holds true, except if the neurovascular status of the injured body part is immediately compromised. The importance of splinting is summed up in the following quote:

> Not only should the technical use (of splints) be appreciated by men, but it should also be appreciated that all unnecessary handling of the injured part without splinting should be avoided. It cannot be too strongly emphasized that a wound which may be of moderate seriousness may become greatly increased in importance by careless or incompetent handling in the transport to or from the hospital.[3]

A splint will often be chosen as the initial immobilization device, especially on the playing field, where the application of a cast would be technically and logistically more difficult. Aside from being more convenient, a splint also allows for soft-tissue swelling, which typically occurs with acute fractures. When soft-tissue swelling is constricted by an unyielding cast, it can result in compartment syndrome and permanent neurologic and tissue damage. Hence, splints are often used for the first 10 to 14 days, thereby allowing the swelling to subside.

Although the ease of application is an advantage of splinting, the ease of splint removal poses a problem for noncompliant, active, or pediatric patients. When a concern about removal exists and a loss of immobilization would result in a bad outcome, a cast could be appropriately chosen as the initial method of immobilization. In this case, to accommodate for anticipated swelling, the cast can be univalved (plaster cut along one side) or bivalved (plaster cut down two sides). Univalved or bivalved casts may be wrapped loosely in an elastic bandage to maintain light soft-tissue compression and optimal immobilization, if desired.

FRACTURE DESCRIPTION

An essential component of fracture management is having a systematic method for describing fractures. An accurate description is paramount when communicating with other providers, and it can be vital in the determination of when, where, and how the patient should be managed. At a minimum, fracture description should include the name and the side of the bone that is injured, the condition of the soft tissue overlying the fracture site, the regional location of where the fracture is on the bone, and the course and direction of the fracture line. Other terms that are commonly used when describing fractures that can be equally important are *angulation, displacement*, and *comminution*.

Location

Fracture description should always start with the name and the side of the injured bone. After this has been established, the provider can go on to discuss what part of the bone is damaged. Regional descriptions of long bones include the epiphysis, the metaphysis, and the diaphysis **(Figure 15.1)**. When describing a fracture of the epiphysis, the physician should note whether it is intra-articular; if it is, the physician should describe how much of the articular surface is involved. If the bone diaphysis is fractured, it is important to note whether it is the proximal, middle, or distal third.[4] When speaking about metaphyseal fractures, the physician should make note of whether the fracture travels to include the epiphyseal or diaphyseal regions (see Chapter 31). When appropriate, more descriptive anatomic terms may be useful. Wording such as "fracture of the femoral neck" reveals more than "proximal femur fracture," and "supracondylar fracture" is more descriptive than "fracture of the distal humerus." A list of some descriptive terms and eponyms that are commonly used to describe fractures is included in **Table 15.1**.

Open versus closed

An open fracture is one in which there is communication between the bone and the outside environment. This can range from a small skin laceration or puncture overlying the fractured bone to the extreme case of a bone protruding through the skin. Open fractures usually cause more morbidity than closed fractures do, and they can be associated with soft-tissue loss, compartment syndromes, neurovascular injuries, and greater degrees of displacement or bony comminution.[5] It must be recognized that an open fracture is an orthopedic emergency that requires immediate intervention, including operative irrigation, debridement, and stabilization to decrease the incidence of osteomyelitis and other complications.[6]

Direction of fracture line/fragments

Transverse, oblique, and *spiral* are common terms used when describing the direction that a fracture travels. A transverse fracture runs at right angles to the long axis of the affected bone, and it is often the result of a bending force or a direct blow. Oblique and spiral fractures cross the shaft of the bone at an angle, and they are often the result of a twisting or rotary force. Oblique and spiral fractures are usually associated with less injury to the surrounding structures[7] **(Figure 15.2)**.

When more than two fracture segments are present, the injury is said to be *comminuted*. Because the degree of comminution or

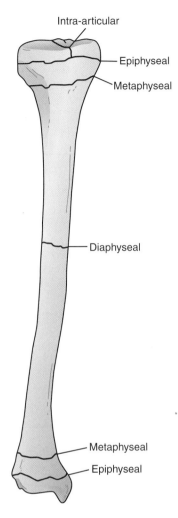

Figure 15.1 Regional descriptions of long bones, including the epiphysis, the metaphysis, and the diaphysis. (From Rakel RE [ed]: Textbook of Family Practice. Philadelphia, WB Saunders, 2002, p 926.)

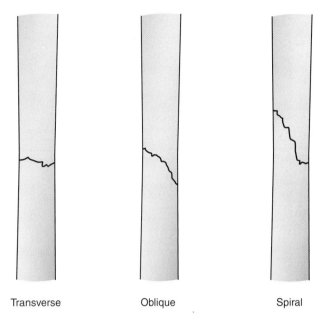

Transverse   Oblique   Spiral

Figure 15.2 A transverse fracture runs at right angles to the long axis of the affected bone, and it is often the result of a bending force or a direct blow. Oblique and spiral fractures cross the shaft of the bone at an angle, and they are often the result of a twisting or rotary force. (From Rakel RE [ed]: Textbook of Family Practice. Philadelphia, WB Saunders, 2002, p 926.)

the number of fracture fragments relates directly to the force of the injury, high degrees of comminution should raise the index of suspicion for significant injuries to the surrounding tissue. If there are two separate, complete fractures that divide a bone into three large fragments, the fracture is said to be *segmental*.[8]

Displacement/angulation

When a fracture is out of normal anatomic alignment, it is typically either displaced or angulated. The term *displacement* refers to the position of the fracture fragments in relation to either an anterior/posterior or medial/lateral plane. *Angulation* refers to the relationship of the fracture fragments to the longitudinal axis of the bone. By convention, the physician notes the movement of the distal end in relation to the proximal end when describing displacement. It is important to note the direction (anterior versus posterior or lateral versus medial) that the distal end has shifted as well as to describe the distance that the bone has shifted, which can be reported in terms of millimeters or the percentage of apposition in relation to the proximal fragment **(Figures 15.3 and 15.4)**. Angulation is best described in relation to the direction of the apex of the angle formed by the two fragments, and it is often reported in degrees[1] **(Figure 15.5)**. Fractures that are displaced or angulated are more likely associated with injuries to surrounding structures than those fractures that remain anatomically aligned.

After describing and communicating the specific characteristics of a fracture, a treatment plan can be formulated that best suits the injury. The management of specific fractures will be discussed by anatomic region in the following chapters of this section. However, there are some general principles and goals to note when dealing with fracture healing.

FRACTURE HEALING

After the patient is stabilized and a treatment plan has been determined, providers should remember that the goal is to have the

Table 15.1 Fracture Terms

Descriptive Term	Anatomic Description
Mallet finger	Avulsion fracture of the dorsal surface of the proximal portion of the distal phalanx
Jersey finger	Avulsion fracture of the volar surface of the proximal portion of the distal phalanx
Radial head fracture	Proximal radius fracture
Femoral neck fracture	Proximal femur fracture
Supracondylar fracture	Distal humerus fracture
Styloid fracture	Distal radius or ulna fracture
Colles' fracture	Distal radius fracture with dorsal and proximal displacement of the distal fragment
Smith's fracture	Distal radius fracture with volar and proximal displacement of the distal fragment
Boxer's/fifth metacarpal neck fracture	Fracture of the distal portion of the fifth metacarpal
Jones fracture	Fracture of the metaphyseal–diaphyseal region of the fifth metatarsal

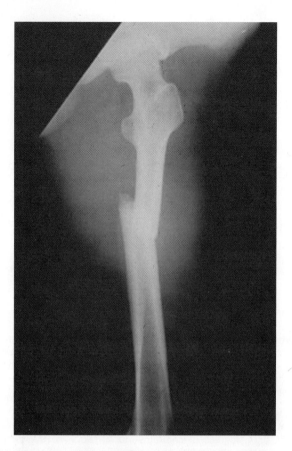

Figure 15.3 Distal fragment displaced approximately 50% medially.

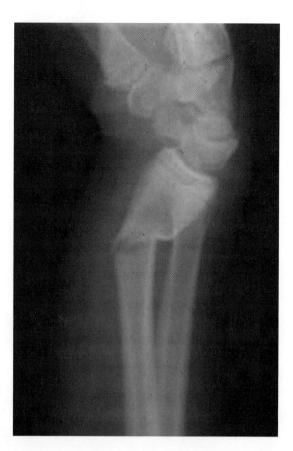

Figure 15.5 Thirty degrees of apex volar angulation.

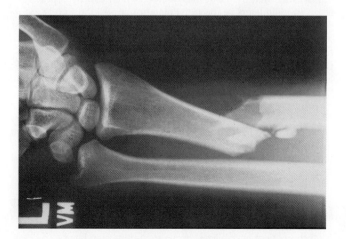

Figure 15.4 Distal fragment displaced 100% in ulnar direction.

injured bone heal in a position in which function and cosmesis are least impaired. It is also desirable that patients return to their activity as soon as is safely possible.[9] To ensure the best possible fracture outcomes, a basic understanding of the phases of bone healing is necessary.

The inflammatory phase of fracture healing is essential for attracting the building blocks that are necessary for bone and cartilage formation. After a bone is fractured, the structures around the fracture begin to bleed; a hematoma forms, and this attracts inflammatory mediators to the fracture site to begin the inflammatory phase of bone healing. There is a transformation of multipotential cells into osteoprogenitor cells, and these osteoprogenitor cells help form the callus.[10] During this time, the patient experiences signs of inflammation, including swelling, erythema, bruising, pain, and impaired function.[11]

Chemotactic factors released during the inflammatory phase stimulate the reparative phase of fracture healing.[11] During this phase, new blood vessels develop, and cartilage formation begins.[10] A soft callus forms and acts to stabilize the fracture site. Over the next 2 to 3 weeks, the soft callus will be replaced by bone as a hard callus forms[11]; clinical union of the fracture occurs during this phase. When the fracture does not move while it is being examined, when attempts to move the fracture do not cause pain, and when radiographs begin to show bone bridging across the fracture site, then clinical union has occurred.[10]

The last phase of fracture healing is the remodeling phase. During this phase, irregular, immature bone is replaced with mature bone. Although it is apparent on radiographs within months, this phase can take several years to complete.[11]

These three phases of fracture healing have variable time courses, depending on the location of the fracture, the patient's nutritional status, and other individual patient factors. In addition to having variable time courses, the phases of fracture healing can overlap. The reparative phase begins as the inflammation phase subsides, and the remodeling phase begins as the reparative phase subsides[12] **(Figure 15.6).**

CONCLUSION

With an understanding of clinical fracture evaluation, emergent fracture management, fracture description, and the physiology of fracture healing, the sports medicine provider will be better equipped to safely treat participants in the acute care setting and

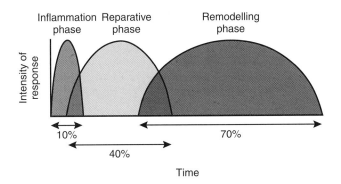

Figure 15.6 An approximation of the relative intensities and the duration of inflammation, repair, and remodeling in fracture healing. (From Rockwood CA, Green DP [eds]: Fractures in Adults, Vol. 1. Philadelphia, Lippincott-Raven, 1996.)

to ensure that correct choices are made throughout the course of fracture care.

REFERENCES

1. Giederman JM: General principles of orthopedic injuries. In Marx JA (ed): Rosen's Emergency Medicine: Concepts and Clinical Practice. Philadelphia, Mosby, 2006, pp 552-564.
2. Eiff MP (ed): Fracture Management for Primary Care. Philadelphia, WB Saunders, 1998, p 20.
3. Rakel RE (ed): Textbook of Family Practice. Philadelphia, WB Saunders, 2002, p 925.
4. Harkess JW, Ramsey WC, Harkess JW: Principles of fractures and dislocations. In Rockwood CA, Green DP (eds): Fractures in Adults, Vol. 1. Philadelphia, Lippincott-Raven, 1996, p 27.
5. Behrens FF, Sirkin MS: Fractures and soft tissue injuries. In Browner BD (ed): Skeletal Trauma: Basic Science, Management, and Reconstruction. Philadelphia, Saunders, 2003, pp 293-316.
6. Auerbach PS (ed): Wilderness Medicine. St. Louis, Mosby, 2001, p 510.
7. Rakel RE (ed): Textbook of Family Practice. Philadelphia, WB Saunders, 2002, p 926.
8. Grainger RG, Allison DA (eds): Diagnostic Radiology: A Textbook of Medical Imaging. London, Churchill Livingstone, 2001, pp 1785-1786.
9. Harkess JW, Ramsey WC, Harkess JW: Principles of fractures and dislocations. In Rockwood CA, Green DP (eds): Fractures in Adults, Vol. 1. Philadelphia, Lippincott-Raven, 1996, p 29.
10. Jones ET: Skeletal growth and development as related to trauma. In Green NE (ed): Skeletal Trauma in Children. Philadelphia, Saunders, 2003, pp 4-5.
11. Eiff MP (ed): Fracture Management for Primary Care. Philadelphia, WB Saunders, 1998, pp 5-6.
12. Buckwalter JA, Einhorn TA, Marsh JL: Bone and joint healing. In Rockwood CA, Heckman JD (eds): Fractures in Adults, Vol. 1. Philadelphia, Lippincott Williams & Wilkins, 2001, p 247.

Splinting and Casting

Timothy J. Mazzola, MD

KEY POINTS

- A working knowledge of the principles and applications of splinting and casting is essential for the sports medicine provider.
- Splints better accommodate swelling than casts do and are preferred for the initial immobilization of many fractures.
- Traditional plaster splints are being replaced by fiberglass and polyester splinting materials.
- Two brands of waterproof cast padding are now available: Gore Procel and 3M Scotchcast Wet or Dry Cast Padding.

INTRODUCTION

When the decision has been made to immobilize an injured body part, one must choose which type of splint or cast to use. Which type of immobilization to use depends on the injury, the patient, and the activities that the patient will be performing. Immobilization of an acute fracture is different than that of overuse tendinitis. Likewise, a fracture in a skeletally immature patient must be considered differently from one in the same bone of an adult. Perhaps most relevant to the sports medicine provider is that the proper immobilization of a metacarpal fracture during a football game is different than what might be done when treating a non-athlete in the clinical setting. The goals of this chapter will be to help clinicians understand the principles of splinting and casting, to decide when to use specific splints and casts, and to know how to properly apply and care for those splints and casts.

PRINCIPLES OF SPLINTING

Indications for splinting

Indications for the use of splints include the following:

- The temporary immobilization of fractures to decrease pain, blood loss, risk of fat emboli, and risk for neurovascular injury and to maintain fracture position.
- The temporary immobilization of injured ligaments or tendons, whether as a result of trauma or overuse, to facilitate the healing process and stabilize the injured tissues.

Advantages of splinting versus casting

The main advantages of splinting over casting are as follows:

- Noncircumferential splints better accommodate the swelling that is expected during the initial days after an acute fracture.
- Splints carry a lower risk of skin and vascular complications than do circumferential casts, and they allow for the earlier and easier diagnosis of these complications when they do occur.
- Splints are typically easy to apply.
- Removable splints allow for skin care, improved hygiene, and early range of motion, if desired.

Materials for splinting

Traditionally, splints have been made using plaster of Paris, but any rigid material can be used effectively as long as the splint can be safely secured to protect the injured body part. Military self-aid and buddy care training has emphasized this for years, promoting the use of "splints of opportunity" such as pieces of wood, rolled magazines, unloaded rifles, or cardboard and fixing them securely with bandages. For the purposes of the office-based physician and team clinician, our choices of splinting material are more familiar but no less varied.

Splint materials include plaster, fiberglass, malleable aluminum, and off-the-shelf splints, which are usually made of plastic and Velcro. Air and vacuum splints are also available. Plaster has a rich history in splint and cast fabrication as a result of its excellent rigidity and moldability, but because of its slow set time, high exothermic reaction, heavy weight, relative mess, and propensity for breakdown, plaster is gradually being replaced by newer materials. The OCL plaster splinting roll is one product that has simplified the making of plaster splints.

Fiberglass has the advantage of being lighter, quicker setting, stronger, and more breathable than plaster. Prepadded rolls of fiberglass splinting material such as OrthoGlass or 3M Scotchcast are now the initial splint of choice for many clinics as a result of their ease of use, comfort, and consistent results.[1] Newer still is OCL Polylite, which is made of a polyester substrate. It is used essentially in the same way as a fiberglass splint. Purported advantages of the OCL Polylite are that it is more radiolucent and that it does not have the sharp edges of fiberglass.

Off-the-shelf splints are made for almost every body part and/or type of injury imaginable. Because they are removable, these splints can be an advantage for hygiene and range of motion, although they may be a liability when it comes to the need for continuous, rigid immobilization. Although they can be used reliably for certain applications (e.g., as a thumb spica, interphalangeal joint splint, ankle stirrup, or knee stabilizer), they often lack a custom fit, which makes results variable **(Figure 16.1).** One of the most used off-the-shelf splints in my sports medicine practice is the walking boot with a locked ankle. This is useful for stable fractures, severe soft-tissue injuries, and overuse tendinitis, and it provides the benefits of early range of motion in combination with excellent immobilization to foster healing **(Figure 16.2).**

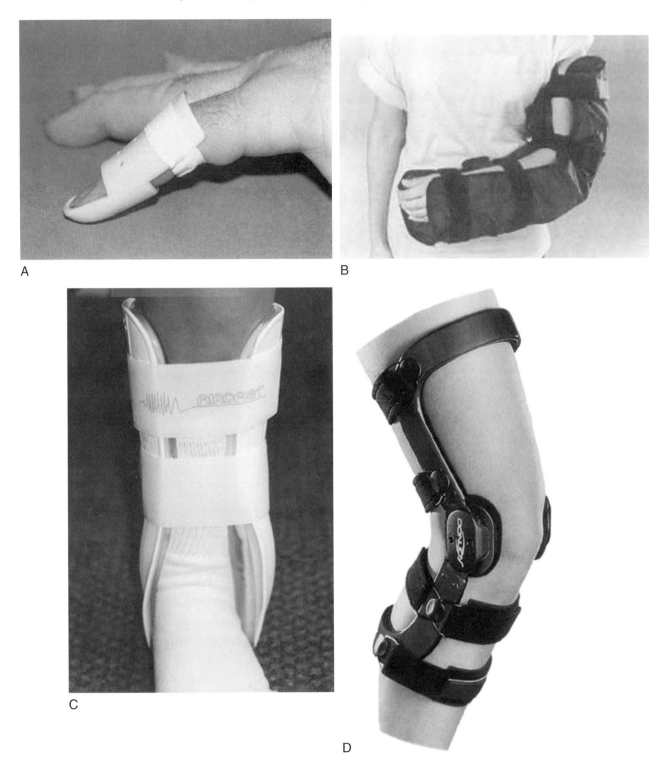

Figure 16.1   Common off-the-shelf braces have inherent advantages and disadvantages in fracture care. *A,* Stack splint. *B,* Arm vacuum splint. *C,* Ankle stirrup brace. *D,* Functional knee brace. (*A,* From Canale ST: Campbell's Operative Orthopaedics, 10th ed. Philadelphia, Mosby, 2005; *B,* from Roberts JR, Hedges JR: Clinical Procedures in Emergency Medicine, 4th ed. Philadelphia, Saunders, 2004; *C* and *D,* from DeLee JC, Drez D: Orthopedic Sports Medicine, 2nd ed. Philadelphia, Saunders, 2003.)

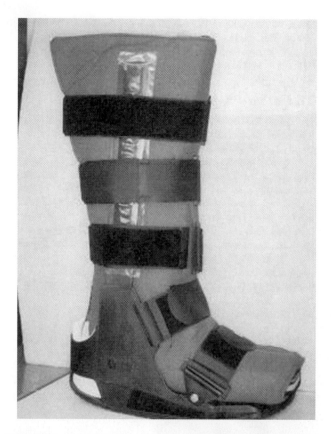

Figure 16.2 A walking boot or fracture boot is very useful for a wide range of ankle and foot injuries. (From Noble J: Textbook of Primary Care Medicine, 3rd ed. St. Louis, Mosby, 2000.)

Finally, for emergent and short-term splinting needs, malleable aluminum, air splints, and vacuum splints have been used. Malleable aluminum (or SAM splints) can be fabricated to emergently stabilize almost any body part. They are extremely light, they can be folded or rolled, and they are easy to store and transport in emergency packs. Air splints can provide excellent immobilization, but they are not used often as a result of the fact that, at the pressures needed for adequate immobilization, vascular compromise is not uncommon.[2] Vacuum splints are more recent additions to the athletic trainer's toolkit, and they provide excellent immobilization for acute unstable injuries on the sideline (see Figure 16.1B). Although they are expensive, bulky, and require a pump to remove air from the system, they are malleable before application, and they can be made rigid in almost any configuration, usually within a few seconds.

Guidelines for splint fabrication

The first rule of splinting must be the satisfactory immobilization of the injured body part. Consider immobilizing the joint above and/ or below the injured site, if indicated. After immobilization is ensured, the prevention of skin breakdown is the second priority. Depending on the injury, hygiene and range of motion are also potentially important goals.

Prepadded rolls of splint material are the easiest and quickest splints to apply, although they do not generally mold as well as a traditional plaster splint.[3] Simply unroll the splint material, cut it to the appropriate length to accommodate folded ends for skin protection, make any customized cuts as appropriate, squirt with water, dry the excess water, apply the splint, and bandage it in place. Hold it in place for a few minutes while it hardens, and your splint is complete.

Customized, handmade splints from fiberglass or plaster involve a similar approach. Options include wrapping the limb circumferentially with Webril and then applying the splint to one side of the extremity or creating a "burrito" splint, which involves padding and splint material stuffed within a tube of stockinette that is then applied the extremity.

For certain indications, a nonremovable splint is desirable. The key points involved in the fabrication of this type of splint are shown in **Figures 16.3 and 16.4.** After gathering the appropriate materials and making measurements, wrap Webril circumferentially around the limb, and then place the moistened splint material directly against the Webril. Immediately wrap the splint with an elastic bandage; as the splint hardens, it will bond to the elastic bandage, which will make it very difficult to remove.

To make an easily removable "burrito" splint, cut a piece of stockinette a few inches longer than what will be needed for the final splint. Next, stuff the stockinette as if stuffing a burrito; first with a couple of layers of padding, which will be placed next to the skin, and then with in the appropriate number of layers of moistened plaster or fiberglass necessary to make a stable splint. Excess moisture is removed, and the plaster or fiberglass is stuffed into the stockinette and smoothed out. Next, the splint is applied to the extremity, with the padding side next to the skin. The ends of the stockinette are then folded up to protect the skin from the splint edges, and an elastic bandage is applied to keep it in place. Upper-extremity splints usually require 8 to 10 layers of plaster, whereas-lower extremity splints generally need perhaps 12 to 15 layers, depending on how much force the splint will be expected to withstand.[4]

Complications of splinting

Although complications arising from appropriately fashioned splints are uncommon, certain pitfalls need to be avoided. Primarily, the alignment of a reduced fracture must be maintained. Radiographs taken immediately after splinting are essential to ensure that the reduction was not lost. Follow-up radiographs in 3 to 7 days will help determine whether the reduction has been preserved. Skin irritation and breakdown are more common if setting plaster burns the skin or if rough fiberglass splint edges contact and abrade the skin. Good splinting technique and doctor–patient communication should help minimize such complications. Lastly, inappropriate motion in an injury that requires continuous or rigid immobilization is a potential problem with splinting that could be avoided with casting. The classic example is whether one should treat a vigorous young boy with a removable splint when a circumferential cast might be more appropriate to ensure compliance. Alas, we not only treat the injury: We must always treat the patient.

PRINCIPLES OF CASTING

Indications for casting

The dual goals of casting are bone healing and good functional outcome. Although one might believe that the complete absence of bony motion is desirable, Sarmiento and colleagues have demonstrated that, in some fractures, limited motion is actually desirable. This limited motion, which may also be called *micromotion*, promotes callus formation as well as functional recovery during the early phases of healing.[5] Nonetheless, rigid casting is still the definitive treatment of choice for most closed, nondisplaced fractures, with a few notable exceptions. Casting allows the normal early bony healing process (external periosteal callus formation) to proceed in a protected environment.[6]

Casting is also indicated as a means of definitive immobilization after initial posttraumatic swelling has resolved, usually 5 to 7 days

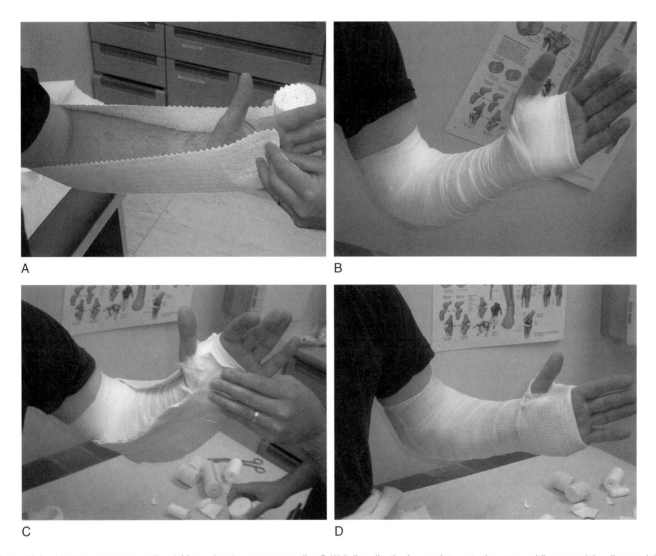

Figure 16.3   Making a sugar tong splint. *A*, Measuring the sugar tong splint. *B*, Webril application is complete; note the extra padding around the elbow and the tear to accommodate the thumb. *C*, Wet plaster placed against the Webril. *D*, Sugar tong splint complete.

after injury. If the fracture is inherently unstable or required reduction, the transition from splint to cast must be done with great caution. In such instances, postcasting radiographs are mandatory to ensure that adequate positioning of the fracture has been maintained.

Advantages of casting versus splinting
The main advantages of casting over splinting are as follows:

- Casts more definitively immobilize the injured part.
- Patients are less able to remove casts than splints, thus increasing compliance in cases that require continuous immobilization.
- Certain casting materials can get wet so that patients can bathe, swim, and wash out their casts. This may allow swimmers and other athletes to continue their training or rehabilitation despite immobilization.

Materials for casting
The two most common cast-making materials are plaster and fiberglass. The relative differences between plaster and fiberglass were discussed previously. Although historically casting has been accomplished with plaster, there is an increasing use of fiberglass. Plaster has the advantage of being cheaper and more moldable, whereas fiberglass is lighter, quick-setting, and more durable. A newer fiberglass-free casting tape called Dynacast P^{II} is more radiolucent than standard fiberglass, and it tends to have smoother edges while maintaining good strength.

Cast padding plays an important part in cast comfort and function, and it has evolved in recent years. Historically, cast padding was made from rolls of comfortable cotton Webril. More recently, synthetic Webril has been used. Although it is less easy to work with and less comfortable against the skin, it does facilitate better moisture transport away from the skin. Changing the mantra of keeping casts dry, there are now two manufacturers of cast padding that not only allow but even encourage their patients to get their casts wet. Their products are the Gore Procel Cast Liner **(Figure 16.5)** and the 3M Scotchcast Wet or Dry Cast Padding. In both cases, the cast needs to be able to drain water, so caution must be used for casts that might trap water, such as a long arm or walking cast. The Scotchcast product is applied and removed just like synthetic Webril, but the Gore product is different. The Gore Procel liner is applied without a stockinette, it has a different feel to work with, and it does not resist the cast saw as well as Webril does. As a result, with the Gore product, some kind of guard

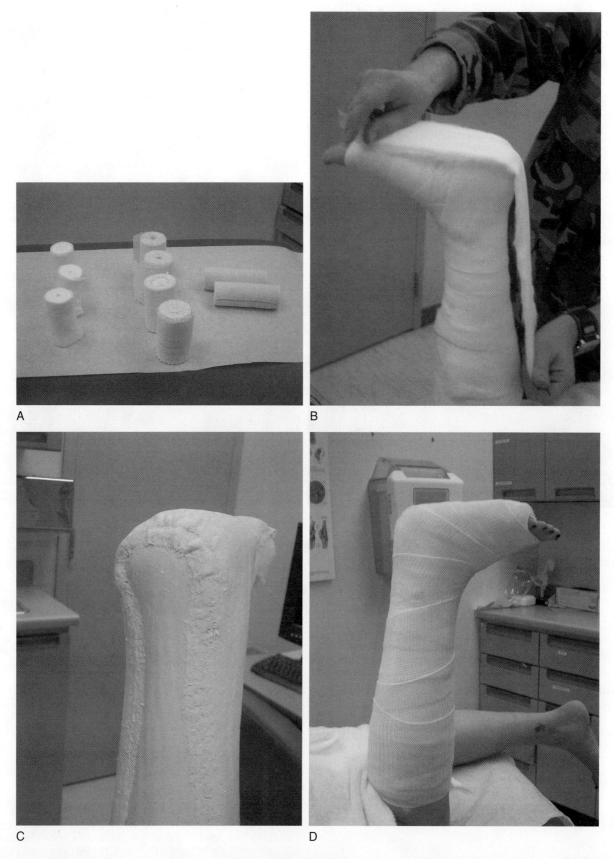

Figure 16.4 Making an AO splint (combined posterior/stirrup splint). *A,* Gather all of the appropriate materials first. *B,* Webril application for the AO splint is complete, and posterior/plantar plaster stirrup is applied. *C,* Posterior view of the AO splint with plaster in place; note the manually smoothed edges of the plaster to maximize strength and comfort. *D,* AO splint complete, with elastic bandage over plaster.

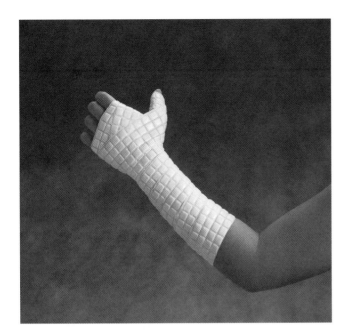

Figure 16.5 With a nonabsorbent and breathable padding like Gore Procel Cast Liner, patients can routinely immerse their cast in water and expect adequate drying times that avoid an increased risk of skin complications. (Image courtesy of W.L. Gore & Associates, Inc.)

must be used when removing the cast to prevent injury to the patient's skin. Patient satisfaction with both cast liners has been high.[7]

Guidelines for cast making

As with splinting, the primary goals with casting must be adequate immobilization in combination with the prevention of complications. To this end, the concept of a three-point cast deserves mention. To maintain the alignment of potentially unstable fracture fragments, three-point molding has been shown to be critical. The point of compression should be at the apex of the fracture, with its direction of force opposite the direction that the bony fragments want to destabilize. Two other points of pressure are then needed on either side of the fracture site, with force applied and maintained in the opposite direction until the cast has time to set up. The key here is using the palms and heels of the hands (rather than the fingers) to achieve the desired result. Using the palms and heels of the hands minimizes the creation of cast pressure points that could lead to skin irritation.[8]

Figures 16.6 and 16.7 highlight the key steps in making both a thumb spica and a short-leg walking cast. The first step in cast fabrication is selecting the appropriate tape (casting material) width and the correct padding materials. Generally, 2-inch tape is preferable around the hand; 3-inch tape should be used for the forearm, and 4-inch tape works well for the upper arm and the lower extremity. Next is determining which type of stockinette and padding will be used. Standard stockinette is cotton, but synthetic materials are now available. Likewise, Webril has historically been made of cotton, but it is now produced in synthetic and water-repellant fabrics.

Stockinette width is selected on the basis of the size of the limb to be casted and then cut slightly longer than the cast will be to allow for the edges to be folded back. Next, the appropriate width and type of Webril padding is rolled over the area to be casted, overwrapping each layer by approximately 50%. Working distal to proximal, additional Webril should be placed over bony prominences that could be sites for skin breakdown. To provide enough padding without

reducing immobilizing effectiveness, usually one to two layers of padding are used for the upper extremity, whereas three to four layers are more appropriate for the lower extremity.

Next, the casting tape is moistened enough to wet all layers of the tape to ensure adequate lamination of the casting material. Recommended water temperatures are tepid or room temperature for plaster and cold for fiberglass applications. Cooler water tends to increase the set time, but it minimizes the exothermic reaction. Warmer water shortens set time and increases the exothermic reaction. Because fiberglass sets so much more quickly than plaster, cooler water is recommended for fiberglass.

The casting tape is then rolled over the padding from distal to proximal. Special cuts can be made, especially around the thumb, to minimize bulk and increase patient comfort. After two or three well-molded layers are applied, this "base" cast is molded well to ensure adequate immobilization. At this point, it is wise to remember the principles of three-point fixation and the beneficial hydraulics of an elliptical or oval-shaped cast versus a round cast.[9] After the base cast is well applied, the ends of the stockinette are folded over, and a final layer of casting tape is applied to give the cast an extra layer of strength while providing a clean, finished appearance. The final step is to ensure that the cast is well laminated and that the final edge adheres to the rest of the cast. Lubrication lotions or gels can be applied to the exterior of the fiberglass cast to help ensure adequate lamination. Recommendations for layers of casting tape on a finished cast are as follows:

- *Upper extremity:* three layers for long-arm casts, two layers for short-arm casts
- *Lower extremity:* three layers for non–weight-bearing casts, four layers for weight-bearing casts

Complications of casting

Although casts are very useful, as with all medical interventions, one must be cognizant of the risks involved in their use. Most complications can be avoided by the proper application and care of the cast. Plaster sores can result from the improperly applied or improperly padded cast. Burns as a result of heat injury have occurred, and they are more likely when plaster is moistened with hot water.[10] Thus, tepid or room temperature water is recommended for moistening plaster casting tape. Particular care must be used when casting a body part that is insensate. Without sensation, patients are helpless to defend themselves from cast-related sores or burns, which are normally heralded by pain or discomfort. Burns or sores naturally result in skin breakdown, which then predisposes patients to another complication: skin infection. If using cotton stockinette and/or Webril, wet casts should be removed as soon as possible to prevent skin maceration, breakdown, and the resultant complications.

Tight casts can also be a problem. Whether they are fitted too snugly or the tightness is a result of soft-tissue swelling after cast application, the results of overly tight casts can be devastating. Vascular compromise of the skin as a result of "hot spots" can quickly lead to skin breakdown in a matter of hours. More concerning is the potential for compartment syndrome, vascular compromise, and compression neuropathy. As such, any complaints of pain or burning in the newly casted patient must be taken seriously and evaluated expeditiously.

Lastly, although perhaps not caused by casting itself but from the resulting immobility, deep venous thrombosis and thromboembolism are more likely seen in the casted patient.[10] As a result, in some countries, it is standard practice to prophylactically administer low-molecular-weight heparin to the casted patient. Consideration must also be given to how long a joint can be immobilized before the risks associated with the loss of joint motion outweigh the benefits of further casting.

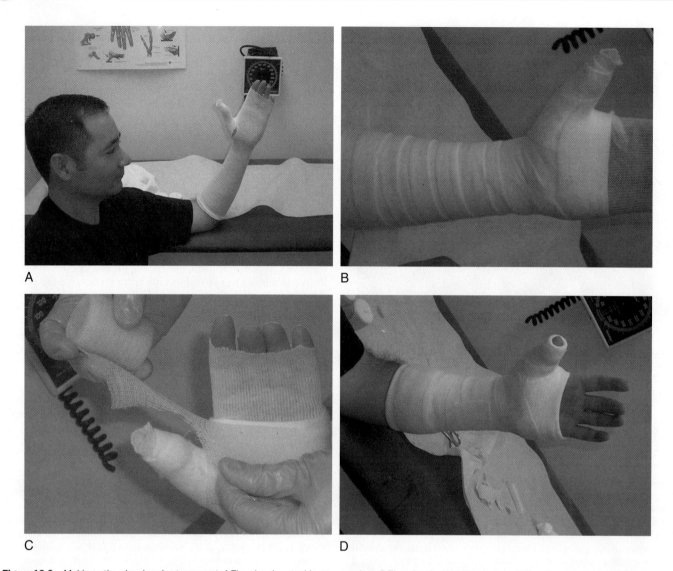

Figure 16.6 Making a thumb spica short arm cast. *A*, Thumb spica stockinette complete. *B*, Thumb spica Webril complete. *C*, Thumb spica casting tape being cut to accommodate the thumb. *D*, Thumb spica cast complete.

Table 16.1 Upper Extremity Splints

Region	Splint/Brace Type	Indications	Application Tips
Fingers	Buddy tape	IP and MCP sprains (second through fifth digits)	Tape the two digits above and below the injured joint. Pad between the digits.
	Aluminum splints	IP and MCP sprains (second through fifth digits)	Dorsal application is more functional than volar application.
	Stack splints	DIP injuries, tuft fx, mallet finger	Finger should be kept in extension on a flat surface if and when the splint is removed or changed.
	Oval 8 splints	DIP or PIP injuries	Simply slide splint over the injured joint. Note DIP precautions above.
Finger/hand	Radial gutter splint	Suspected phalangeal or MC fx (second/third digits)	Splint in an anatomic position (e.g., the "holding a can" position).
	Ulnar gutter splint	Suspected phalangeal or MC fx (fourth/fifth digits)	Splint in an anatomic position (e.g., the "holding a can" position).
Thumb	Thumb spica splint	Thumb fx, first MCP ulnar collateral ligament injury, possible scaphoid fx, and de Quervain's tenosynovitis	Extra padding at the snuff box of de Quervain's region avoids irritation and injury by the splint.
Wrist/hand	Volar wrist splint	Wrist sprains and suspected metacarpal fractures	A dorsal splint may also be applied for increased strength and improved stability.

Table 16.1 Upper Extremity Splints—cont'd

Region	Splint/Brace Type	Indications	Application Tips
Hand	Orthoplast, RTV 11	Hand contusions and metacarpal injury	Orthoplast is light and durable, and its edges should be trimmed. Apply RTV 11 in layers (this is approved by the NCAA).
Fingers/thumb/ hand	Club, soft elastic band orthosis	Finger sprains, dislocations, and thumb injuries	Do not isolate the thumb; this is not a good option if grasping is essential for the player.
Wrist/forearm	Sugar tong splint	Distal radius/ulnar fx, midshaft forearm fx	Extend the splint to the distal MCP necks; this limits pronation and supination.
Wrist/forearm/ elbow	Double sugar tong splint	Distal radius/ulnar fx, mid/proximal forearm fx; elbow fx/dislocations	This is the best immobilizer; it limits pronation/ supination and elbow flexion/extension.
Elbow/arm	Long arm posterior splint	Proximal forearm, elbow or distal humerus fx	This is best if it is used with a sling; the double sugar tong splint providers better stability.
Shoulder	Sling ± swath	Dislocation/subluxation, sprain, AC joint injury, suspected proximal humerus fx, and scapular injury	This is easily fashioned with a triangular bandage or by pinning the sleeve to the shirt with safety pins.
	Brace: harness or dynamic	Recurrent dislocation or subluxation/instability (restricts abduction and external rotation)	A harness is useful if overhead motion not needed; a dynamic brace is not as effective as a harness, but it may help if overhead motion is required.

AC, acromio-clavicular; DIP, distal interphalangeal; fx, fractures; IP, interphalangeal; MC, metacarpal; MCP, metacarpophalangeal; NCAA, National Collegiate Athletic Association; PIP, proximal interphalangeal; RTV, room temperature vulcanizing silicone rubber splinting material.
Adapted from Honsik K, Boyd A, Rubin AL: Curr Sports Med Rep 2003;2(3):147-154.

Contractures of the elbow and hand, for example, are known complications of prolonged continuous immobilization[11] **(Tables 16.1, 16.2, and 16.3).**

SPLINT AND CAST CARE AND REMOVAL

Although certain casts that involve the use of waterproof materials can and should get wet, traditional plaster and fiberglass splints and casts should not get wet. Patients should receive education about proper cast and splint care. An example of a patient handout for how to care for a broken bone and cast is provided in **Box 16.1**. Finally, it is important to complete splint and/or casting care with the competent removal of the brace. Most splints can be removed by simply unwrapping the elastic bandage and gently prying the splint off of the injured body part. Cast removal requires much more finesse and skill, particularly when a pediatric patient is involved. The appropriate use of a cast saw requires enough pressure to cut through the cast material without burning or abrading the patient's skin (see Figure 16.5). Although difficult to cut skin with a cast saw, it is possible. When cutting through a Gore-Procel lined cast, a plastic guide is inserted next to the skin to

Table 16.2 Lower Extremity and Back Splints

Region	Splint/Brace Type	Indications	Application Tips
Back	Spine board, mattress vacuum splint	Any disabling injury to the thoracic or lumbar spine	Practice and training are needed to properly use backboards and splints.
Hips/pelvis	Spine board, crutches, mattress vacuum splint	Hip dislocation and pelvic fx	If possible, early hip reduction may decrease the risk of AVN.
Femur	Traction splint	Suspected femur fx	Early traction decreases pain and potential space for hematoma formation.
Knee	Long leg posterior splint	Knee dislocation or a completely unstable knee	This type of splint is too big for a kit; speak with the trainer about having it available at events.
	Knee immobilizer brace	Knee sprain, suspected patellar fx, and patellar dislocation/subluxation	Sidebars may be bent to be more comfortable before the brace is applied.
	Hinged knee brace	ACL/PCL/MCL/LCL injuries	Many models are adjustable and can block the knee within a specific ROM; this is the best choice if early ROM will speed recovery.
Ankle/leg/foot	Posterior ankle splint, stirrup splint, or posterior/stirrup combination splint	Distal tibia/fibula fx, ankle dislocation/ sprain, tarsal or metatarsal fx, and Achilles tendon injury/rupture	Splint in the equinus position for Achilles injuries, but splint other at 90 degrees. The stirrup is the best choice for early return to play.
	Walking boot	Stable distal tibia/fibula fx, ankle sprain/tendinitis, and tarsal or metatarsal fx	This splint is easy to apply, although the affected joint may initially need to not bear weight.

ACL, anterior cruciate ligament; AVN, avascular necrosis; fx, fractures; LCL, lateral collateral ligament; MCL, medial collateral ligament; PCL, posterior cruciate ligament; ROM, range of motion.
Adapted from Honsik K, Boyd A, Rubin AL: Curr Sports Med Rep 2003;2(3):147-154.

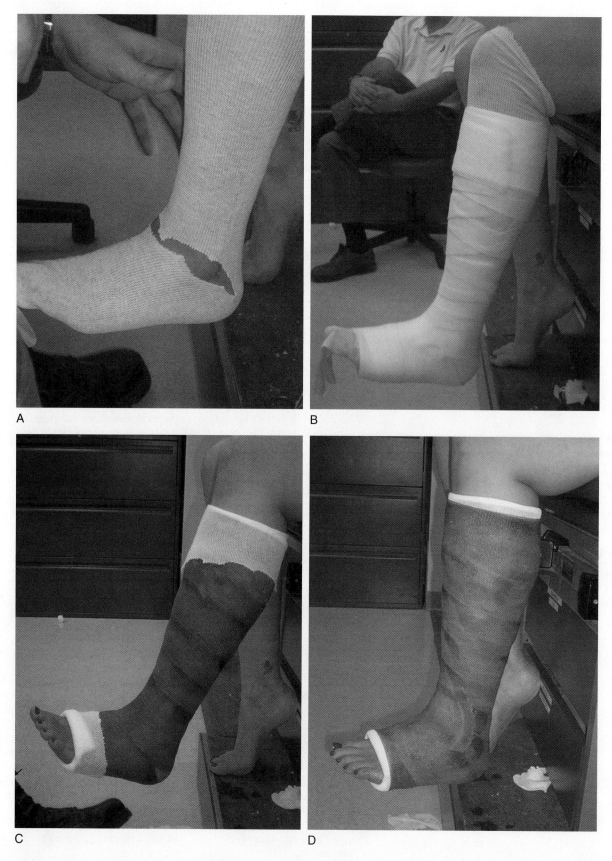

Figure 16.7 Making a short leg walking cast. *A*, Short leg cast with stockinette complete. *B*, Short leg cast Webril complete. (Note extra padding around metatarsul heads, malleoli, and fibular head.) *C*, Short leg with base layer complete before final cosmetic layer. *D*, Short leg cast completed with final outer layer.

Table 16.3 National Collegiate Athletic Association Rules Regarding Protective Equipment

Sport	National Collegiate Athletic Association Rules
Baseball	None.
Basketball	Elbow, hand, finger, wrist, or forearm guards, casts, or braces made of fiberglass, plaster, metal, or any other nonpliable substance shall be prohibited. Pliable (flexible or easily bent) material covered on all exterior sides and edges with no less than 0.5-inch thickness of a slow-rebounding foam shall be used to immobilize and/or protect an injury. The prohibition of the use of hard-substance material does not apply to the upper arm, shoulder, thigh, or lower leg if the material is padded so that it does not to create a hazard for other players. Equipment that could cut or cause an injury to another player is prohibited, without respect to whether the equipment is hard. Equipment that, in the referee's judgment, is dangerous to other players may not be worn.
Fencing	None.
Field hockey	Players shall not wear anything that may be dangerous to other players. Players have the option of wearing soft headgear that is subject to game official approval.
Football	Illegal equipment includes the following:
	1. Equipment worn by a player, including artificial limbs, that would endanger other players.
	2. Hard, abrasive, or unyielding substances on the hand, wrist, forearm, or elbow of any player, unless the substance is covered on all exterior sides and edges with closed-cell, slow-recovery foam padding no less than 0.5-inch thick or with an alternative material of the same minimum thickness and similar physical properties. Hard or unyielding substances are permitted, if covered, only to protect an injury. Hand and arm protectors (covered casts or splints) are permitted only to protect a fracture or dislocation.
	3. Thigh guards of any hard substances (unless all surfaces are covered with material such as closed-cell vinyl foam that is at least 0.25-inch thick on the outside surface and at least 0.375-inch thick on the inside surface and the overlaps of the edges).
	4. Shin guards (unless covered on both sides and all edges with closed-cell, slow-recovery foam padding at least 0.5-inch thick or with an alternative material of the same minimum thickness having similar physical properties).
	5. Therapeutic or preventive knee braces (unless worn under the pants and entirely covered from direct external exposure).
	6. Projections of metal or other hard substance from a player's person or clothing.
Gymnastics	None.
Ice hockey	1. The use of pads or protectors made of metal or any other material that is likely to cause injury to a player is prohibited.
	2. The use of any protective equipment that is not injurious to the player wearing it or to other players is recommended.
	3. Jewelry is not allowed, except for religious or medical medals, which must be taped to the body.
Women's lacrosse	Protective devices that are required on genuine medical grounds must be approved by the umpires. Close-fitting gloves, nose guards, eye guards, and soft headgear may be worn by all players. These devices must create no danger to other players.
Men's lacrosse	1. A player shall not wear any equipment that, in the opinion of the official, endangers the individual or others.
	2. The special equipment worn by the goalkeeper shall not exceed standard equipment for a field player plus standard goalkeeper equipment, which includes shin guards, chest protectors, and throat protectors
Riflery	None.
Soccer	1. A player shall not wear anything that is dangerous to another player.
	2. Knee braces are permissible provided that no metal is exposed.
	3. Casts are permitted if they are covered and not considered dangerous.
	4. A player shall not wear any jewelry, including earrings, chains, charms, watches, hair clips, bobby pins, tongue studs, or items associated with piercing (visible or not visible). Exceptions are medical alert bracelets or necklaces, which may be worn but must be taped to the body.
Skiing	None.
Softball	Casts, braces, splints, and prostheses must be well padded to protect both the player and the opponent, and they must be neutral in color. If they are worn by the pitcher, they cannot be distracting on the nonpitching arm. If they are worn on the pitching arm, they may not cause a safety risk or an unfair competitive advantage.
Swimming and diving	None.
Track and field	1. No taping of any part of the hand, thumb, or fingers will be permitted in the discus and javelin throws or in the shot put except to cover or protect an open wound. In the hammer throw, the taping of individual fingers is permissible. Any taping must be shown to the head event judge before the event starts.
	2. In the pole vault, the use of a forearm cover to prevent injuries is permissible.
Volleyball	1. It is forbidden to wear any object that may cause an injury or give an artificial advantage to the player, including but not limited to headgear, jewelry, and unsafe casts or braces. Religious medallions or medical identifications must be removed from chains and taped or sewn under the uniform.
	2. All jewelry must be removed. Earrings must be removed. The taping of earrings or other jewelry is not permitted.
	3. Hard splints or other potentially dangerous protective devices worn on the arms or hands are prohibited, unless they are padded on all sides with slow rebounding foam that is at least 0.5-inch thick.
Water polo	None.
Wrestling	1. Anything that does not allow normal movement of the joints and that prevents one's opponent from applying normal holds shall be barred.
	2. Any legal device that is hard and abrasive must be covered and padded. Loose pads are prohibited. It is recommended that all wrestlers wear a protective mouth guard.
	3. Jewelry is not allowed.

Adapted from National Collegiate Athletic Association: Guideline 4a, Protective Equipment, Revised June 2002.

Box 16.1: How to Care for Your Broken Bone

Keep it elevated and get out the ice!

Icing and elevation are the best remedies for decreasing swelling that can cause pain and slow down the healing process around your broken bone. For the first 2 to 3 days after your injury, keep the broken bone elevated as much as possible to at least the level of your heart, and restrict movement of the injured area. During the first 24 hours after your injury, put an ice pack directly on the splint or cast over the area of the broken bone for 20 to 30 minutes every 1 to 2 hours while you are awake. On the second day, apply the ice for 20 to 30 minutes at least four times per day. Avoid getting the splint or cast wet unless it is a cast that is designed to get wet.

What about the pain?

It is normal to have some pain after breaking a bone. Icing and elevation should help relieve some of the pain. The cast or splint also helps reduce pain by keeping the injured area immobile. Pain should gradually decrease each day. If the pain becomes worse after a cast has been applied or if you start having pain in a different area, the cast may be too tight. Notify your doctor right away (or go to the emergency room), and elevate the cast until your doctor reexamines you.

How do I care for my cast?

Casts may be made of either fiberglass or plaster. Ask your doctor which kind of cast you have. Unless your cast is designed to get wet, it is best to avoid getting the cast wet. If the cast is not designed to get wet, before bathing, put a plastic bag over the cast, and attach the bag to the cast with a rubber band. If the cast gets wet, try drying it by blowing air through the outside of the cast with a blow dryer that is adjusted to a low setting. If the padding under the cast does not dry, call your doctor to get a new cast as soon as possible. You should also have your cast replaced if it softens, cracks, or breaks. Avoid using knitting needles, rulers, or other devices to scratch an itch under the cast because this can lead to skin breakdown and infections. Instead, try tapping or slapping the cast to relieve the itch.

Call your doctor immediately if you have any of the following:

- Increased numbness or tingling under the cast
- A change in the color of your fingers or toes
- A sensation that your cast may be too tight or that there is an area of irritation

Adapted from Eiff MP: General principles of fracture management. In Eiff MP, Hatch R, Culmbach WL: Fracture Management for Primary Care, 2nd ed. Philadelphia, Saunders, 2003, p 20.

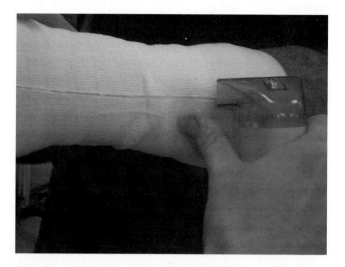

Figure 16.8 How to use a cast saw. Note thumb placement to anchor and stabilize the hand operating the saw.

cast to use can be the source of significant consternation. Likewise, fabrication of comfortable, effective splints and casts can be challenging to the uninitiated. This brief review will help improve providers' confidence and skill in both facets of care. In the end, excellent patient/athlete outcomes should rightly remain the ultimate mutual goal.

protect the skin from the cast saw. Remember: Gore-Procel padding does not resist the cast saw as well as traditional padding material does **(Figure 16.8).**

CONCLUSION

Splinting and casting are common treatments in the care of the injured athlete. Although these materials are commonplace in training rooms and clinics alike, the choice of which splint or

REFERENCES

1. Honsik K, Boyd A, Rubin AL: Sideline splinting, bracing and casting of extremity injuries. Curr Sports Med Rep 2003;2:147-154.
2. Harkess JW, Ramsey WC, Harkess JW: Principles of fractures and dislocations. In Rockwood CA, Green DP (eds): Rockwood and Green's Fractures in Adults, 4th ed. Philadelphia, Lippincott-Raven, 1996, p 28.
3. Itoman EM: Case based pediatrics for medical students and residents. Department of Pediatrics, University of Hawaii, John A. Burns School of Medicine. Chapter XIX.2 Splinting (Web site): Available at http://hawaii.edu/medicine/pediatrics/pedtext/ s19c02.html. Accessed May 2, 2007.
4. Carlson DW: Splinting of musculoskeletal injuries. In Fleisher GR, Ludwig S (eds): Textbook of Pediatric Emergency Medicine, 4th ed. Philadelphia, Lippincott Williams & Wilkins, 2000, pp 1386-1458.
5. Connolly JF, Mendes M, Browner BD: Principles of closed management of common fractures. In Browner BD, Jupiter JB, Levine Am, et al (eds): Skeletal Trauma, Volume 1. Philadelphia, WB Saunders, 1992, pp 219-220.
6. Connolly JF, Mendes M, Browner BD: Principles of closed management of common fractures. In Browner BD, Jupiter JB, Levine Am, et al (eds): Skeletal Trauma, Volume 1. Philadelphia, WB Saunders, 1992, pp 215-216.
7. Selesnick H, Griffiths G: A waterproof cast liner earns high marks. Phys Sportsmed 1997;25(9):67-72.
8. Connolly JF, Mendes M, Browner BD: Principles of closed management of common fractures. In Browner BD, Jupiter JB, Levine Am, et al (eds): Skeletal Trauma, Volume 1. Philadelphia, WB Saunders, 1992, pp 222-227.
9. Connolly JF, Mendes M, Browner BD: Principles of closed management of common fractures. In Browner BD, Jupiter JB, Levine Am, et al (eds): Skeletal Trauma, Volume 1. Philadelphia, WB Saunders, 1992, pp 222-225.
10. Harkess JW, Ramsey WC, Harkess JW: Principles of fractures and dislocations. In Rockwood CA, Green DP (eds): Rockwood and Green's Fractures in Adults, 4th ed. Philadelphia, Lippincott-Raven, 1996, pp 48-53.
11. Hardy MA: Principles of metacarpal and phalangeal fracture management: a review of rehabilitation concepts. J Orthop Sports Phys Ther 2004;34:718-799.

CHAPTER 17

Radiographic Lines and Angles

Peter H. Seidenberg, MD, FAAFP

INTRODUCTION

In sports medicine, radiographs are often required during the evaluation of the injured athlete. It is advisable that clinicians review all of the films that they order and not rely solely on the radiologist's report. The sports medicine physician has the distinct advantage of the clinical examination coupled with the radiographs, whereas the radiologist only has the films. Thus, it is in the patient's best interest that the physician be adept at reading such studies. The physician's ability to differentiate the (at times) subtle difference between normal and abnormal x-ray findings will greatly enhance his or her ability to accurately determine what therapeutic interventions are appropriate and whether or not it is safe for the athlete to continue to participate. This chapter includes some important lines and angles that are used by musculoskeletal physicians and radiologists while they are reviewing films. The normal values should be taken into consideration during fracture reductions. Although the list is not exhaustive or necessarily evidence based, it is another tool in the physician's sports medicine bag for clinical evaluations.

CERVICAL SPINE: LATERAL

Retropharyngeal space[1] (Figure 17.1)
- Distance from the posterior pharyngeal wall to the anteroinferior aspect of C2
- Normal: less than 7 mm

Retrotracheal space[1] (see Figure 17.1)
- Distance from the posterior wall of the trachea to the anteroinferior aspect of C6
- Normal in adults: less than 22 mm
- Normal in children: less than 14 mm

Anterior vertebral line[1] (see Figure 17.1)
- Drawn along the anterior margins of the vertebral bodies
- Should run smoothly without angulation or disruption

Posterior vertebral line[1] (see Figure 17.1)
- Drawn along the posterior margins of the vertebral bodies
- Outlines anterior margin of the spinal canal
- Should run smoothly without angulation or disruption

Spinolaminar line[1] (see Figure 17.1)
- Drawn along the anterior margins of the bases of the spinous processes at the junction with the lamina
- Outlines the posterior margin of the spinal canal
- Should run smoothly without angulation or disruption

Posterior spinous line[1] (see Figure 17.1)
- Drawn along the tips of the spinous processes from C2 to C7
- Should run smoothly without angulation or disruption

Clivus—odontoid line[1] (see Figure 17.1)
- Drawn from the dorsum sellae along the clivus to the anterior margin of the foramen magnum
- Should point to the junction of the anterior and middle thirds of the tip of the odontoid process

Torg ratio[2] (Figure 17.2)
- Used to check for the presence of developmental cervical stenosis
- Spinal-canal-to-vertebral-body ratio
- (Distance of the spinolaminar line to the posterior aspect of the vertebral body)/(Diameter of the vertebral body)
- Normal: greater than 1.0
- Abnormal: less than 0.8

McRae's line[1] (Figure 17.3)
- Diameter of line drawn through the foramen magnum opening
- Normal: tip of odontoid process of axis should be at or below McRae's line

Chamberlain's line[1] (Figure 17.4)
- Posterior edge of the foramen magnum to the most posterior aspect of the hard palate
- Normal: odontoid tip 3 mm above Chamberlain's line
- Greater than 6.6 mm above this line signifies cranial settling

McGregor's line[1] (Figure 17.5)
- Most posterior aspect of the hard palate to the lowest border of the posterior skull
- Normal: tip of odontoid process less than 4.5 mm above McGregor's line

LATERAL CERVICAL SPINE LANDMARKS

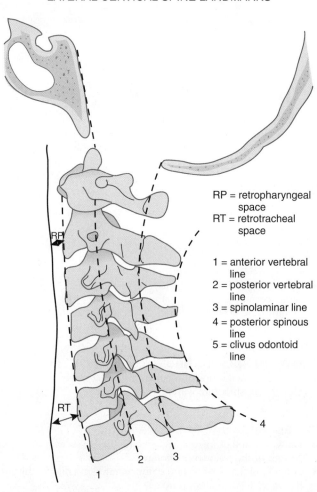

RP = retropharyngeal
space
RT = retrotracheal
space

1 = anterior vertebral
line
2 = posterior vertebral
line
3 = spinolaminar line
4 = posterior spinous
line
5 = clivus odontoid
line

Figure 17.1 Lateral cervical spine (From Greenspan A: Orthopedic Radiology: A Practical Approach, 3rd ed. Philadelphia, Lippincott Williams & Wilkins, 2000, p 335.)

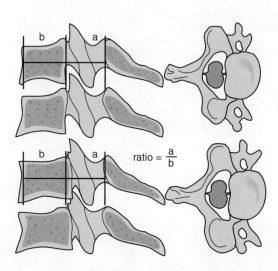

Figure 17.2 Torg ratio. (From McAlindon RJ: Clin Sports Med 2002;21[1]:1-14.)

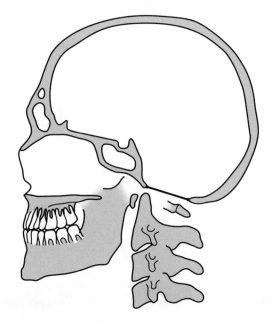

Figure 17.3 McRae's line. (From Greenspan A: Spine. In Orthopedic Radiology: A Practical Approach, 3rd ed. Philadelphia, Lippincott Williams & Wilkins, 2000, p 336.)

Space available for cord[3] (Figure 17.6)

- Also known as *spinal canal width*
- Posterior aspect of odontoid process or vertebral body to the nearest posterior structure
- Normal at the craniocervical junction: 13 to 14 mm
- Normal below C2: 12 mm
- Significance: cord compression

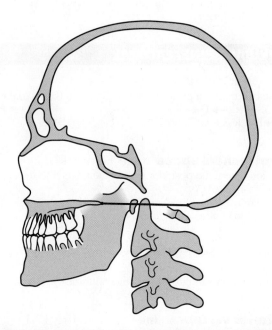

Figure 17.4 Chamberlain's line. (From Greenspan A: Spine. In Orthopedic Radiology: A Practical Approach, 3rd ed. Philadelphia, Lippincott Williams & Wilkins, 2000, p 336.)

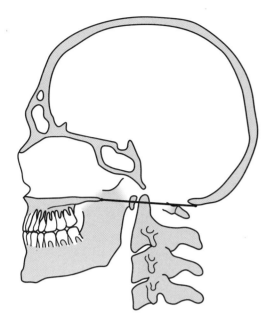

Figure 17.5 McGregor's line. (From Greenspan A: Spine. In Orthopedic Radiology: A Practical Approach, 3rd ed. Philadelphia, Lippincott Williams & Wilkins, 2000, p 336.)

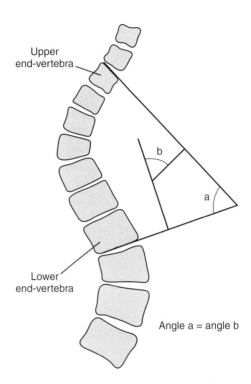

Figure 17.7 Cobb angle, anteroposterior view of spine. (From Greenspan A: Spine. In Orthopedic Radiology: A Practical Approach, 3rd ed. Philadelphia, Lippincott Williams & Wilkins, 2000.)

Atlantal dens interval[3] (see Figure 17.6)

- Distance from anterior border of the odontoid to the posterior border of the atlantal ring
- Normal in adults: less than 3 mm
- Normal in children: less than 4 mm
- Significance: atlantoaxial instability
- If 10 to 12 mm, all ligaments ruptured

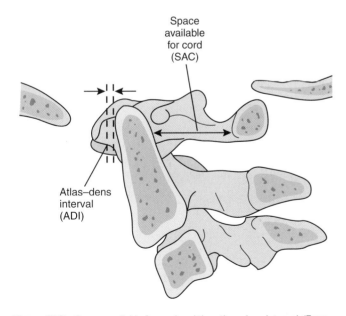

Figure 17.6 Space available for cord and the atlas–dens interval. (From Herman MJ, Pizzutillo PD: Orthop Clin North Am 1999;30[3]:457-466.)

THORACIC AND LUMBAR SPINE

Cobb angle[1] (Figure 17.7)

- Degree of scoliotic curvature on anteroposterior radiograph
- Select vertebrae most tilted from horizontal above and below apex of curve
- Line drawn along superior surface of upper vertebra and along lower surface of lower vertebra
- Method 1:
  - Perpendiculars are drawn to each line
  - Cobb angle is where perpendiculars intersect
- Method 2:
  - Cobb angle is where lines drawn along the superior surface of the upper vertebra and along the lower surface of the lower vertebra intersect
- Both methods produce equivalent angles
- Normal: 0 degrees
- Can use same method to measure kyphosis and lordosis on lateral films

Central sacral line[1]

- Drawn through the center of the sacrum and perpendicular to the line connecting the tops of the iliac crests
- Patient must be standing, with the pelvis level
- Normal: line passes through each vertebrae up the spine
- Vertebrae bisected by this line in scoliosis patients are considered stable
- Used for scoliosis corrective surgery

Harrington stable zone lines[1]

- Parallel lines through lumbrosacral facets
- Normal: all vertebrae fall between these lines
- Vertebrae within these zones are stable

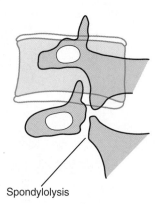

Figure 17.8 Spondylolysis and the Scottie dog. (From Wimberly RL, Lauerman WC: Clin Sports Med 2002;21[1]:133-145.)

- Used during consideration for scoliosis surgery for rod placement

Scottie dog[4] (Figure 17.8)
- Used for the diagnosis of spondylolysis on oblique views of the lumbar spine
- The neck of the "Scottie dog" appears to have a collar on it
- Signifies fracture of the pars interarticularis

Sacral inclination[3,4] (Figure 17.9)
- Relationship of the sacrum to the vertical plane
- Method of measuring the lumbosacral kyphosis in patients with higher degrees of spondylolisthesis

Slip angle[3,4] (see Figure 17.9)
- Angle between the intersection of lines drawn along the posterior border of S1 and the inferior end plate of L5
- Method of measuring the lumbosacral kyphosis in patients with higher degrees of spondylolisthesis
- Used to evaluate and describe L5-S1 spondylolisthesis
- Normal: less than 0 degrees
- Patients with greater than 45 degrees have a higher risk of slip progression

Percentage slip[4] (see Figure 17.9)
- Percentage of anterior displacement of the superior vertebra on the lower body
- Used to evaluate, describe, and grade spondylolisthesis
- Grade I slip: 0% to 25% displaced
- Grade II slip: 25% to 50% displaced
- Grade III slip: 51% to 75% displaced
- Grade IV slip: 76% to 100% displaced
- Grade V slip: greater than 100% displaced

SHOULDER, CLAVICLE, AND PROXIMAL HUMERUS

Acromial type[1] (Figure 17.10)
- Useful for the evaluation of rotator cuff impingement
- Describes morphology of acromium as viewed on outlet view of plain radiographs or T1 coronal oblique view of magnetic resonance imaging
- Type 1: flat

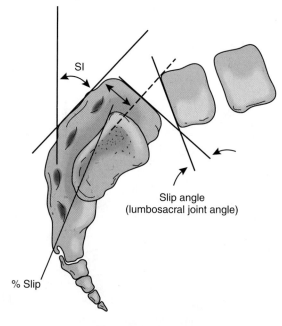

SI = sacral inclination

Figure 17.9 Sacral inclination, percentage slip, and slip angle. (From Wimberly RL, Lauerman WC: Clin Sports Med 2002;21[1]:133-145.)

- Type 2: curved
- Type 3: hooked

Acromiohumeral interval[5,6] (Figure 17.11)
- Anteroposterior shoulder with humerus in neutral rotation
- The minimum distance between the inferior surface of the acromion and the articular cortex of the humerus
- Normal: 7 to 11 mm
- Patients with less than 7 mm thought to be at risk for impingement of the rotator cuff tendons; this is an indicator of a possible rotator cuff tear

Width of acromioclavicular joint space[1] (Figure 17.12)
- Normal: 0.3 to 0.8 mm
- If greater than 0.8 mm, consider the following:
  - Acromioclavicular separation
  - Osteolysis of the distal clavicle

Coracoclavicular distance[1] (see Figure 17.12)
- Normal: 1.0 to 1.3 cm
- If greater than 1.3 cm, consider grade II or higher acromioclavicular separation
  - Grade I: 1.0 to 1.3 cm
  - Grade II: 1.0 to 1.5 cm
  - Grade III: greater than or equal to 1.5 cm

Angle between the humeral head and the humeral shaft[7] (Figure 17.13)
- The angle formed between a line bisecting the shaft of the humerus and a line bisecting the head of the humerus
- Normal: 135 degrees

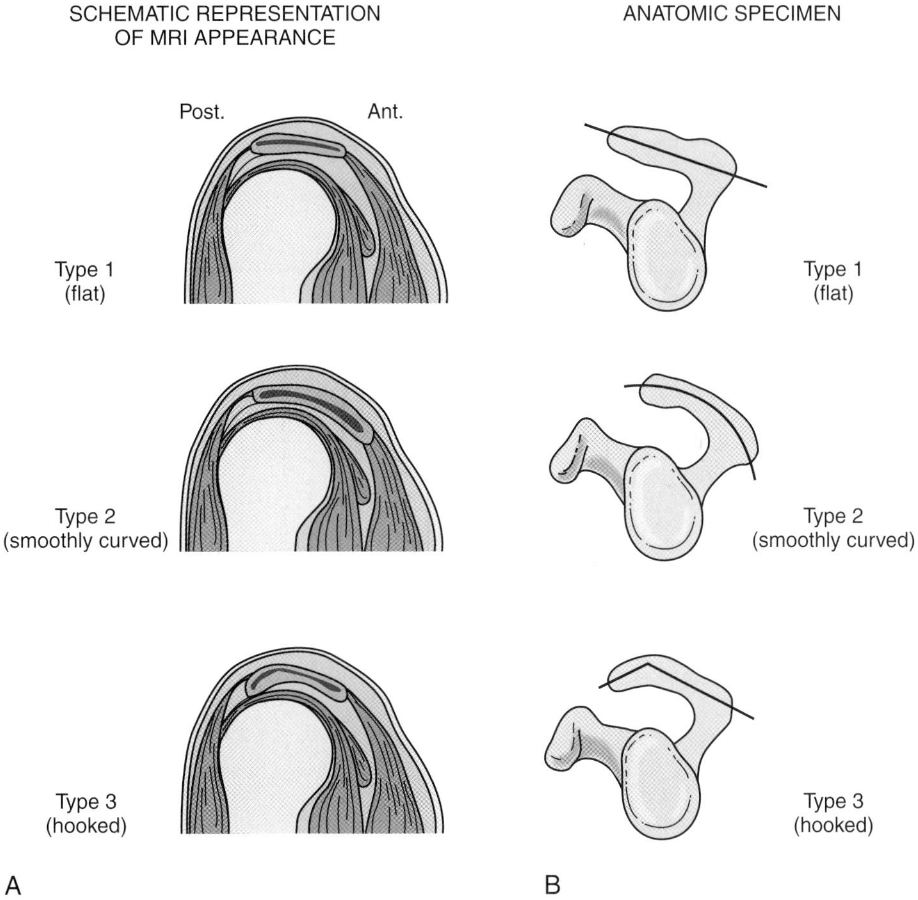

SCHEMATIC REPRESENTATION
OF MRI APPEARANCE

ANATOMIC SPECIMEN

Post.   Ant.

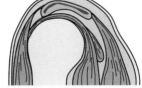

Type 1
(flat)

Type 2
(smoothly curved)

Type 3
(hooked)

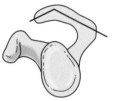

Type 1
(flat)

Type 2
(smoothly curved)

Type 3
(hooked)

Figure 17.10   Bigliani classification of acromial morphology. Ant, anterior; MRI, magnetic resonance imaging; Post, posterior. (From Greenspan A: Upper limb I: shoulder girdle and elbow. In Orthopedic Radiology: A Practical Approach, 3rd ed. Philadelphia, Lippincott Williams & Wilkins, 2000, p 102.)

A   **B**

- An angle of greater than or equal to 90 degrees or greater than 180 degrees signifies a fracture that may require surgical reduction

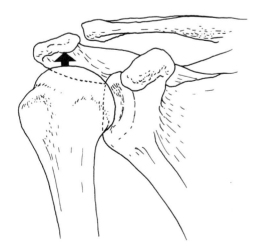

Figure 17.11   Acromiohumeral interval. (From Magee DJ: Shoulder. In Orthopedic Physical Assessment, 3rd ed. Philadelphia, WB Saunders, 1997, p 231.)

DISTAL HUMERUS, ELBOW, AND PROXIMAL FOREARM

Baumann angle[8] (Figure 17.14)
- Anteroposterior view of elbow
- Used to evaluate suspected elbow fractures in skeletally immature patients
- The angle of the distal lateral humeral condylar physis relative to the metaphysis
- Normal: 8 to 20 degrees
- The absolute number of degrees is not as significant as the difference from the contralateral side

Carrying angle[8] (Figure 17.15)
- Anteroposterior view of elbow
- Longitudinal axis of the humerus to the forearm
- Normal in children less than 4 years old: 15 degrees
- Normal in adults: 17.8 degrees
- No significant difference between males and females

Humeral–lateral condylar angle[8] (Figure 17.16)
- Lateral view of elbow
- Longitudinal axis of the humerus relative to the axis of the lateral condyle
- Normal: symmetric, 40 degrees
- If abnormal, consider supracondylar fracture

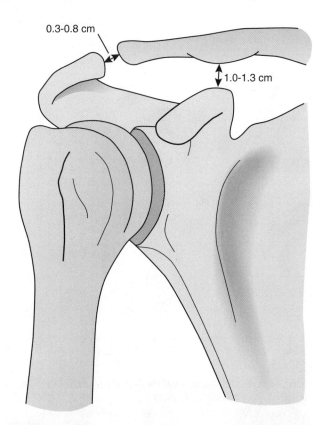

Figure 17.12 Width of acromioclavicular articulation and coracoclavicular distance. (From Greenspan A: Upper limb I: shoulder girdle and elbow. In Orthopedic Radiology: A Practical Approach, 3rd ed. Philadelphia, Lippincott Williams & Wilkins, 2000, p 121.)

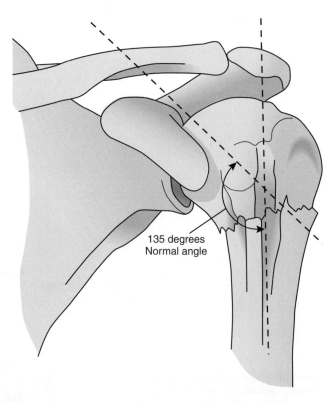

Figure 17.13 Angle between humeral head and shaft. (From Simon RR, Koenigsknecht SJ: Proximal humerus. In Emergency Orthopedics. East Norwalk, NJ, Appleton & Lange, 1987, p 160.)

Anterior humeral line[8] (see Figure 17.16)
- Lateral view of elbow
- Line down anterior humerus through lateral condyle
- Normal: line should pass through the middle third of the lateral condyle ossification nucleus
- If abnormal, suspect supracondylar fracture

Anterior fat pad[1] (Figure 17.17)
- Lateral elbow radiograph
- Normally a thin radiolucent line over the coronoid fossa
- If displaced anteriorly from the fossa, suspect capsular distention as a result of a fracture causing a hemarthrosis

Posterior fat pad[1] (see Figure 17.17)
- Lateral elbow radiograph
- Over the olecranon fossa
- Not normally present
- If seen, consider diagnostic of an intra-articular elbow fracture
- Only seen with significant hemarthrosis of the joint

Radiocapitellar line[7] (Figure 17.18)
- Lateral elbow radiograph
- A line drawn bisecting the long axis of the radius and the head of the radius should intersect the capitellum, regardless of the degree of elbow flexion or extension
- If it does not, suspect the fracture of the proximal radius or the distal humerus

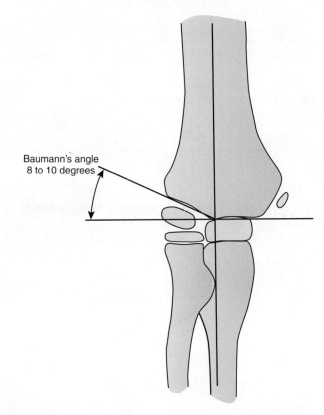

Figure 17.14 Baumann's angle. (From Hak DJ, Gautsch TL: Am J Orthop 1995;24(8):590-601.)

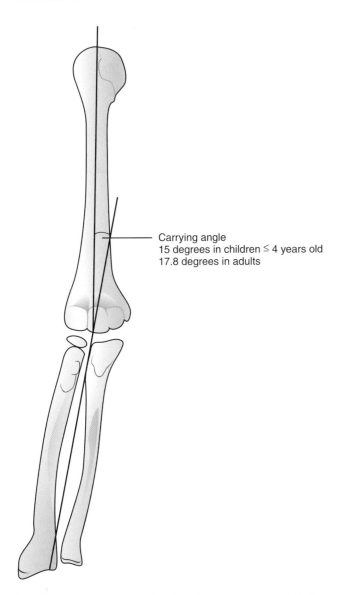

Figure 17.15 Carrying angle of the elbow. (From Hak DJ, Gautsch TL: Am J Orthop 1995;24(8):590-601.)

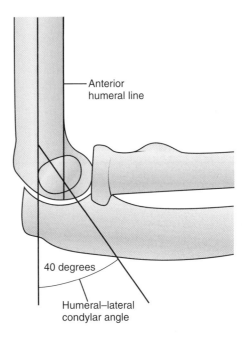

Figure 17.16 Humeral–lateral condylar angle and the anterior humeral line. (From Hak DJ, Gautsch TL: Am J Orthop 1995;24(8):590-601.)

General rules of the radial, lunate, and capitate axes[9]

- All three should form one line on the lateral wrist view
- If the lunate is subluxed:
  - The line of the axes of the radius and the capitate will not bisect the lunate

HAND AND WRIST: LATERAL WRIST RADIOGRAPHS

Radial axis[9,10] (Figures 17.19 and 17.23)
- Longitudinal axis of the radius
- Runs through the center of the medullary canal at 2 and 5 cm proximal to the radiocarpal joint

Lunate axis[9] (Figure 17.20)
- Bisector of the lunate
- Runs perpendicular to the tangent of the two distal poles

Capitate axis[9] (Figure 17.21)
- Longitudinal axis of the capitate
- Bisects the proximal and distal poles

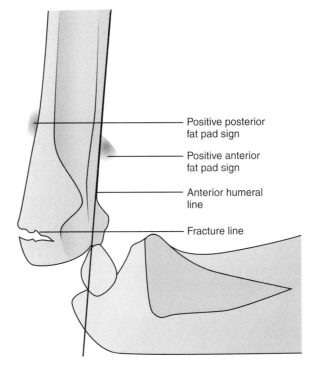

Figure 17.17 Anterior and posterior fat pads. (From Greenspan A: Upper limb I: shoulder girdle and elbow. In Orthopedic Radiology: A Practical Approach, 3rd ed. Philadelphia, Lippincott Williams & Wilkins, 2000, p 135.)

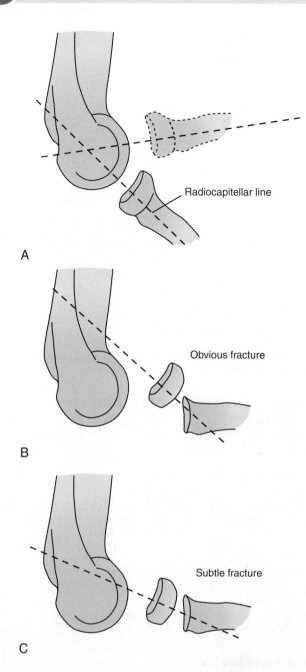

A

Radiocapitellar line

B

Obvious fracture

C

Subtle fracture

Figure 17.18 Radiocapitellar line. (From Simon RR, Koenigsknecht SJ: Proximal humerus. In Emergency Orthopedics. East Norwalk, NJ, Appleton & Lange, 1987, p 103.)

- The radial and capitate axes will transect only a small portion or none of the lunate
- With extension, the capitate and the lunate should both extend relative to the radial axis

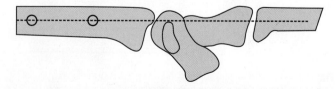

Figure 17.19 Radial axis. (From Larsen CF, Mathiesen FK, Lindequist S: J Hand Surg [Am] 1991;16[5]:888-893.)

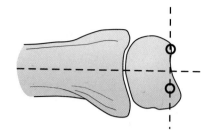

Figure 17.20 Lunate axis. (From Larsen CF, Mathiesen FK, Lindequist S: J Hand Surg [Am] 1991;16[5]:888-893.)

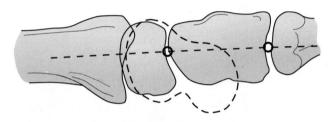

Figure 17.21 Capitate axis. (From Larsen CF, Mathiesen FK, Lindequist S: J Hand Surg [Am] 1991;16[5]:888-893.)

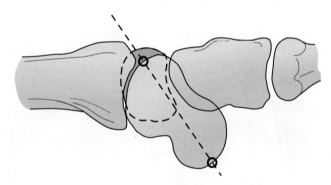

Figure 17.22 Scaphoid axis. (From Larsen CF, Mathiesen FK, Lindequist S: J Hand Surg [Am] 1991;16[5]:888-893.)

- With flexion, the capitate and the lunate should both flex relative to the radial axis
- Asynchronous movement with flexion or extension suggests carpal instability

Scaphoid axis[9,10] (Figures 17.22 and 17.23)
- Bisector of the scaphoid
- Bisects the proximal and distal poles

Radiolunate angle
- Long axis of the radius to the long axis of the lunate
- Normal: 0 degrees
- Greater than 15 degrees of flexion results in volar intercalated segment instability
  - Triquetrolunate dissociation
  - May also occur with scapholunate (less likely than dorsal intercalated segment instability)
- Greater than 10 degrees of extension results in dorsal intercalated segment instability
  - Scapholunate dissociation

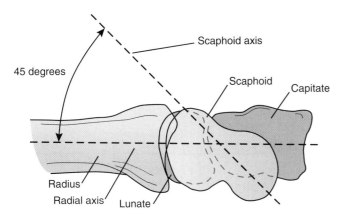

Figure 17.23 Scapholunate angle. (From Eiff MP, Hatch RL, Calmbach WL: Fracture Management for Primary Care. Philadelphia, WB Saunders, 1998, p 67.)

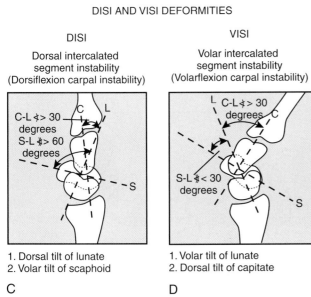

Figure 17.24 Dorsal intercalated segment instability (DISI) and volar intercalated segment instability (VISI). (From Greenspan A: Upper limb II: distal forearm, wrist and hand. In Orthopedic Radiology: A Practical Approach, 3rd ed. Philadelphia, Lippincott Williams & Wilkins, 2000, p 187.)

Scapholunate angle[1,10] (Figures 17.23 and 17.24)

- Scaphoid axis to lunate axis
- Normal: 30 to 60 degrees
- If there is a scaphoid fracture and an angle of greater than 60 degrees, there is internal fixation
- If the angle is greater than 80 degrees with dorsiflexion, dorsal intercalated segment instability is present

Capitolunate angle[1] (see Figure 17.24)

- Intersection of the capitate and lunate axes
- Normal: 0 to 30 degrees
- If greater than 30 degrees, there is carpal instability

Dorsal intercalated segment instability[1] (see Figure 17.24)

- Scapholunate angle: greater than 60 degrees
- Capitolunate angle: greater than 30 degrees
- Significant for ligamentous instability of the carpal bones of the wrist

Volar intercalated segment instability[1] (see Figure 17.24)

- Scapholunate angle: less than 30 degrees
- Capitolunate angle: greater than 30 degrees
- Significant for ligamentous instability of the carpal bones of the wrist

Radiocarpal joint angle[7] (Figure 17.25)

- The volar tilt of the radiocarpal joint
- The angle between a line drawn 90 degrees to the radial axis and a line along the distal volar and dorsal tips of the radius
- Normal: 1 to 23 degrees
- Important for the reduction of distal radius fractures
  - Greater than 5 mm of shortening or a dorsal angle of greater than 20 degrees results in a poor outcome if not surgically managed

ANTEROPOSTERIOR WRIST

Ulnar variance[6] (Figure 17.26)

- Measured in mm
- Normal: 0 mm
- Positive ulnar variance: the articular surface of the ulna is more distal than the articular surface of the radius
- Negative ulnar variance: the articular surface of the radius is more distal than the articular surface of the ulna
- Positive ulnar variance is believed to be a risk factor for triangulofibrocartilage complex tear

Radial inclination[7] (Figure 17.27)

- The line from the ulnar to the lateral side of the distal radius and the line perpendicular to the axis of the radius
- Normal: 15 to 30 degrees

Scapholunate space[6] (Figure 17.28)

- Normal: less than 2 mm
- Greater than 2 mm suggests scapholunate dissociation

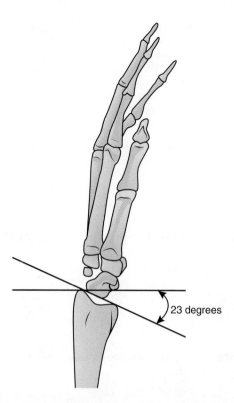

Figure 17.25 Radiocarpal joint angle. (From Simon RR, Koenigsknecht SJ: Proximal humerus. In Emergency Orthopedics. East Norwalk, NJ, Appleton & Lange, 1987, p 115.)

- The clenched fist view may be necessary to bring out the widening of the space
- Compare with the unaffected side

FINGER

V sign of joint incongruity[10] (Figure 17.29)

- Used when investigating for proximal interphalangeal joint subluxation
- Lateral view of the finger
- Normal: parallel congruity between the dorsal base of the middle phalanx and the head of the proximal phalanx
- If the middle phalanx is dorsally subluxed onto the proximal phalanx, the incongruity will result in a "V" between the two articular surfaces

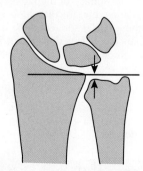

Figure 17.26 Ulnar variance. (From Keats TE, Sistrom C: Upper extremity. In Atlas of Radiologic Measurement. St. Louis, Mosby, 2001, p 188.)

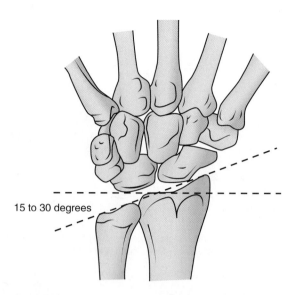

Figure 17.27 Radial inclination. (From Simon RR, Koenigsknecht SJ: Radius and ulna: proximal forearm fractures. In Emergency Orthopedics. East Norwalk, NJ, Appleton & Lange, 1987, p 115.)

HIP AND PELVIS

Angle of the femoral neck[1] (Figure 17.30)

- Angle formed between a line bisecting the femoral diaphysis and a line bisecting the femoral head
- Normal: 125 to 135 degrees
- If less than 125 or greater than 135 degrees, suspect femoral neck fracture

Iliopectineal line[1] (Figure 17.31)

- Also known as the *iliopubic* or *arcuate line*
- Most medial border of the pelvic ring
- Normal: cortical continuity
- Disruption of cortical continuity results in a fracture of the anterior column of the acetabulum

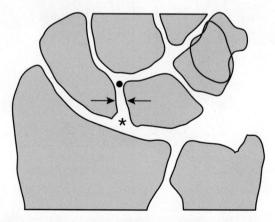

Figure 17.28 Scapholunate space. (From Keats TE, Sistrom C: Upper extremity. In Atlas of Radiologic Measurement. St. Louis, Mosby, 2001, p 192.)

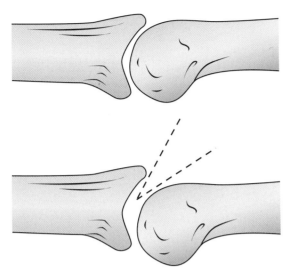

Figure 17.29 V sign of joint incongruity. (From Eiff MP, Hatch RL, Calmbach WL: Fracture Management for Primary Care. Philadelphia, WB Saunders, 1998, p 39.)

a = Iliopectineal line
b = ilioischial line
c = teardrop
d = roof of acetabulum
e = anterior rim of acetabulum
f = posterior rim of acetabulum

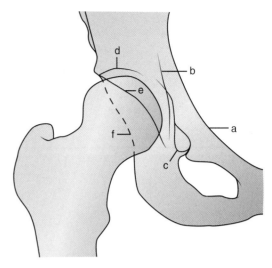

Figure 17.31 Lines of the anteroposterior hip. (From Greenspan A: Lower limb I: pelvic girdle and proximal femur. In Orthopedic Radiology: A Practical Approach, 3rd ed. Philadelphia, Lippincott Williams & Wilkins, 2000, p 208.)

Ilioischial line[1] (see Figure 17.31)

- From the most distal juncture of the ischium and sacrum to the border of the ischium and the ischial tuberosity to the distal juncture of the ischium with the pubic ramus
- Defines the medial border of the posterior column of the acetabulum
- Formed by the posterior portion of the quadrilateral plate of the iliac bone
- Normal cortical continuity
- Disruption is a result of a fracture of the posterior column of the acetabulum

Teardrop[1] (see Figure 17.31)

- Vertical teardrop-shaped line from the medial to the femoral head
- Cortical border of the quadrangular plate
- Normal: teardrop shape
- Disruption is a result of a fracture or penetration through the acetabulum into the pelvis
- A femoral head that is greater than 5 to 8 mm lateral teardrop is a result of the lateral displacement of the femoral head from the osteophyte or from the intra-articular loose body

Perkins' vertical line[5] (Figure 17.32)

- Vertical line drawn through the upper outer rim of the acetabulum

Hilgenreiner's line[5] (see Figure 17.32)

- Horizontal line drawn between the inferior parts of the ilium
- The femoral head ossification center should lie in the distal medial quadrant formed by the Hilgenreiner's and Perkins' lines

Shenton's line[5] (see Figure 17.32)

- Traces the arc of the obturator foramen and the medial femoral neck
- Disrupted when the hip is dislocated
- May not appear intact in normal children until 1 year of age

Acetabular index (Hilgenreiner's angle)[5]
(see Figure 17.32)

- Line drawn along the roof of the acetabulum; intersects with Hilgenreiner's line **(Table 17.1)**

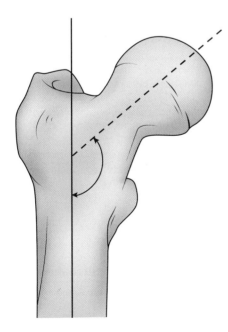

Figure 17.30 Normal angle of the femoral neck. (From Greenspan A: Lower limb I: pelvic girdle and proximal femur. In Orthopedic Radiology: A Practical Approach, 3rd ed. Philadelphia, Lippincott Williams & Wilkins, 2000, p 198.)

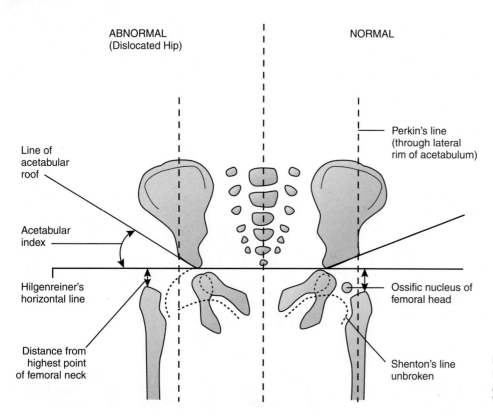

Figure 17.32 Pelvic lines and angles. (From Magee DJ: Shoulder. In Orthopedic Physical Assessment, 3rd ed. Philadelphia, WB Saunders, 1997, p 495.)

- Patients with angles greater than the above are at risk for progressive dysplasia

Epiphyseal angle

- Line along the proximal femoral epiphysis that intersects with Hilgenreiner's line
- Normal: less than 25 degrees
- Developmental coxa vara: 40 to 70 degrees

Wilberg's center edge angle[1] (Figure 17.33)

- Formed by two lines originating from the center of the femoral head
  - One perpendicular to a line connecting the centers of the two femoral heads, drawn superiorly into the baseline of the acetabulum
  - One connecting the center of the femoral head with the superior femoral lip
- Decreased in patients with dysplasia of the acetabulum **(Table 17.2)**

Kline's line

- Line drawn along the superior femoral neck
- Normal: symmetric on the right and left sides

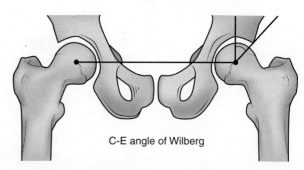

C-E angle of Wilberg

Figure 17.33 Wilberg's center edge (C-E) angle. (From Greenspan A: Anomalies of the upper and lower limbs. In Orthopedic Radiology: A Practical Approach, 3rd ed. Philadelphia, Lippincott Williams & Wilkins, 2000, p 860.)

- If the line transects less of the femoral physis on one side, this suggests a slipped capital femoral epiphysis

KNEE

Q angle

- Anterior superior iliac spine (ASIS) to the center of the patella and the tibial spine to the center of the patella
- Normal in males: less than 10 to 15 degrees
- Normal in females: less than 15 to 20 degrees

Table 17.1 Acetabular Index

Age	Girls	Boys
Birth	< 36 degrees	< 30 degrees
6 months	< 28 degrees	< 25 degrees
1 year	< 25 degrees	< 24 degrees
7 years	< 19 degrees	< 18 degrees

Table 17.2 Dysplasia of the Acetabulum

Age	Lowest Normal Center Edge Angle Value
5 to 8 years	19 degrees
9 to 12 years	12 to 25 degrees
13 to 20 years	26 to 30 degrees

FEMOROPATELLAR RELATIONSHIP

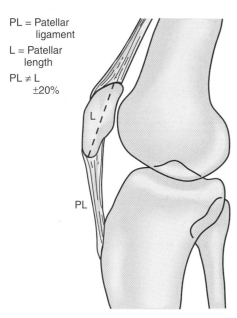

PL = Patellar ligament

L = Patellar length

PL ≠ L ±20%

Figure 17.34 Insall ratio: patellofemoral relationship. (From Greenspan A: Lower limb II: knee. In Orthopedic Radiology: A Practical Approach, 3rd ed. Philadelphia, Lippincott Williams & Wilkins, 2000, p 230.)

Insall ratio[1] (Figure 17.34)

- Lateral x-ray with knee flexed 30 degrees
- Ratio of length of patella to length of patellar tendon
- Normal: 1:1
- Ratio of less than 0.8: patella alta
- Ratio of greater than 1.2: patella baja

Sulcus angle[1] (Figure 17.35)

- On merchant or sunrise view
- Line across the lowest part of the intracondylar sulcus to the highest points on the medial and lateral condyles
- Normal: 126 to 150 degrees
- Larger angles associated with patellar subluxation/dislocation

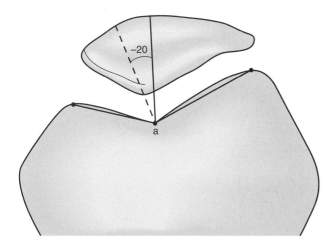

Figure 17.35 Sulcus and congruence angles. (From Greenspan A: Lower limb II: knee. In Orthopedic Radiology: A Practical Approach, 3rd ed. Philadelphia, Lippincott Williams & Wilkins, 2000, p 232.)

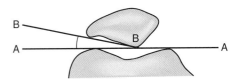

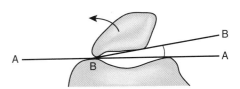

Figure 17.36 Lateral patellofemoral angle. (From Keats TE, Sistrom C: Lower extremity. In Atlas of Radiologic Measurement. St. Louis, Mosby, 2001, p 267.)

Congruence angle[1] (see Figure 17.35)

- On merchant or sunrise view
- Line from the apex of the sulcus angle to the lowest point of the patellar articular ridge and a line that bisects the sulcus angle
- Normal in males: −6 degrees
- Normal in females: −10 degrees
- Greater than 15 degrees is abnormal and associated with patellar subluxation/dislocation

Lateral patellofemoral angle[6] (Figure 17.36)

- On merchant or sunrise view
- Line drawn down the lateral surface of the patella and line drawn along the medial and lateral femoral condyles
- Normal: angle opens laterally
- Parallel or medial opening associated with patellar subluxation/dislocation

Meniscal tear on magnetic resonance imaging[1] (Figure 17.37)

- Various descriptions are given to meniscal tears seen on magnetic resonance imaging
- It is helpful to attempt to visualize the meniscus to best understand the location of the tear

FOOT AND ANKLE

Bohler's angle[10] (Figure 17.38)

- Lateral foot/ankle
- Angle formed by the intersection of a line drawn from the posterosuperior margin of the calcaneal tuberosity and a line drawn from the tip of the posterior facet through the superior margin of the anterior process of the calcaneus
- Used in the evaluation of possible calcaneal fractures
- Normal: 20 to 40 degrees

Gissane's angle[10] (see Figure 17.38)

- Lateral view of the foot/ankle
- Angle of the articulation of the talus and the calcaneus
- Used in the evaluation of possible calcaneal fractures with subsequent subtalar instability
- Normal: 120 to 145 degrees

Intermetatarsal angle[11] (Figure 17.39)

- Anteroposterior view of the foot

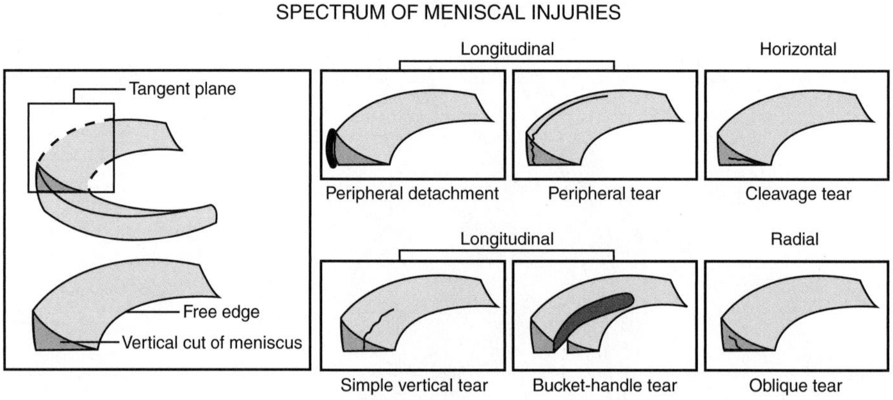

Figure 17.37 Description of meniscal tears on magnetic resonance imaging. (From Greenspan A: Lower limb II: knee. In Orthopedic Radiology: A Practical Approach, 3rd ed. Philadelphia, Lippincott Williams & Wilkins, 2000, p 260.)

SPECTRUM OF MENISCAL INJURIES

- Line drawn through axis of first and second metatarsals
- Normal: less than 9 degrees
- If greater than 15 degrees and correcting hallux valgus, proximal metatarsal osteotomy may be required

First metatarsal angle[11] (see Figure 17.39)
- Anteroposterior view of the foot
- Line drawn through axis of the first metatarsal and the proximal phalanx
- Normal: less than 20 degrees
- Increased in hallux valgus

Anteroposterior talocalcaneal angle (Kite's anteroposterior angle)
- Anteroposterior view of the foot
- Longitudinal axis of the talus and longitudinal axis of the calcaneus
- Normal: 20 to 40 degrees
- Decreased in patients with clubfoot and hindfoot varus

Anterior drawer stress radiograph[12] (Figure 17.40)
- Anterior ankle drawer is performed by the examiner
- Radiograph is taken during "stress" of the anterior drawer
- Comparison is made with the unaffected ankle
- Measure the shortest distance between the talar dome and the posterior margin of the tibial articular surface
- Anterior translation greater than 8 mm or 5 mm greater than the unaffected side is considered positive

Talar tilt stress radiograph[12] (Figure 17.41)
- Talar tilt is performed by the examiner
- Radiograph is taken during "stress" of the talar tilt
- Comparison is made with the unaffected ankle

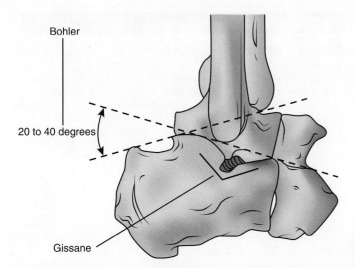

Figure 17.38 Bohler's and Gissane's angles. (From Eiff MP, Hatch RL, Calmbach WL: Fracture Management for Primary Care. Philadelphia, WB Saunders, 1998, p 212.)

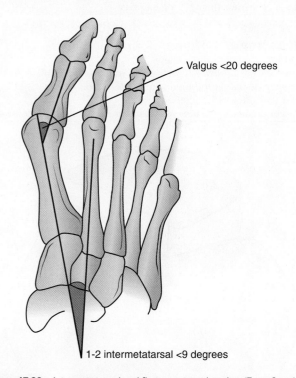

Figure 17.39 Intermetatarsal and first metatarsal angles. (From Coughlin MJ: Conditions of the forefoot. In DeLee JC, Drez D Jr, Miller MD [eds]: DeLee & Drez's Orthopaedic Sports Medicine: Principles and Practice, 2nd ed. Philadelphia, WB Saunders, 2003, p 2487.)

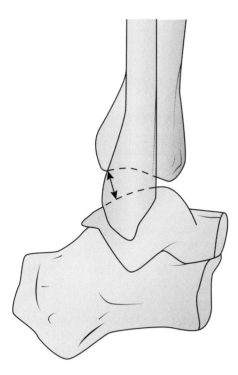

Figure 17.40 Anterior drawer stress radiographs. (From Casillas MM: Ligament injuries of the foot and ankle in adult athletes. In DeLee JC, Drez D Jr, Miller MD [eds]: DeLee & Drez's Orthopaedic Sports Medicine: Principles and Practice, 2nd ed. Philadelphia, WB Saunders, 2003, p 2332.)

- Angle is measured between the two lines drawn along tibial plafond and the talar dome
- Normal: less than 15 degrees or a difference of less than 10 degrees as compared with the normal side

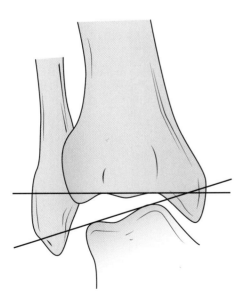

Figure 17.41 Talar tilt stress radiographs. (From Casillas MM: Ligament injuries of the foot and ankle in adult athletes. In DeLee JC, Drez D Jr, Miller MD [eds]: DeLee & Drez's Orthopaedic Sports Medicine: Principles and Practice, 2nd ed. Philadelphia, WB Saunders, 2003, p 2331.)

REFERENCES

1. Greenspan A: Orthopedic Radiology: A Practical Approach, 3nd ed. Philadelphia, Lippincott Williams & Wilkins, 2000.
2. McAlindon RJ: On field evaluation and management of head and neck injured athletes. Clin Sports Med 2002;21(1):1-14.
3. Herman MJ, Pizzutillo PD: Cervical spine disorders in children. Orthop Clin North Am 1999;30(3):457-466.
4. Wimberly RL, Lauerman WC: Spondylolisthesis in the athlete. Clin Sports Med 2002;21(1):133-145.
5. Magee DJ: Orthopedic Physical Assessment, 3rd ed. Philadelphia, WB Saunders, 1997.
6. Keats TE, Sistrom C: Atlas of Radiologic Measurement. St. Louis, Mosby, 2001.
7. Simon RR, Koenigsknecht SJ: Emergency Orthopedics. East Norwalk, NJ, Appleton & Lange, 1987.
8. Hak DJ, Gautsch TL: A review of radiographic lines and angles in orthopedics. Am J Orthop 1995;24(8):590-601.
9. Larsen CF, Mathiesen FK, Lindequist S: Measurements of carpal bone angles on lateral wrist radiographs. J Hand Surg [Am] 1991;16(5):888-893.
10. Eiff MP, Hatch RL, Calmbach WL: Fracture Management for Primary Care. Philadelphia, WB Saunders, 1998.
11. Coughlin MJ: Conditions of the forefoot. In DeLee JC, Drez D Jr, Miller MD (eds): DeLee & Drez's Orthopaedic Sports Medicine: Principles and Practice, 2nd ed. Philadelphia, WB Saunders, 2003.
12. Casillas MM: Ligament injuries of the foot and ankle in adult athletes. In DeLee JC, Drez D Jr, Miller MD (eds): DeLee & Drez's Orthopaedic Sports Medicine: Principles and Practice, 2nd ed. Philadelphia, WB Saunders, 2003.

Wrist and Hand Fractures

Stephen J. Titus, MD, and W. Scott Deitche, MD

KEY POINTS

- Scaphoid or navicular fractures account for 70% of all carpal fractures,[2] and timely diagnosis and treatment are critical. A delay can result in adverse outcomes such as nonunion and avascular necrosis.

- Determining the correct mechanism of injury and performing a proper physical examination are essential for establishing the index of suspicion for a scaphoid fracture. Knowledge of the key anatomic features of the scaphoid bone (especially its blood supply) is critical to understanding the conservative treatment approach for this area.

- Fifth metacarpal neck fractures account for 20% of all hand fractures.[21] Up to 40 degrees of apex dorsal angulation can be accepted; however, efforts should be made to minimize the angulation (LOE: B).[2,29,30]

- Although they are less common than other metacarpal fractures, first metacarpal fractures deserve special note because the first carpal—metacarpal joint is pivotal to hand function. Therefore, all intra-articular fractures involving the first carpal—metacarpal joint should be referred to an orthopedic surgeon.[26]

- During the first 48 hours after hand and wrist fractures, the frequent application of ice and the maintenance of hand elevation above the level of the heart are critical to controlling pain and reducing edema (LOE: D).[2,33]

INTRODUCTION

In life as well as in sports, the wrist and hand are inherently vulnerable to injury. Concern for disabling injury and the overall complexity of the bony articulations can make managing fractures of the wrist and hand a daunting task. Clinicians are often quick to refer to a specialist for assistance when treating these injuries. The goals of this chapter are to aid the clinician with diagnosing and managing common fractures involving the wrist and hand bones and to highlight scenarios in which referral is indicated. These recommendations are to be used with—and not in place of—good clinical judgment.

A solid understanding of the anatomy is needed when addressing wrist and hand fractures **(Figures 18.1 and 18.2).** The wrist contains eight carpal bones that are arranged in a proximal row and a distal row. The proximal row articulates directly with the distal radius. Along the distal ulnar aspect, a direct articulation does not occur. Between the distal ulna and its associated carpal bones resides a nest of ligaments and an articular disc called the triangular fibrocartilaginous complex (TFCC). The distal row articulates with the five metacarpal bones, which articulate with the bones of the fingers or phalanges. The phalanges of the fingers are made up of a proximal, a middle, and a distal phalanx; the thumb has only a proximal and distal phalanx. Further explanation describing specific articular movements and findings during the clinical examination will be covered later in this chapter.

The wrist has two primary arteries for its blood supply: the ulnar artery and the radial artery **(Figure 18.3).** These arteries meet distally to create the palmar radiocarpal arch, the palmar intercarpal arch, and the superficial and deep carpal arches. From these arches, the digital arteries arise and extend to the most distal aspects of the fingers. With this rich blood supply, one would not consider fracture healing a problem. However, the problem arises in the scaphoid, lunate, and capitate carpal bones. These bones rely on a relatively small single blood vessel that enters the bone at the distal aspect. This leaves the middle and proximal areas of these bones at risk for poor fracture healing and avascular necrosis (AVN). Thus, a missed fracture in these bones has a high likelihood of resulting in nonunion **(Figure 18.4),** AVN **(Figure 18.5),** osteoarthritis, or disability.[1]

Important to any injury evaluation is an accurate history and physical examination. Neurovascular function should be confirmed. Specifically, the patient should have intact two-point discrimination at the tip of the fingers. Normal 2-point discrimination is 5 mm; are typically calipers or a paper clip used for testing. Key points in the history include the position of the wrist and hand during injury, the activity or sport during which the injury occurred, the type and direction of forces, and where the pain localizes on examination. The absence of intense pain and signs of related injuries should not minimize the investigator's efforts to locate an occult wrist fracture. Wrist fractures often present with subtle signs and symptoms, with the classic example being a scaphoid fracture. This carpal bone is the most frequently fractured bone in the wrist, accounting for 70% of all carpal bone fractures.[2,3] It is also the most frequently misdiagnosed wrist fracture.

To improve diagnostic accuracy, plain radiographs are cost-efficient, and they should be considered even when a wrist sprain is high in the differential (LOE: B).[4-6] Often the overlapping carpal and metacarpal bones make the interpretations of

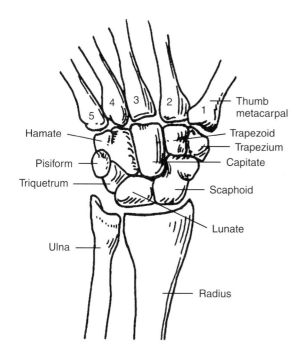

Figure 18.1 Normal carpal bones. (From Barkin RM, Rosen P [eds]: Emergency Pediatrics: A Guide to Ambulatory Care, 6th ed. Philadelphia, Mosby, 2004.)

radiographs difficult. For this reason, the use of multiple views cannot be overstated. The views should include a posteroanterior (PA; equivalent to an anteroposterior), a true lateral, and an oblique. In addition, a scaphoid view with ulnar deviation should be done if a scaphoid fracture is suspected, and a carpal tunnel view should be obtained when a hamate or pisiform fracture is considered. As a result of the multifaceted articulations of the carpal, metacarpal, and phalange bones, bony overshadowing may prevent the clinician from identifying a fracture. To aid the clinician with identifying wrist and hand fractures, several views of a focal area are often indicated. Even with seemingly normal radiographs, a fracture may still be present.

Not to be overlooked is the fact that hand elevation above the level of the heart and gentle ice compression during the acute treatment stage of hand fractures reduces pain and edema. The application of an ice pack for 20 to 30 minutes every 1 to 2 hours while the patient is awake should be done for the first 24 hours. It can then be spaced to three or four times a day for the following day and then discontinued (LOE: D).[2]

FRACTURES OF THE CARPAL BONES

Scaphoid fractures

Of all of the carpal bones, the scaphoid is the most frequently fractured.[2-4,7] It is also the most commonly misdiagnosed carpal fracture. One of the largest carpal bones, the scaphoid articulates directly with the distal radius, and it spans the proximal and distal carpal rows (see Figures 18.1 and 18.2). This positioning makes this bone a major stabilizing structure of the wrist, but it also

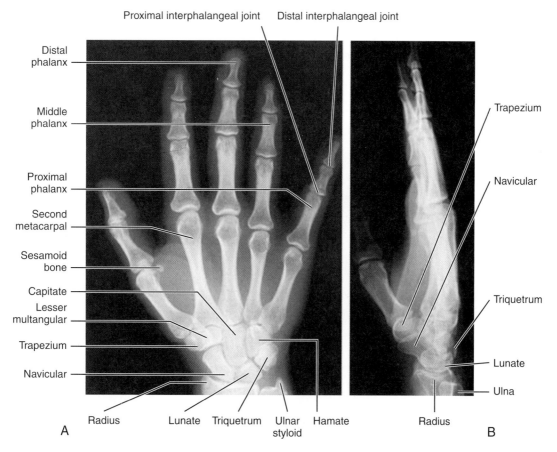

Figure 18.2 Normal anatomy of the hand and wrist in the posteroanterior (A) and lateral (B) projections. (From Mettler FA: Essentials of Radiology, 2nd ed. Philadelphia, WB Saunders, 2005.)

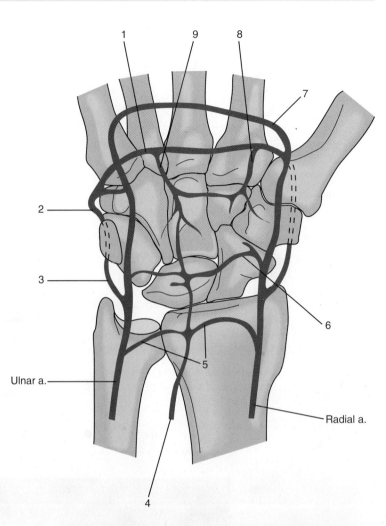

Figure 18.3 The two main arteries of the forearm anastomose to form two primary vascular arches in the palm. Most frequently, the ulnar artery will chiefly supply the superficial palmar arch, and the radial artery will chiefly contribute to the deep palmar arch. 1, Deep palmar arch; 2, branch of ulnar artery to deep arch; 3, medial branch of ulnar artery; 4, palmar branch of intermediate artery; 5, palmar radiocarpal arch; 6, palmar intercarpal arch; 7, superior palmar arch; 8, radial recurrent artery; 9, ulnar recurrent artery. (From DeLee JC, Drez D Jr, Miller MD [eds]: DeLee and Drez's Orthopaedic Sports Medicine: Principles and Practice, 2nd ed. Philadelphia, WB Saunders, 2003.)

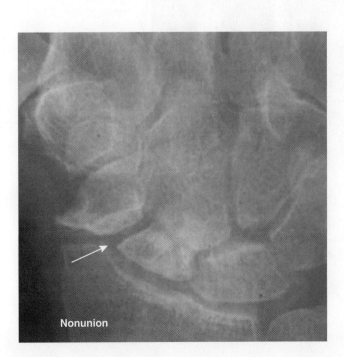

Figure 18.4 Nonunion of a scaphoid fracture. (Photo courtesy of Timothy G. Sanders, MD.)

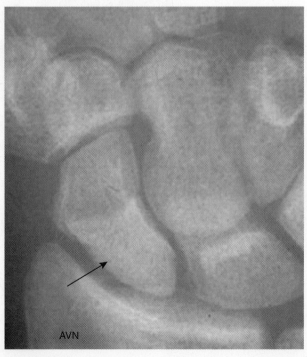

Figure 18.5 Avascular necrosis (AVN) of the scaphoid. (Photo courtesy of Timothy G. Sanders, MD.)

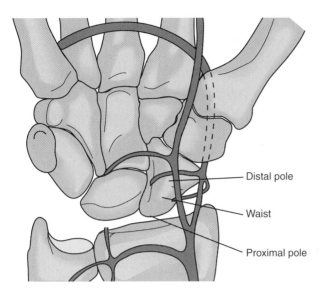

Figure 18.6 Retrograde blood supply arising at the distal aspect of the scaphoid. (Photo courtesy of Timothy G. Sanders, MD.)

predisposes the bone to injury. It has a retrograde blood supply that arises from its most distal aspect from a single interosseus branch of the radial artery **(Figure 18.6).** This predisposes the scaphoid to poor fracture healing and AVN.[1-4] When considering a scaphoid fracture, it is helpful to remember that four common proximal scaphoid fracture patterns exist. The first and most common is at the waist or mid portion; this accounts for 65% to 80% of scaphoid fractures.[2,8] The next most common fracture is a proximal scaphoid injury. Less frequently seen are fractures at the distal articular region, and the least commonly seen scaphoid fractures may occur at the tuberosity.

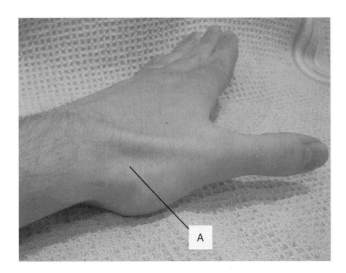

Figure 18.7 Anatomic snuffbox (indicated by A).

Mechanism of injury

When falling, the body's natural reflex is to place the hands forward in an outstretched position to prevent bodily injury. This positioning reflex often results in hand and wrist ailments that are commonly referred to as *FOOSH injuries*, with "FOOSH" being an acronym for "fall on outstretched hand." The FOOSH mechanism commonly results in a carpal ligamentous sprain or a carpal fracture. Other less common injury mechanisms that result in a scaphoid fracture include a direct blow or crushing injury.

Risk factors

Scaphoid fractures are most common among teens and young adults. Young children suffer distal radius (often "buckle") fractures from falls on outstretched hands. The distal radius is also the weakest link of the FOOSH chain in older adults. However, FOOSH fractures in teenagers and young adults most commonly involve the scaphoid.

Clinical features

A patient with a scaphoid fracture will typically describe a FOOSH injury such as a fall from a bike or skateboard. They may present hours, days, or weeks after the injury complaining of pain with wrist movement. Pain is commonly localized to the distal radial aspect at the floor of the anatomic snuffbox. The anatomic snuffbox is a depression that is located between the tendons of the abductor pollicis longus and the extensor pollicis longus when the thumb is abducted **(Figures 18.7 and 18.8).** Tenderness on palpation of the snuffbox is 90% sensitive but only 40% specific for a scaphoid fracture.[9] Scaphoid tubercle tenderness, which is accomplished by extending the patient's wrist with one hand and applying pressure to the tuberosity at the proximal wrist crease with the opposite hand,[4] is 87% sensitive and 57% specific.[9] Pain in the snuffbox with pronation of the wrist followed by ulnar deviation had a 52% positive predictive value and a 100% negative

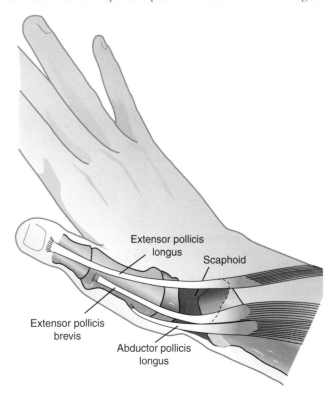

Figure 18.8 The scaphoid (navicular) bone sits in the anatomic snuffbox of the radial aspect of the wrist. (From Auerbach PS: Wilderness Medicine, 4th ed. Philadelphia, Mosby, 2001.)

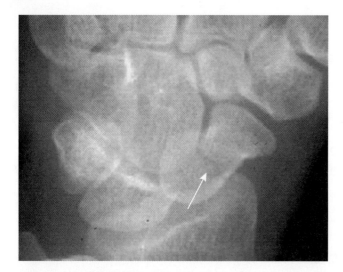

Figure 18.9 Scaphoid waist fracture *(arrow)* seen in the anteroposterior view. (Photo courtesy of Timothy G. Sanders, MD.)

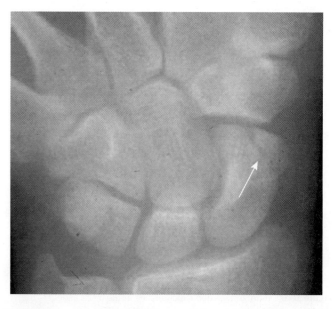

Figure 18.10 A scaphoid revealing a tuberosity fracture *(arrow)* extending into the distal articular surface. (Photo courtesy of Timothy G. Sanders, MD.)

predictive value.[4,10] An additional test that can be helpful is the scaphoid compression test. This is accomplished by axially loading the scaphoid by compressing the patient's thumb in line with the first metacarpal.[2,11] It is important to always compare the affected side with the contralateral one because each individual's pain tolerance differs.

Diagnosis

As mentioned previously, wrist radiographs should include a wrist PA **(Figure 18.9),** scaphoid view **(Figure 18.10),** an oblique view, and a lateral view. An additional PA view with a clenched fist may further aid in the identification of a scaphoid fracture. This view may also aid with the identification of damage to the ligament between the scaphoid and the lunate. A scapholunate gap of more than 3 mm suggests a serious ligamentous injury **(Figure 18.11).**

Diagnosis can be obtained via two scenarios: fractures seen on initial radiographs and those suspected with negative initial radiographs. For fractures that are identified initially, most can be safely managed by an experienced primary care physician. However, if there is displacement (more than 1 mm), angulation, comminution, or scapholunate dissociation, the patient should promptly be referred to an orthopedic surgeon.

Treatment

Nondisplaced Distal third fractures should be placed in a short-arm thumb spica cast or splint.[2,3,12,13] Middle third or proximal fractures should be placed in a long-arm thumb spica cast or splint. At the first follow-up visit in 1 to 2 weeks, radiographs should be repeated to evaluate for displacement or angulation.

Figure 18.11 Scapholunate disassociation. *A,* A posteroanterior view of the wrist demonstrates a widened space between the navicular (N) and the lunate (L) *(arrows)* as a result of ligamentous disruption from an impaction injury. *B,* A normal wrist shows that the typical distance between the navicular and the lunate *(arrows)* should be about the same as that between the navicular and the radius. (From Mettler FA: Essentials of Radiology, 2nd ed. Philadelphia, WB Saunders, 2005.)

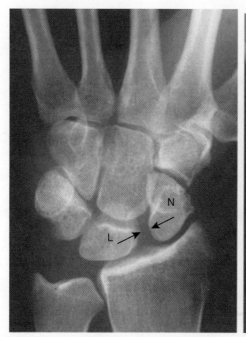

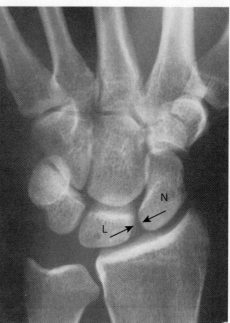

A

B

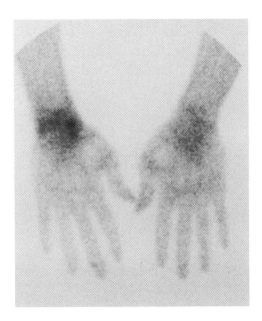

Figure 18.12 Bone scan demonstrating increased uptake over the scaphoid. (From DeLee JC, Drez D Jr, Miller MD [eds]: DeLee and Drez's Orthopaedic Sports Medicine: Principles and Practice, 2nd ed. Philadelphia, WB Saunders, 2003.)

If a splint was used initially, it should be replaced with a cast during this visit. Radiographs and evaluation should be repeated every 2 to 3 weeks until union is seen radiographically. It is recommended that radiographs should be obtained with the cast off (out of plaster) to avoid obscuring evidence of nonunion.[2] Radiographic evidence of union takes approximately 6 to 8 weeks for distal third fractures and 12 to 14 weeks for middle third or proximal fractures. If at any time during follow-up signs of AVN, nonunion, displacement, or angulation are noted on a radiograph, the patient should be referred to an orthopedic surgeon.

Suspected fractures If initial radiographs are negative but clinical suspicion suggests a possible fracture, then the patient should be placed initially in a short-arm thumb spica cast or splint. The patient should have repeat radiographs in 2 weeks. If a fracture is seen at this point, the treatment course should follow that outlined previously. If radiographs are negative, the patient's snuffbox needs to be examined. If tenderness in the snuffbox has resolved, then the patient suffered a wrist sprain and should be managed as such. If tenderness persists in the snuffbox, then the short-arm thumb spica cast or splint should be continued; advanced imaging is usually obtained to further evaluate for fracture. Advanced imaging options include a bone scan **(Figure 18.12),** computed tomography (CT), and magnetic resonance imaging (MRI). MRI was shown to be equivalent to bone scan for detecting a fracture; however, MRI was better for detecting significant ligamentous and carpal instabilities (LOE: B).[14] If advanced imaging studies show no fracture but patients continue to show persistent snuffbox pain, then a ligamentous injury is likely, and consultation with a hand specialist is recommended.[15,16] If advanced imaging reveals a fracture, then treatment should follow the course discussed previously.

Indications for specialty referral

Displacement, angulation, comminution, scapholunate disassociation, late fracture presentation, lack of experience with carpal fracture treatment, or deviation from expected healing times are all indications for referral to an orthopedic or hand surgeon.

Return to sport

Because the primary treatment of a scaphoid fracture involves immobilization, muscular atrophy and decreased range of wrist motion naturally ensue. Return to sport should be considered after a period of supervised physical rehabilitation of 6 to 8 weeks. At this point, an assessment of strength and function should be performed before sports participation is considered. Generally, if strength is at 80% of that of the unaffected wrist, the athlete may return to his or her sport with a sport-specific orthosis. The orthosis should be worn for 3 to 6 months. After this period, if strength and function have fully returned, then the athlete may be allowed to participate without the orthosis (LOE: D).[2]

Lunate fracture

The lunate bone articulates with the scaphoid, the distal radius, and the TFCC. A fracture to the lunate may also be associated with injury to the TFCC. Like the scaphoid bone, the lunate also has a tenuous retrograde blood supply off of an interosseus arterial branch, and it has the same inherent risk of poor healing and AVN after injury.

Mechanism of injury

The FOOSH mechanism is the most common with a lunate fracture, just as it is with a scaphoid fracture. Other scenarios exist that involve heavy lifting or pushing events in which the wrist is placed in extreme dorsiflexion and significant force is applied to its volar aspect.

Risk factors

The length of a patient's distal ulna is an important factor in lunate injury. When the distal ulna is closer to the proximal carpals or "taller" than the distal radius, one is said to have "positive ulnar variance." "Negative" ulnar variance occurs when the distal ulna is farther from the proximal carpals or "shorter" than the distal radius (see Figure 19.4 in Chapter 19 that illustrates ulnar variance). The patient is "ulnar neutral" if the distal radius and the distal ulna are equidistant from the carpals. Fractures of the lunate occur more commonly in individuals with positive ulnar variance. AVN of the lunate (Kienbock's disease) is more commonly found in individuals with negative ulnar variance **(Figure 18.13).**

Clinical features

Often the patient will present with progressive pain or pain that is remotely related to an earlier FOOSH injury. The pain is most often localized distal to Lister's tubercle. Lister's tubercle may be identified at the prominence of the distal radius in line with the third metacarpal. Pain may be elicited by the resisted extension of the third finger. Patients may also present with wrist stiffness or carpal tunnel symptoms.

Diagnosis

The timing of the radiographs in relation to the initial injury will often determine the findings. In the setting of AVN, the diagnosis is often made late in the disease course. Radiographs are notoriously falsely negative in fractures or in AVN, especially during the early phases of disease processes. Classically, the only early x-ray finding in AVN may be an ulnar-negative alignment on PA wrist films **(Figure 18.14).** However, if clinical suspicion is high, a CT scan or MRI should be performed, regardless of normal initial x-rays.[17]

Treatment

In the case of lunate injuries, multiple factors are involved that favor the nonunion of a fracture as well as the lunate's propensity for AVN. Immobilization with a long-arm thumb spica cast should be the initial treatment when a fracture is suspected. In the light of the complications related to lunate fractures, early consultation with an orthopedic surgeon is recommended.[18] Treatment efforts

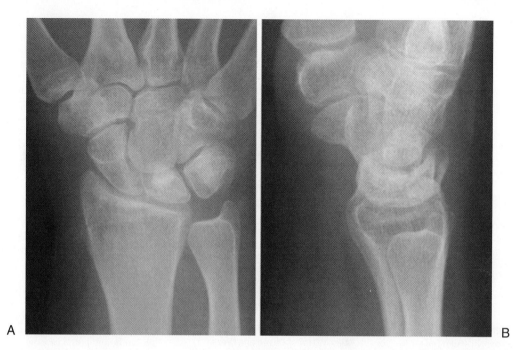

Figure 18.13 A and B, Kienböck's disease. Lunate collapse is present. Ulnar negative variance, as seen here, is a typical feature. (From Browner BD: Skeletal Trauma: Basic Science, Management, and Reconstruction, 3rd ed. Philadelphia, WB Saunders, 2003.)

A

B

employed by orthopedic surgeons are aimed at minimizing compressive forces on the lunate by either lengthening the ulna or shortening the radius to correct an ulnar minus variant. The ultimate surgical goals are to reduce stress on the lunate and to facilitate adequate blood supply to allow for normal bone healing.

Indications for specialty referral
As noted previously, lunate fractures should be referred to an orthopedic surgeon as a result of the high rate of nonunion and the need for frequent follow-up.

Return to sport
Return to sports participation after a lunate fracture is largely determined by the individual's recovery. After removal of the cast, a period of supervised physical therapy rehabilitation focusing on

strength and range of motion should result in function and strength that is nearly equal to that of the unaffected wrist. An orthosis should be worn for a minimum of 3 months after rehabilitation. Return to sport without the orthosis is based on individual performance.

Triquetrum fracture
The triquetrum is the second most commonly fractured carpal bone after the scaphoid. Nondisplaced triquetral fractures usually heal well, without complication.[2] The triquetrum bone articulates with the lunate and resides deep to the pisiform. During radial wrist deviation, it also articulates with the capitate. As with the lunate, a fracture of the triquetrum may be associated with injury to the neighboring TFCC.

Figure 18.14 Transverse lunate fracture. A and B, Plain radiographs demonstrate some irregularity of the lunate. C and D, Axial and sagittal computed tomography images demonstrate the transverse fracture. (From Browner BD: Skeletal Trauma: Basic Science, Management, and Reconstruction, 3rd ed. Philadelphia, WB Saunders, 2003.)

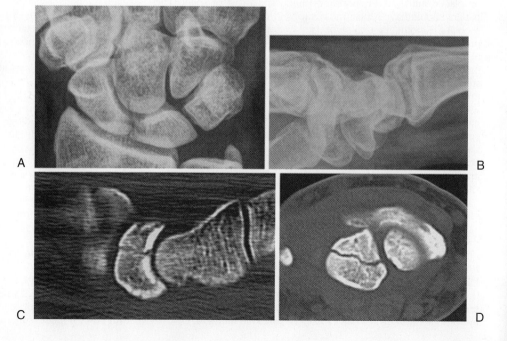

A

B

C

D

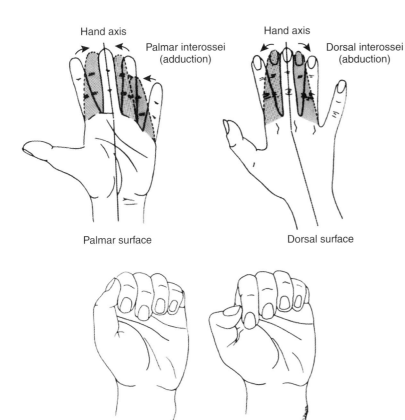

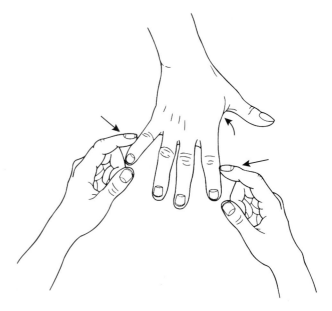

Figure 18.15 Ulnar nerve testing. The weakness of intrinsic muscle is revealed by adduction *(A)* and abduction *(B)* when there is ulnar nerve injury. When ulnar innervation to the adductor pollicis *(C)* is intact, Froment's test reveals a normal pinch. Injury to ulnar nerves results in an abnormal pinch *(D)*; this can only be performed by using the flexor pollicis longus, which is innervated by the median nerve. (From Noble J: Textbook of Primary Care Medicine, 3rd ed. St. Louis, Mosby, 2001.)

Mechanism of injury

Three mechanisms of injury exist that result in different triquetral injury patterns. In a FOOSH injury in which the wrist is hyperextended with ulnar deviation, a fragment typically shears off of the dorsal radial aspect of the triquetrum adjacent to the hamate. With a direct blow, the body of the triquetrum may be fractured. Finally, in the setting of a forceful hyperflexion injury, a bony ligamentous avulsion of the dorsal radiotriquetral ligament may occur. Associated injuries may include perilunate dislocation and injury to the deep motor branch of the ulnar nerve.

Clinical features

Patients present with ulnar wrist pain, and tenderness is typically localized just distal to the ulnar styloid. If the ulnar nerve is injured, neurologic deficits may be present **(Figures 18.15 and 18.16)**. Triquetrum fractures almost never present with significant swelling or bruising.

Diagnosis

Initial x-ray views should include a wrist PA view, a true lateral view, and an oblique view. If an avulsion fracture is present, the findings may be subtle **(Figure 18.17)**. In the setting in which x-rays are negative but a fracture of the triquetrum is clinically suspected, the wrist should be placed in a volar splint until CT scanning or MRI can be performed.

Treatment

Initially the wrist should be supported in slight extension in a volar splint. Initial follow up should be done in 2 weeks. Definitive treatment for avulsion and nondisplaced, transverse fractures should include a short-arm cast that extends to the distal palmar crease with the wrist in slight extension and the metacarpophalangeal (MCP) joints free to flex. Immobilization should be maintained for 6 weeks, with routine scheduled follow-up examinations with radiographs performed every 2 weeks to evaluate for proper healing. Any complications or delay in healing should prompt immediate evaluation by an orthopedic surgeon or a hand specialist.

Figure 18.16 Testing for intrinsic (ulnar) motor weakness (fanning the fingers against resistance). Always look for atrophy of the first dorsal interosseus *(curved arrow)* when ulnar nerve lesions are suspected. (From Mercier LR: Practical Orthopedics, 5th ed, St. Louis, Mosby, 2000. In Ferri FF: Ferri's Clinical Advisor 2007: Instant Diagnosis and Treatment, 9th ed. St. Louis, Mosby, 2007.)

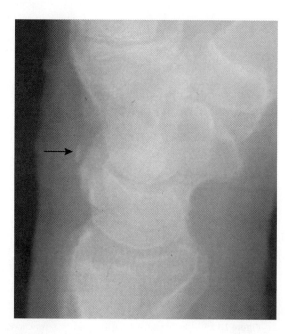

Figure 18.17 Lateral view of a triquetral fracture *(arrow)*. (Photo courtesy of Timothy G. Sanders, MD.)

Indications for specialty referral

Ulnar nerve injury, displaced triquetral fractures, ligamentous damage, concomitant injury to the TFCC, concomitant pisiform fracture, or a symptomatic nonunion after 6 weeks of immobilization should prompt referral to an orthopedic surgeon or a hand specialist. If ulnar nerve injury is suspected, immediate orthopedic consultation is indicated. For fractures with intact neurovascular function, patients should be seen within 72 hours.

Return to sport

After the immobilization period, supervised physical therapy rehabilitation efforts should focus on regaining extension, flexion, hand function, and grip strength. When strength and pain-free function near that of the uninjured hand, return to sports participation is allowed with a protective orthosis until full function returns.

Hamate fracture

The hamate bone is located in the distal carpal row, and articulates with the triquetrum, the capitate, and the fourth and fifth metacarpal bones. The hamate at its distal aspect projects a bony tubercle toward the volar surface. This structure is called the "hook of the hamate." Key anatomic structures in this region are branches of the ulnar nerve. A fracture in this region could affect the ulnar nerve distribution to the entire fifth phalanx and the ulnar side of the fourth phalanx **(Figure 18.18)**.

Mechanism of injury

Injuries to the hamate typically involve the hook of the hamate. Its volar projection and superficial depth make this structure vulnerable to contusion injuries. Sports involving the grasping and swinging of clubs, rackets, and bats are commonly associated with fractures of the hook of the hamate. Direct force on the hamate as generated throughout the swing may significantly increase when the athlete's technique is incorrect. Cyclists may also be at risk for these type of fractures when performing off-road riding. A FOOSH may cause a fracture at the hook. Although they are rarely seen, hamate body fractures are most commonly associated with crush injuries.

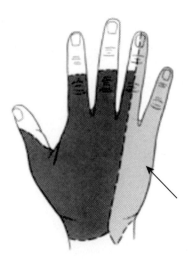

Figure 18.18 Patients with injury or pathology of the ulnar nerve complain of decreased sensation in the ulnar nerve distribution *(light gray area, arrow)*. (From Frontera WR: Essentials of Physical Medicine and Rehabilitation, 1st ed. Philadelphia, Hanley and Belfus, 2002.)

Clinical features

Fractures of the hook of the hamate often present with pain on palpation directly over the hamate, with localized swelling. To locate the hook of the hamate, the examiner should place the interphalangeal joint of his or her thumb over the over the base of the hypothenar eminence of the examined hand. In this position, the examiner's interphalangeal joint is directly over the pisiform. With the tip of the examiner's thumb pointing toward the web of the thumb and index finger of the examined hand, deep palpation with the examiner's thumb tip identifies the hook of the hamate. Hamate body fractures may exhibit pain with axial loading of the fifth metacarpal. As mentioned earlier, ulnar nerve deficits may be associated with hamate injuries. Testing and documenting ulnar nerve function is critical (see Figures 18.15, 18.16, 18.18, and **18.19**).

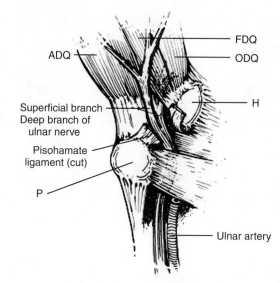

Figure 18.19 Branches of the ulnar nerve lie in close proximity to the hamate and can be injured in hamate fractures. ADQ, abductor digiti quinti; FDQ, flexor digiti quinti; H, hamate; ODQ, opponens digiti quinti; P, pisiform. (From DeLee JC, Drez D Jr, Miller MD [eds]: DeLee and Drez's Orthopaedic Sports Medicine: Principles and Practice, 2nd ed. Philadelphia, WB Saunders, 2003.)

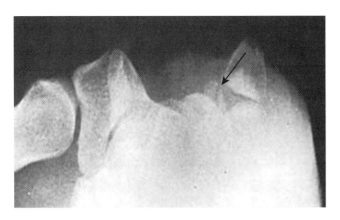

Figure 18.20 Radiograph of the carpal tunnel demonstrating a split fracture of the hook of the hamate *(arrow)*. Lateral tomography and oblique x-ray films might not show this fracture. (From Browner BD: Skeletal Trauma: Basic Science, Management, and Reconstruction, 3rd ed. Philadelphia, WB Saunders, 2003.)

Diagnosis
PA, lateral, oblique, and carpal tunnel wrist views should be initially obtained. The best view to reveal a fracture of the hook of the hamate is the carpal tunnel view **(Figure 18.20).** Hamate body fractures are often identified with oblique carpal x-ray views. If a hook or hamate body fracture is clinically suspected despite normal x-rays, a CT scan may aid in the identification of fractures.

Treatment
A volar splint can be used for initial stabilization. Hamate body fractures, if they are nondisplaced, should be immobilized in a short-arm thumb cast for 4 to 6 weeks. Hook of the hamate fractures have a high complication rate, and they are associated with poor healing and chronic pain.

Indications for specialty referral
Any displaced fractures and hook fractures should be referred to an orthopedic surgeon or a hand specialist for surgical management after immobilization with a volar splint (LOE: D).[19] Ulnar nerve findings in the setting of any hamate fracture require immediate referral to a surgical specialist.

Return to sport
After surgical repair of fractures of the hook of the hamate, athletes may often return to sports after 6 to 8 weeks. Generally, if strength is at 80% of that of the unaffected wrist, the athlete may return to sports participation with a sport-specific orthosis until full function has returned. In surgically repaired hamate body fractures, return to sport is often individually tailored. Usually, return to sport can be anticipated 4 to 6 weeks after the repair if the strength is at 80% of that of the unaffected wrist. The athlete may return to sport with a sport-specific orthosis until full function has returned. Athletes with nondisplaced hamate body fractures may return to sports participation immediately with a semirigid synthetic cast.

Capitate fracture
The capitate bone is the largest of the carpal bones. It resides in the second row, and it articulates with the scaphoid, the lunate, and the third and forth metacarpal bones. Like the scaphoid bone, injury identification may be elusive, and it may require repeat x-rays after 7 to 10 days of immobilization. The capitate's blood supply is also similar to that of the scaphoid, with retrograde flow to the distal aspect leaving the proximal aspect vulnerable to nonunion and AVN. Capitate fractures are typically seen with

associated scaphoid fractures, distal radial fractures, or lunate injuries; they are rarely seen in isolation.

Mechanism of injury
The injury pattern may involve a crush injury, a FOOSH injury **(Figure 18.21),** or a direct blow to the dorsal aspect of the wrist. The latter mechanism frequently occurs when a baseball batter is struck by a pitch on the dorsal aspect of the hand.

Clinical features
The patient will often describe dorsal wrist pain with corresponding tenderness to palpation over the dorsal aspect of the wrist. Pain may also be produced with axial loading of the third metacarpal. Care should be taken to review the surrounding anatomy for additional injures.

Diagnosis
Initial PA, lateral, and oblique views may appear normal. The immobilization of suspected capitate fractures for 7 to 10 days followed by repeat radiographs may identify a fracture or evidence of fracture healing. CT scanning, MRI, or bone scanning may assist with the diagnosis of acute or subacute capitate fractures.

Treatment
As with the scaphoid bone, any suspicion of a capitate fracture should prompt the clinician to immobilize the wrist in a short-arm thumb spica splint or cast and to arrange for more definitive imaging studies or repeat examination and radiographs in 10 to 14 days. Immobilization should continue for 6 to 8 weeks.

Indications for specialty referral
Any identification of fracture displacement or multiple injuries should prompt immediate referral to an orthopedic surgeon for surgical evaluation and repair with the wrist immobilized in a short-arm thumb spica splint or cast.[20]

Return to sport
In the nonsurgical case, the athlete may return to sports participation after a semirigid synthetic cast is applied. In the cases of a surgical repair, participation is restricted while the athlete is immobilized in a cast for a minimum of 4 to 6 weeks. Thereafter, protective splinting is employed for an additional 3 months. Supervised physical therapy should be undertaken until strength and function nears that of the uninjured wrist. Upon full recovery, sport participation may be allowed without a protective splint.

Pisiform fracture
The pisiform bone is a sesamoid bone that is enveloped within the flexor carpi ulnaris tendon and that is superficial to the triquetrum on the volar surface. It is rarely fractured, and it is even more rarely displaced when it is fractured.

Mechanism of injury
A pisiform fracture is often the result of a direct blow to the hypothenar eminence region, or it may result from a FOOSH injury.

Clinical features
Pain is often detected with palpation over the hypothenar eminence. Because it resides in close proximity to the ulnar nerve, nerve deficits in the forth and fifth finger may be present. In the setting of ulnar nerve deficits (see Figures 18.15, 18.16, 18.18, and 18.19), injury to structures bordering Guyon's canal (volar carpal ligament, hamate, and pisohamate ligament) should be investigated.

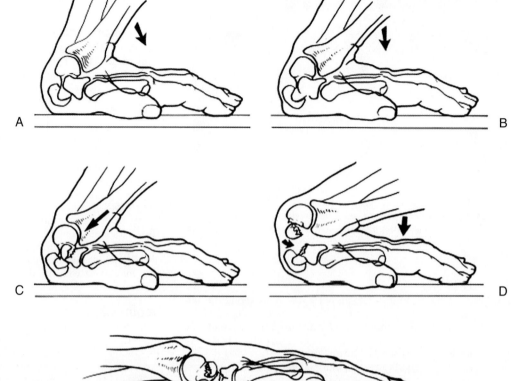

Figure 18.21 The mechanism of carpal fractures from falls on an outstretched hand with the wrist going into marked dorsiflexion. *A,* Wrist in marked dorsiflexion. Note that the capitate is at a 90-degree angle to the radius. *B,* Scaphoid fractures as a result of increased dorsiflexion at the midcarpal joint. *C,* The dorsal lip of the radius strikes the capitate, causing it to fracture. *D,* The proximal fragment of the capitate is rotated 90 degrees. *E,* Return of the wrist to a neutral position. Note that the proximal fragment of the capitate is now rotated 180 degrees. (From Stein F, Siegel MW: J Bone Joint Surg 1969;51A:391. In Canale ST: Campbell's Operative Orthopaedics, 10th ed. Philadelphia, Mosby, 2003.)

Diagnosis

PA and lateral views often do not reveal a fracture to the pisiform bone. Fractures are best seen on oblique PA views with 30 degrees of rotation or with a carpal tunnel view.

Treatment

Pisiform fractures are traditionally managed with short-arm thumb spica casts for 3 to 6 weeks.

Indications for specialist referral

If pain persists after immobilization, further studies can be done to possibly identify a nonunion. In the case of nonunion, surgical removal of the pisiform is the recommended treatment (LOE: D).[2,17]

Return to sport

Protective synthetic semirigid casting, tape, or wrapping can be done in an effort to reduce the pain. If the athlete is pain free with any of these modalities, sports participation can resume. Recurrence of pain may be the result of arthritic processes caused by poor healing. In this setting, referral to an orthopedic surgeon for excision of the pisiform should be considered.

Trapezium fracture

Fractures of the trapezium are uncommon, and they account for less than 5% of carpal bone fractures. Three classic bony injury patterns may be identified: an avulsion fracture of the trapezial ridge, a vertical fracture of the body, and comminuted fractures.

Mechanism of injury

The patient may give a history of a FOOSH, which may yield an avulsion to the trapezial ridge. A direct blow or a forcefully abducted thumb may result in a vertical or comminuted fracture pattern.

Clinical features

Pain and swelling are typically located over the base of the thenar eminence. Pain is also reported with thumb movements and axial loading of the thumb.

Diagnosis

PA, lateral, and oblique views usually provide adequate visualization of a fracture. Carpal tunnel views may aid in the identification of trapezial ridge fractures.

Treatment

Nondisplaced vertical fractures of the trapezium respond very well to conservative treatment, and they may be managed without orthopedic consultation. These fractures should be immobilized in a short-arm thumb spica cast for 4 to 6 weeks. Periodic follow-up evaluations every 2 weeks with x-rays to monitor healing progress should be performed.

Indications for specialty referral

If displacement or multiple fragments are evident, referral to an orthopedic surgeon or a hand specialist is indicated for open reduction and surgical repair.

Return to sport

After the immobilization period, supervised physical therapy rehabilitation efforts should focus on regaining extension, flexion, hand function, and grip strength. After strength and pain-free function nears that of the uninjured hand, return to sports participation is allowed with a protective orthosis. The orthosis should be used during athletic activity for an additional 4 weeks.

Trapezoid fracture

Fractures of the trapezoid are uncommon. This bone is well supported in the distal carpal row by the scaphoid, the capitate, and the trapezium.

Mechanism of injury
Fractures to the trapezoid may occur with axial loading forces from the second metacarpal.

Risk factors
There are no particular risk factors for this type of injury.

Clinical features
Patients usually present with pain and swelling over the dorsal aspect of the hand. Pain may be reported with movements and axial loading of the index finger.

Diagnosis
PA, lateral, and oblique views should be obtained. However, owing to the location of the trapezoid and the adjacent carpal bones, routine x-ray views may not demonstrate a fracture. A CT scan should be performed when a trapezoid fracture is clinically suspected.

Treatment
Nondisplaced fractures of the trapezoid may be managed with immobilization in a short-arm thumb spica cast for 4 to 6 weeks. Periodic follow-up evaluations every 2 weeks with x-rays to monitor healing progress should be performed.

Indications for specialty referral
Displaced fractures or fracture dislocations warrant referral to an orthopedic surgeon or a hand specialist for surgical repair.

Return to sport
After the immobilization period, supervised physical therapy rehabilitation efforts should focus on regaining extension, flexion, hand function, and grip strength. When strength and painless function near that of the uninjured hand, a return to sports participation is allowed.

FRACTURES OF THE METACARPALS

Metacarpal fractures are not at all unique to athletics; they are commonly seen in the emergency department and primary care settings, and they account for up to one third of all hand fractures.[21,22] As a result of their unique implications and management, first metacarpal fractures are considered separately from fractures of the second through the fifth metacarpals. All metacarpal fractures are further classified by the fracture location within the metacarpal bone. These classes include fractures of the metacarpal base, shaft, neck, and head.

The second through the fifth metacarpals have differing degrees of motion, with the fourth and fifth metacarpal bones being capable of the most motion (15 to 25 degrees in the anteroposterior plane). This motion is evident when one observes his or her own hand in a loosely closed fashion and then progresses to a tightly clenched fist. During the same maneuver, one may also recognize that the second and third metacarpals remain fixed. This exercise helps illustrate how the metacarpal motion relies on a fixed center (metacarpals two and three) that provides the remaining metacarpal bones with the mobility to generate stability and grip strength. This difference in mobility dictates the allowable amount of fracture angulation when managing metacarpal fractures.

Although varying degrees of metacarpal angulation may be tolerated, rotational malalignment is not. To recognize when a

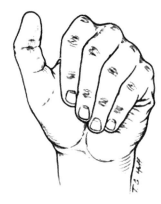

Figure 18.22 In flexion, the digits should all point to the scaphoid tuberosity. (From Browner BD: Skeletal Trauma: Basic Science, Management, and Reconstruction, 3rd ed. Philadelphia, WB Saunders, 2003.)

rotational fracture deformity is present, one should be familiar with normal finger positioning. Normally, the second through fifth fingertips point toward the scaphoid tubercle when the fingers are flexed so that the pads of the fingertips approximate the volar surface **(Figure 18.22)**. Additionally, with the fingers flexed in this position, the fingernails of all digits should reside in the same plane; this is called the *convergence test* **(Figure 18.23)**. Any deviation from this finger orientation should alert the examiner of a possible rotational malalignment.

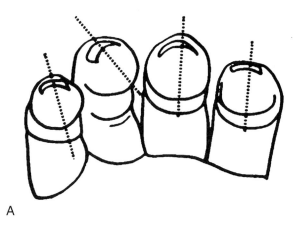

A

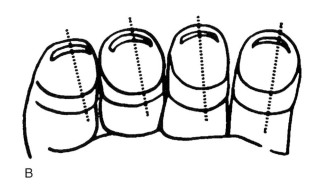

B

Figure 18.23 Flexed fingertips should be checked for rotational alignment. A, Rotational malalignment of the fourth finger caused by metacarpal or phalangeal fracture. B, Normal alignment. (From Noble J: Textbook of Primary Care Medicine, 3rd ed. St. Louis, Mosby, 2001.)

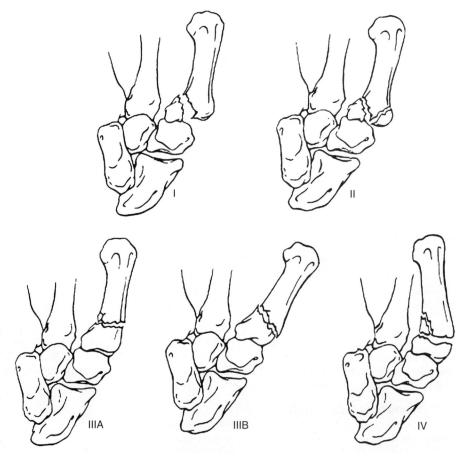

Figure 18.24 Four types of fractures of the base of the first metacarpal. Type I (Bennett's fracture-dislocation) and type II (Rolando's fracture) are intra-articular. Type III fractures are extra-articular and either transverse (III A) or oblique (III B). Type IV fractures are only seen in children, and they involve the proximal epiphysis. (From Eiff MP, Hatch RL, Calmbach WL: Fracture Management for Primary Care, 2nd ed. Philadelphia, WB Saunders, 2003.)

First metacarpal fractures

Fractures of the first metacarpal are not as common as other metacarpal fractures. However, they are important because the first metacarpal is crucial to grip strength and hand function. Extra-articular shaft fractures are the most common and the simplest to treat.[2] Three primary fracture patterns exist in adults (types I, II, and III A/B), and only one is seen in children (type IV) **(Figure 18.24).** Type I (Bennett's fracture) was first described in 1882 by E.H. Bennett, MD[23]; it is an oblique intra-articular base fracture-dislocation[24] **(Figure 18.25).** Type II (Rolando's fracture) is an intra-articular comminuted fracture of the base that can be T- or Y-shaped[25] **(Figure 18.26).** An extraarticular fracture localized to the shaft can be horizontal (type III A) or oblique (type III B) **(Figure 18.27).**

Mechanism of injury

The injury is likely the result of direct contact, a forced hyperabduction, or an axial load against a partially flexed thumb. Another mechanism of injury may be from torsion of the thumb. Any of these mechanisms may yield a fracture either at the base or the shaft.

Clinical features

The patient will complain of pain localized to the base of the first metacarpal, the anatomic snuffbox, or the distal radius. Grip strength is weakened as a result of pain, and pain is worsened with attempted thumb movements. The range of motion will be limited. Swelling and bruising occur more commonly on the dorsal aspect.

Diagnosis

PA and lateral views of the first metacarpal will often identify a fracture at the shaft. Oblique views are frequently needed to

identify an intra-articular fracture. In some cases in which an intra-articular fracture is suspected but not detected on x-ray, CT scanning can be helpful.

Treatment

Type III A fractures are commonly managed without orthopedic referral. Fractures resulting in an angulation of less than 30 degrees do not require reduction. Healing will usually result without any deformity or functional limitations. However, those resulting in

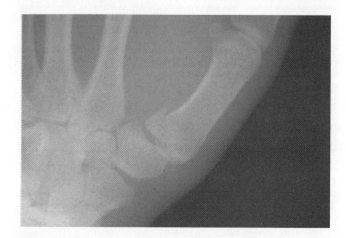

Figure 18.25 An oblique intra-articular base fracture-dislocation of the first metacarpal (Bennett's fracture) in the anteroposterior view. (From Browner BD: Skeletal Trauma: Basic Science, Management, and Reconstruction, 3rd ed. Philadelphia, WB Saunders, 2003.)

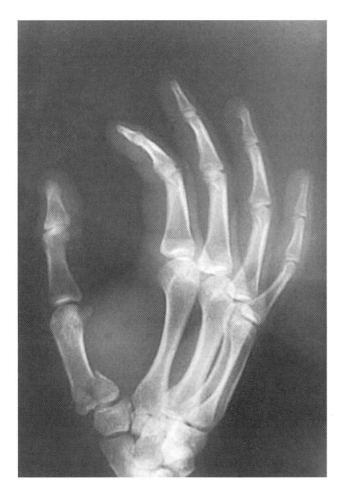

Figure 18.26 A three-part Rolando fracture. (From Browner BD: Skeletal Trauma: Basic Science, Management, and Reconstruction, 3rd ed. Philadelphia, WB Saunders, 2003.)

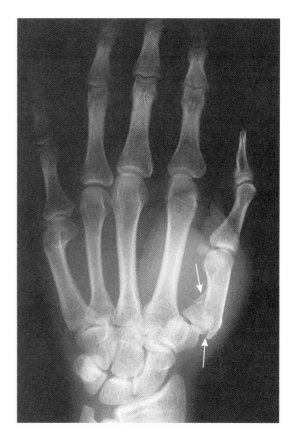

Figure 18.27 Extra-articular fracture of the first metacarpal base. An oblique fracture is seen at the metacarpal base *(arrows)* but without extension into the joint space. If extension into the joint space with a single linear fracture had occurred, this would be a Bennett's fracture; if it were a comminuted fracture extending into the joint space, it would be a Rolando's fracture. (From Browner BD: Skeletal Trauma: Basic Science, Management, and Reconstruction, 3rd ed. Philadelphia, WB Saunders, 2003.)

more than 30 degrees of angulation will require closed reduction with local anesthesia.[2] The angle reduction can be performed by applying longitudinal traction while simultaneously applying force to the fracture apex. Post reduction x-rays should confirm a reduction in angulation to less than 30 degrees before splinting or casting. The inability to obtain adequate angulation reduction requires specialist referral.

After any necessary reduction, the patient should be splinted in a thumb spica splint with the wrist in 30 degrees of extension, and the arm should then be placed in a sling to maintain upright elevation. Care should be taken to not hyperextend the thumb when forming the splint. Splinting (as opposed to casting) during the acute stages accommodates the anticipated swelling. Follow-up at 48 to 72 hours should include assessment for swelling and for motor and sensory function.

Definitive treatment involves a short-arm thumb spica cast with care taken to not hyperextend the thumb and wrist positioning at 30 degrees of extension. Cast immobilization should be maintained for 4 weeks. Follow-up examinations at 2-week intervals should be done with radiographs to evaluate for proper healing and placement.

Indications for specialty referral

Patients identified as having type I or II fractures require immediate referral to an orthopedic surgeon or a hand specialist,[22,26,27] and their injuries should be treated with a thumb spica splint

(as described previously for type III A fractures). Early diagnosis and treatment of these fractures are crucial to preventing carpal–metacarpal arthritis and maintaining normal function (LOE: D).[25,28] Type III B oblique fractures are prone to being unstable, and this results in a rotational malalignment; patients with this type of injury should also be immediately referred. In addition, evidence of nonunion or subluxation or the inability to maintain less than 30 degrees of angulation after the reduction of a type III A fracture should be referred.

Return to sport

After the 4-week immobilization period, supervised rehabilitation efforts should focus on regaining extension, flexion, hand function, and grip strength. Again, the athlete should be reminded that bone healing of the fracture is still in progress during these early rehabilitation stages. When strength and pain-free function near that of the uninjured hand, return to sports participation is allowed with a protective orthosis until full function returns.

Metacarpal base fractures of the second through the fifth metacarpals

Fractures at these locations are not as common as fractures of other metacarpal locations.

Mechanism of injury

The injury is often related to a direct blow, to a torsion force from a digit, or to a crush injury. In rare circumstances, injury here may be related to a poorly delivered punch or to a FOOSH injury.

Risk factors

There are no particular risk factors for this type of injury.

Clinical features

The patient will present with pain and swelling localized to the base of the second through the fifth metacarpals that increases with flexion and extension of the wrist. The examiner should look for deformities that include signs of a rotation. Injury to the motor branch of the ulnar nerve may be associated with fractures at the base of the forth and fifth metacarpals. A relative inability to actively abduct and adduct the fingers or weakness of the intrinsic hand muscles may aid in the identification of injuries to the motor branch of the ulnar nerve (see Figures 18.15 and 18.16).

Fracture dislocations of the second and third metacarpal bases are rare as a result of their relatively fixed positioning. By contrast, dislocations of the fifth metacarpal followed by dislocations of the fourth metacarpal are more common as a result of their enhanced mobility.

Diagnosis

Standard wrist PA, lateral, and oblique views of the metacarpal bones should be performed. The lateral view is helpful for identifying a metacarpal dislocation. CT scanning or MRI may be used to identify fractures that are not evident on plain films.

Treatment

The acute management of uncomplicated fractures of the second through the fourth metacarpal bases should include immobilization with dorsal and volar splints. In the splinted position, the wrist should be maintained in 30 degrees of extension, with the MCP joints left free and the patient instructed to perform ice application and elevation. Initial follow up at 5 to 7 days should include assessing swelling status and motor and sensory function. Definitive treatment is with the application of a short-arm cast with the wrist maintained in 30 degrees of extension. Cast immobilization should be maintained for 4 to 6 weeks. Weekly follow-up examinations with radiographs to evaluate for proper healing and positioning are needed for 3 weeks. Follow up can then be every 2 weeks thereafter.

Indications for specialty referral

Fractures associated with injury to the ulnar nerve, crush injuries with extensive soft-tissue trauma, rotational malalignment, injury to flexor or extensor tendons, fracture-dislocations, and fractures of the base of the fifth metacarpal require orthopedic consultation or evaluation by an orthopedic hand specialist. Fractures of the base of the fifth metacarpal are unique in that they are very unstable and often require internal fixation (LOE: D).[21,27] Any complication or delay in healing noted during the treatment course of fractures of the bases of the second to fourth metacarpals should prompt immediate evaluation by an orthopedic surgeon or a hand specialist.

Return to sport

After the immobilization period, supervised rehabilitation efforts should focus on regaining extension, flexion, hand function, and grip strength. The patient should be reminded that bone healing of the fracture is still in progress during these early stages. The purpose of removing the casting material before full healing is to minimize the formation of adhesions and weakness related to immobilization. When strength and pain-free function near that of the uninjured hand, return to sports participation is allowed with a protective orthosis, which should be used for an additional 4 to 6 weeks.

Metacarpal shaft fractures of the second through the fifth metacarpals

Fractures of the shaft region present in three forms: transverse, oblique, and comminuted. They are often the result of a direct blow or of a crushing or torsion injury. Associated with the metacarpal shaft are three volar and four dorsal interosseous muscles, which are innervated by a motor branch of the ulnar nerve. Originating at the metacarpal shaft, they insert on the corresponding phalanx, aid in the flexion of the metacarpophalangeal joint, and extend the interphalangeal joints. Independently, the volar interossei adduct the fingers, whereas the dorsal interossei abduct them. The third metacarpal and its corresponding phalanx lack a palmar interosseous muscle. Knowing the function of these muscle aids in the understanding of the forces applied to the fragments of a metacarpal shaft, neck, and head fracture, and it explains the inherent instability of some metacarpal fractures **(Figure 18.28)**.

Transverse fractures often result in apex dorsal angulation **(Figure 18.29)** (see Chapter 15 for a discussion of angulation conventions), whereas oblique fractures result in foreshortening of the metacarpal bone. Functionally the metacarpal shaft acts as a lever arm. Angulated fractures (especially in more proximal shaft fractures) disproportionately displace the head of the metacarpal further to the volar aspect. Failure to reduce a metacarpal shaft fracture increases the chances of developing a deformity called *pseudoclawing* (see Figure 18.28). Because of the risk of deformity and loss of function, rotation and angulation are relatively unacceptable in metacarpal shaft fractures. Oblique fracture fragments tend to slide over each other, and this accounts for a length reduction of the metacarpal bone. Length reductions of up to 5 mm are acceptable and will often heal without functional limitations.[2]

Figure 18.28 Transverse metacarpal shaft fractures will angulate with the apex pointing dorsally as a result of the pull of the interosseous muscles. (From Browner BD: Skeletal Trauma: Basic Science, Management, and Reconstruction, 3rd ed. Philadelphia, WB Saunders, 2003.)

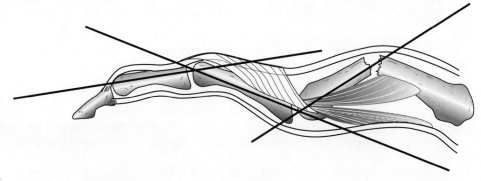

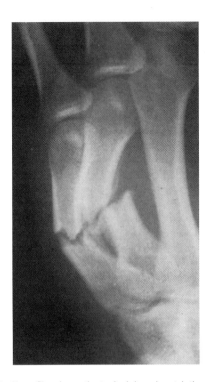

Figure 18.29 X-ray film shows the typical dorsal angulation of fractures of the metacarpal shafts. These fractures are usually the result of a direct blow, and they generally angulate dorsally as a result of the interosseous muscles exerting a volar force. (From DeLee JC, Drez D Jr, Miller MD [eds]: DeLee and Drez's Orthopaedic Sports Medicine: Principles and Practice, 2nd ed. Philadelphia, WB Saunders, 2003.)

Mechanism of injury

Transverse fractures are usually the result of a direct blow. Oblique fractures are often the result of torsion injuries. Comminuted fractures are associated with forceful crush injuries.

Clinical features

Patients presenting with metacarpal shaft fractures will have pain and swelling over the dorsal aspect of the affected metacarpal. Finger flexion tests of the injured hand need to be performed to aid with the identification of a rotational malalignment (see Figures 18.22 and 18.23). Sensory and motor deficits as a result of nerve injuries are rare.

Diagnosis

PA, lateral, and oblique views of the metacarpals are usually all that is required to identify a fracture (see Figure 18.29). Evidence of a rotational malalignment may present with two fracture fragments with differing diameters. Acceptable angulation deformities are less than 10 degrees for the second and third metacarpals and less than 20 degrees for the forth and fifth metacarpals.[2]

Treatment

Acutely, nondisplaced, uncomplicated, transverse metacarpal shaft fractures should be placed in a gutter splint. The wrist should be positioned at 30 degrees of extension, with the MCP joint at 90 degrees. The proximal interphalangeal (PIP) and distal interphalangeal (DIP) joints are maintained in extension. Displaced fractures should be reduced to acceptable ranges (less than 10 degrees for the second and third metacarpals and less than 20 degrees for the fourth and fifth metacarpals). Techniques used are the same as those used for the reduction of

metacarpal neck fractures (described later). If finger traps are available, they can be useful to help with the reduction. A gutter splint (described previously) should be placed and postreduction radiographs obtained to confirm fracture position. Initial follow-up should be done in 5 to 7 days with repeat radiographs. Definitive treatment involves casting in the same splint positioning for 4 weeks. Evaluations are needed every 2 weeks, with radiographs taken to monitor for proper fracture healing and position. Evidence of incomplete healing at 4 weeks requires additional immobilization for another 2 weeks. Beyond this period, if healing is not progressing, an evaluation by an orthopedic surgeon or a hand specialist should be obtained.

Indications for specialty referral

The following conditions required orthopedic consultation or evaluation by a hand specialist: complicated fractures associated with nerve injury; crush injuries with extensive soft-tissue trauma; multiple metacarpal fractures; rotational malalignment; angulations that cannot be reduced to acceptable ranges; length reductions of more than 5 mm; comminuted, spiral, and oblique fractures; and injury to flexor or extensor tendons.

Return to sport

After radiographic evidence of healing is documented and the casting material is removed, supervised physical therapy rehabilitation efforts should focus on regaining extension, flexion, hand function, and grip strength. When strength and pain-free function near that of the uninjured hand, return to sports participation is allowed with a protective orthosis until full function returns.

Metacarpal neck fractures of the second through the fifth metacarpals

Similar to those of the metacarpal shaft, fractures involving the neck may result in angulation and rotation. These fractures are most commonly transverse, and they often have some degree of angulation. The likely angulation is apex dorsal, which forces the head into the volar plane.

Anatomic angle reduction is critical to normal healing and function when dealing with fractures of the second and third metacarpal neck. This intolerance of angulation is the result of the relatively fixed nature of these two bones. These strict tolerances do not apply to the fourth and fifth metacarpal necks. Angulations of up to 30 degrees for the fourth metacarpal neck and 40 degrees for the fifth metacarpal neck are well tolerated, and they heal with a minimal loss of function.

Mechanism of injury

Accounting for 50% of metacarpal fractures and 20% of hand fractures, a fifth metacarpal neck fracture is the most common.[21] This fracture has earned the name "boxer's fracture," because it often results from a poorly delivered punch.

When the punch lands in the region of the mouth, this fracture may be associated with soft-tissue trauma from an impacting tooth, which adds the name "fight bite" to the injured area of broken skin over the MCP joint (see Chapter 19).

Clinical features

Lacerations of the skin over the MCP joint may be present. In some cases, tooth fragments or wall debris may reside in the lesion. The MCP joint may appear abnormally depressed from the neighboring MCP joints. The patient will complain of pain at the MCP joint, and he or she may present with pseudoclawing (see Figure 18.28). Swelling on the dorsal aspect with bruising may be appreciated. Care must be taken to identify signs of rotational malalignment.

Diagnosis

PA, lateral, and oblique metacarpal radiographs will usually identify a fracture at the metacarpal neck **(Figure 18.30)**. As mentioned previously, a foreign body may be present in the wound. Films with an obvious fracture should be scrutinized to rule out foreign bodies.

Treatment

If lacerations are present, these wounds should be carefully examined and irrigated. Antibiotics should be initiated, and tetanus status should be verified and treated as necessary on the basis of the immunization history. Immediate orthopedic intervention is required for fractures with foreign bodies or lacerations because these injuries are considered open fractures, and they typically require operating room exploration and irrigation (see Chapter 19).

Nondisplaced and nonangulated fractures of the second or third metacarpal necks should be placed in a radial gutter splint with the MCP joint in 70 to 90 degrees of flexion and the PIP and DIP joints in partial flexion. Nondisplaced and nonangulated fractures of the fourth or fifth metacarpal neck should be placed in an ulnar gutter splint. Fractures of the fourth metacarpal with up to 30 degrees of apex dorsal angulation and fractures of the fifth metacarpal with up to 40 degrees of apex dorsal angulation can be accepted; however, efforts should be made to reduce the fracture to a more acceptable range (LOE: B).[2,29,30] Reduction techniques are described later in this chapter. Patients with fractures of the second or third metacarpal will require follow-up in 4 to 5 days, with radiographs taken to confirm fracture position. Patients with fractures of the fourth or fifth metacarpal should be seen within 7 to 10 days. Immobilization should be continued for 3 to 4 weeks in the gutter splint, with evaluations performed every 7 to 14 days to monitor alignment, rotation, angulation, and healing progression.

Patients with fractures of the fourth and fifth metacarpals with angulations exceeding those limits outlined previously or patients with pseudoclawing on examination must have closed reduction attempted. Local anesthesia can be achieved via ulnar nerve block or hematoma block. Finger traps help disimpact fracture fragments, and they can be useful if they are available. One of two methods can be used for the closed reduction. With the first method, the patient's wrist is extended, and the MCP is maximally flexed. The shaft of the proximal phalanx is grasped and used as a lever to push the metacarpal head dorsally. Simultaneously, the clinician uses his or her other hand to apply counterpressure just proximal to the fracture on the dorsum of the metacarpal.[2] With the second method, which is also called the 90/90 *method*, the patient's MCP, PIP, and DIP are flexed at 90 degrees **(Figures 18.31 and 18.32)**. Pressure is applied dorsally to the volarly displaced metacarpal head using the patient's PIP, while counterpressure is applied to the proximal fracture fragment.[29] Immediate application of the ulnar gutter splint (as described previously) is critical to maintaining the reduction. As with all reductions, postreduction radiographs must be obtained. Treatment course then follows in the same way as it does for nondisplaced, nonangulated fractures, as described previously.

Indications for specialty referral

Referral to an orthopedic surgeon or a hand specialist should be performed for the following situations: open fractures, fractures of the second or third metacarpal neck with any angulation, evidence of rotational malalignment, or reductions of the forth and fifth metacarpals that fail to achieve acceptable angles. Before referral, these fractures should be splinted in an ulnar or radial gutter splint with the MCP joint in 90 degrees of flexion and the PIP and DIP joints in partial flexion. In addition, any evidence of poor healing or increasing angulation should prompt referral.

Return to sport

After the immobilization period, an additional 4 to 6 weeks of supervised physical therapy rehabilitation should focus on regaining extension, flexion, hand function, and grip strength. The patient should be reminded that he or she may have persistent asymmetric-appearing knuckles. Bone healing of the fracture is

Figure 18.30 *A*, Anteroposterior view of a fracture through the neck of the fifth metacarpal, with apparent modest angulation. *B*, The same metacarpal fracture seen in a lateral view in 10 degrees of supination. The true amount of angulation is much better appreciated in this view. (From DeLee JC, Drez D Jr, Miller MD [eds]: DeLee and Drez's Orthopaedic Sports Medicine: Principles and Practice, 2nd ed. Philadelphia, WB Saunders, 2003.)

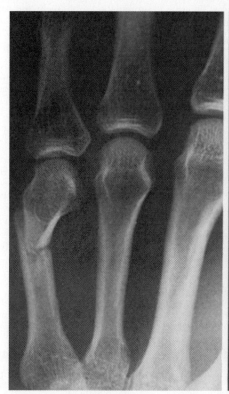
A

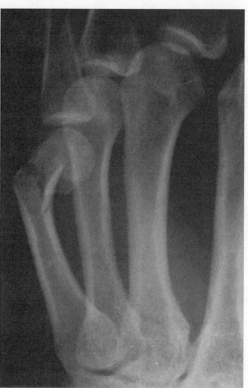
B

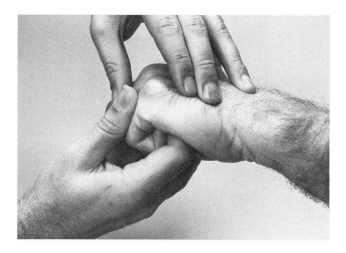

Figure 18.31 The 90–90 method of metacarpal neck fracture reduction. (From Marx JA: Rosen's Emergency Medicine: Concepts and Clinical Practice, 6th ed. Philadelphia, Mosby, 2006.)

still in progress during these early stages. When strength and pain-free function approach that of the uninjured hand, a return to sports participation is allowed with a protective orthosis, which is worn until full function returns.

Metacarpal head fractures of the second through the fifth metacarpals

Metacarpal head fractures are rare and account for only 4% to 5% of metacarpal injuries.[17] The second metacarpal is the head that is the most likely to be injured. Anatomically, it is important to remember that the eccentric, hemispheric design of the metacarpal head allows for greater flexion while limiting extension of the MCP joint.

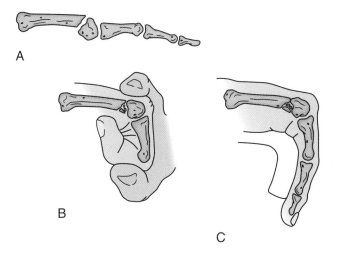

Figure 18.32 A displaced metacarpal neck can be reduced by flexing the metacarpophalangeal joint to 90 degrees and using the proximal phalanx to control rotation and as a lever to push the metacarpal head up. *A*, A displaced neck fracture is generally associated with comminution on the volar surface. *B*, Fracture reduction was accomplished by using the proximal phalanx to push the metacarpal head up. *C*, Immobilization in plaster should place the metacarpophalangeal joint in 70 to 90 degrees of flexion and the proximal interphalangeal joints in close to full extension. (From Browner BD: Skeletal Trauma: Basic Science, Management, and Reconstruction, 3rd ed. Philadelphia, WB Saunders, 2003.)

Mechanism of injury
Like metacarpal neck fractures, metacarpal head fractures can be the result of direct trauma from delivering a punch. Other possible mechanisms include axial trauma and crush injuries, with a crush injury being most likely to yield a comminuted fracture.

Clinical features
Usually pain and swelling will be localized to the involved MCP, and there will also be a limited range of motion. Axial loading of the corresponding phalanx will result in increased pain. The need to clinically evaluate the injured hand for rotation is crucial. Just as with boxer's fractures, these injuries can be associated with lacerations or other soft-tissue injuries, and a careful inspection should be made.

Diagnosis
PA, lateral, and oblique views should be obtained. With more subtle fractures, 10 degrees of supination and/or pronation may help with the identification of a metacarpal head fracture. Careful inspection for foreign bodies should be done for injuries that are associated with a laceration.

Treatment
If lacerations are present, treatment should follow that prescribed for metacarpal neck fractures with lacerations, which was discussed previously. These injuries are considered open fractures, and they require immediate referral to an orthopedic surgeon.

In the absence of an open fracture, immobilization with a ulnar or radial gutter splint with 30 degrees of wrist extension, flexion of the MCP joint at 70 to 90 degrees, and DIP flexion of 5 to 10 degrees should be applied. Ice, analgesics, and elevation should be initiated to help minimize pain and swelling.

Indications for specialty referral
Metacarpal head fractures require early consultation and definitive treatment by an orthopedic surgeon or a hand specialist because these fractures are intra-articular by definition. Open fractures should be immediately referred to a specialist, and closed fractures need to be evaluated by an orthopedist within 1 week.

Return to sport
A return to sports participation is often related to the severity of the fracture. Fractures that require surgical repair are usually given 6 to 8 weeks of immobilization, and this is followed by 4 to 6 weeks of supervised physical therapy before the athlete can return to participation. In less complicated, nondisplaced fractures, the immobilization period is 2 to 3 weeks, with subsequent rehabilitation focusing on range of motion, hand function, and grip strength. Total healing time can take 4 to 6 weeks. When strength and pain-free function nears that of the uninjured hand, a return to sports participation is allowed, with a protective orthosis. When full function returns, participation without the orthosis is possible. For cases in which the injury was minimal and good healing occurred, buddy taping may be sufficient support during the early stages of return.

PHALANX FRACTURES

Proximal and middle phalanx fracture
Fractures that present at the proximal and middle phalanx include greenstick, transverse, oblique, and comminuted fractures. The transverse, oblique, and comminuted fractures may present with some degree of displacement, angulation, or rotational malalignment. The fracture may be isolated to the shaft, or it may include the proximal or distal articular aspects as well. Volar angulations commonly occur as a result of the interaction of distal extensor

forces with mid-shaft flexor forces. These forces can result in rotational deformity, which is most commonly seen with oblique fractures.

Mechanism of injury

Often the injury is the result of a direct blow or of torsion. In the case of a direct blow, a transverse fracture may result. In the case of a torsion injury, a greenstick injury, or an injury involving more force, an oblique fracture may occur. A reduction in bone length is often associated with oblique fracture as a result of the two fragments sliding over each other **(Figure 18.33).** A crush injury often results in a comminuted fracture pattern.

Clinical features

The skin should be carefully examined for skin lacerations. Vascular, sensory (two-point discrimination), and motor function should be assessed. The patient will present with pain, swelling, and often bruising over the fracture region. The fingers should be examined for malrotation (see Figures 18.22 and 18.23). Examining both the injured and uninjured hands may further aid in the determination of the patient's normal amount of rotation. No degree of rotation should be tolerated with these fractures.[21,22,24]

Diagnosis

PA, lateral, and oblique finger views will often identify the fracture type and angulation. Diameter differences in the two fracture fragment ends suggest a rotational malalignment. Apex volar angulation is most common **(Figures 18.34 and 18.35).** It should be noted that some degree of angulation can be anatomically normal in the phalanges. An x-ray of the uninjured hand may aid in the identification of anatomic angulation from a traumatic fracture.

Treatment

Nondisplaced, nonangulated shaft fractures may be managed by buddy taping the injured finger to an adjacent finger at the proximal and middle phalanx or by aluminum splinting. Aluminum splinting

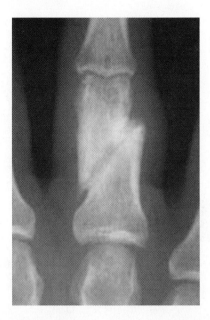

Figure 18.33 Long oblique proximal phalanx fracture allowed to heal after closed treatment with shortening and rotational deformity. (From Browner BD: Skeletal Trauma: Basic Science, Management, and Reconstruction, 3rd ed. Philadelphia, WB Saunders, 2003.)

should include the joint proximal and distal to the fracture, and it should maintain the joints in 30 degrees of flexion.[24] Repeat follow-up examination with radiographic evaluation to assess bone healing should be done after 7 to 10 days. Immobilization should continue for at least 2 to 3 more weeks, with weekly examinations and radiographs. Buddy taping with activities should then continue until the patient is free of pain.

Figure 18.34 Angulation of fractures of the proximal phalanx may be clinically less apparent at the base than at the mid-diaphyseal (midshaft) level. (From Browner BD: Skeletal Trauma: Basic Science, Management, and Reconstruction, 3rd ed. Philadelphia, WB Saunders, 2003.)

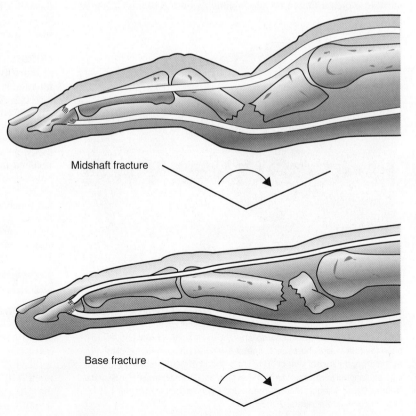

Midshaft fracture

Base fracture

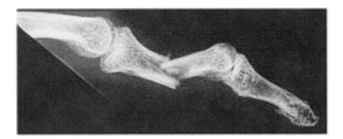

Figure 18.35   Middle phalanx fracture. (From Townsend CM Jr: Sabiston Textbook of Surgery, 17th ed. Philadelphia, WB Saunders, 2004.)

Angulated transverse fractures of the shaft of the proximal and middle phalanx should undergo closed reduction. Local anesthesia can be achieved using a digital nerve block. Longitudinal traction is applied, and the distal fragment is manipulated to align it with the proximal fragment.[1] Acceptable reduction involves less than 6 mm of shortening, less than 20 degrees of angulation, and no malrotation.[21,22] While reduction is maintained, an ulnar or radial gutter splint with the wrist in 30 degrees of extension and the MCP joint flexed to 90 degrees should be placed. The PIP and DIP are partially flexed to 45 degrees for proximal phalanx fractures, whereas the PIP and DIP at partial flexed to 5 to 10 degrees for middle phalanx fractures. The splint should start at the proximal forearm and extend to the fingertips. Postreduction radiographs are needed to confirm the stability of the reduction. An initial follow-up at 7 days with radiographs to evaluate for positioning and healing should be performed. Immobilization should last for 4 weeks, with weekly follow-up to ensure proper healing.

Small avulsion fractures at the PIP or DIP joint **(Figure 18.36)**, which occur with volar plate or central slip injuries, should follow those respective treatment recommendations as outlined in Chapter 19, Soft-Tissue Injuries of the Hand and Wrist.

Indications for specialty referral
Intra-articular fractures **(Figure 18.37)** on one or both condyles; comminuted, malrotated, oblique, and spiral fractures; or angulated fractures that cannot be corrected or maintained should be evaluated by an orthopedic surgeon within 72 hours after splinting. Open fractures and those with evidence of neurologic or vascular comprise require immediate orthopedic evaluation.

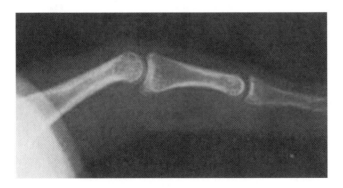

Figure 18.36   Small chip fractures avulsed off of the base of the middle phalanx by the volar plate are not uncommon after dorsal proximal interphalangeal joint dislocations. These do not affect the routine management of the dislocation. (From DeLee JC, Drez D Jr, Miller MD [eds]: DeLee and Drez's Orthopaedic Sports Medicine: Principles and Practice, 2nd ed. Philadelphia, WB Saunders, 2003.)

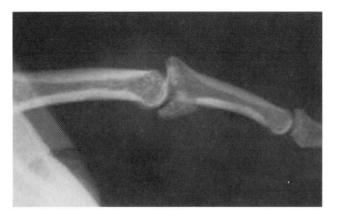

Figure 18.37   Fracture-dislocation (more correctly called *fracture-subluxation*) of the proximal interphalangeal joint. The volar base of the middle phalanx is crushed (usually comminuted), and it generally involves 30% or more of the articular surface. The remaining base of the middle phalanx is subluxated dorsally. (From DeLee JC, Drez D Jr, Miller MD [eds]: DeLee and Drez's Orthopaedic Sports Medicine: Principles and Practice, 2nd ed. Philadelphia, WB Saunders, 2003.)

Return to sport
After the initial immobilization, supervised physical therapy rehabilitation efforts should focus on regaining extension, flexion, hand function, and grip strength. The patient should be reminded that the fracture is in the healing stages during these early stages. When strength and pain-free function near that of the uninjured hand, a return to sports participation is allowed with a protective orthosis until full function returns. For nondisplaced fractures, buddy taping may be used during sporting events.

Distal phalanx fractures
The distal phalanx is the most commonly fractured bone in the hand.[31] Fractures to the distal phalanx may result in one of three forms: longitudinal, transverse, and comminuted[32] **(Figure 18.38)**. These fracture patterns may reside either at the articular, middle, or distal aspect. The flexor profundus tendon inserts at the proximal and middle volar surface, and the terminal extensor tendon inserts proximal on the dorsal surface. Fibrous septa extend from the volar aspect of the distal phalanx to the skin. Knowledge of these structures provides information that accounts for stabilizing and destabilizing forces applied to distal phalanx fracture fragments.

Mechanism of injury
The most common injury to this aspect is a crush injury that results in a comminuted fracture; these are often referred to as *tuft fractures* **(Figure 18.39)**. Lesser trauma affecting the very tip of the distal phalanx may result in a single-appearing fragment of small bone. Nail injuries are often associated with distal phalanx fractures.

Clinical findings
As mentioned previously, the nail is often affected, and this may present with a subungual hematoma. Pain and tense swelling with bruising may also be present. Two-point discrimination, DIP flexion, and extension function should be assessed.

Diagnosis
PA, lateral, and oblique views should be obtained to aid in ruling out any degree of angulation or displacement.

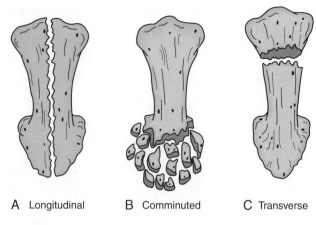

A Longitudinal   B Comminuted   C Transverse

Figure 18.38 Kaplan's classification of distal phalangeal fractures. *A,* Longitudinal. *B,* Comminuted. *C,* Transverse. (From Browner BD: Skeletal Trauma: Basic Science, Management, and Reconstruction, 3rd ed. Philadelphia, WB Saunders, 2003.)

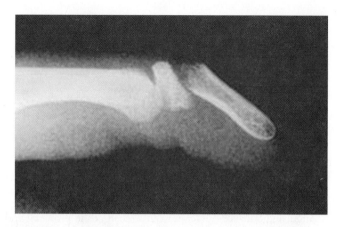

Figure 18.40 Fractures of the base of the distal phalanx tend to be unstable, and they will angulate with the apex pointing dorsally. (From Browner BD: Skeletal Trauma: Basic Science, Management, and Reconstruction, 3rd ed. Philadelphia, WB Saunders, 2003.)

Treatment

During the acute stages, efforts to reduce pain and swelling should include ice applications, analgesics, and elevation. Symptomatic subungual hematomas should be relieved; this can easily be done by burning a hole in the nail with a cautery unit or a paper clip.[2] In the event of angulation **(Figure 18.40),** a closed reduction may be attempted with a hematoma block or a digital nerve block. All fractures of the distal phalanx should be placed in a padded aluminum hairpin or a "U" splint with the DIP in extension, leaving the PIP and MCP free. Care should be demonstrated

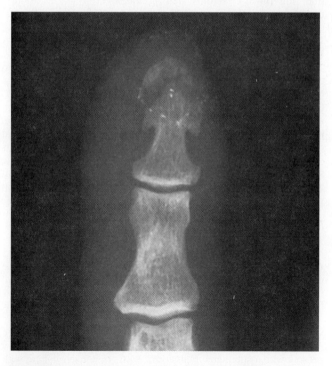

Figure 18.39 Tuft fracture of the distal phalanx of the thumb, anteroposterior view. This radiograph reveals the comminuted displaced fracture fragments and some radiopaque foreign material on the substance of the nail. (From Marx JA: Rosen's Emergency Medicine: Concepts and Clinical Practice, 6th ed. Philadelphia, Mosby, 2006.)

during the splint application to avoid excessive compression of the distal finger and to accommodate for swelling. In the successfully reduced or the nondisplaced, nonangulated fracture, initial follow up should be in 7 to 14 days. Radiographs should be obtained to assess bone healing and position if initial reduction was needed. Splinting may be maintained for 4 weeks or until the finger is no longer tender to impact.

Indications for specialty referral

Failed closed reductions and angulated or displaced transverse fractures should be promptly referred to an orthopedic surgeon. Evidence of nonunion or pain that persists for 6 months after treatment should also be referred.

Return to sport

In patients with healing fractures that do not require orthopedic referral, return to sports participation may be considered with the use of a protective splint when pain allows for participation. Splints may be worn for several months to avoid incidental impact because one of the complications of distal phalanx fractures is hypersensitivity.

CONCLUSION

A solid understanding of wrist/hand anatomy and function provides the primary care clinician with the ability to care for a multitude of wrist and hand fractures. Scaphoid fractures are the most common of all carpal fractures and can often present with symptoms similar to a wrist sprain. With scaphoid fractures and other fractures of the carpal bones, delays in diagnosis and treatment can lead to nonunion and avascular necrosis. When evaluating fractures of the phalanges and metacarpals, verificiation of neurovascular status and acceptable alignment (rotation, angulation, comminution) is essential. Good clinical judgement should always be used, especially when deciding to refer for specialty care and when to return to sport.

REFERENCES

1. Greene WB: Essentials of Musculoskeletal Care, 2nd ed. Rosemont, IL, American Academy of Orthopaedic Surgeons, 2001, pp. 252-254.

2. Eiff MP, Hatch RL, Calmbach WL: Fracture Management for Primary Care, 2nd ed. Philadelphia, WB Saunders, 2003, pp. 40-115.

3. Geissler WB: Carpal fractures in athletes. Clin Sports Med 2001;20:167-188.

4. Phillips TG, Reibach AM, Slomiany WP: Diagnosis and management of scaphoid fractures. Am Fam Physician 2004;70:879-884.

5. Tiel-van Buul MM, van Beek EJ, Borm JJ, et al: The value of radiographs and bone scintigraphy in suspected scaphoid fracture. A statistical analysis. J Hand Surg [Br] 1993;18:403-406.

6. Tiel-van Buul MM, Broekhuizen TH, van Beek EJ, et al: Choosing a strategy for the diagnostic management of suspected scaphoid fracture: a cost-effectiveness analysis. J Nucl Med 1995;36:45-48.

7. Tay BK-B, Coleman WW, Berven S, et al: Chapter 42: Orthopedics. In Doherty GM, Way LW (eds): Current Surgical Diagnosis and Treatment, 12nd ed. Norwalk, CT: Appleton & Lange, 2006.

8. Seitz WH Jr, Papandrea RF: Fractures and dislocations of the wrist. In Bucholz RW, Heckman JD (eds): Rockwood and Green's Fractures in Adults, 6th ed. Lippincott Williams & Wilkins, 2005.

9. Freeland P: Scaphoid tubercle tenderness: a better indicator of scaphoid fractures? Arch Emerg Med 1989;6:46-50.

10. Powell JM, Lloyd GJ, Rintoul RF: New clinical test for fracture of the scaphoid. Can J Surg 1988;31:237-238.

11. Chen SC: The scaphoid compression test. J Hand Surg [Br] 1989;14:323-325.

12. Rettig ME, Dassa GL, Raskin KB, et al: Wrist fractures in the athlete. Distal radius and carpal fractures. Clin sports Med 1998;17:469-489.

13. McCue FC III, Bruce JF Jr, Koman JD: Chapter 24: Wrist and hand. In DeLee JC, Drez D Jr, Miller MD (eds): DeLee and Drez's Orthopaedic Sports Medicine: Principles and Practice, 2nd ed. Philadelphia, WB Saunders, 2003.

14. Thorpe AP, Murray AD, Smith FW, et al: Clinically suspected scaphoid fracture: a comparison of magnetic resonance imaging and bone scintigraphy. Br J Radiol 1996;69:109-113.

15. Bond CD, Shin AY, McBride MT, et al: Percutaneous screw fixation or cast immobilization for nondisplaced scaphoid fractures. J Bone Joint Surg [Am] 2001;83-A:483-488.

16. Atkinson LS, Baxley EG: Scapholunate dissociation. Am Fam Physician 1994;49:1845-1850.

17. Meyer FN: Upper extremity and hand injury. In Moore EE, Feliciano DV, Mattox KL (eds): Trauma, 5th ed. New York, McGraw-Hill, 2004.

18. Lourie GM: Carpal fractures. In Light TR (ed): Hand Surgery Update 2, 2nd ed. Rosemont, IL: American Academy of Orthopaedic Surgeons, 1999, p 107.

19. Walsh JJ 4th, Bishop AT: Diagnosis and management of hamate hook fractures. Hand Clin 2000;16:397-403.

20. Canale ST: Campbell's Operative Orthopaedics, 10th ed. Philadelphia, Mosby, 2003, p 3579.

21. Peterson JJ, Bancroft LW: Injuries of the finger and thumb in the athlete. Clin Sports Med 2006;25:527-542.

22. Lee SG, Jupiter JB: Phalangeal and metacarpal fractures of the hand. Hand Clin 2000;1:323-332.

23. Bennett EH: Fractures of the metacarpal bones. Dublin Med Sci J 1882;73:72-75.

24. Hong E: Hand injuries in sports medicine. Prim Care 2005;32:91-103.

25. Palmer RE: Joint injuries of the hand in athletes. Clin Sports Med 1998;17:513-531.

26. Ashkenaze DM, Ruby LK: Metacarpal fractures and dislocations. Orthop Clin North Am 1992;23:19-33.

27. Walsh JJ: Fractures of the hand and carpal navicular bone in athletes. South Med J 2004;97:762-765.

28. Rosner JL, Zlatkin MB, Clifford P, et al: Imaging of athletic wrist and hand injuries. Semin Musculoskelet Radiol 2004;8:57-79.

29. Leggit JC, Meko CJ: Acute finger injuries: part II. Fractures, dislocations, and thumb injuries. Am Fam Physician 2006;73:827-834.

30. Statius Muller MG, Poolman RW, van Hoogstraten MJ, et al: Immediate mobilization gives good results in boxer's fractures with volar angulation up to 70 degrees: a prospective randomized trial comparing immediate mobilization with cast immobilization. Arch Orthop Trauma Surg 2003;123:534-537.

31. Browner BD: Skeletal Trauma: Basic Science, Management, and Reconstruction, 3rd ed. Philadelphia, WB Saunders, 2003.

32. Kaplan L: The treatment of fractures and dislocations of the hand and fingers. Technic of unpadded casts for carpal, metacarpal, and phalangeal fractures. Surg Clin North Am 1940;20:1695-1720.

33. Buckwalter JA, Einhorn TA, Bolander ME, et al: Healing of the musculoskeletal tissues. In Bucholz RW, Heckman JD (eds): Rockwood and Green's Fractures in Adults, 6th ed. Lippincott Williams & Wilkins, 2005.

Soft-Tissue Injuries of the Hand and Wrist

MAJ Chad Asplund, MD, and MAJ Christopher D. Meyering, DO

KEY POINTS

· The complex anatomy of the hand and wrist can make diagnosis a challenging task, but the correct pathoanatomic diagnosis can reduce morbidity and speed up return to play.

· The management of soft-tissue injuries of the hand and wrist requires balancing the athlete's desire to return to sports participation with proper treatment that allows healing and that prevents long-term complications of the injury.

· Any question about the instability of a joint in the hand or wrist warrants urgent surgical consultation.

· The physical examination of any injury should include an evaluation of active and passive range of motion verifying the stability of the joints involved, a neurovascular examination, and an inspection of the nail when the digits are injured.

· All jersey finger injuries require surgery, whereas most mallet finger injuries do not.

INTRODUCTION

Injuries of the wrist and hand are common in sports. The complex anatomy of the hand and wrist can make diagnosis a challenging task **(Figure 19.1).** A thorough assessment and a thoughtful differential diagnosis may reveal various injuries or syndromes. Proper diagnosis and rehabilitation will lead to decreased morbidity and faster return to sports participation.

HAND

Mallet finger

A mallet finger injury occurs when there is disruption of the extensor mechanism into the distal phalanx as a result of tendon rupture or fracture **(Figure 19.2).** The injury results in the incomplete extension of the distal interphalangeal (DIP) joint or extensor lag.

Mechanism of injury

Mallet fingers typically occur as a result of the impact of the fingertip on a ball or another object. The athlete is typically attempting to extend the DIP joint (e.g., preparing to catch the ball or extending the hand to grasp on object) when the DIP joint is forcibly flexed by the impact from the ball or the other object. The resulting force overloads the extensor mechanism of the DIP joint. Less commonly, mallet fingers can result from a combination of voluntary extension and an applied axial load force.

Bony fracture and tendon rupture are both common. Fractures through a large amount of the articular surface may result in acute or late subluxations, which can develop into malunion and arthrosis.

Risk factors

Mallet fingers are common in ball sports; sports involving hand-to-hand combat; and in activities requiring rapid, explosive hand movements. No specific brace or guard has been shown to reduce the incidence of mallet fingers.

Diagnosis

A careful physical examination (as mentioned in the Key Points) should be performed in addition to evaluating collateral stability, extensor lag, and digit rotation. Holding the proximal interphalangeal (PIP) joint in a fixed position and then asking the patient to extend the finger is the most effective method to establish the diagnosis. Rotation of the affected digit should be assessed by looking down the long axis of the fingers flexed to 90 degrees at the metacarpophalangeal (MCP) joint and comparing this with the result of the unaffected side. The PIP joint may rarely be involved and should also be assessed (LOE: C).[1]

Radiographs are advisable in all cases to assess whether there is an accompanying fracture or overt joint subluxation. Obtain lateral and posteroanterior radiographs before treatment to assess injury and after splinting to verify positioning.

Treatment

Treatment for mallet finger varies according to the type of injury, but splinting is almost always applied. In a recent meta-analysis of more than 1000 injuries, Geyman and colleagues found that conservative treatment was safe and effective for more than 80% of mallet finger injuries (LOE: B).[2] A Stack splint (see Figure 16.1*A*) is commonly used; however, a modified dorsal splint **(Figure 19.3)** is also sufficient.[3] Splinting is very effective if the joint is stable and if the patient follows instructions about its use for the entire treatment period. The Stack splint should be worn 24 hours a day for 6 weeks for a fracture and for 8 weeks for tendon failure. Patients can maintain the DIP joint in extension when the splint is removed for skin care by placing the finger on a flat surface and sliding the

ANATOMY OF THE FINGER JOINTS

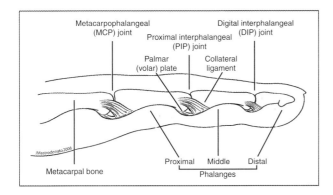

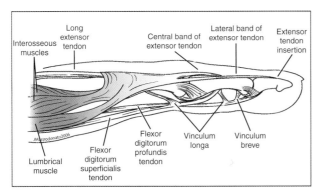

Figure 19.1 Anatomy of the finger joints. Each joint has a collateral ligament, a joint capsule, and a palmar plate.

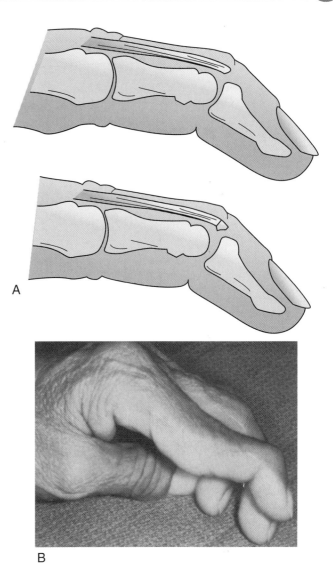

A

B

Figure 19.2 *A,* The two most common types of mallet finger. The tendon may be avulsed cleanly from the base of the distal phalanx (*top*), or the tendon may pull a small fragment of bone with it (*bottom*). Treatment for these two types is identical. *B,* Severe flexion deformity of the distal interphalangeal joint as a result of a mallet finger may lead to swan-neck deformity. This is particularly likely to occur in patients with lax proximal interphalangeal joints. (From DeLee JC, Drez D Jr, Miller MD [eds]: DeLee & Drez's Orthopedic Sports Medicine: Principles and Practice, 2nd ed. Philadelphia, WB Saunders, 2003.)

splint out from underneath the finger. If flexion of the DIP joint occurs during the treatment period, it has been recommended that the treatment should be started over (LOE: C).[4]

For late-presenting mallet fingers, success has been demonstrated with conservative treatment up to 3 months after the injury (LOE: B).[5,6] Patients who have residual lag should be observed for up to 6 months after splinting because considerable improvement can occur during this time period (LOE: B).[4] If residual functional deformity exists for more than 6 months despite appropriate treatment with immobilization, surgical intervention may be considered.

Return to play
Return to play is allowed immediately after injury if the athlete is comfortable and can safely return to participation with a splinted DIP joint. Otherwise, the athlete can return to play when there is pain-free, sport-specific range of motion.

Jersey finger
A jersey finger results from the loss of bony or ligamentous attachment of the flexor mechanism into the distal phalanx that results in a loss of flexion at the DIP joint. Although mechanistically this sounds like the opposite of a mallet finger, the management of these injuries is very different.

Mechanism of injury
Avulsion of the flexor digitorum profundus at its insertion on the distal phalanx results from the forced extension of the DIP joint while the patient is grasping. This is often referred to as "jersey finger" in football because it can occur when a player catches a finger on another player's jersey. The ring and middle fingers are most commonly affected.[7]

Risk factors
Any sport that would result in an actively flexing finger being forced into extension at the DIP joint (e.g., tackling sports, martial arts, and rock climbing) can be a risk.

Clinical features
Jersey finger should be suspected in all injuries to the DIP joint in players of most sports. The patient will have pain at the volar aspect of the DIP joint and the inability to fully flex the joint.[8]

Diagnosis
The physical examination again involves the evaluation of active and passive range of motion, a neurovascular examination, and an

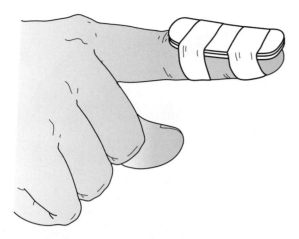

Figure 19.3 Splinting a mallet finger. The dorsal splint immobilizes only the distal interphalangeal joint, which allows for use of the finger. Hyperextension of this joint predisposes the patient to skin sloughing and should be avoided. The patient should be advised to not flex the joint during splint changes. (From Roberts JR: Clinical Procedures in Emergency Medicine, 4th ed. Philadelphia, WB Saunders, 2004.)

inspection of the nail. The flexor digitorum profundus is examined by holding the PIP joint straight and asking the patient to flex the DIP joint. However, an ability to slightly flex the DIP joint does not rule out avulsion of the tendon. The vinculum and synovial layers around the tendon usually remain attached to the palmar plate of the DIP joint, and, thus, some flexion force can be transferred to the distal phalanx without the tendon itself having a bony attachment.

Radiographs should be obtained in all potential jersey finger injuries and should consist of posteroanterior, lateral, and oblique views. These views may reveal an avulsed fragment of the distal phalanx, and they can help localize the amount of tendon retraction. Leddy[8] describes three types of profundus avulsions: (1) type 1, the tendon retracts into the palm and substantial blood supply is lost; (2) type 2, the profundus attachment to the distal phalanx retracts to the PIP joint, with some preservation of blood supply; and (3) type 3, a bony fragment avulses from the distal phalanx, with preserved blood supply.

Treatment

All jersey finger injuries require surgery. The greater the degree of tendon retraction, the more urgent surgery is required. Type 1 injuries should be repaired as soon as possible, whereas type 3 avulsions may be repaired up to 2 months after injury, although early surgery is advised (LOE: B).[9,10]

Return to play

Postoperative rehabilitation protocols vary to some degree, but they usually involve controlled motion in a custom-made splint for 6 weeks to allow for tendon healing (but to maintain tendon excursion). Return to contact sports and those sports that require the use of the affected hand may be anticipated at 4 to 6 months after surgery. Return to play is much earlier for those who participate in sports that do not place the hand at risk for further injury.

Skier's or gamekeeper's thumb

Skier's or gamekeeper's thumb is an ulnar collateral ligament rupture at the thumb MCP joint. The injury may involve the bone, the ligaments, or both, and it can result in a weak or a painful pincer grip. Although the injury was first associated with gamekeepers, who acquired the injury as a result of repeated abduction forces on

the ulnar collateral ligament, it is now almost exclusively seen after trauma.

Mechanism of injury

Injury is caused by the forced abduction and hyperextension of the thumb, and it is commonly seen in skiing and contact collision sports. The rupture of the ligament can be proximal or distal to the joint line, and it may include bony avulsion. The ligament may become trapped outside of the adductor aponeurosis, with more extensive angulation and distal disruption resulting in a Stener lesion **(Figure 19.4).** The same injury on the radial side of the joint results in a "reverse gamekeeper's thumb." The management of this injury differs because it does not produce a Stener lesion and only requires a thumb spica cast, without surgery.

Clinical features

Patients will complain of ulnar-sided pain and swelling at the thumb MCP joint. Physical findings that indicate Stener lesions include the presence of a mass over the ulnar side of the MCP

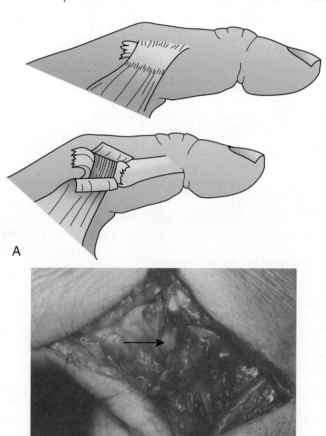

A

B

Figure 19.4 Stener's lesion seen in gamekeeper's (skier's) thumb. *A*, The distal end of the ulnar collateral ligament has been ruptured off the base of the proximal phalanx and is turned 180 degrees, facing proximally. The adductor tendon then becomes interposed between the torn end of the ligament and its site of insertion. *B*, At operation, the torn end of the avulsed ligament is seen end on, just proximal to the adductor aponeurosis (beneath the *arrow*). Healing cannot occur until the tendon is repositioned into the base of the proximal phalanx. (From DeLee JC, Drez D Jr, Miller MD [eds]: DeLee & Drez's Orthopedic Sports Medicine: Principles and Practice, 2nd ed. Philadelphia, WB Saunders, 2003.)

joint and a lack of an end point to ulnar stress at both full extension and flexion at 30 degrees (LOE: B).[11]

Diagnosis

Any patient with these complaints or physical findings coupled with an appropriate mechanism should have posteroanterior, lateral, and oblique plain films taken. Stress radiographs may be helpful for the identification of a Stener lesion if no fracture is seen on initial plain films, but they are not always recommended because displacement of a nondisplaced fracture can occur (LOE: C).[4]

To obtain stress films, flex the joint maximally, and apply radially directed stress to the injured thumb's MCP joint. The degree of joint opening should be compared with that of the opposite (and hopefully unaffected) side. The joint is considered stable if it opens less than 35 degrees, and it is considered unstable if it opens more than that.[7] Patients may have too much pain to tolerate this maneuver, and they may require a digital block before the stress views. Be sure to evaluate for neurologic status before injection.

Some investigators have suggested that the palpation of a mass proximal to the joint confirms a Stener lesion and that an absence of this finding determines that conservative therapy is appropriate (LOE: C).[4,12] However, it has been suggested that any instability (with or without a mass) requires surgical intervention as a result of the potential for chronic instability and the difficulties associated with delayed surgery on a Stener lesion (LOE: C).[4]

Treatment

If the ligament is not relocated and surgically repaired, the injury can result in chronic instability.[13] The initial treatment of any injury to this area should include analgesics as needed and immobilization with a thumb spica splint. Definitive treatment varies with the extent of injury. Injuries with either a nondisplaced fracture or a stable joint without fracture are treated with a thumb spica cast for 6 weeks. Those injuries that involve a displaced avulsion fracture or that have no fracture but that are unstable with a displaced ulnar collateral ligament outside of the adductor aponeurosis (Stener lesions) require surgical intervention.

Return to play

Return to play is allowed after the injured thumb is comfortable and protected in a splint. If thumb immobilization does not allow for participation, then return is delayed until healing has taken place and the joint is stable.

Proximal interphalangeal joint collateral ligament injuries

The PIP joint is one of the most commonly injured joints in sports, and its main stabilizers are the collateral ligaments and the volar plate **(Figure 19.5)**.

Mechanism of injury

Collateral ligament injuries of the PIP joint are quite common and result from axial loading and valgus or varus stress on the joint. Any sport that involves a moving ball or moving people in close contact with each other can potentially cause this very frequent injury. Fingers may be "jammed" while catching or deflecting a ball, or they may get caught in a player's facemask or jersey.

Risk factors

Risks for this type of injury include collision, contact, and ball sports.

Clinical features

Patients will complain of pain and swelling of the lateral or medial aspects of the affected joint. Not all patients may be able to relay

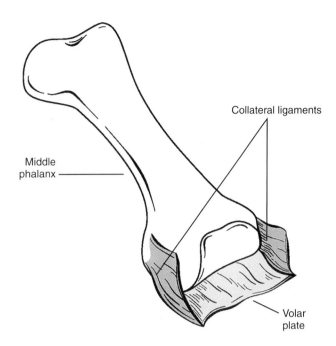

Figure 19.5 The proximal interphalangeal joint is stabilized by a three-dimensional ligament box complex that consists of the collateral ligaments and the thick volar (or palmar) plate.

the exact mechanism of injury to the joint as a result of the intensity of sport participation. Self or on-field reduction of a dislocation may have occurred and should be specifically queried.

Diagnosis

Evaluate the PIP joint as previously described in the Key Points section, and check for other ligamentous ruptures. The evaluation of active flexion and extension may reveal some joint instability. Isolate the PIP joint, and place a valgus and varus stress on the joint. Most injuries to the collateral ligaments are incomplete ruptures with minimal instability. In incomplete ruptures, physical exam findings may be limited to tenderness to palpation that is maximal along one or both of the collateral ligaments. If stress testing results in more than 20 degrees of deviation, the injury is a complete rupture. Obtain posteroanterior and lateral x-rays because they help evaluate for concomitant fracture, the percentage of the articular surface involved, and joint displacement, if present.

Treatment

Splinting or simple buddy taping of the PIP joint in full extension generally treats isolated incomplete collateral ligament injuries. Incomplete injuries with a mild amount of pain and swelling at the joint may be treated with buddy taping until symptoms subside. Injuries with increased pain and swelling with some mild laxity should be immobilized with a splint. The splint should be worn constantly for 7 to 10 days, after which buddy taping can be used and range-of-motion exercises started.[14] If moderate laxity is still present, splinting may be needed for up to 21 days.

Treatment for complete collateral ligament injuries at the PIP joint is the subject of some debate.[14,15] Indications for surgical repair include dynamic instability or an inability to achieve a reducible position. Initial management should be a full-finger splint followed by referral to an orthopedist or a hand surgeon within 5 days. Complete collateral ligament instability on the radial side of the index finger is more aggressively treated because

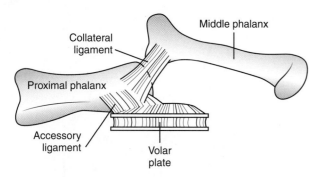

Figure 19.6 A dorsal proximal interphalangeal joint dislocation may involve rupture of the volar plate itself or avulsion of varying amounts of bone from the middle phalanx. If a large fragment is avulsed, the dislocation is unstable. The collateral ligaments can also tear in varying degrees and should be assessed with stress testing after reduction. (Redrawn from Roberts JR [ed]: Clinical Procedures in Emergency Medicine, 4th ed. Philadelphia, Saunders, 2004.)

this ligament is highly stressed with pinching, and instability can be painful. Collateral ligament injuries coupled with volar plate injuries will be discussed in the PIP dislocation section **(Figure 19.6).**

Return to play
Before returning an athlete with a collateral ligament injury to play, several variables must be considered. First, the sport must allow for a splint to be worn during play. If a splint is not allowed, then the athlete should not participate until buddy taping will provide adequate protection. Also, all athletes should be warned that significant swelling may persist at the injury site and that a faster transition to buddy taping and playing may worsen the cosmetic results. Individuals who need more function of their digits (e.g., musicians, archers, shooters) may opt for more conservative approaches with longer bracing and therapy before returning to play. For seasonal athletes, it is traditionally recommended to continue buddy taping throughout the remaining season to prevent recurrent injury.

Proximal interphalangeal joint dislocations
PIP joint dislocations are the most common ligamentous injury of the hand, and they can occur in athletes participating in any sport that involves a moving ball or players in contact with each other.[16]

Mechanism of injury
The most frequent mechanism is hyperextension of the PIP joint, which causes dorsal or lateral dislocation. Rarely, the PIP can dislocate in a volar direction when it is in a flexed position and struck by a rotational or hyperextension force. Dislocation produces a disruption of the volar plate from the base of the middle phalanx with or without bony avulsion, and it is frequently accompanied by a tear of the collateral ligaments **(Figure 19.7).**

Risk factors
Activities that expose the PIP joint to hyperextension, such as volleyball, football, and basketball, are risks for this type of injury.

Clinical features
The patient will present with pain and swelling in the PIP joint with or without obvious deformity. The finger and specifically the PIP joint may be in varying degrees of hyperextension, with maximal tenderness over the volar aspect of the PIP. As previously mentioned with PIP collateral ligament injuries, not all patients may recall the mechanism of injury, and they may have had a dislocation that was reduced on the field or court.

Diagnosis
Always be sure to evaluate the neurovascular status of the finger before giving any treatment. Posteroanterior and lateral radiographs will reveal a dorsally or volar displaced middle phalanx with some retraction, and they may show a degree of fracture in the articular surface. The majority of the examination occurs after the reduction of the dislocation.

Treatment
The reduction of a dorsal or lateral dislocation is accomplished through gentle traction on the distal phalanx with direct pressure over the dislocated base. The joint should be examined after reduction for the loss of active flexion and extension and for any collateral ligament instability. If there is significant pain during the evaluation, a digital block can be applied,

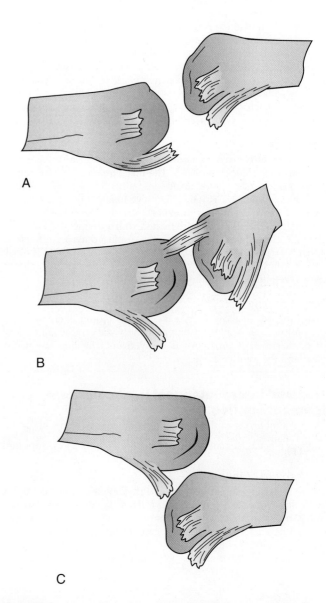

Figure 19.7 Dislocations in the hand are classified by the position of the distal skeletal unit in relation to its proximal counterpart. A, Dorsal proximal interphalangeal joint dislocation. B, Lateral proximal interphalangeal joint dislocation. C, Palmar proximal interphalangeal joint dislocation. (Redrawn from Browner: Skeletal Trauma: Basic Science, Management and Reconstruction, 3rd ed. Philadelphia, WB Saunders, 2003.)

but only after assessing neurovascular status. Rarely, operative reduction may be needed if closed reduction is unsuccessful.

Dorsal and lateral dislocations that do not involve a fracture and that maintain reduction should be placed in a dorsal splint, typically at 30 degrees of flexion. Immobilization is brief (only 3 to 5 days), with close x-ray follow-up[4] or follow-up until the immediate swelling has subsided (LOE: B). These injuries are typically stable, and most long-term difficulties stem from stiffness rather than instability (LOE: B).[14,17] After splinting, ROM exercises with buddy taping should begin and continue for 3 to 4 weeks.

PIP dislocations with a stable fracture involving less than 40% of the articular surface can be treated with an extension block splint, with the PIP in 30 to 60 degrees of flexion for 3 weeks.[4]

If the fracture involves more than 40% of the articular surface, is unstable, or cannot maintain reduction, the patient should be referred for surgical evaluation. Volar dislocations should be referred to a hand surgeon or an orthopedist who has experience with these injuries. If faced with a neurovascular compromise and delayed specialist evaluation, reduction may be attempted by placing the wrist in extension and the MCP and PIP joints in flexion, followed by a rotation and traction force.[4] If reduction is successful, the PIP joint should be placed immediately in full-extension immobilization.

Return to play

Return-to-play guidelines are similar to those described for collateral ligament injuries. Athletes with stable dislocations that are amenable to treatment with immediate range of motion may return to sports participation immediately after relocation (LOE: C).[17] Return to play is allowed as the athlete tolerates it, with immobilization or buddy taping to protect the injured volar plate and collateral ligaments while the healing of these tissues takes place. Ensure that the athlete is aware that earlier return to play may worsen a cosmetic outcome.

Extensor mechanism injuries (central slip rupture and boutonniere deformity)

The term *boutonniere deformity* refers to the rupture of the central slip of the extensor mechanism at its insertion into the base of the middle phalanx. In this deformity, the head of the phalanx may "buttonhole" up through the defect.

Mechanism of injury

Injury can occur with forced flexion of the middle phalanx when the athlete is attempting to extend the joint. Rarely, this injury can also include palmar dislocation of the PIP joint, during which the extensor mechanism attachment to the middle phalanx is ruptured **(Figure 19.8)**.

Risk factors

Collision and contact sports increase the likelihood of this type of injury.

Clinical features

Athletes will complain of pain and swelling over the PIP joint. The classic deformity of flexion at the PIP joint coupled with extension at the DIP joint is rarely seen immediately after injury.[18] Typically, the PIP is in 15 to 30 degrees of flexion, and patients will have decreased strength with extension.

Diagnosis

Start with the basic examination. The simplest clue that the central slip is injured is acute, maximal local tenderness over the dorsum of the PIP joint. In some complete avulsions, a defect in the tendon

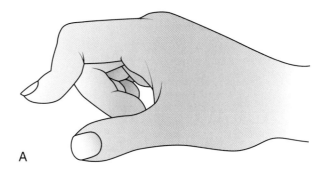

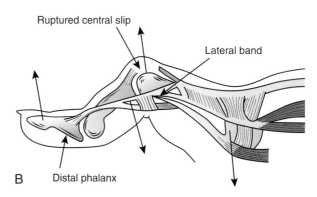

Figure 19.8 An established boutonniere deformity or flexion deformity of the proximal interphalangeal joint *(A)* is caused by a combination of pathologic forces *(B)*. A loss of active extension from the ruptured central slip as well as the deforming force of the lateral bands, which now pass volar to the axis of the proximal interphalangeal joint, cause the PIP joint to migrate dorsally. Additionally the pull of intrinsic finger/hand muscles through the lateral bands leads to hyperextension of the distal interphalangeal joint. (Redrawn from DeLee JC, Drez D Jr, Miller MD [eds]: DeLee & Drez's Orthopedic Sports Medicine: Principles and Practice, 2nd ed. Philadelphia, WB Saunders, 2003.)

can be palpated. When extensor mechanism injury is suspected, the degree of injury must be completely assessed. A digital block is often helpful if there is significant pain after neurovascular assessment. After the finger is anesthetized, full active extension of the PIP joint should be attempted. Limited active extension indicates that the fibers of the extensor tendon mechanism that attach to the proximal dorsal aspect of the middle phalanx (the central slip) have been partially or completely detached. Posteroanterior and lateral x-rays may show an avulsion injury to the dorsal base of the middle phalanx.

Treatment

Closed injuries can often be treated by nonoperative means if the extensor injury is an isolated finding. The PIP joint is splinted in full extension, whereas the DIP joint is allowed to flex actively using a safety-pin splint **(Figure 19.9)**. This motion at the DIP allows the lateral bands to resume their normal position.[18] A 6-week period of intermittent splinting usually follows the 6 weeks of continuous splinting. The presence of a small articular fracture does not usually require surgical intervention.[18] Leddy and colleagues[8] suggest that the only indication for the surgical repair of acute central slip injuries is a nonreducible PIP joint dislocation or a large, displaced intra-articular fracture.[8,18] Operative treatment for these injuries does not decrease the time that is necessary for splinting.

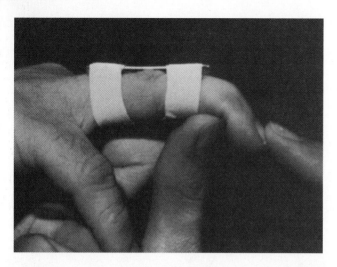

Figure 19.9 Appropriate treatment of a boutonniere deformity involves two elements: 1, continuous immobilization of the proximal interphalangeal joint in full extension for 6 weeks; and 2, passive stretching of the distal interphalangeal joint into flexion. (From DeLee JC, Drez D Jr, Miller MD [eds]: DeLee & Drez's Orthopedic Sports Medicine: Principles and Practice, 2nd ed. Philadelphia, WB Saunders, 2003.)

Return to play

Splinting for up to 12 weeks may be necessary, and rehabilitation can be complicated and prolonged. An experienced therapist or trainer who knows how best to advance rehabilitation while minimizing swelling is very important for a good result and for timely return to play. Athletes may return to play if their sport allows the wearing of the splint, although additional padding may be required for protection.[18]

Fight bite
Mechanism of injury

A clenched-fist injury that occurs when one person strikes another person's mouth is referred to as a "fight bite."

Risk factors

Collision and contact sports are risk factors for this injury.

Clinical features

This is a serious injury with an annual estimated incidence of 11.8 per 100,000 persons.[19] A tooth typically penetrates the dorsum of the hand over the third or fourth MCP joint.

Diagnosis

Although initial findings may reveal a small, seemingly innocuous puncture, the penetration often injures the soft tissue, the extensor tendon, and the sheath, and it may disrupt the MCP joint. In a study of 191 patients with clenched-fist injuries, 75% had an injury to tendon, bone, joint, or cartilage.[20] Radiographs are recommended to exclude foreign bodies, to identify fractures, and to assess for possible soft-tissue damage. *Staphylococcus* and *Streptococcus* bacteria are frequently cultured from these injuries. *Eikenella corrodens*, which is a less common pathogen, is also found in these injuries and will not respond to treatment with a first-generation cephalosporin.

Treatment

Recommended antibiotic prophylaxis includes amoxicillin–clavulanate potassium (Augmentin) or ampicillin–sulbactam (Unasyn).[21] The wound should be irrigated and covered.

Surgical intervention with irrigation and debridement vastly improves prognosis. Wound exploration and treatment in the operating room are necessary if deep structures, joints, or tendons have been penetrated (LOE: B).[22] If these structures are not involved, the wound can be allowed to heal by secondary intention and closely followed. The wound should be rechecked after 24 hours because infections can spread to deep structures and lead to osteomyelitis.[22]

Return to play

Athletes may return to play if they have been on antibiotics for 24 hours, if they have no constitutional symptoms (i.e., fever, chills, and malaise), and if they have adequate range of motion with minimal discomfort. In addition, because these wounds should not be closed with sutures, any draining fluids need to be adequately contained before return to play.

Flexor tenosynovitis
Mechanism of injury

A puncture wound over the flexor tendons may result this type of injury.

Risk factors

Rock climbing, mountaineering, and collision and contact sports are all risks for flexor tenosynovitis.

Clinical features

Flexor tenosynovitis is an infection within the flexor tendon sheath in the hand. When infected, the sheath fills with pus. This injury can rapidly progress to a deep palmar infection with necrosis and destruction of the flexor mechanism.

Diagnosis

Primary care physicians should have a high index of suspicion for flexor tenosynovitis. Kanavel described four cardinal signs of flexor sheath infection: (1) tenderness over the flexor tendon; (2) symmetric swelling of the digit; (3) pain with passive extension; and (4) flexed posturing of the digit.[23]

Treatment

These infections are an emergency. An immediate discussion of the case with an orthopedist or a hand surgeon is warranted so that treatment with incision and irrigation can be initiated.

Return to play

Because most of these injuries will be treated with surgical intervention, the return to play is dictated mostly by pain and the amount of surgical involvement. Athletes who have not received surgery must have been on antibiotics for at least 24 hours before return to play can be considered. Usually pain and decreased ROM will severely limit any attempts to return to athletic participation.

WRIST INJURIES

Soft-tissue injuries to the wrist may be the result of either acute trauma or overuse. Overuse syndromes such as de Quervain's tenosynovitis, extensor carpi ulnaris tendinitis, and sprains of the pisotriquetral ligament are associated with throwing and racquet sports.[24] Dislocation of the distal radioulnar joint, midcarpal instability, and triangular fibrocartilage complex (TFCC) tears can occur as a result of a traumatic fall or repetitive twisting motions, as seen in gymnasts. Carpal dislocation typically requires significant force, such as a collision while playing football or a fall from a height while cheerleading.

Carpal tunnel syndrome

Carpal tunnel syndrome is the most common overuse injury of the wrist, occurring in about 3% of all adults, and it is three times more common in women than in men.[25] It is common in gymnasts, throwing athletes, wheelchair athletes, and those that participate in sports that require gripping.[26]

Mechanism of injury

Overuse injury from repetitive wrist motion results in compression of the median nerve at the wrist.

Risk factors

Sports involving repetitive wrist motion, such as rowing and racquet sports, are risk factors for carpal tunnel syndrome. Alterations in fluid balance may predispose pregnant women to this condition.

Clinical features

The classic symptoms of carpal tunnel syndrome are pain, numbness, and tingling in the distribution of the median nerve **(Figure 19.10),** although numbness in all fingers may be a more common presentation. Symptoms are usually worse at night, and they can awaken patients from sleep. To relieve the symptoms, patients often "flick" their wrists as if shaking down a thermometer (flick sign).

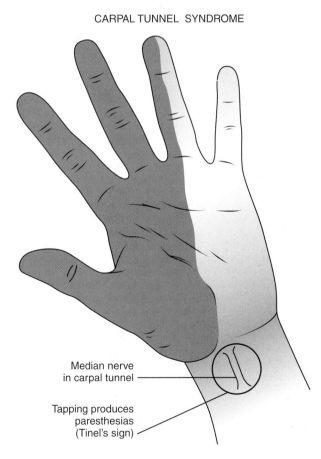

CARPAL TUNNEL SYNDROME

Median nerve in carpal tunnel

Tapping produces paresthesias (Tinel's sign)

Figure 19.10   Distribution of pain and/or paresthesias *(dark-shaded area)* when the median nerve is compressed by swelling in the wrist (carpal tunnel). (Redrawn from Ferri FF: Ferri's Clinical Advisor: Instant Diagnosis and Treatment, 8th ed. St. Louis, Mosby, 2006.)

Diagnosis

The most highly predictive findings of carpal tunnel syndrome are symptom location (i.e., a classic or probable pattern marked on hand symptom diagrams; positive predictive value, 0.59), hypalgesia (diminished sensitivity to pain along the palmar aspect of the index finger; positive predictive value, 0.55), and weak thumb abduction.[27] The principal clinical tests for carpal tunnel syndrome are Phalen's maneuver and Tinel's sign. Phalen's maneuver is positive when flexing the wrist to 90 degrees for 1 minute elicits symptoms in the median nerve distribution. Tinel's sign is positive when tapping over the carpal tunnel elicits symptoms in the distribution of the median nerve. Two-point discrimination, vibration, and monofilament testing may also elicit sensory findings in patients with carpal tunnel syndrome. Two-point discrimination can be tested with a special pair of calipers or a bent paper clip and alternating between touching the patient with one or both points. The minimal separation (in millimeters) at which the patient can distinguish these stimuli should be recorded.

Treatment

Initial conservative treatment consists of activity modification, the avoidance of aggravating activities, nonsteroidal anti-inflammatory drugs, and wrist splints (see Chapter 38 for a discussion of evidence supporting bracing for carpal tunnel syndrome) Stretch and massage techniques may also be effective; these involve the placement of the wrist at 90 degrees of extension with the application of steady pressure on the flexor retinaculum starting centrally and massaging laterally and medially. There is strong evidence that local corticosteroid injection and, to a lesser extent, oral corticosteroids give short-term relief to patients with this condition (LOE: A).[28,29] However, although steroid injection is the most effective nonsurgical treatment, it can result in possible complications of nerve injury, scarring, infection, allergic dermatitis, hypopigmentation, soft-tissue atrophy, and tendon rupture. Similarly, oral corticosteroids can cause adverse reactions such as nausea, anxiety, acne, menstrual irregularities, insomnia, headaches, and mood swings.[30] Although it is less beneficial than local corticosteroid injection, iontophoresis shows benefit without the risks of local or systemic steroids (LOE: B).[28] Carpal tunnel release surgery should be considered for patients with refractory or more severe cases and for patients who have progressive slowing of nerve conduction on electromyogram testing (LOE: B).[31,32]

Return to play

Return to play is allowed as the athlete tolerates it, with immobilization or sport-specific, pain-free range of motion. Return to work (with or without job modification) should be tried in most people. If symptoms worsen or reappear after return to work, reevaluation of both the patient and the work environment may be needed.

Ulnar nerve compression (Guyon canal syndrome)

Mechanism of injury

Repetitive wrist extension or palmar pressure causes compression of the relatively superficial distal ulnar nerve within the ulnar tunnel (Guyon canal) of the wrist.

Risk factors

Sports with excessive pressure on the palmar–ulnar side of the wrist, such as cycling, racquet sports, hockey goalies, and weight lifting, may be risk factors for this type of injury.

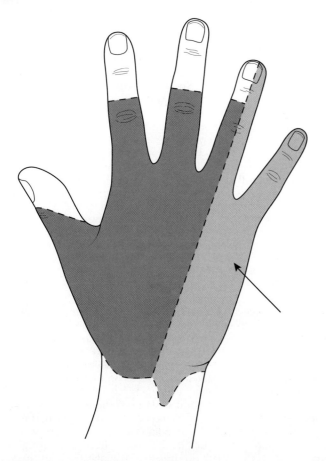

Figure 19.11 Patients with injury or pathology of the ulnar nerve complain of decreased sensation in the ulnar nerve distribution *(light gray area, arrow)*. (Redrawn from Frontera WR, Silver JK: Essentials of Physical Medicine and Rehabilitation, 1st ed. Philadelphia, Hanley and Belfus, 2002.)

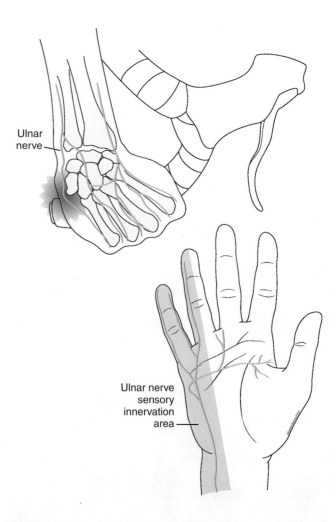

Figure 19.12 Pressure proximal to the bifurcation of the ulnar nerve will result in both sensory and motor findings.

Clinical features

Entrapment neuropathy of the ulnar nerve in the Guyon canal is much less common than carpal tunnel syndrome, but it is particularly apt to occur in cyclists, and it has been also called "handlebar palsy."[33] The cause in this case is direct pressure, and the syndrome is characterized by paresthesia in the ulnar nerve distribution **(Figure 19.11)**. Compression may also occur as a result of ganglia, lipomas, anatomic abnormalities, carpal fractures, local inflammation, or ulnar arterial thrombosis.[34]

Diagnosis

Symptoms caused by compression vary with the location of the lesion. Pressure proximal to the bifurcation of the ulnar nerve will result in both sensory and motor findings **(Figure 19.12)**. Sensation is decreased in the ring and little fingers, and intrinsic muscle weakness or atrophy of the hypothenar eminence may be noted. Tinel's test may cause paresthesias into the little and ring fingers. Conversely, a lesion distal to the bifurcation of the nerve will result in findings that are limited to either motor or sensory changes, depending on whether the deep motor branch or the superficial sensory branch is most affected. Electromyograms are useful for confirming the diagnosis, and they will demonstrate denervation potentials in the interosseous muscles. Nerve conduction velocity studies will reveal prolongation of the motor latency to the first dorsal interosseous. A difference of more than 1 msec is considered significant. These changes aid in localizing the lesion to the Guyon canal as opposed to a more proximal area of compression.

Treatment

Conservative treatment consists of splinting, anti-inflammatory medication, and modification of activity. Off-the-shelf splints can be used, and it is recommended that they be worn both at night and as tolerated during the day. The splint may be removed as needed for essential activity. The local injection of a corticosteroid into the carpal tunnel or the Guyon canal may be effective. Cases refractory to conservative management should be referred to a hand surgeon. Padded gloves and handlebar grips as well as changing hand position while riding may help prevent the condition from occurring.[35]

Return to play

Most athletes with ulnar nerve entrapment can continue to participate in sport. The treatments described previously can help with symptoms control.

Triangular fibrocartilage complex injuries and distal radioulnar joint stability
Mechanism of injury

Injuries to the TFCC **(Figure 19.13)** occur with repetitive ulnar loading (e.g., bench pressing and racquet sports) or acute

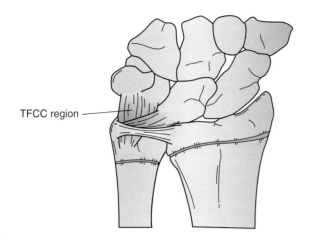

Figure 19.13 The triangular fibrocartilage complex (TFCC) consists of the triangular fibrocartilage and the ulnocarpal ligaments. It provides the articular surface for the carpus and a flexible mechanism for stable rotational movements of the radius and ulna, it suspends the ulnar carpus from the radius, and it cushions the forces that are transmitted through the ulnocarpal axis. (Redrawn from Green: Skeletal Trauma in Children, 3rd ed. Saunders, 2003.)

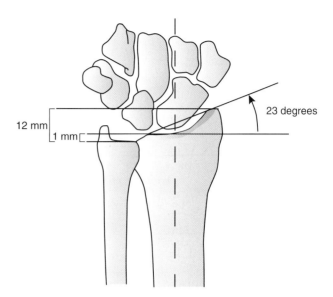

Figure 19.14 Measurements of radiographic parameters of the distal radius and ulna. Radial inclination, which is measured off the perpendicular to the radial shaft, averages 23 degrees. Radial length is the difference in length between the ulnar head and the tip of the radial styloid (average, 12 mm). Ulnar variance depicts the difference in length between the ulnar head and the ulnar aspect of the distal radius (shown as 1 mm ulnar negative). (Redrawn from Browner BD, Jupiter JD, Levine AM, et al: Skeletal Trauma: Basic Science, Management and Reconstruction, 3rd ed. Philadelphia, WB Saunders, 2003.)

traumatic axial load with rotational stress (e.g., a fall on an out-stretched hand). TFCC injuries are commonly seen in athletes who participate in sports such as gymnastics, hockey, racquet sports, boxing, and pole vaulting.[36]

Risk factors

Collision or contact sports, gymnastics, rodeo, parachuting, mountain climbing, and skiing are risk factors for TFCC injuries. TFCC injuries are also associated with positive ulnar variance **(Figure 19.14).**

Clinical features

Patients with TFCC injuries complain of ulnar-sided wrist pain with associated clicking, which is exacerbated by forearm rotation. They may describe a past wrist injury that has since healed except for residual pain and clicking in the TFCC region.

Diagnosis

Examination will reveal point tenderness palmar to the extensor carpi ulnaris tendon and just distal to the ulna. A TFCC compression test, in which the wrist is axially loaded and then deviated to the ulnar side, is positive if it reproduces the ulnar-sided pain with clicking. It is important to differentiate between a TFCC injury and a distal radioulnar joint injury. Injury to the TFCC is suspected when tenderness and crepitus are palpated between the ulna and the triquetrum. Pain that is relieved by the manual stabilization of the distal radioulnar joint may be an indicator of distal radio-ulnar joint instability. It is important to assess the stability of the distal radioulnar joint, and this can be done using the piano key and the shuck tests. To perform the piano key test, the patient's hand is pronated, and the examiner presses down on the distal ulna as if pressing on a piano key. If little resistance occurs as the ulna moves volarly, the test is positive. For the shuck test, the examiner holds the radius with one hand and the ulna with the other and moves the distal radius dorsally against the head of the ulna **(Figure 19.15).** Laxity should be compared with that of the other wrist.

Plain film radiography is used only to evaluate ulnar variance. Positive ulnar variance is when the distal ulna extends farther than the distal plateau of the radius. Negative ulnar variance is when the distal ulna is shorter than the distal radius (see Figure 19.14 for an example of positive ulnar variance). This variance affects the axial load that is borne by the ulna. A normal load distribution is approximately 82% across the radius and 18% across the ulna. A negative ulnar variance of 2.5 mm reduces the axial force across the ulna to 4%, whereas a positive ulnar variance of 2.5 mm increases the ulnar load to 42%.[37] Also, the thickness of the TFCC varies inversely with positive ulnar variance. In positive ulnar variance, the TFCC is thinner and has more forces directed through it, thus making it more susceptible to injury.[38]

TFCC injuries traditionally have been diagnosed with wrist arthrography, but high-resolution magnetic resonance imaging and wrist arthroscopy are increasingly used for this purpose.

Treatment

Initial treatment for the acute TFCC injury without distal radial joint instability is immobilization for 4 to 6 weeks in slight flexion and ulnar deviation. Injection of the ulnar carpal space with a corticosteroid and a local anesthetic may be helpful for both diagnosis and treatment (see Chapter 48).

If a stable wrist remains symptomatic and pain persists despite immobilization as described previously, then arthroscopy is indicated. Surgical options for TFCC tears include the debridement of localized defects, the decompression of the ulnar carpal space, and the arthroscopic repair of the TFCC.[39] For the active patient with a long-standing tear and positive ulnar variance, ulnar shortening should be incorporated into the operative procedure.

Return to play

Athletes typically return to play 2 to 3 weeks after splinting or 6 to 12 weeks after arthroscopic treatment. Open TFCC procedures may cause the athlete to miss up to 6 months of athletic participation.[40]

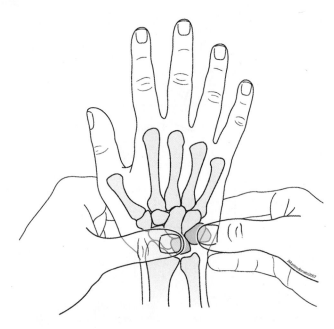

Figure 19.15 Reagan shuck test.

Dorsal ganglion cysts

Ganglions are benign tumor masses filled with viscous fluid that originate from the joint capsule or tendon sheath. Ganglion cysts may arise in any location in the wrist, but they are usually adjacent to joints or tendons. Of these, dorsal wrist ganglions account for 60% to 70% of these cysts, and they most commonly arise from the dorsal scapholunate ligament. The volar wrist ganglion arises from the distal aspect of the radius and accounts for about 20% to 25% of ganglia; flexor tendon sheath ganglia make up the remaining 10% to 15%. These cystic structures are found near or are attached to tendon sheaths and joint capsules. The cyst is filled with soft, gelatinous, sticky, mucoid fluid.

Mechanism of injury

Ganglions are probably induced by trauma, which allows fluid to pass through a weakness in the joint capsule or tendon sheath and to produce a cyst. There is an individual predisposition to ganglia, but repetitive trauma or overuse may increase development.

Risk factors

Repetitive microtrauma to the wrist and individual predisposition may increase the risk of this condition.

Clinical features

Localized tenderness and maximum aggravation of pain occur during flexion and result in motion limitations and a weak grip. Occult dorsal wrist ganglia can produce chronic wrist pain, which may be constant or associated only with activity. A history of trauma is often missing in these patients.

Diagnosis

Ganglions typically present as soft-tissue masses adjacent to ligaments or tendons. Clinically, they are often 1 cm to 2 cm in size, slightly mobile, and translucent. For patients who have occult ganglia, the initial examination should include evaluation for carpal or scapholunate instability.

Treatment

Most patients require reassurance that the cyst is not serious. For patients with limitations in their function, initial treatment consists of activity modification with immobilization, nonsteroidal anti-inflammatory drugs, and aspiration, with or without injection. Traditional methods of traumatic rupture of the cyst with a direct blow (i.e., "bible bump") have lost favor. Treatment for persistent or limiting cysts includes one corticosteroid injection followed by immobilization in a cock-up wrist splint for 7 to 10 days. If this conservative therapy fails, operative treatment may be initiated.

Return to play

Dorsal ganglion cysts are not a contraindication to sports participation or vocational activities. However, pain from the cysts might make these activities uncomfortable. It is reasonable to restrict activity for a short period of time (no more than 2 to 3 weeks) to allow inflammation from ruptured or growing cysts to subside.

de Quervain's tenosynovitis

Inflammation or relative narrowing of the extensor pollicis brevis and abductor pollicis longus tendons, which make up the first dorsal compartment, is known as *de Quervain's tenosynovitis* **(Figure 19.16)**. This is the most common tendinopathy of the wrist in athletes.

Mechanism of injury

Repetitive ulnar deviation is most commonly implicated as the cause of this syndrome.[38]

Risk factors

Activities involving the repetitive use of the thumb or forceful grasping coupled with ulnar deviation predispose athletes to this condition. Predisposing sports include golf, fly fishing, and certain racquet sports, such as squash and racquetball. de Quervain's tenosynovitis is also classically described in postpartum women and breastfeeding mothers.

Clinical features

Patients frequently complain of pain over the thumb side of the wrist as the main symptom. The pain may appear either gradually or suddenly. It is felt in the wrist, and it can travel up the forearm. The pain is usually worse with the use of the hand and thumb, especially during forcefully grasping or twisting the wrist.

Diagnosis

On examination, localized tenderness is present over the first dorsal compartment, and performing the Finkelstein test reproduces symptoms. The Finkelstein test is a diagnostic maneuver in which the patient folds the thumb under the fingers and the examiner ulnarly deviates the wrist **(Figure 19.17)**. The test is positive if the ulnar deviation causes radial-sided pain. The Finkelstein test can cause discomfort even in the normal wrist. Hence, in patients with unilateral symptoms, the pain caused by the Finkelstein test should be significantly more severe on the affected side. In individuals with bilateral symptoms, the examiner must determine if the pain is greater than would be expected during a normal examination.[41]

Treatment

Initial treatment classically consists of thumb spica splinting, nonsteroidal anti-inflammatory drugs, and physical therapy for 2 to 4 weeks, with a corticosteroid injection into the first dorsal compartment being considered after 10 to 14 days if there has been no significant improvement. However, results of a recent meta-analysis showed that there was an 83% cure rate with injection alone.[42] Given the immediacy of relief with injection,

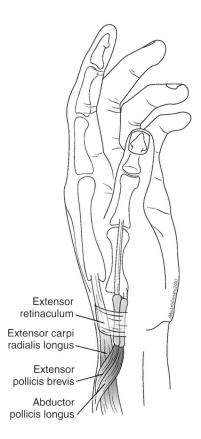

Figure 19.16 de Quervain's tenosynovitis involves relative narrowing of the tendons that make up the first dorsal compartment: the extensor pollicis brevis and the abductor pollicis longus. (From DeLee JC, Drez D Jr, Miller MD [eds]: DeLee & Drez's Orthopedic Sports Medicine: Principles and Practice, 2nd ed. Philadelphia, WB Saunders, 2003.)

Labels on figure:
Extensor retinaculum
Extensor carpi radialis longus
Extensor pollicis brevis
Abductor pollicis longus

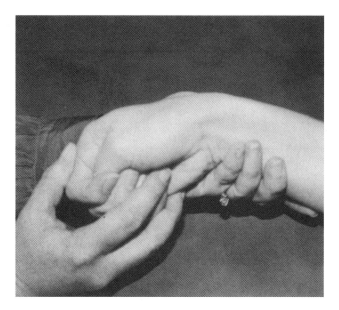

Figure 19.17   The Finkelstein test. (From DeLee JC, Drez D Jr, Miller MD [eds]: DeLee & Drez's Orthopedic Sports Medicine: Principles and Practice, 2nd ed. Philadelphia, WB Saunders, 2003.)

the high cure rate, and the very low risk of complications, many musculoskeletal physicians use steroid injection as their first-line treatment for this very common syndrome. Many providers place the affected wrist in a removable splint after the injection to immobilize the thumb and to prevent further irritation and inflammation, but a recent clinical trial showed no additional benefit from post-injection splinting.[42a]

Repeat injection may be required for those with recalcitrant symptoms, especially those with chronic tenosynovitis, a condition in which inflammation has resulted in thickening and stenosis of the fibro-osseous tunnel. Some surgeons advocate repeated steroid injections, noting that the results of surgical release can be unpredictable.[43] However, surgical decompression may be required for chronic symptoms that do not respond to conservative treatment.

Return to play

Sport-specific, pain-free range of motion, adequate strength, and the need for protective bracing determine an athlete's return to sport. Most cases of de Quervain's tenosynovitis should not result in long-term disability or restricted participation.

Intersection syndrome
Mechanism of injury

The syndrome is caused by the overuse of the radial wrist extensors.

Risk factors

Intersection syndrome occurs in athletes who are exposed to repetitive wrist extension, such as rowers, players of racquet sports, weight lifters, and canoeists.[44]

Clinical features

Intersection syndrome is similar to de Quervain's tenosynovitis, and it involves the junction at which the first dorsal compartment (the abductor pollicis longus and the extensor pollicis brevis tendons) crosses under the second compartment (the extensor carpi radialis longus and brevis tendons).

Diagnosis

Athletes complain of dorsoradial pain and tenderness proximal to the wrist. They may have swelling or crepitus that is 4 to 6 cm proximal to the Lister tubercle.[34] Crepitation or squeaking can be heard with passive or active motion, which has led to the term "squeaker's wrist."

Treatment

Initial treatment consists of rest, splinting, anti-inflammatory medication, and corticosteroid injection; conservative treatment is successful 95% of the time (LOE: C).[34,45] For rare cases that do not respond to conservative treatment, surgical management includes release of the second dorsal compartment, release of the fascia of the abductor pollicis longus and the extensor pollicis brevis muscles, and debridement of the bursa.[46]

Return to play

A graduated return to sports participation is recommended after symptoms have been relieved.

Extensor carpi ulnaris tendinopathy

The sixth dorsal compartment, which houses the extensor carpi ulnaris (ECU) tendon, is the second most common site of tenosynovitis after de Quervain's tenosynovitis.[47]

Mechanism of injury

Overuse injury from repetitive ulnar deviation seems to cause this condition.

Risk factors

ECU tendinopathy is common in players of racquet sports, baseball, golf, and rowing as a result of the repetitive ulnar deviation involved. ECU tendinitis may also be the result of underlying wrist pathology, such as a TFCC injury.[48]

Clinical features

Patients who have ECU tenosynovitis have pain and tenderness over the tendon, especially with ulnar deviation. Athletes may also complain of pain and swelling distal to the ulnar head that is worsened by resisted wrist extension.

Diagnosis

The ECU becomes prominent when the wrist is supinated and ulnar deviated. Recurrent painful subluxation can be detected by a palpable snap when the forearm is actively supinated with the wrist flexed and ulnarly deviated. When stenosing tenosynovitis is present, the tendon is tender to palpation and swollen. Occasionally, crepitus may be noted within the swollen ECU subsheath. Symptoms are reproduced with resistance to dorsiflexion and ulnar deviation.

Treatment

Treatment consists of avoiding aggravating activities, using a wrist splint, taking nonsteroidal anti-inflammatory drugs, and receiving physical therapy for 2 to 4 weeks. A one-time local corticosteroid injection after 10 to 14 days of symptoms should be considered. If an injection is given, a splint is recommended as well as complete rest from sports participation for 7 to 10 days following the injection.[49] Athletes should also modify sports technique by limiting excessive ulnar–radial deviation and flexion of the wrist.

Return to play

Athletes may return to competition when they have sport-specific, pain-free ROM.

Extensor carpi ulnaris tendon subluxation
Mechanism of injury

ECU tendon subluxation is caused by acute forceful supination, palmar flexion, and ulnar deviation of the wrist.

Risk factors

This injury can be seen in tennis players who hit a low forehand and in baseball players at the end of a swing. It has also been reported in golfers, weight lifters, and rodeo riders.[46]

Clinical features

ECU tendon subluxation has symptoms and causes that are similar to those of tenosynovitis, and it occurs when disruption of the compartment sheath allows the ECU tendon to subluxate. This condition should be suspected when the patient has clicking on the ulnar side of the forearm with pronation and supination. A painful snap may be elicited as subluxation of the ECU occurs with supination and ulnar deviation of the wrist.

Treatment

Patients with acute ECU subluxation may be treated with long-arm casting with the wrist in full pronation and slight dorsiflexion. However, some argue that surgical correction offers a more predictable outcome.[50]

Return to play

For those athletes in casts, return to play is usually about 6 weeks. With chronic ECU subluxation, surgical reconstruction of the fibrous rim shows excellent results, with a return to sports participation in 3 months.[46]

Scaphoid impingement syndrome
Mechanism of injury

Scaphoid impingement syndrome occurs as a result of repetitive, forced hyperextension of the wrist that causes the proximal scaphoid and the radius to abut. This leads to damage of the proximal capsule, the ligament, or the articular surface.[51]

Risk factors

Repetitive wrist dorsiflexion sports such as weight lifting and gymnastics are risk factors for this condition.

Clinical features

Patients with this condition experience dorsal wrist pain that is increased with dorsiflexion.

Diagnosis

Physical examination reveals tenderness dorsally between the proximal scaphoid and the radius, with the wrist slightly flexed and in ulnar deviation. In chronic cases, lateral radiographs can show a hypertrophic ridge on the scaphoid rim.

Treatment

Initial management includes activity modification, ice, and splinting to limit wrist dorsiflexion. Lion-paw and tiger-paw braces are very helpful for gymnasts. If initial management is unsuccessful, steroid injection along the dorsal rim of the scaphoid may be helpful. Recalcitrant cases may require surgery.

Return to play

Athletes may return to competition when they have sport-specific, pain-free range of motion. Bracing with future gymnastic practice and competition is recommended to avoid recurrent symptoms.

Dorsal impingement syndrome
Mechanism of injury

Dorsal impingement syndrome occurs as a result of repetitive loading of the wrist in maximum extension. The shear forces created by this action may lead to a localized synovitis or even osteophytes on the dorsum of the scaphoid, the lunate, or the capitate.[52]

Risk factors

This condition occurs most frequently in gymnasts, especially during floor exercises and horse routines.

Clinical features

Athletes commonly complain of pain and tenderness on the mid dorsum of the wrist, at the projection of the lunocapitate joint.

Diagnosis

Lateral radiographs may show bony hypertrophy of the dorsal rim of the scaphoid or the dorsal border of the lunate as a result of impingement with the capitate during hyperextension. The clinician must be careful not to misdiagnose radial growth plate injury as dorsal impingement syndrome in skeletally immature gymnasts.

Treatment

A splint that restricts wrist dorsiflexion (e.g., a lion- or tiger-paw brace) and wrist-flexion–strengthening exercises are first-line treatments. Often, 2 to 3 weeks of rest with or without immobilization may be required to decrease daily symptoms. A steroid injection into the hypertrophied synovium has also been found helpful for recalcitrant daily pain. After pain resolves, wrist flexor strengthening is begun for 3 to 4 weeks. After wrist strengthening is well established, a lion-paw brace can be used as athletes slowly return to play. In refractory cases, wrist arthroscopy may be needed.

Return to play

Athletes can return to play when they have sport-specific, pain-free range of motion. These athletes should be counseled, however, that return to the same activity (especially without protective bracing) will likely result in a recurrence of symptoms.

Scapholunate dissociation
Mechanism of injury

Scapholunate dissociation occurs as the ligamentous support of the proximal pole of the scaphoid is disrupted and the scaphoid rotates into palmar flexion. It typically occurs after a fall onto the hand while the wrist is extended and ulnar deviated.

Risk factors

Risk factors for scapholunate dissociation include contact and collision sports as well as motor vehicle accidents.

Clinical features

The patient usually has a history of a fall, a motor vehicle accident, or another trauma along with pain, swelling, and decreased motion. The greatest pain is typically over the dorsal scapholunate area, and this is accentuated with dorsiflexion. Swelling is usually minimal, but pressure applied over the scaphoid tuberosity will elicit further pain. In the absence of an associated scaphoid fracture, these injuries can be missed unless there is a high index of suspicion and unless radiographs (especially of the lateral wrist) are carefully interpreted.

Diagnosis

The scaphoid shift test described by Watson and colleagues[53] is a provocative maneuver to elicit scapholunate instability. With this maneuver, the wrist is brought from ulnar to radial deviation while the scaphoid tuberosity is stabilized with the examiner's thumb. A click with associated pain is considered a positive test **(Figure 19.18)**. The associated click is the result of subluxation of the proximal pole of the scaphoid over the dorsal rim of the radius.

Further evaluation of scapholunate instability includes routine posteroanterior and lateral x-rays of the wrist. Scapholunate instability is associated with a widening of the scapholunate interval of more than 3 mm on the anteroposterior view, which is also known as the Terry Thomas or David Letterman sign. A cortical ring sign may also be noted in which the scaphoid tuberosity is seen in profile as a result of the flexed position of the scaphoid **(Figure 19.19)**. Normally, the proximal carpal row will form a smooth arc on the neutral anteroposterior view. A step off in the contour of the scapholunate interval may indicate an instability pattern, or it may be a normal variant.[54] To evaluate dynamic instability, obtain an anteroposterior clenched-fist view to axially load the wrist while evaluating for a widened scapholunate gap. Correct interpretation of the lateral wrist radiograph is essential to properly diagnose scapholunate pathology. On the lateral view, the normal scapholunate angle is between 30 and 60 degrees.

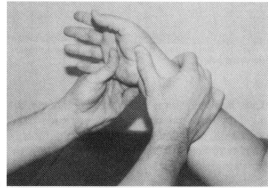

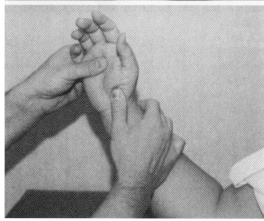

Figure 19.18 The Watson test for scapholunate instability. *A*, The scaphoid is stabilized with the thumb over the volar pole. *B*, When the hand is brought from ulnar to radial deviation, pain results. (From DeLee JC, Drez D Jr, Miller MD [eds]: DeLee & Drez's Orthopedic Sports Medicine: Principles and Practice, 2nd ed. Philadelphia, WB Saunders, 2003.)

A scapholunate angle of more than 70 degrees is consistent with scapholunate dissociation **(Figure 19.20)**. In patients with scapholunate instability, the scaphoid is flexed while the lunate and the triquetrum will lie extended in a dorsal intercalary segment instability pattern[55] **(Figure 19.21)**.

Treatment

If the patient has extreme tenderness over the scapholunate joint with no radiographic evidence of separation or carpal malalignment, the injury should be treated as a severe ligament sprain with a splint or a short-arm cast for 6 weeks. However, if evidence of scapholunate dissociation exists or if there are any other concerns, the patient should be referred to a hand surgeon.

With prompt diagnosis and appropriate referral, the success rate for treating scapholunate dissociation is high. Unfortunately, most injuries are initially unrecognized or misdiagnosed. Reduction is often possible as long as 3 months after injury, but the delay results in a much poorer long-term prognosis.[56]

Return to play

The athlete can return to play when he or she has sport-specific, pain-free ROM. This typically occurs in 3 months for those who are conservatively managed. A high-level athlete whose sport cannot tolerate wrist immobilization may miss the remainder of the season.

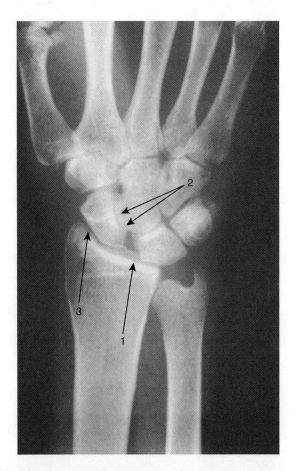

Figure 19.19 Radiographic findings of scapholunate dissociation: 1, widening of the scapholunate interval; 2, shortened appearance of the scaphoid; and 3, the "ring sign" of the cortical projection of the distal pole. (From DeLee JC, Drez D Jr, Miller MD [eds]: DeLee & Drez's Orthopedic Sports Medicine: Principles and Practice, 2nd ed. Philadelphia, WB Saunders, 2003.)

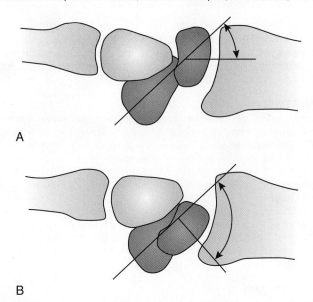

Figure 19.20 The normal scapholunate angle is 30 to 60 degrees (A). A scapholunate angle of more than 70 degrees (B) suggests scapholunate dissociation. (From DeLee JC, Drez D Jr, Miller MD [eds]: DeLee & Drez's Orthopedic Sports Medicine: Principles and Practice, 2nd ed. Philadelphia, WB Saunders, 2003.)

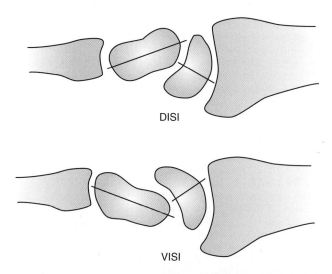

Figure 19.21 Patterns of carpal instability. Dorsal intercalated segmental instability (DISI) is present when the lunate lies volar to the capitate but is flexed dorsally. Volar intercalated segmental instability (VISI) is present if the lunate lies dorsal to the capitate and is flexed volarly. (Redrawn from DeLee JC, Drez D Jr, Miller MD [eds]: DeLee & Drez's Orthopedic Sports Medicine: Principles and Practice, 2nd ed. Philadelphia, WB Saunders, 2003.)

CONCLUSION

In conclusion, injuries of the hand and wrist are common. Although the diagnosis may be challenging, a thorough and thoughtful assessment may reveal the correct diagnosis. Striving to achieve the proper diagnosis will lead to the appropriate rehabilitation program, which will decrease morbidity and speed return to play.

REFERENCES

1. Bach AW: Finger joint injuries in active patient. Phys Sportsmed 1999;27(3):89-104.
2. Geyman JP, Fink K, Sullivan SD: Conservative versus surgical treatment of mallet finger: a pooled quantitative literature evaluation. J Am Board Fam Pract 1998;11(5):382-390.
3. Hart RG, Kleinert HE, Lyons K: The Kleinert modified dorsal finger splint for mallet finger fracture. Am J Emerg Med 2005;23(2):145-148.
4. Lairmore JR, Engberger WD: Serious, often subtle, finger injuries: avoiding diagnosis and treatment pitfalls. Phys Sportsmed 1998;26(6):57-69.
5. McFarlane RM, Hampole MK: Treatment of extensor tendon injuries of the hand. Can J Surg 1973;16:366-375.
6. Stern PJ, Kastrup JJ: Complications and prognosis of treatment of mallet finger. J Hand Surg [Am] 1988;13:329-334.
7. Manske PR, Lesker PA: Avulsion of the ring finger flexor digitorum profundus tendon: an experimental study. Hand 1978;10:52-55.
8. Leddy JP, Parker JW: Avulsions of the flexor digitorum profundus. Hand Clin 1985;1:77-83.
9. St. Pierre P: Hand and wrist injuries. In Lillegard WA, Butcher JD, Rucker KS (eds): Handbook of Sports Medicine: A Symptom-Oriented Approach, 2nd ed. Boston, Butterworth-Heinemann, 1999, pp 181-194.
10. Rettig AC, Coyle MP, Hunt TR: Hand and wrist problems in the athlete. Am Orthop Soc Sports Med Instr Course 108: AOSSM 28th Annual Meeting, Orlando, FL 2002.
11. Melone CP, Beldner S, Basuk RK: Thumb collateral ligament injuries: an anatomic basis for treatment. Hand Clin 2000;16:345-357.
12. Abrahamsson SO, Sollerman C, Lundborg G, et al: Diagnosis of displaced ulnar collateral ligament of the metacarpophalangeal joint of the thumb. J Hand Surg [Am] 1990;15(3):457-460.
13. Stener B: Displacement of the ruptured ulnar collateral ligament of the MCP joint of the thumb. J Bone Joint Surg Br 1962;44:869-879.
14. Arora R, Lutz M, Fritz D, et al: Dorsolateral dislocation of the proximal interphalangeal joint: close reduction and early active motion or static splinting; a retrospective study. Arch Orthop Trauma Surg 2004;124(7):486-488. Epub 2004 June 3.

15. McCue FC, Honner R, Johnson ME, et al: Athletic injuries of the proximal interphalangeal joint requiring surgical treatment. J Bone Surg 1970;52A:937-956.
16. Green DP (ed): Operative Hand Surgery, 3rd ed. New York, Churchill Livingstone, 1993.
17. Palmer RE: Joint injuries of the hand in athletes. Clin Sports Med 1998;17(3):513-531.
18. Aronowitz ER, Leddy JP: Closed tendon injuries of the hand and wrist in athletes. Clin Sports Med 1998;17(3):449-467.
19. Perron AD, Miller MD, Brady WJ: Orthopedic pitfalls in the ED: fight bite. Am J Emerg Med 2002;20:114-117.
20. Patzakis MJ, Wilkins J, Bassett RL: Surgical findings in clenched-fist injuries. Clin Orthop 1987;220:237-240.
21. Sanford JP: Guide to Antimicrobial Therapy, 35th ed. Antimicrobial Therapy Inc. Hyde Park, VT, 2005, p 35.
22. Harrison BP, Hilliard MW: Emergency department evaluation and treatment of hand injuries. Emerg Med Clin North Am 1999;17:793-822.
23. Kanavel AB: Infections of the Hand. A Guide to the Surgical Treatment of Acute and Chronic Suppurative Processes in the Fingers, Hand, and Forearm, 7th ed. Philadelphia, Lea & Febiger, 1939.
24. Mirabello SC, Loeb PE, Andrews JR: The wrist: field evaluation and treatment. Clin Sports Med 1992;11:1-25.
25. Atroshi I, Gummesson C, Johnsson R, et al: Prevalence of carpal tunnel syndrome in a general population. JAMA 1999;282:153-158.
26. Izzi J, Dennison D, Noerdlinger M, et al: Nerve injuries of the elbow, wrist, and hand in athletes. Clin Sports Med 2001;20(1):203-217.
27. Katz JN, Larsen MG, Sabra A, et al: The carpal tunnel syndrome: diagnostic utility of the history and physical examination findings. Ann Intern Med 1990;112(5):321-327.
28. Gokuglu F, Findikoglu G, Yorgancioglu ZR, et al: Evaluation of iontophoresis and local corticosteroid injection in the treatment of carpal tunnel syndrome. Am J Phys Med Rehabil 2005;84(2):92-96.
29. Dammers JW, Veering MM, Vermeulen M: Injection with methylprednisolone proximal to the carpal tunnel: a randomized double blind trial. BMJ 1999;319(7214):884-886.
30. Goodyear-Smith F: What can family physicians offer patients with carpal tunnel syndrome other than surgery? A systematic review of nonsurgical management. Ann Fam Med 2004;2(3):267-273.
31. Gerritsen AA, Uitdehaag BM, van Geldere D, et al: Systemic review of randomized clinical trials of surgical treatment for carpal tunnel syndrome. Br J Surg 2001;88(10):1285-1295.
32. Scholten RJ, Gerritsen AA, Uitdehaag BM: Surgical treatment options for carpal tunnel syndrome. Cochrane Database Syst Rev 2004;(4):CD003905.
33. Mellion MB (ed): Bicycling. Team Physicians Handbook, 3rd ed. Philadelphia, Hanley & Belfus, 2002, p 688.
34. Plancher KD, Peterson RK, Steichen JB: Compressive neuropathies and tendinopathies in the athletic elbow and wrist. Clin Sports Med 1996;15:331-371.
35. Taylor KS: Prevention of handlebar palsy with an experimental handlebar and glove. Clin J Sport Med 2006;6(5):434.
36. Palmer AK, Werner FW: Triangular fibrocartilage complex ow the wrist: anatomy and function. J Hand Surg 1981;6(2):153-162.
37. Loftus JB, Palmer AK: Disorders of the distal radioulnar joint and triangular fibrocartilage complex: an overview. In Lichtman DM, Alexander AH (eds): The Wrist and Its Disorders, 2nd ed. Philadelphia, WB Saunders, 1997, pp 385-414.
38. Rettig AC: Wrist and hand overuse syndromes. Clin Sports Med 2001;20:591-611.
39. Steinberg B: Acute wrist injuries in the athlete. Orthop Clin North Am 2002;33(3):535-545.
40. Nagel DJ: Triangular fibrocartilage complex tears in the athlete. Clin Sports Med 2001;20(1):155-166.
41. Rettig AC: Wrist problems in the tennis player. Med Sci Sports Exerc 1994;26(10):1207-1212.
42. Richie CA, Briner WW: Corticosteroid injection for treatment of de Quervain's tenosynovitis: a pooled quantitative literature evaluation. J Am Board Fam Pract 2003;16(2):102-106.
42a. Richie CA 3rd, Briner WW Jr. Corticosteroid injection for treatment of de Quervain's tenosynovitis: a pooled quantitative literature evaluation. J Am Board Fam Pract 2003;16(2):102-106.
43. DeQuervain's disease. In: Duke Orthopaedic presents Wheeless' Textbook of Orthopaedics (textbook online): Available at www.wheelessonline.com/ortho/dequervains_disease. Accessed May 14, 2007.
44. Wood MB, Dobyns JH: Sports related extra-articular wrist syndromes. Clin Orthop 1986;202:93-102.
45. Pantukosit S, Petchkura W, Stiens SA: Intersection syndrome in Burriam hospital: a 4-yr prospective study. Am J Phys Med Rehabil 2001;80:656-661.
46. Rettig AC: Athletic injuries of the wrist and hand: part II: overuse injuries of the wrist and traumatic injuries to the hand. Am J Sports Med 2004;32(1):262-273.
47. Howse C: Wrist injuries in sport. Sports Med 1994;17(3):163-175.
48. Osterman AL, Moskow L, Low DW: Soft tissue injuries of the hand and wrist in racquet sports. Clin Sports Med 1988;7:329-348.
49. Montalvan B, Parier J, Cousteau JP, et al: Clinical aspects of extensor carpi ulnaris (ecu) injuries in the professional tennis player. Society for Tennis Medicine and Science 2001;6(4). P. Cousteau, D. le Viet, French Tennis Federation, Paris.
50. Aronowitz ER, Leddy JP: Closed tendon injuries of the hand and wrist in athletes. Clin Sports Med 1998;17(3):449-467.
51. Rettig AC: Athletic injuries of the wrist and hand part I: traumatic injuries of the wrist. Am J Sports Med 2003;31(6):1038-1048.
52. Linscheid RL, Dobyns JH: Athletic injuries of the wrist. Clin Orthop Relat Res 1985;198:141-151.
53. Watson HK, Ashmead D, Makhlouf V: Examination of the scaphoid. J Hand Surg [Am] 1988;13:657-660.
54. Peh WCG, Gilula LA: Normal disruption of carpal arcs. J Hand Surg [Am] 1996;21:561-566, 1996.
55. Bozentka DJ: Scapholunate instability. U Penn Orthop J 1999;12:27-32.
56. Blatt G, Tobias B, Lichtman DM: Scapholunate injuries. In Lichtman DM, Alexander AH: The Wrist and Its Disorders, 2nd ed. Philadelphia, WB Saunders, 1997.

Elbow Injuries

Mark A. Slabaugh, MD

KEY POINTS

- Radial head fractures without mechanical block should never be immobilized for more than 3 days to avoid significant arthrofibrosis.
- The key to differentiating lateral epicondylitis from entrapment neuropathies is the proximity of the tenderness to the epicondyle.
- Elbow dislocations require emergent reduction to avoid potentially disastrous complications.
- The key to diagnosing unstable olecranon fractures is the inability to extend the elbow against gravity.
- The failure to palpate an intact biceps tendon with the arm actively flexed is pathognomonic of a distal biceps tendon rupture.

INTRODUCTION

Elbow injuries in adults are commonly grouped into two major categories: traumatic and nontraumatic (i.e., overuse). Traumatic injuries are very common in individuals who have sustained a fall onto an outstretched hand (FOOSH). Any patient who has sustained such a fall requires a good elbow examination to ensure that an occult elbow fracture is not missed. As a result of the intra-articular nature of most elbow fractures, treatment often requires orthopedic intervention. Alternatively, overuse elbow injuries are often the result of subacute injury, and they are best treated with a variety of conservative therapies, with only the refractory cases warranting orthopedic referral. Knowledge of the mechanism of injury, anatomy, clinical examination, and treatment will help sports medicine physicians to appropriately treat these injuries.

ELBOW ANATOMY

The elbow is composed of three joints: the ulnohumeral joint, the radiohumeral joint, and the proximal radioulnar joint. The first two are responsible for elbow flexion and extension, and the last one is responsible for forearm pronation and supination. The bony architecture of the elbow is quite complex, and it allows for a maximal range of motion while maintaining a stable joint **(Figure 20.1).**

The distal humerus is configured in a two-column construct (medial and lateral), with the articular portion of the elbow connecting these two columns **(Figure 20.2).** The lateral column is composed of the lateral condyle and the lateral epicondyle. The lateral epicondyle serves as the attachment site of the wrist extensor muscles, whereas the lateral condyle is composed of the capitellum and the origin of the lateral stabilizing ligaments, the lateral ulnar collateral ligament, and the lateral collateral ligament **(Figure 20.3).** The medial column is composed of the medial condyle and the medial epicondyle. The medial condyle consists of the trochlea and the origin of the medial stabilizing ligaments **(Figure 20.4),** whereas the medial epicondyle serves as the attachment for the wrist flexor and the forearm pronator muscles **(Figure 20.5).** In between the triangle of the two columns and the articular surface is a wafer thin piece of bone that separates the olecranon fossa posteriorly and the coronoid fossa anteriorly (see Figure 20.1). These fossas allow for full flexion and extension, and they engage the olecranon process and the coronoid process, respectively.

The articular surface is composed of two major portions: the capitellum and the trochlea. The capitellum is the convex, almost rounded extension of the lateral condyle, and it articulates with the convex proximal radius. The trochlea is spool shaped, with two convex articulations and a central ridge separating the two. This complex architecture serves to create inherent stability while providing for maximal range of motion.

The proximal ulna is composed of two processes: the olecranon and the coronoid. In between the two processes is a semilunar shaped biconcave articulation that engages the trochlea and that allows for elbow flexion and extension. The olecranon is easily palpated along the posterior elbow. As a result of its superficial nature, the olecranon has a bursa overlying it to reduce the friction that is inherent in elbow flexion and extension. The olecranon also serves as the attachment site for the broad insertion of the triceps muscle, which is responsible for elbow extension. The ulnar nerve is just medial to the olecranon in a recess between its tip and the medial epicondyle. The coronoid process is a triangular structure at the anteriormost portion of the olecranon, which lends stability to the elbow in flexion. The proximal ulna also has a concave notch (sigmoid notch) that allows the proximal radius to rotate with respect to the ulna with forearm pronation and supination (see Figure 20.1). Just distal and posterior to the coronoid process is a small process called the sublime tubercle, where the medial collateral ligament attaches (see Figure 20.4).

The elbow portion of the proximal radius is composed of the head, the neck, and the bicipital tuberosity. The radial head

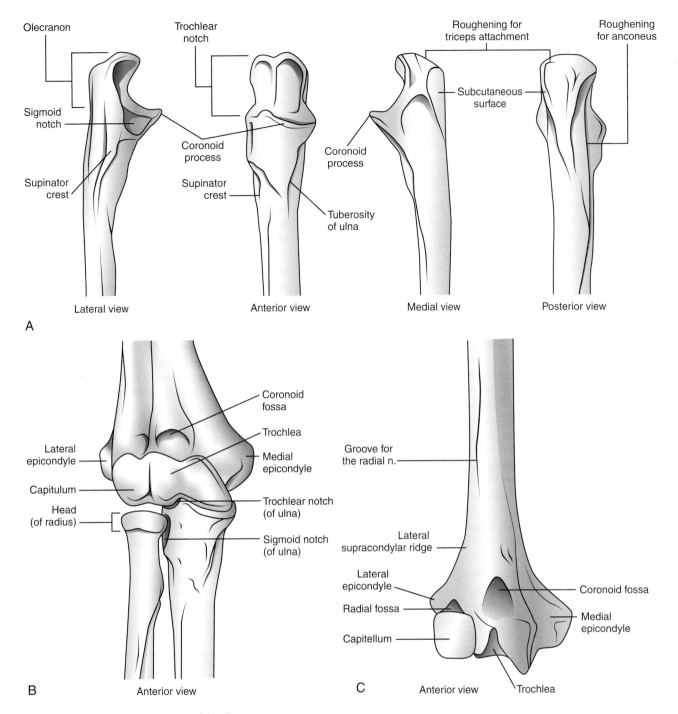

Figure 20.1 *A, B, C,* and *D,* Bony anatomy of the elbow.

is a rounded, bulbous structure that is concave at its tip to allow it to articulate with the capitellum portion of the distal humerus. Just distal to the articulation with the capitellum, the radial head is circular and covered circumferentially with cartilage to allow for articulation with the proximal ulna in the sigmoid notch, thus allowing for forearm rotation. Around the radial neck is a thick, almost circumferential ligament called the annular ligament, which keeps the radial head located under the capitellum (see Figure 20.3). This ligament is an actual thickening of the lateral collateral ligament. Just distal to the radial head is a narrowing called the radial neck. A large protuberance rests on

the proximal radius and serves as the insertion for the biceps, which is a strong forearm supinator. This tuberosity will be positioned posteriorly with forearm pronation, and it will rotate anteriorly with forearm supination. The radial head can be easily palpated on the lateral side of the arm by rotating the forearm through pronation and supination and feeling for the structure that rolls during this maneuver. The radial head lies posterior to the wrist extensors about 1 to 2 cm distal to the lateral epicondyle.

Armed with a good knowledge of elbow anatomy, an astute clinician can localize and confirm a clinical differential diagnosis

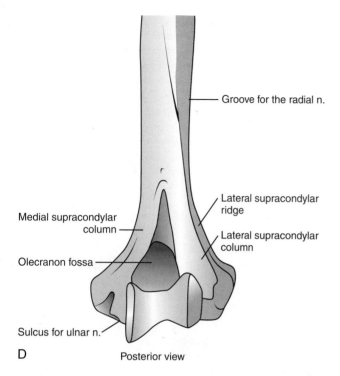

D — Posterior view

Figure 20.1 cont'd

when presented with a patient who is complaining of either traumatic or nontraumatic elbow pain.

ELBOW FRACTURES

Radial head and neck fractures
Mechanism of injury
Patients with fractures of the radial neck and head typically sustain a fall on a FOOSH. Typically, this FOOSH has a valgus moment that causes the radial head to impact on the capitellum.

Signs and symptoms
Patients who have sustained a radial head or neck fracture typically have minimal swelling of the elbow unless there are other associated fractures. The patients will typically complain of pain over the lateral aspect of their elbows, and they will often

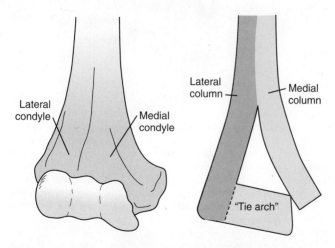

Figure 20.2 Lateral column, medial column, and tie arch.

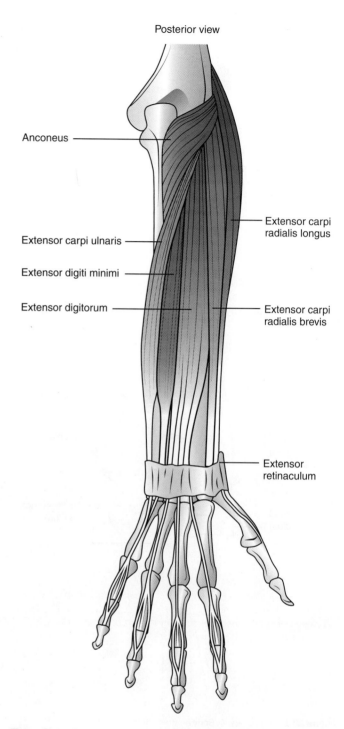

Figure 20.3 Superficial layer of muscles in the posterior compartment of the forearm.

complain of the inability to move or to fully extend the joint. The physical examination shows localized swelling over the lateral aspect of the proximal forearm. Occasionally, there will be a traumatic effusion. Patients will not be tender except with direct palpation over the radial head or neck. Patients are very hesitant to move the elbow, and the examination is more difficult than one would expect from the radiographic findings. Flexion and extension are often limited to avoid the terminal ranges of motion, which place more pressure on the radial head. Additionally, forearm rotation is difficult to assess. With patients in whom it is difficult

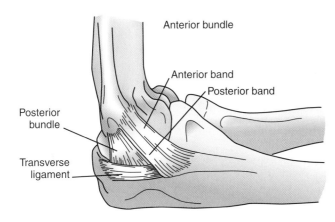

Figure 20.4   The anatomy of the medial collateral ligament of the elbow. (From Green D, Hotchkiss R, Pederson W, Wolf S: Green's Operative Hand Surgery, 5th ed. Philadelphia, WB Saunders, 2005.)

to assess range of motion of the elbow, it is important to determine the cause of the restricted range of motion. This finding is caused by one of two things: pain or a mechanical block. To differentiate between the two, a diagnostic injection with lidocaine and, occasionally, aspiration of the hemarthrosis can be very helpful. The procedure is performed as detailed in **Box 20.1.**

Radiographic findings
Two views of the elbow are always required when suspicion of an elbow fracture exists. Radial head and neck fractures are often nondisplaced and thus difficult to see on plain films. In this situation, an additional radiocapitellar view (with the forearm in a neutral position and an x-ray beam with 45 degrees of cephalad tilt) is superb for noting these nondisplaced fractures.

Patients who have a radial neck or head fracture will often have a fat pad or "sail sign" either anteriorly or posteriorly that indicates the displacement of the fat pad by an effusion or hemarthrosis in the coronoid or olecranon fossas, respectively. Fractures of the radial head will show articular incongruity if they are displaced with either a step off, displacement, and/or diastasis. X-rays must be closely inspected for patients who have a mechanical block for evidence of a loose body or a fragment incarcerated in the joint. Radial neck fractures should be carefully assessed for angulation, rotation, and displacement because these are important for determining treatment options. Occasionally, a computed tomography scan must be obtained to better define articular congruity for patients in whom x-ray is not adequate. Additional images of the forearm or wrist should be obtained if the clinical examination raises concern for another fracture. Care should be taken to identify patients with a radial head/neck fracture and tenderness at the wrist joint. These patients have most likely injured the interosseous membrane between the ulna and the radius, thus making the forearm unstable and susceptible to proximal migration.

Treatment
The treatment of radial head and neck fractures is determined by the degree of fracture displacement.

Nondisplaced (less than 2 mm) radial head/neck fractures
Initial treatment: For patients who have a nondisplaced fracture of the radial head or neck (defined as an articular step off or diastasis of less than 2 mm), a sling for comfort can be prescribed for the first 3 days **(Figure 20.7).**

Definitive treatment: Early range of motion is essential to avoid the complication of arthrofibrosis. Occasionally, the hemarthrosis must be aspirated to provide patient comfort and to allow the

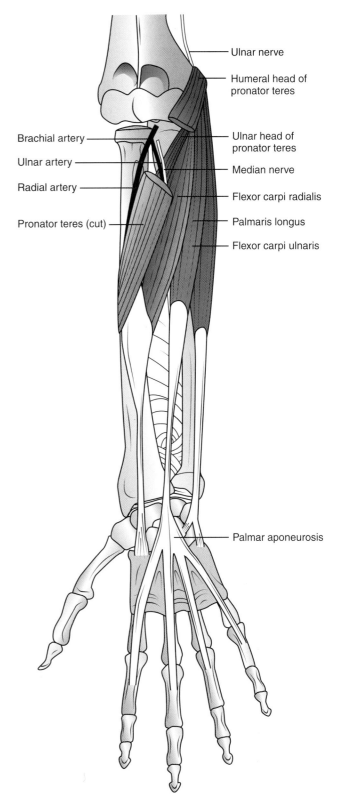

Figure 20.5   Superficial layer of the forearm muscles.

patient to start early range-of-motion exercises (see Box 20.1). Patients should be instructed to work on obtaining full flexion, extension, pronation, and supination as well as range of motion at the wrist. Splints, slings, and other immobilizing devices should be avoided to encourage patients to use the affected extremity.

Box 20.1: How to Perform an Elbow Joint Injection/Aspiration

- Sterilize the lateral aspect of the elbow with betadine.
- Insert an 18-gauge needle using sterile technique in the center of the triangle that is formed by the tip of the olecranon, the lateral epicondyle, and the center of the radial head **(Figure 20.6).**
- Aspirate any hemarthrosis, if it is present.
- Inject 3 to 5 mL of 1% lidocaine into the joint without removing the prior needle.
- Allow the patient to sit for 5 minutes for the lidocaine to take effect.
- Reexamine the patient, concentrating on elbow flexion/extension and pronation/supination to determine if any mechanical block is felt or if any step off in the radial head is felt.
- If the patient has a mechanical block, note at what degree of motion this occurs; also note whether any crepitus is felt and at what degree of motion this happens.

Follow-up should be accomplished at the 2-week point. In patients who are not making progress, a consultation with an occupational or physical therapy is warranted to facilitate the range of motion. Repeat radiographs should be obtained at this time to ensure that the fracture is stable and that there is no change in the alignment of the fracture. Full range of motion is typically obtained by about 3 weeks; occasionally, however, a patient will have a loss of full extension. If this loss is not more than 30 degrees, it will typically not affect the patient's function.

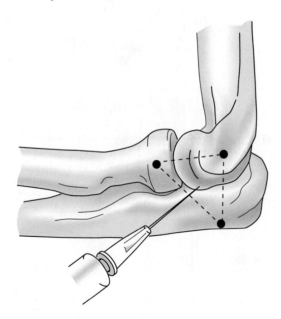

Figure 20.6 Aspiration of the elbow. Under sterile technique with the forearm maintained in pronation, a needle is introduced into the center of the triangle that is formed by the lateral epicondyle, the radial head, and the tip of the olecranon. The hemarthrosis is aspirated, and a local anesthetic is injected. An improvement in rotation is suggestive of pain-limiting motion, whereas a persistent restriction of rotation is suggestive of a mechanical block that requires surgical management. (From Green D, Hotchkiss R, Pederson W, Wolf S: Green's Operative Hand Surgery, 5th ed. Philadelphia, WB Saunders, 2005.)

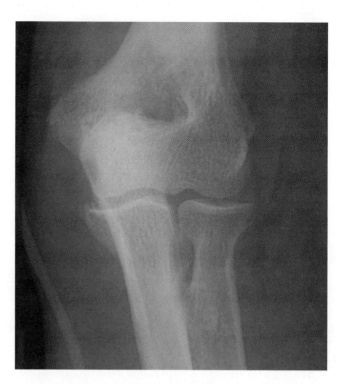

Figure 20.7 Nondisplaced radial head fracture.

Displaced (greater than 2 mm) or comminuted radial head fractures *Initial treatment:* A sling for comfort is used just as it is for nondisplaced radial head fractures as long as there is not a concomitant elbow dislocation.

Definitive treatment: Patients with radial head/neck fractures in which there is articular incongruity, significant angulation/comminution, or mechanical block warrant an orthopedic referral within 24 to 48 hours.[1] In addition, any patient who has a radial head/neck fracture with other associated injuries (e.g., nerve injury or elbow dislocation) should also have an immediate consult placed. These patients are typically best treated with open reduction and internal fixation; only occasionally can these injuries be treated with closed reduction in younger patients. For those fractures in which there is a significant amount of comminution and the radial head is not reconstructable, radial head arthroplasty has been shown to offer good pain relief with very little loss of function.[2] Radial head arthoplasty is especially helpful for cases in which there is damage to the interosseous ligament.[3]

Olecranon fractures
Mechanism of injury

Olecranon fractures can occur by several mechanisms. In patients who have osteoporotic bone, forceful eccentric contraction of the triceps may result in an olecranon avulsion fracture. Additionally, a direct blow with the elbow slightly flexed can cause an olecranon fracture. Indirect trauma when a patient sustains a FOOSH injury may also precipitate an olecranon fracture.

Signs and symptoms

Patients who have sustained an olecranon fracture have a varied clinical picture. With small avulsion fractures or fractures in which there is minimal displacement and no articular incongruity, swelling is minimal. The most significant clinical finding is tenderness to direct palpation over the olecranon. It is important in these patients to ascertain whether their triceps mechanism is intact, which is done by having the patient try

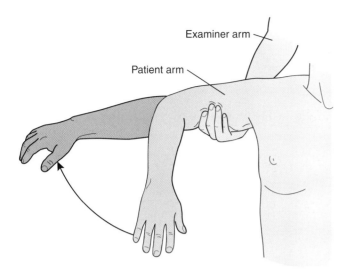

Figure 20.8 Active elbow extension test. The examiner stands behind the patient and holds the patient's shoulder and arm at 90 degrees of abduction (away from the body), letting the patient's elbow and forearm relax. The patient is then instructed to actively extend the elbow and to bring the forearm parallel to the level of the shoulder and arm. An inability to perform this active extension indicates a significant disruption in the triceps extensor mechanism.

to extend his or her elbow against gravity **(Figure 20.8).** Occasionally, an intra-articular injection of lidocaine is necessary before performing this test (see Box 20.1 for injection/aspiration procedures).

By contrast, for those patients with a more forceful injury, swelling is significant, with a large hemarthrosis and often a sympathetic bursitis. If significant triceps damage has occurred, the posterior aspect of the arm may have ecchymosis that extends far proximal and distal to the site of injury. Patients who have fractures with displacement will also have a palpable defect at the fracture site. A detailed neurologic examination is critical and should be performed and documented immediately, because subsequent pain and swelling often limit this examination. The neurologic examination should focus on the ulnar nerve (sensation in the ring and small fingers and motor by crossing of the fingers) as a result of its proximity to the fracture. As with all trauma, a thorough skin inspection should be done to look for any open injuries that would necessitate an emergent orthopedic referral. Other areas such as the wrist, hand, and shoulder should also be examined to ensure that an associated injury is not missed.

Radiographic findings
Again, as with all elbow fractures, anteroposterior (AP) and lateral x-rays are crucial to determine treatment. The olecranon is more easily identified on the lateral radiograph because it is in more profile with this view. It is crucial to obtain a good lateral radiograph to determine any articular incongruity. Radiographs should be repeated if an inadequate lateral is obtained. Radiographs should be inspected for diastasis (gapping at the fracture site), comminution, or any step off at the fracture site. Most olecranon fractures are articular by their nature, except for the rare avulsion fractures in which the triceps is not intact. Patients who have a nondisplaced fracture on a true lateral image require repeat radiographs with the elbow flexed to 90 degrees to ensure that the fracture will be stable with the elbow in the position of immobilization. Radiographs should also be inspected for any displacement of the radial head.

Olecranon fractures are classified as either nondisplaced and stable or displaced and unstable. Unstable fractures can be subclassified on the basis of the orientation of their fracture line: transverse, oblique, or comminuted. Avulsion fractures are also considered unstable fractures because the triceps mechanism is typically disrupted in this type of fracture, which requires the triceps to be repaired back down to the olecranon.

Treatment
Treatment of olecranon fractures is based on the stability of the fracture **(Figure 20.9).**

Stable fractures *Initial treatment:* Fractures of the olecranon that are stable and nondisplaced on the lateral radiograph can be treated in a long-arm cast with the elbow in 90 degrees of flexion. It is imperative that the patient can actively extend the elbow against gravity and that the fracture be nondisplaced on a lateral x-ray with the elbow in 90 degrees of flexion.

Definitive treatment: These patients should be seen in 1 week for an x-ray out of the cast to ensure that the fracture has not displaced. If the fracture continues to be stable, the patient is then treated in a long-arm cast for 4 weeks. Active range-of-motion exercises are then permitted up to 90 degrees of flexion until there is evidence of bony union on x-ray. Full pronation and supination are allowed at 4 weeks.

Unstable fractures *Initial treatment:* Unstable olecranon fractures are those with any comminution, diastasis of greater than 2 mm, incongruity of greater than 2 mm, or an inability to extend the elbow against gravity (see Figure 20.9). These patients should have an urgent (within 24 hours) consultation with an orthopedist. These injuries should be placed in a long-arm splint for comfort and swelling control. Open injuries and other associated fractures and dislocations warrant an emergent consultation.

Definitive treatment: For patients with an unstable olecranon fracture, the treatment of choice is some internal fixation construct. If the unstable fracture is just an avulsion fracture with the triceps mechanism, the triceps is typically repaired down to bone through drill holes in the olecranon or with anchors. Unstable intra-articular fractures are treated with open reduction and internal fixation.

Distal humerus fractures
Mechanism of injury
Fractures of the distal humerus are produced with an axial load (direct impact) with the elbow flexed beyond 90 degrees. This mechanism typically will produce an intra-articular fracture. In patients who have severe osteoporosis, fractures can occur with hyperextension and a FOOSH injury. This mechanism will more often produce a transcondylar fracture that is more analogous to the pediatric supracondylar fracture.

Signs and symptoms
Patients with distal humerus fractures have a more marked presentation and physical examination. Typically, the force needed to produce these fractures is much more than that needed for the previously discussed fractures; therefore, the patients are in much more pain, and the physical examination is much more difficult. Swelling around the elbow is marked, and it often can extend quite distally, even to the point where compartment syndrome of the forearm must be kept in mind. These patients have impressive tenderness to palpation in most areas of the elbow, and crepitus is felt with any attempted flexion or extension. Because of their proximity to the major neurovascular bundles anteriorly, distal humerus fractures often have associated injuries to the

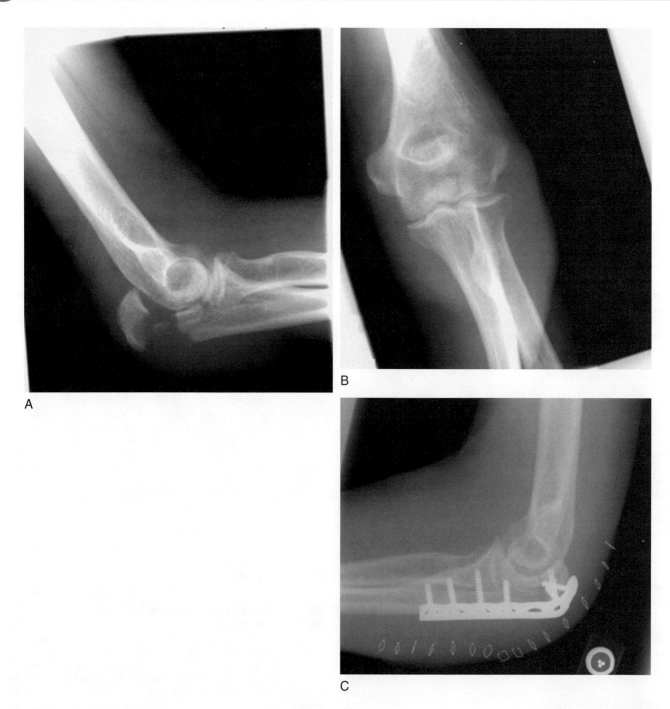

A

B

C

Figure 20.9 *A, B,* and *C,* Olecranon fractures.

vessels or nerves. This often is the result of the fracture pattern that is produced with these injuries. The nerves or vessels are either tented, entrapped, or lacerated by the fracture ends. Thus, it is imperative that a detailed neurovascular examination be performed to document the motor, sensory, and vascular examinations. It is rare that these fractures are open, but good inspection of the skin must be performed to ensure that an open injury is not missed.

Radiographic findings

For these injuries, AP and lateral images of both the elbow and the entire humerus are required. There will often be extension of the fracture into the diaphysis of the humerus with the most distal

humerus fractures **(Figure 20.10).** Occasionally, oblique x-rays are needed to determine if there is a nondisplaced fracture of the supracondylar region of the distal humerus.

There are three types of distal humerus fractures: supracondylar, intercondylar, and condylar. Fractures that do not extend into the articular surface are often transverse or short oblique fractures; these are called *supracondylar fractures*. Supracondylar fractures are best appreciated on the AP radiograph, but the lateral radiograph is the key to determining treatment. Often the fracture appears to be well aligned on the AP image, but the lateral image will typically demonstrate posterior displacement. The lateral image must be closely inspected to inspect the anterior humeral line (see Chapter 17). This line is an extension of the anterior

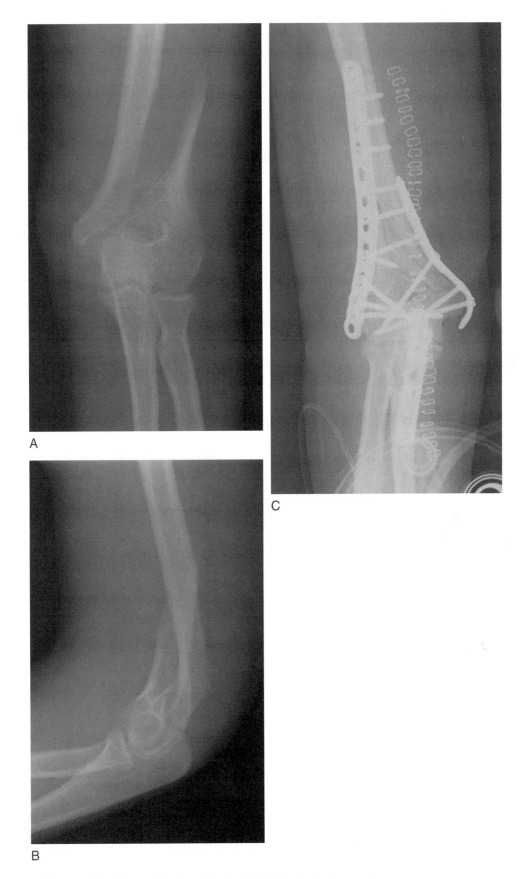

A

B

C

Figure 20.10 *A, B,* and *C,* Displaced distal humerus fracture with extension into the diaphysis.

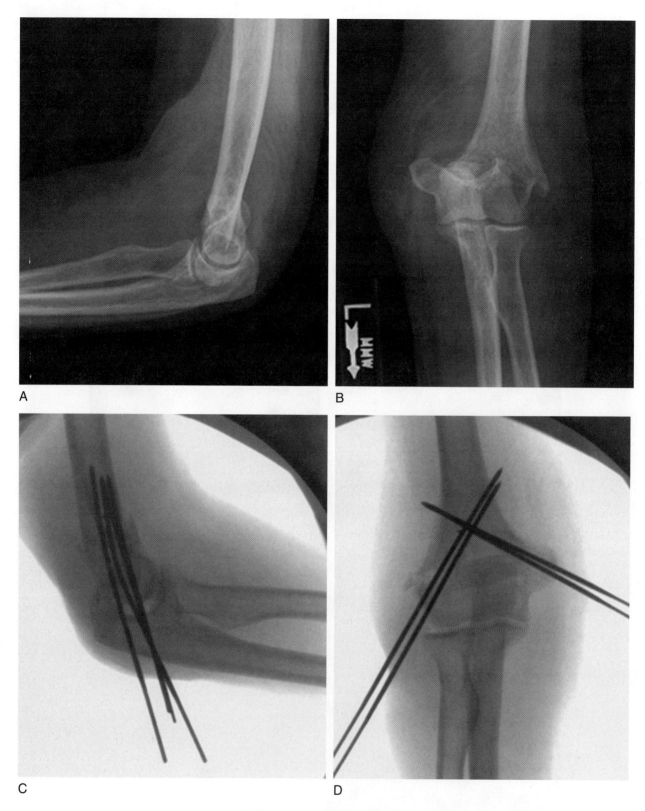

A

B

C

D

Figure 20.11 *A, B, C,* and *D,* Supracondylar fracture (trochlear fracture).

cortex, and it should bisect the capitellum through the medial third of this structure. If the anterior humeral line is anterior to the capitellum, this indicates that the fracture is posteriorly displaced and that it needs internal fixation **(Figure 20.11).** This posterior displacement is very common because the radial head forces the capitellum and the supracondylar fracture posterior with the axial load imparted during the FOOSH injury.

Intercondylar fractures are any fracture that extends across the distal humerus and that has extension into the articular surface. These intercondylar fractures are very unstable, and they often have significant displacement and rotation. Intracondylar fractures typically look like a "T" on the AP radiograph. Again, both images must be inspected carefully for any displacement and articular incongruity. With significant injuries, the two condyles will be displaced medially and laterally, with the supracondylar region impacted into the proximal ulna. Intercondylar fractures are classified on the basis of their displacement and rotation; however, all of these fractures are unstable and required an urgent orthopedic referral. Isolated capitellar or trochlear fractures are very rare, intra-articular fractures. These fractures will best be seen on the lateral radiograph, where only a sliver of bone will be visualized. This sliver is often displaced anteriorly on the lateral radiograph, and it may be mistaken for a loose body. The "sliver" of bone appearance is deceiving because the fragment will have a large portion of articular cartilage attached to it that is not appreciated on an x-ray.

Condylar fractures are very infrequent in the adult population. Adult condylar fractures typically involve one fracture line extending from the supracondylar area into the joint. These fractures can be subclassified as either medial or lateral condyle fractures.

Treatment

Initial treatment After evaluation, these injuries should be placed in long-arm posterior splints.

Definitive treatment Almost all distal humerus fractures need urgent (within 24 hours) orthopedic referral because it is only the exceptional distal humerus fracture that is amenable to nonoperative treatment. The only distal humerus fracture that can possibly be treated without surgery is the truly nondisplaced nonarticular fracture. Typically, these are the rare supracondylar fractures in elderly osteoporotic individuals. Even after the decision for nonoperative treatment is made, these rare cases must be followed very closely to ensure that they remain nondisplaced as a result of the high forces that act on them. This involves weekly follow up with good AP and lateral radiographs until fracture union has been achieved. All intra-articular and displaced fractures should be treated with open reduction and internal fixation with a variety of fixation options.

Elbow dislocations
Mechanism of injury

The most common types of elbow dislocations are posterior followed distantly by anterior. The type of dislocation is described by the position of the ulna/radius with regard to the distal humerus. Posterior elbow dislocations are usually sustained via a FOOSH. For patients with posterior dislocations, the elbow is typically partially flexed so that the olecranon is not engaged in the olecranon fossa. A posterior directed force is also necessary to tear or fracture the anterior structures. If the elbow is fully locked in extension, this transmits the injury force into the distal humerus, which results in distal humerus fractures.

Anterior dislocations are a result of a direct fall onto a partially flexed elbow. Several anatomic structures contribute to the stability of the elbow and resist elbow dislocation. The radial head as well as the coronoid resist posterior dislocations, whereas the olecranon resists anterior dislocations.[4]

Signs and symptoms

Patients who present with an elbow dislocation are very tentative to move the elbow, and they complain of significant pain and deformity. When suspicion of an elbow dislocation is high, the first priority is not the relocation of the elbow. Rather, a detailed neurovascular examination must be performed before radiographs or relocation occurs to ensure that patient is neurologically intact before the reduction. This is paramount because neurovascular

structures can be entrapped during the reduction. If a detailed examination is not performed before the reduction and there is a postreduction neurovascular deficit, there will be questions as to whether the dislocation or the relocation caused the deficit, which can cause difficulty with continuing treatment decisions. The most common nerves that are injured are the median and ulnar nerves, and the brachial artery is frequently injured as well. Physical examination is impressive for the deformity and the soft-tissue injury. The elbow is significantly swollen and tender to palpation. If the dislocation is posterior, the elbow is typically flexed, with a large bony protuberance posteriorly and with divots medially and laterally where the concave portion of the olecranon can be felt. Anterior dislocations present with an extended elbow, a shortened arm, and a lengthened supinated forearm.

Radiographic findings

X-rays readily show anterior and posterior elbow dislocations. The key is to recognize any concomitant fractures that will affect the stability of the reduction or the postreduction treatment options. As usual, standard AP and lateral radiographs of the elbow are needed as well of the humerus and the forearm to ensure that no other associated fractures are missed. Radiographs will show whether the elbow is posteriorly or anteriorly dislocated **(Figure 20.12).** Medial, lateral, or divergent dislocations may rarely occur as well.

With elbow dislocations, there are often associated fractures. The most common is the radial head or neck fracture. Additionally, the coronoid is often sheared off with a posteriorly directed force. Small avulsion fractures of the medial or lateral epicondyle can be visualized on the AP image, and they are an indication of possible valgus or varus instability, respectively. In patients who have significant instability of the elbow after reduction, a computed tomography scan may be helpful for further delineating any associated fractures and their locations.

Treatment

Prompt reduction is the key to treating elbow dislocations because the longer the elbow is allowed to remain dislocated, the more difficult the reduction is to perform and the higher the risk of neurovascular injury.[4] Reduction maneuvers differ for the different types of dislocation.

Initial treatment Posterior elbow fractures (even with associated fractures) should be reduced by the primary care physician if an orthopedic surgeon is not immediately available. This should be performed in a monitored environment with the ability to give intravenous sedation and analgesia. The reduction maneuver for a posterior dislocation is detailed in **Box 20.2** on page 227.

Definitive treatment Elbow dislocations that have no associated fractures or concomitant injuries and that are completely stable through all ranges of motion after reduction can be treated by primary care physicians. These dislocations should be splinted for 3 to 5 days for soft-tissue rest and then begun on an aggressive range-of-motion protocol with physical therapy. The splint should be discontinued at this time to encourage patients to regain function in the elbow. Radiographs should be repeated if patients complain of any instability or clicking in the elbow. Patients should be followed every 3 weeks to ensure that they are progressing in their physical therapy.

Patients who have any associated fractures with the elbow dislocation or residual instability after reduction should be referred to an orthopedist within 24 hours or immediately if the elbow cannot be kept reduced in a splint. One associated fracture that is known for its instability is the terrible triad of the elbow. This triad is composed of a radial head fracture, a coronoid fracture, and a medial collateral ligament tear.

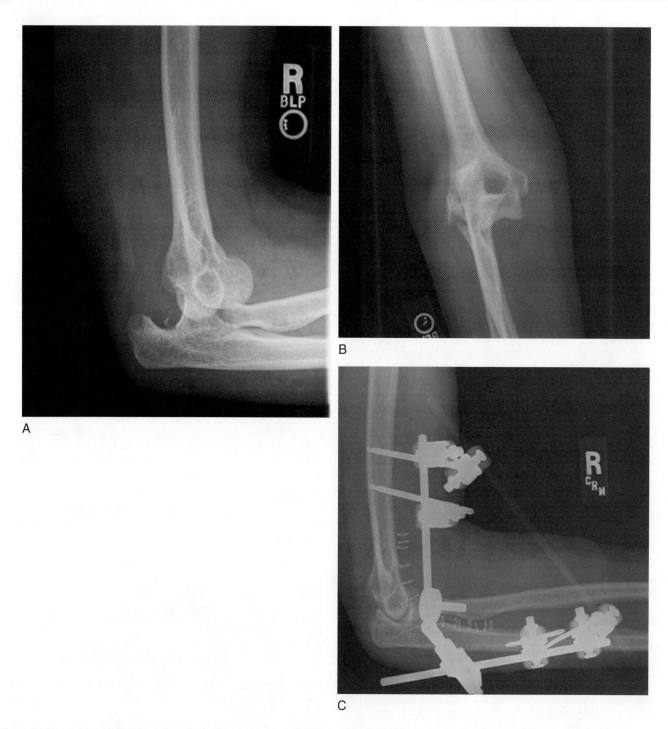

Figure 20.12 *A, B,* and *C,* Posterior elbow dislocation with associated radial head/neck fracture.

ELBOW OVERUSE INJURIES

Lateral epicondylitis (tennis elbow)
Mechanism of injury

Lateral epicondylitis is sustained with repetitive motions that stress the origin of the wrist extensors. Classically, eccentric contraction of the wrist extensors with the backstroke in tennis was taught as the typical mechanism, hence the term *tennis elbow*. However, only a minority of patients that are seen with this condition are tennis players. More often, there is an overuse of the wrist extensors, especially the extensor carpi radialis brevis (ECRB).[5] Occasionally, lateral epicondylitis can be seen with direct trauma to the origin of the wrist extensors. Contributing factors include an area of hypovascularity in the ECRB just distal to the lateral epicondyle or possibly a history of fluoroquinolone use.[6] The typical patient with lateral epicondylitis is at least 40 years of age at the time of presentation.

Signs and symptoms

Patients with lateral epicondylitis typically present with vague lateral forearm pain that radiates down to the wrist and that is exacerbated by forearm extension.[7] Patients most often describe the

Box 20.2: Elbow Dislocation

To reduce a posterior elbow dislocation, apply longitudinal traction to the forearm with the forearm in supination. Gentle force with one's thumb is placed over the posterior tip of the olecranon while the arm is flexed.[4] After the elbow is felt to reduce, it is taken through a range of motion from full extension to maximal flexion, full pronation, and supination to ensure stability. Varus and valgus stability should also be checked. If the elbow redislocates, it should be noted in which position this occurs. Reduction is then repeated, and the elbow is splinted in 90 degrees of flexion, with the forearm in a neutral position. Orthopedic consultation is then obtained within 24 hours. If the elbow cannot be reduced, then an emergent referral is necessary.

After the elbow is reduced, repeat radiographs are obtained, with the elbow splinted to document that the elbow is in fact reduced. Repeat neurovascular examination is paramount to ensure that no neurovascular structures are entrapped within the joint.

Anterior dislocations are treated with posterior-directed pressure over the proximal forearm while maintaining longitudinal traction. The elbow is slowly taken from flexion to extension. After the elbow is felt to relocate, the same examination and radiographs are performed and documented to ensure stability, neurovascular function, and concentric reduction **(Figure 20.13)**.

pain as gradually worsening; however, occasionally a patient might recall a specific traumatic injury or a specific episode of blatant overuse. Patients will complain of weakness in the arm and difficulty carrying something in the associated hand without dropping it or feeling fatigued.

The physical examination should be directed at the lateral aspect of the elbow. Typically, patients with lateral epicondylitis will have a full range of motion. However, the range of motion of the elbow with both flexion/extension and pronation/supination should be checked to rule out other conditions. The elbow will have tenderness to palpation with direct palpation just distal to the lateral epicondyle. Occasionally, in severe cases, this tenderness will be present on the lateral epicondyle and distal to the musculotendinous junction. Provocative maneuvers include resisted wrist extension with the elbow fully extended. This maneuver stresses the diseased muscle (ECRB) and causes pain that is localized to the lateral elbow. Additionally, passive full flexion of the wrist with the elbow extended places the involved muscle on maximum stretch and reproduces the characteristic pain at the lateral elbow. Grip strength with a dynamometer is measured with the patient's elbow flexed and then fully extended. Grip strength will be significantly less with the elbow extended as compared with it flexed.[8] A detailed neurologic examination is crucial and should focus on the posterior interosseous nerve because radial tunnel syndrome is often confused with tennis elbow. Posterior interosseous nerve syndrome as well as radial tunnel syndrome, osteoarthrosis, capitellar chondral defects, and loose bodies in the lateral gutter are the main differential diagnoses to address when considering lateral-sided elbow pain **(Table 20.1)**.

Radiographic evaluation

Radiographs are almost always normal in patients with lateral epicondylitis. Only in rare cases may some mineralization in the area of the ECRB tendon origin be seen. However, normal radiographs effectively rule out concomitant pathology, so they are often obtained. In patients who have recalcitrant lateral epicondylitis, calcification at the origin of the wrist extensors may be seen, especially if the tendon has been avulsed. On the T2-weighted images, magnetic resonance imaging (MRI) will show edema in the ECRB origin and in the tendon in acute cases, but MRI is seldom needed for the diagnosis and management of lateral epicondylitis. More chronic disease will be associated with more attritional changes in the ECRB tendon.

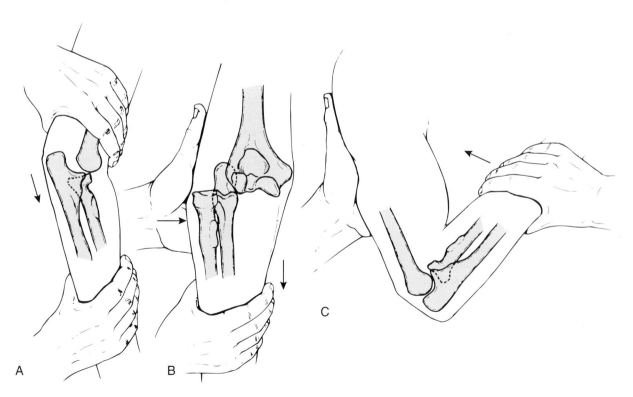

Figure 20.13   A, B, and C, Reduction of posterior elbow dislocation. (From Bowner B, Jupiter J, Levine A, Trafton P: Skeletal Trauma: Basic Science, Management, and Reconstruction, 3rd ed.)

Treatment

The majority of patients with lateral epicondylitis can be treated with nonoperative therapy (LOE: expert opinion).[9] Activity modification, anti-inflammatory medications, and ice and bracing with a counterforce brace are the mainstays of treatment. Knowing the pathophysiology of lateral epicondylitis, patients should be counseled to immediately stop all offending activities, including sports that cause pain in the lateral elbow. It has been shown that relapses or a failure of treatment is most often the result of continuation of the offending activity (LOE: E).[10] Patients who have symptoms with sports should examine their equipment and technique to ensure that they do not have a recurrence after symptoms have subsided. Recurrent episodes of epicondylitis in athletes should trigger an investigation into the proper sizing of equipment and the proper mechanics of their technique. Racquet sports especially require proper sizing of the grip handle, proper tension of the strings, appropriate size of the racquet head, and the correct number of strings on the racquet head to reduce vibration and force transmission to the lateral elbow.

Bracing is begun during the early stages of lateral epicondylitis to decrease the force that acts on the pathologic areas. Braces should be worn at all times when the patient has symptoms. Additionally, if a patient can wear the brace and return to sport without symptoms, he or she can be allowed to participate in sports. Instead of acting on the ECRB origin, the muscle contraction exerts its pull up to the brace, thereby allowing the origin to rest and heal itself. Walther and colleagues[11] have shown that a brace placed distal to the lateral epicondyle significantly reduces the load on the lateral epicondyle (LOE: C).

Additionally, physical or occupational therapy is helpful in refractory cases that have failed the above treatments. Therapists focus on nonpainful stretching, strengthening, and modality treatment. Therapy has been shown more effective than injections for long-term control of pain (>6 weeks) (LOE: C).[12] One of the modalities that therapists employ for recalcitrant lateral epicondylitis is iontophoresis, during which a steroid cream is introduced through the skin with the aid of ultrasound. Nirschl and colleagues[13] have found that the iontophoresis of dexamethasone is superior to placebo in the acute setting and that it remains efficacious at 1 month of follow up (LOE: A).[15]

If these treatments fail, then injection with cortisone is attempted.[16] Dexamethasone may be preferred because it is water soluble and does not leave steroid deposits. This area of maximal tenderness to palpation is marked before prepping. Depending on the site of attrition, this could be right at the tip of the lateral epicondyle to 4 cm distal to the lateral epicondyle. The lateral elbow is then sterilely prepped over the area of maximal tenderness. Typically, 1.5 mL of dexamethasone and 1.5 mL of 1% lidocaine are drawn up and injected at this site. The needle is advanced until a small pop is felt, which indicates that the fascia overlying the wrist extensors has been entered. The solution is then injected into this area, with an effort made to pepper the injection diffusely around the point of maximal tenderness. If resistance is met, then the tendon has been entered, and the needle should be withdrawn until the injection flows freely. Typically, a 21- or 22-gauge needle is used. Patients are then instructed about the pathology of their condition and educated about activity modifications. Hay and colleagues[14] have shown that steroid injections are superior to oral nonsteroidal anti-inflammatory drugs and placebo in a randomized, controlled trial (LOE: B). In this study, 92% of patients treated with a steroid injection had full or improved relief of symptoms at 4 weeks. Additionally, the steroid injection remained efficacious in 85% of patients at 1 year of follow up. Other studies have not yielded such good long-term results. Price and colleagues[17] demonstrated that about 90% of patients will experience temporary pain relief with this type of injection. However, the patients in this study did not demonstrate long-term efficacy of cortisone injections, with up to 54% of patients suffering a recurrence (LOE: A).[17]

If patients obtain relief with the first injection but the effects are temporary, they can be reinjected twice before the treatment should be considered a failure. In these refractory cases, the patients should be referred to an orthopedist for operative treatment to cure this condition. Surgical debridement of the involved ECRB is currently the gold standard. This technique has been shown to result in an improvement of symptoms in more than 97% of patients, with 85% returning to full function. Rehabilitation from this surgery is typically 6 weeks, with immobilization for less than 1 week.

Medial epicondylitis
Mechanism of injury

As with lateral epicondylitis, medial epicondylitis is an overuse injury of the muscles that originate from the medial epicondyle. This overuse results in the microtearing of the flexor and pronator

Table 20.1 Evaluating and Treating Elbow Overuse Injuries

	History	Examination	Treatment
Lateral epicondylitis	Overuse injury causing lateral elbow pain that is worsened with gripping activities	Tenderness at or just distal to the lateral epicondyle; pain with resisted extension of the wrist	Activity modification, occupational/physical therapy counterforce braces, steroid injection
Radial tunnel syndrome	Vague and often diffuse pain distal to the lateral epicondyle; no motor symptoms	Pain with middle finger resisted extension or resisted supination	Activity modifications, occupational therapy, steroid injection
Posterior interosseous nerve compression syndrome	Like radial tunnel syndrome with motor symptoms	Weakness in muscles that are innervated by the posterior interosseous nerve, such as the extensor pollicis longus	Activity modifications, steroid injection
Osteoarthrosis	Deep ache in lateral elbow that is worse with movements; restricted range of motion	Crepitus; tenderness over joint line; restricted range of motion	Activity modifications, nonsteroidal anti-inflammatory drugs
Capitellar osteochondritis dissecans	Trauma in a younger patient or a young gymnast	Pain over the joint line only laterally	Restriction of impact activities, occupational therapy
Loose bodies	Catching or locking of elbow	Effusion with restricted range of motion	Surgical removal

muscles of the forearm. The body attempts to repair these tears; however, as a result of repetitive stress, it is unable to complete the reparative process, and an angiofibroblastic tendinosis ensues. Initially, there may be inflammatory cells that can be mediated by a nonsteroidal anti-inflammatory drug, but, as the disease progresses, there is an insufficient vascular response that leads to a fibroblastic condition.[18] The end-stage disease is not an inflammatory condition as was once previously thought; it is now understood as an incomplete reparative process that is caused by chronic overload. The most frequent muscle groups that are injured are the pronator teres and the flexor carpi radialis, which are more radial and anterior than the other flexor muscle groups.[19] Common activities that elicit stress on the medial epicondyle origin are those that involve eccentric contraction of the wrist flexors and pronators, such as golf, javelin, racquetball, and bowling.[19] Additionally, manual laborers like plumbers, electricians, and carpenters who repetitively pronate or flex their forearms will present with symptoms of medial epicondylitis.

Signs and symptoms

Patients with medial epicondylitis present with an insidious onset of medial elbow pain that is exacerbated by repetitive motion of the elbow and forearm. As a result of the proximity of the ulnar nerve, patients also may complain of numbness and a vague weakness down the medial forearm into the small and ring fingers. Weakness when gripping and holding objects is often a chief complaint of patients with this diagnosis.

Physical examination begins with the range of motion, which is most likely normal unless the condition has been untreated for a prolonged period of time. Patients have mild swelling over the medial aspect of the elbow. Tenderness varies, but it is most often more anterior over the medial epicondyle. Tenderness should not be more than 1 cm from the medial epicondyle, where the musculotendinous junction of the flexor/pronator mass begins.[20] Resistance testing reproduces pain in the same place where tenderness was elicited. Patients should have pain with resisted flexion of the wrist and pronation of the forearm. Occasionally, patients will also have pain with stretch of the flexor/pronator origin when the wrist is brought into full extension with the forearm in supination.

A neurologic examination that focuses on the ulnar nerve is key to not missing a concomitant ulnar neuritis (cubital tunnel syndrome). Two-point discrimination in the ulnar nerve is checked as well as intrinsic strength. Typically these tests are normal, and the only findings indicating ulnar neuritis are a positive Tinel's sign at the cubital tunnel with a positive compression test and elbow flexion test. The elbow flexion test is performed by having the patient maximally flex and pronate the elbow for 30 seconds. Paresthesias in the small and ring fingers would indicate a positive test.

For patients who are overhead athletes, it is very important to assess the stability of the medial collateral ligament. The elbow must be flexed to around 30 degrees to disengage the olecranon from its fossa, and the elbow is then stressed with a valgus moment. Clinical instability has been associated with only 1 mm of opening.[21] Often the clinical examination is more positive with regard to pain than to opening with valgus stressing.

As always, when obtaining a detailed history and performing an examination for medial elbow pain, a differential diagnosis list must be kept in mind so that other conditions are not missed. The differential diagnosis for medial elbow pain is medial epicondylitis, ulnar neuritis, olecranon stress fracture, posterior medial stress overload, and ulnar collateral ligament insufficiency.

Radiographic evaluation

Radiographs should be obtained in cases of recalcitrant medial epicondylitis, especially chronic cases. Often calcification will be seen just distal to the medial epicondyle. MRI is rarely obtained for this diagnosis.

Treatment

As with lateral epicondylitis, initial treatment for medial epicondylitis is conservative. Activity modifications, bracing with a counter-force brace, nonsteroidal anti-inflammatory drugs, ice, and rest are effective initially. Because medial epicondylitis is less common than lateral epicondylitis and the disease process is virtually similar to lateral epicondylitis, many treatment modalities have not been rigorously scrutinized or validated for medial symptoms. Many of the treatments for medial epicondylitis are extrapolated from the literature that addresses lateral epicondylitis.

Initial treatment begins with the physician counseling the patient to immediately cease all activities that cause pain at the medial elbow. Nonresistive range-of-motion exercises are allowed to avoid atrophy of the affected muscles. If sports are the provocative activity, they must either be eliminated until pain-free resumption is possible or modified by using a different technique or equipment to eliminate pain.

Anti-inflammatory medications are prescribed for a short course (about 1 month) to help alleviate any inflammatory process (if caught early). Additionally, nonsteroidal anti-inflammatory drugs are thought to be effective because they relieve pain that arises from a compensatory synovitis of the elbow joint.[13] However, despite the widespread use of anti-inflammatory medications, there is a paucity of studies that show either their efficacy or ineffectiveness.

Bracing is also initiated during the first visit with patients. The pathophysiology of medical epicondylitis is tension and microtears of the wrist flexor muscles. Bracing attempts to move the origin of these muscles from the medial epicondyle to under the brace. Patients must be educated about the proper wearing of the brace. It should be placed approximately 4 cm distal to the elbow flexion crease and then tightened for comfort. Patients should be counseled that overtightening of the brace can lead to either vascular or neurologic deficits. To date, there are no studies that show the effectiveness of bracing for medial epicondylitis, despite its prevalent use and presumed effectiveness (LOE: expert opinion).

Therapy for medial epicondylitis should also be instituted early for cases of medial epicondylitis. Initially, therapists work with patients to help them regain full painless range of motion. After this is achieved, therapists work on stretching and strengthening the involved muscles within the confines of pain-free exercises. If therapy is not progressing as it should be, therapists can employ modalities to help alleviate pain. This most often includes iontophoresis or the introduction of a steroid cream into the affected area with the use of ultrasound. The short-term effectiveness of this modality has been shown by Nirschl and colleagues,[22] with good results obtained in more than 50% of patients (as compared with approximately 30% of patients who were given placebo) (LOE: A). However, the long-term effectiveness remains similar to placebo at 1 month follow-up.

Patients who are not managed effectively with conservative treatment can be injected with cortisone. This injection is performed by locating the area of maximal tenderness to palpation, which is typically just distal to the medial epicondyle. A sterile injection using lidocaine and dexamethasone is performed using the same technique as previously described for the treatment of lateral epicondylitis. After the injection, the patient is told to avoid any type of inciting activity for the next 3 to 4 days. To date, there has only been one study that demonstrated the efficacy of steroid injections for medial epicondylitis. Stahl and Kaufman[22] showed that pain relief was statistically better at 6 weeks in those patients who received a cortisone injection as compared with those who received placebo. However, there was no difference between the two groups when they were examined at 3 months and 1 year

(LOE: A).[22] If injection provides some relief and symptoms recur, reinjection can be performed. However, if the second injection is not effective, the patient should be referred to an orthopedist to discuss surgery.

Surgical treatment typically consists of debridement of the diseased tendon, which is very similar to the treatment of lateral epicondylitis. Studies show that nearly 90% of patients experience pain relief after this surgery. Additionally, the results of pain relief can be expected to last for up to 6 to 7 years of follow-up (LOE: B).[23,24] Patients who are involved in sports can expect to go back to their preinjury function approximately 80% of the time (LOE: B).[25]

Biceps rupture
Mechanism of injury
Distal biceps tendon rupture occurs typically during the sixth or seventh decade of life, and males are much more commonly affected than females. Classically, patients present with a history of a single traumatic event to a flexed and supinated elbow.[26] Eccentric contraction of the biceps tears the biceps tendon off of the radial tuberosity. Occasionally, patients recall prodromal pain in the anterior elbow that was exacerbated with elbow flexion, which indicates that they had prior tendinopathy of the biceps. Anabolic steroid use has also been implicated as a risk of biceps rupture (LOE: E).[27]

Signs and symptoms
Patients with a distal biceps tendon rupture present with pain in the anterior aspect of the elbow. However, patients describe the pain as being much less than that of the initial injury. A tearing sensation or pop is commonly elicited from patient's history with this injury.[26] Occasionally, if there has been a long period between the injury and presentation, patients will complain of weakness in the arm with flexion or supination. On examination, the elbow is often held flexed, and obvious ecchymosis is evident over the cubital fossa. Range of motion is normal, and strength testing reveals decreased elbow flexion and supination strength. Patients will have tenderness in the antecubital fossa with palpation. If the lacertus fibrosis is also avulsed with the biceps tendon, a palpable defect will be felt in the distal portion of the antecubital fossa. However, if the lacertus is intact, often the biceps is mistakenly thought to be intact. Occasionally, the tendon stump is palpable about 2 cm above the elbow crease, and it is more pronounced with attempted elbow flexion.

Radiographic evaluation
Radiographs are usually obtained only for ruling out other diagnoses. Very infrequently, the ruptured tendon will have a small avulsion fracture from the radial tuberosity.[28] For cases in which there is a high clinical suspicion for a ruptured biceps and the clinical examination is equivocal, MRI can be helpful to differentiate a torn biceps with an intact lacertus from a partial tear of the biceps.[29]

Treatment
The treatment of distal tendon biceps injuries is most commonly surgical, with the reattachment of the biceps stump back to the bicipital tuberosity.[30] However, for patients with multiple medical problems who are not good surgical candidates, nonoperative treatment is encouraged. Occasionally, patients who have low functional demands and who would not miss decreased arm flexion and forearm pronation strength can also be treated nonoperatively. Patients are counseled that they will lose about 30% of their flexion strength and 40% of their pronation strength (LOE: D).[31,32] Results of surgical repair of a torn distal biceps are superior to nonoperative treatment with regard to the recovery of both supination and flexion strength. Patients who were treated operatively in a study by Morrey and colleagues[30] had a recovery of 97% of their flexion strength and 95% of their supination strength (LOE: D). Stiffness, temporary neuropraxia, and radioulnar synostosis are the most common complications.

Osteochondritis dissecans
Mechanism of injury
The exact mechanism that causes causing osteochondritis dissecans (OCD) in the elbow is currently unknown. However, OCD is thought to be the result of a combination of microtrauma and a tenuous blood supply to portions of the elbow.[33] As a result of the anatomic constraints of the ulnohumeral joint and the relative mobility/decreased congruity of the radiocapitellar joint, the capitellum is virtually always the affected portion of the elbow. This injury is seen most commonly in young throwing athletes. The throwing mechanism places a valgus compression load onto the capitellum during the cocking phase of throwing[34] **(Figure 20.14)**. Additionally, in the growing child, the vascular anatomy of the capitellum predisposes this portion of the elbow to injury.[35] During development, the rapidly growing capitellum receives its blood supply from two epiphyseal arteries instead of the rich metaphyseal arterial system like the medial condyle. This tenuous blood supply is enough to support regular growth;

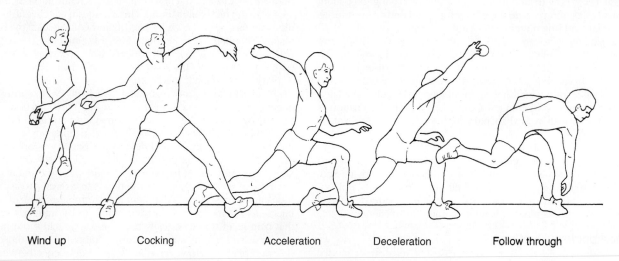

Wind up   Cocking   Acceleration   Deceleration   Follow through

Figure 20.14 Stages of throwing. (From Miller D: Review of Orthopaedics, 4th ed. Philadelphia, PA, Saunders, 2004.)

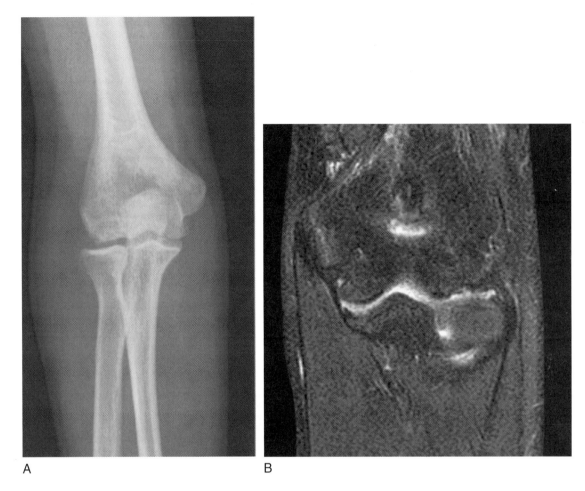

A   B

Figure 20.15   Images of a patient with osteochondritis dissecans of the capitellum. *A*, Radiograph showing a loose body behind the capitellum and subtle joint space narrowing, which indicates the origin of the loose body. *B*, Magnetic resonance image showing significant osteochondritis dissecans of the capitellum, with corresponding cartilage loss.

however, in the face of trauma, the vascular supply is not enough to support regeneration if the subchondral bone is damaged.

Signs and symptoms

The clinical presentation of OCD is the insidious onset of activity-related pain in the dominant arm of a young athlete. The typical age of patients presenting with this condition is 10 to 16 years.[36] Baseball, football, and other throwing sports as well as gymnastics are the most common sports in which young athletes develop OCD lesions. Lateral elbow pain that is exacerbated by activity during sports participation and that is relieved with rest is the most common complaint. Occasionally, if the disease process has been allowed to progress to fragmentation of the OCD, mechanical symptoms such as locking, catching, and loss of range of motion can be seen in patients who have a loose body. Clinical examination reveals occasional swelling over the anterolateral aspect of the elbow, with focal tenderness to palpation in the same area. Range of motion is most often normal, except in those patients who presenting late in whom the typical finding is a mild (less than 10 degrees) loss of extension. Occasionally, in patients with mechanical symptoms, a larger loss of range of motion can be expected as well as a positive catch with range of motion. Actively stressing the elbow with a valgus load while pronating and supinating the forearm will elicit pain in most patients.

One uncommon condition that is often mistaken for OCD of the capitellum is Panner disease, which is a self-limiting disease that is the result of vascular interference of the blood supply to the growing epiphysis. Often the signs and symptoms are similar to OCD of the capitellum, with one key difference: patients with Panner disease most often present at an age that is younger than that of those with OCD. Typically, patients with Panner disease are less than 10 years of age, whereas those with OCD of the capitellum are teenagers between 10 and 16 years of age. The radiographic appearance of Panner disease is very similar to that of OCD of the capitellum, except Panner disease shows characteristic improvement with the tincture of time and follow-up radiographs **(Figure 20.15).**

Radiographic evaluation

Evaluation should start with standard AP and lateral x-rays, which often show a focal lucency in the capitellum. In more advanced cases, collapse and fragmentation with obvious loose bodies can be seen on plain films. For patients in whom the history and physical examination are indicative of an OCD lesion and plain films are negative, MRI should be ordered. MRI is invaluable for formulating a treatment plan as a result of its superior visualization of the articular cartilage. MRI will show whether the articular cartilage is intact, the extent of the lesion, any fragmentation, subchondral collapse, loose bodies, and cyst formation.

Treatment

A treatment plan is formulated by taking into consideration the patient's symptoms, the physical examination, and the radiographic findings. Practicing the art of medicine (as compared with the science of medicine) is indeed necessary for the clinician who is dealing with this injury. The clinical presentation and the status of the articular cartilage are the keys to determining the treatment. Patients who are minimally symptomatic and who have no pain when they are not involved in impact activities should be treated with activity modifications. Additionally, if the MRI shows an intact articular surface with no evidence of collapse, then observation is warranted.[37] Patients must be kept out of the offending sport until they are completely asymptomatic and there is evidence of radiographic healing. This is typically several years, which presents a dilemma when trying to limit the activities of active teenagers for such an extended period of time. Nonoperative treatment has been postulated to be better for patients who present at an earlier age and who have less severe symptoms and pain that is relieved with rest (LOE: expert opinion).[38]

If there is any incongruity of the articular surface, loose bodies, fragmentation, collapse, or fissuring of the cartilage or if patient has failed nonoperative treatment, then surgical treatment is warranted.[39] Referral to a physician who is experienced in the treatment of juvenile elbow OCDs is warranted for all cases of OCD in the capitellum. Surgical treatment includes the removal of loose bodies, the fixation of loose but stable cartilage injuries, and occasionally, the microfracture of the underlying subchondral bone. These procedures have high success rates for relieving preoperative symptoms. Baumgarten and colleagues,[40] in their study of surgically treated OCD of the capitellum, found that all 14 patients in their series were pain free at 2 years after surgery (LOE: C). Alternatively, at follow up 2 years after surgery, McManama and colleagues found that 86% of patients who were treated surgically had returned to sports participation (LOE: C).[39] However, these short-term results are called into question when long-term results of the natural history of osteochondritis of the capitellum have shown that patients have restricted range of motion, pain with activities, and advanced arthrosis of the capitellum 50% of the time.[41,42]

CONCLUSION

Due to the complex anatomy of the elbow and the multiple structures that cross the elbow, most patients who present to a primary care clinic with elbow-related complaints will have an overuse syndrome. Armed with knowledge of the anatomy of the elbow and a good history and physical, primary care physicians can easily treat and initially diagnose both traumatic and overuse injuries. The majority of elbow conditions can be treated with activity modifications, physical therapy, anti-inflammatory medications, and bracing. It is essential to have a clear differential diagnosis when presented with a patient who has an elbow complaint. Understanding the above conditions and their treatments will help the primary care sports medicine provider treat the majority of patients with elbow complaints.

REFERENCES

1. Curtis RJ Jr, Corley FG Jr: Fractures and dislocations of the forearm. Clin Sports Med 1986;5(4):663-680.
2. Calfee R, Madom I, Weiss AP: Radial head arthroplasty. J Hand Surg [Am] 2006;31(2):314-321.
3. Edwards GS Jr, Jupiter JB: Radial head fractures with acute distal radioulnar dislocation. Essex-Lopresti revisited. Clin Orthop Relat Res 1988;234:61-69.
4. Mehta JA, Bain GI: Elbow dislocations in adults and children. Clin Sports Med 2004;23(4):609-627, ix.
5. Nirschl R: Muscle and tendon trauma: tennis elbow. In Morrey BF (ed): The Elbow and Its Disorders. WB Saunders; 1985, pp 537-552,
6. Ribard P, Audisio F, Kahn MF, et al: Seven achilles tendinitis including 3 complicated with rupture during fluoroquinolone therapy. J Rheumatol 1992;19:1479-1481.
7. Whaley AL, Baker CL: Lateral epicondylitis. Clin Sports Med 2004;23(4):677-691, x.
8. De Smet, L Fabry G: Grip force reduction in patients with tennis elbow: influence of elbow position. J Hand Ther 1997;10(3):229-231.
9. Nirschl RP, Ashman ES: Elbow tendinopathy: tennis elbow. Clin Sports Med 2003;22(4):813-836.
10. Jobe FW, Ciccotti MG: Lateral and medial epicondylitis of the elbow. J Am Acad Orthop Surg 1994;2(1):1-8.
11. Walther M, Kirschner S, Koenig A: Biomechanical evaluation of braces used for the treatment of epicondylitis. J Shoulder Elbow Surg 2002;11:265-270.
12. Newcomer KL, Laskowski ER, Idank DM, McLean TJ, Eyan KS: Corticosteroid injection in early treatment of lateral epicondylitis. Clin J Sport Med 2001;11(4):214-222.
13. Nirschl RP, Rodin DM, Ochiai DH, Maartmann-Moe C: Iontophoretic administration of dexamethasone sodium phosphate for acute epicondylitis. A randomized, double-blinded, placebo-controlled study. Am J Sports Med 2003;31(2):189-195.
14. Hay EM, Paterson SM, Lewis M, et al: Pragmatic randomised controlled trial of local corticosteroid injection and naproxen for treatment of lateral epicondylitis of elbow in primary care. BMJ 1999;319(7215):964-968.
15. Nirschl RP, Pettrone FA: Tennis elbow. The surgical treatment of lateral epicondylitis. J Bone Joint Surg Am 1979;61(6):832-839.
16. Altay T, Gunal I, Ozturk H: Local injection treatment for lateral epicondylitis. Clin Orthop Relat Res 2002;(398):127-130.
17. Price R, Sinclair H, Heinrich I, Gibson T: Local injection treatment of tennis elbow—hydrocortisone, triamcinolone and lignocaine compared. Br J Rheumatol 1991;30(1):39-44.
18. Ciccotti MC, Schwartz MA, Ciccotti MG: Diagnosis and treatment of medial epicondylitis of the elbow. Clin Sports Med 2004;23(4):693-705.
19. Regan W, Wold LE, Coonrad R, Morrey BF: Microscopic histopathology of chronic refractory lateral epicondylitis. Am J Sports Med 1992;20(6):746-749.
20. Ciccotti MC, Schwartz MA, Ciccotti MG: Diagnosis and treatment of medial epicondylitis of the elbow. Clin Sports Med 2004;23(4):693-705, xi.
21. Williams RJ 3rd, Urquhart ER, Altchek DW: Medial collateral ligament tears in the throwing athlete. Instr Course Lect 2004;53:579-586. Review.
22. Stahl S, Kaufman T: The efficacy of an injection of steroids for medial epicondylitis. A prospective study of sixty elbows. J Bone Joint Surg Am 1997;79(11):1648-1652.
23. Gabel GT, Morrey BF: Operative treatment of medical epicondylitis. Influence of concomitant ulnar neuropathy at the elbow. J Bone Joint Surg Am 1995;77(7):1065-1069.
24. Vangsness CT Jr, Jobe FW: Surgical treatment of medial epicondylitis. Results in 35 elbows. J Bone Joint Surg Br 1991;73(3):409-411.
25. Ollivierre CO, Nirschl RP, Pettrone FA: Resection and repair for medial tennis elbow. A prospective analysis. Am J Sports Med 1995;23(2):214-221.
26. Boucher PR, Morton KS: Rupture of the distal biceps brachii tendon. J Trauma 1967;7(5):626-632.
27. Visuri T, Lindholm H: Bilateral distal biceps tendon avulsions with use of anabolic steroids. Med Sci Sports Exerc 1994;26(8):941-944.
28. Vidal AF, Drakos MC, Allen AA: Biceps tendon and triceps tendon injuries. Clin Sports Med 2004;23(4):707-722, xi.
29. Fritz RC, Steinbach LS: Magnetic resonance imaging of the musculoskeletal system: Part 3. The elbow. Clin Orthop Relat Res 1996;(324):321-339.
30. Rantanen J, Orava S: Rupture of the distal biceps tendon. A report of 19 patients treated with anatomic reinsertion, and a meta-analysis of 147 cases found in the literature. Am J Sports Med 1999;27(2):128-132.
31. Morrey BF, Askew LJ, An KN, Dobyns JH: Rupture of the distal tendon of the biceps brachii. A biomechanical study. J Bone Joint Surg Am 1985;67(3):418-421.
32. Baker BE, Bierwagen D: Rupture of the distal tendon of the biceps brachii. Operative versus non-operative treatment. J Bone Joint Surg Am 1985;67(3):414-417.
33. Cain EL Jr, Dugas JR, Wolf RS, Andrews JR: Elbow injuries in throwing athletes: a current concepts review. Am J Sports Med 2003;31(4):621-635.
34. Tullos HS, King JW: Lesions of the pitching arm in adolescents. JAMA 1972;220(2):264-271.
35. Haraldsson S: On osteochondrosis deformas juvenilis capituli humeri including investigation of intra-osseous vasculature in distal humerus. Acta Orthop Scand Suppl 1959;38:1-232.
36. Rudzki JR, Paletta GA Jr: Juvenile and adolescent elbow injuries in sports. Clin Sports Med 2004;23(4):581-608, ix.
37. Yocum LA: The diagnosis and nonoperative treatment of elbow problems in the athlete. Clin Sports Med 1989;8(3):439-451.
38. Kobayashi K, Burton KJ, Rodner C, et al: Lateral compression injuries in the pediatric elbow: Panner's disease and osteochondritis dissecans of the capitellum. J Am Acad Orthop Surg 2004;12(4):246-254.
39. McManama GB Jr, Micheli LJ, Berry MV, Sohn RS: The surgical treatment of osteochondritis of the capitellum. Am J Sports Med 1985;13(1):11-21.
40. Baumgarten TE, Andrews JR, Satterwhite YE: The arthroscopic classification and treatment of osteochondritis dissecans of the capitellum. Am J Sports Med 1998;26:520-523.
41. Takahara M, Ogino T, Sasaki I, et al: Long term outcome of osteochondritis dissecans of the humeral capitellum. Clin Orthop Relat Res 1999;363:108-115.
42. Bauer M, Jonsson K, Josefsson PO, Linden B: Osteochondritis dissecans of the elbow: a long-term follow-up study. Clin Orthop 1992;284:156-160.

CHAPTER 21

Injuries of the Shoulder and Arm

Part A SOFT-TISSUE SHOULDER INJURIES

Patrick St. Pierre, MD, and MAJ Rodney Gonzales, MD

KEY POINTS

- There are many causes of rotator cuff syndrome; however, nonoperative treatment is usually effective for controlling the pain and rehabilitating the rotator cuff muscles.
- Rotator cuff tears often require surgical repair, but small tears may be successfully treated nonoperatively.
- Shoulder dislocations are very common among young people, and the recurrence rate is very high. The risk of recurrent dislocation after a first-time dislocation diminishes with age.
- Rehabilitation is an extremely important part of the treatment of shoulder injuries. Restoring motion as well as strengthening the lower rotator cuff and periscapular stabilizers are the hallmarks of nonoperative or postoperative rehabilitation.
- Biceps tendinopathy is a common source of shoulder pain, and it may be the result of an acute injury or repetitive overuse. Biceps injuries range from tendinosis to frank tears within the tendon or at its insertion on the superior labrum.

INTRODUCTION

The shoulder girdle is made up of four articulations (sternoclavicular, acromioclavicular, glenohumeral, and scapulothoracic) and three bones (clavicle, scapula, and humerus). These articulations allow the shoulder girdle to provide a large range of motion for the hand to locate itself maximally in space. Shoulder injuries are frequent because of the increased vulnerability of the shoulder while providing this motion. Chronic shoulder injuries are often seen in overhead athletes; however, shoulder girdle injuries are also commonly caused by activities of daily living that involve repetitive overhead motions or in contact sports that involve direct trauma. Regardless of the mechanism, these injuries are evaluated and treated equally in all patients. Specific return-to-sport therapeutics may be added for patients who have special needs for certain sports.

ROTATOR CUFF SYNDROME AND IMPINGEMENT SYNDROME

Charles Neer, II, first proposed the term *impingement syndrome* when discussing pain that involved the subacromial bursa and the superior rotator cuff.[1] Impingement syndrome usually will start with some mild inflammation of the bursa and the rotator cuff tendons, which may in time progress to chronic pain, decreased range of motion, and rotator cuff weakness. Severe cases may lead to partial-thickness or full-thickness rotator cuff tears. Multiple causes not involving impingement have been described as leading to these symptoms, but all causes involve diminished rotator cuff function. Thus the term *rotator cuff syndrome*, which is inclusive of a combination of bursitis and rotator cuff tendinosis, may be a more appropriate to use to refer to these types of injuries.

Mechanism of injury

Patients with rotator cuff syndrome occasionally will recall a specific fall or injury to the shoulder as the start of their symptoms. However, many often do not recall a specific event or trauma that caused their symptoms to begin. Pain will frequently develop hours or even a day after the inciting overuse event. Other nontraumatic activities may be associated with the onset of symptoms, such as moving boxes, carrying luggage, or being involved in a weekend sports tournament. Typically, patients will complain of pain with overhead activities whether they are throwing, reaching into a high cabinet, or combing their hair. They may also complain of pain when sleeping on the affected side that will often awaken them at night. Itoi and colleagues[2] found that pain with motion is more commonly a feature of cuff tendinopathy than of having rest pain or night pain; they also reported that pain is most commonly located to the anterior or lateral portions of the shoulder.

Regardless of the cause of the symptoms, the final pathway of rotator cuff syndrome is identical. The chronic pain triggers atrophy of the rotator cuff muscles, which results in superior migration of the humeral head, first with activity and later with rest. The humeral head then compresses the subacromial bursa and the rotator cuff tendons against the acromion, which causes the impingement. This compression leads to greater inflammation of the subacromial bursa and of the rotator cuff tendon, which causes greater pain. Thus, the cycle of impingement continues, even when the patient may be doing everything possible to "baby" the affected shoulder. With continued compression, the rotator cuff tendon injury may progress to a partial or complete tear.

Risk factors

Risk factors for rotator cuff syndrome may be both intrinsic and extrinsic. Extrinsic risk factors include type III (or hooked) acromion, subacromial osteophyte formation, acromioclavicular joint arthritis that leads to inferior osteophytes, and coracoacromial ligament calcification. Each of these factors causes a decrease in the space between the acromion and the humeral head.

Intrinsic factors are typically a result of subtle instability leading to subacromial impingement with repetitive use of the arm above the horizontal plane. This may occur with traumatic instability that results in shoulder subluxation instead of dislocation.

The cause may also be atraumatic in nature and result from repetitive-use injuries in baseball, swimming, racquet sports, and weight lifting. However, there are non–sports-related activities that commonly lead to the symptoms of rotator cuff syndrome, such as painting, automotive or mechanical work, and lifting. Constant repetitive overhead activity of any type may lead to rotator cuff fatigue, which then leads to superior migration of the humeral head and the symptoms of rotator cuff syndrome.

Clinical features

Patients with rotator cuff syndrome will often complain of anterior–lateral shoulder pain. The pain will often radiate from the anterior–lateral aspect of the acromion distally to the deltoid insertion on the humerus. When the pain is felt at the distal deltoid insertion, it is the result of referred pain from the inflamed subacromial bursa. This inflamed bursa causes irritation to the deep portion of the deltoid, which then refers the pain to the distal insertion. Occasionally, when the infraspinatus is involved, pain will be noted posteriorly in the infraspinatus fossa.

The shoulder examination is described earlier in this book; however, there are some specific findings on examination that aid in the diagnosis of rotator cuff syndrome. Patients may have a painful arc of motion on forward flexion at varying degrees of elevation, and this is often even more noticeable with abduction. During the active range-of-motion part of the examination, the examiner should be attentive to abnormalities or asymmetries in scapular motion, and these should be assessed from both the front and back of the patient. Hiking of the scapula and anterior tilt of the acromion cause greater subacromial compression forces that lead to increased rotator cuff symptoms **(Figure 21A.1)**.

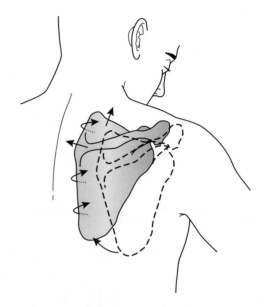

Figure 21A.1 Compensatory scapular rotation seen with chronic rotator cuff syndrome. (Redrawn from Frontera WR, Silver T: Essentials of Physical Medicine and Rehabilitation. Philadelphia, Hanley & Belfus, 2001.)

Strength testing should include the rotator cuff muscles as well as the deltoid, biceps, and triceps muscles. The supraspinatus muscle is best tested with a full-can test[3] rather than an empty-can test.[4] The infraspinatus and teres minor muscles can be examined by testing external rotation strength with the arm at the side. The subscapularis muscle is best tested by performing the lift-off test.[5] When internal rotation behind the back is not obtainable, the Napoleon or belly-press test may be used.[6]

Special tests when looking for rotator cuff syndrome include the Neer's impingement sign and test[1,7] and the Hawkins' sign.[8] When performing the Neer's impingement sign, the examiner stands to the side or just behind the seated patient. The arm is held in a maximal internal rotation, and then the arm is raised while scapular rotation is prevented by the examiner. This maneuver causes the greater tuberosity to rotate below the acromion, and this elicits pain if there is injury to the tendons or the bursa. Pain with this maneuver is a positive Neer's impingement sign. The Neer's impingement test is positive if, after a subacromial injection of a local anesthetic such as xylocaine, the pain is relieved with the same maneuver **(Figure 21A.2)**.

Hawkins and Kennedy[8] described the Hawkins' sign as an indicator of impingement. The examiner forward flexes the arm of the

Figure 21A.2 Neer's impingement sign and impingement test. (Redrawn from Marx JA, Hockberger R, Walls RM, et al: Rosen's Emergency Medicine: Concepts and Clinical Practice, 6th ed. Philadelphia, Mosby, 2005.)

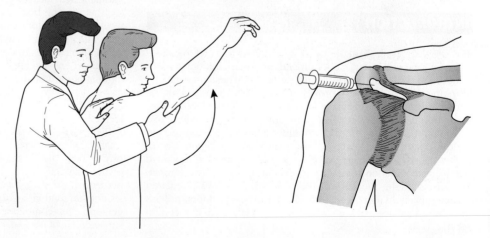

patient to 90 degrees and then forcibly internally rotates the shoulder. This maneuver causes the greater tuberosity to be drawn under the coracoacromial ligament. When this maneuver elicits pain, the sign is positive. Valadie and colleagues[9] showed that, if the examiner applies a downward pressure at the elbow with the patient resisting, the sensitivity of the examination is improved.

Diagnosis

The most common differential diagnosis for rotator cuff syndrome includes cervical spine pathology, calcific tendinitis, adhesive capsulitis, acromioclavicular joint degenerative joint disease, shoulder instability, and biceps tendinitis. Certain radiographs can help eliminate the possible causes of the pain, or they may reveal anatomic risk factors that are associated with rotator cuff syndrome.

The standard radiographs for evaluating the shoulder include the anteroposterior and axillary views. This allows diagnoses such as degenerative joint disease at the acromioclavicular joint and the glenohumeral joint, fractures, avascular necrosis, and calcific tendinitis to be evaluated. For patients with expected instability, a West Point view is obtained to assess the glenoid for a bony Bankart lesion. For patients with suspected rotator cuff pathology, the supraspinatus outlet view is used to determine the morphology of the acromion, which may possibly be causing an extrinsic risk factor that is involved with the rotator cuff syndrome.

Although magnetic resonance imagining (MRI) may be an excellent tool to assess rotator cuff pathology, it is often not needed during the early clinical evaluation and treatment of rotator cuff syndrome. If the patient has a full range of motion, normal radiographs, and no signs of instability, one should attempt nonoperative care first. If nonoperative care fails to improve the symptoms, then one can consider obtaining an MRI at a later evaluation. For patients with a more severe presentation, MRI may be ordered initially to evaluate for a rotator cuff tear **(Figure 21A.3)**. Plain radiographs should always be obtained first to rule out bony pathology.

The diagnosis of rotator cuff syndrome can be made after a careful history and physical examination that are consistent with the diagnosis. The examination and radiographs should also help eliminate other causes of the shoulder pain.

Treatment

The initial management of rotator cuff syndrome includes activity modification, pharmacologic modalities, and physical therapy. The treatment of rotator cuff syndrome is usually nonoperative; however, this type of treatment may not be effective for a small percentage of patients, and surgical intervention may then be required.

Initially, treatment consists of activity modification to avoid aggravating activity, pain control, and rehabilitation. Depending on the patient, acetaminophen or nonsteroidal anti-inflammatory drugs (NSAIDs) may initially be used to control pain and to allow for protective rehabilitation without pain. NSAIDs may have an added benefit of treating the inflammation in the subacromial bursa and reducing swelling. However, these typical pain relievers are often ineffective for providing pain relief for subacromial pain, especially when they are used in isolation.

Rehabilitation should be directed at improving pain-free range of motion and increasing rotator cuff strength. Morrison and colleagues[10] reported good results with nonoperative treatment of rotator cuff syndrome using NSAIDS and physical therapy modalities. Physical therapy was initially directed at soft-tissue stretching and range-of-motion exercises. As the patients progressed, only strengthening of the infraspinatus, teres minor, and subscapularis were added. These rotator cuff muscles were strengthened first because of the effect that they have with humeral head depression. After the patient developed full, pain-free motion, strengthening of the deltoid and supraspinatus were added. This treatment resulted in 67% of patients having excellent or good results; 28% had no improvement and later required surgical intervention. The remaining 5% had no improvement but refused additional treatment.

Rehabilitation should also be directed at strengthening the stabilizers of the scapula. Simple exercises such as squeezing the shoulder blades together and doing scapular rows can help with this. The effectiveness of this can be monitored by watching scapulothoracic motion. If this fails to improve, then one should consider other causes that lead to scapular winging, such as long thoracic nerve palsy. Tightness in the anterior shoulder (subscapularis and pectoralis minor muscles) can also lead to scapular dysfunction: hence the importance of a primary goal of rehabilitation being to restore full range of motion.

The second phase of treating pain and inflammation is the use of subacromial injections. Subacromial injections are performed with 1 to 3 mL of a corticosteroid with an additional 7 to 9 mL of local anesthetic. (See Chapter 48 for a complete discussion of injections.) The subacromial injection helps provide pain relief and decreases inflammation in the bursa, thus allowing patients to continue progression through rehabilitation. Subacromial injections are usually used after a failure of NSAIDs to control pain in patients who are unable to take NSAIDs or for severe acute pain that the provider does not think will respond to NSAIDs. Blair and colleagues[11] showed that, although patients who received subacromial steroid injections had greater increases with range of motion, they had no difference in functional status as compared with patients who did not receive injections. Initially, one can consider doing the steroid injection as part of the Neer's impingement test, thus confirming the diagnosis and starting treatment. The number of injections should be individualized on the basis of response, but most providers would limit the number of injections to three in patients who are surgical candidates.

If nonoperative therapy fails or if there is abnormal anatomy that causes a physical impingement, referral is indicated for possible surgical intervention. Neer[1] originally described an open subacromial decompression that involved removing spurs on the acromion, removing the inflamed bursa, and releasing the

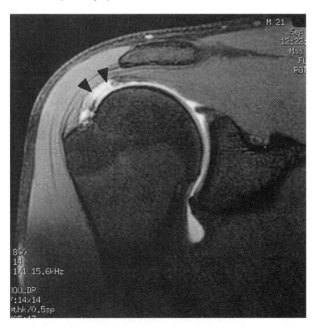

Figure 21A.3 Magnetic resonance imaging view of a retracted rotator cuff tear. (From Harris ED Jr: Kelley's Textbook of Rheumatology, 7th ed. Philadelphia, WB Saunders, 2005.)

coracoacromial ligament. However, current treatment is directed toward the cause of the syndrome because changes to the acromion are a secondary phenomenon and are thus not always present. With the development of arthroscopic techniques, subacromial decompression can be performed with a less invasive approach. Acromioplasty should be directed at removing only the bony excrescences and not injuring the body of the acromion. If the acromion is normal, a bursectomy alone is performed.[12] An intra-articular and bursal inspection is performed to treat associated pathology. Sachs and colleagues[13] showed that, although patients who undergo arthroscopic subacromial decompression have less pain and an earlier return to normal function, after a year, there in no significant difference in function between arthroscopic and open subacromial decompression.

Return to play

As part of the rehabilitation program, after the patient has restored pain-free range of motion, he or she can begin sport-specific exercises and rehabilitation. Return to full activity is allowed after the return of full motion and full strength without associated pain.

SHOULDER INSTABILITY AND LABRAL TEARS

In younger athletes, shoulder instability is a common problem. The exact incidence is not well described because there are a variety of presentations and because some athletes are able to adapt dynamically to mild instability. These patients have symptoms of recurrent dislocation, subluxation, and/or apprehension. *Apprehension* is the feeling of impending instability; *subluxation* is the sensation of the shoulder popping out and back into place; and *dislocation* is the disassociation of the glenohumeral joint. Some patients may have some laxity of the glenohumeral joint but without symptoms; this is commonly observed in patients with generalized joint laxity, and it may be normal for those patients. The physical finding of normal laxity should not be confused with the pathologic process of instability. Instability can also be described by the direction that the humeral head slides in relation to the glenoid fossa: anterior, posterior, inferior, superior, or multidirectional. Instability is usually divided into traumatic and atraumatic causes. Atraumatic instability may be the result of acquired microinstability or atraumatic multidirectional instability. This usually results in the stretching of the glenohumeral ligaments without detachment of the glenoid labrum. Traumatic dislocations usually result in a Bankart lesion (an avulsion of the anterior labrum from the glenoid) and possibly a Hill–Sachs lesion (an impaction fracture of the posterior humeral head).

Mechanism of injury

Unidirectional traumatic instability is usually described by direction, with anterior dislocations accounting for more than 90% of dislocations. Anterior instability is when the humeral head shifts anteriorly on the glenoid fossa. Dislocations are not usually caused by a direct blow to the shoulder but rather by a combination of forces that stress the anterior glenohumeral ligaments and force the humeral head out of the glenoid fossa. Characteristically, the arm is abducted and externally rotated when the force is applied to the arm. The force can be from falling on the ground in that position or from contact with another athlete or object that causes a posterior directed force on the arm that leads to the anterior displacement of the humeral head.

Anterior dislocations may cause detachment of the anterior labrum from the glenoid; this is also referred to as a *Bankart lesion*. Taylor and Arciero[14] report that 97% of their college-aged, first-time, traumatic dislocation patients had Bankart lesions

during arthroscopy. Anterior dislocations may also extend to the superior labrum, thus creating associated superior labrum anterior posterior tears.

With posterior instability, the arm receives a force that causes posterior displacement of the humeral head with respect to the glenoid fossa. This typically occurs with the arm forwardly elevated, internally rotated, and adducted, and it can occur by an athlete falling on an outstretched arm or receiving a blow from another athlete while having the arm in the position described previously. If the mechanism of injury is unknown or unwitnessed, one should consider seizures or electrical shock as possible causes of posterior dislocations.

Acquired microinstability is caused from the repetitive stretching of the shoulder ligaments as a result of activity. This can be seen in the overhand throwing athlete when excessive external rotation in the cocking position can lead to the subtle instability of the anterior capsule and glenohumeral ligaments. This slight anterior instability can lead to internal impingement with which the tendons of the supraspinatus and infraspinatus are impinged against the posterior superior labrum. This internal impingement has been described as leading to rotator cuff tears or labral tears.[15]

Patients with multidirectional instability, by definition, have instability in more than one direction. These patients may present with a history of multiple subluxations or dislocations that often can be self-reduced. However, the presenting complaint may be shoulder pain or numbness without knowledge of instability. The history of injury will help determine if the patient's primary complaint is anterior, posterior, or inferior instability. With anterior instability, the problems occur when the patient has the arm abducted and externally rotated. Posterior instability will cause symptoms when the arm is forward flexed and the patient is pushing an object. Inferior instability will lead to pain when carrying heavy objects at the side while the arms are straight down the side of the body. One direction usually dominates, but treatment should address all aspects

Risk factors and shoulder biomechanics

Some forms of instability are traumatic in nature; thus, participation in activities that lead to contact with the arm in positions that may cause traumatic instability is a risk factor. The shoulder has both static and dynamic stabilizers. Abnormalities or injuries to these structures increase the risk for instability.

The static stabilizers of the shoulder are made up of bone, cartilage, and ligaments **(Figure 21A.4)**. The scapula provides the base for the glenoid and sets up the orientation for the glenohumeral joint. The version of the scapula in relationship to the thorax and the version of the glenoid in relationship to the scapula are important factors in shoulder stability. The glenoid is a fossa that provides some stability, although it is limited as a result of not having a deep cavity. The labrum is the cartilaginous rim that provides additional stability to the humeral head by completely surrounding the glenoid and deepening the fossa for the humeral head to rest. It acts as a block to prevent the humeral head from sliding out, and it is the attachment of the glenohumeral ligaments. The inferior glenohumeral ligament complex looks like a hammock that rotates around the humeral head to provide support and that limits the excursion of the humeral head in relationship to the glenoid. It is deficiency of these ligaments, either by stretching or tearing, that leads to most forms of instability **(Figure 21A.5)**.

The dynamic stabilizers of the shoulder include the rotator cuff muscles (supraspinatus, infraspinatus, teres minor, and subscapularis), the long head of the biceps, and the scapular stabilizers (rhomboids, serratus anterior, trapezius, and levator scapulae). The role of the rotator cuff is essentially to keep the humeral head centered in the glenoid during normal use **(Figure 21A.6** on page 238). The scapula stabilizers ensure the proper version of the

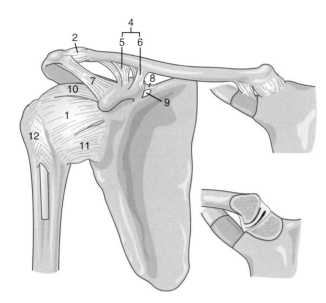

Figure 21A.4 Ligaments of the shoulder joint. 1, Capsule blends with rotator cuff tendon; 2, acromioclavicular ligament; 4, coracoclavicular ligament; 5, trapezoid ligament; 6, conoid ligament; 7, coracoacromial ligament or arch; 8 and 9, superior and inferior transverse ligament; 10, coracohumeral ligament; 11, glenohumeral ligament; and 12, transverse humeral ligament. (From Noble S: Textbook of Primary Care Medicine, 3rd ed. St. Louis, Mosby, 2001.)

scapula, and they provide for the proper motion of the scapula on the thorax during elevation. Injury to these dynamic stabilizers leads to shoulder dysfunction and further injury. Rehabilitation of these muscles is essential for the treatment of any type of shoulder injury.

The final mechanical factors that assist with shoulder stability are negative intra-articular pressure and the viscosity of the synovial fluid. Rotator cuff tears or shoulder instability may lead to the loss of these factors, thus compounding the symptoms.

Clinical features

The clinical features at presentation will depend on the type of instability present. Patients with anterior instability complain about the sensation of the shoulder slipping out with the arm abducted and externally rotated. With acute traumatic anterior instability, the patient is often in acute distress as a result of the anterior dislocation. The arm may be held in abduction and external rotation. Typically, the patient will try to support the arm in a neutral position. Movement of the arm at the glenohumeral joint causes considerable pain. Upon inspection, there is a loss of the deltoid contour and a prominent acromion that squares off the shoulder. Recurrent dislocations may cause the patient to have apprehension with overhead activity. Instability will be noted on examination by a positive apprehension test and a positive anterior load-and-shift test **(Figure 21A.7)**.

Patients who have posterior instability will complain of pain with pushing heavy objects (e.g., a door) with the arm forward flexed. In acute traumatic posterior instability, the arm is adducted and internally rotated. An anterior dimple may be appreciated on examination. The posterior aspect of the shoulder may appear rounded. The patient will be unable to externally rotate the arm as a result of the dislocation.

Patients with acquired microinstability have anterior capsule laxity. The patient may present with a vague complaint of pain. On examination, there is excessive external rotation; however, the arc of motion will typically be normal at 180 degrees, thus having decreased internal rotation. With anterior translation of the humerus on the glenoid, the patient may have some pain or apprehension.

Patients with atraumatic multidirectional instability typically have vague pain complaints. They may complain of having a sensation that the shoulder wants to slip out, but this may not be a presenting complaint. The physician should also inquire if the patient is able to self-dislocate the shoulder and in which direction. The classic signs on physical examination include a positive sulcus sign and generalized ligamentous laxity. The sulcus sign tests for inferior joint laxity, whereas the apprehension test will examine the anterior instability, and the jerk test checks for posterior instability. The examiner should also check for the laxity of other joints, including hyperextension of the knees and elbows.

Diagnosis

Acute traumatic instability can typically be determined on the basis of the history and the physical examination, as described previously. However, one should obtain radiographs, including the

Figure 21A.5 Inside view of the shoulder joint showing the relationship between the rotator cuff biceps tendon and the static stabilizers, including the superior, middle, and inferior glenohumeral ligaments. (From DeLee JC, Drez D Jr, Miller MD [eds]: DeLee & Drez's Orthopaedic Sports Medicine: Principles and Practice, 2nd ed. Philadelphian, WB Saunders, 2003.)

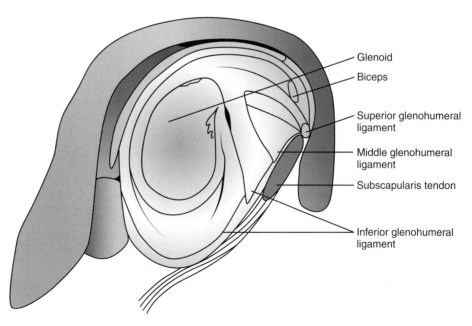

- Glenoid
- Biceps
- Superior glenohumeral ligament
- Middle glenohumeral ligament
- Subscapularis tendon
- Inferior glenohumeral ligament

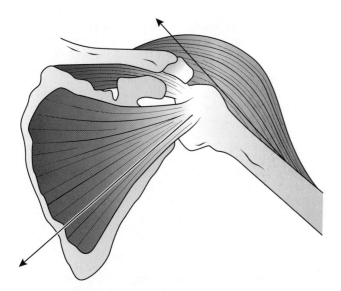

Figure 21A.6 The rotator cuff acts as a dynamic stabilizer, resisting the shear forces exerted on the glenohumeral joint by the larger muscles, including the deltoid, the pectoralis major, and the latissimus dorsi. (From DeLee JC, Drez D Jr, Miller MD [eds]: DeLee & Drez's Orthopaedic Sports Medicine: Principles and Practice, 2nd ed. Philadelphia, WB Saunders, 2003.)

anteroposterior view, the scapular Y view, and the West Point view. The anteroposterior view may incorrectly give the impression that the humeral head is reduced, and one view of the shoulder is not enough. The scapular Y view can assist with determining the direction of dislocation if there is any doubt after examination **(Figure 21A.8).**

The West Point view allows visualization of the anterior glenoid to determine if there are any bony fragments, as with a bony Bankart lesion. An additional view that can be obtained is the Stryker notch view, which documents humeral head impaction fractures (the Hill–Sachs lesion). Although immediate MRI is not necessary,

if labral injury is suspected, one may obtain an MRI study or a magnetic resonance arthrogram of the shoulder to look for labral tears or a Bankart lesion **(Figure 21A.9** on page 240).

Acquired microinstability is diagnosed by history and physical examination. No additional radiographic examination is necessary unless additional injury is suspected or the patient fails to respond to rehabilitation. MRI or magnetic resonance arthrogram can help determine if the microinstability has progressed to a labral tear or if there are any avulsions of the glenohumeral ligaments.

Atraumatic multidirectional instability is diagnosed by history and physical examination. Radiographic examination is not necessary unless the diagnosis is in doubt or other causes of shoulder pain are being evaluated.

Treatment

Acute traumatic instability should initially be treated by reduction of the dislocation. Before reduction of the dislocated shoulder, it may be necessary to premedicate the patient with intravenous pain medication and an anxiolytic. One may also consider the intra-articular injection of a local anesthetic. There are multiple methods that have been described for the reduction of anterior shoulder dislocations.

The Rockwood method is a two-person method in which one person wraps a sheet around the torso to stabilize the chest and to provide counter traction. The second person applies gentle traction of the affected arm in slight abduction. Internal and external rotation can be used to help disengage the humeral head. The Stimson method **(Figure 21A.10** on page 241) has the patient lying prone on a table. The affected arm is allowed to hang over the edge, with about 5 to 10 lb of weight providing gentle traction. This will cause the muscles to gradually relax, and then reduction will occur. The scapular manipulation technique also has the patient lying prone, with the arm flexed. A 5-lb to 15-lb traction is placed at the elbow. The scapula is then rotated medially by pushing the inferior tip toward the spine. With the Milch method, the patient lies supine. The arm is elevated, and then gentle abduction with external rotation is applied while the humeral head is pushed into place.

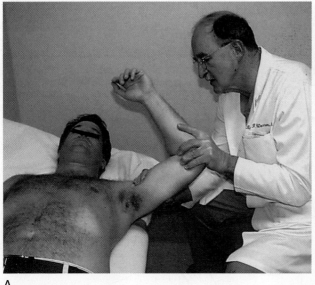
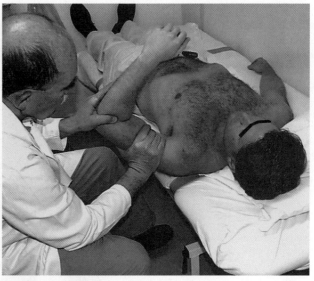

A   B

Figure 21A.7 *A,* The anterior apprehension test for anterior instability, with the patient supine. The arm is abducted 90 degrees, and the shoulder is increasingly externally rotated to stress the anterior capsule. *B,* The axial load test is performed with the patient supine and the arm abducted 90 degrees and in neutral rotation. While one hand applies an axial load, crepitation and translation are noted when the other hand applies an anteriorly and posteriorly directed force to the shoulder joint. (From DeLee JC, Drez D Jr, Miller MD [eds]: DeLee & Drez's Orthopaedic Sports Medicine: Principles and Practice, 2nd ed. Philadelphia, WB Saunders, 2003.)

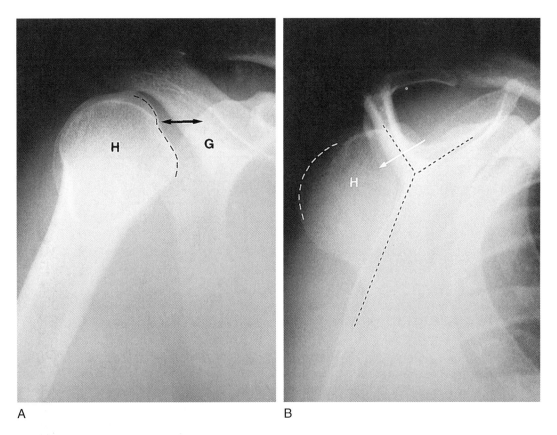

A B

Figure 21A.8 Posterior dislocation of the humeral head. *A,* An anteroposterior view of the shoulder initially looks fairly normal. However, an increased space *(double-ended arrow)* is present between the humeral head *(H)* and the glenoid *(G);* the fact that the humeral head is not spherical *(dotted line)* is another clue. *B,* On the Y view of the shoulder, the humeral head *(H)* can clearly be seen as displaced posteriorly relative to the central portion of the Y formed by the scapula. (From Mettler FA Jr: Essentials of Radiology, 2nd ed. Philadelphia, WB Saunders, 2005.)

The senior author's preferred method is one that has not been previously described, and it has been coined the *fulcrum method.* This has been developed from that author's technique for arthroscopic entry using the beach-chair position. With the patient in a sitting position, the practitioner's fist is placed in the injured shoulder's axilla to act as a fulcrum to separate the humeral head from the glenoid. Using the other hand to apply gentle internal and external rotation, a counter adduction force is applied to the patient's elbow using the practitioner's abdomen or with the help of an assistant. After the Hill-Sachs lesion is disengaged, internal rotation is applied to the humerus, thus placing the head within the glenoid. This technique has been used successfully on many occasions and is particularly useful in the acute setting. A reduction can be obtained quite easily without the use of narcotics and even with football shoulder pads still in place **(Figure 21A.11).**

For posterior shoulder dislocations, reduction can be performed with the patient lying in the supine position. Traction is applied to the arm in line with the deformity; the arm is flexed with internal rotation. It may be necessary during the traction to have lateral traction on the proximal humerus to allow the humeral head to disengage from its locked position. External rotation of the arm should be avoided **(Figure 21A.12 on page 242).**

After reduction, radiographs should be obtained to look for any bony pathology and to confirm the reduction. It is also important to perform a neurovascular examination before and after the reduction to evaluate for neurologic injury during the initial injury or reduction. Axillary nerve injury is a common complication of anterior shoulder dislocations, but this injury may also occur during the reduction. Axillary nerve function should be documented before and after reduction by checking sensation over the

deltoid (see the information about the badge sign in Chapter 9). Sling immobilization after reduction is recommended, although multiple authors have stated that the immobilization does not seem to affect the outcome in that recurrent dislocations are not decreased.[16-21] However, a recent study by Itoi and colleagues[22] suggests that immobilization with the arm in 30 degrees of external rotation reduces the recurrence rate by allowing better approximation of the labrum's Bankart lesion to the glenoid. This may in fact be true; however, it is very difficult to have a patient maintain this position for the required 4 to 6 weeks that are required for healing.

Patients who are less than 25 years old who have sustained a traumatic, first-time dislocation should be evaluated for the consideration of acute arthroscopic stabilization to reduce the high risk of recurrent dislocation. All patients meeting this criteria or who have had recurrent dislocation should be referred to an orthopedic surgeon for possible surgical repair.[19]

After immobilization, the patient should begin a rehabilitation program that is directed at strengthening the dynamic stabilizers of the shoulder. The rehabilitation program works on restoring the full range of motion by advancing a patient through passive range of motion to active assisted range of motion and then finally to full active range of motion. Rehabilitation will also focus on strengthening the muscles of the shoulder girdle. Strengthening of all of the dynamic stabilizers of the shoulder, including the rotator cuff and the scapula stabilizers, is an important part of instability rehabilitation.

Finally, braces may also be used to help protect the arm from being placed in a position of apprehension or potentially causing a recurrent dislocation. Multiple off-the-shelf braces exist to include the Shoulder Subluxation Inhibitor brace by Boston

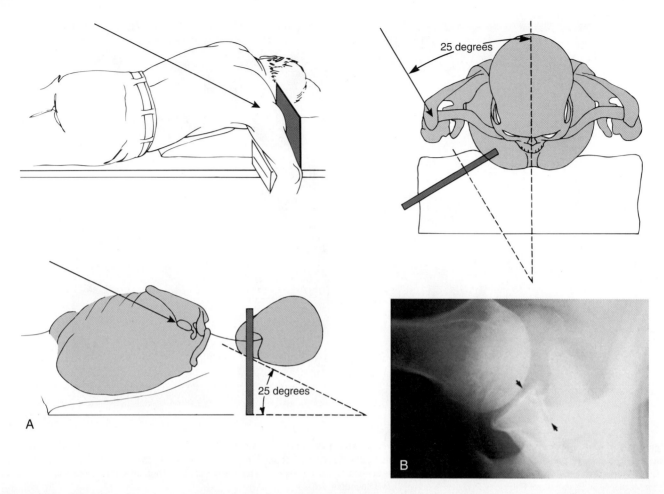

Figure 21A.9 West Point axillary view to visualize the anteroinferior glenoid rim for evidence of labral detachment or a rim fracture. *A,* Radiographic evaluation. *B,* Anteroinferior rim fracture *(arrows)* after anterior dislocation. (From Canale ST: Campbell's Operative Orthopaedics, 10th ed. Philadelphia, Mosby, 2003.)

Brace International, which limits the motion of the shoulder and which also provides some protection against direct blows. The Sawa Shoulder Brace by Brace International provides anterior support and adds a check rein to limit motion. DeCarlo and colleagues[23] found that the Shoulder Subluxation Inhibitor brace was more effective for limiting anterior shoulder subluxation; however, the Sawa brace was considered more comfortable. Braces are most helpful when trying to assist a player with finishing a season or for postoperative protection.

For acquired microinstability and multidirectional instability, rehabilitation is the mainstay of treatment. The patient's rehabilitation program is similar to that described previously. The focus will be on strengthening the dynamic stabilizers of the shoulder. For these patients, range of motion is usually less of an issue. Protective bracing is usually not necessary unless there are concerns about acute dislocations during activity. With acquired microinstability, surgery should be considered if rehabilitation fails. For patients with multidirectional instability, surgery should only be considered if rehabilitation is not effective and symptoms are preventing desired activity.

Return to play

Several factors must be considered before returning a player with a history of instability to sports participation. McCarty and colleagues[15] proposed their "ideal criteria" to determine whether an athlete is safe to return to play without an increased risk of injury. The "ideal criteria" involves six factors: (1) little or no pain; (2)

patient subjectivity; (3) near-normal range of motion; (4) near-normal strength; (5) normal functional ability; and (6) normal sports-specific skills. When most or all of these factors are met, then it is possible to begin returning the athlete to play. Play should be gradually introduced, especially for contact sports. A physician may also consider having the athlete wear a protective brace to help prevent him or her from getting into a position of risk.

BICEPS AND SUPERIOR LABRAL PATHOLOGY

The biceps muscle has two proximal origins and one distal attachment. Proximally, the long head of the bicep originates from the superior labrum. It exits the shoulder and passes through the bicipital groove between the greater and lesser tuberosities of the humerus. The short head of the biceps originates from the coracoid process. These two tendons join together just beyond the bicipital groove to form the belly of the biceps muscle. The distal attachment of the biceps is at the radial tuberosity. The biceps brachialis is the primary supinator of the forearm as well, and it assists with humeral elevation and flexion of the forearm. When the arm is externally rotated, the biceps assists with depressing the humeral head. The long head of the biceps is most susceptible to injury within the shoulder. Injury to this tendon includes biceps tendinosis, subluxation or dislocation of the biceps tendon, and biceps tendon rupture. Injury to the superior labrum may occur with biceps pathology or independently. The same mechanisms are often involved with the injuries that

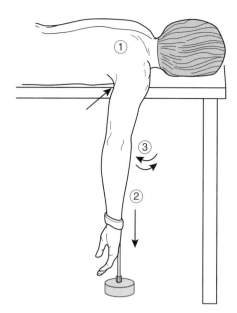

Figure 21A.10 Stimson technique. This technique is often tried first because it is the least traumatic if the patient can relax the shoulder muscles. 1, The patient is lying prone on the edge of the table. The physician must be careful that the sedated or intoxicated patient does not fall off the table. Belts or sheets can be used to secure the patient to the stretcher. 2, 5-kg weights are attached to the arm, and the patient maintains this position for 20 to 30 minutes, if necessary. 3, Occasionally, gentle external and internal rotation of the shoulder with manual traction aids reduction. (From Roberts JR, Hedges JR: Clinical Procedures in Emergency Medicine, 4th ed. Philadelphia, WB Saunders, 2004.)

were initially classified by Snyder and colleagues[24] and that are described in **Figure 21A.13.** Superior labrum anterior-posterior tears will often need surgical treatment if the symptoms continue after a short course of rest and rehabilitation.

Mechanism of injury

Biceps tendinosis can develop within the long head of the biceps tendon. The tendinosis develops in the tendon at the bicipital groove as a result of repetitive movements such has overhead

throwing and lifting. The tendinosis usually begins as microscopic tearing and fraying and then causes inflammation within the tendon.[25] Curtis and Snyder[26] found that these lesions tend to extend proximally and that they are commonly associated with other shoulder pathology, such as rotator cuff syndrome.[26]

Biceps tendon subluxation or dislocation as an isolated phenomenon is uncommon. If it occurs, the site of instability will be medially along the bicipital groove,[27] and it is often associated with a tear of the subscapularis tendon. Less frequently, there is an associated tear of the supraspinatus tendon.

Biceps tendon tears typically occur in the long head portion of the tendon. Long head tendon ruptures account for 96% of all bicep ruptures, with distal attachment accounting for 3% and short head accounting for 1%.[27] Tears occur at the labral attachment, within the bicipital groove or at the muscle tendon junction. Although a history of tendinosis within the biceps tendon can increase the risk of rupture within the substance of the tendon, ruptures at the muscle tendon junction tend to be caused by a traumatic event. Garrett and colleagues[28] showed that abrupt eccentric contraction of the biceps muscle can cause a tear of the long head biceps tendon at the muscle tendon junction.

Risk factors

Major risk factors for biceps tendinosis include repetitive overhead activities such as overhead throwing and weight lifting. Acute traumatic injuries may also occur. Because of its association with rotator cuff syndrome, having additional shoulder pathology is likely to increase the risk of developing biceps tendinosis. Risk factors for subluxation or dislocation of the biceps tendon are disruptions in supporting capsular ligaments or rotator cuff tendons. Levinsohn and Santelli[29] showed that having a shallow bicipital groove also increases the risk for medial subluxation of the biceps tendon. Increased risk for biceps tendon rupture includes a history of recurrent biceps tendinosis, contralateral biceps tendon rupture, a history of rotator cuff tear, older age, poor conditioning, and rheumatoid arthritis.

Clinical features

Patients with biceps tendinopathy will typically complain of pain in the anterior aspect of the shoulder. However, the location and quality of pain may be vague. The patient may have a snapping or clicking sensation, especially with biceps subluxation; this may be

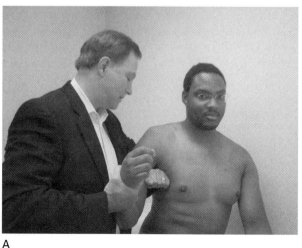

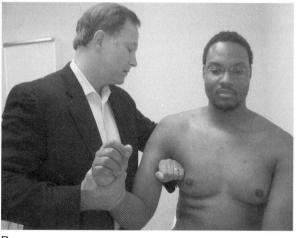

A   B

Figure 21A.11 The fulcrum method of shoulder reduction uses the fist in the axilla and pressure on the elbow to disengage the Hill-Sachs lesion. Gentle rotation of the shoulder with the other hand reduces the head into the glenoid fossa.

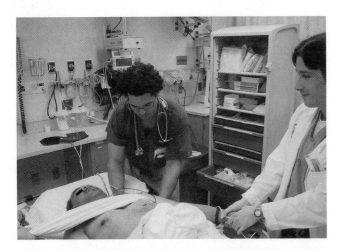

Figure 21A.12 Reduction of a posterior shoulder dislocation. With countertraction being applied, traction on the internally rotated and adducted arm is combined with posterior pressure on the humeral head to effect reduction. (From Roberts JR, Hedges JR: Clinical Procedures in Emergency Medicine, 4th ed. Philadelphia, WB Saunders, 2004.)

exacerbated with external rotation. Because of the potentially associated impingement syndrome, the patient may also have signs and symptoms that are consistent with impingement syndrome. Having localized tenderness over the bicipital groove can help distinguish biceps tendinopathy from pure impingement syndrome. With biceps tendon ruptures, the patient may report having sudden pain in the upper arm that was associated with a snap. This can be followed by a muscle bulge developing in the arm from the contraction of the biceps muscle.

On physical examination, with biceps tendinosis, subluxation, or dislocation, the appearance of the shoulder and arm may be normal. However, with biceps tendon ruptures of the long head, the presence of a bulge in the distal arm as a result of retraction of the biceps muscle is common. In acute cases, the patient may also have ecchymosis tracking down the arm. If the patient attempts to contract the biceps against resistance, the muscle bulge will become more prominent. The Ludington test is a maneuver that can be done to help accentuate the asymmetric appearance of the biceps muscle as compared with the contralateral side. The patient interlocks the fingers of both hands behind the head and then flexes the biceps muscle.[26] Patients with biceps tendon ruptures may have weakness that is appreciated when doing strength testing of the biceps; however, many may have normal strength to manual testing.

Another important physical examination is Speed's test. Speed's test is done by the examiner providing resistance to arm flexion while the patient has the arm extended and supinated at the elbow. Pain localized to the bicipital groove is considered a positive test.[26] This test is not specific for biceps tendinitis. Bennett showed that it had a specificity of 14% and sensitivity of 90% from inflammation of the biceps tendon and superior labrum anterior-posterior lesions.[31] Yergason's sign was originally described as the "supination sign" in 1931. Yergason's observations showed that this sign is positive with biceps tendinosis but negative with supraspinatus tendon tears. Yergason's sign is performed by having the patient flex at the elbow to 90 degrees while having the arm pronated. Resistance is then applied while the patient attempts to actively supinate the forearm. Pain localized to the bicipital groove is considered a positive test.[30] With biceps tendon subluxation, it is possible to palpate the tendon subluxation by putting the shoulder in about 80 to 90 degrees of abduction and then alternately rotating the arm internally and externally.[25]

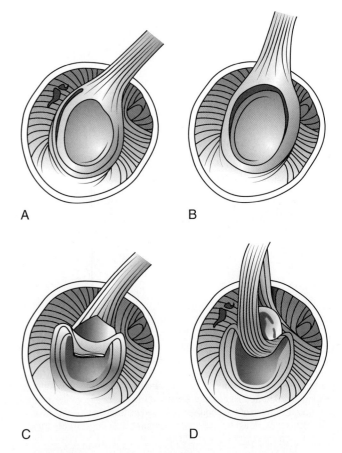

Figure 21A.13 The original Snyder classification of superior labrum anterior-posterior lesions. *A*, Type I has degenerative superior labrum tearing but attached biceps. *B*, Type II has detachment of the superior labrum/biceps tendon complex from the superior glenoid. *C*, Type III has a bucket handle tear of a meniscoid superior labrum but attached biceps. *D*, Type IV has tearing of the superior labrum up into the biceps tendon. Variable amounts of the biceps are left attached. (From DeLee JC, Drez D Jr, Miller MD [eds]: DeLee & Drez's Orthopaedic Sports Medicine: Principles and Practice, 2nd ed. Philadelphia, WB Saunders, 2003.)

Diagnosis

Biceps tendinopathy can be diagnosed on the basis of the history and the physical examination; however, there are many other diagnoses that can produce the same set of symptoms. The examiner must look for other shoulder pathology (e.g., rotator cuff syndrome) because it is not uncommon to have other problems in the shoulder with biceps tendinopathy. Although radiographic imaging is not necessary for the diagnosis of biceps tendon injury, it is helpful for ruling out other conditions. Radiographs should include the anteroposterior, axillary, outlet, and bicipital groove views.

MRI provides an anatomic view of the biceps tendon. MRI also helps diagnose rotator cuff tears and superior labrum anterior posterior lesions, which may be associated with biceps tendon injuries. Magnetic resonance arthrogram has been shown to be more accurate than MRI alone for evaluating biceps and superior labral pathology.[31] The transverse cuts demonstrate the biceps tendon's relationship to the bicipital groove as well as the presence of swelling within the tendon sheath and tendinosis within the tendon. Oblique coronal views best demonstrate the superior labrum and the presence of superior labrum anterior–posterior tears.

Treatment

Biceps tendon injuries are first treated with rehabilitation. Because biceps tendon injuries are often associated with other shoulder pathology such as rotator cuff syndrome, the rehabilitation and treatment should focus on the primary diagnosis. Modalities include rest, NSAIDs, analgesics, rehabilitation, and counter-force bracing. Rehabilitation should focus not only on the biceps tendon but also on any other associated shoulder pathology. Counter-force bracing can be used proximally to the biceps muscle belly. Injections are often helpful for the diagnosis and treatment of biceps injuries in a way that is similar to that described previously for the subacromial bursa. If the patient does not respond to conservative measures, then surgical options can be considered. Surgery should also focus on the primary diagnosis.

When true biceps tendon subluxation or dislocation is diagnosed, the patient is unlikely to fully recover with nonoperative treatment. However, if there is a contraindication for surgery or if the patient desires a trial period of nonoperative treatment, therapy for rotator cuff and scapular stabilization should be attempted. If conservative measures fail or the injury is limiting desired activities, then surgical treatment options should be considered. A primary repair aims to stabilize the biceps tendon within the bicipital groove. Repairing the transverse humeral ligaments and addressing tears of the subscapularis tendon can achieve this. A more common option is a biceps tenotomy or tenodesis to the humerus. This can be achieved arthroscopically as well as with the use of open techniques.

For biceps tendon tears, the treatment should be individualized for each patient. Most authors agree that, with older, sedate individuals, even complete tears of the biceps tendon can be treated nonoperatively and with rehabilitation. Results have shown that patients have minimal to no functional loss, and patients are often satisfied with their results.[26,32] With a younger, more active patient, surgical options are favored; these usually provide better cosmesis and strength.[26,33] With tenotomy, the tendon is debrided, and the damaged tendon is released to retract distally. With tenodesis, the biceps tendon is reattached to a different location, such as the proximal humerus or the surrounding rotator cuff.[34]

Return to play

A patient may return to activity after biceps tendon injury when their symptoms of pain and weakness have improved. The rehabilitation program is similar to that previously described and should include building up to sport-specific or occupational-specific activities. Other associated shoulder pathology should also be treated during this rehabilitation.

REFERENCES

1. Neer CS II: Anterior acromioplasty for the chronic impingement syndrome in the shoulder: a preliminary report. J Bone Joint Surg 1972;54A:41-50.
2. Itoi E, Minagawa H, Yamamoto N, et al: Are pain location and physical examinations useful in locating a tear site of the rotator cuff? Am J Sports Med 2006;34(2): 256-264.
3. Kelly BT, Kadrmas WR, Speer KP: The manual muscle examination for rotator cuff strength: an electromyographic investigation. Am J Sports Med 1996;24:581-588.
4. Jobe FW, Moynes DR: Delineation of diagnostic criteria and a rehabilitation program for rotator cuff injuries. Am J Sports Med 1982;10:336-339.
5. Gerber C, Krushell RJ: Isolated rupture of the tendon of the subscapularis muscle. J Bone Joint Surg 1991;73B:389-394.
6. Gerber C, Hersche O, Farron A: Isolated rupture of the subscapularis tendon. J Bone Joint Surg 1996;78A:1015-1023.
7. Neer CS II: Impingement lesions. Clin Orthop 1983;173:70-77.
8. Hawkins RJ, Kennedy JC: Impingement syndrome in athletes. Am J Sports Med 1980;8:151-158.
9. Valadie AL III, Jobe CM, Pink MM, et al: Anatomy of provocative tests for impingement syndrome of the shoulder. J Shoulder Elbow Surg 2000;9:36-46.
10. Morrison DS, Frogameni AD, Woodworth P: Non-operative treatment of subacromial impingement syndrome. J Bone Joint Surg 1997;79A:732-737.
11. Blair B, Rokio AS, Cuomo F, et al: Efficacy of injections of corticosteroids for subacromial impingement syndrome. J Bone Joint Surg 1996;78A:1685-1689.
12. Budoff JE, Rodin D, Ochiai D, et al: Arthroscopic rotator cuff debridement without decompression for the treatment of tendinosis. Arthroscopy 2005;21:1081-1089.
13. Sachs R, Stone ML, Devine S: Open vs. arthroscopic acromioplasty: a prospective, randomized study. Arthroscopy 1994;10:248-254.
14. Taylor DC, Arciero RA: Pathologic changes associated with shoulder dislocations. Arthroscopic and physical examination findings in first-time, traumatic anterior dislocations. Am J Sports Med 1997;25:306-311.
15. McCarty EC, Ritchie P, Gill HS, et al: Shoulder instability: return to play. Clin Sports Med 2004;23:335-351.
16. Rowe CR: Prognosis in dislocations of the shoulder. J Bone Joint Surg 1956;38A:957-976.
17. Henry JH, Genung JA: Natural history of glenohumeral dislocation—revisited. Am J Sports Med 1982;10:135-137.
18. Simonet WT, Cofield RH: Prognosis in anterior shoulder dislocation. Am J Sports Med 1984;12:19-24.
19. Wheeler JH, Ryan JB, Arciero RA, et al: Arthroscopic versus nonoperative treatment of acute shoulder dislocations. Arthroscopy 1989;5:213-217.
20. Hovelius L, Augustini BG, Fredin H, et al: Primary anterior dislocation of the shoulder in young patients. A ten-year prospective study. J Bone Joint Surg 1996;78A: 1677-1684.
21. Kralinger FS, Golser K, Wischatta R, et al: Predicting recurrence after primary anterior shoulder dislocation. Am J Sports Med 2002;30:116-120.
22. Itoi E, Hatakeyama Y, Kido T, et al: A new method of immobilization after traumatic anterior dislocation of the shoulder: a preliminary study. J Shoulder Elbow Surg 2003;12:413-415.
23. DeCarlo M, Malone K, Geric B, et al: Evaluation of shoulder instability braces. J Sports Rehabil 1996;5:143-150.
24. Snyder SJ, Karzel RP, Del Pizzo W, et al: SLAP lesions of the shoulder. Arthroscopy 1990;6:274-279.
25. Neviaser R: Lesions of the biceps and tendinitis of the shoulder. Orthop Clin North Am 1980;11:343-348.
26. Curtis AS, Snyder SJ: Evaluation and treatment of biceps tendon pathology. Orthop Clin North Am 1993;24:33-43.
27. Aldridge JW, Bruno RJ, Strauch RJ, et al: Management of acute and chronic biceps tendon rupture. Hand Clin 2000;16:497-503.
28. Garrett WE Jr Safran MR, Seaber AV, et al: Biomechanical comparison of stimulated and nonstimulated skeletal muscle pulled to failure. Am J Sports Med 1987;15:448-454.
29. Levinsohn E, Santelli ED: Bicipital groove dysplasia and medial dislocation of the biceps brachii tendon. Skeletal Radiol 1991;20:419-423.
30. Crenshaw AH, Kilgore WE: Surgical treatment of bicipital tenosynovitis. J Bone Joint Surg 1966;48A:1496-1502.
31. Bennett WF: Specificity of the Speed's test: arthroscopic technique for evaluating the biceps tendon at the level of the bicipital groove. Arthroscopy 1998;14:789-796.
32. Yergason RM: Supination sign. J Bone Joint Surg 1931;13:160.
33. Mariani EM, Cofield RH, Askew LJ: Rupture of the tendon of the long head of the biceps brachii: surgical versus nonsurgical treatment. Clin Orthop 1998;228: 233-239.
34. Gill TJ, McIrvin E, Mair SD, et al: Results of biceps tenotomy for treatment of pathology of the long head of the biceps brachii. J Shoulder Elbow Surg 2001;10:247-249.

Part B SHOULDER FRACTURES AND CLAVICULAR JOINT INJURIES

Patrick St. Pierre, MD, and MAJ Rodney Gonzales, MD

KEY POINTS

- Acromioclavicular joint injuries (shoulder separations) are very common and can often be treated nonoperatively; however, they may lead to late arthritis.

- The medial clavicular growth plate is the last physis in the body to fuse, and sternoclavicular joint injuries in patients who are in their late teens or early 20s may actually be growth plate fractures or dislocations.

- Midshaft clavicle fractures in adults were thought to be best treated nonoperatively. However, closer evaluation of clinical results reveals the possibility of significant morbidity, and newer operative techniques may result in improved outcomes.

- Scapula fractures are best treated nonoperatively unless the fracture extends into the glenoid or alters the orientation of the glenoid significantly.

- Proximal humerus fractures may be treated nonoperatively if there is minimal displacement; however, if displacement is noted on radiographs, operative consideration is indicated.

INTRODUCTION

There are three bones that make up the shoulder girdle: the clavicle, the scapula, and the humerus. Soft-tissue injuries, as described in the previous section, are more common; however, contact sports often result in injury to the bone and joint structures of the shoulder. Injury to the glenohumeral joint was described with shoulder instability in the previous section. The sternoclavicular (SC) and acromioclavicular (AC) joints are also susceptible to injury, and they are covered in this chapter. Fractures can also occur in all three bones of the shoulder girdle. Common athletic injuries also include fractures of the clavicle and the proximal humerus.

STERNOCLAVICULAR JOINT ARTHROPATHIES

The SC joint is the only true joint that links the axial skeleton and the upper extremity. The SC joint has the least amount of bony stability as compared with other joints in the body; however, it is infrequently injured. The SC joint is stabilized by the joint capsule and the costoclavicular ligaments **(Figure 21B.1).**

Three main arthropathies occur at the SC joint: subluxation, dislocation, and degenerative arthritis. The first two are included in the grading of SC sprains, whereas the latter is a chronic condition of the SC joint. The patient's medial growth physis of the clavicle is the last growth physis to close, and it may not do so until approximately 23 to 25 years of age.

Mechanism of injury

Despite having minimal bony stability, injury to the SC joint takes a significant amount of force. This force may be applied directly to the shoulder and clavicle, such as what occurs with a direct blow anteriorly from trauma during a contact sport or a motor vehicle accident. However, injury to the SC joint is most often the result of an indirect force, such as an athlete falling on the lateral aspect of the shoulder, perhaps during a football tackle. Subluxations or dislocations typically occur as the result of a single traumatic event. However, chronic subluxations may be a result of repeated events that are not severe enough to cause a true dislocation. Degenerative arthritis of the SC joint is usually seen in individuals that have had previous traumatic injury to the SC joint.

Dislocations of the SC joint are described by the direction that the clavicle disassociates from the sternum. Anterior dislocations are much more common than posterior dislocations. Nettles and Linscheid[1] revealed that 95% of the cases that they reviewed were anterior dislocations. Posterior dislocations are more serious due to the risk of injury to the great vessels and the airway by the medial portion of the clavicle.

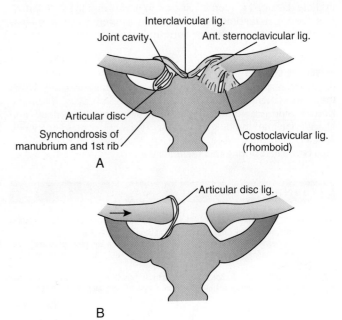

Figure 21B.1 *A,* Normal anatomy around the sternoclavicular joint. Note that the articular disk divides the sternoclavicular joint cavity into two separate spaces and inserts onto the superior and posterior aspects of the medical clavicle. *B,* The articular disk ligament (lig.) acts as a checkrein for a medial displacement of the proximal clavicle. (Redrawn from DeLee JC, Drez D Jr, Miller MD [eds]: DeLee & Drez's Orthopaedic Sports Medicine: Principles and Practice, 2nd ed. Philadelphia, WB Saunders, 2003.)

Risk factors

Participation in contact sports such as football or rugby has an inherently increased risk of injury. SC injury can also be seen with falls and motor vehicle accidents. Postmenopausal women have an increased risk of developing spontaneous arthritis of the SC joint, but the mechanism behind this relationship is not clearly understood.

Clinical features

Injury to the SC joint is typically graded I, II, or III on the basis of the degree of injury. With grade I SC sprains, there is stretching and partial tearing of the sternoclavicular ligaments. The costoclavicular ligament is usually not involved. This usually does not cause any instability, but it may result in late arthritis. With grade II SC sprains, there is a complete tear of the SC ligaments and the SC joint capsule. The costoclavicular ligament may be stretched or have partial tearing. Instability of the SC joint is present, with possible subluxation. Grade III SC sprains involve a dislocation of the SC joint, either anteriorly or posteriorly. There is complete tearing of the SC and costoclavicular ligaments.

Patients will typically present with pain over the SC joint. However, as a result of the significant force necessary to cause injury to the SC joint, the patient may have other traumatic injury that distracts both the patient and the examiner from the SC joint injury. The patient may present with other life-threatening injuries that warrant immediate attention. Conversely, when one suspects injury to the SC joint (especially a posterior dislocation), one must ensure that the patient is stable. Checking for difficulty with breathing or swallowing and for possible choking will help determine if the posterior dislocation may have caused injury to other vital organs.

With grade I SC sprains, the patient will often present with pain at the SC joint that increases with arm movement. On examination, there may be some slight swelling and tenderness; however, no instability of the SC joint will be appreciated. With a grade II SC sprain, the patient will also complain of pain that is increased with arm movement. On examination, the patient will also have subluxation of the SC joint. This can occur both anteriorly and posteriorly.

With grade III anterior SC joint dislocations, the patient will have severe pain. Any movement of the shoulder will increase the pain. The patient prefers to sit and keep the arm on the affected side, supported across the trunk by the unaffected arm. When lying supine, the patient will complain of worsening of the pain as a result of the stress across the SC joint. The medial end of the clavicle at the SC joint is visibly prominent in grade III anterior injuries.

With grade III posterior SC joint dislocation, the patient will also have severe pain that increases with any arm movement. The arm position will be similar to anterior dislocation because the patient will support it with the unaffected side, and he or she will prefer to sit up. The prominence of the medial aspect of the clavicle is not visible. On palpation, the medial aspect of the clavicle will be posteriorly displaced. Careful examination of the upper extremity, the neck, and the cardiac and respiratory systems must be done to evaluate for vital organ damage.

Diagnosis

When an athlete has an injury near the SC joint, it is important to rule out fracture of the medial clavicle. In the differential diagnosis for the skeletally immature athlete is a physeal injury to the medial growth plate of the clavicle. When an SC joint injury is suspected, radiographs should be obtained immediately. Routine anteroposterior (AP) and lateral views of the chest may not show dislocations, even when present. A cephalic tilt view, which is an AP view with approximately 45 degrees of cephalic tilt, will better reveal anterior and posterior displacement at the clavicle.

A computed tomography (CT) scan is often helpful for making the diagnosis and determining the degree of injury. The CT scan will help determine displacement, and it allows for the evaluation of the physis in the skeletally immature patient. Some authors advocate obtaining a CT scan for all SC joint injuries.[2] With posterior dislocations, a CT scan will also help with the evaluation for possible injury to other vital organs. Magnetic resonance imaging is not usually necessary unless the physician is attempting to evaluate adjacent soft-tissue injury.

Treatment

The treatment of SC joint injuries depends on the severity of the injury. Grade I and II SC sprains will often heal completely, without any residual effects. Grade I SC sprains are often treated effectively with rest, ice, and a sling for about 4 to 5 days. Grade II SC sprains are treated in a similar fashion, and the duration of immobilization is directed by symptoms, taking up to 4 to 6 weeks. For both grades, the gradual resumption of activity through a rehabilitation program follows rest and immobilization.[3]

For acute grade III anterior SC joint dislocations, an attempt at reduction should be made. Reduction can be done with the patient lying supine, with a bolster under the thoracic spine and the arm abducted 90 degrees. The arm is extended 10 to 15 degrees with gradually increased traction, whereas the medial end of the clavicle is pushed posteriorly.[2] Although the reduction is usually successful, it is generally unstable, and it may redislocate. After reduction, the extremity should be immobilized with a figure-of-eight harness and sling for 4 to 6 weeks. After the period of immobilization, the athlete should only participate in light to moderate activity for 2 weeks before progressing to more strenuous activity. If the reduction is not successful or if the injury redislocates after reduction, one should treat it as a grade II SC sprain and seek orthopedic consultation. Despite the dislocation, most patients are able to have painless function of the extremity.[1,4] Operative treatment of anterior SC dislocations is controversial; however, most agree to avoid metallic transfixion of the SC joint as a result of the risk of pin migration.[5] Anterior dislocations that have been present for more than 7 to 10 days should be treated conservatively. If symptoms continue beyond 6 to 12 months, then surgery may be considered.

Grade III posterior SC joint dislocations should be reduced as soon as possible. Other life-threatening associated injuries, such as a pneumothorax, may require treatment and stabilization before the reduction. If the patient is otherwise stable and the dislocation is less then 7 to 10 days old, closed reduction should be attempted. The patient lies supine with a bolster under the thoracic spine, the arm is abducted to 90 degrees, and then the arm is extended 10 to 15 degrees, with traction applied. The reduction may spontaneously occur; however, it may be necessary to try and manually pull the medial clavicle anteriorly with either the fingers or a towel clip[2] **(Figure 21B.2).**

As a result of the risk of injury to the underlying vital organs, immediate reduction is necessary. If closed reduction fails, an orthopedic surgeon should evaluate the patient for open reduction. After successful reduction, the patient should be placed in a figure-of-eight harness and sling for 6 weeks. After 6 weeks, strenuous activity should be avoided for an additional 2 weeks while gradual rehabilitation and return to activity begins. If a patient presents with a posterior dislocation of more than 7 to 10 days duration, open reduction is the preferred treatment option.[5]

For patients who are less than 23 to 25 years of age and thus whose medial growth plate may not closed, both anterior and posterior dislocations may be conservatively managed. In these

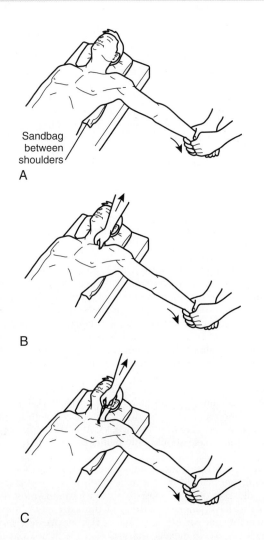

Sandbag
between
shoulders

A

B

C

Figure 21B.2 Technique for closed reduction of the sternoclavicular joint. *A*, The patient is positioned supine with a sandbag placed between the two shoulders. Traction is then applied to the arm against countertraction in an abducted and slightly extended position. With an anterior dislocation, direct pressure over the medial end of the clavicle may reduce the joint. *B*, For a posterior dislocation, in addition to the traction, it may be necessary to manipulate the medial end of the clavicle with the fingers to dislodge the clavicle from behind the manubrium. *C*, In a stubborn posterior dislocation, it may be necessary to sterilely prepare the medial end of the clavicle and use a towel clip to grasp around the medial clavicle to lift it back into position. (From Rockwood CA Jr, Green DP, Bucholz RW [eds]: Rockwood and Green's Fractures in Adults, 3rd ed. Philadelphia, JB Lippincott, 1991.)

patients, the injury is usually a physeal injury, and, as a result of the potential for remodeling, expectant management is often all that is necessary. If symptoms indicate risk to the underlying vital structures, then operative management should be considered.

Return to play

After the athlete has completed the immobilization period, rehabilitation is initiated to work toward full, painless motion. With grade I injuries, the athlete is often able to return within a week. Grade II injuries often require 6 weeks before the athlete is able to begin rehabilitation. Grade III injuries also typically require 6 to

8 weeks before return to play is an option. With posterior dislocations, contact sports should be avoided for 3 months after injury to avoid recurrent dislocation.[2] Return-to-play criteria for all grades is full, pain-free range of motion with normal strength of the upper extremity.

STERNOCLAVICULAR JOINT DEGENERATIVE ARTHRITIS

Damage to the sternoclavicular joint may lead to osteoarthritic changes with time. Often these are a result of low-grade sprains, and they do not involve instability at the time of original injury. These injuries present with chronic pain at the SC joint that is aggravated by increased upper extremity activity. Commonly, there is crepitus at the SC joint with motion and a grinding with palpation. As with other arthritic conditions, this condition should be treated with analgesics or anti-inflammatory drugs. When severe pain persists despite nonoperative treatment, surgical resection of the proximal clavicle may be performed.[1,5] This procedure is very reliable for pain relief, but often the patient may feel a loss of strength because of the loss of the medial buttress that the SC joint provides.

ACROMIOCLAVICULAR JOINT ARTHROPATHIES

A large percentage of shoulder girdle injuries occur at the AC joint. The ligaments that stabilize the AC joint are the acromioclavicular ligaments and the coracoclavicular ligaments (trapezoid and conoid ligaments). The AC joint is the second most commonly dislocated major joint, with the glenohumeral joint being the most common. Much like the SC joint, the main injuries of the AC joint are instability and degenerative disease. Although the AC joint has less mobility than the SC joint, it is more frequently injured, and it can be injured with much less force. Chronic irritation or injury of the AC joint can lead to degenerative changes within the joint that cause significant disability, especially with overhead activity and lifting. An AC sprain is commonly referred to as a "shoulder separation."

Mechanism of injury

Most AC joint injuries result from a fall on the point of the shoulder with the arm adducted, such as falling to the side and striking the ground with the lateral shoulder. The impact with the ground causes an inferior and medially directed force along the acromion. This drives the acromion medially, causing superior displacement of the clavicle and disruption of the lateral clavicular ligaments.[5] These ligaments often have an injury pattern that is sequential, with the first ligaments injured being the acromioclavicular ligaments **(Figure 21B.3).** The injury may begin as a stretch or partial tear to the ligament, but if the force is severe enough, a complete tear can occur. Next, the coracoclavicular ligaments are injured, beginning with the trapezoid and then progressing to the conoid ligament. If the force is severe enough, both the acromioclavicular and the coracoclavicular ligaments can be torn.[6] This renders the distal clavicle completely unstable.

Risk factors

The risk of injury to the AC joint is increased in those that play contact sports. It is also a more common injury among male athletes. Athletes who fall from bicycles or horses, ski jump, or participate in other noncontact sports that may involve falls have a high incidence of AC joint injury.

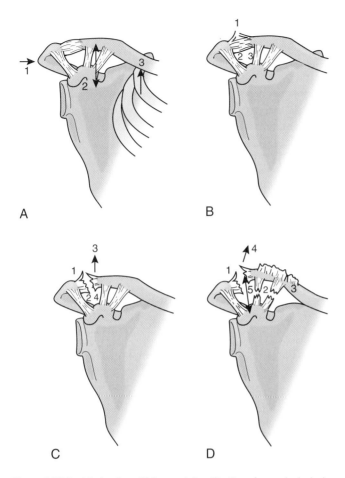

A   B

C   D

Figure 21B.3 Mechanism of injury and classification of acromioclavicular joint injuries. *A*, The direct force is applied to the point of the shoulder (1); the scapula and the attached clavicle are forced downward and medially; the clavicle approaches the first rib (2). If the force continues, the first rib abuts the clavicle, thus producing a counterforce (3). Depending on the magnitude of the force, a grade I, II, or III sprain may occur. *B*, Grade I sprain. A few fibers of the acromioclavicular ligament stretch, and a few tear (1); the acromioclavicular joint is stable (2); and the coracoclavicular ligament is intact (3). *C*, Grade II sprain (subluxation). The capsule and the acromioclavicular ligament rupture (1); the joint is lax and unstable (2); the end of the clavicle rides upward, usually less than half of the width of the end of the clavicle (3); the coracoclavicular ligament remains intact (4); and the attachments to the trapezius and deltoid remain intact. *D*, Grade III sprain (dislocation). The capsule and acromioclavicular ligaments rupture (1); the coracoclavicular ligament ruptures (2); the insertions of the trapezius and deltoid tear away (3); the clavicle rides upward (4); and the interval between the clavicle and the coracoid process is greatly increased (5). (From DePalma AF: Surgery of the Shoulder, 3rd ed. Philadelphia, JB Lippincott, 1983. In Marx JA, Hockberger R, Walls RM: Rosen's Emergency Medicine, 6th ed. Philadelphia, Mosby, 2006.)

Clinical features

The patient's typical complaint with AC injury is pain over the AC joint area. Pain will increase with overhead or cross-body motion. The patient with acute injury will typically present with the uninjured arm supporting the injured arm in a splint-type fashion. Even if it is a more severe injury with displacement of the distal clavicle, there may not be any obvious deformity as a result of the swelling of the injury. On inspection, the patient may have abrasions over the lateral aspect of the shoulder as evidence of the fall that led to the injury. Palpation of the AC joint will cause pain.

AC sprains have been subcategorized into six types of injuries. A type I AC injury involves a sprain of the acromioclavicular

ligament without tearing or rupture of the ligament. On examination, there will be minimal tenderness over the AC joint and no palpable displacement of the distal clavicle. There is no instability of the distal clavicle. The crossover test may reveal minimal to no pain.

With a type II AC injury, the AC ligament is torn, including the joint capsule, and there is a sprain of the coracoclavicular ligaments without tearing. The patient may have snapping of the AC joint on shoulder motion. Pain will be more intense, and there will be more swelling in the area of the AC joint. There will be appreciable asymmetry as compared with the unaffected side. On palpation, instability of the distal clavicle will be noted. Much like type I injuries, the patient may be able to do a crossover test and to resist downward pressure on the elbow with minimal to no pain.

Type III and VI AC joint injuries involve the complete disruption of the AC ligaments and the coracoclavicular ligaments. The patient will have marked swelling and pain over the AC joint, and there will be asymmetry as compared with the uninjured side. Pain will be exacerbated with movements of the shoulder. The patient will often try to support the arm against the body and elevate it in attempt to reduce the pain. The patient will have severe pain or be unable to perform a crossover test. Distinction between types III, IV, V, and VI AC injuries is made by the direction of the displacement of the distal clavicle.

A type III AC injury means that the distal clavicle is displaced superiorly up to 100% of the clavicular height. On examination, the patient will have a distal clavicular prominence. Type IV AC injuries indicate that the distal clavicle is posteriorly displaced. The distal end of the clavicle may be into or through the trapezius muscle. Type V AC injuries have a distal clavicle that is superiorly displaced by 100% to 300% in relation to the acromion. There may be significant tenting of the skin, and patients will have significant asymmetry as a result of the anterior displacement. With a type VI AC injury, the distal clavicle is inferiorly displaced in a subcoracoid position, and the normal contours of the shoulder may appear flattened.[6] Very few type VI injuries have been described in the literature. A complete neurovascular examination of the affected extremity should be performed to rule out brachial plexus or vascular injury as a result of the displacement.

Diagnosis

AC sprains are first diagnosed on the basis of the history and the physical examination. However, it is still imperative to obtain radiographs to help classify the type of sprain and to rule out fractures. AP and axillary views are essential. The AP view should be a bilateral view that has both AC joints on a single image for comparison. It is important to let the technician know that you are looking at the AC joint because standard radiographs may overexpose the AC joint, thus making the evaluation more difficult.[6] Traditionally, stress views were obtained with the patient holding weights in each hand. However, these stress views have been shown to be of little diagnostic benefit.[7]

Type I AC injuries often have normal radiographs. With a type II injury, the AC joint may be slightly wider on the injured side, and the clavicle will be superiorly displaced slightly more than the unaffected side. Type III AC injuries show a gross displacement of the distal clavicle as compared with the acromion. The coracoclavicular interspace is increased by 30% to 100%. Type IV injuries are best appreciated on the axillary view, where there will be posterior translation of the distal clavicle. The AP view may show some slight increase in the coracoclavicular space. Type V injuries are similar to type III injuries, except the coracoclavicular interspace is increased by 100% to 300% as compared with that of the uninjured side. Type VI injuries will show a distal clavicle that is inferior to the acromion or coracoid, and there will be a decrease in the coracoclavicular interspace.

Although other radiographs are not necessary, occasionally a CT scan may help determine the degree of displacement, especially with type IV injuries. Magnetic resonance imaging is usually not necessary; however, for in-season contact athletes, it may help evaluate the extent of ligamentous injury and thus assist with making a determination about return to sports participation.

Treatment

The treatment of AC injuries depends on the type of injury. The controversy surrounds the type III injuries. Most authors agree that types I and II should be treated nonoperatively and that types IV, V, and VI should be treated operatively. However, the medical literature contains articles that support both the nonoperative and the operative treatment of type III injuries.[8-12]

For nonoperative therapy, treatment is initiated with rest, ice, and immobilization with a sling. Immobilization for type I injuries should be for about a week. Range-of-motion exercises can begin even after 24 to 48 hours. After about a week, gradual return to activity can be part of the rehabilitation program. For type II injuries, the time in the sling may be closer to 2 to 3 weeks. Also, heavy lifting should be avoided for at least 6 weeks.[11] Although there is little support for primary operative therapy, one might consider later operative interventions for a patient who has failed conservative treatment and who is having significant limiting symptoms.[6] This is usually the result of degenerative changes in the joint.

As mentioned previously, for type III AC injuries, some authors suggest operative treatment, and some suggest nonoperative therapy. Surgical intervention should be considered for younger patients, for throwing athletes, for patients with manual labor jobs that require repetitive lifting, and for patients in whom the deformity is not visually acceptable.[6] Patients who carry loads on their shoulders, such as backpackers and parachutists, are often unable to return to their desired activity without surgery. Some argue that if the patient is an athlete in a contact sport in which the injury is likely to recur, then nonoperative treatment may be better until the playing career is over. At that time, if symptoms still persist, operative treatments could be considered. Nonoperative therapy for these injuries is similar to that for type II injuries, except the duration of sling immobilization is 2 to 4 weeks.

For all type IV, V, and VI AC injuries and if there is doubt about the type III injury, then referral an orthopedic surgeon is indicated. There are multiple operative techniques described in the literature, which are beyond the scope of this book.

Return to play

As with SC injuries, return to play after an AC injury is based on having full, pain-free range of motion. Type I injuries typically require a week of rest before more aggressive rehabilitation can begin. This typically results in a total of 2 weeks before the athlete is able to return to full, unrestricted athletic participation. For type II and III injuries that are treated nonoperatively, 2 to 3 weeks of rest are often required before rehabilitation can begin. Although some activities may be cleared earlier, heavy lifting and contact sports should be avoided for 8 to 12 weeks. Certain circumstances may require the athlete to return to sports sooner than recommended. In these cases, a padded donut can be fabricated to protect the joint under standard padding. Intra-articular injections of local anesthetic may also be used at the discretion of the team physician.

After operative therapy, the patient will typically be in a sling for 4 to 6 weeks. Their rehabilitation will start working them toward simple activities of daily living for about 6 weeks. If a metallic fixation device is used, it may need to be removed, after which another 6 weeks of rehabilitation will follow.

Rehabilitation may be modified on the basis of sport-specific activities. After full, painless range of motion and near-normal strength have returned, the patient may return to play. This may take 4 to 6 months.

ACROMIOCLAVICULAR JOINT DEGENERATIVE CHANGES

The most common long-term complication of AC joint sprains is degenerative arthritis. This may take years to develop, and because of its insidious onset, a direct correlation with a specific injury is often not possible. Degenerative changes may also occur after high-level repetitive use; these are commonly found among weight lifters, swimmers, throwers, and tennis players.

Diagnosis

The patient presents with a complaint of pain in the shoulder, especially with overhead activity or weight lifting. There is tenderness to palpation at the AC joint, and pain may be elicited with cross-arm adduction. As compared with subacromial bursal inflammation, which usually causes pain that radiates distally to the deltoid insertion, AC joint pain often radiates proximally to the neck. The diagnosis is confirmed with radiographs, and it is usually easily seen on a standard AP radiograph of the shoulder. The severity of disease noted on the radiograph is very predictable with regard to the effectiveness of nonoperative treatment. Magnetic resonance imaging is not necessary to make the diagnosis, but it is often obtained to evaluate for associated injuries. A recent study indicated that edema within the distal clavicle is a better predictor of symptomatic pathology and that it may be an indication for operative intervention.[13]

Treatment

Nonoperative treatment is the mainstay of treatment, and it consists of the standard use of analgesics and nonsteroidal anti-inflammatory drugs. When pain continues despite medical treatment and rest, intra-articular injections may be attempted. The effectiveness of the injection is often directly related to the amount of pathology, and it is not as effective in the presence of severe degenerative changes. If nonoperative treatment fails, operative intervention is very reliable for pain relief and return of function. Because the clavicle is stabilized by the medially based coracoclavicular ligaments, a distal clavicle resection is an excellent option for chronic AC arthritis. This can be accomplished either by an open direct technique (the Mumford procedure) or an arthroscopic technique. Arthroscopic techniques provide a better opportunity to evaluate the glenohumeral joint and the subacromial space for associated pathology and to treat it appropriately.[14] The subacromial approach allows for the preservation of the AC ligaments, which are critical for the AP stability of the joint.

Return to play

Return to play is predicated on the patient having full, painless range of motion. Guidelines are identical to those of AC joint injuries, and they have been detailed previously in this chapter. Return to play after operative treatment will be managed by the surgeon's assessment of healing and recovery.

CLAVICLE FRACTURES

Fractures of the clavicle are a common injury. A Swedish study revealed that clavicle fractures represented 4% of all fractures and

35% of all fractures in the shoulder girdle.[15] The incidence of clavicle fractures seems to be rising, a fact that some attribute to increased participation in sports.[16]

Mechanism of injury

Clavicle fractures are the result of high-energy injury during play, usually from a fall that causes a lateral impaction on the point of the shoulder at the acromion.[6,16] Although it is less common, a clavicle fracture can also occur in a fall on an outstretched arm. Direct trauma causing clavicle fractures is uncommon, except in high-energy injuries such as motor vehicle accidents.[17]

Risk factors

Risk factors for clavicle fractures include participation in contact sports. Men also have an increased incidence of clavicle fractures.[16] Sports in which a stick is used and can be struck against another player, such as hockey and lacrosse, also increase the risk for clavicle fractures.[17]

Clinical features

A patient with a clavicle fracture will typically remember the event that causes the injury. They may report hearing a crack or snap at the time of the injury and having immediate pain. The clavicle area will typically swell immediately. Patients will report a worsening of their pain with any arm motion; thus, they tend to self-support the injured arm with the uninjured arm in a sling-type position. The clinician also needs to ask about other associated injury symptoms, such as shortness of breath, which may result from pneumothorax, and paresthesias in the extremity as a result of brachial plexus injury, which may occur with high-energy, direct trauma.

On physical examination, the patient usually has an obvious lump at the fracture site, and there will be tenderness at that site. The skin may be tented, and the physician needs to rule out the presence of an open fracture. It is also important to assess for associated injuries. Chest auscultation should be done to rule out a pneumothorax. A careful neurologic examination should be performed to rule out brachial plexus injuries, especially the distribution of the medial cord (ulnar nerve) of the brachial plexus. Injury to a subclavian vessel can be checked by examining pulses and by looking for swelling in the affected extremity.[18]

Clavicle fractures are typically classified by groups according to the site of the fracture on the clavicle. Group I fractures are middle third fractures, group II fractures are distal third fractures, and group III fractures are medial third fractures.[19] Group I fractures account for 80% of clavicle fractures, whereas group II and III fractures account for 15% and 5% of clavicle fractures, respectfully. Neer describes two types of distal clavicle fractures.[19] Type I fractures are lateral to the coracoclavicular ligaments, and they are usually stable as a result of the nondisruption of these ligaments. Type II fractures are medial to the coracoclavicular ligaments, and they are usually unstable.[19] Since Neer's description, further subtyping has been added to include type III fractures, which are distal to the ligaments and involve the AC joint. Although type III fractures are usually nondisplaced as a result of the joint involvement, they may predispose an individual to posttraumatic AC arthritis.

Diagnosis

Although the diagnosis of a clavicle fracture is usually not much of a dilemma with the appropriate history and examination, radiographs should always be obtained. To evaluate trauma to the shoulder and to rule out other possible injuries, radiographs should include AP and axillary views. As a result of the shape of the clavicle, it is not possible to get true orthogonal views (two pictures at 90 degrees to each other), so an AP view with a 45-degree cephalic tilt is obtained to determine the AP displacement of the fracture. The AP view alone may not show any displacement. The axillary view will help if there is posterior displacement of the clavicle's medial fragment **(Figure 21B.4).**

Although further imaging is usually not necessary, when the radiographs are normal and a proximal clavicle fracture is suspected, advanced modalities may be required. In this situation, a CT scan may be necessary to completely rule out proximal clavicle fracture. The CT scan will also help rule out a SC joint injury, which could also coexist with or masquerade as a clavicular fracture.

Treatment

Most clavicle fractures can be treated successfully with nonoperative techniques, and this is almost universally true in the pediatric patient. Clavicle fractures that are nondisplaced or that are minimally displaced will usually heal well with relative rest, pain control, and immobilization. Immobilization can be in a sling or in a figure-of-eight harness; studies have shown no difference in treatment outcomes with these two immobilization techniques.[20,21] However, the devices themselves do offer quality-of-life differences. The figure-of-eight harness is awkward to put on and difficult to keep under the proper tension, and it may apply pressure over the fracture site. However, it frees up the use of both extremities for performing daily activities. The sling is less awkward to wear; however, not only does it limit the use of the affected arm, it also brings the affected arm into internal rotation, which provides a compressive force to the clavicle that may cause shortening and rotation of the fracture. Regardless of the immobilization

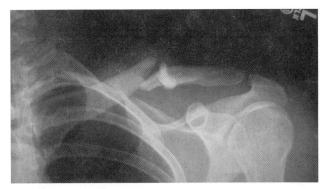

A

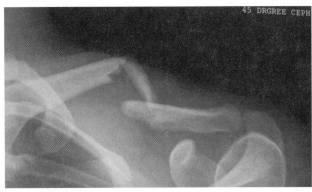

B

Figure 21B.4 *A* and *B*, A 45-degree cephalad view of a midshaft clavicle fracture demonstrates the actual amount of displacement and shortening that is not apparent on a standard anteroposterior view.

technique used, the arm should not be allowed to do overhead activity for 4 to 6 weeks or until radiographic and clinical healing are noted. At that point, range-of-motion exercises can begin, and rehabilitation can be started to progress activity. Patients who fail conservative therapy and who have a painful fracture nonunion should be referred to an orthopedist for possible operative treatment.

Operative treatment should be considered when there is neurovascular compromise or when there is an open fracture. Another indication for surgery is significant fracture displacement or shortening of 20 mm or greater with middle third clavicle fractures. Although some of these fractures may heal, there may be significant impact on range of motion of the shoulder after healing. The healed fracture callus is often undesirably prominent, and the shortening of the clavicle can cause symptomatic restriction of shoulder motion. Therefore, in skeletally mature patients with significant shortening and displacement, surgical treatment will usually result in a better functional result. In the skeletally immature patient, the lump will usually remodel with growth, and it may not be noticeable.

Type II distal clavicle fractures have been shown to have a high nonunion rate when they are treated nonoperatively, so a patient with a type II distal clavicle fracture should be considered for surgical treatment.[19] Other indications for surgery include coexisting conditions or diseases that prevent or preclude immobilization. A patient with a floating shoulder in whom there is also a fracture of the scapular neck should be referred for operative treatment. The forms of operative treatment are beyond the scope of this book, but they include intramedullary devices and plating **(Figure 21B.5)**.

Return to play

For patients who undergo nonoperative therapy, it is important to maintain immobilization for 4 to 6 weeks. Initially, there should be no forward flexion beyond 90 degrees or any overhead activity until radiographic and clinical fracture healing. At that point, rehabilitation should begin with range-of-motion exercises and progress to incorporate sport-specific therapy. Final return to

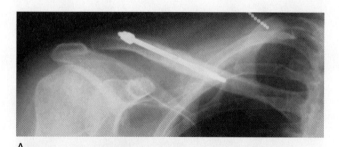

A

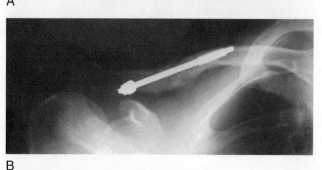

B

Figure 21B.5 *A* and *B*, Intramedullary fixation provides for anatomic reduction and the restoration of length and alignment.

play is based on complete radiographic healing, no pain at the fracture site, and full painless motion. It is important to tell the patient that this may take 3 to 6 months.

After operative treatment, a sling is used for only a short time to provide comfort. The patient is otherwise under the same limitations as the nonoperative patient. If the patient had an intramedullary fixation, the device is typically removed about 12 to 16 weeks postoperatively, after confirmation of fracture healing. Contact sports may be resumed 4 to 6 weeks after the device is removed. However, the patient must also have full, painless motion and radiographic healing before return to play.

PROXIMAL HUMERUS FRACTURES

Proximal humerus fractures are an uncommon sports injury, and most are related to high-energy sports, such as alpine skiing. Kocher and Feagin[22] looked at injuries over a three-season period at an alpine skiing resort. Their data showed that only 11.4% (393 of 3451) of injuries were shoulder injuries; of these injuries, only 6.9% (27) were greater tuberosity fractures, and 1.0% (4) were humeral head fractures. Outside of the sports population, most proximal humerus fractures occur in the elderly.

Mechanism of injury

Although the exact mechanisms for proximal humerus fractures are variable, most sports-related injuries occur as the result of high-energy trauma. Some believe the injury is the result of a direct force trauma to the shoulder and an associated muscle contraction of the rotator cuff muscles.[16] These fractures may be associated with dislocations of the glenohumeral joint. Fractures of the greater tuberosity may accompany anterior glenohumeral dislocations, and lesser tuberosity fractures may accompany posterior glenohumeral dislocations **(Figure 21B.6)**.

Risk factors

The incidence of proximal humerus fractures in sports is extremely small. However, participation in high-energy sports such as alpine skiing and snowboarding increase the risk to the athlete. Most proximal humerus fractures occur in the elderly, who also have an increased risk of osteoporosis. Patients with osteoporosis can sustain proximal humerus fractures even with low-intensity trauma.[23]

Clinical features

The patient with a proximal humerus fracture will typically have a recent history of a high-energy traumatic event. Pain and swelling may be diffuse, and other associated injuries must be evaluated and ruled out. As a result of the high-energy trauma, the patient may also have an associated glenohumeral dislocation, a distal clavicle fracture, or an AC injury. Patients will typically present with the uninjured arm holding the affected arm in a self-splinting fashion.

Examination may show extensive ecchymosis and swelling, and any movement of the arm or shoulder will cause pain. Dislocations may be associated with an anterior bulge for anterior dislocations and a posterior bulge and anterior dimple for posterior dislocations. It is important to do a good neurovascular examination to rule out associated nerve or vascular injury. The motor neurologic examination may be difficult as a result of the pain associated with the fracture, and the examiner may need to depend on the sensory examination.

Neer[24] described the proximal humerus as being composed of four major segments: the articular segment, the lesser tuberosity,

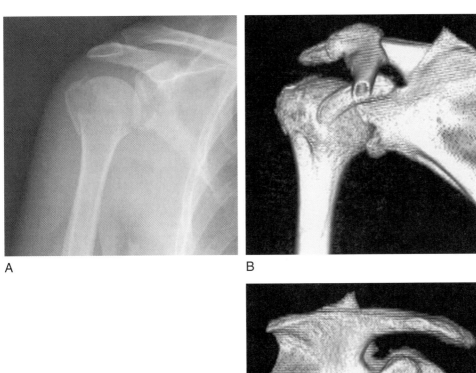

Figure 21B.6 *A,* A 38-year-old man slipped on icy ground and sustained a stable, well-aligned fracture of the proximal end of the humerus and a fracture of the anterior margin of the glenoid. *B,* Three-dimensional computed tomography verified good alignment of the proximal end of the humerus and glenohumeral joint. *C,* Subtraction of the humerus showed that the glenoid fragment was very small. (From Browner BD, Jupiter JB, Levine AM, et al: Skeletal Trauma, 3rd ed. Philadelphia, WB Saunders, 2003.)

the greater tuberosity, and the humeral shaft **(Figure 21B.7).** He then described proximal humerus fractures as occurring in four main locations on the basis of these segments: the anatomic neck, the surgical neck, the greater tuberosity, and the lesser tuberosity. Proximal humeral fractures are then described on the basis of the number of parts in the resultant fractured humerus; thus, fractures are typically classified as two-, three-, or four-part.[24] A "part" is defined by a displaced fragment of at least 10 mm or rotated at least 45 degrees. Three-part fractures can also be described with the associated tuberosity (e.g., three-part greater tuberosity or three-part lesser tuberosity. There have been recent challenges to the interobserver reliability of this classification system, but it remains the gold standard for describing these fractures.

Diagnosis

To diagnose a proximal humerus fracture, it is important to obtain proper radiographs. Radiographs should include a true AP of the glenohumeral joint with both internal and external rotation of the arm and an axillary view. If an axillary view is not successful, then a scapular Y view should be done. The external rotation view helps to visualize the greater tuberosity. The axillary view will help to determine whether there is an associated dislocation, and it also allows the examiner to view the anterior and posterior glenoid rim. Although it is uncommon to require further imaging to diagnose a proximal humerus fracture, some authors argue that a

CT scan may help better define the fracture and determine the type of treatment.[25] Magnetic resonance imaging is rarely necessary in the acute setting. If vascular injury is a concern, then one may consider obtaining an angiogram.

Treatment

The treatment of a proximal humerus fracture depends on the type of fracture, the amount of displacement, the associated injuries, and the level of activity of the patient. Most fractures of the proximal humerus are minimally displaced and can be treated with nonoperative modalities; the most common proximal humerus fracture is a fracture of the greater tuberosity. Minimal displacement is defined as less than 10 mm. Some authors report that they will use 5 mm of displacement as their cutoff for patients when the injury is in the dominant hand and the patients' occupations or sports involve overhead activities.[16] Patients with displaced fractures or three-part or four-part fractures should be referred to an orthopedic surgeon for possible operative treatment.

Nonoperative treatment includes immobilization of the affected extremity with a sling. Limited rehabilitation will be started nearly immediately. The patient should be encouraged to work on active range of motion of the fingers, wrist, and elbow. Pendulum exercises and passive range of motion of the arm should be initiated when the patient is able to tolerate the motion. Aggressive passive motion should be avoided until there is evidence of clinical and radiographic healing. When follow-up radiographs start to reveal

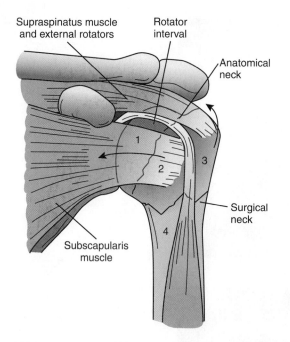

Figure 21B.7 Rotator interval, the ligamentous area between the tendons of the supraspinatus and the subscapularis, and four major fragments of proximal humeral fractures. 1, Head; 2, lesser tuberosity; 3, greater tuberosity; 4, shaft. The retraction of both tuberosities tears the rotator interval and involves both the surgical and anatomic necks of the humerus. (Redrawn from Canale ST: Campbell's Operative Orthopaedics, 10th ed. Philadelphia, Mosby, 2003.)

union of the fracture, active range of motion can be initiated. As the patient progresses in rehabilitation, strengthening exercises can be added. Use of a sling is continued until fracture union is appreciated radiographically. The patient continues rehabilitation even after removal of the sling because he or she will need to continue to work on range of motion and strength. In many cases, the patient will not regain full motion.

Return to play

Most available studies about proximal humerus fractures involve an older population. Outcome measures are often based on functional assessment rather than a return to the previous activity level. Also, many of the studies have addressed operative management rather than the more common nonoperative management. Patients should not be allowed to return to play until they have full painless range of motion. The strength should be normal to near normal, and the rehabilitation should also focus on sport-specific activities.

REFERENCES

1. Nettles JL, Linscheid R: Sternoclavicular dislocations. J Trauma 1968;8:158-164.
2. Bicos J, Nicholson GP: Treatment and results of sternoclavicular joint injuries. Clin Sports Med 2003;22:359-370.
3. Yeh GL, Williams GR: Conservative management of sternoclavicular injuries. Orthop Clin North Am 2000;31:189-203.
4. DeJong KP, Sukui DM: Anterior sternoclavicular dislocation: a long-term follow-up study. J Orthop Trauma 1990;4:420-423.
5. Rudzki JR, Matava MJ, Paletta GA: Complications of treatment of acromioclavicular and sternoclavicular joint injuries. Clin Sports Med 2003;22:387-405.
6. Clarke HD, McCann PD: Acromioclavicular joint injuries. Orthop Clin North Am 2000;31:177-187.
7. Bossart PJ, Joyce SM, Manaster BJ, et al: Lack of efficacy of "weighted" radiographs in diagnosis acute acromioclavicular separations. Ann Emerg Med 1988;17:20-24.
8. Bjerneld H, Hovelius L, Thorling J: Acromio-clavicular separations treated conservatively: a 5-year follow-up study. Acta Orthop Scand 1983;54:743-745.
9. Eskola A, Vainionpaa O, Korkala S, et al: Four year outcome of operative treatment of acute acromioclavicular dislocation. J Orthop Trauma 1991;5:9-13.
10. Galpin RD, Hawkins RJ, Grainger RW: A comparative analysis of operative versus nonoperative treatment of grade III acromioclavicular separations. Clin Orthop 1985;193:150-155.
11. Lemos MJ: The evaluation and treatment of the injured acromioclavicular joint in athletes. Am J Sports Med 1998;26:137-144.
12. Phillips AM, Smart C, Groom AF: Acromioclavicular dislocation: conservative or surgical therapy. Clin Orthop 1998;353:10-17.
13. Shubin-Stein BF, Ahmad CS, Pfaff CH, et al: A comparison of magnetic resonance imaging findings of the acromioclavicular joint in symptomatic versus asymptomatic patients. J Shoulder Elbow Surg 2006;15(1):56-59.
14. Robalais RD, McCarty E: Surgical treatment of symptomatic acromioclavicular joint problems. Clin Orthop 2007;455:30-37.
15. Nordqvist A, Petersson C: The incidence of fractures of the clavicle. Clin Orthop 1994;300:127-132.
16. Brunelli MP, Gill TJ: Fractures and tendon injuries of the athletic shoulder. Orthop Clin North Am 2002;33:497-508.
17. Fowler AW: Fractures of the clavicle. J Bone Joint Surg 1962;44B:440.
18. Allman FL Jr: Fractures and ligamentous injuries of the clavicle and its articulation. J Bone Joint Surg 1967;49A:774-784.
19. Neer CS II: Fractures of the distal third of the clavicle. Clin Orthop 1968;58:43-50.
20. Andersen K, Jensen PO, Lauritzen J: Treatment of clavicular fractures: figure-of-eight bandage versus a simple sling. Acta Orthop Scand 1987;58:71-74.
21. McCandless DN, Mowbray MA: Treatment of displaced fractures of the clavicle: sling versus figure-of-eight bandage. Practitioner 1979;223:266-267.
22. Kocher MS, Feagin JA: Shoulder injuries during alpine skiing. Am J Sports Med 1996;24:665-669.
23. McKoy BE, Bensen CV, Hartsock LA: Fractures about the shoulder: conservative management. Orthop Clin North Am 2000;31:205-216.
24. Neer CS II: Displaced proximal humeral fractures. I. classification and evaluation. J Bone Joint Surg 1970;52A:1077-1089.
25. Castagno AA, Shurman WP, Kilcone RF, et al: Complex fractures of the proximal humerus: role of CT in treatment. Radiology 1987;165:759-762.

CHAPTER 22

Craniomaxillofacial Injuries

Allyson S. Howe, MD

KEY POINTS

- An athlete with hemotympanum, Battle sign (bruising noted behind the auricle of the ear), raccoon eyes. clear otorrhea, or clear rhinorrhea should be thoroughly evaluated for a skull fracture.
- Visual acuity is "the vital sign of the eye" and must be assessed with any eye injury.
- Clean scalp wounds do not require irrigation prior to closure with sutures or staples (LOE: B). Dirty or contaminated scalp wounds should be copiously irrigated before closure (LOE: D).
- All patients with an acute onset of photopsia (flashing lights) or floaters should be referred for ophthalmologic retinal evaluation. The early treatment of retinal tears and fissures can stop progression to retinal detachment, and it may also save vision (LOE: A).
- Avulsed teeth that are replanted within 30 minutes have a greater than 90% chance of survival. A delay of more than 2 hours results in a tooth survival rate of only 5% (LOE: A).
- One gentle but firm attempt at reducing a dislocated mandible may be attempted on the field if there is no facial deformity or other sign of bony fracture. If this initial attempt is not successful, the athlete should be transported to the emergency department for imaging and definitive care (LOE: D).

INTRODUCTION

Injuries to the craniomaxillofacial area during sports are a cause of significant morbidity for athletes and a common cause of concern for medical personnel. Injuries to the eye or its orbit have the potential to result in visual deficits, and facial injuries carry a cosmetic concern. Dental and oral injuries may affect the stability of the airway. Injuries to the ears can affect hearing as well as the cosmetic appearance of the auricles. Unfortunately, the best evidence for the treatment of craniomaxillofacial injuries comes by way of observational studies rather than randomized comparison trials. The rapid recognition and proper treatment of craniomaxillofacial injuries improves patient morbidity and cosmetic outcomes.

INTRACRANIAL BLEEDING

Within the cranium, bleeding can occur in the parenchyma of the brain or in the layers of tissue that surround the brain. The brain is lined by three layers of tissue: the pia mater, the arachnoid mater, and the dura mater. Bleeding can occur within the brain (intraparenchymal hematoma) **(Figure 22.1)**, beneath the arachnoid mater (subarachnoid hemorrhage), beneath the dura mater (subdural hematoma), or between the dura mater and the cranium (epidural hematoma).

Subarachnoid hemorrhage
With traumatic subarachnoid bleeding, damage is usually to the superficial vessels of the brain, and it involves a small amount of bleeding. The traumatic rupture of cerebral aneurysms or arteriovenous malformations may involve more serious bleeding. Common symptoms include a sudden, severe headache that may or may not lateralize, nausea, vomiting, and a brief loss of consciousness. Irritation from the blood may precipitate seizure activity. Mortality rates have been reported at 51%[1] **(Figure 22.2).**

Subdural hematoma
Subdural bleeding tends to come from damage to venous structures. Damage may be to veins that connect the dura to the brain or from diffuse brain surface injury. In either case, injury to the underlying brain structures can occur. Disruption in the level of consciousness is common and may begin with a complete loss of consciousness. As with epidural hematomas, the athlete can regain consciousness, but he or she may not reach a fully normal mental status. Common signs and symptoms with subdural hematomas are neck stiffness and pain, behavior changes, and pupillary abnormalities. Treatment involves consultation with a neurosurgeon. While awaiting care, hyperventilation with intubation, mannitol, and loop diuretics may help decrease intracranial pressure to temporarily stabilize the patient. Mortality is generally high, but rates improve with early recognition and neurosurgical intervention **(Figure 22.3).**

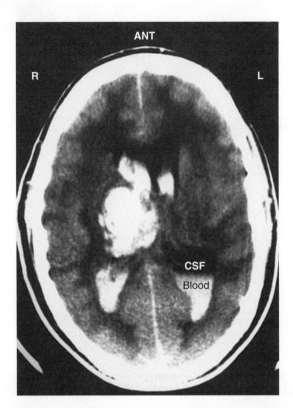

Figure 22.1 Intracerebral hematoma. In this hypertensive patient with an acute severe headache, the noncontrasted computed tomography scan shows a large area of fresh blood in the region of the right thalamus and the anterior and posterior horns of the lateral ventricles. (From Mettler FA: Essentials of Radiology, 2nd ed. Philadelphia, WB Saunders, 2005.)

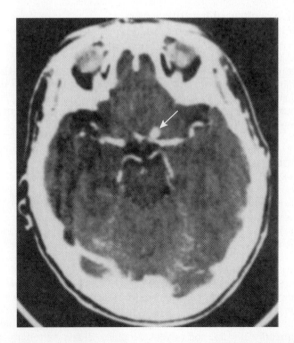

Figure 22.2 Subarachnoid hemorrhage. (From Cwinn AA, Grahovac SZ: Emergency CT scans of the head: a practical atlas. St. Louis, 1998, Mosby. In Noble J: Textbook of Primary Care Medicine, 3rd ed. St. Louis, Mosby, 2001.)

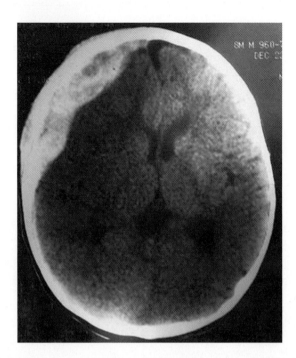

Figure 22.3 Subdural hematoma. Large right frontotemporal subdural hematoma in a child tackled during a football game. (From DeLee JC, Drez D Jr, Miller MD [eds]: DeLee and Drez's Orthopaedic Sports Medicine: Principles and Practice, 2nd ed. Philadelphia, WB Saunders, 2003.)

Epidural hematoma

Epidural bleeding is generally fast arterial bleeding. This classically occurs with the tearing of the middle meningeal artery with fracture or trauma to the temporal bones. Although patients with epidural hematomas can present with normal or altered level of consciousness, the classic presentation includes an immediate loss of consciousness followed by a return of consciousness (lucid interval). After this is a progressive decrease in the level of consciousness and a relatively rapid lapse into a comatose state. Treatment by surgical decompression as soon as possible is indicated **(Figure 22.4)**.

SCALP LACERATION

Definition

A scalp laceration is an interruption of the integrity of the scalp. The scalp is made up of five layers. From external to deep, these are the skin, the superficial fascia, the galea aponeurotica, the subaponeurotic areolar connective tissue, and the periosteum. The first three are so intimately adhered that they function as one layer.

Mechanism of injury

Scalp lacerations occur after direct trauma with a hard object (e.g., a hockey stick) or from shearing forces.

Risk factors

The lack or improper wear of headgear when playing a contact sport can leave the scalp susceptible to laceration. At the same time, a correctly and firmly fitted helmet that gets forcibly moved during competition can lead to scalp injury from shearing forces.

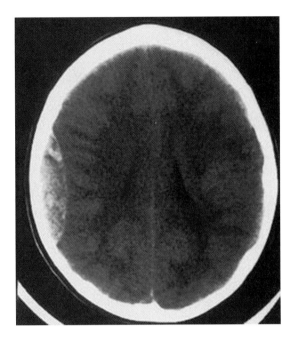

Figure 22.4 Epidural hematoma. Classic lentiform epidural hematoma in a child who struck a tree while skiing. (From DeLee JC, Drez D Jr, Miller MD [eds]: DeLee and Drez's Orthopaedic Sports Medicine: Principles and Practice, 2nd ed. Philadelphia, WB Saunders, 2003.)

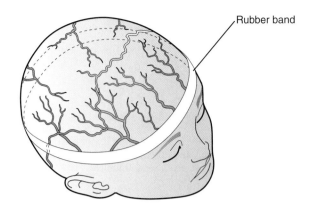
Rubber band

Figure 22.5 Scalp laceration. A wide, tight, sterilized rubber band or Penrose drain may be placed around the forehead and occiput to compress the arterial supply to the scalp. (From Roberts JR: Clinical Procedures in Emergency Medicine, 4th ed. Philadelphia, WB Saunders, 2004.)

Clinical features

Extensive bleeding is common and can hinder diagnosis. This is mostly the result of the rich blood supply of the scalp and the tendency for scalp vessels to be held open by the fibrous subcutaneous fascia that surrounds them. Lacerations will either remain fairly well approximated or splay open, depending on whether or not the galea is disrupted. An athlete with a scalp laceration may also have other injuries of the head and neck, so care should be taken to evaluate these areas.

Diagnosis

Most large scalp lacerations are obvious disruptions of scalp integrity. However, smaller lesions can be hidden by matted hair. Discovering one lesion should prompt a search for other lacerations. Further identifying the quality of the laceration(s) will help with treatment decisions. A scalp wound can only gape open if all three of the superficial layers (the skin, the superficial fascia, and the galea aponeurotica) are disrupted. If the wound does not gape open, the galea is intact. Before closure of the wound, visual examination of the skull and palpation of the wound are necessary to rule out occult scalp fractures. If bone is exposed, the risk of bony necrosis or osteomyelitis increases because the uncovered bone may become a nidus for infection.[2]

Treatment

Initially, the wound should be grossly decontaminated with sterile saline and covered with a clean dressing (sterile, if available). Forceful irrigation of a clean scalp wound is not necessary because it has not been shown to reduce the risk of infection and could lead to tissue damage or cosmetic failure. Closure of the wound at the field site (in the training room, ideally, and if supplies are available) or transport to the nearest emergency room for treatment should happen expediently. In the case of exposed bone, repair will help prevent bone death by restoring blood supply.

Scalp wounds that interrupt the subgaleal layer involve a higher risk for infection of the meninges and the intracranial tissues as a result of the potential of the emissary vein flow to deliver bacteria to these areas. Closing the galeal layer first helps to stop bleeding and reduce the risk of infection.

As mentioned previously, bleeding is an obstacle that is common to scalp laceration treatment. Having an assistant hold direct pressure over the wound during repair is preferable to tying off blood vessels because the latter rarely provides effective hemostasis.[2] A common and useful procedure is to place a wide, tight, sterilized rubber band around the forehead and occiput to decrease flow **(Figure 22.5)**. The use of lidocaine with epinephrine for local anesthesia may help to control bleeding around the wound.

Simple scalp lacerations can be closed with 3-0 nonabsorbable suture or staples. The use of blue suture and leaving long suture tails will aid with subsequent removal. In the case of galea disruption, it may not be necessary to close the galea separately; however, a separate galeal closure can be helpful to decrease wound tension if the laceration is large. As with any potentially contaminated wound, tetanus status should be evaluated and prophylaxis given if the patient has not had a booster shot for 5 years.

Return to play

Scalp sutures should stay in place for at least 5 to 7 days. Staples may be removed after 5 days if the wound appears well approximated and dry. After the removal of sutures or staples, the athlete can return to play, but consideration should be given to covering the wound until complete healing is observed. In the case of potential trauma to the wound by a helmet, delaying return by a few days or padding the newly healing wound may be beneficial.

Controversies

The decision to irrigate a clean scalp wound in patients presenting to an emergency department setting was challenged in a recent study. The authors cited possible tissue injury leading to tissue damage, infection, or cosmetic failure from high-pressure wound irrigation. They hypothesized that natural host defenses would be sufficient to prevent infection. At the time of suture/staple removal, there was no significant difference between the incidence of wound infection in wounds treated after irrigation and the incidence in those treated without irrigation. Wounds that were clearly contaminated were not entered into the study[3] (LOE: B).

SKULL FRACTURE

Mechanism of injury

Skull fractures usually occur after blunt trauma to the head.

Risk factors

Playing a sport without the proper headgear (improper fit, poor construction, or lack of use) could lead to head injury. Sports played with sticks and hard objects could lead to skull fracture if contact between the head and an object occurs. Contact with other players may also rarely result in skull fractures.

Clinical features

After blunt head trauma, complaint of severe headache, nausea, and disorientation should prompt evaluation for skull fracture. Palpation of the scalp may reveal a step off or a depression in the tissues, which indicates disruption of the periosteum. In the case of extensive soft-tissue injury, it may be difficult to determine if a skull fracture is present as a result of profuse bleeding from the scalp.

The presence of these physical findings increases the clinical suspicion of skull injury[4]:

- Hemotympanum (blood behind the tympanic membrane)
- Battle sign (bruising noted behind the auricle of the ear)
- Raccoon eyes (periorbital ecchymosis)
- Clear otorrhea
- Clear rhinorrhea

Diagnosis

Imaging is necessary when evaluating for a skull fracture. A computed tomography (CT) scan is useful to determine the presence or extent of the fracture. CT scanning may also be helpful to identify bony fragments that are in contact with or embedded in brain tissue. If underlying brain tissue injury is suspected, magnetic resonance imaging may offer more information.

Treatment

Recognition of a skull fracture must prompt evaluation for more serious injury to the underlying parenchyma of the brain. Intracranial bleeding, infection by way of contamination of the wound, and bone fragments that migrate to the underlying brain tissue are concerns with every skull fracture. Consultation with a neurosurgeon is necessary in every case of skull fracture.

Return to play

Before returning to full athletic competition, the confirmation of fracture healing and the absence of associated neurologic symptoms (nausea, light-headedness, confusion, weakness) are mandatory. Consultation with and clearance by a neurosurgeon should be strongly considered as well.

EYE INJURIES

Eye injuries can threaten eyesight temporarily or permanently. Sports account for more than 40,000 eye injuries in the United States annually, and about 90% of these are considered preventable.[5] Correctly identifying particularly dangerous eye conditions, symptoms, and signs can lead to appropriately timed referral to an ophthalmologist and can also be sight saving **(Figure 22.6).**

Attempts to prevent eye injuries have resulted in modifications to protective equipment. Some sports have recently instituted requirements for higher levels of protective gear—such as women's lacrosse, which now requires eye guards for all players. Other sports have been able to demonstrate higher safety with protective gear (e.g., facial guards in youth baseball), but implementing their routine use has been challenging. Local attitudes and player beliefs are difficult to overcome.

Examination

Visual acuity is the vital sign of the eye, and must be obtained after any eye injury. If necessary, to correct for myopia in the case of lost/missing glasses or contacts, a pinhole examination can be used. This is accomplished by giving the athlete a piece of paper with a small pinhole punched through it to look through. The pinhole examination should correct the vision of myopic athletes to at least 20/40. Failure to correct this level may indicate serious damage to the eye and warrants immediate referral for further examination.

During examination, pressure on the acutely injured globe should be avoided in the event that there has been a globe rupture. Check pupillary response to light individually and with consensual response. The swinging flashlight test can rule out intracranial damage to the optic nerve and the brain. To perform this test, shine a penlight into one eye to attain maximum pupil constriction, then quickly switch the light source to the other eye and back again. Normally, the second eye should respond with the same pupillary constriction as the first eye as a result of a consensual response. If the eye does not respond at all to the light source (i.e., the pupil is dilated and does not change), then there should be concern about damage to the efferent pupillary reflex. Acutely, this is most commonly seen with damage to the third cranial nerve by herniation of the temporal lobe. A pupil that dilates in response to light during the swinging flashlight test is known as a *Marcus Gunn pupil*, and it indicates injury to the optic nerve or the retina. In this situation, the consensual response to light in the affected eye will be intact.[6]

The use of a penlight will be helpful to examine the eyelids and the orbit for lacerations or foreign bodies. Extraocular muscle control should be evaluated. Palpation of the orbital rims will help to evaluate for step-off lesions and tenderness that are indicative of

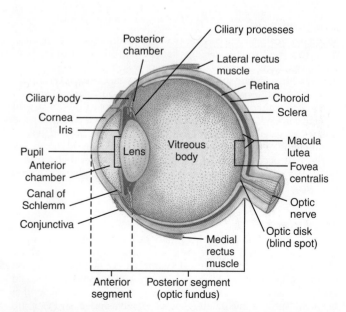

Figure 22.6 Eye anatomy. (From Ignatavicius DD, Workman ML, Mishler, MA: Medical-Surgical Nursing Across the Health Care Continuum, 3rd ed. Philadelphia, WB Saunders, 1999.)

orbital fracture. The documentation of facial sensation to light touch may be helpful to exclude nerve injuries. Infraorbital or supraorbital nerve injuries are associated with orbit fractures, and they may present with numbness of the skin around the eye.

If possible, a slit-lamp examination to evaluate the sclera, the conjunctiva, the cornea, the anterior chamber, and the iris is recommended. Fluorescein can be helpful to identify lesions of the cornea or the conjunctiva. Cloudy or opaque fluid in the anterior chamber may indicate a more serious eye injury. Fundoscopic evaluation may demonstrate damage to the retina, the optic nerve, or the macula.

Corneal abrasion
Definition
Corneal abrasion involves superficial injury to the cornea (the transparent layer of tissue that covers the iris). Corneal abrasions account for up to 10% of new patients visits in eye emergency units of the United Kingdom. In primary care offices where eye complaints account for 2% of patient visits, 8% of eye patients are diagnosed with abrasions.[7]

Mechanism of injury
A scratch or superficial contact with an object that drags across the eye causes this type of injury. In sports, this is commonly the finger of an opposing player that pokes into the unprotected eye.

Risk factors
Playing sports in which no protective eye gear is worn may put an athlete at increased risk of corneal abrasion. Contact lens wearers are at higher risk of corneal abrasions due to improperly fitted or cleaned lenses.

Clinical features
The nerves of the cornea come from the trigeminal nerve, and they are among the most sensitive in the body. An athlete with a corneal abrasion will complain mostly of pain in the eye. He or she may note blurry vision and the feeling that a foreign object is in the eye, and he or she may recall trauma to the eye. On examination, there may be copious tearing, pain with opening the eye fully, or photophobia. The eye may be red or have an injected sclera (a prominence of superficial blood vessels seen through the sclera).

Diagnosis
Definitive diagnosis is paramount to a good outcome. The use of a topical anesthetic in the eye (e.g., tetracaine eye drops) may be necessary for the patient to tolerate examination. Fluorescein dye should be used to stain the corneal epithelium. Use of a Wood lamp or a cobalt blue filter during a slit-lamp examination can highlight corneal damage because the accumulation of fluorescein at the site of injury will be visible under this special lighting.

Treatment
Simple corneal abrasions should heal in 2 to 3 days, with no long-term complications.[8] Topical antibiotic coverage is indicated for most patients with a corneal abrasion to prevent secondary bacterial infection. This treatment has not been well studied, but it is commonly used to help prevent tragic complications. Antibiotic choices are listed in **Box 22.1**. The decision for tetanus toxoid administration is controversial. Superficial or uncomplicated corneal abrasions do not require a booster, but tetanus toxoid may be protective in the case of penetrating eye trauma.[9] Patching the eye has not been shown to decrease pain or shorten healing times (LOE: B).[8] Treatment with nonpatched eyes improves compliance with medications and treatment (LOE: B).[8] Contact lens wearers should be told to avoid use of their contact lenses during treatment and healing.

Box 22.1: Antibiotic Choice for Corneal Abrasion

- Bacitracin ointment, four times daily
- Erythromycin ointment, four times daily
- Sulfacetamide ointment, four times daily
- Ofloxacin 0.3% solution, 2 drops, four times daily
- Ointment is preferred to solutions because ointments offer lubrication to the corneal epithelium.
- Daily follow-up examination is necessary until healing occurs, even with antibiotic coverage.
- Begin antibiotic treatment on the day that injury occurs, and continue it through the healing course (usually 3 to 5 days of antibiotic therapy).
- The use of steroids and aminoglycosides is contraindicated for corneal abrasions.

At the time of initial diagnosis, the lesion size should be measured. Close follow-up examination within 24 hours to assess for healing is important, and subsequent daily examinations are necessary until resolution. Any corneal abrasion that does not demonstrate a daily decrease in size or that has not healed after 3 days should be referred to an ophthalmologist. A corneal abrasion can progress to a corneal ulceration, which is a devastating injury that requires urgent specialty consultation with an ophthalmologist if it is suspected. A patient should never be sent home with a topical anesthetic because these medicines may inhibit wound healing or lead to further corneal injury in the patient who has an occult foreign body (see Box 22.1).

Return to play
An athlete may return to play after the abrasion has fully healed and visual acuity has returned to normal.

Controversies
Tetanus toxoid has not been shown to be necessary, but it is often given in cases of corneal abrasion. An animal study demonstrated a greater need for tetanus toxoid if penetrating eye injury has occurred but no need for tetanus in the case of superficial, uncomplicated injury.[9] Eye patches are not recommended for the treatment of corneal abrasions that are not infected and that are not related to contact lens trauma because their use may retard healing and negatively affect compliance with therapy (LOE: B).[8]

Foreign body in the eye
Definition
Any foreign object that gets lodged in the superficial portion of the eye or trapped under the eyelid is considered a foreign body.

Mechanism of injury
The risk of eye injury by foreign body is high during outdoor athletics. Dirt, small pebbles, and pellets from turf fields are common sources.

Risk factors
Athletes who play sports on turf and in outdoor venues may have an increased risk of a foreign body in the eye. Casual exercise can be risky as well. Foreign body injuries while walking and running along a roadway are common.[10]

Clinical features

The patient will likely feel the sensation that something is "stuck" in his or her eye. The eye will water, it will be painful, and it may appear red.

Diagnosis

The use of fluorescein may reveal several linear lesions along the cornea that are made as the lid opens and closes over the foreign object. The superior lid must be reflected back to determine whether a foreign body is trapped inside the upper lid. To assess this area, grasp the eyelashes, and evert the eyelid. Most foreign bodies will be seen against the mucosal surface of the lid or the eye.

Treatment

If it is safe to do so, removing a superficial foreign body is indicated as early as possible. Contact lenses should also be removed right away. Topical anesthetic will help the patient tolerate the procedure. The use of sterile irrigating solution running over the eye or a moistened sterile swab are the most commonly accepted methods of foreign body removal, and they are generally safe.[5,11] A needle should not be used to remove objects because of the potential for further injury. If the object is removed, apply antibiotic ointment to the eye, and ensure that follow up occurs in 24 hours. At that visit, reevaluation for the presence of a foreign body or a corneal abrasion may be indicated. If the foreign body cannot be removed, immediate referral to a specialist is indicated.[5]

Return to play

If there is no corneal abrasion associated with the injury and symptoms resolve completely, the athlete may return to play in the same contest. Otherwise, return to play is safe after the foreign body has been removed and the symptoms have resolved.

Controversies

The use of a needle to remove an object is not recommended as a result of the needle's to cause further injury.

Black eye (ecchymosis)
Definition

Ecchymosis is a contusion of the soft tissues surrounding the eye (not the eye itself) after trauma to the eye or nose.

Mechanism of injury

This condition generally results from trauma to the face. A blow to the nose can cause the swelling of both eyes because fluid tends to collect in the loose soft tissue of the eyelids. Recall that injury to the basilar skull can result in bilateral black eyes, which are called "raccoon eyes" and which can be very serious. Postsurgical changes to the face can also lead to one or two black eyes.

Risk factors

Contact sports carry a higher risk for black eyes to occur because of the potential for trauma related to contact. Sports that do not require protective eye gear may also have a higher incidence of this type of injury.

Clinical features

When this injury occurs after trauma, there is usually a complaint of pain and swelling around the eye. Swelling may inhibit visual acuity or prohibit the full opening of the eye. The pain will usually resolve before the ecchymosis. Because the condition usually results from trauma, athletes with black eyes should be evaluated for evidence of concussion. A simple black eye is just that: simple. There should not be significant visual changes, altered consciousness, inability to move the eye, blood or clear fluid from nose or ears, blood on the surface of the eye, or strong headache. If any of these symptoms are present, consider a more serious diagnosis.

Diagnosis

A full evaluation of the eye that includes direct observation, the examination of extraocular muscle movement, and a determination of visual acuity should be done, along with the palpation of orbital bones and an assessment for sensory deficits. Ecchymosis can appear quickly as the surrounding soft tissue expands with traumatic fluid. Evaluation at the time of injury is most helpful.

Treatment

Ice to the affected eye for 20-minute intervals should occur for the first 24 hours. Pain control with over-the-counter medications may be necessary, but it is rarely needed after the first 2 days.

Return to play

The athlete's return to play is delayed only by visual deficits that are caused by swelling or by pain that is not easily controlled with over-the-counter medications. If return is delayed for any reason beyond 2 to 3 days, reevaluation for a more serious diagnosis is necessary.

Subconjunctival hemorrhage
Definition

Blood in the superficial subconjunctival layer of the eye characterizes this type of injury.

Mechanism of injury

Although blunt eye trauma can cause this injury, something as innocuous as a coughing spell or a big sneeze can also result in a subconjunctival hemorrhage. When direct eye trauma is present, evaluation for further injury is necessary.

Risk factors

Athletes who regularly and forcefully perform the Valsalva maneuver during exercise (e.g., wrestlers, weight lifters, and synchronized swimmers) may be at increased risk. Athletes with atherosclerotic vessels and/or hypertension may have a higher risk of presenting with a subconjunctival hemorrhage.[11]

Clinical features

Blood will be seen clearly under the area that is covered by the conjunctiva. Because the conjunctiva ends at the limbus, which is in the transition zone between the sclera and cornea, blood will not cover the cornea[12] (**Figure 22.7**).

Diagnosis

The hemorrhage will appear as a bright red area that covers the sclera but that does not cross the cornea. The size of the hemorrhage varies, but visual acuity should be normal. If there is a history of direct trauma to the eye, evaluation to rule out penetrating eye injury or a surface foreign body is needed.

Treatment

This injury is self-limited and, in the absence of other eye injuries, it will tend to resolve completely without treatment in 2 to 3 weeks.

Return to play

An athlete with normal vision and no evidence of further injury can participate in sports while having a subconjunctival hemorrhage.

Hyphema
Definition

Hyphema is the presence of layered blood in the anterior chamber of the eye (**Figure 22.8**).

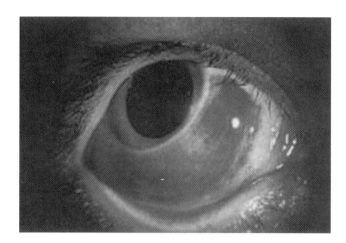

Figure 22.7 Subconjunctival hemorrhage. (From Auerbach PS: Wilderness Medicine, 4th ed. St. Louis, Mosby, 2001.)

Mechanism of injury

A hyphema usually results from blunt trauma to the eye from a ball, playing equipment, or another player.

Risk factors

Playing a contact sport without sufficient eye protective gear is a risk for this type of injury. Noncontact sports that are played with a ball (e.g., tennis and racquetball) can also lead to hyphema if direct trauma to the eye occurs.

Clinical features

Athletes with hyphema generally complain of vision changes and eye pain. Symptoms may range from blurred vision to frank loss of vision after trauma. Signs of hyphema include the appearance of layered blood in the anterior chamber of the eye. With a severe hyphema, the blood can fill the entire anterior chamber, which results in a condition known as an *8-ball hyphema.*

Diagnosis

If hyphema is suspected, an eye examination including fundoscopic evaluation is necessary. A ruptured globe must be ruled out, and care should be taken to protect the eye during transport to a facility where an ophthalmologist is available. Given the level of trauma that is often associated with hyphema, a CT scan is advisable to rule out orbital fractures.

Treatment

Hyphema is a medical emergency. Permanent vision impairment is likely if the condition is not treated because the blood level in the anterior chamber can stain the cornea permanently if it is not rapidly removed. The presence of blood can also increase the intraocular pressure in the eye, thus leading to glaucoma and optical nerve damage. Covering the eye with a shield during transport is recommended. The vessels that bled to produce the hyphema remain fragile, and rebleeding is a significant concern. Transport should occur with the patient in the upright position so that gravity does not increase intraocular pressure. Often a patient with hyphema will be admitted to the hospital for the monitoring and treatment of increased intraocular pressure and so that the clot in the eye can be stabilized. Pain control should be considered.

Return to play

After vision and intraocular pressure have returned to normal and an ophthalmologist determines that no active bleeding is present, return to play may be possible. The athlete should be encouraged to wear eye protection during competition.

Globe rupture
Definition

The globe is the spherical structure that is bound by the eye wall and that sits in the orbit. Any break in the integrity of the eye wall is considered a rupture of the globe, and this requires surgical treatment.

Mechanism of injury

Direct trauma to the eye precedes globe rupture. Penetrating trauma can pierce the external integrity of the eye. Blunt trauma can increase intraocular pressure and cause the rupture of the eye wall.

Clinical features

In the case of a ruptured globe, there will be eye pain and vision loss if the patient is conscious. The red reflex may be obscured. The signs of globe rupture include subconjunctival hemorrhage, hyphema, irregular or peaked pupil, corneal lacerations, shallow anterior chamber, low intraocular pressure, or intraocular contents being noted outside of the globe.[6]

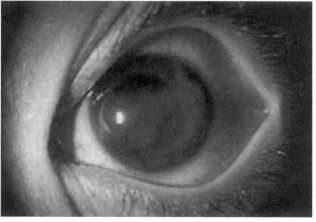

A

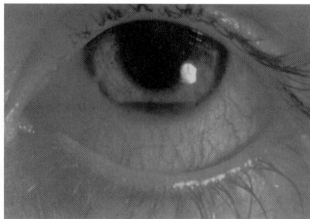

B

Figure 22.8 *A,* Hyphema. *B,* Small hyphema layering out in the inferior portion of the anterior chamber. (*A,* From Auerbach PS: Wilderness Medicine, 4th ed. St. Louis, Mosby, 2001; *B,* from Marx JA: Rosen's Emergency Medicine: Concepts and Clinical Practice, 6th ed. St. Louis, Mosby, 2006.)

Diagnosis

The evaluation is limited in the case of globe rupture. A slit lamp or penlight may be helpful to see intraocular contents outside of the eye or to notice a break in the eye wall. If intraocular foreign body or orbital fracture is suspected, a CT scan may be helpful in the evaluation. Pressure should not be placed on the eye during examination in case the globe has ruptured. With pressure, the intraocular contents can displace and cause further hemorrhage, retinal detachment, lens displacement, and permanent visual loss.

Treatment

The placement of a metal shield over the eye during transport is recommended to protect the eye from further trauma. If a ruptured globe is suspected, emergent transfer to a medical center with an ophthalmologist is indicated. The patient should be transported sitting up, and nothing should be given by mouth considering the high likelihood of immediate surgery upon arrival. Further examination of the eye can be delayed until the patient is under general anesthesia.

Tetanus toxoid booster (if indicated) and intravenous antibiotics should be given. The use of antiemetic medications may be helpful to prevent emesis, which would significantly increase intraocular pressure.

Surgical treatment is necessary in all cases of globe rupture. The prognosis is serious, and patients should be counseled regarding the possible need for enucleation (the removal of eye and its contents) if repair is not possible. A very serious reaction to penetrating eye trauma is called *sympathetic ophthalmia*, which is the immunologic rejection of the unaffected eye. Enucleating the injured eye within the first 2 weeks after injury significantly reduces the risk of sympathetic opththalmia.[6]

Return to play

Functionally one-eyed or monocular athletes should be cautioned about the risk of losing vision in their remaining eye. Serious consideration regarding the use of eye protection (e.g., goggles and masks) should be discussed with the athlete.

Orbital fracture
Definition

This injury involves the fracture of any bone that defines the bony orbit. This may be an orbital rim bone (the prominent bones that surround the eye) or a bone within the orbit that supports the globe itself. Portions of the maxillary, zygomatic, frontal, ethmoid, palatine, sphenoid, and lacrimal bones make up the orbit. Nearly a third of orbital fractures occur during athletic play.[13,14] Only assault is more common than athletic participation as a cause for orbital fracture.

Mechanism of injury

During sports, virtually all orbital fractures result from trauma from an object or a human body part. In 19 fractures of professional football players, 74% were caused by digital poke, and the other 26% were caused by blunt trauma.[15]

There are two main classes of orbital bone fractures: orbital rim fractures and orbital wall fractures. Orbital rim fractures are usually the result of a direct blow to the bony rim. Orbital wall fractures are more commonly seen after globe trauma, such as when a ball directly strikes the globe. In this latter case, intraocular pressure increases, and it is transmitted to the orbital walls. The thinnest, weakest, and, therefore, the most vulnerable portion of the wall is located posteromedially. Fracture of the posteromedial orbit allows for the dissipation of sudden, rapid increases in intraocular pressure, and it may be somewhat vision protective.

Orbital fractures often create a moveable bony fragment that leads to a "trapdoor effect" for the soft tissues of the orbit.[16] Of particular concern with orbital wall fractures is the entrapment of eye muscles, orbital fat, and fibrous connective tissue septa between the fracture fragments. In the posteromedial fracture, the inferior rectus muscle is at highest risk. If the fracture site opens, entraps soft tissue, and then seals again, then the soft tissue may become incarcerated, lose its blood supply, and become necrotic. Hence, soft-tissue entrapment is an emergent situation that requires immediate ophthalmologic consultation for surgical decompression **(Figure 22.9).**

Risk factors

In the United States, the sports that are the most associated with orbital fractures are baseball, football, basketball, and racquet sports.[15,16] In the United Kingdom, soccer, rugby, and cricket playing result in the highest incidence of these fractures.[13]

Clinical features

Patients with orbital fractures will commonly complain of eye pain, double vision, numbness of the cheek (from damage to the infraorbital nerve), and nausea. There may be gross bony deformity of the orbit. A sideline physical examination should include the assessment of extraocular muscle function, pupillary reaction, fundoscopic examination, and visual acuity. It may be easier to complete this initial examination in the training room, or injured athletes may need to be referred directly to the emergency department when field-side conditions are not optimal.

Physical examination signs that are indicative of orbital fracture include periorbital ecchymosis, hypesthesia in the cranial nerve V2 distribution, restricted eye movements (particularly limitation of the lateral or upward gaze), enophthalmus (eye depression as compared with the normal side), and orbital emphysema. With inferior rectus muscle entrapment, the patient will be unable to maximally elevate the eye when asked to look up. If the medial rectus muscle is impinged, the patient will exhibit decreased lateral gaze. Trismus (pain with opening of the mouth) commonly occurs with lateral wall fractures.

Any patient with significant orbital trauma warrants rapid evaluation for globe rupture and further imaging to rule out orbital fracture. The concern for serious injury is heightened in the presence of hyphema, monocular diplopia, or corneal laceration.

Diagnosis

Athletes with cosmetic defects around the eye, pain or deformity along the orbital rim, enophthalmus, extraocular muscle dysfunction, infraorbital anesthesia, or significant vision changes warrant further imaging to evaluate for orbital fracture or globe injury.

Plain films may be obtained when the technology is readily available, but the high likelihood that an occult fracture will be missed makes this a poor imaging choice.[16] In a study of 59 patients with orbital wall fractures, 26 had plain films done for diagnostic purposes. Of these plain films, 50% were falsely negative, and only 5 (19%) were truly positive. In the same population, 51 CT scans were ordered, and all 51 demonstrated truly positive results.[14] CT scanning can be used to confirm suspected fracture or to rule out fracture in high trauma situations.[15] A standard CT scan with 2 mm coronal cuts is sufficient to fully evaluate the size and location of an orbital fracture.[14]

Magnetic resonance imaging does not provide adequate bony detail, and, hence, it is not very useful for the evaluation of orbital fractures.[14] Ultrasound may prove helpful for the imaging evaluation.[17] With experienced operators, ultrasound findings were shown to correlate with the presence of orbital floor fracture 86% of the time as compared with CT and direct evaluation with surgery, and the overall sensitivity was 85%. For a patient in whom CT evaluation may have risks (e.g., a pregnant patient or one with metal fragments near the eye, which can distort images),

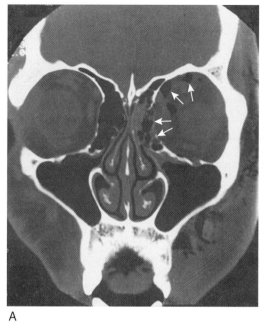
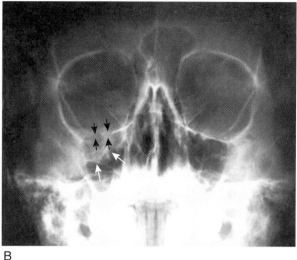

Figure 22.9   *A,* A fracture of the medial orbital wall with hemorrhage into the left ethmoid sinus *(large arrows).* Air within the orbit is seen in this case. *B,* Inferior blowout fracture of the orbit. An anteroposterior view of the face shows discontinuity of the floor of the right orbit *(black arrows)* as well as a soft-tissue mass hanging down from the orbit into the maxillary atrium *(white arrows).* (From Mettler FA: Essentials of Radiology, 2nd ed. Philadelphia, WB Saunders, 2005.)

ultrasound can be used to confirm a fracture. However, if the ultrasound is negative, it still may be prudent to proceed to CT scanning or surgery if a fracture is highly suspected.

Treatment

The initial treatment of orbital fractures includes the recognition of significant injury and protection of the eye during transport to a higher level of care. Cold compresses can be applied to the eye, but care must be taken to not put pressure on the globe or orbit with the application of the compress. The head of the bed should be elevated, and nasal decongestant medications should be considered. Aspirin should be avoided, if possible. The injured player should be instructed to not blow his or her nose, because there is a risk of air passage from the sinuses into the orbit, which leads to orbital emphysema. If there is significant travel time to a facility with a higher level of care, there should be a consideration of prophylactic antibiotics. If an ophthalmologist can be contacted before care is given, corticosteroids should be considered by the treating physician and the consultant to assist with decreasing soft-tissue swelling and subsequent pressure.[6,14]

All orbital fractures should be immediately referred to an ophthalmologist for definitive care, which often involves surgery. Conservative care has also been shown to produce satisfactory results in appropriate clinical scenarios. Conditions that are likely to lead to surgical intervention include inferior rectus muscle entrapment, large fractures (>50% of the orbital floor), globe malposition, or early enophthalmus of more than 2 mm.[14,16] Of note is that diplopia is not an early indication for surgery because it tends to improve after swelling and neuropraxia resolve. If surgery is indicated, surgical exploration within 5 days of injury may produce the best results.[16]

Return to play

Return-to-play decisions depend greatly on any residual effects of the orbital injury. Persistent diplopia, visual acuity loss, or eye pain can produce unsafe conditions for a player to return to contact sports. If visual loss is severe, an athlete may be considered functionally "one eyed" and thus require counseling regarding the risk of injury to the unaffected eye for any sport.

Generally, an athlete is allowed to begin light weightlifting 3 weeks after surgery. If they wear protective eyewear, most athletes can return to most sports by 6 weeks.[18] In a small study of professional football players with orbital fractures, 89% of players (17 of 19) returned to football participation. Fifteen of these players underwent surgical correction, whereas the other 4 were treated nonoperatively. Nearly half of all of the injured players reported persistent diplopia with upward gaze.[15]

An athlete with persistent visual deficits should be encouraged to wear eye protection during athletic play. Obviously, an athlete with a complete resolution of symptoms from an orbital fracture may still prefer and should be encouraged to wear eye protective gear to help prevent recurrence.

Controversies

The decision of whether to treat an athlete operatively or nonoperatively remains a difficult one. Many patients with mild symptoms and no cosmetic defects do very well with conservative (nonoperative) management. Indications for surgery include muscle entrapment, large fractures, and globe malposition.

Traumatic lens dislocation
Definition

Traumatic lens dislocation involves the subluxation or dislocation of the lens of the eye as a result of disruption of the ciliary body zonules that hold the lens in place. The condition is also known as *ectopia lentis.*

Mechanism of injury

Blunt trauma to the eye can damage the tiny zonules and result in an unstable lens.

Risk factors

Athletes with Marfan syndrome and high degrees of myopia are at a higher risk for lens disruption. Other genetic conditions such as Ehlers-Danlos syndrome, congenital glaucoma, and aniridia also confer higher risk. In genetic situations, the condition is frequently bilateral.

Clinical features

A complete dislocation will result in an immediate loss of vision in the affected eye because the focusing power of the lens (up to a third of the total focus) will be acutely lost. Alternatively, a subluxed lens may not be noticed by the athlete until it completely dislocates. Generally, there is no pain associated with the injury because the lens lacks sensory innervation. If a lens dislocation blocks aqueous drainage from the eye, there may be an acute rise in intraocular pressure. If this occurs, the patient may complain of nausea, intense eye pain, headache, vomiting, and blurred vision.[12]

Diagnosis

Lens subluxations or dislocations may not be noticed until the pupil is dilated for examination.

Treatment

Definitive treatment is surgical. If signs of elevated pressure are present, urgent ophthalmology referral is indicated. After acute treatment, investigation for a genetic predisposition should be considered.

Return to play

Clearance for play is likely to come from the treating or team ophthalmologist. The speed at which treatment occurred, the extent of dislocation, and the presence of permanent visual deficits will play a large role in determining the athlete's ability to return to play.

Rentinal detachment
Definition

The separation of the inner layers of the retina from the underlying retinal pigment epithelium or choroids defines a retinal detachment. The retina is a neurosensory tissue with rods and cones that help change light images into nerve impulses for the optic nerve. The blood supply is found in the retinal pigment epithelium; thus, disruption can lead to ischemia of the delicate retinal tissue.[19,20]

Mechanism of injury

Retinal detachments in athletes most commonly result from trauma. During direct globe trauma, rapid compression and decompression can generate vitreoretinal traction, which can lead to a tear of the retinal tissue.[20] Retinal detachment as a result of head or periocular trauma is relatively uncommon, but it must be recognized early to prevent a loss of vision.

Risk factors

Athletes with a high level of myopia are at a higher risk for retinal injury. In addition, a history of a retinal detachment in one eye leads to a higher risk of the occurrence in the other eye. Among patients who are younger than 45 years of age, men are more commonly affected than women.[21] Older athletes may be at higher risk because advancing age leads to molecular breakdown and the shrinkage of the vitreous humor.[20]

Clinical features

Flashing lights, floaters, wavy vision, and vision loss are possible visual deficits. Generally, floaters from retinal detachment occur abruptly and dramatically.[20] Patients may describe a shadow that forms and that begins to cover more and more of the visual field, much like a curtain. This visual loss often begins in the periphery of the visual field and progresses centrally.

Diagnosis

All patients with an acute onset of flashing lights (photopsia) or floaters should be referred to an ophthalmologist for further evaluation within 1 week. Visual field loss warrants an urgent referral. When available, referral to a retinal specialist may be preferable.[20]

Treatment

Surgical treatment by a retinal specialist is often needed in acute settings. It is important to note that a retinal tear may occur initially and then progress to a retinal detachment. Prompt treatment is highly effective for preventing the progression to detachment.[20] Laser or cryogenic burns to create a chorioretinal scar will prevent fluid from passing behind the retina, and they can prevent progression of detachment in 95% of patients.[22]

Team physicians and medical staff can offer treatment in the form of prevention. Protective eyewear is important for all contact sports, but especially for patients with myopia. In addition, the referral of any patient (either urgently or routine) with visual complaints after trauma is recommended. Specialist examination may reveal retinal tears or posterior vitreous detachments that otherwise may not have become clinically apparent for months.

Return to play

Clearance for play is likely to come primarily from the treating ophthalmologist. The speed at which treatment occurred, the extent of the lesion, and the presence of permanent visual deficits will play a large role in determining an athlete's ability to return to play.[21]

NASAL INJURIES

Nasal trauma commonly occurs during sporting events. Direct trauma to the nose may be with a blunt object, such as an elbow or the head of an opposing player, or with an object that provides a penetrating blow, such as a stick while playing ice hockey. As a general rule, injuries to the nose are medically uncomplicated, but they hold a high potential for cosmetic deformity if they are not treated adequately. At times, nasal pathology may mask a more serious injury, such as an orbital wall fracture from a strong blow to the nasal bones. Additionally, posterior bleeding from injuries to the nose might not be obvious after trauma. Very serious nasal injuries can transmit force to and cause a fracture of the cribriform plate. In these cases, cerebrospinal fluid may be discovered and thus provide a critical clue about the severity of the injury.

Epistaxis
Definition

Epistaxis, or nosebleed, is a common problem; 60% of adults have experienced an episode of this condition.[23] Bleeding from the nose is further characterized into anterior and posterior epistaxis, so named for the location of the vessels that are bleeding. Anterior bleeding is far more common (>90%) and easier to recognize and control. Posterior bleeding constitutes a serious situation because extensive bleeding can occur without significant symptoms and may therefore be overlooked (**Figure 22.10**).

Mechanism of injury

Blunt trauma from an object (e.g., a ball, puck, or bat) or from another player (e.g., a head, elbow, or knee) can lead to nasal bleeding.

Risk factors

History of epistaxis episodes, dry weather, seasonal allergies, chronic sinusitis, topical nasal corticosteroids, and sports without facial protection all put an athlete at a higher risk for traumatic epistaxis.

Clinical features

Most athletes with nasal trauma will not have epistaxis. When it is present, it is usually obvious because blood drips—or seemingly pours—out of the anterior nose. Because the bleeding can come on quickly, the source of bleeding may initially be obscured. After bleeding is localized to the nasal structures, the most likely injury is to the anterior vessels. Posterior bleeding may occur with trauma, and it generally presents with difficult-to-control bleeding with airway concerns (e.g., choking or coughing).

Diagnosis

The presence of epistaxis requires further evaluation. Direct nasal visualization may offer clues about the location of the bleeding (i.e., either anterior or posterior). However, if the bleeding is active, visualization is unlikely to be possible. Direct pressure to the nose by compression between the thumb and first finger and the administration of topical nasal decongestants may allow for better visualization after about 15 minutes. If possible, plugging the affected nostril with a gauze soaked in nasal decongestant may be helpful to identify the bleeding vessels. Anterior bleeding begins at the Kiesselbach plexus, which is a series of arterial anastomoses located on the nasal septum. Posterior bleeding occurs behind the middle turbinate or at the roof of the nasal cavity, and it often originates from the sphenopalatine artery.[24] Posterior bleeding may be subtle, and it may not initially be recognized. If it is left untreated, a patient is likely to present with nausea and hematemesis or hemoptysis. Posterior bleeding can, in rare situations, be very brisk and life-threatening.

Nasal bleeding from trauma warrants an evaluation for nasal fracture. Palpation of the bony structures is likely to reveal tenderness in the presence of a fracture. Deformity of these structures is often notable, and it is suggestive of the diagnosis of fracture. Evaluating extraocular muscle movements and checking for stability of the teeth are also prudent to rule out concomitant orbital or maxillary bone fracture.

In traumatic epistaxis, a ring test should be performed to rule out the presence of cerebrospinal fluid in the bloody discharge. This is done by holding a piece of clear gauze or tissue paper under the patient's nose. A drop of blood is allowed to fall on the paper. If cerebrospinal fluid is present, it will form a clear ring around the blood spot (i.e., a "halo"). The presence of CSF indicates a medical emergency because the injury communicates with the central nervous system, and the patient should be transported immediately to an emergency department for evaluation and treatment.

Treatment

Nearly all nasal injuries will improve with ice, direct pressure, elevation, and topical nasal decongestants. Leaning the patient's head forward slightly prevents blood from pooling in the posterior pharynx. With anterior bleeding, compressive pressure with the fingers should be focused at the approximate location of the Kiesselbach plexus.

Topical decongestants can be very helpful to get bleeding under control. This can be accomplished by direct administration if a nasal spray is available or with the placement of a gauze soaked with decongestant. After bleeding has slowed, visualization and cautery of the bleeding site with silver nitrate sticks or handheld cautery can be useful.. Treatment should be carefully limited to superficial vessels to avoid penetrating injury of the nasal structures.

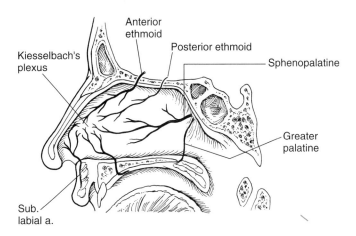

Figure 22.10 Anterior epistaxis is most commonly caused by trauma to kiesselbach's plexis. Posterior epistaxis is due to damage to the larger posterior vessels, most commonly the sphenopalatine artery. (From Emanuel JM: Epistaxis. In: Cummings CW et al [eds]: Otolaryngology: Head and Neck Surgery, 3rd ed. St. Louis, Mosby, 1998.)

If the bleeding still does not stop, packing of the nose should be considered. Anterior packing can be accomplished with a multitude of products, including gauze soaked in petroleum jelly, cellulose, nasal tampons, and specialty pledgets that are specially made to control epistaxis.[25]

Posterior epistaxis requires rapid triage and transport to a medical facility. Most of these patients will need some sort of packing to their nose to slow bleeding or to prevent rebleeding. The removal of the clot followed by the immediate inhalation of topical decongestant, until expectoration of the decongestant from the oral cavity if possible, will be successful in most cases.[26] Any patient that requires nasal packing should be sent for further evaluation by an otorhinolaryngologist.

Return to play

An athlete with active bleeding should not play until the bleeding comes under control. With current precautions against body fluid exposure, it is unlikely that referees will allow play until a person's bleeding is controlled and contaminated parts of the uniform have been cleaned or changed. After the cessation of bleeding, return to play requires clinical judgment on the part of the medical staff. An athlete with an easily controlled episode without concomitant fracture can probably return to play during the same event after counseling regarding the risk of reinjury and the potential for cosmetic and functional impairment.

Nasal fracture
Definition

Nasal fracture involves the disruption of the bony segments of the nose. The bony portion of the nose is the proximal half of the nasal structure. Centrally, the nasal bones are paired, and they connect laterally to the frontal processes of the maxilla.[27] Distal to the bones is cartilage that provides support and that makes up the nasal shape. Nasal fractures account for 40% of traumatic facial bone injuries.[28]

Mechanism of injury

Nasal fractures often result from direct trauma to the nose. During athletic events, this is often caused by contact with another player's head, fist, elbow, or knee. The nasal fracture may occur in the setting of significant trauma, and it can mask a more severe injury, such as a closed head injury, a cervical spine injury, or a more serious facial injury.

Risk factors

The anterior prominence of the nose makes it the facial bone most likely to be fractured. Those who have had prior rhinoplasty are at higher risk of nasal fracture, even if full healing has occurred.[29]

Clinical features

The vector of the nasal trauma may help to determine the location and extent of injury.[28] A direct frontal blow may lead to inward displacement of the nasal bones. A lateral blow often shifts the bones away from the original impact.

If some time has passed since the time of injury, ecchymosis and edema are likely to obscure the initial examination. The patient is likely to have tenderness over the nasal bridge, and he or she may have difficulty breathing out of one or both nostrils if significant deformity or a septal hematoma is present. A septal hematoma is seen on intranasal examination, appearing either as a dark purple or bluish area of fluctuance lying against one or both of the septa. A septal hematoma must be cared for urgently because untreated septal hematomas can result in a saddle deformity of the nose that will require surgical correction **(Figure 22.11)**.

Concerning features that warrant immediate referral to an emergency department are the drainage of clear cerebrospinal fluid from the nares, new malocclusion of the teeth, mental status changes, subcutaneous emphysema, or an abnormal evaluation of the extraocular muscles.[28]

Diagnosis

The diagnosis of nasal fracture is primarily made from the physical examination. Taking pictures from multiple angles of the injured nose may be helpful for evaluating the effects of treatment and for medicolegal purposes to document the level of cosmetic disruption.[27]

After ensuring that the airway is patent and stable, that the cervical spine has been cleared, that an evaluation for concussion has occurred, and that no other life-threatening injuries are present, evaluation of the nose by observation may be revealing. Deformity of the nasal structures is often obvious. In cases of subtle deformity, having the patient look at his or her nose in a mirror may help to determine if a change has occurred. Looking at a picture of the athlete taken before the trauma may help as well. The presence of epistaxis, nasal swelling, or periorbital ecchymosis warrants further evaluation for nasal fracture.[27]

In the event of a nasal fracture, the palpation of the other bony structures of the face is necessary to ensure that concomitant fractures are not present. The evaluation of the ocular muscles can reveal a subtle orbital fracture if limitations in movement are present. Checking the teeth for abnormal movement and tenderness should be done to rule out maxillary fracture.

Plain films are unlikely to offer any additional information to assist with treatment, but they are often obtained. One investigation demonstrated a 66% false-positive rate with plain x-rays resulting from the misinterpretation of normal suture lines.[30] Old fractures heal by callus formation only 15% of the time, so it is nearly impossible to distinguish new from old fractures on plain films.[31] If there is concern about further injury to facial bones, CT scanning is the most helpful to assess for bony injury.

Treatment

Nondisplaced nasal fractures with either no defect or a small cosmetic defect that is acceptable to the patient should be monitored and treated with observation alone. Fractures that are displaced and/or that have resulted in cosmetic defects should be considered for reduction. Fracture reduction is best accomplished when

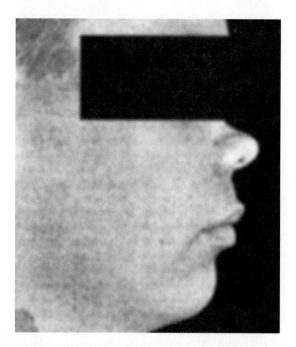

Figure 22.11 Saddle nose. (From De Weese DD, Saunders WH: Textbook of Otolaryngology, 4th ed. St. Louis, Mosby, 1973.)

swelling is minimal. Hence, unless the fracture can be reduced immediately after the injury, reduction is typically best performed 5 to 10 days after the injury, when the bruising and swelling have diminished. Patients with nasal fractures who present for care 2 to 72 hours after injury should be scheduled for reexamination around day 5, with reduction planned on day 5 to 10. Fractures should optimally be reduced by day 10, before bony adhesion has occurred.

Closed reduction is indicated for unilateral, minimally displaced nasal fractures. A team physician with sufficient training in treating nasal fractures may decide to perform the reduction, although most reductions are now performed by otorhinolaryngologists for the best cosmetic results. Even in the most experienced hands, the aesthetic result of closed reduction may not be acceptable for the patient; nasal reconstruction surgery may be necessary in these cases.

As previously mentioned, septal hematomas commonly occur in conjunction with nasal fractures, and they must be treated as soon as possible. Septal hematomas are caused by blood collecting between the cartilage and the supporting perichondrium. The blood can become infected, or it may lead to permanent saddle nose deformity from pressure necrosis of the cartilage. Recommended treatments include aspiration with a large-gauge needle or incision of the hematoma with drainage and packing. Consultation with an otorhinolaryngologist should be considered for follow-up care. Concern about the reaccumulation of the hematoma warrants daily evaluation of the athlete until definitive treatment occurs **(Figure 22.12)**.

Return to play

The criteria for return to competition takes into account the type of treatment used for the fracture. Any athlete who has had packing or splinting should not return until these have been removed (usually after 3 to 7 days for packing and 7 to 10 days for splints). During the convalescent period, discussion with the athlete regarding the risk of recurrent injury leading to failure of the reduction should occur. A full face shield will allow for an early return to sports participation, generally 1 to 2 weeks after treatment.[27] The shield should be worn for the remainder of the season (at least 8 weeks) or longer, if the athlete prefers.

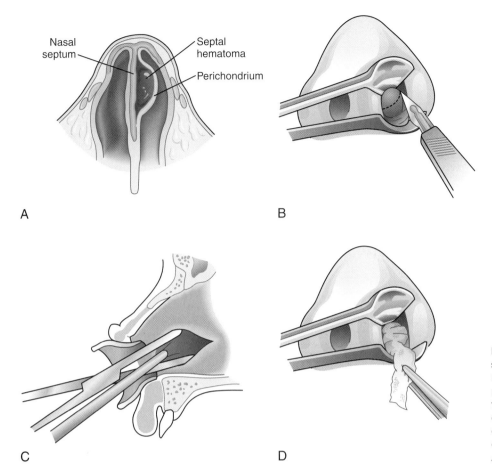

A

B

C

D

Figure 22.12   Septal hematoma. *A,* Cross-sectional view of a septal hematoma, showing blood accumulation between the septum and perichondrium. Treatment involves anesthesia that is followed by incision using a hemostat *(B),* drainage of the hematoma *(C),* and the insertion of sterile gauze to prevent the reaccumulation of blood *(D).* (From Kucik CJ, Clenney T, Phelan J: Am Fam Physician 2004;70[7]:1315-1320.)

EAR INJURIES

Auricular hematoma
Definition
Auricular hematoma is a collection of blood between the ear perichondrium and the cartilage after trauma. The condition is also known as *cauliflower ear.*

Mechanism of injury
A hematoma results from a shearing force or a direct blow to the ear, at which time blood collects between the perichondrium and the cartilage.[32] Wrestling is most commonly associated with this injury, but it can occur during any sport that involves the possibility of ear trauma.

Risk factors
Headgear in wrestling has helped to decrease the incidence of this injury, but it has not eliminated it completely.[33] Many wrestlers who develop a hematoma will report noncompliance with headgear. In a survey of 537 division I collegiate wrestlers, only 35% reported compliance with headgear during practice.[34] Prior injury may increase the incidence of future events.

Clinical features
The pinna will appear deformed at the time of presentation, and there is usually a history of trauma to the ear. Pain may be present, but it is usually not severe.

Diagnosis
The diagnosis is made by the evaluation of the ear after known trauma. The pinna will demonstrate a mass that the athlete may recall as having either gradually or rapidly expanded since the time of injury. The mass will be moderately firm, and it may have a fluctuant nature.

Treatment
The hematoma must be evacuated completely to allow for the reapproximation of the perichondrium and the cartilage. The most common techniques are aspiration and incision.

Aspiration of the hematoma is best performed under sterile technique using a large-bore needle (18 or 20 gauge). The needle is placed into the largest portion of the hematoma, and blood is "milked" toward the needle until the entire hematoma is evacuated. A pressure dressing should be applied immediately after drainage to prevent reaccumulation. If the blood does reaccumulate, reaspiration is recommended. The athlete should be evaluated daily for 1 week to monitor for recurrence.

The incision technique aims to evacuate the hematoma fully by opening the layers of the perichondrium to allow for direct evacuation. The technique works best if it is done within 7 days of hematoma formation. After a local anesthesia (without epinephrine) is used, an incision should be made with a no. 15 blade scalpel along the natural curvature of the pinna. The overlying skin and perichondrium can be peeled off of the hematoma. Remove the hematoma completely, and irrigate the pocket with normal saline. The wound should be reapproximated, and antibiotic ointment should be spread over the incision. A pressure dressing should be placed within minutes after the procedure. The goal of a compressive pressure dressing is to firmly approximate the perichondrium and cartilage to allow for healing and to prevent the reaccumulation of the hematoma. However, care should be taken to avoid pressure necrosis from a dressing that is too tight. Two common types of pressure dressings used are a gauze dressing and a dental roll with sutures. **(Figures 22.13 and 22.14).**

Infection of the perichondrium can occur after the auricular hematoma and as a complication from drainage. Both the physician and the patient should be vigilant when examining the wound for signs of infection and/or necrosis from vascular occlusion.

Return to play

The athlete should not compete while wearing the compression dressings. For the best cosmetic result, return to play should be delayed until the dressing is removed and the reapproximation of the perichondrium and the cartilage has been confirmed.

DENTAL INJURIES

Dental injuries are common in sports. A knowledge of dental anatomy and physiology can help improve morbidity. The teeth have unique tissues: the enamel and dentin of the teeth are the hardest tissues in the body, and they are not able to repair themselves.[35] The two main portions of the tooth are the root and the crown. The crown is made up of soft dentin (yellowish color), which is covered by enamel; this is the portion of the tooth that is visible above the gums. The pulp of the tooth underlies the dentin and extends into the root of the tooth. The pulp holds the neurovascular bundle of the tooth, and it is contained within the pulp chamber and the root canals. The root attaches to the socket by periodontal ligaments[36] **(Figure 22.15).**

Dentoalveolar trauma occurs most frequently during skateboarding, gymnastics, swimming, ice sports, inline skating, squash, and bicycling.[37] With the exception of ice hockey, these sports do not require mouth guards, which may contribute to the higher incidence of dental trauma.

Prevention
Mouth guards

The safety of mouth guards has been firmly established. The mouth guard functions to protect the teeth and soft tissues during contact sports. The functions of a mouth guard are listed in **Box 22.2.**

Tooth luxation
Definition

Tooth luxation is the loosening of a tooth. Luxated teeth occur along a spectrum, from slight loosening without displacement (subluxation) to intrusion (a tooth driven into its socket) to extrusion (tooth dislocation with tearing of the neurovascular bundle) to complete avulsion **(Figure 22.16).**

Any luxated tooth should be evaluated by a dental provider. Splinting may be required. Of the conditions listed previously, only tooth avulsion constitutes a dental emergency. However, the others require urgent dental consultation for recommendations of care. One of the most helpful clinical clues to tooth disruption is the athlete's sense that the teeth do not fit correctly. Care should be taken to evaluate for the segmental mobility of multiple teeth, which could indicate the fracture of the maxillary or mandibular bone.

Tooth intrusion
Definition

Tooth intrusion is the forceful impaction of a tooth into its alveolar socket.

Mechanism of injury

Direct trauma may cause intrusion. Typically, this is from an object striking a tooth (e.g., a stick or a puck). Indirect trauma occurs when the forceful closure of the teeth occurs as a result of impact elsewhere on the head.

Risk factors

Improperly fitting mouth guards or the failure to wear a mouth guard during participation in a contact sport leaves the teeth relatively unprotected.

Clinical features

The athlete is likely to complain of pain around the area of the intruded tooth, and he or she may feel a sense of malalignment of the teeth.

Diagnosis

The affected tooth will appear shorter than the surrounding teeth because it has been forced into the socket.

Treatment

The intruded tooth should not be reduced in the field. More than likely, the dental provider will allow the tooth to re-erupt on its own. The patient will need to be followed by a dental provider because the erupted tooth is likely to need splinting. Treatment should be sought urgently but not emergently.

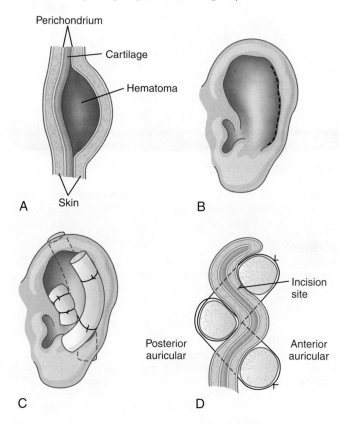

Figure 22.13 *A,* Hematoma separating the perichondrium from the cartilage. *B,* Incision made along the skin curvature at the posterior edge of the hematoma. The hematoma is evacuated, and the area is irrigated. *C,* Two anterior dental rolls are secured with sutures to a posterior dental roll to maintain the normal anatomy of the pinna. *D,* A side view illustrates the position of sutures and dental rolls in relation to the incision site. Note that the perichondrium is apposed to the cartilage. (From Clemons JE, Seveneid LR: Otohematoma. In Cummings CW [ed]: Otolaryngology: Head and Neck Surgery, 2nd ed. St Louis, Mosby, 1993.)

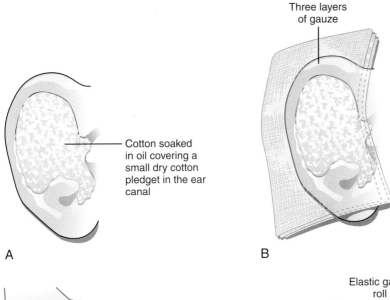

Three layers
of gauze

Cotton soaked
in oil covering a
small dry cotton
pledget in the ear
canal

A   B

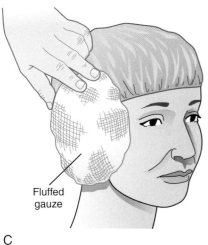

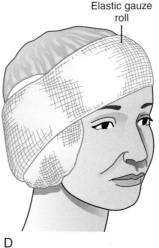

Elastic gauze
roll

Fluffed
gauze

C   D

Figure 22.14 Compression dressing of the ear. After the successful aspiration of an auricular hematoma, a compression dressing is used to prevent the reaccumulation of the hematoma or fluid. *A*, Dry cotton is first placed into the ear canal. A conforming material is then carefully molded into all of the convolutions of the auricle. One may use Vaseline gauze or cotton soaked in mineral oil or saline. *B*, When the convolutions are fully packed, a posterior gauze pack is placed behind the ear. A V-shaped section has been cut from the gauze to allow it to fit easily behind the ear. *C*, Multiple layers of fluffed gauze are placed over the packed ear, and the entire dressing is held in place with Kling gauze or an elastic gauze roll. *D*, The ear is thus compressed between two layers of gauze, and the packing ensures even distribution of pressure to all parts of the auricle. (From Roberts JR: Clinical Procedures in Emergency Medicine, 4th ed. Philadelphia, WB Saunders, 2004.)

Return to play

The athlete may return to full competition after the dental splints are removed and healing has occurred (usually 3 to 6 weeks). Before removal of the splints, only light training is recommended.

Tooth avulsion
Definition

Tooth avulsion is the complete dislocation of a tooth from the alveolar bone and soft-tissue socket.

Mechanism of injury

Tooth avulsion requires contact with enough force to disrupt the affected tooth from its periodontal ligament as it is cradled in the alveolar socket. Many patients with tooth avulsion will suffer a concussion at the time of injury.

Risk factors

The absence of an appropriate mouth guard leaves the teeth open for injury. Contact sports have a higher incidence of head and neck trauma.

Clinical features

The athlete will likely have a vacant area along the gum line, and a dislocated tooth may be obvious. There may be bleeding at the affected socket. Rinsing the mouth with saline or sterile water may make the vacancy more apparent. After trauma, the vacancy may be seen without an apparent avulsed tooth. A search for the tooth in the nearby area as well as in the clothing of the other athletes involved in the contact will often reveal the tooth. If the tooth is not found, x-rays or other imaging modalities are necessary to ensure that the athlete has not aspirated the avulsed tooth **(Figure 22.17)**.

Diagnosis

A complete tooth avulsion is generally apparent readily at the time of injury. Care must be taken to ensure that the tooth has avulsed completely and that it has not fractured at the base.

Treatment

A primary tooth (i.e., a "baby tooth") need not be reimplanted. A permanent adult tooth should be reimplanted as soon as possible. Time is critical to the success of reimplantation. If a tooth can be replanted within 30 minutes, there is a greater than 90% chance of saving the tooth. Delay of greater than 2 hours results in a tooth survival rate of only 5%.[35] The avulsed tooth should be cleaned by rinsing in saline, cool running tap water, sterile water, or milk, but it should not be scrubbed. Hanks' balanced salt solution is often available in sports medicine kits to assist with the cleansing and transfer of the avulsed tooth.

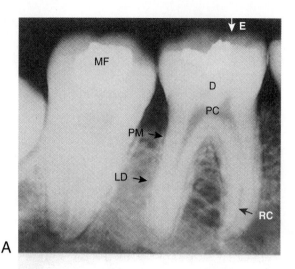

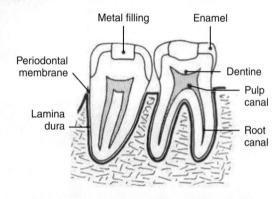

Figure 22.15 Tooth anatomy. *A*, A periapical radiograph labeled to show a tooth and its supporting structures. *B*, Corresponding line diagram. E, Enamel; D, dentine; LD, lamina dura; MF, amalgam filling; PC, pulp; PM, periodontal membrane (periodontal ligament space); RC, root canal. (From Grainger & Allison's Diagnostic Radiology: A Textbook of Medical Imaging, 4th ed. Churchill Livingstone, 2001.)

Box 22.2: Functions of a Mouth Guard

1. To provide a barrier between the teeth and lips to prevent lacerations and contusions
2. To distribute forces from the front of the teeth to the entire mouth, thereby cushioning any blow and limiting trauma to the anterior teeth
3. To assist with the prevention of forceful contact of the maxillary and mandibular teeth
4. To absorb damaging forces that otherwise have the potential to fracture the jaw
5. To prevent concussion by inhibiting the upward and backward motion of the mandible and the base of the skull
6. To offer support to edentulous spaces
7. To allow athletes to compete in athletics with less concern about dental injuries

Adapted from Kerr IL, Bigsby GA, Haeseler GA, et al: Compendium 1993;14(9):1142-1156.

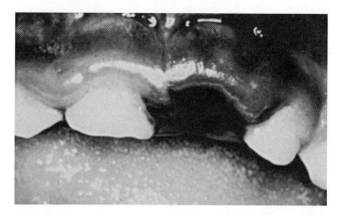

Figure 22.16 Tooth luxation. (From Behrman RE: Nelson Textbook of Pediatrics, 17th ed. Philadelphia, Saunders, 2004.)

Hold the tooth by the crown so as not to disrupt the root or the periodontal ligament. The viability of this ligament determines the success of reimplantation. Injury to the ligament will result in the resorption of the tooth and the probable loss of the tooth.

The reimplantation process begins at the time of avulsion. After lightly cleaning the tooth with rinsing, an attempt should be made to identify the front and back of the tooth. Ideally, the tooth should be reimplanted in the correct anterior-to-posterior orientation. Replacing a tooth in a backward position is not recommended, but it is preferable to not replacing it at all. Minimal pressure is used to put the tooth back into its original position.

If replacement of the tooth is not possible, it can be stored inside the patient's cheek at the level of the gums during transport. Keep in mind that an avulsed tooth may compromise the airway if it is placed in the mouth of an athlete with altered consciousness. In this situation, other acceptable transfer methods are wrapping the tooth in gauze and storing it in milk or storing it in normal saline. The tooth should not be stored in another person's mouth or in dry gauze. Immediate transfer to dental care for splinting offers the best chance for tooth survival. Definitive care ultimately results in root canal treatment. Antibiotic prophylaxis with penicillin and evaluation of tetanus status are recommended.

Return to play

The athlete may return to full competition after the dental splints are removed and healing has occurred (usually 3 to 6 weeks). Before the removal of the splints, only light training is recommended.[38]

Tooth fracture
Definition
Partial breaks in tooth congruity occur at either the root or crown level. The injuries are further characterized into simple (no pulp involvement) and complex (pulp involved) **(Figure 22.18)**.

Mechanism of injury
Tooth fracture can result from indirect trauma in which a part of the face or head other than the mouth is struck and the bones of the jaw strike each other with transmitted force.[35]

Risk factors
Improper wearing of or a lack of sufficient mouth protection can lead to tooth fractures.

Clinical features
The fractured segment may be obvious or subtle (lodged in the soft-tissue structures or lost outside of the mouth). Pulp involvement is likely to cause significant pain and irritation when there is contact with liquids, air, or temperature changes.[36]

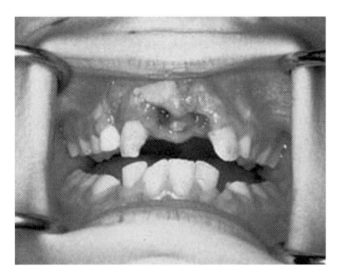

Figure 22.17 Tooth avulsion. (From Cummings CW: Otolaryngology: Head and Neck Surgery, 4th ed. Philadelphia, Mosby, 2005.)

Diagnosis

The diagnosis of pulp involvement is critical to determining the severity of the fracture. A bleeding site or a pinkish-red dot in the middle of the yellowish dentin indicates pulp involvement.[36]

Treatment

Tooth fractures can lead to significant cosmetic impairment, and tooth death is common. Any available portion of the tooth should be sent with the athlete to the dentist, although it is unlikely to be of use.[36] To help with pain control, gently biting on a gauze or towel will decrease outside exposure to air, saliva, or the tongue and gums. If available, covering the exposed nerve with cyanoacrylate (i.e., Superglue) may relieve discomfort. It should be noted that the US Food and Drug Administration does not currently endorse cyanoacrylate for these purposes, but it has been endorsed as a dental cement.[39] If pain is well controlled, immediate dental care is not necessary.

Return to play

Definitive treatment and clearance will depend on the extent of the original injury. Proper wearing of a mouth guard is recommended for the remainder of the athlete's career to help prevent further damage to the tooth.

JAW INJURIES

The prominence of the jaw leaves it vulnerable to injury during athletics. The mandible is one of the most commonly fractured bones of the face.[40]

Temporomandibular joint dislocation
Definition

The connection between the mobile mandible and the temporal bone of the skull is primarily ligamentous and cartilaginous. Injury to these soft-tissue structures or to the bony portion of the joint can occur with sports.

Mechanism of injury

Direct blunt trauma to the jaw or deceleration injuries may lead to temporomandibular joint (TMJ) injury.[35] Many patients report being struck on a partially open jaw.[41]

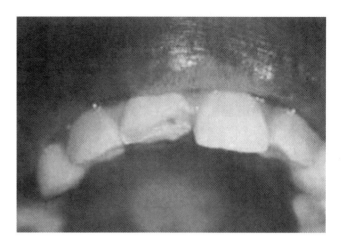

Figure 22.18 A complex tooth fracture. (From Roberts JR: Clinical Procedures in Emergency Medicine, 4th ed. Philadelphia, Saunders, 2004.)

Risk factors

Athletes with shallow mandibular fossa in the temporal bone or underdeveloped mandibular condyles are at a higher risk for TMJ dislocation. Marfan syndrome and Ehlers–Danlos syndrome put a patient at higher risk as a result of increased compliance of the ligamentous structures.[41] An athlete with history of prior dislocation is at higher risk of recurrence.

Clinical features

With dislocation of the TMJ, a patient may have pain, and the jaw may appear malformed. Dislocation happens both unilaterally and bilaterally. An athlete with a bilateral dislocation may appear to have an underbite as the mandible dislocates anteriorly. Spasm of the masseter and pterygoid muscles results in trismus, and speaking may be difficult.[41] Reduction of the injury is generally simple, and it can occur on the field.

Diagnosis

The use of plain radiography or CT scanning is indicated in dislocation injuries of the TMJ to rule out fracture. Plain films of the mandible are often sufficient to diagnose the fractures accurately.

Treatment

Before reduction, the stability of the airway should be confirmed. In instances of violent trauma or if there is any doubt about the presence of a fracture, x-rays or CT scanning should precede any attempted reduction.

Reduction of the dislocation can be accomplished by facing the affected athlete. With gloved hands, the tips of the thumbs are placed along the buccal aspect of the last molar teeth, and the fingers are placed along the inferior surface of the mandible. Reduction requires the exertion of considerable firm downward pressure on the mandible to allow the condyle to be released from its entrapment anterior to the auricular eminence. Next, the mandible should be allowed to migrate posteriorly to return to anatomic alignment. If reduction is successful, the teeth will close correctly, and the patient may feel a "clunk" as the mandible slides back into place.[41] A single attempt to reduce the jaw is prudent at the time of injury if no significant facial deformity is present (which indicates possible fracture). If the first attempt is unsuccessful, consider transport to an emergency department for conscious sedation and a repeat effort. Postreduction films should be taken to confirm proper alignment.

The delayed or inappropriate treatment of TMJ disorders can lead to chronic pain, chewing difficulties, and chronic subluxations of the jaw. Wiring the teeth together may be required to immobilize the joint and allow healing.[35]

Return to play

These injuries can be quite painful, and the athlete is typically unable to continue competition. In less painful situations, the malformation of the jaw and the inability to close the mouth fully may lead the athlete to pull himself or herself from competition. Return to play after a healed dislocation depends on the presence of fractures and other injuries.

Controversies

Reduction on the field should be undertaken gently and with caution because iatrogenic condyle fracture is possible.

Mandibular fracture
Definition

There are multiple possible locations for jaw fracture; this overview is focused on the recognition of injury and referral for definitive care **(Figure 22-19).**

Mechanism of injury

In a study of more than 5000 mandible fractures in active-duty army members, athletic participation accounted for 13.6% of the injuries. Blunt trauma causes a majority of the fractures.[42] In this military population, more than a third of the sports-related injuries occurred while playing football, followed by basketball and softball. The frequency of mandibular fractures from sports ranges from 4% to 14%.[37,40,42]

Mandibular fractures are further characterized by their location: condylar, coronoid, ramus, angle, parasymphysis, symphysis, alveolar, or combination fractures.

Risk factors

The improper wearing of head protection or face guards while playing American football or ice hockey may lead to jaw injury. Having a lower third molar may double the risk of having a mandibular angle fracture.[40]

Clinical features

Numbness or dysesthesia of the lower lip may be seen, especially with displaced fractures, because these are more likely to disrupt the inferior alveolar nerve. The face may appear malformed when the mandible fractures, and malposition of the teeth on biting is likely. Asking the patient to bite down may produce premature contact of the molars and cause the anterior teeth to be unable to make contact, which results in an "anterior open bite."

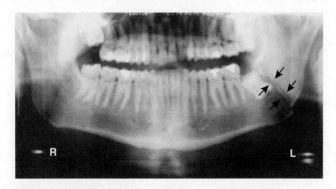

Figure 22.19 Mandibular fracture. A panoramic x-ray view shows a fracture (arrows) through the left mandibular angle. (From Mettler FA: Essentials of Radiology, 2nd ed. Philadelphia, Saunders, 2004.)

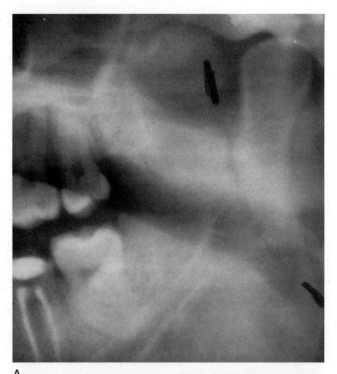

A

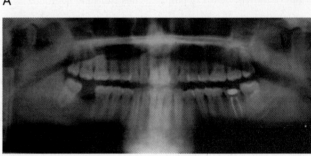

B

Figure 22.20 A and B, A nondisplaced mandibular body and angle fracture in a boxer who was injured by a punch during a fight.

Diagnosis

First and foremost, patients with facial trauma must have an evaluation of airway patency and airway stability before the treatment of fractures or lacerations. Mandibular fractures require a relatively high level of force, and they tend to occur in association with other injuries. Some of these associated injuries may be subtle: for example, vertebral artery dissection and basilar skull fracture have been reported in conjunction with mandibular fracture.

If fracture of the mandible is suspected, plain radiographs (lateral–oblique, occlusal, posteroanterior, and periapical views) along with a panorama view of the mandible are preferred. CT scanning may be helpful to diagnose displacement or comminution of the fracture as well as to identify other bony injuries.

Treatment

Closed reduction is preferred when possible because of the increased infection risk of open reduction. Soft diet, pain control, and close observation are recommended in these cases. Mandibular fractures tend to heal slowly, and they can show radiographic fracture lines for months after the acute event.

Indications for open reduction include displaced fractures, the presence of multiple facial fractures, and significant malocclusion. After surgical treatment, antibiotics and pain medications are given. The jaw is usually wired closed for splinting purposes, so nutritional issues may arise.[43] Because mandibular fractures typically occur in conjunction with other serious injuries and because of the risk for serious complications, these fractures should be referred to a provider who is experienced with the management of mandibular trauma **(Figure 22.20).**

Return to play

If open reduction is required, the athlete will likely have jaw wiring for at least 4 to 6 weeks. After this, sufficient time for improving nutrition and increasing physical stamina should be allowed before return to competition.

CONCLUSION

Sports-related injuries to the craniomaxillofacial region can be cosmetically devastating and occasionally life threatening. Rapid evaluation and triage will identify the most serious injuries, allow for rapid initial treatment, and prompt timely referral to specialists when indicated. Use of protective equipment (e.g., mouth guards, headgear) has been shown to effectively prevent many severe injuries to the face and head. Sports medicine providers should encourage their athletes in the proper wear of these proven-effective appliances.

REFERENCES

1. Hop JW, Rinkel GJ, Algra A, van Gijn J: Case-fatality rates and functional outcome after subarachnoid hemorrhage: a systematic review. Stroke 1997;28(3):660-664.
2. Roberts JR, Hedges JR, Chanmugam AS, et al: Clinical Procedures in Emergency Medicine, 4th ed. Philadelphia, WB Saunders, 2004.
3. Hollander JE, Richman PB, Werblud M: Irrigation in facial and scalp lacerations. Does it alter outcome? Ann Emerg Med 1998;31:73-77.
4. Mihata LCS: Chapter 37: Head injuries. In Birrer RB, O'Connor FG (eds): Sports Medicine for the Primary Care Physician, 3rd ed ed. Boca Raton, FL, 2004, CRC Press, pp 419-430.
5. Rodriguez JO, Lavina AM, Agarwal A: Prevention and treatment of common eye injuries in sports. Am Fam Physician 2003;67(7):1481-1488.
6. Harrison A, Telander DG: Eye injuries in the young athlete: a case-based approach. Pediatr Ann 2002;31(1):33-40.
7. Jacobs DS: Corneal abrasions and corneal foreign bodies (Web site): Available at www.uptodateonline.com. Accessed November 7, 2006.
8. Kaiser PK: A comparison of pressure patching versus no patching for corneal abrasions due to trauma or foreign body removal. Corneal Abrasion Patching Study Group. Ophthalmology 1995;102:1936-1942.
9. Benson WH, Snyder IS, Granus V, et al: Tetanus prophylaxis following ocular injuries. J Emerg Med 1993;11(6):677-683.
10. Jaycock PD, Poon W, Wigley F, et al: Three cases of intraocular foreign bodies as a result of walking or running along roadways. Am J Ophthalmol 2004;137(3):585-586.
11. Wirbelauer C: Management of the red eye for the primary care physician. Am J Med 2006;119:302-306.
12. Mihata LCS: Chapter 38: Eye injuries. In Birrer RB, O'Connor FG (eds): Sports Medicine for the Primary Care Physician, 3rd ed. Boca Raton, FL, 2004, CRC Press, pp 431-441.
13. Jones NP: Orbital blowout fractures in sport. Br J Sports Med 1994;28:272-275.
14. Brady SM, McMann MA, Mazzoli RA, et al: The diagnosis and management of orbital blowout fractures: update 2001. Am J Emerg Med 2001;19:147-154.
15. Williams RJ 3rd, Marx RG, Barnes R, et al: Fractures about the orbit in professional American football players. Am J Sports Med 2001;29(1):55-57.
16. Petrigliano FA, Williams III RJ: Orbital fractures in sport. Sports Med 2003;33(4):317-322.
17. Jenkins CN, Thuau H: Ultrasound imaging in assessment of fractures of the orbital floor. Clin Radiol 1997;52(9):708-711.
18. Zafar A, Penne RB: Orbital fracture, medial wall (Web site): Available at www.emedicine.com/oph/topic762.htm. Accessed March 21, 2006.
19. Weber TS: Training room management of eye conditions. Clin Sports Med 2005;24:681-693.
20. Gariano RF, Kim CH: Evaluation and management of suspected retinal detachment. Am Fam Physician. 2004;69(7):1691-1698.
21. Larkin GL: Retinal detachment (Web site): Available at www.emedicine.com/emerg/topic504.htm. Accessed December 5, 2006.
22. Smiddy WE, Flynn HW Jr, Nicholson DH, et al: Results and complications in treated retinal breaks. Am J Ophthalmol 1991;112:623-631.
23. Alter H: Approach to the adult with epistaxis (Web site): Available at www.uptodateonline.com. Accessed December 22, 2006.
24. Kucik CJ, Clenney T: Management of epistaxis. Am Fam Physician. 2005;71(2):305-311.
25. Webb CW, Birrer RB: Chapter 40: Nasal injuries. In Birrer RB, O'Connor FG (eds): Sports Medicine for the Primary Care Physician, 3rd ed ed. Boca Raton, FL, 2004, CRC Press, pp 443-447.
26. Stackhouse T: Onsite management of nasal injuries. Phys Sportsmed 1998;26(8).
27. Cummings CW, Flint PW, Haughey BH, et al (eds): Chapter 41: Nasal fractures. In Otolaryngology: Head & Neck Surgery, 4th ed. Philadelphia, Mosby, 2005.
28. Kucik CJ, Clenney T, Phelan J: Management of acute nasal fractures. Am Fam Physician 2004;70(7):1315-1320.
29. Guyuron B, Zarandy S: Does rhinoplasty make the nose more susceptible to fracture? Plast Reconstr Surg 1994;93:313-317.
30. de Lacey GJ: The radiology of nasal injuries: problems of interpretation and clinical relevance. Br J Radiol 1977;50:412-414.
31. Illum P: Legal aspects in nasal fractures. Rhinology 1991;29:263-266.
32. Roberts JR, Hedges JR, Chanmugan AS, et al (eds): Chapter 65: Otolaryngologic procedures. In Clinical Procedures in Emergency Medicine, 4th ed. Philadelphia, WB Saunders, 2004.
33. Bowers MG, Howard TM: Chapter 95: Wrestling. In O'Connor FG, Sallis KE, Wilder RP, et al (eds): Sports Medicine: Just the Facts. New York, McGraw-Hill, 2005, pp 553-558.
34. Schuller DE, Dankle SK, Martin M, Strauss RH: Auricular injury and the use of headgear in wrestlers. Arch Otolaryngol Head Neck Surg 1989;115(6):714-717.
35. Kerr IL, Bigsby GA, Haeseler GA, et al: Prevention and emergency first-aid treatment for sports-related dentofacial injuries. Compendium 1993;14(9):1142-1156.
36. Roberts WO: Field care of the injured tooth. Phys Sportsmed 2000;28(1):101-102.
37. Tuli T, Hachl O, Hohlrieder M, et al: Dentofacial trauma in sports accidents. Gen Dent 2002;50(3):274-279.
38. Allen JE: Chapter 41: Injuries to facial bones and teeth. In Birrer RB, O'Connor FG (eds): Sports Medicine for the Primary Care Physician, 3rd ed ed. Boca Raton, FL, 2004, CRC Press, pp 449-452.
39. US Food and Drug Administration: Guidance for industry and FDA staff: cyanoacrylate tissue adhesive for the topical approximation of skin—premarket approval applications (Web site): Available at www.fda.gov/cdrh/ode/guidance/1233.pdf. Accessed May 24, 2007.
40. Soule WC, Fisher LH: Mandible, fractures (Web site): Available at www.emedicine.com/radio/topic423.htm. Accessed December 26, 2006.
41. Newton E, McClung CD: Dislocations, mandible (Web site): Available at www.emedicine.com/emerg/topic147.htm. Accessed December 26, 2006.
42. Boole JR, Holtel M, Amoroso P, Yore M: 5196 mandible fractures among 4381 active duty army soldiers, 1980 to 1998. Laryngoscope 2001;111:1691-1696.
43. Barrera JE, Batuello SG: Mandibular body fractures (Web site): Available at www.emedicine.com/ent/topic415.htm. Accessed March 21, 2006.

CHAPTER

Cervical Spine Injuries

Barry P. Boden, MD

KEY POINTS

· The sports with the highest risk of catastrophic spinal injuries are football, ice hockey, wrestling, diving, skiing, snowboarding, and rugby.

· Acute brachial plexus injuries (i.e., "burners") are common among players of American football, and they involve only one extremity. Any individual with neurologic symptoms in more than one extremity has a spinal cord injury until proven otherwise.

· Axial compression forces to the top of the head can lead to cervical fracture and quadriplegia in players of any sport.

· Any medical personnel covering team sports should have a plan for the stabilization and transfer of an athlete with a cervical spine injury.

· The role of methylprednisolone for the treatment of acute spinal cord injuries remains controversial; it requires evaluation with additional evidence-based clinical studies.

INTRODUCTION

Most cervical spine injuries that are incurred during sports participation are stable injuries that require careful nonoperative treatment. These injuries include cervical strains and transient brachial plexopathy. Catastrophic spine injuries in sports are rare but tragic events that may lead to permanent disability. The sports with the highest risk of catastrophic spinal injuries are football, ice hockey, wrestling, diving, skiing, snowboarding, rugby, cheerleading, and baseball. A common mechanism of injury for all at-risk sports is an axial compression force to the top of the head with the neck slightly flexed. The author reviews the spectrum of cervical spine injuries in the athletic population, the common mechanisms of injury, the on-field management of the athlete with a cervical spine injury, and the sport-specific injuries in the at-risk sports.

BRACHIAL PLEXUS INJURIES

Brachial plexus injuries are rare in most sports except football, ice hockey, and wrestling. Most sports-related brachial plexus injuries are compression or traction neuropraxias, which have a favorable prognosis. The differential diagnosis of a brachial plexus injury should include transient brachial plexopathy (TBP), acute brachial neuropathy, root avulsion or neurotmesis, disc herniation, cervical cord neuropraxia, and cervical spine fracture.

TRANSIENT BRACHIAL PLEXOPATHY

Most brachial plexus injuries occur in American football players, and they are referred to as "burners" or "stingers." The single season incidence of TBP in American college football players has been reported to be between 6.9% and 50%.[1-4] One study revealed that 65% of 201 National Collegiate Athletic Association division III football players had a history of a TBP.[4]

Athletes with TBP typically present with acute unilateral upper extremity radicular symptoms from the supraclavicular region to the fingertips. TBP must be differentiated from cervical cord neuropraxia, which is defined as injury to the spinal cord with neurologic symptoms in at least two extremities. This important clinical point cannot be overemphasized: burners occur in a *single* arm. Athletes with neurologic symptoms bilaterally or in more than one extremity should be considered to have a spinal cord injury until it is proven otherwise. On the sidelines, the player with TBP initially presents shaking his or her arm or holding it at his or her side as a response to paresthesias and dyesthesias. Weakness is often associated with the injury, and it may occur on a delayed basis hours to days after the injury.[2,5] Neurologic deficits, if present, usually occur at the C5 and C6 levels, and they are manifested by shoulder abduction (deltoid) and elbow flexion (biceps) weakness. In most instances, the neurologic symptoms only last for several minutes, but, in 5% to 10% of athletes, they persist for days to months.[6] Prolonged symptoms are more common among athletes with multiples episodes. Physical examination usually reveals a normal, painless cervical range of motion.

Three causes of TBP have been proposed: traction, extension compression, and direct compression. Traction is the most frequently hypothesized mechanism to explain the burner phenomenon, and it usually occurs in younger athletes. The injury mechanism involves a tackling maneuver when the shoulder is depressed, with lateral neck flexion to the contralateral side. The extension–compression mechanism typically involves older players with degenerative changes of the cervical spine. The cervical spine is in extension, compression, and rotation toward the affected arm, similar to the Spurling maneuver position. Foraminal narrowing and/or degenerative disk disease have been implicated as causing impingement on the C5 and C6 nerve roots.[7,8] Lastly, the injury may occur as a result of direct compression at the Erb point, where the brachial plexus is most superficial.

Diagnosis of TBP is usually made by performing a thorough history and physical examination. Electrodiagnostic studies are not indicated for routine cases of TBP because the study often reveals persistent abnormalities, even after complete clinical resolution. Rather, electrodiagnostic evaluation is warranted in athletes who have had symptoms for more than 3 weeks or for those with multiple episodes. The treatment of TBP involves symptomatic measures. Physical therapy may be helpful to strengthen the affected muscles. Athletes should not be allowed to return to contact sports until full painless neck range of motion and complete neurologic recovery are achieved. The prevention of TBP should include a review of tackling techniques and instructing the athlete not to tackle with the shoulder dropped and the head laterally rotated toward the contralateral side. Using a neck roll or other equipment to limit neck extension may reduce the incidence of TBP, but this is controversial because the cervical spine in placed in a more vulnerable position for axial forces.

ACUTE BRACHIAL NEUROPATHY

Acute brachial neuropathy, which is also referred to as *Parsonage–Turner syndrome, brachial neuritis*, and *acute brachial radiculitis*, is a condition that is associated with acute shoulder and neck pain that may spread to the forearm region. The painful phase typically lasts between several hours and 3 weeks, and it is followed by varying degrees of weakness. Weakness may be mild or severe, and it usually involves the C5 and C6 distributions, especially the deltoid, supraspinatus, and infraspinatus muscles. Signs that should alert the clinician to acute brachial neuropathy are an onset of symptoms with no trauma, pain that continues despite rest, and dominant arm predominance.[9] The cause of this disorder is unknown, but it may involve an inflammatory process, such as a viral or autoimmune cause. Treatment during the early painful phase involves rest, a sling, and analgesics. After the pain has subsided, a course of physical therapy that concentrates on passive range of motion and strengthening[10] should be instituted. Most cases are self-limiting and resolve over the course of several months or years.[11] Upper plexus lesions have a more favorable prognosis.[12]

NERVE ROOT INJURIES AND NEUROTMESIS

Nerve root avulsions and neurotmesis injuries are rare among athletes, but they may occur in high-velocity sporting events.[13] Most injuries occur as a result of severe downward pressure on the shoulder with head flexion to the contralateral side. If the arm is at the side or adducted, injury typically occurs to the upper trunk region; hyperabduction often leads to injury at the lower trunk. Diagnosis is confirmed by computed tomography (CT) myelography. Cervical or shoulder fractures and vascular injuries may be sustained in conjunction with the nerve disruption as a result of the violent forces that are necessary to produce this injury. Immediate sensory and motor loss are evident in the affected distribution. Immediate surgical intervention is recommended for patients with a vascular injury or penetrating trauma. In most other cases, surgery is postponed for 3 to 6 months to allow for maximum healing. If significant functional deficits persist, muscle transfer procedures and nerve exploration with direct repair, nerve grafting, and/or neurolysis may be helpful.[14] The prognosis for athletes with root avulsions is poor, and the likelihood of returning to competitive sports is low.

COMMON CERVICAL SPINE INJURIES

The most common athletic injury to the cervical spine is a strain or sprain. Although whiplash injuries with a sudden extension–flexion mechanism are common, any low-grade force to the cervical spine may cause a sprain. Athletes present with paravertebral muscle spasm, occasional limited neck range of motion, and normal neurologic examination. Plain radiographs may reveal a loss of normal lordosis. The vast majority of cervical spine strains resolve uneventfully with conservative modalities, including relative rest, anti-inflammatory medications, muscle relaxants, and physical therapy.

Compression fractures of the cervical spine usually occur at the lower levels. In addition to plain radiographs, flexion–extension radiographs, CT scanning, and/or magnetic resonance imaging may be helpful to exclude a more serious injury. Isolated fractures with less than 25% anterior compression can be managed conservatively with a cervical orthosis. Compression fractures with greater than 50% anterior compression may be associated with posterior ligamentous disruption, and they may result in instability that may require surgical stabilization. A CT scan is recommended to rule out fracture of the posterior aspect of the vertebra or of the posterior elements because these injuries may compromise spinal stability.

Avulsion injuries to the spinous process are also known as *clay shoveler's fractures* (**Figure 23.1**). The injuries usually occur in football players and power lifters, and they usually occur at the C7 level. The proposed mechanism of injury of clay shoveler's

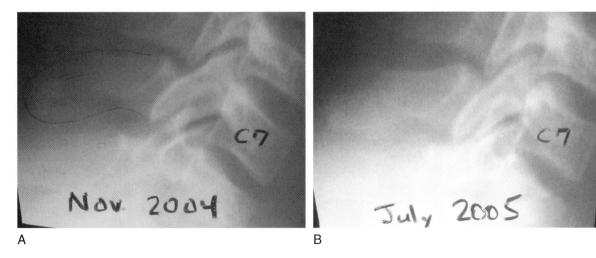

A   B

Figure 23.1   *A*, C7 spinous process fracture. *B*, Healed spinous process fracture.

fractures is the forceful flexion of the cervical spine or the abrupt contraction of the trapezius and rhomboid muscles. These fractures are stable, and they can be treated with a cervical orthosis and symptomatic measures. Patients with stable, healed compression or spinous process avulsion fractures who have full, painless cervical range of motion and no neurologic deficits have no contraindications to participate in contact sports.

Cervical disk herniations **(Figure 23.2)** may occur in athletes who participate in any sport. Symptoms typically include neck pain, restricted cervical motion, radicular symptoms, and sensory and motor deficits. Although neurologic examination can localize the site of the lesion, magnetic resonance imaging is helpful to confirm the diagnosis. Many athletes with a cervical herniated disc respond to nonoperative modalities such as rest, anti-inflammatory agents, a Medrol dose pack, physical therapy, and, occasionally, epidural steroid injections. When these measures fail or the athlete has a progressive neurologic deficit, surgical decompression is indicated. For far lateral disc herniations, a minimally invasive posterior foraminotomy can adequately decompress the nerve root; otherwise, an anterior cervical diskectomy with instrumented fusion is the standard of care. In rare cases, athletes may develop transient quadriplegia or long-tract findings from a large central disk herniation. Anterior diskectomy and interbody fusion is recommended for this condition on an urgent basis.

CATASTROPHIC CERVICAL SPINE INJURIES

In the United States, approximately 7% of all new cases of spinal cord injury are related to athletic activities.[15] Sports injuries are the second most common cause of spinal cord injury during the first 30 years of life.[16] Permanent spinal cord injury is much more likely to result from cervical spinal injury than thoracic or lumbar trauma. In a 3-year nationwide survey of all sports in Japan, the incidence of spinal injury was 1.95 per million per year, with a mean age at injury of 28.5 years and 88% of injuries occurring in males.[17] Sports that have been identified as placing the participant at high risk for spinal cord injury include football, ice hockey, wrestling, diving, skiing, snowboarding, rugby, cheerleading, and baseball.[18] Information about catastrophic injuries in athletes is provided by the National Center for Catastrophic Sports Injury Research, the National Spinal Cord Injury Statistical Center, the US Consumer Product Safety Commission, and other organizations **(Table 23.1).**

The spectrum of catastrophic cervical spine injuries in sports includes unstable fractures and dislocations, cervical cord neuropraxia (transient quadriplegia), and intervertebral disk herniation.[19] Unstable fractures and dislocations are the most frequent causes of catastrophic cervical spine injury, resulting in permanent neurologic sequelae; they typically occur in the lower cervical spine, especially at the C5-C6 level. The spinal cord occupies less than half of the canal's cross-sectional area at the level of the atlas, but it occupies close to 75% at the lower cervical levels.[20]

The mechanism associated with most catastrophic cervical injuries that result in quadriplegia is an axial force to the top of the head with the neck slightly flexed.[21] When the neck is in a neutral position, the cervical spine is in a lordotic or extended position, and most energy is dissipated by the paravertebral muscles and the intervertebral discs. However, when the neck is flexed 30 degrees, the cervical spine becomes straight, and the forces are transmitted to the segmented cervical column. After the maximum compressive deformation is

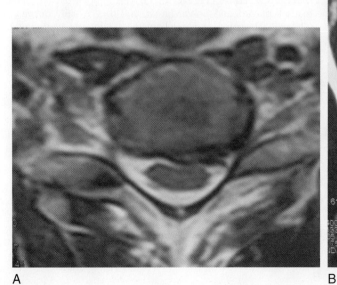

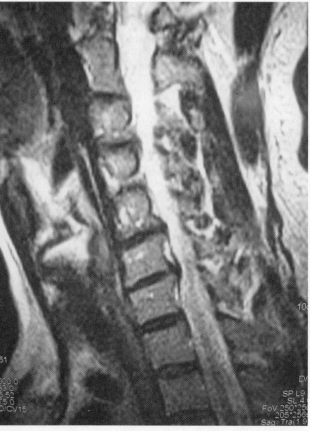

A

B

Figure 23.2 Axial (*A*) and sagittal (*B*) magnetic resonance imaging of patient with C6-C7 left-sided disk herniation.

Table 23.1   Sources of Information about Sports Safety

American Association of Cheerleading Coaches and Advisors: www.aacca.org

Consumer Product Safety Commission: www.cpsc.gov

National Collegiate Athletic Association: www.ncaa.org

National Catastrophic Center Sports Injury Research: www.unc.edu/dept/nccsi/

National Spinal Cord Injury Statistical Center: www.ncddr.org

National Center of Injury Prevention and Control, Centers for Disease Control and Prevention: www.cdc.gov/ncipc

National Federation of State High School Associations: www.nfhs.org

National Operating Committee on Standards for Athletic Equipment: www.nocsae.org

USA Baseball: www.usabaseball.com

reached, the spine fails in either a flexion (flexion teardrop) **(Figure 23.3)** or pure compression (burst fracture) **(Figure 23.4)** mode with a resultant fracture, dislocation, or subluxation. Spinal fragments or the intervertebral disc may retropulse into the spinal canal, thereby causing spinal cord damage.

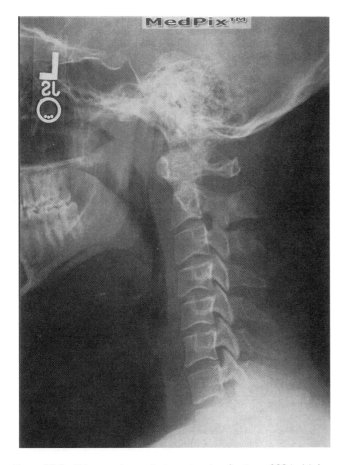

Figure 23.3   This x-ray demonstrates a teardrop fracture of C2 (axis). A transverse fracture of the C7 spinous process (i.e., a "clay shoveler's fracture") is also seen. (Courtesy of Dr. Tehar.)

MANAGEMENT OF THE ATHLETE WITH A CERVICAL SPINE INJURY

Cervical spine trauma can lead to devastating neurologic consequences. Improper care of the athlete's cervical spine on the playing field or during transportation can worsen any spinal cord damage. Therefore, the on-site medical team must be prepared to act in an efficient, organized manner. This is best accomplished by a well-trained, rehearsed group of medical personnel. The proper early care of the athlete with cervical trauma can lead to improved outcomes.[22,23]

Planning and preparation

There are several principles that should be adhered to by the medical staff responsible for immobilizing and transporting an athlete with a cervical spine injury to the hospital:

- An individual, such as the team physician or trainer, should be designated as the leader responsible for supervising the on-field management of the injured athlete.
- The leader must ensure that all emergency equipment is available at the site of the potential injury. Necessary equipment includes a spine board, straps to secure the athlete to the spine board, a facemask removal kit, communication devices, and a cardiopulmonary resuscitation kit.
- An ambulance and hospital that are properly equipped and staffed to handle catastrophic cervical spine injuries should be selected in advance of the sporting event.
- The medical team should practice proper techniques in a mock situation to be fully prepared for an on-field emergency.
- A decision should be made before the event as to which member of the sports medicine team will accompany the athlete during transport.

Removal of protective equipment

The National Athletic Trainers' Association formed the Inter-Association Task Force for Appropriate Care of the Spine-Injured Athlete in 1998 to develop guidelines for the proper management of the athlete with a severe spine injury.[24] The task force recommended that, in the majority of cases of cervical spinal cord injury, the helmet and shoulder pads should not be removed before arrival at an emergency department. Studies of both football and ice hockey players have demonstrated that the removal of the helmet or shoulder pads can result in a significant change from the neutral cervical position.[25,26]

In rare circumstances, it may be necessary to remove the helmet or shoulder pads before transporting the athlete to a hospital. Situations that warrant helmet or shoulder pad removal in the injured athlete are summarized in **Table 23.2**. It is always best to remove both the helmet and the shoulder pads together if either requires removal.[25]

On-field assessment and treatment

Any suspected injury should be treated as if there is a true cervical spine injury until proper radiographs can be obtained. The first step in managing the athlete with a cervical spine injury is to immobilize the head and neck in a stable position. The initial evaluation of the injured athlete should assess for any life-threatening conditions using the ABCDE sequence of trauma care (airway, breathing, circulation, disability or neurologic status, and exposure of the athlete).[22] If a life-threatening problem is identified or suspected, the emergency medical system should be activated. Any unconscious athlete should be assumed to have a cervical spine injury.

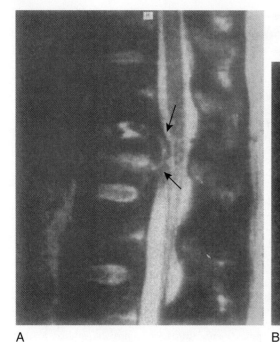

A

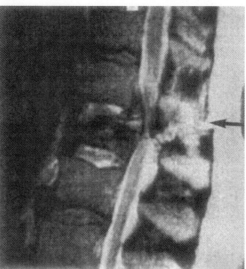

B

Figure 23.4 In a burst fracture, the vertebral body fails in flexion, thereby causing the fragments to retropulse posteriorly into the spinal cord. *A,* A T2-weighted (5000/90) turbo spin echo sagittal image of a stable burst fracture. The *arrows* point to an intact posterior longitudinal ligament, which drapes the retropulsed fragment and the small epidural hematoma. *B,* A T2-weighted (3500/103) turbo spin echo sagittal image of a stable burst fracture. (From Petersilge CA, Emery SE: Semin Ultrasound CT MR 1996;17[2]:105-113.)

Normal mental status without cardiorespiratory compromise

The most common scenario is an athlete with a cervical injury who is breathing and who has a normal mental status. In this situation, the mouth guard should be removed and the airway maintained. The facemask need not be removed initially unless the airway is threatened. If the athlete is breathing and has a normal pulse, the neurologic status and level of consciousness should be assessed. The prone athlete should be carefully logrolled to a supine position, with the head and trunk being moved as a single unit **(Figure 23.5).** The leader maintains immobilization of the head by applying slight traction and using the crossed-arm technique. This technique allows for the constant immobilization of the head and neck without the leader's arms becoming entangled during the logroll maneuver. In addition to the leader, at least three medical personnel should be available to maintain body alignment during the logroll maneuver. The designated leader controls the head and gives the command for turning.

After the athlete is logrolled onto the spine board, the torso of the athlete is secured to the backboard using Velcro straps. The straps are firmly secured, allowing enough room for chest movement during breathing. With the leader maintaining cervical stabilization, the facemask is then removed. Removal of the facemask depends on the type of helmet that the athlete is wearing. A cordless screwdriver should be available, because it allows for quick removal with minimal helmet motion[27] **(Figure 23.6).** The medical team should also be prepared with bolt cutters for the older single- and double-bar masks as well as a sharp knife or scalpel to detach any plastic loops. Although there is currently no standard for loop straps, the Shockblocker loop strap allows for more efficient facemask removal than other currently available devices.[27] After the facemask is fully removed, the head is firmly stabilized to the backboard. On the leader's count, the spine board is then lifted with a minimum of four assistants, and the patient is placed in the ambulance for evacuation to an emergency department.

Cardiovascular compromise

If the athlete is not breathing at initial evaluation or stops breathing, an airway must immediately be established. Respiratory distress can be caused by upper cervical spinal cord injury with paralysis of the

diaphragm. Access to the airway must be accomplished without causing further injury to the spine. The prone athlete is carefully logrolled into a supine position. After the facemask has been removed, rescue breathing according to the standards of the American Heart Association should be initiated. If the athlete's airway is not open, then a gentle jaw-thrust maneuver without cervical traction is performed. This is accomplished by grasping the angles of the victim's lower jaw and lifting to move the tongue away from obstructing the airway. The head-tilt maneuver should be avoided as a result of the potential for altering cervical alignment. In the athlete who is

Table 23.2 Equipment Removal Guidelines

The following situations warrant on-site helmet removal for the injured athlete:

- If, after a reasonable period of time, the facemask cannot be removed to gain airway access
- If the design of the helmet and chinstrap is such that, even after the removal of the facemask, the airway cannot be controlled or ventilation provided
- If the helmet and chinstrap do not hold the head securely such that immobilization of the helmet does not also immobilize the head
- If the helmet prevents immobilization for transport in an appropriate position
- If the shoulder pads require removal

The following situations warrant on-site shoulder pad removal for the injured athlete:

- If there are multiple injuries that require full access to the shoulder area
- If ill-fitting shoulder pads result in the inability to maintain spinal immobilization
- If cardiopulmonary resuscitation requiring access to the thorax is inhibited by the shoulder pads
- If the helmet requires removal

Adapted from Kleiner DM, Almquist JL, Bailes J, et al: Prehospital Care of the Spine-Injured Athlete. Dallas, TX, National Athletic Trainers' Association, 2001.

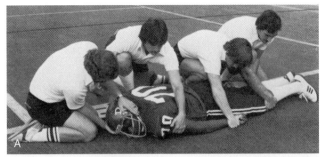

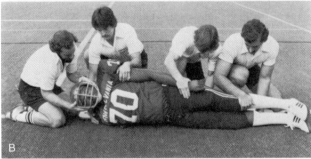

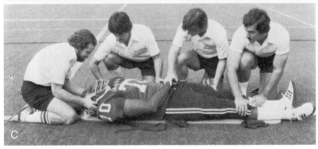

Figure 23.5 Proper logrolling technique. A minimum of four individuals is required. The leader uses the crossed-arm technique to immobilize the head as the athlete is turned from a prone to supine position onto the spine board. (Reprinted with permission from Torg JS, Gennarelli, TA: Chapter 14: Head and Cervical Spine Injuries. In DeLee JC, Drez D Jr [eds]: Orthopaedic Sports Medicine: Principles and Practice, vol. 1. WB Saunders, 1994.)

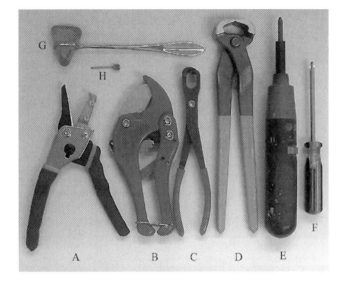

Figure 23.6 Essential equipment that should be available to remove the facemask. *A,* Facemask extractor; *B,* polyvinyl chloride pipe cutter; *C,* trainer's angel; *D,* wire cutter; *E,* electric screwdriver; *F,* manual screwdriver; *G,* reflex hammer (used to pry away cheek pads); *H,* air pump needle (used to deflate the helmet air bladder). (Reprinted with permission from Waninger KN: Am J Sports Med 2004;32:1331-1350.)

unresponsive, an oral airway may be necessary to prevent occlusion of the oropharynx.

Emergency department management

After the athlete has been transported to a stable setting in the hospital, care is transferred to the emergency medical staff. The team physician or athletic trainer should assist with the removal of equipment because emergency medical personnel often are not familiar with the protocol. After reevaluating the ABCDEs, radiographs should be performed. Although the traditional protocol was to perform plain radiographs before the removal of equipment, this practice has recently been called into question. Football helmets and shoulder pads interfere with radiographic visualization of the cervical spine, and this often leads to undetected pathology.[28] Although controversial, the current trend is that head and shoulder protective gear should be cautiously removed before cervical spine radiographic imaging or that, at a minimum, they should be removed if radiographs are obscured by protective equipment[29] (LOE: B). In addition, several studies have documented that cervical spine radiographs miss up to 45% of injuries (especially at the upper cervical levels) as compared with CT scanning for trauma victims (LOE: B)[30,31] **(Figure 23.7).** Therefore, helical CT scans are

recommended for the complete evaluation of the cervical spine in any athlete with suspected cervical injury **(Box 23.1).**

Equipment removal

Before the removal of the helmet, the chinstrap should be unfastened and discarded, the cheek pads should be removed, and/or the air bladder should be deflated. Equipment removal is best accomplished with a minimum of three medical personnel to minimize the motion of the cervical spine.[32] The athlete's head is then supported at the occiput by one member of the medical staff while the leader removes the helmet in a straight line with the spine.

The shoulder pads should be removed at the same time as the helmet to avoid excessive flexion or extension of the spine. As the athlete's head and neck are secured, medical personnel gently flex the trunk at the hips approximately 30 degrees so that the shoulder pads can be removed. Next, a hard collar is applied to the neck for immobilization. The front of the shoulder pads should be removed to allow for cardiopulmonary resuscitation and defibrillation, if necessary. Further imaging studies such as a complete cervical spine series, magnetic resonance imaging, or CT scanning are then performed on the basis of the clinical findings. In conclusion, a clearly defined and coordinated treatment algorithm can improve the outcome of a catastrophic cervical injury.

SPORT-SPECIFIC CONSIDERATIONS FOR SPINE INJURIES

Football
Quadriplegia

Football is associated with the highest number of severe cervical injuries per year among high school and college sports in the United States.[35-37] Although the incidence of head-related fatalities declined during the early 1970s, the number of cases of permanent cervical quadriplegia started to rise. This is likely because the improved helmets allowed tacklers to strike an opponent using the crown of the head with less fear of self-induced injury.

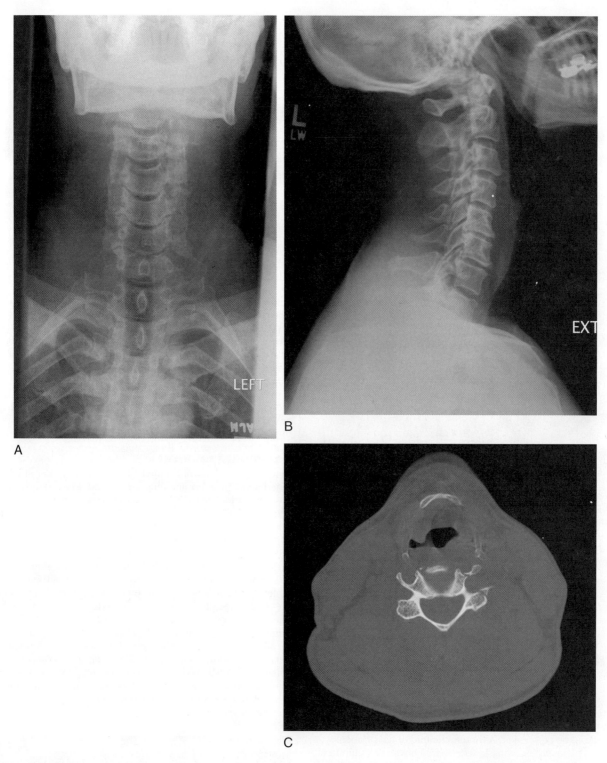

Figure 23.7 Anteroposterior (A) and lateral (B) radiographs reported as normal in a patient with neck pain. The patient returned to the emergency department 2 days later, at which time a computed tomography scan revealed fractures to the left transverse foramina (C) at C5 and C6. The patient also suffered a vertebral artery injury.

Torg and colleagues were instrumental in reducing the rate of quadriplegic events by demonstrating that spearing or tackling a player with the top of the head is the major cause of permanent cervical quadriplegia[38] **(Figure 23.8).** The vast majority of spear tackling injuries occur to defensive players, especially defensive backs (LOE: B).[39,40] A disproportionate number of injuries also occur to players on special teams, in which the speed of collision is extremely high.[40] In 1976, spearing was banned, and the rate of catastrophic cervical injuries dramatically dropped.[21] From 1976 to 1987, the rate of traumatic quadriplegia in football decreased by approximately 80%.[21] Other than a spike of 13 quadriplegic injuries during the 1989-1990 academic year, the incidence of injuries

Box 23.1: The Role of High-Dose Steroids

Since the early 1990s, the use of high doses of methylprednisolone for the treatment of acute spinal cord injury has become the standard of care. In a clinical study by Bracken and colleagues,[33] it was found that patients with acute spinal cord injuries who were treated with high-dose methylprednisolone within the first 8 hours of injury had significant neurologic improvement at the 6 months of follow up as compared with a placebo group.[33] The recommended dose of methylprednisolone is an intravenous bolus of 30 mg per kilogram of body weight over 1 hour, followed by infusion at 5.4 mg per kilogram per hour for 23 hours. Although high-dose methylprednisolone for acute spinal cord injury has traditionally been the standard of care, this practice has recently been questioned. One evidence-based analysis of the published literature about methylprednisolone revealed serious flaws in data analysis and conclusions, with no clear support for the use of methylprednisolone in patients with acute spinal cord injury.[34] In fact, several studies showed a higher incidence of infectious and respiratory complications with methylprednisolone. Until further reliable data is available, the use of high-dose methylprednisolone for acute spinal cord injury remains controversial. Each patient or the patient's family should be consulted about the risks and benefits of the medication before use.

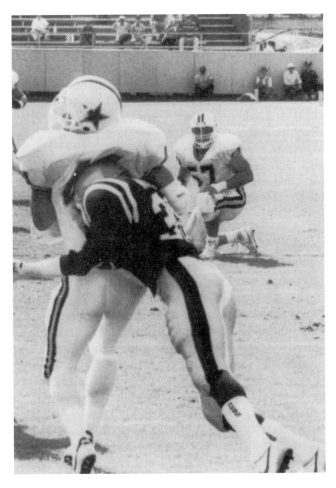

Figure 23.8 Photograph of an athlete spear tackling with the top of his head. (Reprinted with permission from Torg JS, Guille JT, Jaffe S: J Bone Joint Surg Am 2002;84:112-122.)

continued to decline through the 1990s.[40] The rate of quadriplegic injuries at the high school and college levels remained fairly steady during the 1990s and the early 2000s at 5.19 per 1 million participants or 1 injury per 192,000 participants.[40]

In an effort to reduce the number of quadriplegic injuries, the National Collegiate Athletic Association strengthened its rule banning spear tackling (effective during the 2005-2006 academic year). The revision removes the word "intentional" from the rule, which makes it easier for referees to call spearing penalties. Under the previous rule, intent was difficult for referees to assess on the field, and the penalty was rarely called. Among the National Collegiate Athletic Association's efforts to publicize its spearing rule change, the association has produced a poster for locker rooms, a PowerPoint presentation, and a video addressing the risks, the mechanism of injury, the concept of axial loading, and the prevention of injury by adopting safe tackling techniques (LOE: B).[41] Future epidemiologic data will reveal if this new rule can further reduce the incidence of quadriplegia in football.

The identification of spear tackling as the primary culprit leading to quadriplegic injuries has had a profound effect on reducing this catastrophic injury. Coaches must continually reinforce proper tackling techniques with the head up; players should never be allowed to tackle with the head down.

Cervical cord neurapraxia

Cervical cord neurapraxia (CCN) is an acute, usually transient neurologic episode associated with sensory changes with or without motor weakness or complete paralysis in at least two extremities.[21,42,43] The cervical area is usually pain free at the time of injury, with full painless range of motion. The prevalence has been estimated to be 7 per 10,000 football participants.[21] Complete recovery usually occurs within 10 to 15 minutes, but it may take longer. Cervical stenosis is believed to be the primary causative factor that predisposes an individual to CCN (LOE: B).[43] The hypothesized mechanism is either hyperflexion or hyperextension of the neck causing a pincer-type compression injury to the spinal cord.[21] New data reveal that there is no one position that particularly predisposes an individual to a CCN episode and that a variety of mechanisms (including axial forces) can lead to CCN (LOE: B).[40]

The classification of CCN is based on the neurologic deficit, the duration of the neurologic symptoms, and the pattern of injury.[44] The neurologic deficit may involve motor and/or sensory abnormalities. The grade of injury is based on the duration of neurologic symptoms: grade I, less than 15 minutes; grade II, 15 minutes to 24 hours; and grade III, longer than 24 hours. The pattern of injury is classified as quad, upper only, lower only, or hemi.

An episode of CCN is not an absolute contraindication to return to football. It is unlikely that athletes who experience CCN are at risk for permanent quadriplegia with return to play. Rather, playing technique in which the athlete employs the top of the head for tackling is the primary factor that results in cervical quadriplegia. There are no known reports of an athlete with a CCN injury returning to football and sustaining a quadriplegic event. However, the number of athletes returning to play after a CCN episode is too low to make a definitive conclusion. Permanent neurologic deficits after a CCN episode are uncommon, but they can occur.[45,46] Athletes must be counseled on an individual basis about the known and potential risks of injury with return to football after a CCN injury.

The overall risk of a recurrent CCN episode with return to football participation is just over 50%, and it is correlated with the canal diameter size; the smaller the canal diameter, the greater the risk of recurrence (LOE: B).[43] Athletes with ligamentous instability, neurologic symptoms lasting more than 36 hours, multiple episodes, or magnetic resonance imaging evidence of cord defect, cord edema, or minimal functional reserve should not be allowed to return to contact sports.[21]

Screening

The Pavlov–Torg ratio was developed as a method to assess cervical spinal stenosis that eliminates the need to correct for radiographic magnification.[21] The ratio is measured as the diameter of the spinal canal divided by the anteroposterior width of the vertebral body at the midpoint on the lateral radiograph. A ratio of less than 0.8 was proposed as indicating significant spinal stenosis. The ratio has been found to have a high sensitivity for detecting significant spinal stenosis, but it is a poor predictor of which players will suffer a CCN episode. In one study, 40 of 124 (32%) professional football players had a ratio of less than 0.8.[47] Many football players have large vertebral bodies with normal canal dimensions that may bring the ratio below 0.8.[48] Therefore, the ratio is a poor screening tool for athletic participation. "Functional" spinal stenosis, which is defined as a loss of cerebrospinal fluid around the spinal cord as documented by magnetic resonance imaging or CT myelography, is a more accurate method of determining spinal stenosis and a risk for CCN.[49] There is currently no cost-effective tool to screen for athletes who are at risk for CCN; however, all athletes who experience an episode of CCN should undergo appropriate imaging studies to evaluate their risk of recurrence. Preparticipation physicals should specifically address whether an athlete has had a previous neck injury so that appropriate counseling and return-to-play decisions can be made.

Ice hockey

Although the number of catastrophic injuries in high school and college ice hockey players is low as compared with those in other sports, the incidence per 100,000 participants is high.[35] The majority of spinal injuries in ice hockey are reported to occur to the cervical spine, especially between levels C5 and C7.[50] The most common mechanism of injury is checking from behind and being hurled horizontally into the boards[50,51] **(Figure 23.9).** Contact with the boards typically occurs to the crown of the player's head, thereby subjecting the neck to an axial load.[51] Biomechanical studies have shown that impact velocities as low as 1.8 m/s provided compressive forces from C3 through C5 to 75% of their failure loads in axial compression.[52] It has been demonstrated that skating speeds often reach 12 m/s and that the speed of a sliding skater on ice is approximately 6.7 m/s.[53] Both situations are well above the speeds necessary to cause failure in axial compression.

A Canadian survey from 1966 to 1993 reported a total of 241 spinal fractures and dislocations in ice hockey.[51] The incidence of major spinal injuries worldwide in ice hockey started to increase significantly during the early 1980s.[54] Data from the SportSmart registry revealed an average of 17 cases a year, with a peak of 26 injuries in 1995.[54] In 1994, the rule against pushing or checking from behind was adopted into the International Ice Hockey Federation rules book[55] **(Figure 23.10).** As a result of this rule change, the incidence of severe spinal injuries has dramatically decreased since the late 1990s.[54] Padding the boards is an alternative preventive strategy that may also be effective. Although it has been suggested that head and facial protection lead to an increased risk of catastrophic spinal injuries, this has never been substantiated.[56] Aggressive play and fighting in hockey should also be discouraged.

Wrestling

Cervical fractures or major cervical ligament injuries constitute the majority of traumatic catastrophic wrestling injuries.[57] There is a trend toward more spine injuries in the low and middleweight classes. Most injuries occur in match competitions, in which intense, competitive situations place wrestlers at a higher risk.[57] The position that is most frequently associated with spinal injury in wrestling is the defensive posture during the takedown maneuver **(Figure 23.11),** followed by the down position (kneeling) and the

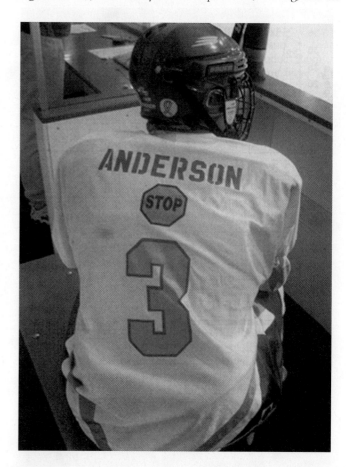

Figure 23.10 SafetyToward Other Players (STOP) patch worn on the back of an amateur hockey player as a visual reminder for players to not hit an opponent from behind. (Reprinted with permission from Waninger KN: Am J Sports Med 2004;32:1331-1350.)

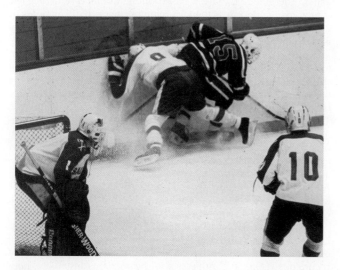

Figure 23.9 Photograph of an ice hockey player checked from behind and thrown into the boards headfirst. (Courtesy of J. S. Torg, MD, Philadelphia, PA.)

lying position.[57] There is no clear predominance of any one type of takedown hold that contributes to cervical injuries in wrestling. The athlete is typically injured by one of three scenarios:

1. The wrestler's arms are in a hold such that he or she is unable to prevent himself or herself from landing on his or her head when thrown to the mat;
2. The wrestler attempts a roll but is landed on by the full weight of his or her opponent; and
3. The wrestler lands on the top of his or her head, sustaining an axial compression force to the cervical spine.

General prevention strategies for catastrophic spine injuries in wrestling rely on the referees and coaches. Referees should strictly enforce penalties for slams, and they should gain more awareness of dangerous holds. There is particular vulnerability for the defensive wrestler who may be off balance, who has one or both arms held, and who then has his or her opponent land on top of him of her. Stringent penalties for intentional slams or throws are encouraged. The referee should have a low threshold of tolerance to stop the match during potentially dangerous situations. Coaches can prevent serious injuries by emphasizing safe, legal wrestling techniques such as teaching wrestlers to keep their heads up during any takedown maneuver to prevent axial compression injuries to the cervical spine. Proper rolling techniques, with an avoidance of landing on the head, must be emphasized during practice sessions.

Diving

Most catastrophic spinal swimming injuries are related to the racing dive into the shallow end of the pool.[35] The injury occurs when a swimmer dives headfirst into the shallow end of a pool and sustains an axial compression injury to the cervical spine **(Figure 23.12)**. The national high school and collegiate associations have implemented rules to prevent injuries during the racing dive. At the high school level, swimmers must start the race in the water if the water depth at the starting end is less than 3.5 feet. If the water depth is 3.5 feet to less than 4 feet at the starting end, the swimmer may start in the water or from the deck. If the water depth at the starting end is 4 feet or more, then the swimmer may start from a platform up to 30 inches above the water surface. College rules require a minimum water depth of 4 feet at the starting end of the pool. During practice sessions in which platforms may not be available, swimmers are advised to only dive into the deep end of the pool or to jump into the water feet first.

Many recreational diving injuries go unreported, hampering attempts at improving awareness and water safety. In a retrospective review of patients with traumatic spinal cord injuries presenting to a trauma center in Germany, 7.7% were caused by diving accidents.[58] Ninety-seven percent of the injured patients were male. Inadequate supervision, alcohol use, shallow water, and lack of experience with diving are all risk factors for injury.[59] Diving head first into shallow or unknown waters was the reported cause in most cases. Many recreational aquatic centers have removed the high board in favor of a waterslide to reduce the incidence of spinal cord injuries.

Downhill skiing/snowboarding

Although the injury rate in skiing is 1.5 to 4 per 1000 skier-days, the incidence of serious spinal cord injury is 0.01 injuries per 1000 skier-days.[60] The location of spinal injuries is fairly evenly

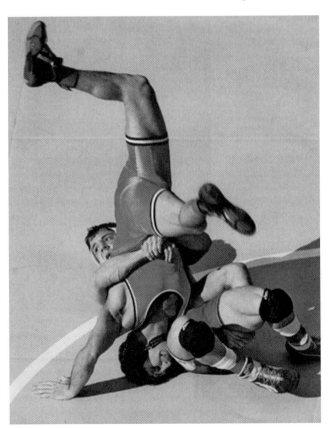

Figure 23.11   A wrestler landing on the top of his head during a takedown maneuver. (From *Sports Illustrated*.)

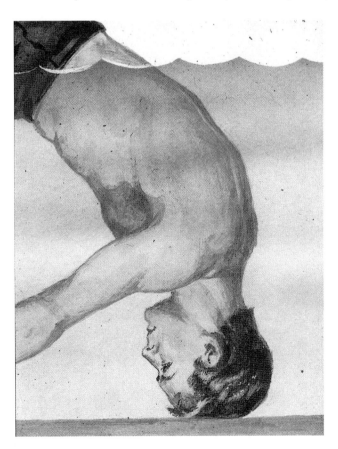

Figure 23.12   An illustration of a diver landing on the top of his head while diving into the shallow end of a pool. (Courtesy of J. S. Torg, MD, Philadelphia, PA.)

distributed between the cervical, thoracic, and lumbar levels.[61] Spinal injuries appear to have increased among skiers over the last 20 years, and they tend to occur predominantly among young males. The primary causes of injury are falls caused by poorly groomed slopes, equipment failure, unfavorable weather conditions, overcrowding (with skier-skier or skier-snowboarder collisions), skier error, or high speeds with loss of control. The injury rates increase at the end of the day, which suggests a link with skier fatigue. Fatality rates for downhill skiers have been estimated to be 1 per 1.5 million skier-days.[60] Most fatalities result from reckless skiers colliding with a stationary object, especially a tree.[60] Although most fatalities are caused by severe head injuries, spinal injuries have also been documented.[60] The enforcement of responsible safe skiing by the ski patrol is an important factor in the prevention of injuries.

The incidence of spinal injury in snowboarding has been reported to be four times higher than that seen in skiing.[62] Jumping is the primary cause of injury in snowboarding, and it contributes up to 80% of the injuries, with most occurring in the thoracolumbar region.[61,62] Prevention strategies include regulating the downhill runs so that snowboarders do not overcrowd the slopes and separating snowboarders from skiers on the slopes. Snowboarders should also be made aware of the potentially deleterious effects of high-risk jumping practices.

Rugby

The lack of protective gear and aggressive style of play in rugby has resulted in a high rate of cervical injury. Scher[63,64] reported that 10% of serious injuries in rugby involve the cervical spine, with spinal cord contusions constituting one fourth of the spinal injuries. Cervical spine injuries most frequently occur during the scrum, when the opposing packs of tightly bound players come together (engagement).[65] The hooker or central player on the front row suffers the most injuries **(Figure 23.13)**. During engagement, the 8-person scrum may generate forces of up to 1.5 tons: the hooker may encounter almost 50% of this force. If engagement does not occur properly or the hooker employs his or her head as a weapon with the neck flexed during contact, a severe cervical injury may result. Preventive methods include avoiding a mismatch in the physical size of the hookers, not allowing unskilled players to participate on the front row, and changing the rules of engagement. Sequential engagement or having the front rows engage separately from the pack prevents the second and third rows from thrusting unprepared front-row players into their opponents. An uncontested scrum in which the

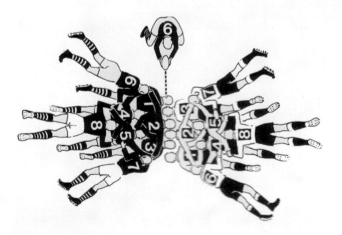

Figure 23.13 Diagram of scrum positions. The hooker for each team is in position 2. (Reprinted with permission from Wetzler MJ, Akpata T, Laughlin W, et al: Am J Sports Med 1998;26:177-180.)

offensive team is allowed to win the scrum has also been shown to be an effective preventive strategy.[65] There is insufficient data to determine whether protective headgear changes the rates of cervical spine injury.

Cheerleading

During the past 20 years, cheerleading has evolved into an activity that demands high levels of skill, athleticism, and complex gymnastic maneuvers. As compared with other sports, cheerleading has a low overall incidence of injuries but a high risk of catastrophic injuries. At the college and high school levels, cheerleading accounts for more than half of the catastrophic injuries that occur among female athletes.[35] College athletes are more likely to sustain a catastrophic injury than their high school counterparts, which is likely the result of the increased complexity of stunts at the college level.[66] In 2000, the US Consumer Product Safety Commission estimated a total of 1814 neck injuries in cheerleaders of all ages; 76 of these were cervical fractures.[67]

The most common stunts that result in catastrophic injury are the pyramid, with the cheerleader at the top of the pyramid being the most frequently injured, and the basket toss.[66] A basket toss is a stunt in which a cheerleader is thrown into the air, often to a height of between 6 and 20 feet, by either three or four tossers. Less common mechanisms include advanced floor tumbling routines, participating on a wet surface, and performing a mount. The majority of injuries occur when an athlete lands on an indoor hard gym surface.[66]

The high school and college associations have attempted to reduce pyramid injuries by limiting the height and complexity of a pyramid and by specifying positions for spotters. Height restrictions on pyramids are limited to two levels in high school and two-and-a-half body lengths in college. The top cheerleaders are required to be supported by one or more individuals (base) who are in direct weight-bearing contact with the performing surface. Spotters must be present for each person who is extended above shoulder level. The suspended person is not allowed to be inverted (head below horizontal) or to rotate on the dismount.

Safety measures have also been instituted for the basket toss, such as limiting the basket toss to four throwers, starting the toss from the ground level (no flips), and having one of the throwers behind the top person during the toss. The top person (flyer) is trained to be directed vertically and to not allow the head to drop backward out of alignment with the torso or below a horizontal plane with the body. Because several injuries have been reported during rainy weather, all stunts should be restricted when wet conditions are present. Floor tumbling injuries can be prevented by proper supervision, progression to complex tumbling only when simple maneuvers are mastered, and the use of spotters as necessary. Small trampolines, springboards, and any other apparatuses used to propel a participant have been prohibited since the late 1980s.

During practices, cheerleading coaches must spend the same amount of time and attention on the technique and attentiveness of spotters as they do on the athletes' performance of the stunts. Pyramids and basket tosses should be limited to experienced cheerleaders who have mastered all other skills; they should not be performed without qualified spotters and landing mats.[66]

Baseball

Similar to cheerleading, baseball has a low rate of noncatastrophic injuries but a relatively high incidence of catastrophic injuries as compared with other sports. Severe head injuries are more frequent than spine injuries. The most common mechanism of catastrophic spine injury in baseball is a collision between a base

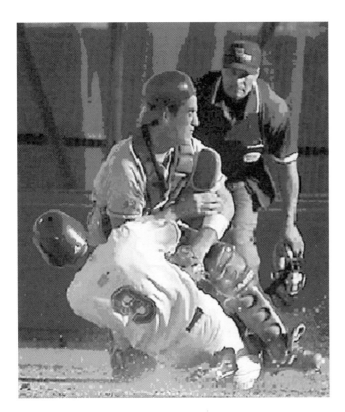

Figure 23.14 The most common mechanism for cervical spine injury in baseball is the collision of a base runner with the catcher. (Courtesy of *Daily Nexus*.)

runner and a fielder,[68] and these collisions often also involve the catcher **(Figure 23.14).** A typical scenario is a base runner who dives headfirst into a catcher and sustains an axial compression cervical injury.[68] Baseball rules state that the runner should avoid the fielder, who has the right to the base path. Unfortunately, this rule is not always enforced when a base runner is racing toward home plate. Because the risk of injury from the collision of a base runner and a catcher is significant and because the speed of head-first sliding has been shown to not be statistically different from feetfirst sliding, it may be that the use of the headfirst slide must be reassessed at the high school and college levels.[69] In Little League baseball, headfirst sliding is not allowed at any base.

CONCLUSION

It has been clearly documented that physical activity has numerous health-related benefits. Participation in sports is an excellent way to encourage physical activity and to promote teamwork and camaraderie. However, it must be kept in mind that there is an extremely low risk of catastrophic spine injuries in certain organized sports. The cost of catastrophic injury to the injured athlete and to society can be tremendous. In addition to the decreased quality of life for the patient, the lifetime cost for a completely quadriplegic individual can easily surpass $2 million dollars.[70] It has been estimated that the annual aggregate cost of the treatment of spinal cord injuries as a result of sports in the United States in 1995 was close to $700 million.[70] Prevention is the most effective means of reducing the incidence and costs associated with catastrophic spine injuries in sports. Continued research into the causes and mechanisms of catastrophic spine injuries is critical to prevent these injuries.

REFERENCES

1. Markey KI, Di Benedetto M, Curt WW: Upper trunk brachial plexopathy. The stinger syndrome. Am J Sports Med 1993;21:650-655.
2. Robertson WC, Eichman PL, Clancy WG: Upper trunk brachial plexopathy in football players. JAMA 1979;241:1480-1482.
3. Clancy WG Jr, Brand RI, Bergfeld JA: Upper trunk brachial plexus injuries in contact sports. Am J Sports Med 1977;5:209-216.
4. Sallis RE, Jones K, Knopp W: Burners: offensive strategy for an underreported injury. Phys Sportsmed 1992;20:47-55.
5. Bateman JE: Nerve injuries about the shoulder in sports. J Bone Joint Surg Am 1967;49A:785-792.
6. Speer KP, Bassett FH: The prolonged burner syndrome. Am J Sports Med 1990;18:591-594.
7. Kelly JD, Clancy M, Marchetti PA, et al: The relationship of transient upper extremity paresthesias and cervical stenosis. Orthop Trans 1992;16:732.
8. Kelly JD, Aliquo D, Sitler MR, et al: Association of burners with cervical canal and foraminal stenosis. Am J Sports Med 2000;28:214-217.
9. Hershman EB, Wilbourn AJ, Bergfeld JA: Acute brachial neuropathy in athletes. Am J Sports Med 1989;17:655-659.
10. Yang SS, Hershman EB: Idiopathic brachial plexus neuropathy: a review. Crit Rev Phys Rehab Med 1993;5:193-201.
11. Tsairis P, Dyck PJ, Mulder DW: Natural history of brachial plexus neuropathy: report on 99 patients. Arch Neurol 1972;27:109-117.
12. Tracy JF, Brannon EW: Management of brachial plexus injuries (traction type). J Bone Surg 1958;40-A:1031-1042.
13. Taylor PE: Traumatic intradural avulsion of the nerve roots of the brachial plexus. Brain 1962;85:579-601.
14. Kline DG: Perspectives concerning brachial plexus injury and repair. Neurosurg Clin N Am 1991;2:151-169.
15. Mueller FO: Introduction. In Mueller FO, Cantu RC, VanCamp SP (eds): Catastrophic Injuries in High School and College Sports. Champaign, IL: HK Sport Sceince Monograph Sreies, 1996, pp 1-4.
16. Nobunga AI, Go BK, Karunas RB: Recent demographic and injury trends in people served by the model spine cord injury care systems. Arch Phys Med Rehabil 1999;80:1372-1382.
17. Katoh S, Shingu H, Ikata T, et al: Sports-related spinal cord injury in Japan (from the nationwide spinal cord injury registry between 1990 and 1992). Spinal Cord 1996;34:416-421.
18. Boden BP, Prior C: Catastrophic spine injuries in sports. Curr Sports Med Rep 2005;4:45-49.
19. Banerjee R, Palumbo MA, Fadale PD: Catastrophic cervical spine injuries in the collision sport athlete, part 1: epidemiology, functional anatomy, and diagnosis. Am J Sports Med 2004;32:1077-1087.
20. Parke WW: Correlative anatomy of cervical spondylotic myelopathy. Spine 1988;13:831-837.
21. Torg JS, Guille JT, Jaffe S: Current concepts review: injuries to the cervical spine in American football players. J Bone Joint Surg Am 2002;84:112-122.
22. Banerjee R, Palumbo MA, Fadale PD: Catastrophic cervical spine injuries in the collision sport athlete, part 2: principles of emergency. Am J Sports Med 2004;32:1760-1764.
23. Torg JS, Gennarelli TA: Head and cervical spine injuries. In DeLee JC, Drez D Jr (eds): Orthopaedic Sports Medicine: Principles and Practice. Philadelphia, WB Saunders, 1994, pp 417-462.
24. Kleiner DM, Almquist JL, Bailes J, et al: Prehospital Care of the Spine-Injured Athlete. Dallas, TX, National Athletic Trainers' Association, 2001.
25. Palumbo MA, Hulstyn MJ, Fadale PD, et al: The effect of protective football equipment on alignment of the injured cervical spine. Radiographic analysis in a cadaveric model. Am J Sports Med 1996;24:446-453.
26. LaPrade RF, Schnetzler KA, Broxterman RF, et al: Cervical spine alignment in the immobilized ice hockey player: a computed tomographic analysis of the effects of helmet removal. Am J Sports Med 2000;28:800-803.
27. Swartz EE, Norkus SA, Cappaert T, et al: Football equipment design affects face mask removal efficiency. Am J Sports Med 2005;33:1210-1218.
28. Griffen MM, Frykberg ER, Kerwin AJ, et al: Radiographic clearance of blunt cervical spine injury: plain radiograph or computed tomography scan? J Trauma 2003;55:222-227.
29. Davidson RM, Burton JH, Snowise M, et al: Football protective gear and cervical spine imaging. Ann Emerg Med 2001;38:26-30.
30. Babra CA, Taggert J, Morgan AS, et al: A new cervical spine clearance protocol using computed tomography. J Trauma 2001;51;652-657.
31. Nunez DB, Zuluaga A, Fuentes-Bernando DA, et al: Cervical spine trauma: how much more do we learn by routinely using helical CT? Radiographics 1996;16:1307-1318.
32. Peris MD, Donaldson WF III, Towers J: Helmet and shoulder pad removal in suspected cervical spine injury: human control model. Spine 2002;27:995-998; discussion 998-999.

33. Bracken MB, Shepard MJ, Collins WF, et al: A randomized, controlled trial of methyl-prednisolone or naloxone in the treatment of acute spinal-cord injury: results of the second national acute spinal cord injury study. N Engl J Med 1990;322:1404-1411.

34. Hulbert RJ: The role of steroids in acute spinal cord injury: an evidence-based analysis. Spine 2001;26:539-546.

35. Mueller FO, Cantu RC: National Center for Catastrophic Sports Injury Research: Twentieth Annual Report, Fall 1982-Spring 2002. Chapel Hill, NC, National Center for Catastrophic Sports Injury Research, 2002, pp 1-25.

36. Cantu RC, Mueller FO: Catastrophic football injuries: 1977-1998. Neurosurgery 2000;47:673-677.

37. Boden BP: Direct catastrophic injury in sports. J Am Acad Orthop Surg 2005;13:445-453.

38. Torg JS, Vegso JJ, O'Neill MJ, et al: The epidemiologic, pathologic, biomechanical, and cinematographic analysis of football-induced cervical spine trauma. Am J Sports Med 1990;18:50-57.

39. Torg JS, Pavlov H, Genuario SE, et al: Neuropraxia of the cervical spinal cord with transient quadriplegia. J Bone Joint Surg Am 1986;68:1354-1370.

40. Boden BP, Tacchetti RL, Cantu RC, et al: Catastrophic cervical injuries in high school and college football players. Am J Sports Med 2006;34:1223-1232.

41. National Collegiate Athletic Association: NCAA health and safety (Web site): Available at www.ncaa.org/health-safety. Accessed May 26, 2007.

42. Torg JS, Pavlov H, Genuario TA et al: Neuropraxia of the cervical spinal cord with transient quadriplegia. J Bone Joint Surg Am 1986;68:1354-1370.

43. Torg JS, Naranja Jr. RJ, Pavlov H, et al: The relationship of developmental narrowing of the cervical spinal canal to reversible and irreversible injury of the cervical spinal cord in football players. An epidemiological study. J Bone Joint Surg Am 1996;78:1308-1321.

44. Torg JS, Corcoran TA, Thibault LE, et al: Cervical cord neurapraxia: classification, pathomechanics, morbidity, and management guidelines. J Neurosurg 1997;87:843-850.

45. Brigham CD, Adamson TE: Permanent partial cervical spinal cord injury in a professional football player who had only congenital stenosis. J Bone Joint Surg 2003;85-A:1553-1556.

46. Cantu RV, Cantu RC: Guidelines for return to contact sports after transient quadriplegia. J Neurosurg 1994;80:592-594.

47. Odor JM, Watkins RG, Dillin WH, et al: Incidence of cervical spinal stenosis in professional and rookie football players. Am J Sports Med 1990;18:507-509.

48. Herzog RJ, Wiens JJ, Dillingham MF, et al: Normal cervical spine morphometry and cervical spinal stenosis in asymptomatic professional football players: plain film radiography, multiplanar computed tomography, and magnetic resonance imaging. Spine 1991;16:S178-S186.

49. Cantu RC: Functional cervical spinal stenosis: a contraindication to participation in contact sports. Med Sci Sports Exerc 1993;25:1082-1083.

50. Molsa JJ, Tegner Y, Alaranta H, et al: Spinal cord injuries in ice hockey in Finland and Sweden from 1980 to 1996. Int J Sports Med 1999;20:64-67.

51. Tator CH, Carson JD, Edmonds VE: Spinal injuries in ice hockey. Clin Sports Med 1998;17:183-194.

52. Bishop PJ, Wells RP: Cervical spine fractures: mechanism, neck load, and methods of prevention. In: Castaldi CR, Hoerner EF (eds): Safety in ice hockey. Volume 2, ASTM STP 1050. Philadelphia, American Society for Testing and Materials, 1989, pp 71-83.

53. Sim FH, Chao EY: Injury potential in modern ice hockey. Am J Sports Med 1978;15:30-34.

54. Biasca N, Wirth S, Tegner Y: The avoidability of head and neck injuries in ice hockey: an historical review. Br J Sports Med 2002;36:410-427.

55. International Ice Hockey Federation: Official Rule Book 1994. Zurich, International Ice Hockey Federation, 1994.

56. Stuart MJ, Smith AM, Malo-Ortiguera SA, et al: A comparison of facial protection and the incidence of head, neck, and facial injuries in junior A hockey players: a function of individual playing time. Am J Sports Med 2002;30:39-44.

57. Boden BP, Lin W, Young M, et al: Catastrophic injuries in wrestlers. Am J Sports Med 2002;30:791-795.

58. Schmitt H, Gerner HJ: Paralysis from sport and diving accidents. Clin J Sports Med 2001;11:17-22.

59. Cooper MT, McGee KM, Anderson DG: Epidemiology of athletic head and neck injuries. Clin Sports Med 2003;22:427-443.

60. Morrow PL, McQuillen EN, Eaton LA Jr, et al: Downhill ski fatalities: the Vermont experience. J Trauma 1998;28(1):95-100.

61. Levy AS, Smith RH: Neurologic injuries in skiers and snowboarders. Semin Neurol 2000;20:233-245.

62. Tarazi F, Dvorak MF, Wing PC: Spinal injuries in skiers and snowboarders. Am J Sports Med 1999;27(2):177-180.

63. Scher AT: Rugby injuries to the cervical spine and spinal cord: a 10 year review. Clin Sports Med 1998;17(1):195-206.

64. Scher AT: Rugby spinal cord concussion in rugby players. Am J Sports Med 1991;19(5):485-488.

65. Wetzler MJ, Akpata T, Laughlin W, et al: Occurrence of cervical spine injuries during the rugby scrum. Am J Sports Med 1998;26:177-180.

66. Boden BP, Tacchetti R, Mueller FO: Catastrophic cheerleading injuries. Am J Sports Med 2003;31:881-888.

67. US Consumer Product Safety Commission home page (Web site): Available at www.cpsc.gov. Accessed May 26, 2007.

68. Boden BP, Tacchetti R, Mueller FO: Catastrophic injuries in high school and college baseball players. Am J Sports Med 2004;32:1189-1196.

69. Kane SM, House HO, Overgaard KA: Head-first versus feet-first sliding: a comparison of speed from base to base. Am J Sports Med 2002;30:834-836.

70. DeVivo MJ: Causes and costs of spinal cord injury in the United States. Spinal Cord 1997;35:809-813.

CHAPTER 24

Thoracic and Lumbar Spine Injuries

Charles W. Webb, DO, FAAFP, and CPT Richard Geshel, DO

KEY POINTS

- The majority of injuries to the lower back are self-limiting, soft-tissue injuries that resolve without the need for specific treatment.
- Most athletes respond well to conservative treatment, including rest, heat/ice modalities, nonsteroidal anti-inflammatory drugs, analgesics, physical therapy, and manipulative therapy.
- Imaging is not usually needed for the initial evaluation and treatment, unless red flags are present.
- Typically discogenic pain is worse with flexion and eases slightly with extension of the lumbar spine.
- When training exceeds 15 hours per week, the risk of injury increases from 13% to 57%.
- If night pain, nonmechanical pain, and constitutional symptoms are present, the clinician must be suspicious of a tumor, an inflammatory process, or an infection as the cause of the athlete's pain.
- The majority of worrisome causes of back pain can be successfully ruled out with a negative basic physical examination that includes a seated straight leg-raise test, patellar and Achilles reflexes, strength testing of the foot and ankle, and symmetric fine touch of the lower leg and foot.

INTRODUCTION

Lower back pain (LBP) is defined as pain, muscular tension, or stiffness that is localized between the costal margins and the inferior gluteal folds, with or without leg pain (i.e., sciatica).[1] LBP is a symptom that is caused by either intrinsic or extrinsic factors and that is often not associated with any identifiable structural abnormality; it is not a diagnosis.[2]

This chapter will discuss the more common sports-related injuries of the lumbar region, including their epidemiology, risk factors, mechanisms of injury, treatments, return-to-play guidelines, and prevention techniques.

The conditions discussed do not fit nicely within a box. Many of these conditions lead to the development of others, and they underscore the interrelatedness of the human body.

CAUSES AND EPIDEMIOLOGY

LBP afflicts millions throughout the world. The reported lifetime prevalence of LBP approaches 85% to 90% in the general population, and it is the most common cause of disability among people who are less than 45 years of age.[3] A sports-related mechanism is the cause of LBP in between 6% and 13% of affected athletes.[4] Back injuries in young athletes are estimated to occur in 10% to 15% of participants.[5] Certain sports predispose the athlete to a higher prevalence rate of back-related injuries (59% in wrestlers, 79% in elite gymnasts).[2] LBP is a common reason for lost playing time. In a study documented by Bono, the complaint of LBP accounted for the sidelining of 30% of college football players.[2] However, this problem is quite rare in the prepubescent population, occurring with an incidence rate of 1% among 7-year-old children and 6% of 10-year-old children.[6]

The incidence of back pain varies from 1.1% to 30%,[2-4] depending on the specific sporting activity involved, with some sporting activities approaching 50% (football lineman).[4] LBP accounts 10% to 15% of sports injuries.[3] Approximately 90% of those afflicted with LBP cannot remember the cause, and the cause is thus designated as nonspecific.[1]

Back pain in athletes results from one of two events: acute, traumatic events or overuse/overtraining in which repetitive activity leads to fatigue injuries.[4,5] Of the two, overuse injuries far outnumber acute trauma, despite most overuse incidents going unreported. For the majority of athletes, injuries to the lower back are self-limiting, soft-tissue injuries that resolve without the need for specific treatment. Most athletes respond well to conservative therapy: rest, heat/ice modalities, anti-inflammatory drugs, analgesics, manipulation, and physical therapy. For those who suffer more serious injuries or spinal derangement (e.g., herniated nucleus pulposus, discitis, or spondylolysis/spondylolisthesis), a prolonged treatment plan may be required. An aggressive but appropriate treatment plan ensures adequate healing while making sure that the athlete returns to play as soon as he or she is safely capable or doing so.

RISK FACTORS

See **Table 24.1.**

Table 24.1 Lower Back Pain Risk Factors

History	Individual and family history of lower back pain outweighs all other considerations and is the most significant prognostic risk factor for future back pain.[2*†‡]
Growth	Elongation of the skeleton predisposes the adolescent to pain and injury. Linear growth is a painful event that does not subside until a new linear length set point is attained after growth acceleration. Those with an increased linear growth rate (greater than 5 cm within 6 months) are three times as likely to report back pain.[7]
	Different growth rates for vertebrae and for the surrounding musculotendinous and ligamentous tissue increase the likelihood of somatic imbalances. These imbalances correspond with the increased incidence of injury during the adolescent growth spurt.[7]
Training regimen	A sudden increase in the intensity or frequency of training may lead to back pain.
	Pain is usually encountered at the initiation of a new season or during a heightening of training intensity.[3]
	Overtraining predisposes the female athlete to injury because the catabolic process of bone demineralization progresses faster than anabolic remodeling, thereby decreasing cortical bone and increasing the rate of stress fracturing.[§]
Poor conditioning	Poor condition is found among returning athletes who did not maintain a level of fitness.[5]
	Decreased core stability results in straining ligaments, poor functioning of the trunk musculature (the normal trunk extension-to-flexion strength ratio is 1.3:1),[3,4] and inefficient neuromuscular control, which leads to overcompensation to maintain balance.[6,7]
Improper technique and equipment	Pain may result from blocking from an erect stance while playing football.[3]
	Excessive lordosis while performing a military press during weightlifting may also lead to pain.[3]
	Being seated in a flexed position from an excessively high seat while cycling can cause back pain as well.[3] Adjusting the seat to a neutral lumbar position has been shown to decrease symptoms by 70%.
	A difference in saddle type (traditional as compared with Western) among equestrians decreased the prevalence of low back pain from 72% to 33% among women and from 33% to 6% among men.
	Improper or ill-fitting footwear[5] will lead to changes in posture that cause the paraspinal and postural muscles to fatigue in an attempt to maintain pelvic balance.
Flexibility	Hamstring tension,[5] femoral anteversion, thoracolumbar fascia tightness, genu recurvatum body habitus, thoracic kyphosis, and inflexibility of the iliopsoas muscles increase lumbar lordosis,[6,10] whereas hip extensors (iliopsoas) act to decrease the normal lumbar lordotic curve.[5]
	Proper balance between these opposing forces must be maintained for the spine to withstand the stresses of axial loading.
Female athletes	Malalignment syndrome involves increased hip bitrochanteric width, hip varus angulation, femoral anteversion, genu valgum, and foot pronation affecting the spine and pelvis in a closed-chain pattern.
	Inference of core back strengthening exercise on low back pain found that female athletes with weaker left hip abductors had a significant probability of developing lower back pain.[*]
	In addition, the same author found right hip extensor weakness among female athletes with a history of and in those who developed low back pain.
	A forced decrease in caloric ingestion leads to diminished estrogen production, thereby resulting in an inadequacy of calcium stores. This leads to irreversible osteopenia and stress fracturing.[¶]
Nonspecific	Life dissatisfaction, neuroticism, hostility, anger, extroversion, and poor sleep quality have also been found to be risk factors for back pain.[2,9]

[*]Radebold A, Cholewicki J, Panjabi MM, Patel TC: Spine 2000;25(8):947-954.
[†]Greene HS, Cholewicki J, Galloway MT, et al: Am J Sports Med 2001;29(6):795-800.
[‡]O'Kane JW, Teitz CC, Lind BK: Am J Sports Med 2003;31(1):80-82.
[§]Arendt EA: Clin Orthop Relat Res 2000;372:131-138.
[¶]Nadler SF, Malanga GA, Bartoli LA, et al: Med Sci Sports Exerc 2002;34(1):9-16.

HISTORY

The single most important portion of the office visit is the medical history. Questions regarding the time of pain onset (acute versus gradual), the inciting incident, the duration of symptoms, the frequency and intensity of pain, the worsening of pain at specific time (e.g., at rest, with exertion, or daytime versus nighttime), the type of pain, and the associated radiation of pain[7] should be asked at every visit. A complete history of the athlete's specific sport or sports—including the number of hours per week of training and participation as well as the training intensity and frequency[8]—is instrumental in determining the cause of the pain and the steps necessary for treatment.[7] A menstrual history of all female patients should include the age of menarche, the number of cycles that occurred within the preceding 12 months, and the length of each cycle. Dietary habits and self-perception of body image should also be addressed.

PHYSICAL EXAMINATION

A full and comprehensive physical evaluation is required for any athlete who complains of LBP rendering him or her unable to perform training and specific sports-related activities for more than 10 days.[9] Initially, notice the patient's position of comfort: sitting midline, leaning to one side, shifting in the seat, sitting against the back of chair, leaning forward, or standing. Note any gait abnormalities or any evidence of pelvic asymmetry.[7] Take note of any abnormalities in the patient's body contours from the posterior and lateral views, with attention paid to lumbar lordosis, thoracic kyphosis, or evidence of scoliosis.[7] Ascertain the exact location of tenderness, the radiation of pain, or paresthesias. Palpate the spine, the paraspinal musculature, and the sacroiliac (SI) joints, noting any points of tenderness, tissue texture changes, warmth, or abnormalities of the lumbosacral mechanics. Lastly, ask the patient to perform flexion/extension, side bending, and rotational maneuvers, and note any restriction or asymmetry of motion **(Figure 24.1).**

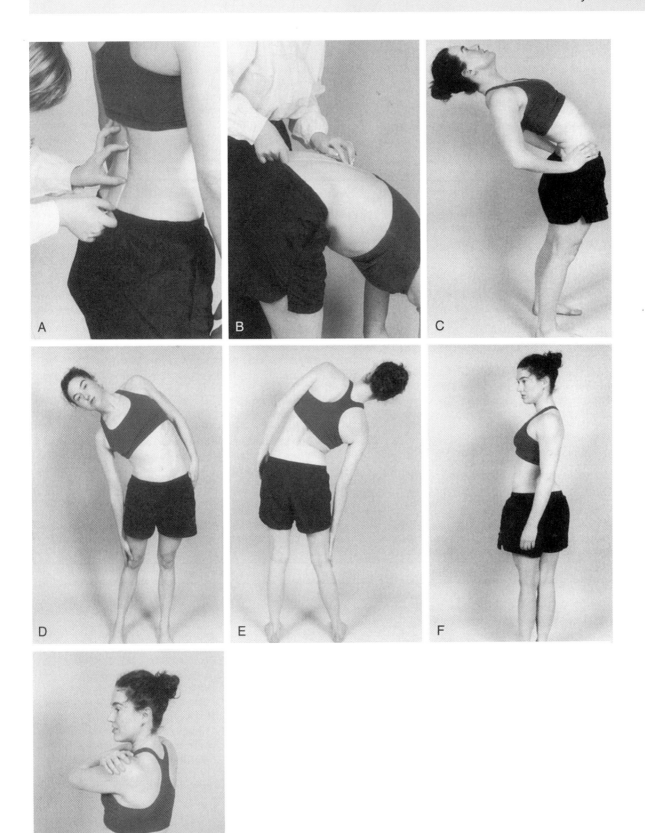

Figure 24.1 Active movements of the lumbar spine. *A* and *B*, Measuring forward flexion using tape measure. *C*, Extension. *D*, Side flexion (anterior view). *E*, Side flexion (posterior view). *F*, Rotation (standing). *G*, Rotation (sitting). (From Magee: Orthopedic Physical Assessment, 4th ed. Philadelphia, WB Saunders, 2002.)

A complete neurologic evaluation is required. Important components include examination of hip flexor, hamstring, tibialis anterior, peroneal, and extensor hallicus longus strength; patellar and Achilles deep tendon reflexes; dermatomal sensory, vibratory, and two-point discrimination; and Babinski's sign.

IMAGING MODALITIES

The imaging study of choice is dependent on the athlete's presentation and their response to treatment. Imaging studies of LBP are indicated by the following criteria[10]:

- Patient reports of the presence of true radicular symptoms
- Findings on the physical examination of nerve root irritation (positive straight leg test) or findings that are indicative of surgical candidacy
- Conservative treatment of the patient has not been successful for 3 to 6 weeks
- Patient presents with clinical features that raise suspicion of a malignant or infectious process or a worsening of neurologic symptoms
- History includes trauma, a fall, a hit in the back (e.g., during football or soccer), or a motor vehicle accident

Radiographs are the initial imaging studies to obtain because they are the most readily available and cost-effective. If radiographs are indicated, anteroposterior, lateral, and oblique images should be obtained. Radiographs should be reviewed for evidence of bony abnormalities, deformity, fracture, degenerative changes, and loss of spinal curves.

Scintigraphy demonstrates the metabolic activity that occurs within bone, either from a neoplastic, infectious, or inflammatory condition. Single photon emission computed tomography (SPECT) also provides information about bony metabolic activity; however, it is more specific because it provides for the localization of pathologic findings within the bone.

Magnetic resonance imaging (MRI) is more specific for visualizing soft-tissue abnormalities, including disc pathology, neoplasms, and anatomic anomalies. MRI is indicated when an athlete presents with neurologic deficiencies in conjunction with back pain.[11]

The clinician should always bear in mind that abnormalities seen on imaging studies should correlate with the athlete's clinical presentation[2] and physical findings.

DIFFERENTIAL DIAGNOSIS

See **Table 24.2.**

CAUSES OF LOW BACK PAIN

Specific causes of LBP can be subdivided by the position of the spine at the time of injury: neutral, flexion, or extension. Neutral conditions will be discussed first. These are defined as injuries or pain syndromes of the lower back that occur while the lumbar spine is in a neutral position.

Sprains, strains, and somatic dysfunction

Sprain, strains, and somatic dysfunction are the predominant reasons that an athlete seeks assistance from a sports medicine professional. Sprains are ligamentous derangements that result from injury, whereas strains involve derangements of the muscles and tendons.[2,3] Somatic dysfunction is an osteopathic term implying "impaired or altered function of related components of the somatic (body framework) system: skeletal, arthrodial, myofascial structures and related vascular, lymphatic and neural elements."[12] Somatic dysfunction encompasses lower back sprain or strain, idiopathic or mechanical LBP, and similar terminology.

Table 24.2   Differential Diagnosis of Low Back Pain[2,9,32]*

Anatomic	Neoplastic	Infectious
Muscle spasm/trigger points	Primary: multiple myeloma, sarcoma, lymphoma/leukemia, oligodendroglioma	Osteomyelitis/discitis
Nerve compression		Abscess (paraspinal, epidural)
Arthritis	Secondary: prostate, lung, breast	Herpes zoster (shingles)
Degenerative joint disease	**Rheumatologic**	Tuberculosis (Pott's disease)
Vertebral/sacral fracture	Rheumatoid arthritis	Visceral: pyelonephritis, prostatitis, gastrointestinal, appendicitis
Facet syndrome	Scleroderma	**Viscerogenic**
Spondylolysis/spondylolisthesis	Reiter's syndrome	Irritable bowel syndrome, uterine fibroids, endometriosis, renal
Congenital malformations	Beçhet's	**Vasculogenic**
Sacroiliac dysfunction	Polymyalgia rheumatica	Aortic aneurysm, spinal claudication
Pelvic outlet syndrome	Fibromyalgia	**Metabolic**
Psoas syndrome	Ankylosing spondylitis	Osteoporosis, Paget's disease, diabetes
Herniated/bulging disc	Psoriatic arthritis	**Psychogenic**
Coccygodynia		Somatization
Hip pathology		
Trochanteric bursitis		
Scoliosis		
Spina bifida		
Bertolotti's syndrome		
Iliosacral syndrome		

*Deyo RA, Weinstein JN: N Engl J Med 2001;344(5):363-370.

Epidemiology and risk factors

No specific epidemiologic information exists concerning the incidence or prevalence of lumbosacral somatic dysfunction per se. However, lumbar strain, a related ailment, accounts for 70% of all LBP cases. Risk factors remain the same as for most other lumbosacral conditions: growth, overuse/overtraining, poor overall conditioning, and an imbalance of opposing muscular structures. Overuse injuries cause somatic dysfunction in 26% of male and 33% of female athletes with previous back injury.[5]

Pathogenesis and mechanism of injury

Somatic dysfunction arises as a result of sudden loading or shearing forces on the spine, its ligamentous stabilizing framework, and/or the attached musculotendinous structures. These forces overload muscle fibers, causing a stretch of the collagen makeup of the tendons, muscles, and fascia and resulting in the release of inflammatory cytokines. This causes the perception of pain, muscular hypertonicity, microscopic tendinitis, and minute fascial herniations that, with continued injury, may result in the derangement of normal physiologic motion and function.

History and physical

A specific painful event or injury leading to a lumbosacral somatic dysfunction may not be immediately recalled by the athlete who, in most circumstances, may report the pain only after a period of rest or after the resumption of training or activity. Patients may present with nonspecific back pain that was intermittent but that has now become persistent.

Physical examination may reveal areas of point tenderness or paraspinal tightness, and these areas may be erythematous and warm. Tender points may be found in regions of bony stress: the iliac crest, the thoracolumbar spinous processes, and along the muscle bellies of the paraspinal muscles and quadratus lumborum. Additionally, myofascial strain patterns may develop as a result of fascial stress along the paraspinal musculature, the thoracolumbar fascia, and the sacrum.

Treatment

Generally, minor lumbosacral dysfunction will resolve with conservative treatment of rest, ice/heat modalities, anti-inflammatory drugs, analgesics, soft-tissue manipulation, and physical therapy. Osteopathic manipulative medicine techniques such as counter strain, facilitated positional release, and myofascial release techniques may alleviate the athlete's pain and restore myofascial, musculotendinous, and ligamentous motion (LOE: C).[13-17]

Return to play

When the athlete is able to perform sports-specific requirements and activities with little discomfort at full speed, he or she may return to competition.[7]

Psoas spasm/syndrome[18]

Psoas spasm (contracture) and psoas syndrome can cause SI joint pain and LBP that insidiously become associated with sciatic neuritis. However, this malady is not well documented in the current literature.[13,18] Overall, psoas spasm and its associated syndrome may lead to more disability than any other muscular spasm of the back.[18]

Risk factors include prolonged, explosive hip flexion as is seen among athletes who run hurdles or who perform step aerobics or full sit-ups. Additionally, diseases of the sigmoid colon (including retrocecal appendicitis[19]) or the ureter may cause psoas irritation and spasm via viscerosomatic reflexes. Athletes who are most prone to developing this condition participate in track events (e.g., hurdlers), rowing, cycling, and the performance of multiple sit-ups for conditioning (e.g., boxers) **(Figure 24.2)**.

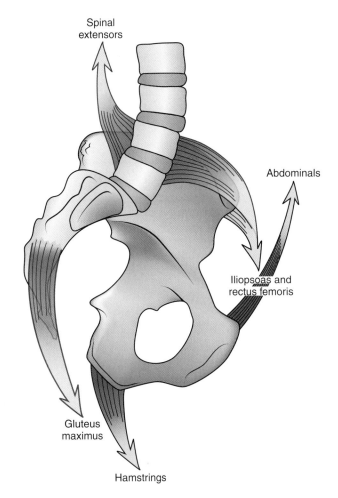

Figure 24.2 Muscles "balancing" the pelvis. Spasm of the iliopsoas may result in an anterior pelvic tilt and malalignment of the sacroiliac and lumbar spine. (Redrawn from Magee: Orthopedic Physical Assessment, 4th ed. Philadelphia, WB Saunders, 2002.)

Psoas syndrome is defined by certain key findings **(Figure 24.3)** (1) nonneutral, side bending L_{1-2} ipsilaterally, (2) a nonneutral rotation with associated side bending of the sacrum on an opposite oblique axis on the side of pain, followed by (3) opposite hip shift, which causes (4) irritation and spasm of the piriformis, and then (5) sciatic pain.[11]

History and physical

Patients complaining of LBP or SI pain have an inability to extend their backs without pain. They usually feel more comfortable sitting or lying with their knees up or their hips flexed.

Initial observation may demonstrate a patient who is slightly flexed and bent toward the side of the psoas spasm. Additionally, an anteriorly rotated pelvis may be noted on the involved side. Other physical findings include paraspinal tightness opposite from the psoas spasm, a shallow sacral sulcus ipsilateral to the psoas spasm with a deepened inferior lateral angle contralaterally and a mid-belly tender point in the contralateral piriformis muscle. Tender points may be noted along the origination sites (T_{12}-L_4 transverse processes) of the psoas on the involved side. The patient may also have a physiologically shortened and externally rotated thigh as a result of the psoas contracture. The athlete usually will demonstrate a positive Thomas' test.

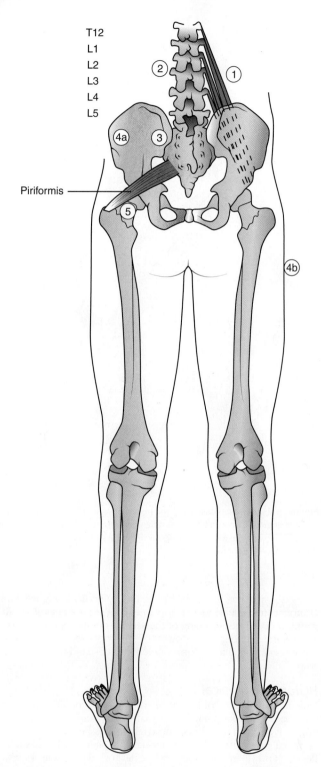

Figure 24.3 Physical findings in right psoas syndrome. 1, Contracture of the psoas. 2, Right rotation and side bending of T12-L4 with lumbar flattening. 3, Left rotation of sacral base leading to a prominent base on the left, sunken base on the right. 4a and 4b, Pelvic shift to the left occurs, causing right femur external rotation, and, 5, increased left piriformis irritation and force.

Treatment (LOE: C)[12,14,17,18,20,21]

Rest, ice, anti-inflammatory agents, and muscle relaxants may provide initial relief of discomfort and pain. An effective means of treatment is to counter strain the affected iliopsoas by flexing, abducting, and externally rotating the hip to "soften" the anterior iliopsoas tender points. This same technique, with a compressive force translated to the proximal lumbar spine, may be used for the facilitated positional release technique. Other osteopathic techniques to consider include Still's technique (an articulatory technique that involves passing through the restrictive barrier), muscle energy, and facilitated myofascial release. If the spasm is found before syndrome development, a lumbar high-velocity/low-amplitude technique may be attempted to rapidly restore the nonneutral dysfunction.

Piriformis (pelvic outlet) syndrome[22-25]

The piriformis muscle is unique in its relative location posterior to the sciatic nerve. All neurovascular structures that innervate or provide blood supply to the buttock region run through the greater sciatic notch, passing either superior to, inferior to, or directly through the piriformis. Trauma, spasm, and hypertonicity of this muscle may lead to the development of sciatic-type pain and paresthesia of the ipsilateral lower extremity in a distribution that is normally distal to the knee and posterior the fibular head **(Figure 24.4)**.

Piriformis syndrome was first described in 1947 by Robinson[22] as a "type of sciatica which is due to an abnormal condition of the piriformis muscle, usually traumatic in origin." This particular condition may be considered an entrapment syndrome. A primary condition that is intrinsic to the piriformis occurs after a fall in which the individual forcibly strikes the ground while bent forward or flexed at the torso (e.g., hockey and football players, gymnasts, and cheerleaders). Primary injury also occurs in a near fall when the piriformis violently contracts to maintain balance. A secondary condition includes piriformis irritation caused by SI joint dysfunction. Because of the piriformis muscle's unique orientation and because it is the only muscle to cross the SI joint, the piriformis plays a large role in SI joint pain. In addition, any lesion or dysfunction of the SI joint can release inflammatory cytokines, which induces a paracrine inflammatory response on the piriformis muscle and its fascia and predisposes to spasm.

The cardinal features of this syndrome include a history of trauma to the SI and gluteal regions; regional pain localized to the SI joint, the greater sciatic notch, and the piriformis muscle that extends down the limb; acute exacerbation of pain by stooping and lifting; a palpable tender myofascial point within the involved piriformis muscle; a positive Lasegue sign (straight leg raise) with prolonged hypertonicity or irritation; and gluteal atrophy as a result of compression of the superior and inferior gluteal nerve(s). The most notable hallmark of this condition is the development of sciatic neuritis.

Epidemiology and risk factors[1,3-7,9]

The incidence rate of piriformis syndrome ranges from 0.33% to 6%, with a female-to-male preponderance ranging from 3:1 to 6:1. Aside from direct trauma, causative physical activities are extremes of running, hiking long distances, or climbing. Each of these activities requires the athlete to perform numerous, repetitive hip extension maneuvers (e.g., Eco Challenge, triathlons, marathons, and speed skating).

History and physical

A history of a fall or another related direct trauma to the gluteal region as well as activities that cause a prolongation or exacerbation of hip rotation/extension will normally be reported by the athlete. Complaints of buttock pain with or without radiation to the posterior thigh, knee, and calf are usually present. Hip adduction and

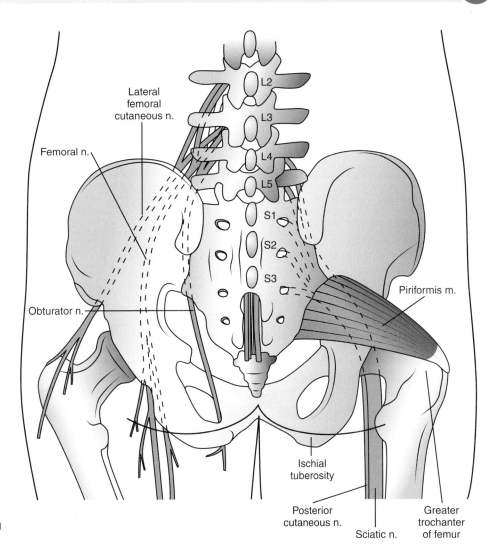

Figure 24.4 Sciatic nerve (n.) anatomy: posterior view. (From Brown: Atlas of Regional Anaesthesia, 3rd ed.)

internal rotation activities increase the symptoms as a result of the stretch placed on the piriformis. Patients may complain of pain while performing either hip extension and/or flexion as a result of the unique biomechanics of this muscle. As the hip is flexed, the piriformis contracts, which aids in the flexion. Likewise, when the hip extends, the piriformis also contracts, thus assisting with this motion. The key clinical characteristic is the complaint of sitting intolerance because sitting places direct pressure on the spasming muscle. In addition, because of the proximity of the piriformis to the lateral pelvic wall, patients may also complain of dyspareunia or pain with bowel movements, resulting from the activation of the pelvic splanchnic nerve. One major distinction between this condition and other sciatica-producing conditions (e.g., herniated nucleus pulposus) is the lack of true radiculopathy in piriformis syndrome.[24]

Physical examination findings that are indicative of piriformis syndrome include a palpable tender point within the muscle belly, origin, or insertion. Painful resisted active external rotation of the hip while seated and in the fully internally rotated position is considered the most specific test for differentiating this condition from other causes of pain.[23] Patients with a long history of piriformis syndrome may develop gluteal atrophy as a result of the entrapment of the peritoneal branch of the sciatic nerve. This gluteal atrophy is more commonly found in the elder athlete with a positive Trendelenburg sign and motor weakness along the S_1 myotome.

Imaging

As a result of the associated neural involvement with this condition, all necessary studies should be performed to rule out spinal causes of sciatica and SI joint or hip pathology. Computed tomography (CT) scanning, MRI scanning, and scintigraphy with technitium-99m bone scanning rarely demonstrate any identifiable piriformis abnormality.[23] However, neurophysiologic testing has proven helpful.[23] The peritoneal branch of the sciatic nerve and the internal gluteal nerve may demonstrate signs of denervation from the compression of a hypertrophied piriformis. Nerve conduction studies will demonstrate delays in the H reflexes of these nerves.[23]

Treatment

Conservative treatment consists of rest, the use of nonsteroidal anti-inflammatory nonnarcotic analgesics, and muscle relaxants.[23] Additionally, osteopathic manipulative treatment with indirect (e.g., counter strain and facilitated positional release) and direct (e.g., Still's technique, facilitated myofascial release, and muscle energy) techniques are useful adjuncts.[24] Trigger point injections with an analgesic or a corticosteroid can be tried in those patients whose conditions are resistant to conservative therapy.[23] Surgery should only be considered when patients fail to improve with conservative treatment[23] and when they have intractable pain or neurologic deficits (e.g., gluteal atrophy or foot drop).

Sacral torsion/shear and sacroiliac joint dysfunction

Some of the most common and significant sources of LBP include sacral torsion, shear of the sacrum, or derangement of the SI joint (Figures 24.5 and 24.6).

Because of the biomechanics and load translation that occur through this joint, the dysfunction or loss of sacral motion will cause pain and dysfunction elsewhere (e.g., in the lumbosacral segments or the hip joint) as the body attempts to maintain normal function.[26] Additionally, distant anatomic or mechanical alterations such as physiologic leg-length discrepancy, muscle imbalance (predominately the contralateral gluteus maximus and the latissimus dorsi in an attempt to stabilize the incompetent joint[14]), trunk or hip flexibility, or improper sport-specific technique may lead to sacral and SI joint mechanics that result in injury and pain.[26] Of the three transverse axes of the sacrum (superior, middle, and inferior), the middle axis is primarily involved in sacral dysfunctions.[13,25] A sacral shear is a nonphysiologic dysfunction that occurs as a result of a sudden downward force of the sacrum in combination with an equal or greater upward force on the ipsilateral leg. A key to discriminating a sacral shear from a simple SI joint dysfunction is the lack of pain referred above the L_5 level in sacral dysfunction.[20,27]

Epidemiology and risk factors

Training and sporting events that require repetitive unidirectional pelvic shear and torsional forces (e.g., skating, gymnastics, and bowling) increase the risk of developing sacral and SI joint dysfunction. A sacral shear is commonly caused by a runner who unexpectedly steps in a hole or in an Olympic

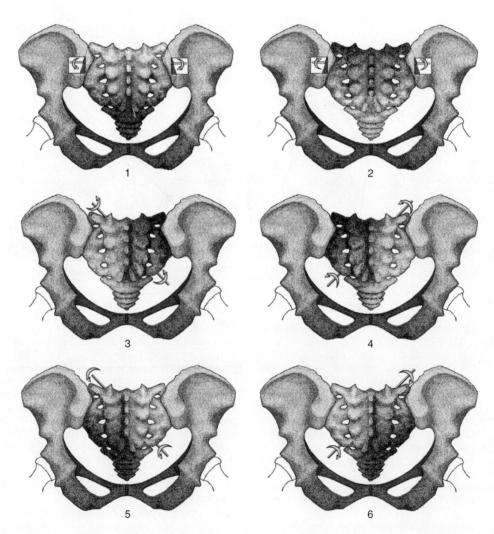

Figure 24.5 Illustrative representations of some common physical examination findings of the sacrum with the patient in the prone position. 1, Sacral base posterior. Findings include a shallow sacral sulci bilaterally and an anterior-inferior lateral angle bilaterally. The sacral base will resist springing anteriorly. Posterior superior iliac spines (PSISs) are level. Sacral apex is anterior. Sacrotuberous ligaments are lax bilaterally. 2, Sacral base anterior. Findings include deep sacral sulci bilaterally, posterior sacral inferior lateral angles (ILAs) bilaterally. Sacral base will spring anteriorly. PSISs are level. Sacral apes is posterior. Sacrotuberous ligaments are tight bilaterally. 3, Left-on-left sacral torsion. Left ILA is posterior and slightly inferior. PSIS is low on the left and high on the right. Right sacral sulcus is deep. Left sacrotuberous ligament is tight. Anterior superior iliac spines (ASIS) is high on the left and low on the right. 4, Right-on-right sacral torsion. Right ILA is posterior and slightly inferior. PSIS is low on the right and high on the left. Left sacral sulcus is deep. Right sacrotuberous ligament is tight. ASIS is high on the right and low on the left. 5, Right-on-left sacral torsion. Left ILA is slightly anterior. PSIS is low on the right. Right sacral sulcus is shallow. Left sacrotuberous ligament is loose. ASIS is elevated on the right. 6, Left-on-right oblique axis sacral torsion. Right ILA is anterior and inferior. Left PSIS is low. Left sacral sulcus is shallow. Right sacrotuberous ligament is loose. ASIS is high on the left.

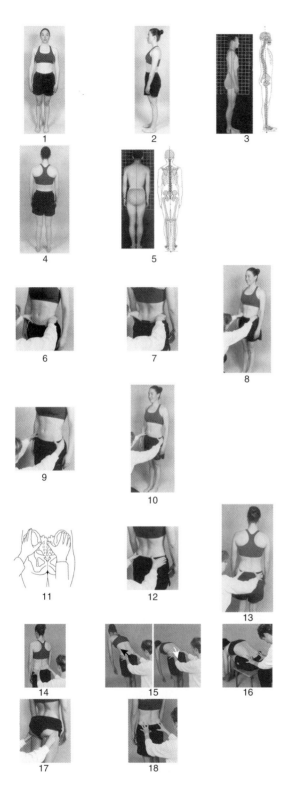

Figure 24.6 Pictographic representations of some common physical examination findings. 1, Posture standing anterior view. 2 and 3, Posture standing lateral view. 4 and 5, Posture standing posterior view. 6, 7, and 8, Standing iliac crest height. 9 and 10, Position of ASIS. 11, 12, and 13, Position of PSIS. 14, 15, and 16, Flexion test: positive side PSIS will catch and continue to move superiorly as patient forward bends. Standing and seated. 17, Ischial tuberosity positions. 18, Positions of the sacral sulci and ILAs. (From Magee: Orthopedic Physical Assessment, 4th ed. Philadelphia, WB Saunders, 2002.)

weight lifter whose weight suddenly shifts and causes a buckling of the opposite knee while the ipsilateral leg remains locked in place.

Biomechanics
The function of the SI joint is stability, which facilitates a safe load transfer[15] through the lumbosacral–pelvic complex. Any muscle imbalance in this region can lead to SI joint dysfunction, which can result in a torsion or shear.

History and physical
Athletes will normally complain of pain in the SI joint, with pain focused around the posterior superior iliac spine and the sacral sulcus. Pain may be exacerbated during repetitive overload activities, transitional movements, or unsupported sitting.[18] The patient may sit on the opposite buttock in an attempt to alleviate his or her symptoms. A patient who is found to have a sacral torsion or shear may complain of pain in the SI region contralaterally as well as pain in the mid back or even the neck **(Figure 24.7),** resulting from spinal compensation for an unleveled base as the body attempts to keep the eyes level with the horizon.

The physical examination of a sacral torsion consists of both the seated and standing flexion tests to determine if an SI or iliosacral dysfunction exists. Next, the examiner must determine the rotation and axis of the dysfunction by bilaterally palpating the sacral sulcus (base) with his or her thumbs: the thumb that is more anterior by palpation is the deeper sulcus. Next, he or she must palpate the inferior lateral angles of the sacrum: the thumb that is more posterior and, by convention of sacral mechanics, more inferior is the posterior inferior lateral angle. Innominate compression can be performed with the patient lying supine: the innominate that does not move freely or that elicits pain at the SI joint when equal, posterior force is placed on the anterior superior iliac spines is the dysfunctional side. Using this information, the physician can determine the athlete's type of sacral dysfunction. Figure 24.5 is a pictographic representation of some common physical examination findings.

To test for a sacral shear, the practitioner places his or her thumbs on the soft tissue below the gluteus on either side of the coccyx and pushes cephalad with light pressure until the thumbs strike the caudal surface of the sacrum on each side of the coccyx: the more inferiorly displaced inferior lateral angle is ipsilateral to the sacral shear. In addition, in sacral shear dysfunction, no motion will be felt at the ipsilateral inferior pole of the

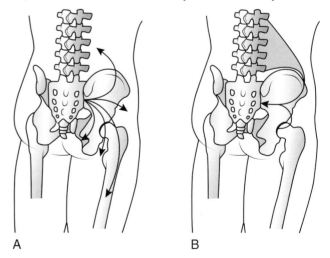

Figure 24.7 Referred pain from the sacroiliac joint (A) and to the sacroiliac joint (B). (Redrawn from Magee: Orthopedic Physical Assessment, 4th ed. Philadelphia, WB Saunders, 2002.)

SI joint.[18] Palpation of the ipsilateral sacrotuberous ligament will reveal it to be lax as a result of the bony approximation of the sacrum and the ischium. Finally, to test gross SI joint motion, the patient is placed prone with the affected side leg flexed to 90 degrees at the knee. While one hand abducts the athlete's leg, the other monitors for gapping of the SI joint just medial to the posterior superior iliac spine ipsilaterally. The side with the sacral shear will not gap.[18]

The physical examination of the SI joint is extensive, and numerous tests have developed that induce shearing or rotational forces to stress inflamed structures, thus provoking pain. The most common provocation and motion tests for the sacrum and SI joint include the compression test; the distraction (gapping) test; the Gaenslen sign[27]; the flexed, abducted, externally rotated (FABER) test (i.e., Patrick's or figure four test); the flexed, adducted, internally rotated (FADIR) test; Gillet's test[14]; the Lesegue sign; the posterior shear (POSH) test[27]; the resisted abduction (REAB) test[27]; the Wilson–Barstow test[28]; and the Yeoman test.[13,18] However, for SI joint assessment, a combination of the FABER, POSH, and REAB tests has a high predictive value in diagnosing SI joint dysfunction, with a sensitivity ranging from 77% to 87% and a specificity approaching 100% (LOE: B).[16]

Imaging

All types of imaging studies (plain radiographs, CT scanning, MRI, bone scintigraphy, and SPECT) have proven to be of little value for diagnosing SI joint and sacral dysfunctions (LOE: B).[26] However, if an infectious, metabolic, fracture, or neoplastic condition is suspected, or if symptoms persist after a trial of conservative and manipulative treatment, imaging of the SI joint should be performed.[26]

Treatment

The conservative modalities of rest, heat/ice, anti-inflammatory drugs, analgesic medications, and muscle-relaxing agents may be of benefit on an individual basis (LOE: B).[26] Osteopathic manipulative treatment has been demonstrated to improve function and to decrease the pain associated with this condition (LOE: B).[12,13,17,18,27,29,30] One technique that has been found to be useful acutely is the articulatory technique to free up the SI joint.

Multiple authors[5,20,26] report intra-articular injections, primarily under fluoroscopic guidance, as the gold standard for diagnosing the SI joint dysfunction. However, as beneficial as this modality may be for alleviating the patient's pain, it does not address the sacral or SI joint dysfunction nor does it offer an opportunity to stabilize the incompetent joint or assess the extra-articular structures, muscles, ligaments, and tendons that may be generating symptoms.[18,20] Biomechanic proprioceptive retraining should be done to maintain sacral and SI joint function. Exercises to improve SI joint stabilization should include those that isolate the transverses abdominus, multifidus, and piriformis as well as those that strengthen the coordination between the contralateral gluteus maximus and the latissimus dorsi (LOE: C).[15,17,21,29]

Prolotherapy has recently gained a following as an alternative treatment for back pain. A few studies have demonstrated a substantial effect. Dextrose/glycerin/phenol injections at weekly intervals have been shown in one study to be helpful in treatment; however, all of the patients treated had LBP in addition to SI joint dysfunction, and they were treated with joint stabilization exercises as well as prolotherapy. Further investigation is needed with this therapeutic intervention (LOE: C).[15]

Sacral stress fracture

Wolf's law states that repetitive microtrauma concentrated at a specific bony location will provoke adaptive remodeling.[30,31]

Training within the physiologic range of bone homeostasis results in a positive anabolic response to bone density. Conversely, overtraining results in a catabolic effect of bone density, thus setting up a fracture.[25]

Two forms of sacral stress fractures exist: insufficiency stress fracture, which occurs in those with insufficient bone mineralization who undergo normal stress-type and fatigue-type fracture, in which fractures occur in bone with normal mineralization that is overstressed.[25]

Epidemiology and risk factors

This condition occurs almost exclusively among athletes who are participating in high-level running events such as soccer, track, cross-country, and marathon or triathlon competitions.[2] Sacral stress fractures appear to be more common among female athletes, perhaps as a result of the risk factors discussed in Table 24.1.[2,25]

History and physical

The athlete will commonly report an insidious onset of asymmetric LBP, hip pain, or gluteal pain that, after being intermittent and associated with exercise for weeks, has now become persistent.[4] Usually no acute incident is associated with the pain onset, and the pain may only become problematic after a change in training intensity or at times of prolonged sitting. Examination may reveal point tenderness over the lateral sacrum or the SI joint. Range-of-motion testing may reveal discomfort during hip extension, lateral flexion, and the rotation of lumbosacral spine.[31] The FABER test and the single-leg hop test (standing and hopping on the ipsilateral leg, respectively) may be positive and elicit pain.[2]

Female athletes with suspected stress fractures should be asked about dietary habits and menstrual history.[4] Any female athlete who is amenorrheic, who has evidence of an eating disorder, and who complains of lateral sacral pain should promptly undergo a bone scan or another type of advanced imaging to determine whether a sacral stress fracture has developed.[2]

Imaging[31]

Plain radiographs of the sacrum and the SI joint may be beneficial if bony sclerosis is present. However, the multiple radiographic lines in the normal sacrum make the interpretation of plain films difficult. SPECT scanning attains a greater precision of locating regions of sacral fracturing (**Figure 24.8**). CT scanning proved to be both sensitive and specific for determining sacral fracture location, and it includes findings of cortical disruption and of periosteal, endosteal, and medullary new bone formation (LOE: B).[25,31] MRI is useful for determining sclerotic lesions and areas of bone edema; however, this modality may not be specific for fracture lesions.

Treatment

Treatment begins with rest, the discontinuance of athletic training, and the use of crutches for limited weight bearing. This is followed by incremental (several weeks) increases in weight bearing and mobility. Females found by CT scanning to have a bone density of less than 110 mg/mL should receive daily oral calcium and vitamin D (LOE: C).[31] Water aerobics, water running, and swimming are encouraged after the resolution of pain. Female athletes with insufficiency fractures or with a history of multiple stress fractures should receive both nutritional and psychologic counseling.

Return to play

Pain-free activities of daily living and negative physical findings are a must before impact activities can be initiated. As with all stress fractures, the athlete should be symptom free with daily walking before a gradual walk-to-run program can be initiated. (See Chapter 32 for a more in-depth discussion of general principles of stress fracture rehabilitation.)

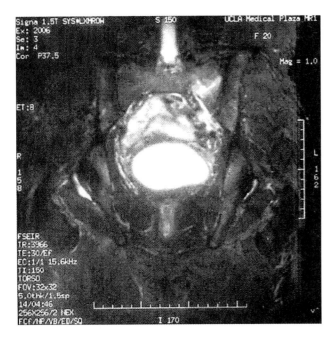

Figure 24.8 MRI of a sacral stress fracture in a young female distance runner. The fracture is seen here as a bright, transverse line across the left sacrum on T2 imaging. (From DeLee JC, Drez D Jr, Miller MD [eds]: DeLee and Drez's Orthopaedic Sports Medicine: Principles and Practice, 2nd ed. Philadelphia, WB Saunders, 2003.)

EXTENSION-RELATED CONDITIONS

Extension-related injuries occur when the lumbar spine is in extension.

Spondylolysis/spondylolisthesis

The term *spondylolysis* is formed from the Greek words *spondylos*, meaning "spine," and *lysis*, meaning "to dissolve".[25] The condition itself is a defect (stress fracture) of the pars interarticularis.[4] However, a defect may occur at any point, from the posterolateral vertebral body, the pedicle, or even the spinous process.[2] This can arise with or without a corresponding spondylo*listhesis* or the anterior slippage of a superior vertebrae on an inferior vertebrae. **Table 24.3** describes the modified Wiltse classification system for spondylolysis.

Most authors describe spondylolysis in an incremental progression that ranges from stress injury of the pars (which may only be seen on MRI or SPECT imaging studies), to a stress reaction, to a stress fracture that is free from gross lucency or sclerosis, to a fully visible fracture with sclerosis, to the classic spondylitic defect of the pars.[11]

Spondylolisthesis, which was first described in 1782 by Herbiniaux,[32] occurs in two forms: the elongation of an intact pars interarticularis or anterior translation as a result of a bilateral spondylolytic defect.

The Meyerding classification of spondylolisthesis offers a grading scale that defines the degree of slippage on the basis of the percentage of anterior translation of the cephalad vertebral body relative to the superior endplate of the next caudad segment.[32] Grades I through IV correspond with 0% to 25%, 26% to 50%, 51% to 75%, and 76% to 99% of slippage, respectively. Grade V injury, or spondyloptosis, is a complete (100%) slippage. It is usually traumatic, and it is a surgical emergency **(Figure 24.9)**.

Spondylolisthesis slippage progression is of great concern for the female athlete. Females have an increased susceptibility to this

Table 24.3 Modified Wiltse Spondylolysis Classification[31]*

Form	Type	Description
Developmental: Occurs to those who undergo linear growth: children and adolescents	Type I: Dysplastic	Congenital as a result of dysplasia of the upper sacrum or the neural arch of the superior vertebrae
	Type II: Isthmic; most common form seen in children	Lesion of the pars interarticularis
Acquired: May occur among members of any age group	Type III: Degenerative	Longstanding intersegmental instability
	Type IV: Traumatic	Fracture of vertebrae other than the pars
	Type V: Pathologic	Results from generalized or localized bone disease
	Type VI[30]: Iatrogenic/postsurgical	Results from a medical procedure or spinal surgery

*Wiltse LL, Newman PH, Macnab I: Clin Orthop Relat Res 1976;117:23-29.

deformity (2:1 to 3:1 female-to-male ratio),[32] an earlier-aged increase in this deformity as a result of growth,[32] an increased risk of severe displacement, and more severe clinical symptoms.[33] The progression of spondylolisthesis most commonly occurs during the adolescent growth spurt.[32] As the vertebrae progress through the cartilaginous, apophyseal, and epiphyseal stages of bony growth, slip progression has been found in 52%, 39%, and 10% of athletes, respectively.[34] Spondylolisthetic progression is uncommon after adolescence, and further slippage is minimal after the attainment of skeletal maturity.[32]

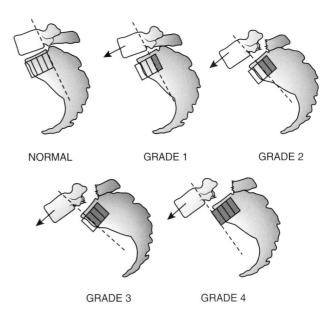

Figure 24.9 Meyerding grading system for slipping in spondylolisthesis. (Redrawn from Magee: Orthopedic Physical Assessment, 4th ed. Philadelphia, WB Saunders, 2002.)

Three measurements have been devised to assist in the determination of spondylolisthetic progression: the lumbar index (the slippage percentage), the slip angle, and the sacral inclination.[35] The slippage percentage is the degree of displacement (equal to a/A × 100%), which is measured as the distance of the posterior wall portion of the vertebral body of the inferior vertebrae (a) in relation to the sagittal length of the sacral plateau (A).[36] The slip angle (or sagittal roll) is the angle that is formed between the end plates of the inferior (or posterior border of the sacrum) and superior vertebrae, and it defines the degree of lumbosacral kyphosis.[35,36] This delineation can predict the risk of future slip progression, which commonly occurs when the angle exceeds 55 degrees.[5,11] Sacral inclination is defined as the angle formed by an imaginary line made by the sacral plateau to the vertical.[35,36] When a decrease of this inclination is documented (steepening of the sacrum), spondylolisthetic progression is also more likely. The definitive documentation of spondylolisthesis progression requires a change of 10% to 15% of slippage or 4 to 5 mm of anterior displacement[32] **(Figure 24.10).**

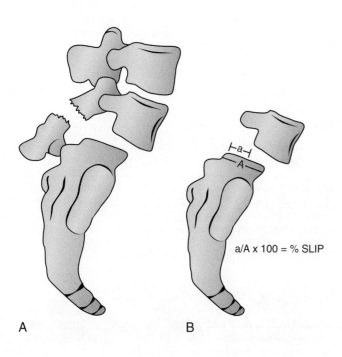

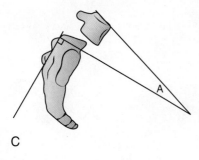

Figure 24.10 *A,* Spondylolisthesis is the anterior translation of one vertebral segment relative to the next caudal segment in association with a bilateral pars defect. *B,* The Meyerding classification is used to quantify the degree of spondylolisthesis. Grade I, 0% to 25% slip; grade II, 26% to 50% slip; grade III, 51% to 75% slip; grade IV, 76% to 100% slip. *C,* The slip angle quantifies the degree of lumbosacral kyphosis. A value of more than 55 degrees correlates with an increased risk for the progression of spondylolisthesis. (From Imhof HI, Mang T: Orthop Clin North Am 2006;37[3]:292.)

Epidemiology and risk factors (Table 24.4)

Spondylolysis and spondylolisthesis are the most common spinal injuries that occur in athletes. They both tend to occur more commonly at the L5-S1 level as a result of the rotational shearing forces applied at this segment.[2,36] The reported incidence rate for spondylolysis among young athletes as compared with the general population is 47% and 5%, respectively.[3]

Certain sports predispose the athlete to the development of spondylolysis that may progress to spondylolisthesis. These include weight lifting, dancing, figure skating, rowing, pole vaulting, wrestling, and volleyball. However, football, diving, gymnastics, and rhythmic gymnastics are considered to carry the highest risk.[11] Numerous studies report incidence rates as high as 32% among gymnasts and 63% among divers,[3] whereas the prevalence rate for spondylolisthesis among football lineman ranges from 48% to 50%.[4] More than 15 hours of training per week predisposes the adolescent athlete to the development of spondylolysis.[3] Sixty-eight percent of patients diagnosed with spondylolysis demonstrate concomitant anterior disc and end plate involvement.[3] Because this condition, when misdiagnosed, can result in back pain well into adulthood, any suspicion of spondylolysis or spondylolisthesis in the adolescent must be actively pursued.

Pathophysiology and mechanism of injury

Spondylolysis commonly develops as a result of repetitive extremes of lordotic hyperextension, which are primarily seen among adolescent athletes who are growing. Normal lumbar biomechanics center the pivot point for motion over the vertebral body. However, when the lumbar spine is placed in extremes of extension, this pivot point becomes centered over the facet joints, thus leading to microtrauma. Certain positions of hyperextension (e.g., back walkovers in gymnastics, the inexperienced rhythmic gymnast performing the back scale[37] and the squatted, lumbar-locked position with an upright torso of the offensive lineman) increase the axial loading and translational forces at the lower lumbar facet joints. To obtain increased lumbar hyperextension beyond the complete closure of the posterior facet, the subsequent extension occurs through the neural arch,[11] beyond the normal physiologic range active motion. Repetitive flexion with hyperextension movements that involve large stress reversals in the pars interarticularis leads to the development of spondylolysis.[38]

Table 24.4 Spondylolysis and Spondylolisthesis Risk Factors

Absolute Risk Factors

Family history: Incidence of 26% reported among first-degree relatives[32]

Indigenous Alaskan ancestry, particularly among those who reside north of the Yukon River[31]; risk increased up to 50%[4]

Relative Risk Factors

Spinal anomalies[30,33]:
  Spina bifida occulta
  Transitional vertebrae
  Scoliosis

Growth as ossification of the lamina progresses posteriorly, becoming congenitally incomplete, particularly at pars interarticularis[6]

Gender differences that may be factors in the differences in sports participation between the sexes during youth:
  Predominance of pars defects in boys
  Predominance of high-grade slippage in girls

Trabecular strength of the pars: Strength of the neural arch increases up to the fourth and fifth decade of life[36]

Extension-related conditions

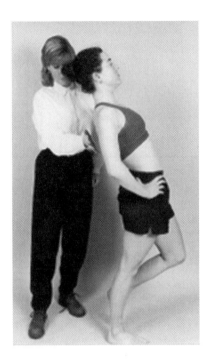

Figure 24.11 One-leg standing lumbar extension test. (From Magee: Orthopedic Physical Assessment, 4th ed. Philadelphia, WB Saunders, 2002.)

History and Physical

Dull, unilateral pain that is usually confined to the lower back is the most common presenting symptom. The onset of pain is insidious and progresses over weeks. Athletes report a worsening of their pain during extension and rotational maneuvers. Conversely, flexion posturing often relieves some of the pain and discomfort. Pain radiating to the buttocks or the posterior thighs is commonly seen from tightened hamstrings or piriformis spasms, which accompany the spondylolysis. Neurologic complaints are not common, but when they are present, they can mimic an L5 radiculopathy.[35]

On examination, a flattened lumbar lordosis is commonly seen in athletes with spondylolysis. Conversely, during the examination of a patient with spondylolisthesis, an exaggeration lumbar lordosis may be found as a result of an increased sacral inclination.[11]

A single-leg hyperextension test **(Figure 24.11)** is a relatively sensitive physical examination finding to detect pars stress fracture (spondylolysis).[39] With increasing spondylolisthetic slippage, a palpable step off between the spinous processes may be felt. Point tenderness may be elicited in some cases of spondylolysis at the affected spinous process.[2]

Imaging

Plain radiography is the least expensive and easiest imaging study to obtain; however, it is also the least sensitive and specific. Standing anteroposterior, lateral, and bilateral oblique views of the lumbosacral region are recommended (LOE: C).[2,11,35] Upright and flexion/extension views may provide additional information to help with the discovery of bony defect. Additionally, a lateral spot view and a 30-degree up-angled anteroposterior view across the lumbosacral junction assists with the viewing of this region.[37] Oblique views at 15 degrees may demonstrate the elongation of the neck of the "Scottie dog of LaChappelle"[11] in spondylolisthesis, whereas the "Scottie dog" may appear to wear a collar in nondisplaced spondylolysis **(Figure 24.12).**

CT scanning is considered best means of defining the defect, and it has the added benefit of demonstrating other forms of spinal pathology,[40] including disc herniation. CT also provides visualization of the vertebral ring **(Figure 24.13)**. If this ring is intact, the exclusion of a pars fracture may be made.[35] However, if an incomplete ring is viewed, a pars fracture is usually present. Callus formation at the site of the fracture is indicative of healing, whereas well-corticated margins indicate an established nonunion.[35] Both standard axial views and reverse-angle gantry images have been found to clearly visualize pars lesions.[37] CT scanning has been shown to be more sensitive than plain radiography; however, the ionizing radiation of nearly 10 times the exposure of radiography[41] makes its use less desirable in some populations.[37]

SPECT is considered to be the imaging modality of choice for this condition because it improves the localization of the spondylolytic lesion by the special separation of overlapping bony structures[2,11,39,42] **(Figure 24.14)**. A negative SPECT scan with normal plain radiography can exclude spondylolysis or spondylolisthesis as the primary cause of back pain.[35,37] The limitation of this imaging modality is the diminution of its specificity as a result of an increased uptake with neoplastic or infectious causes.[7,35,37]

MRI will visualize areas of stress reactivity and fracturing before there is radiographic evidence of spondylolysis. An additional benefit of MRI is the lack of ionizing radiation, which makes it particularly desirable to employ, especially in the adolescent female population.[41]

Treatment

Asymptomatic The incidental finding of an asymptomatic spondylolytic lesion on plain radiography, SPECT, or CT scanning should not be of any great concern to the ordering physician. Although low, the risk of progression to spondylolisthesis warrants the obtainment of annual imaging studies until skeletal maturity is reached to ensure that no further progression ensues. No restriction in activity or sports participation is required.[42]

Symptomatic* Healing is judged clinically by the reduction of symptoms, the return of function, and the radiographic documentation of the trabecular bridging of the pars abnormality.[33] The goal of treatment for an actively healing spondylolysis is the production of a stable bony or fibrous union. Conversely, in those who have evidence of a well-defined, chronic spondylitic defect (nonunion), the goal of treatment focuses on symptom improvement and return of function.[33] The staging of spondylolysis is important for determining treatment initiation and educating the patient about the success of treatment outcomes and returning to sports participation **(Table 24.5).**

Bracing with an antilordotic lumbosacral orthosis (Boston Brace or modified Boston Overlap Brace, Warm-n-Form orthosis, or Risser cast) **(Figure 24.15)** is the primary means of stabilizing a spondylolytic defect. There is a conflict in the literature regarding the length of wear, with one study returning the athlete to sports participation after 4 to 6 weeks,[42] but most suggest continued use of braces from 4 to 6 months. The brace is molded at 0 degrees of posterior alignment or lordosis, with 15 degrees[23] of anterior cavitation[42] to assist with unloading the posterior facets and decreasing shear stress across the pedicle. The brace is worn until the athlete is pain free during the performance of full sports-specific activities during brace wear, whereupon weaning may begin at a rate of 1 less hour per day per week.[11,42] A limited CT scan to determine

---

*Many different algorithms exist for treatment of symptomatic spondylolysis with little evidence to support the superiority of one method over another. An alternative approach to diagnosis and treatment of spondylolysis is discussed in Chapter 31.

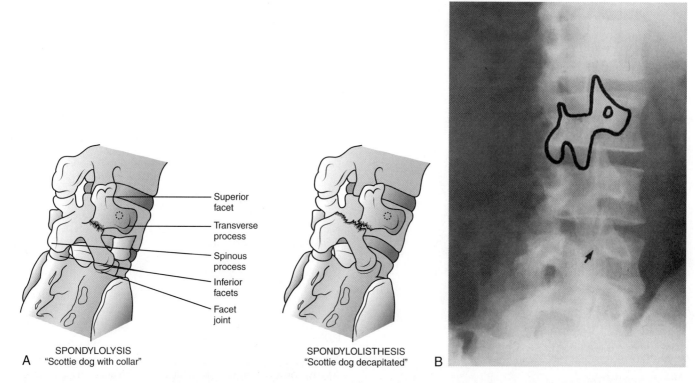

Superior
facet

Transverse
process

Spinous
process

Inferior
facets

Facet
joint

A   SPONDYLOLYSIS
"Scottie dog with collar"

B   SPONDYLOLISTHESIS
"Scottie dog decapitated"

Figure 24.12 *A*, Diagrammatic representation (posterior oblique view) of spondylolysis and spondylolisthesis. *B*, Posterior oblique film showing "Scottie dog" at L2. L4 shows Scottie dog with a "collar" *(arrow)*, which indicates spondylolysis. (Redrawn from Magee: Orthopedic Physical Assessment, 4th ed. Philadelphia, WB Saunders, 2002.)

healing progression is recommended at 4 months.[7,42] The athlete, the parents, and the coaches must be counseled regarding the fact that therapy may last 6 to 9 months before the athlete returns to full activity.

An isometric trunk stabilization program should be initiated after the abatement of symptoms. William's flexion-type and Richardson draw-in transversus abdominis exercises should be incorporated into the treatment program to improve the abdominal musculature and inner core strength (LOE: D).[11,17] Hamstring and hip flexor stretching are also emphasized. Between 75% and 83% of athletes diagnosed with a spondylolysis who undergo nonoperative treatment achieve the treatment goals of lesion stabilization and return to full function.[39] Osteopathic manipulative techniques such as counter strain, facilitated positional release, and myofascial release may decrease pain levels and reduce structural stresses on the fractured area.[12] The use of high-velocity, low-amplitude techniques is contraindicated because the force required to articulate the vertebrae may actually result in the further separation of the pars defect and exacerbate the patient's condition.[12]

Surgery is indicated for persistent pain that has failed at least 6 months of conservative treatment,[2] to include bracing. However, surgery should be delayed for at least 1 year[11] to allow time for the body to heal and for growth to continue, particularly in the setting of an adolescent growth spurt. Surgery for spondylolisthesis may become necessary if the slippage is beyond 50% (grade III) at time of initial presentation or if evidence of progression exists, even in the asymptomatic patient.

Continued clinical examination at 6-month intervals is highly encouraged in the growing athlete until he or she is skeletally mature (by radiographic evidence of epiphyseal plate closure) to detect the rare case of spondylolysis or spondylolisthesis progression and to intervene accordingly if such a change is documented.[32]

Return to play[40]

Athletes are allowed to resume training and competition as long as they have a pain-free full range of motion with sport-specific activities. One study returned athletes to full competition within 4 to 6 weeks of treatment initiation with a lumbar orthosis and pain-free extension.[42] Limiting certain activities that require excessive lordosis, such as backward bends in gymnastics and dead lifts in weightlifting, may decrease recurrence rates.[10]

Athletes who undergo single-level spinal or lumbosacral fusion are usually allowed to return to collision sports 1 year after their procedure, as long as all other functional requirements are met. Athletes who participate in noncontact activities, such as running and tennis, are typically allowed to return to competition 6 months postoperatively.[33]

FLEXION CONDITIONS

Disc degeneration/herniation (herniated nucleus pulposus)
Epidemiology and risk factors

Disc degeneration is predominately seen in the adult population as a result of years of overuse and improper lifting techniques. Degenerative disc changes in preadolescent gymnasts are well described in the literature, with a reported incidence rate

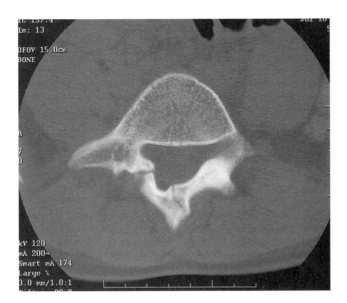

Figure 24.13 Axial computed tomography image of a 17-year-old football player demonstrating unilateral spondylolysis with sclerosis of the contralateral pars. (From DeLee JC, Drez D Jr, Miller MD [eds]: DeLee and Drez's Orthopaedic Sports Medicine: Principles and Practice, 2nd ed. Philadelphia, WB Saunders, 2003.)

of 11% in pre-elite gymnasts, 43% in elite gymnasts, and 64% in Olympic gymnasts.[6] Conversely, this is a relatively uncommon injury among children who do not participate in gymnastics.[9] When training exceeds 15 hours per week, the risk of injury increases from 13% to 57%.[6] Other sports that are associated with disc degeneration are collision sports (e.g., football, lacrosse, and hockey), soccer, bowling, gymnastics, weight lifting, and wrestling.[2] Of all professional sports, golfers have the highest incidence of back injury because of the torsional stress of the golf swing wind up, swing, and follow through.[43] Intrinsic and extrinsic risk factors for degenerative disc disease are listed in **Table 24.6.**

Pathogenesis and mechanism of injury

A number of hypotheses have been developed to clearly define the mechanism of disc degeneration. One of the most convincing is the "wear-and-tear" hypothesis, which proposes that localized microtrauma from repeated lateral bending, rotational torque, and axial loading during repetitive movements of the lumbar region cause injury to the intervertebral disc.[44] In vitro studies have demonstrated that the application of static loads can induce cell apoptosis, alter structural disc properties (thickness, axial compliance, and angular laxity), change matrix content (proteoglycan and type I/II collagen), interfere with metalloproteinase activity, and alter gene expression (aggrecan and collagen II).[45] These factors are exacerbated in the skeletally immature athlete who is undergoing the extrinsic stresses of athletic training and competition and the intrinsic stresses of growth and structural turnover. Excessive extrinsic stress such as repeated high-energy compressive forces, vibration, and pressurization result in the inhibition of protein production during this vulnerable period of growth.[45]

Initially, microscopic circumferential tearing of the inner annular fibers occurs from repeated microtrauma. Next, a focal defect appears in the cartilage end plate, and an increase in the thickness and spacing of collagen fibers occurs. With continued stress, these tears become increasingly larger and coalesce into radial tears that extend beyond the annulus into the nucleus pulposus.[45] As the disc degenerates, the nucleus becomes more consolidated, more fibrous, and less demarcated from the annulus.[45] The continuation of axial loading forces on the nucleus pulposus at the point of least resistance along the weakened inner annulus increases tearing and annular fissuring. With repeated axial loading and flexion/extension movements, desiccation of the nuclear pulposus occurs, and this results in a loss of hydrostatic properties, thereby reducing the tensile strength of the disc.[44] As this layer continues to weaken and tear, the outer layer becomes stressed. Delamination occurs with repeated high interlaminar shear stresses[45] and finally gives way to the extrusion of the nucleus pulposus. Annular tears may occur with as little as 3 degrees of torque rotation.[44] As a result of the extensive innervation of the outer annulus, tremendous pain and paraspinal reflex spasming occur.

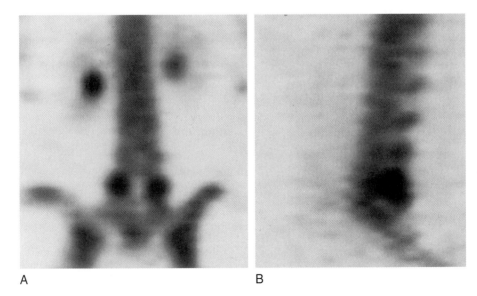

A   B

Figure 24.14 Coronal (A) and sagittal (B) single photon emission computed tomographic images from a 15-year-old boy with uptake in the region of the L5 pars interarticularis. The findings are consistent with spondylolysis. (From DeLee JC, Drez D Jr, Miller MD [eds]: DeLee and Drez's Orthopaedic Sports Medicine: Principles and Practice, 2nd ed. Philadelphia, WB Saunders, 2003.)

Table 24.5 Staging and Progression of Spondylolysis*

Prespondylolysis	Indicative of disease pathology in athletically active adolescents. Repetitive hyperextension movements that causes microtrauma to the pars interarticularis result in the formation of a stress reaction or fracture not radiographically evident but visible on bone scintigraphy (particularly single photon emission computed tomography).
Early spondylolysis	Development of a hairline cortical and trabecular disruption with focal bony absorption evident on computed tomography scanning but may remain equivocal on plain radiography. If caught in this stage of development, athlete may have an excellent outcome with conservative treatment.[37] Results in high healing rates.[35,37]
Progressive spondylolysis	Continued overstressing and hyperextension. Characterized by the creation of radiographic-viewed (obliquely) widening defect of the bony morphology.
Terminal (sclerotic) spondylolysis	Distinguished by a sclerotic nonunion that is now easily identifiable on oblique radiographs. Spondylolytic defect becomes nearly permanent with little or no healing in follow-up studies.[35]

*Ralston S, Weir M: Clin Pediatr (Phila) 1998;37(5):287-293.

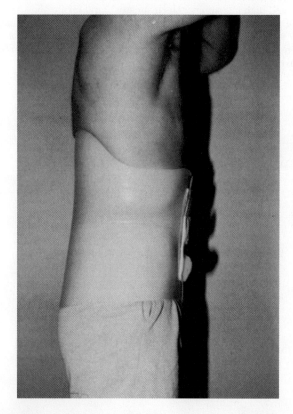

Figure 24.15 Lumbosacral orthosis. (From DeLee JC, Drez D Jr, Miller MD [eds]: DeLee and Drez's Orthopaedic Sports Medicine: Principles and Practice, 2nd ed. Philadelphia, WB Saunders, 2003.)

Table 24.6 Disc Degeneration Risk Factors

Intrinsic

Positive family history,* predominately in a first-degree relative
Morphologic uniqueness of a transitional vertebrae and rounder end plates in both men and women and of end plate size in men[†]

Extrinsic[‡]

Extremes of hyperlordotic positioning and flexion/extension movements, such as back walkovers, flips, and vault dismounts in gymnastics
Repeated axial loads with extreme weight, particularly when lifting above the head during the clean and jerk techniques of weightlifting
Axial and torsional loads of football blocking

*Battie MC, Videman T, Parent E: Spine 2004;29(23):2679-2690.
[†]Harrington J Jr, Sungarian A, Rogg J, et al: Spine 2001;26(19):2133-2138.
[‡]Watkins RG: Clin Sports Med 2002;21(1):147-165.

History and physical

The most common reported symptom is back pain that is aggravated by activity and relieved with rest. The athlete may report feeling a popping or tearing sensation at the moment of initial discomfort.[46] There may be a complaint of inguinal pain if a lower lumbar intervertebral disc is involved.[2,46] Teens complain of back spasms, hamstring tightness, buttock pain, and, occasionally, neurogenic sciatica, although this is seen less frequently than it is among adults. Hamstring tightness and back spasms are usually the initial complaint.[14] Typically, discogenic pain is worse with flexion and eases slightly with extension of the lumbar spine.

Examination reveals reduced lumbar motion, the exacerbation of pain upon flexion and relief upon extension, a positive straight-leg raise test (Lasegue sign) **(Figure 24.16)**; the most common physical finding) and a positive Larson test.[2] If lumbar radiculopathy accompanies the patient's complaints, a potential reduction of both reflexes and strength in the lower extremities may be found[14] **(Figure 24.17)**.

Imaging

Plain anteroposterior and lateral radiographs may or may not show disc space narrowing. This imaging modality is obtained first before other, more expensive studies, but it may prove to be of little value when used early during the course of this condition, without the presence of "red flag" symptoms **(Table 24.7)**.

MRI provides imaging of the intervertebral disc, and it is the imaging study of choice when disc injury is suspected **(Figure 24.18)**. With the desiccation of the nucleus pulposus, MRI findings include decreased signal intensity within the nucleus pulposus on T2-weighted images.[47]

Treatment

Those without noteworthy disc pathology usually have significant improvement in function and pain at 6 months; however, those who are noted to have disc herniation at the time of initial presentation may have persistent symptoms, and they are likely to be less functional at 6 months.[47] An apparently useful predictor of the success of conservative treatment in both short-term and long-term outcomes is the ability to passively extend the lumbar spine.[10]

The Cooke treatment protocol for discogenic lumbar pain **(Table 24.8)** details a five-stage nonoperative treatment program for discogenic lumbar pain.[2,46] Conservative therapy usually consists of rest, ice and heat modalities, anti-inflammatory drugs, and narcotic medication for intolerable pain. Distractive and unloading manipulative techniques can assist with the restoration of the normal biomechanics of the intervertebral segment and influence the alignment of collagen during annular remodeling.[18]

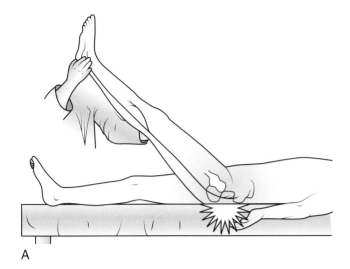

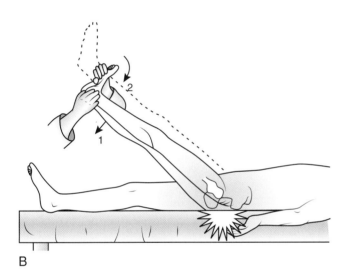

Figure 24.16 Straight leg raising. *A*, Radicular symptoms are precipitated on the same side with straight leg raising. *B*, The leg is lowered slowly until pain is relieved. The foot is then dorsiflexed, causing a return of symptoms; this indicates a positive test. (Redrawn from Magee: Orthopedic Physical Assessment, 4th ed. Philadelphia, WB Saunders, 2002.)

In addition, physical therapy and extension exercises are employed for those patient with less severe pain to promote normal function. If pain is severe and distracting from activities of daily living, epidural injections may be used to turn down the inflammation cascade. An isometric trunk stabilization program should be initiated after the abatement of symptoms. This may be increased to neutral positioning exercises followed by resistant strength training, motion, and aerobic conditioning as the athlete tolerates.

Caution must be considered when determining conservative treatment failure among adolescent athletes, particularly those who are treated during the academic year because they sit in classes from 5 to 6 hours daily.[27] However, if the competitive athlete does not have symptom resolution within 6 weeks after appropriate conservative care, surgical options may be necessary to restore function and decrease symptoms.

Return to play

After the full resolution of symptoms and the performance of trunk stabilization, neutral positioning, and resistance training exercises,

Table 24.7 Red Flags of Low Back Pain

Constitutional symptoms (fever, chills, night sweats)
Recent bacterial infection
Intravenous drug use
Immunosuppression
Night pain
Saddle anesthesia
Bladder and/or bowel incontinence
Acute, severe, or progressive neurologic motor or sensory deficit

From Eck JC, Riley LH: Clin Sports Med 2004;23:367-379.

the athlete may begin sport-specific training and return to practice on an incremental elevation of play.[46]

Return-to-play criteria for an athlete who has undergone single-level microdiscectomy or surgical fusion is not well documented in the literature. Conservatively, return to sports training and play should not take place until the radiographic evidence of spinal fusion is seen and nearly complete to full abatement of pain is attained. Additionally, the athlete should have restored his or her muscular strength, coordination, endurance, and flexibility to near preinjury levels.[47]

Discitis (and vertebral osteomyelitis)[9,33,48-51]

Discitis is a relatively rare inflammatory or infectious state of the vertebral end plate or the intervertebral disc. The most common cause in the preadolescent population is the hematogenous spread of an infective agent from a primary infection site.[9,50] The next most common causes are the sharing of intravenous needles and any form of immunosuppression.

Pathophysiology and mechanism of injury

Discitis is unique to the pediatric athlete, and it has preponderance for the lumbar spine as a result of this region's distinctive blood supply.[9] Blood enters from the segmental artery, passes through to the end arterioles and sinusoidal vessels that traverse the vertebral end plate from the body, and enters into the intervertebral disc, thereby establishing a route for the hematogenous transmission of bacteria. The most commonly identified causative organism is *Staphylococcus aureus*.[9,33,49-51]

History and physical

This condition differs from other inflammatory or infectious states because there are usually no systemic symptoms. The usual presentation is back, hip, or abdominal pain with a refusal to perform lumbar flexion maneuvers or ambulate.[49] Abdominal pain may be the presenting symptom in patients with an infection involving the T8-L1 levels.[9]

Patients are usually afebrile[33] and complain only of point-specific back pain. However, some patients may be febrile, toxic, and irritable on presentation. Palpation of the lumbar spine elicits localized point tenderness over the involved disc. Patients will have a loss of lumbar lordosis with tight hamstrings as a result of an attempt to self-brace to decrease pain with movement. Tension signs (i.e., straight-leg raise) are usually positive. A positive Gowers sign[50,52] (the hands incrementally stepping up the thighs to support the upper torso when rising) may be noted during the early stages of the disease.

Laboratory analysis

Ten percent of patients may present with an elevated white blood cell count. The erythrocyte sedimentation rate and the C-reactive protein level are usually elevated.[9,33,52] An analysis of any

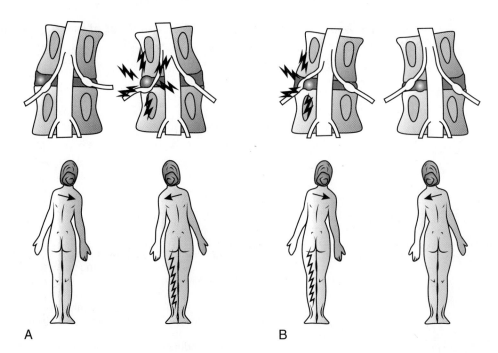

Figure 24.17 Patients with herniated disk problems may sometimes list to one side. This is a voluntary or involuntary mechanism to alleviate nerve root irritation. The list in some patients is toward the side of the sciatica; in others, it is toward the opposite side. A reasonable hypothesis suggests that, when the herniation is lateral to the nerve root (A), the list is to the side opposite from the sciatica because a list to the same side would elicit pain. Conversely, when the herniation is medial to the nerve root (B), the list is toward the side of the sciatica because tilting away would irritate the root and cause pain. (Redrawn from Magee: Orthopedic Physical Assessment, 4th ed. Philadelphia, WB Saunders, 2002.)

Table 24.8   Cooke Treatment Protocol for Discogenic Lumbar Pain[2,45]

Stage 1: *Early protected mobilization* is begun with a brief period of rest and the use of nonsteroidal anti-inflammatory drugs, soft-tissue manipulation, therapeutic modalities (heat and ice), and epidural injections. After pain control has been obtained, an early exercise program to restore lumbar and lower extremity range of motion is begun. The goals of the initial stage include the control of pain and inflammation and the promotion of healing.

Stage 2: *Dynamic spinal stabilization* is centered on exercises that emphasize the cocontraction of the intrinsic core stabilizers and the extrinsic lumbar extensors to stabilize the injured vertebral segment. This work is predominately performed with isometric exercises to retrain core and extrinsic stabilizing muscles to maintain a neutral lumbar position. The goals of this stage are to gain dynamic control of the segmental spine and the kinetic chain forces and to minimize repetitive motion segmental injury to reduce acute dynamic overload.

Stage 3: *The strengthening of the lumbar musculature* is begun, initially through improvements in neuromuscular firing rather than muscular hypertrophy. The main goal is the ability to perform 20 to 30 minutes of aerobic exercise two to three times weekly.

Stage 4: *Return to sports activity* may occur when the following criteria are met: (1) full, painless range of motion is present; (2) the athlete is able to maintain a neutral lumbar position during sports-specific activities; and (3) a return of muscle strength, endurance, and control has occurred. The addition of plyometric exercises (eccentric followed by explosive concentric contraction) is started during this stage.

Stage 5: *A maintenance program* with regular home and warmup exercises is instituted to ensure that the athlete preserves the flexibility, protection, and strength to continue in sports activities while reducing the recurrence of reinjury.

causative agent should be undertaken, and CT-guided needle aspiration of the suspected disc is usually recommended.[33]

Imaging

Plain lumbar radiographs may not demonstrate disc space narrowing or abnormality of the vertebral end plate until late in the disease course. A bone scan or MRI is indicated in the presence of abnormal laboratory results.[9] A technetium bone scan demonstrates inflammatory changes, and it is useful for ascertaining an early diagnosis. However, MRI scanning with and without gadolinium is more specific than a bone scan for demonstrating soft-tissue and bone edema, and it allows for differentiation among discitis, vertebral osteomyelitis, and epidural abscess.[9]

Treatment

Empiric treatment with parenteral antibiotics for 1 week on the basis of Gram staining results followed by oral antibiotic treatment for an additional 4 to 6 weeks provides symptomatic relief in 85% of patients within 2 to 3 weeks of treatment initiation (LOE: B).[9,51] If oral antibiotics do not eradicate the causative organism, an indwelling catheter may be necessary to deliver outpatient intravenous antibiotics.[52] Antibiotic treatment should be continued until the erythrocyte sedimentation rate normalizes.[9] Spinal immobilization or orthotic bracing may help with symptom control for those with severe symptoms.[33]

Atypical Scheuermann kyphosis

Atypical Scheuermann kyphosis usually occurs at the thoracolumbar junction.[4,7] There is a strong association between this condition and degenerative disc disease in adolescent athletes, and it should be considered in young patients who present with LBP.[5,7] The peak incidence is seen among athletes between 15 and 17

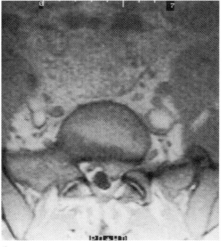 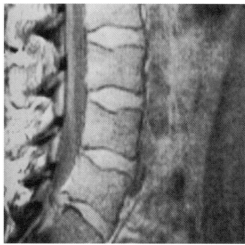

Figure 24.18 Magnetic resonance imaging scans of lumbar disk herniation. *A,* Axial view. *B,* Sagittal view. (From DeLee JC, Drez D Jr, Miller MD [eds]: DeLee and Drez's Orthopaedic Sports Medicine: Principles and Practice, 2nd ed. Philadelphia, WB Saunders, 2003.)

A   B

years of age, with a 2:1 male predominance.[7] Athletes who participate in gymnastics and diving are at an increased risk for developing Scheuermann kyphosis.[7,9]

Pathophysiology and mechanism of injury

This condition presents with similar manifestations of typical Scheuermann kyphosis: disc space narrowing, end plate fracturing, Schmorl nodes, and vertebral apophyseal avulsions.[9]

History and physical

Athletes complain of the insidious onset of moderate to severe pain that worsens with flexion and improves with rest.[7] Physical findings include a flattening of the thoracic spine (a loss of the kyphotic curve) with tightness of both the thoracolumbar fascia and the hamstrings.[7,9] Additionally, a palpable bump may be felt at the affected level.[9]

Treatment

The nonoperative treatment consists of anti-inflammatory and non-narcotic analgesic medications, stretching the thoracolumbar fascia, paraspinal exercises for stabilization, and lordotic bracing at 15 degrees of lordosis with activity reduction. Bracing should be reserved for those patients who have thoracolumbar curves of more than 60 degrees.[4] Curves of more than 75 degrees in patients with this condition require a surgical referral.[4] With symptom abatement, the athlete may return to play in 1 to 2 months.[6]

Slipped vertebral apophysis (apophyseal ring fractures)[9,27]

A unique entity to the adolescent patient population, slipped vertebral apophysis typically occurs among adolescent boys who are younger than 18 years of age.[9] Growth plates are susceptible to compression, distraction, and torsion forces that may culminate in acute apophyseal avulsion because immature ossification centers form the weakest link of the force transfer chain.[7] This condition is closely associated with heavy lifting and vigorous activity,[33] and it most commonly occurs at the inferior apophysis of L4.[9]

History and physical

The historic findings are similar to those of a herniated disc: back, buttock, and posterior thigh pain. Physical examination findings are also similar, but a contralateral straight-leg raise is more frequently positive in a patient with an apophyseal ring fracture than in the patient with a herniated disc.[9]

Imaging

Spinal radiographs may confirm an avulsed fracture fragment within the spinal canal; however, the imaging study of choice is CT scanning.[9]

Treatment

If no neurologic deficits exist, conservative treatment with heat and ice modalities, anti-inflammatory drugs and analgesics, bracing, and physical therapy is usually successful. However, those athletes who experience neurologic deficits usually require the surgical excision of the disc and the apophyseal ring.[9]

Lumbar facet (arthrosis) syndrome

Lumbar facet (arthrosis) syndrome (chondromalacia facetiae), which was described by R.K. Ghormley[2] in 1933, is a chondromalacial condition that occurs at the zygapophyseal joint. This condition most commonly occurs among older athletes, but it can be seen as early as late adolescence, predominantly among football lineman and weight lifters, who subject their spines to tremendous axial and torsional loads.

Pathophysiology and mechanism of injury

Asymmetric angulation of facet joints that are subjected to increased axial loads produces stresses that are sufficient to cause articular cartilage damage. With repeated microtrauma, fracturing of the articular surface occurs, with subsequent erosion of the underlying bony surface (eburnation).

History and physical

No characteristic pain pattern or level-specific signs and symptoms have been found to be specific for the diagnosis of lumbar facet syndrome.[47] Patients commonly present with pain upon rising or when performing lumbar flexion and with point tenderness in the paraspinous region over the affected facet joint. Referred pain, when occassionally present, extends to the thigh but not below the knee.[51,53] Other common findings are tightened hamstrings and a positive Gowers sign (the hands incrementally stepping up the thighs to support the upper torso when rising).[54]

Imaging

Radiographic imaging during the latter stages of this condition demonstrates changes that are indicative of facet arthrosis.[47] However, this finding is relatively uncommon during the early stages of disease, and it is therefore of little diagnostic value. CT scanning provides detailed imaging of the facet joint chondral surfaces, and it can delineate areas of cartilaginous damage.

Treatment

The treatment of choice is direct, intra-articular injection with lidocaine either with or without corticosteroids. However, there are no large controlled trials that cite the efficacy of this treatment.

Internal disc derangement

Internal disc derangement consists of an inner annulus radial tear with an intact outer annulus.[5]

Pathophysiology and mechanism of injury

The cartilaginous (growth) end plate of the spinal body is weaker than the nucleus pulposus, which leads to the extrusion of the nucleus pulposus into the vertebral body.[5]

History and physical

The patient will present with nonradiating LBP. This will be sharp in nature, and it will be limited to the area of the spine that is affected.

Imaging

T2-weighted MRI may detect a high-intensity zone in the posterior annulus.[5]

Treatment

Treatment begins with an extension-based lumbar stabilization program to alleviate symptoms and pulposus irritation. Direct corticosteroid injection within selective nerve roots can be beneficial. In those with persistent, intolerable axial pain or sitting intolerance, discography may be considered for symptom relief.[5]

Thoracolumbar herniation

Thoracolumbar herniation through the superior lumbar (Grainfield–Layshaft) triangle should be considered for those patients complaining of LBP with an area of associated swelling that is predominately lateral to the spine.

Pathophysiology and mechanism of injury

More commonly a nontraumatic or congenital defect of the thoracolumbar fascia, the hernia may increase in size and discomfort and ultimately lead to posterior bowel incarceration. The fascial defect is made more prominent upon spinal extension maneuvers, and often disappears during flexion.[55]

History and physical

Lumbar herniation presents as chronic LBP. Diagnosis is difficult if the there is an absence of swelling in the area of pain. Patients may present with a decrease in bulk of the erector spinae muscles in the area of the herniation.

Imaging

MRI is the imaging of choice. However, it may be difficult to diagnose this condition unless the spine is moved into a position that causes the herniation to be symptomatic.

Treatment

Hernia repair requires surgical intervention. Usually a double breasting repair of the defect is required (LOE: D).[55]

OTHER CONSIDERATIONS

If night pain, nonmechanical pain, and constitutional symptoms are present, the clinician must consider a tumor, an inflammatory process, or an infection as the possible cause of an athlete's pain.

Lastly, referred pain from the hip, leg, abdominal, or reproductive organs (e.g., uterine fibroids, endometriosis, adnometriosis, hematocolpos as a result of an imperforate hymen, gonadal masses[27]) must be considered in the athlete who presents with back pain. These conditions are discussed in other chapters of this book and in other medical textbooks.

CONCLUSION

The lumbar spine is the most commonly injured area of the spine, with mechanical low back pain being the most common musculoskeletal complaint in primary care offices. Lumbar spine injuries are diverse in nature, but all have a common theme in treatment: decrease or stop the offending activity and then strengthen the muscular response to increase stability of the spine. The importance of an adequate and well-practiced physical examination cannot be overstated because most worrisome causes of back pain are ruled out with a negative physical examination that includes assessment of a straight leg raise, patellar and Achilles reflexes, strength testing of the foot and ankle, and fine touch of the lower leg and foot.

REFERENCES

1. Manek NJ, MacGregor AJ: Epidemiology of back disorders: prevalence, risk factors and prognosis. Curr Opin Rheumatol 2005;17(2):134-140.
2. Bono CM: Low-back pain in athletes. J Bone Joint Surg Am 2004;86-A(2):382-396.
3. Trainor TJ, Wiesel SW: Epidemiology of back pain in the athlete. Clin Sports Med 2002;21(1):93-103.
4. Trainor TJ, Trainor MA: Etiology of low back pain in athletes. Curr Sports Med Rep 2004;3(1):41-46.
5. d'Hemecourt PA, Gerbino PG: Back injuries in the young athlete. Pediat Adoles Sports Injuries 2001;19(4):663-679.
6. Taimela S, Kujala UM, Salminen JJ, Viljanen T: The prevalence of low back pain among children and adolescents. A nationwide, cohort-based questionnaire survey in Finland. Spine 1997;22(10):1132-1136.
7. Waicus KM, Smith BW: Back injuries in the pediatric athlete. Curr Sports Med Rep 2002;1(1):52-58.
8. d'Hemecourt PA et al: Spinal injuries in female athletes. Sports Med Arthro Rev 2002;10(1):91-97.
9. Sassmannshausen G, Smith BG: Back pain in the young athlete. Clin Sports Med 2002;21(1):121-132.
10. Kim S: Nonoperative treatment for lumbar disc herniation with radiculopathy and for lumbar spinal stenosis. Curr Opin Orthop 1999;10(2):137-141.
11. Herman MJ, Pizzutillo PD, Cavalier R: Spondylolysis and spondylolisthesis in the child and adolescent athlete. Orthop Clin North Am 2003;34(3):461-467.
12. Ward RC: Foundations for Osteopathic Medicine. Philadelphia, Lippincott Williams & Wilkins, 2003.
13. Van Buskirk RL: The Still Technique Manual: Applications of a Rediscovered Technique of Andrew Taylor Still, MD, (DO). Indianapolis, American Academy of Osteopathy, 2000.
14. Mooney V, Pozos R, Vleeming A, et al: Exercise treatment for sacroiliac pain. Orthopedics 2001;24(1):29-32.
15. O'Sullivan PB: Altered motor control strategies in subjects with sacroiliac joint pain during the active straight-leg-raise test. Spine 2002;27(1):E1-E8.
16. Broadhurst NA, Bond MJ: Pain provocative test for the assessment of sacroiliac joint dysfunction. J Spinal Disord 1998;11(4):341-345.
17. Richardson CA: The relation between the transversus abdominis muscles, sacroiliac joint mechanics and low back pain. Spine 27(4):399-405.

18. Kuchera WA, Kuchera ML: Osteopathic Principles in Practice. Columbus, OH, Greydon Press, 1992, pp 402, 439, 461, 481-498.
19. Drezner JA, Harmon KG: Chronic appendicitis presenting as low back pain in a recreational athlete. Clin J Sports Med 2002;12(3):184-186.
20. Chen YC et al: Sacroiliac joint pain syndrome in active patients. Phys Sportsmed 2002;30(11).
21. Barker KL, Shamley DR, Jackson D: Changes in the cross-sectional area of multifidus and psoas in patients with unilateral back pain: the relationship to pain and disability. Spine 2004;29(22):E515-E519.
22. Robinson DR: Pyriformis syndrome in relation to sciatic pain. Am J Surg 1947;47:355-358.
23. Papadopoulos EC, Khan SN: Piriformis syndrome and low back pain: a new classification and review of the literature. Orthop Clin North Am 2004;35(1):65-71.
24. Steiner C, Staubs C, Ganon M, Buhlinger C: Piriformis syndrome: pathogenesis, diagnosis and treatment. J Am Osteopath Assoc 1987;87(4):318-323.
25. Wimberly RL, Lauerman WC: Spondylolisthesis in the athlete. Clin Sports Med 2002;21(1):133-145.
26. Prather H: Pelvis and sacral dysfunction in sports and exercise. Phys Med Rehabil Clin North Am 2000;11(4):805-836.
27. Zelle BA, Gruen GS, Brown S, George S: Sacroiliac joint dysfunction: evaluation and management. Clin J Pain 2005;21(5):446-455.
28. Nadler SF, Wu KD, Galski T, Feinberg JH: Low back pain in college athletes. A prospective study correlating lower extremity overuse or acquired ligamentous laxity with low back pain. Spine 1998;23(7):828-833.
29. Prather H: Sacroiliac joint pain: practical management. Clin J Sports Med 2002;13(4):252-255.
30. Johnson AW, Weiss CB Jr, Stento K, Wheeler DL: Stress fractures of the sacrum. An atypical cause of low back pain in the female athlete. Am J Sports Med 2001;29(4):498-508.
31. Arendt EA: Stress fractures and the female athlete. Clin Orthop Relate Res 2000;372:131-138.
32. Lonstein JE: Spondylolisthesis in children. Cause, natural history, and management. Spine 1999;24(24):2640-2648.
33. Thompson GH: Back pain in children. J Bone Joint Surg Am 1993;75-A(6):928-938.
34. McTimoney CA, Micheli LJ: Current evaluation and management of spondylolysis and spondylolisthesis. Curr Sports Med Rep 2003;2(1):41-46.
35. Muschik M, Hahnel H, Robinson PN, et al: Competitive sports and the progression of spondylolisthesis. J Pediatr Orthop 1996;16(3):364-369.
36. Standaert CJ, Herring SA: Spondylolysis: a critical review. Br J Sports Med 2000;34:415-422.
37. Hutchinson MR: Low back pain in elite rhythmic gymnasts. Med Sci Sports Exerc 1999;31(11):1686-1691.
38. Sys J, Michielsen J, Bracke P, et al: Nonoperative treatment of active spondylosis in elite athletes with normal x-ray findings: literature review and results of conservative treatment. Eur Spine J 2001;10:498-504.
39. Kraft DE: Low back pain in the adolescent athlete. Pediatr Clin North Am 2002;49:643-653.
40. Standaert CJ, Herring SA, Halpern B, King O: Spondylolysis. Phys Med Rehab Clin N Am 2000;11(4):785-803.
41. Lim MR, Yoon SC, Green DW: Symptomatic spondylolysis: diagnosis and treatment. Curr Opin Pediatr 2004;16(1):37-46.
42. d'Hemecourt PA, Zurakowski D, Kriemler S, Micheli LJ: Spondylolysis: returning the athlete to sports participation with brace treatment. Orthopedics 2002;25(6):653-657.
43. Watkins RG: Lumbar disk injury in the athlete. Clin Sports Med 2002;21(1):147-165.
44. Stokes IA, Iatridis JC: Mechanical conditions that accelerate intervertebral disc degeneration: overload versus immobilization. Spine 2004;29(23):2724-2732.
45. Cooke PM, Lutz GE: Internal disc disruption and axial back pain in the athlete. Phys Med Rehabil Clin N Am 2000;11(4):837-865.
46. Eck JC, Riley LH: Return to play after lumbar spine conditions and surgeries. Clin Sports Med 2004;23:367-379.
47. Modic MT: Degenerative disc disease and back pain. MRI Clin N Am 1999;7(3):481-491.
48. Buoncristiani AM et al: An unusual cause of low back pain. Osteomyelitis of the spinous process. Spine 1998;23(7):839-841.
49. Ring D, Johnston CE 2nd, Wenger DR: Pyogenic infectious spondylitis in children: the convergence of discitis and vertebral osteomyelitis. J Pediatr Orthop 1995;15(5):652-660.
50. Yigal M et al: Gowers' sign in children with discitis of the lumbar spine. J Ped Ortho B 2005;14(2):68-70.
51. Eisenstein SM, Parry CR: The lumbar facet arthrosis syndrome. Clinical presentation and articular surface changes. J Bone Joint Surg Br 1987;69-B(1):3-7.
52. McCuthcen TM: Intervertebral disk space infection. Neurosurg Qu 2001;11(3):209-219.
53. Helbig T, Lee CK: The lumbar facet syndrome. Spine 1988;13(1-4):61-64.
54. Markwalder TM, Merat M: The lumbar and lumbosacral facet-syndrome. Diagnostic measures, surgical treatment and results in 119 patients. Acta Neurochir (Wien) 1994;128(1-4):40-46.
55. Faraj AA, Mehdian H: Thoracolumbar hernia: a rare cause of back pain. Eur Spine J 1997;6(3):203-204.

Pelvic Pain in the Athlete

Adam J. Farber, MD; John H. Wilckens, MD; and MAJ Christopher G. Jarvis, MD, FAAFP

KEY POINTS

- Pelvic pain in the athlete, which may involve musculoskeletal and nonmusculoskeletal causes, requires an accurate history, a detailed physical examination, and a multidisciplinary approach.

- Most acute musculoskeletal injuries respond to rest and physical therapy and rarely require surgery, but they have a high incidence of recurrence with premature return to competition.

- Groin pain in the running endurance athlete should be considered a femoral neck stress fracture until proven otherwise. These athletes require emergent imaging or bone scanning and then surgery if the scans are positive for a displaced or tension-side femoral neck stress fracture.

- A sports hernia may present as insidious-onset groin pain. Patients have localized pain at the superior pubic rami, and they may have a dilated inguinal ring without a frank bulge or hernia. Imaging studies are helpful only to rule out other abnormalities. These patients seldom improve without surgical repair.

- All pediatric/adolescent athletes with groin pain should be examined and should undergo imaging for slipped capital femoral epiphysis. Apophyseal avulsions are common causes of groin pain in the skeletally immature athlete.

INTRODUCTION

Pelvic pain is a common entity among athletes, especially among those who participate in sports that require specific use (or overuse) of the proximal musculature of the thigh and lower abdominal muscles, such as soccer, ice hockey, Australian Rules football, skiing, running, and hurdling.[1] One study found that groin injuries represent approximately 5% of all soccer injuries.[1] Despite the high prevalence of pelvic pain in athletes, the cause of that pain can be difficult to elucidate because of the complex local anatomy and the multitude of differential diagnoses. The anatomic and biomechanical considerations for injuries in these areas are among the most complex in the musculoskeletal system **(Figure 25.1),** thus making the diagnosis and management of these injuries challenging. In addition, the conditions responsible for pelvic pain in the athlete often present with diffuse, insidious symptoms and

uncharacteristic profiles. Many athletes with chronic pelvic pain have more than one condition that accounts for their symptoms.[2] Furthermore, the differential diagnoses include numerous entities that are both orthopedic and nonorthopedic. The most common musculoskeletal causes of pelvic pain include adductor strains and osteitis pubis.[3,4] Other causes of pelvic pain include ilioinguinal neuralgia, tears of the acetabular labrum, avulsion injuries, stress fractures, sports hernias, iliopsoas bursitis, and snapping hip syndrome. Referred pain may come from the lumbar spine, the abdominal and pelvic viscera, and genitourinary problems.

Regardless of the cause of pelvic pain, an accurate sports-specific history and a meticulous physical examination of the groin, abdomen, hips, spine, and lower extremities are the keys to accurate diagnosis, which allows for the initiation of timely and appropriate treatment. The fact that pelvic pain can result from both musculoskeletal and nonmusculoskeletal causes makes it difficult for any one physician to perform a comprehensive assessment of the athlete with pelvic pain. This fact underscores the need for a multidisciplinary approach.

Although the causes of pelvic pain can be classified by anatomic considerations, it is preferable to use the timing of the onset of symptoms (i.e., acute or insidious) for categorization. Acute conditions include musculotendinous strains, contusions, avulsion fractures, hip fractures and dislocations, and acetabular labral injuries. Chronic conditions include sports hernia, osteitis pubis, bursitis, snapping hip syndrome, nerve entrapment syndromes, stress fractures, osteonecrosis, Legg-Calvé-Perthes disease, and osteoarthritis.

In this chapter, some of the more common conditions that are responsible for acute and chronic pelvic pain in the athlete are reviewed, with emphasis on the causes, presentation, clinical and radiographic findings, and treatment options. In addition, a comprehensive list of potential causes of pelvic pain that the sports medicine provider should consider when evaluating the athlete with pelvic pain is provided.

ACUTE-ONSET INJURIES

Muscle strains

Muscle strains, which are the most common athletic-related injuries in the region of the hip and pelvis, result from violent muscular contraction during an excessively forceful muscular stretch (an overloaded eccentric contraction), and they occur most frequently

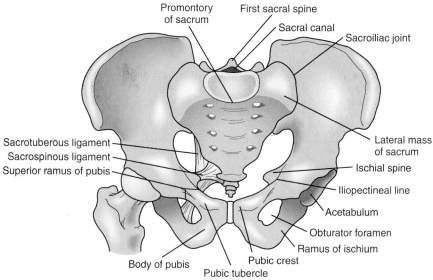

A

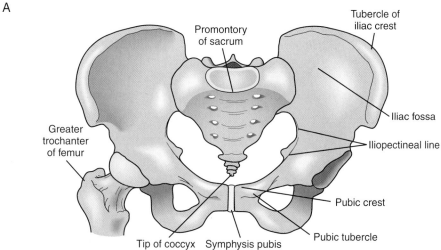

B

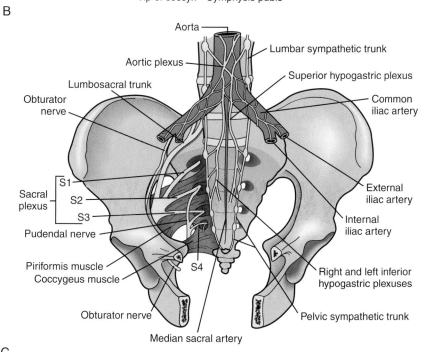

C

Figure 25.1 Anterior view of the male pelvis (A), the female pelvis (B), and the neurologic anatomy of the pelvis and hip (C).

in muscles that cross two joints.[5] Muscle weakness and imbalance are risk factors for developing a strain (especially an adductor strain), and studies have shown that strength training can lower the incidence of muscular strains.[6,7] Strains typically occur at the musculotendinous junction, and they vary in degree and consequent disability, depending on the extent of muscle fiber disruption.[5,8] These injuries typically occur during a specific event that causes a pulling sensation, and they are followed by pain and perhaps swelling.[9] Radiographic workup typically is not necessary; plain radiographs are usually unremarkable. Magnetic resonance imaging (MRI) is the only study that can visualize a muscle strain, which appears as an area of high signal on T2-weighted images, with no evidence of muscle fiber disruption.[10] Partial or complete muscle or tendon tears can be visualized by MRI and ultrasound[10]: on MRI, muscle tears appear as discontinuity of the muscle fibers with increased signal on T2-weighted images[10]; on ultrasound, muscle tears appear as local hypoechoic areas with fiber discontinuity.[10-13] Strains or tears can affect any of the numerous muscle groups that originate or insert on or about the pelvis, including hip flexors, hip adductors, and hip abductors.

Quadriceps

Mechanism of injury Because the quadriceps muscle group spans two joints (the hip and knee), it is subject to more stress than muscles that cross only one joint and consequently to more potential injury. Muscle strains typically happen at the myotendinous junction when a contracted muscle is eccentrically loaded or motion is suddenly blocked.[14,15] Severe quadriceps injuries, which sometimes result in quadriceps rupture, occur while the muscle is stressed with the hip extended and the knee flexed. The muscle may be avulsed from its origin on the pubis or torn in its mid belly. This injury can occur with any sport involving squats, kicking, jumping, or sprinting.[16]

Clinical presentation Swelling, bruising, spasm, and tenderness occur over the anterior thigh or at the anterior inferior iliac spine if the injury occurs at the tendon–bone interface. In these cases, provocative testing of the rectus femoris will elicit pain. In femoris injuries, resisted flexion of the hip and extension of the knee may induce pain superior to the acetabulum.[1,15] Some athletes may have scar-tissue formation within the muscle, and examiners may appreciate an asymmetry or a mass on physical examination.[17,18]

Diagnosis Brown and Brunet[19] classified muscle strains as grade I (mild), grade II (moderate), or grade III (severe, or complete tear). Grade I strains represent small disruptions of the structural integrity at the musculotendinous unit, and they are manifested by local spasm and tenderness. The athlete may not notice the strain until a day after the injury occurs. Grade II strains are partial tears of the muscle with some muscle fibers left intact, and they are diagnosed by a palpable area of tenderness and swelling. Grade III tears are uncommon and severe injuries that result in the complete rupture of the muscle. Strains are differentiated from ruptures by the latter having a complete, palpable muscular defect (typically just proximal to the patella) and an inability to actively extend the knee.[16] Athletes with suspected complete rupture may have it confirmed by MRI.[17,18] Muscular scarring from previous strain and tear injuries can also be seen on MRI imaging.

Treatment The clinical grade of injury guides treatment. Grade I strains are treated with immediate massage and stretching. For grade II strains, passive stretching is usually painful, and initial therapy involves only relative rest, ice, and nonsteroidal antiinflammatory drugs (NSAIDs) followed by massage and stretching. Rehabilitation focuses on the restoration of pain-free range of motion and strength. Concentric and eccentric exercises emphasize low weight and high repetitions. Grade III strains are treated nonoperatively for mid-belly tears and surgically for patellar avulsions or quadriceps tendon ruptures. Nonoperative treatment is effective for most partial mid-belly ruptures; however, some of these patients develop chronic pain and disability as a result of scar tissue within the muscle. Such patients frequently do well with surgical excision of the scar tissue.[17] Complete tears have been reported to require surgical repair.[15,18]

Return to play Although most minor (grade I) quadriceps strains resolve within 2 to 4 weeks, return to athletics can be prolonged by reinjury. Most athletes with grade II strains can return to training within 2 weeks and to competition after 3 to 4 weeks of rest and physical therapy as determined by symptoms. Athletes with grade III injuries usually return to play within several months after the muscle scars and function returns, although strength and flexibility may be permanently compromised. The timing of return to play varies and usually depends on the athlete's compliance with the rehabilitation process. Compliance, especially with massage and physical therapy modalities, may speed healing and return to play. Return to cutting, sprinting, and competition should advance slowly because the risk of reinjury is high.[16]

Hip flexors

The iliopsoas, which originates on the T12-L5 vertebrae and the iliac fossa and inserts on the lesser trochanter, is the strongest hip flexor. Strain of the iliopsoas tendon occurs during resisted hip flexion or passive hyperextension,[1,20,21] which is an injury that occurs frequently in soccer players, often after a kick is blocked.[21,22] This injury is also commonly associated with uphill running and weight lifting.[13] Patients report deep groin pain that is difficult to palpate. Pain is increased with resisted active hip flexion and passive external rotation and extension.[1,20]

The rectus femoris originates on the anterior inferior iliac spine and hip capsule, and it inserts as the patellar tendon on the tibial tuberosity. It functions as a hip flexor and knee extensor. Strains of the rectus femoris muscle commonly result from an explosive hip flexion maneuver, such as sprinting or kicking.[1,20] Injuries to the rectus femoris also occur as a result of eccentric overload as the hip is extended during running, jumping, soccer, or bicycling.[1] Pain from a rectus femoris strain may be felt from the area anterior to the hip, and it may radiate to the thigh and inguinal region.[1,13] Physical examination reveals palpable swelling and tenderness in the anterior thigh 8 to 10 cm below the anterior superior iliac spine (ASIS).[20] Resisted knee extension and hip flexion also are painful.[20,23]

Hip adductors

The hip adductors (the adductor longus, the adductor magnus, and the adductor brevis) **(Figure 25.2)** originate along the inferior pubic rami and insert along the linea aspera of the femur. Of these muscles, the adductor longus is the most frequently injured in athletes.[4] In fact, adductor longus strains are one of the most common causes of groin pain in athletes.[24] One study suggested that 62% of groin injuries were from the adductor longus muscle–tendon unit,[1] and another study suggested that 19% of cases of chronic groin pain in athletes can be attributed to adductor injuries.[3] Adductor injury is caused by forced external rotation of an abducted leg, overuse with repetitive abduction, or forceful eccentric contractions, such as with sharp cutting movements.[13,20,25] This injury is common in hockey, football, rugby, skating, and soccer athletes, especially among veteran players.[6,7,22,23,25,26] Patients report groin and medial thigh pain. On examination, localized tenderness is present along the subcutaneous border of the inferior pubic ramus at the tendinous insertion.[7,20] In addition, swelling may be present;

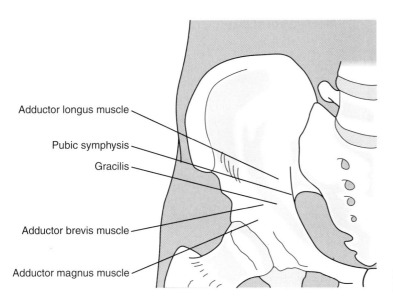

Adductor longus muscle

Pubic symphysis

Gracilis

Adductor brevis muscle

Adductor magnus muscle

Figure 25.2 Bony pelvis with origin of adductor musculature. (From Morelli V, Smith V: Am Fam Phys 2001;64[8]:1405-1414.)

with more severe injuries, a defect may be palpable.[1,23] Pain is elicited with passive hip abduction and resisted active hip adduction.[1,3,20,22,23,25]

Hip abductors

The hip abductors include the gluteus minimus and medius as well as the tensor fascia lata. Gluteus medius strains are common among runners. The mechanism may be related to the repeated tilting action of the pelvis.[22] Patients complain of lateral thigh pain near the greater trochanter. On physical examination, maximum tenderness is just proximal to the trochanter. Pain is elicited by resisted abduction of the hip.[22]

Treatment of hip flexor, adductor, and abductor injuries

Most musculotendinous injuries of these muscles can be treated nonoperatively. Initially, rest, ice, and compression are used to reduce pain and limit inflammation.[20] After the pain subsides, the emphasis is on the range of motion. After full, painless range of motion is achieved, strengthening exercises are started. Return to full activity occurs only when the athlete is pain free.[22,23] This return may take 4 to 8 weeks after an acute musculotendinous strain and up to 6 months for chronic strains. The presence of a functional deficit despite a formal rehabilitation program should be the only indication for surgical intervention. For adductor strains, if nonoperative treatment has failed and other potential causes of groin pain have been excluded, patients may benefit from the resection of abnormal tissue at the adductor origin or the adductor tenotomy.[25,27] Martens and colleagues[25] had good or excellent results in 81% of patients with chronic adductor tendinopathy after percutaneous tenotomy of the gracilis and adductor brevis tendons. Akermark and Johansson[28] reported symptomatic improvement (37%) or complete relief (67%) in all patients with chronic adductor longus pain treated by open adductor longus tenotomy. Complete tears of the tendinous insertion from bone, although rare, generally have better outcomes after surgical repair than after nonoperative intervention.[1,8]

Hamstring muscle group

The hamstring muscle group also spans two joints and therefore is highly susceptible to injury.[14,18] In rugby players, hamstring strains were associated 62% of the time with end of the half and the end of match play, which suggests that fatigue may play a part in injury occurrence.[18,29]

Mechanism of injury and risk factors The literature suggests several predisposing factors for hamstring injury, including insufficient warm up, poor flexibility, muscle imbalances, muscle weakness, neural tension, dyssynergic contraction of the muscle groups, and previous injury.[30] One study showed that the use of a standardized stretching protocol could decrease the rate of hamstring injuries in professional soccer players.[31] It must be remembered that the ischial tuberosity may not fused until the third decade, thus indicating that some hamstring injuries are actually avulsion fractures.[18,23]

Hamstring injuries are common in sprinting, dancing, martial arts, hockey, and kicking sports such as soccer, American football, and Australian football.[32] Hamstring strains comprise 12% of soccer injuries, and approximately half (53%) involve the biceps femoris.[30] In 57% of cases, the injury occurred while running.[30] Certain groups of players, including professional players, outfield players, players of black ethnic origin, and players in the older age groups sustained higher-than-expected rates of hamstring injury.[30] The reinjury rate for a hamstring injury was 12% over the course of the season.[30] Hamstring strain is reported as the most common injury in Australian football, making up 13% of all injuries.[31,33] High hamstring strains, which frequently involve partial avulsion of the muscle from its origin on the ischial tuberosity, occur most commonly among dancers, hurdlers, runners, water-skiers, and other athletes who place excessive stress on the stretched hamstrings[18,34] **(Figure 25.3).**

Because the hamstring provides most of the power for acceleration in sprinting, it is particularly susceptible to strains in such athletes. This predisposition to hamstring injury increases with age, overstriding, and weaknesses around the hip joint.[16] The relative risk associated with an age of more than 23 years in Australian football players is 3.8. However, players with increased quadriceps flexibility are less likely to sustain a hamstring injury (relative risk, 0.3).[32]

Clinical features Careful palpation of the hamstring muscles along their entire length often will yield pain and occasionally a defect in the mid-belly portion in an injured athlete. In high hamstring strains, it is rare to palpate an actual defect in the muscle belly, although ecchymosis and pain may be found at the muscle origin on the ischial tuberosity.[16]

Diagnosis The diagnosis of hamstring strains is clinical. However, should imaging be needed to support the diagnosis, MRI is the

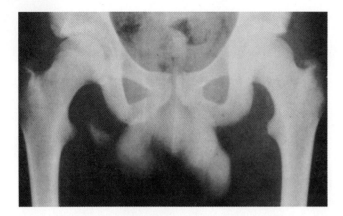

Figure 25.3 Ischial avulsion fracture caused by forceful hamstring contractures in a track athlete. (From DeLee JC, Drez D Jr, Miller MD [eds]: DeLee and Drez's Orthopaedic Sports Medicine: Principles and Practice, 2nd ed. Philadelphia, WB Saunders, 2003.)

imaging modality of choice. It must be remembered that, even with acute injuries, MRIs have an 18% false-negative rate.[18,29] In one study of 83 hamstring injuries recorded with MRIs, the biceps femoris was involved in 81%, and it was the only muscle injured in 47%.[29] A careful physical examination and an MRI should differentiate this injury from ischial tuberosity apophysitis and ischial avulsion fracture.[18,35]

Treatment There is no consensus regarding the optimal rehabilitation of hamstring injuries; management tends to be based on experience and anecdotal evidence rather than on evidence-based medicine.[30,36] Many authors favor a stepwise rehabilitation program that starts with rest, ice, compression, and progression to isometrics, isotonics, isokinetics, and then finally to light running.[19] Strength training rehabilitation after hamstring injuries simulates the loads placed on the hamstring during sports.[37] Concentric hamstring rehabilitation may be detrimental and may predispose the athlete to recurrent injury, whereas eccentric training and sprinting more closely parallel sport-specific activity and better prepare the athlete for to return to play.[16] One small study involving 21 patients with ischial apophyseal avulsion and 14 patients with apophysitis found that two thirds of those who had apophyseal avulsion and all patients with apophysitis responded well to the above-mentioned nonoperative management.[35] However, several authors recommend early surgical repair for all complete ischial tuberosity avulsions, believing that this modality provides the best outcome; a delay in repair of more than 2 months yielded worse outcomes as compared with early repair.[18,34,35] Finally, some evidence suggests that hamstring strengthening programs may be protective against hamstring injuries, but there is no evidence—either for or against—to suggest that strengthening exercises prevent high hamstring injuries.[38]

Return to play As with many other injuries, return to play after hamstring injuries varies with the degree of injury severity and the patient's response to treatment.[16] One study showed that the mean time to recovery from a hamstring strain was 27 days.[29]

Contusions: Hip pointer

Soft-tissue contusions, which are among the most frequent hip and pelvic injuries sustained by competitive athletes, result from direct blows to the soft tissue. The term "hip pointer" is used to describe a contusion to the iliac crest that is associated with a subperiosteal hematoma.[39]

Mechanism of injury

Contusions typically arise from collisions with another player, the player's equipment, or the playing surface. These injuries are common in contact sports such as football. Contusions may be superficial, overlying relatively subcutaneous bone, or deep within a large muscle mass. On occasion, substantial muscular hemorrhage occurs, and this results in prolonged disability. Slow bleeding into the tissues surrounding the area of impact also may occur.[39] Such injuries can lead to a secondary bursitis.[22]

Clinical features and diagnosis

Physical examination reveals point tenderness, ecchymosis, and muscle spasm.[23] Radiographs should be obtained to rule out a fracture. These injuries are often minor and can be handled with symptomatic treatment of short duration, with return to competition as symptoms allow.[40] Early treatment for contusions should be directed at the control of swelling and deep bleeding with ice, compression, and rest.[22,23] Heat, massage, and vigorous physical therapy should be delayed for 48 to 72 hours because they may increase bleeding.[39] For hip pointers, the use of a local anesthetic with or without a corticosteroid injection may help alleviate pain and hasten the return to activity.

Return to play

Rehabilitation is aimed at maintaining flexibility. Muscle use should be restricted until function has returned to normal. Return to full competitive activity should be delayed until full strength and coordination have returned.

Apophyseal and avulsion injuries
Mechanism of injury

A common injury in the skeletally immature athlete is the avulsion fracture. The usual mechanism is either a sudden violent muscular contraction (usually eccentric) or an excessive amount of repetitive muscle action across an open apophysis.[23,40,41] These fractures primarily occur in persons between 14 and 25 years of age, after the appearance of the apophyses but before its fusion.[40] These injuries are most common among sprinters, jumpers, and soccer and football players.[13]

In the pelvis, there are four common sites of avulsion injuries: the ASIS, the anterior inferior iliac spine, the ischium, and the lesser trochanter; the iliac crescan also be aroused **(Figure 25.4).** Avulsion of the ASIS occurs when there is a relative overpull of the sartorius muscle, especially during jumping or running sports.[4,42] Avulsion of the anterior inferior iliac spine occurs with vigorous contraction of the straight head of the rectus femoris. The classic mechanism is a kicking injury, and, therefore, this injury is commonly seen in soccer players.[4,22,42] Avulsion of the ischial apophysis is caused by maximum hamstring contraction with the hip in flexion and the knee in extension. Therefore, this injury is most common among hurdlers, gymnasts, sprinters, cheerleaders, and waterskiers.[43,44] Avulsion of the lesser trochanter results from a sudden contracture of the iliopsoas and should be considered in an athlete who experiences a sudden onset of severe anteromedial hip pain while running or kicking.[22]

Clinical features

On presentation, the athlete may complain of a sudden "pop" that is followed by substantial pain and a sudden loss of function although there was no external trauma.[41,45] Physical examination reveals a limited range of motion, localized tenderness at specific bony sites, swelling, and ecchymosis. Resisted contraction or passive stretch of the involved muscle usually reproduces pain.[23,41]

Diagnosis

Radiographs are useful to confirm the diagnosis. Comparison views with the contralateral side may be necessary to assess the

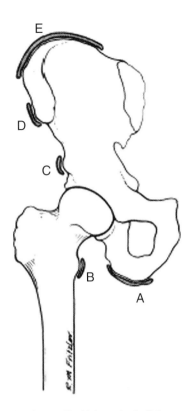

Figure 25.4 The ischium and ischial apophysis (A) is a common site for pediatric avulsion injuries. Other common sites include the lesser trochanter (B), the AIIS (C), and the ASIS (D). The iliac crest (E) is an uncommon site for avulsion injuries. (Redrawn from Canale ST: Campbell's Operative Orthopaedics, 10th ed. St. Louis, Mosby, 2003.)

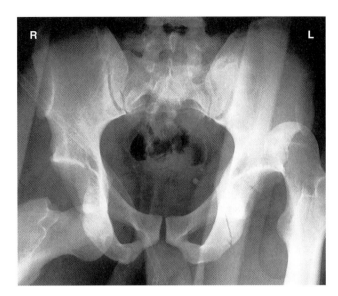

Figure 25.5 Hip dislocation. This patient, who was in a motor vehicle accident, has both an anterior and a posterior dislocation of the hips. Posterior dislocation occurs 90% of the time, and it is seen here on the left, with the femoral head displaced superior and lateral to the acetabulum. On the right, an anterior dislocation appears, with the femoral head displaced inferiorly and medially. (From Mettler FA Jr: Essentials of Radiology, 2nd ed. Philadelphia, WB Saunders, 2005.)

appearance of the normal apophysis in the skeletally immature patient.[41] It is possible to avulse the apophysis before ossification, in which case radiographs would be normal and MRI would be needed for diagnosis.

Treatment

Nonoperative treatment is usually recommended for avulsion fractures of the pelvis: comfortable positioning, rest, protected weight bearing, ice, and analgesics followed by range-of-motion exercises and, finally, strengthening exercises.[23,41] Metzmaker and Pappas[41] described a five-stage rehabilitation program that enabled them to successfully treat 27 athletes with acute avulsion fractures of the hip and pelvis: (1) rest with positioning to relax the involved muscle group, ice, and analgesics for the first 72 hours; (2) gradual increases in the excursion of the injured musculotendinous unit when pain has subsided; (3) the initiation of resistive exercises after full, active range of motion is achieved; (4) integration of the use of the injured musculotendinous unit with other muscle groups of the pelvis and the lower extremity; and (5) a preparation for return to competitive sports.[41] Consideration may be given to surgical fixation if the fragment is of sufficient size to contain hardware and the displacement is ≥2 cm, although reports of poor results with nonoperative treatment are rare.[8,23,44] Some believe that this degree of displacement may be associated with nonunion or fibrous union. Displaced avulsions can be associated with chronic pain, and surgical excision can be considered.[40]

For additional discussion of this topic, see Chapter 31.

Hip dislocation

High-energy trauma directed along the axis of the femur when the hip is in the extremes of its normal range of motion is necessary to cause a hip dislocation. In athletes, this injury tends to occur as a result of a collision during skiing and contact sports.[23] Hip dislocations are classified according to the direction of the dislocation (anterior or posterior). Most (85% to 92%) traumatic hip dislocations are posterior.[46] Plain radiographs, including an anteroposterior view of the pelvis and a lateral view of the hip, should be obtained to confirm the diagnosis and direction of dislocation (**Figure 25.5**). Treatment consists of closed reduction in an emergent manner in an effort to decrease the risk of osteonecrosis and posttraumatic arthritis. If closed reduction is unsuccessful, open reduction must be performed. After reduction, a computed tomography (CT) scan or MRI is recommended to ensure a concentric reduction without loose fragments in the joint.[23] Postreduction treatment depends on the stability of the reduction. Most hip dislocations are stable and require protected weight bearing for 3 to 4 weeks and restriction from vigorous sports for at least 3 months. A follow-up MRI should be performed at 3 months to rule out osteonecrosis.[23]

Acetabular labral tears

The acetabular labrum is a fibrocartilaginous rim that encompasses the circumference of the acetabulum; the labrum serves to deepen the acetabulum and thus to increase the stability of the hip joint.[47,48] The labrum is attached to the bony rim of the acetabulum and to the transverse acetabular ligament.

Mechanism of injury

Trauma to the hip, including minor twisting injuries and major trauma that leads to hip dislocations, is a common cause of acetabular labral tears, but many patients do not recall any trauma.[23,48,49] Labral tears can also be associated with hip dysplasia and degenerative hip disease.[51]

Clinical features

Patients present with pain that is typically precipitated by pivoting or twisting.[50] The pain is mainly in the groin, but it can also occur in the trochanteric and buttock regions.[48-50] Often there is associated catching or audible clicking of the hip and a mild limitation of motion.[23,47-51] Passive movement of the hip during the physical examination reproduces the pain, with or without clicking.[52] According to many authors, the provocative maneuver depends on the location of the labral tear. For anterosuperior labral tears, symptoms are reproduced by moving the hip into flexion, adduction, and internal rotation.[48,49,53,54] Also, acute flexion of the hip with external rotation and full abduction followed by extension, adduction, and internal rotation will elicit pain in patients with anterior labral tears.[50] In addition, pain in patients with posterior labral tears may be reproduced by moving the hip into extension, abduction, and external rotation from a flexed, adducted, and internally rotated position.[48-50,53,54] However, some authors have found that the provocative maneuver does not necessarily correlate with the location of the tear.[52]

Diagnosis

Although plain radiographs will not reveal the labral tear, they frequently will show acetabular dysplasia, arthritis, acetabular cysts, or other intra-articular abnormalities.[48,55] Arthrograms are useful for excluding hip abnormalities other than labral tears, but they are inadequate for making the diagnosis of acetabular labral tears.[47-49,52,53] In the past, MRI alone was considered not sensitive or accurate for the diagnosis of acetabular labral tears.[47,49,50,52,56-58] Traditionally, magnetic resonance arthrography has been considered the diagnostic imaging modality of choice for acetabular labral tears[47] **(Figure 25.6)**. This test is more than 90% sensitive for this diagnosis,[57,59] but the use of magnetic resonance arthrography is limited by its invasive nature and its associated costs.[57] A recent article has suggested that because of improved technology and new pulse sequences, noncontrast MRI can identify labral tears with an accuracy that is similar to that of magnetic resonance arthrography.[60] However, additional research is needed to confirm this claim before magnetic resonance arthrography is abandoned as part of the workup for acetabular labral tears. The presence of a paralabral cyst on MRI is 100% specific for the existence of a labral abnormality; therefore, if a paralabral cyst is present on MRI, magnetic resonance arthrography can be avoided.[61]

Treatment

Intra-articular abnormalities as the source of hip pain may be confirmed by the temporary relief of symptoms with an intra-articular injection of local anesthetic.[23,61] Nonoperative treatment (i.e., protected weight bearing for 4 weeks[23]) is the recommended initial intervention for acetabular labral tears; this treatment is effective in approximately 13% of patients.[50] If nonoperative treatment fails, arthroscopic debridement is the preferred surgical treatment.[47-50] Recent reports have shown that arthroscopic debridement yields good results in 71% of patients without evidence of osteoarthritis.[52]

Proximal femur fracture

Fractures of the proximal femur are unusual injuries in athletes.[23] These injuries typically occur as a result of high-energy mechanisms such as forceful falls or collisions. This injury has also been described in cross-country and alpine skiing, and it has therefore been termed "skier's hip."[62] Patients with this injury present with complaints of severe groin pain after trauma. Plain radiographs will reveal the fracture, and they are adequate for the diagnosis. Displaced femoral neck fractures represent a surgical emergency. Treatment consists of emergent reduction and internal fixation to minimize the risk of osteonecrosis.[23]

INSIDIOUS-ONSET INJURIES

Sports hernia

This condition, which is also called *sportsman's hernia* or *athletic pubalgia*, refers to an occult hernia that is caused by weakness or a tear of the posterior inguinal wall (without a clinically recognizable hernia) that leads to a condition of chronic groin pain[4,8,63,64] **(Figures 25.7 and 25.8)**. This condition occurs almost exclusively in men.[63,65-68] There is often a prolonged course before diagnosis because of its insidious-onset, nonspecific symptoms, and lack of clinical findings.

Mechanism of injury

Several theories exist in the literature regarding the cause of sports hernia, but most theories implicate overuse.[23,63] Hip range of motion and resultant pelvic motion (often from trunk hyperextension and thigh hyperabduction) lead to shearing across the pubic symphysis.[65,67] The shearing forces are theoretically greater among athletes with an imbalance between the strong adductor muscles of the thigh and the relatively weak lower abdominal musculature.[45]

Figure 25.6 Traditionally, the definitive test for hip labral tears is magnetic resonance arthrography, as seen here. *A*, MRI delineates the extent of the labral tear. *B*, Arthroscopic debridement of the torn labrum. (From Canale ST: Campbell's Operative Orthopaedics, 10th ed. St. Louis, Mosby, 2003.)

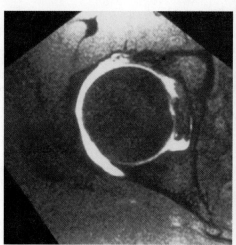

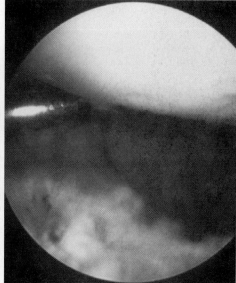

A

B

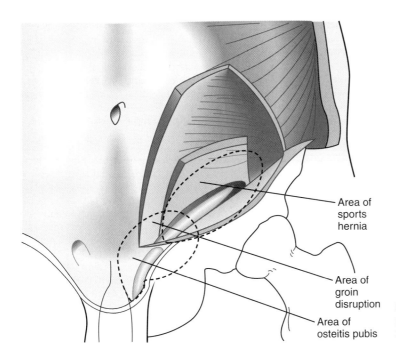

Figure 25.7 Areas of sports hernia, groin disruption, and osteitis pubis. (Redrawn from Morelli V, Smith V: Am Fam Phys 2001;64[8]:1405-1414.)

These forces place stress on the inguinal wall musculature, which ultimately leads to the attenuation of the local soft tissues. Numerous studies have described a variety of abnormal findings, including attenuation or tearing of the transversalis fascia or conjoined tendon, abnormalities at the insertion of the rectus abdominis muscle, avulsion of part of the internal oblique muscle fibers at the pubic tubercle, tearing within the internal oblique musculature,

and abnormalities in the external oblique muscle and aponeurosis.[13,63,67,69-72] The exact incidence of this condition is unknown, but several studies suggest that it is common among athletes with chronic groin pain that is recalcitrant to nonoperative treatment. Lovell[3] reviewed 189 cases of chronic groin pain in athletes and found that sports hernia was the primary diagnosis in 50%. Kluin and colleagues[73] found sports hernias to be the cause of chronic groin pain in 7 of 18 (39%) patients. Polglase and colleagues[69] found deficiency of the posterior wall of the inguinal canal to be present in 61 of 72 (85%) athletes who underwent surgical exploration for chronic groin pain of unknown origin.

Risk factors

The sports hernia is a common injury among athletes who participate in sports that require repetitive twisting and turning at speed, such as ice hockey, soccer, Australian Rules football, tennis, and field hockey.[23,64,69,71]

Clinical features

Patients typically present with an insidious onset of unilateral, deep groin pain, but sudden-onset groin pain may occur in some cases.[13,63,67,70,71,74] The hallmark of the pain is that it is absent during inactivity but that it returns when activity is resumed.[63,65,67,70,74,75] The pain may radiate into the adductor region, the perineum, the rectus muscles, and the testicular area, and it is typically aggravated by sudden movements, coughing, or kicking.[8,45,63,67,69,71] Physical examination reveals no detectable hernia. The most common physical findings include local tenderness over the conjoined tendon, the pubic tubercle, and the mid inguinal region and a tender, dilated superficial inguinal ring.[2,8,63,65,66,68,71,72,74,75] Pain with a resisted sit-up is another common finding during examination.[13,67,68]

Diagnosis

Plain radiographs and bone scans are not useful for establishing this diagnosis, but they can be used to rule out other conditions, such as osteitis pubis, symphyseal instability, osteoarthritis, and tumor. MRI typically reveals nonspecific findings, but it is also useful for ruling out other causes of groin pain, especially stress fractures and osteitis pubis.[11,65,71,74,76] Dynamic high-resolution

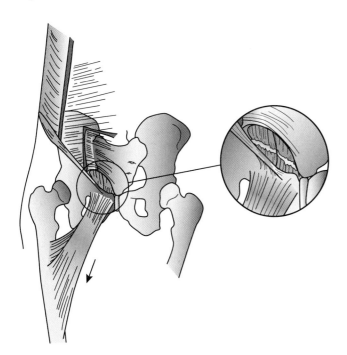

Figure 25.8 This simplified diagram shows a proposed theory of the mechanism of the sports hernia or "athletic pubalgia." An imbalance exists between the strong adductor muscles *(arrow)* and the relatively weak lower abdomen. This condition may lead to attenuation, avulsion, or the tearing of structures of the pelvic floor (as shown in the *inset*). (Redrawn from Anderson K, Strickland SM, Warren R: Am J Sports Med 2001;29[4]:521-533.)

ultrasound can be useful for evaluating sports hernia,[64] but the advantage of its noninvasive nature can be limited by the fact that it is dependent on the operator.[12,64]

Herniography (plain radiographs after the injection of radiopaque dye into the peritoneal cavity) has gained increasing popularity in Europe for the evaluation of chronic groin pain in athletes who are considering undergoing surgical exploration.[74,77] Herniography is intended to decrease the number of unnecessary herniorrhaphies performed by detecting the presence of a sports hernia (or excluding its absence) in patients who potentially carry this diagnosis and who are considering surgical exploration after failure of nonoperative treatment. However, some authors think that herniography study is inadequate for detecting many sports hernias.[74] A recent review reported herniography to have a sensitivity of 82% and a positive predictive value of 89% but a specificity of only 64%.[3] In addition, this procedure does carry some potential risks, such as hollow viscus perforation, vasovagal reaction, infection, abdominal wall hematoma, and reaction to the contrast agent; reported complication rates range from 3% to 5%.[78-80] Therefore, herniography is controversial as a part of the diagnostic workup of sports hernias.[74]

Treatment

Like most other conditions that cause groin pain in the athlete, sports hernias are initially treated with nonoperative methods, such as massage, heat or ice, stretching and strengthening exercises, and physical therapy modalities.[65,72] However, unlike most other causes of groin pain that typically respond to such treatment, sports hernias rarely improve with these modalities. Surgical exploration and repair are considered if nonoperative treatment fails after 6 to 8 weeks and after a careful sports-specific history and physical examination have ruled out other potential sources for the pain.[8,23,65,66,73,81] Surgical repair of the weak posterior inguinal wall with conventional or laparoscopic techniques leads to excellent results, with typical success rates of 85% to 95%.[63,66-69,71-75,81] In the light of the potential underlying pelvic imbalance, the treatment of a contracted or overdeveloped adductor muscle should not be neglected. Therefore, if symptomatic adductor abnormality is present preoperatively, some authors recommend adductor tenotomy in combination with herniorrhaphy.[28,65,68] Postoperatively, most athletes return to sports within 2 to 6 weeks after a laparoscopic repair (as opposed to 1 to 6 months after an open repair).[65,68,70,72,75,81,82]

Gilmore's groin

Gilmore's groin is a variant of the sports hernia that was described by Gilmore.[20] The pathologic features of Gilmore's groin include a torn external oblique aponeurosis, a torn conjoined tendon, a dehiscence between the conjoined tendon and the inguinal ligament, and the lack of a clinically detectable hernia. The condition is common among soccer players.[20] Most patients with this condition are males who present with the insidious onset of groin pain. The pain is typically unilateral and in the inguinal region, but it may occasionally be bilateral or involve the adductor or perineal areas.[20] The symptoms are chronic, they increase with activity, and they are exacerbated by sudden movements, such as sprinting, kicking, coughing, and getting out of bed the day after a game.[20] On physical examination, the only finding is a tender and dilated superficial inguinal ring.[20] As in the case of sports hernia, a radiographic workup is not diagnostic, but it may be useful for excluding other sources of groin pain. Initial treatment is nonoperative, but it is typically unsuccessful. Surgical treatment, which is indicated if nonoperative measures fail, consists of restoring the normal anatomy with a six-layered suture repair. Gilmore[20] has shown a 97% success rate with this procedure among professional soccer players.

Hockey player's syndrome

This condition, which is also called *hockey groin syndrome*, is an entity that is unique to elite hockey players.[13,83] It is the result of overuse and of a tear of the external oblique aponeurosis that is associated with inguinal nerve entrapment.[83,84] Patients present with groin pain that may radiate to the scrotum, the hip, and the back.[84] The pain is gradual in onset and muscular in nature,[84] it is exacerbated by ipsilateral hip extension and contralateral torso rotation,[83,84] and it occurs on the side opposite of the player's forehand slapshot.[83,84] Patients typically report pain during the first few strides of ice skating and during the slap shot motion.[84] Physical examination fails to reveal overt signs of hernia, but pain is often noted on palpation of the superficial inguinal ring.[84] In addition, a palpable gap may occasionally be felt in the external oblique aponeurosis as the supine patient elevates the head or actively flexes the hip against resistance.[83] Imaging studies such as plain radiographs, bone scintigraphy, CT, MRI, and ultrasound fail to reveal the defect.[83,84] Surgical exploration is the only method with which to confirm the diagnosis. Nonoperative treatment is usually unsuccessful. Surgical intervention to repair and reinforce the external oblique aponeurosis with neurectomy of the inguinal nerve is the usual definitive therapy, and it leads to successful outcomes in more than 90% of patients.[83,84]

Osteitis pubis

Osteitis pubis is an inflammatory lesion of the bone adjacent to the pubic symphysis. It is commonly seen in athletes, during or after pregnancy, and after prostate or bladder surgery.[85,86]

Mechanism of injury and risk factors

Although its exact cause is undetermined, in athletes, it is associated with mechanical strain from trauma and repetitive twisting and cutting movements.[13,86] These activities place increased stresses across the pubic symphysis, which can lead to pain and radiographic changes around the joint.[8,87] Osteitis pubis may be associated with instability of the pubic symphysis[20] and a decrease in the hip's range of motion.[88] Osteitis pubis is common among long-distance runners, weight lifters, ice-hockey players, swimmers, fencers, soccer players, and football players.[23,45,85-87]

Clinical features

Patients report an insidious onset of pain in the pubic region that may be unilateral or bilateral.[85,86,88] The pain may radiate into the medial aspect of the thigh, the perineum, the inguinal area, the scrotum, the testicles, or the abdomen.[13,86,89] Fricker and colleages[85] noted that, in 59 patients with osteitis pubis, 80% reported adductor pain, 40% reported pubic symphysis pain, 30% reported lower abdominal pain, 12% reported hip pain, and 8% reported scrotal pain. This pain is associated with kicking, running, jumping, Valsalva maneuvers, or pivoting on one leg.[23,86,87] Tenderness along the subcutaneous border of the pubis and pubic symphysis is present on physical examination, and the lack of this tenderness excludes osteitis pubis.[4,20,85-87,89] Passive abduction and resisted active adduction elicit pain.[13,45,86,87] The impairment of hip rotation may also be seen on physical examination.[85]

Diagnosis

Plain radiographs, including an anteroposterior view of the pelvis, should be obtained, although radiographic findings may not be visible for 2 to 4 weeks after the onset of symptoms.[40,86] These findings include bone resorption of the medial ends of the bilateral pubic bones, widening of the pubic symphysis, and rarefaction or sclerosis along the pubic rami[10,45,86,87,89] **(Figure 25.9).** Instability, symphysis step off, or sacroiliac joint changes also may be seen.[23] Gradual reossification with complete restoration of the

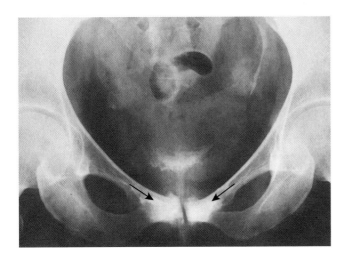

Figure 25.9 Findings of osteitis pubis on a radiograph may not appear for up to 4 weeks after the onset of clinical symptoms. However, classic radiographic findings include bone resorption at the symphysis pubis and sclerosis of the pubic rami. (From Mettler FA Jr: Essentials of Radiology, 2nd ed. Philadelphia, WB Saunders, 2005.)

joint is associated with healing, but it can take several months.[86,89] One-legged standing views (also known as *flamingo views*) are beneficial if instability of the symphysis is suspected.[85,86] Instability is defined as more than 2 mm of height difference between the superior rami of the symphysis.[85,86,90] Bone scintigraphy is also diagnostic. Early during the course of the disease, bone scans show diffuse increased uptake unilaterally or bilaterally in the pubic bones.[13,40,85] MRI shows marrow edema in the pubic bones (often bilaterally) early during the course of the condition, and this is followed by a low signal on T1- and T2-weighted images that is consistent with sclerosis as the disease progresses.[10,11,91] MRI has the diagnostic benefit of also displaying other local soft-tissue abnormalities.[86]

Treatment

Osteitis pubis may be treated nonoperatively with relative rest, ice, NSAIDs, stretching, strengthening, hip range-of-motion exercises, and physical therapy modalities because the condition is considered to be self-limited.[85,86,92] However, despite its self-limited nature, osteitis pubis tends to have a protracted course, and 6 to

9 months or more may elapse before the athlete can return to a preinjury level of functioning.[8,9,86] Therefore, if symptoms persist despite adequate nonoperative treatment, corticosteroid injections may be considered in an attempt to hasten the recovery process.[86,87] Holt and colleagues[87] reported good results after corticosteroid injections into the area of the pubic symphysis. Many of their athletes were able to return to competition within 3 weeks of the injection, but the best results occurred among patients who were treated within 2 weeks of symptom inception.[87] Rarely, in chronic cases that are unresponsive to nonoperative therapy and corticosteroid injections, operative treatment may be indicated.[86] Procedures described in the literature include arthrodesis of the pubic symphysis (if symphyseal instability is present)[89,92] and wedge resection of the symphysis pubis.[89,92]

Bursitis

Bursitis is an inflammation of the saclike cavities, called *bursae*, which are often associated with joints and bony prominences. Although there are at least 13 bursae **(Figure 25.10)** in the hip region, only three are commonly affected: the ischial, the iliopectineal, and the trochanteric bursae.[42]

Mechanism of injury and risk factors

Bursitis in the hip and pelvis typically occurs as a result of trauma or excessive friction, and it is often associated with overuse. Contributing factors to the development of an inflammatory bursitis in this region include excessive training, inadequate shoes, and biomechanical abnormalities such as leg-length inequality and hyperpronation.

Clinical features

Ischial bursitis presents with pain in a sitting position and local tenderness around the ischial tuberosity. This condition typically occurs after trauma to the ischial tuberosity.[42] Iliopectineal bursitis is caused by friction from the iliopsoas tendon.[42] This bursitis occurs with or without associated abnormalities of the iliopsoas tendon.[42] Iliopectineal bursitis presents as severe acute pain over the anterior aspect of the hip.[1] The pain may radiate down the thigh to the knee.[93] This condition is common among runners, jumpers, and soccer players, and it is closely associated with the internal variety of snapping hip.[12,93] With this condition, patients typically assume a position of hip flexion and external rotation to obtain relief.[13] On examination, pain is elicited by passive extension and internal rotation as well as by resisted flexion.[3,12]

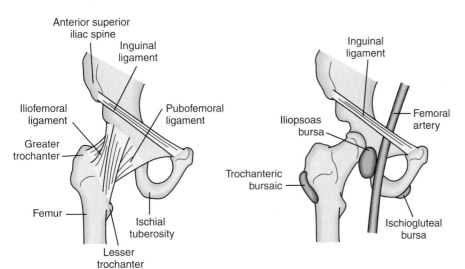

Figure 25.10 Diagram of the relationship of the distended iliopsoas, the trochanteric, and the ischiogluteal bursae to the hip joint and adjacent structures. (Redrawn from Goldman L, Ausiello D: Cecil Textbook of Medicine, 22nd ed. Philadelphia, WB Saunders, 2004.)

A   B

Tenderness to palpation is present distal to the midpoint of the inguinal ligament in the femoral triangle.[93] Trochanteric bursitis typically results from friction of the iliotibial band over the bursa. This condition is associated with maximum tenderness over the greater trochanter that is accentuated with hip adduction and external rotation.[1] Women with a wide pelvis or a prominent trochanter or runners who adduct beyond the midline are at risk for trochanteric bursitis.

Diagnosis

In all locations, physical examination reveals focal tenderness or warmth over the affected bursae. If plain radiographs are obtained, they are typically normal. Bursography can be used to visualize the bursae, but it is typically unnecessary and therefore avoided because of to its invasive nature.[94] Ultrasound can be used to show bursitis, which appears as a fluid collection at the site of a bursa.[10,93] Bursitis is best visualized by MRI, which reveals a well-defined area with high signal at the site of a bursa on T2-weighted images.[10]

Treatment

Symptoms caused by bursitis are usually relatively benign, and they respond to symptomatic treatment such as rest, ice, stretching of the involved tendons, NSAIDs, and attention to training and biomechanical deficits.[4,22,94] Local steroid injections may be necessary, and they should be used as the second line of treatment.[93] Extreme disabling pain is a rare complication, and it may require surgical excision or the release of the overlying tendons if nonoperative treatment fails.[40,95]

Snapping hip syndrome

Snapping hip syndrome, which is also called *coxa saltans,* is a clinical condition in which a usually painful, audible snap occurs during hip flexion and extension. This condition commonly occurs among distance runners, gymnasts, swimmers, and dancers.[94] The cause of the snapping can be external or internal.

External type

The external type of snapping hip is caused by the iliotibial band (most commonly), the tensor fascia lata, or the gluteus maximus tendon sliding over the greater trochanter with hip flexion and extension. This condition is not always painful, but, when pain

is present, it usually is the result of secondary trochanteric bursitis.[95] On physical examination, patients have tenderness over the posterior aspect of the greater trochanter that is consistent with trochanteric bursitis.[95] The snapping can be reproduced during physical examination as the extended hip is brought into full flexion while the patient is in the lateral decubitus position with the hip adducted and the knee extended.[95] When this condition is painful, treatment involves rest, iliotibial band stretching, NSAIDs, and, occasionally, corticosteroid injections.[23,95] The vast majority of patients improve with these measures.[95] Surgical options, which are only required in rare refractory cases, include the excision of the greater trochanteric bursa, the excision of all or part of the iliotibial band, or Z-plasty of the iliotibial band[95,96] **(Figure 25.11).** Zoltan and colleagues[95] reported that surgical excision of an ellipsoid-shaped portion of the iliotibial band overlying the greater trochanter and the removal of the trochanteric bursa yielded good results in patients for whom nonoperative treatment failed. Brignall and Stainsby[96] reported excellent results in 7 of 8 (88%) patients who were treated with Z-plasty of the iliotibial band.

Internal type

The internal variety of snapping hip is commonly caused by the iliopsoas tendon catching on the pelvic brim (iliopectineal eminence), the anterior inferior iliac spine, or the femoral head **(Figure 25.12)** and hip capsule.[94] Other possible causes of internal hip snapping include acetabular labral tears, osteochondral injury, osteitis pubis, osteochondromatosis, hip subluxation, synovial chondromatosis, and loose bodies within the joint.[22,93,95] Subluxation of the iliopsoas tendon is the most common cause of internal snapping hip. This snapping occurs as the hip is extended from a flexed, abducted, and externally rotated position and the tendon travels from a relative anterolateral position to a more posteromedial position.[94] On physical examination, internal snapping is elicited as the hip is passively brought from flexion to extension in the supine patient. Diagnosis is typically based on patient history and physical examination, but dynamic ultrasound during hip motion may show the tendon subluxation as it coincides with pain and audible snapping.[93,94,97] MRI has a limited role in the diagnosis of internal hip snapping, but it may be useful for ruling out other abnormalities.[11,93,97] The treatment of painful internal snapping of the hip is similar to that of the external variety. Activity modification, stretching,

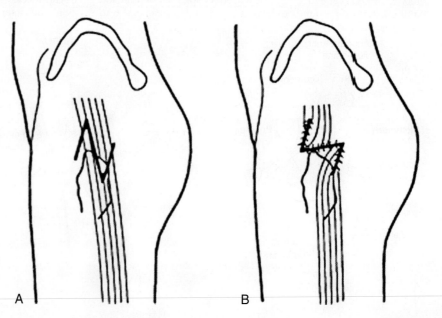

Figure 25.11 Z-plasty of the iliotibial band for snapping hip. *A,* Incision. *B,* Transposition and suture of flaps. (Redrawn from Canale ST: Campbell's Operative Orthopaedics, 10th ed. St. Louis, Mosby, 2003.)

A   B

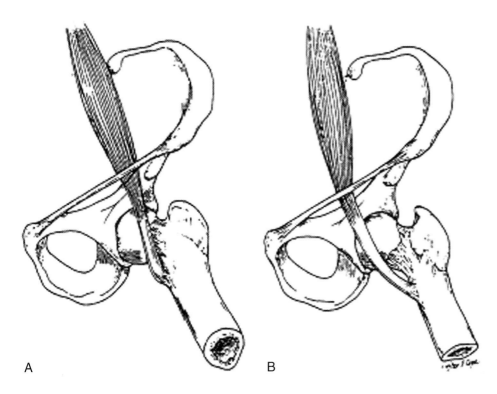

Figure 25.12 *A*, With flexion of the hip, the iliopsoas tendon shifts laterally in relation to the center of the femoral head. *B*, With extension of the hip, the iliopsoas tendon shifts medially in relation to the center of the femoral head. (Redrawn from Canale ST: Campbell's Operative Orthopaedics, 10th ed. St. Louis, Mosby, 2003.)

and NSAIDs are the key treatment modalities. Surgical intervention for internal snapping hip syndrome, which is indicated only if nonoperative measures fail, consists of release versus lengthening of the iliopsoas tendon.[98] Taylor and Clarke[98] reported successful results in 63% of 16 hips treated with iliopsoas tendon release. Jacobson and Allen[94] reported excellent results in 95% of 20 hips after an iliopsoas lengthening procedure.

Proximal iliotibial band syndrome

The iliotibial band (ITB) is a long strap of connective tissue that runs, as the name suggests, from the iliac crest to the lateral tibia. As a result of its complex array of muscular attachments, the ITB lies posterior to the greater trochanter when the hip is extended. Then, as the hip is flexed, the ITB glides over the trochanter, and it is found anterior to the trochanter in hip flexion.

Mechanism of injury and risk factors

Symptoms usually occur at 30 degrees of hip flexion, as in runners during foot strike. Reducing the foot-strike angle, as in downhill running, may make athletes more susceptible to ITB friction syndrome (ITBFS). Track athletes, who train and compete primarily on level surfaces, have greater foot-strike angles and lower incidences of ITBFS. Anything that increases strain on the lateral thigh, including the width of the ITB, excessive pronation, varus alignment of the lower limb, and lateral tilt of the pelvis, may predispose the athlete to ITBFS.[16,99]

Clinical features

Athletes with ITBFS complain of persistent aching pain on the lateral aspect of the upper thigh and knee. Pain onset typically occurs at a predictable point during each run, but it may be sporadic. Long runs or runs over uneven surfaces are particularly inciting. Athletes complain of tenderness and, occasionally, crepitus over the greater trochanter. Compressive forces applied over the lateral proximal thigh sometimes reproduce symptoms.

Diagnosis

A positive Ober's test indicates a tight ITB and suggests ITBFS in symptomatic patients. MRI or ultrasound may identify an inflamed bursa underlying the ITB.[16]

Treatment

A conservative approach with ice, NSAIDs, and electrotherapeutic modalities can be helpful. Treatment of ITBFS emphasizes reducing the stress applied to the ITB, which can be achieved by increasing ITB fascial length through ITB massage and a dedicated ITB stretching program. In addition to stretching, a physical therapy program should also strengthen the lateral stabilizers to reduce pelvic tilt. Patients who do not achieve adequate relief through these measures may benefit from a corticosteroid injection to the bursa underlying the ITB at the femoral trochanter. More recalcitrant cases may require surgical release of the ITB and excision of the inflamed bursa. Certainly, before surgery, functional gait analysis and podiatric assessment may help to correct an underlying biomechanical abnormality and prevent recurrences.[16] Athletes may gradually return to sports participation in 2 to 6 weeks, after they are asymptomatic.

Stress fractures

Among young athletes, stress fractures occur when cumulative stresses exceed the structural strength of the bone.[100] These injuries are common in military recruits and long-distance runners, and they are more common among women, especially those with amenorrhea and eating disorders.[8,101] These injuries are also often associated with a sudden change in training regimen.[22,101]

Femoral neck

Femoral neck stress fractures have been well described in military recruits in basic training and in runners.[102,103] According to one study, femoral neck stress fractures accounted for 7% of all stress fractures in runners.[100]

Risk factors Predisposing factors include coxa vara, training errors, improper footwear, and poor running surfaces.[22,100]

Clinical features The major presenting symptom of a femoral neck stress fracture is pain in the groin, the anterior thigh, or the knee. Typically, the pain is gradual in onset, it is associated with weight bearing or exertion, and it abates with rest.[8,13,42,100] On physical examination, patients often have local tenderness, an antalgic gait, and limited internal rotation of the hip.[4,100] Axial compression of the hip, extreme range of motion of the hip, or percussion of the greater trochanter may also elicit pain.[13,103]

Diagnosis Plain radiographic findings may not develop until 2 to 4 weeks after the initial injury.[45,100,102] If clinical suspicion of this diagnosis is present and plain radiographic findings are not seen, a bone scan or MRI should be obtained.[103] Bone scintigraphy is highly sensitive early during the course of this condition and is positive on presentation; however, bone scintigraphy lacks specificity.[11,13,42,45,100,102] MRI is also highly sensitive, and, unlike bone scintigraphy, it is very specific and allows for the evaluation of other soft-tissue injuries.[11] Shin and colleagues[104] have reported that, in the diagnosis of femoral neck stress fractures, the accuracy of MRI is 100%; the accuracy of bone scintigraphy is only 68%. Early diagnosis is essential to avoid delays in treatment, which could allow for progression to displaced fractures and the potential consequences of displacement, including nonunion and osteonecrosis.[103]

Treatment The treatment of femoral neck stress fractures is based on fracture pattern. Fullerton and Snowdy[102] modified Devas' original classification system[105] and described three types of fracture patterns: compression, tension (or distraction), and displaced fractures of the femoral neck **(Figure 25.13)**. The early radiographic appearance of these fractures is a sclerotic area of internal callus on the inferior cortex of the femoral neck without cortical disruption.[102] Unlike tension fractures, continued stress does not typically cause displacement of the compression fracture pattern. Therefore, nonoperative treatment is considered for this fracture pattern[103]: discontinuation of weight bearing until the patient is pain free, followed by a gradual return to weight bearing.[102] Jogging should be avoided for 4 to 8 weeks. During this time, frequent radiographs are obtained. If there is no response to nonoperative treatment or if widening or displacement is seen at the fracture, the hip is stabilized with internal fixation.[102] Tension fractures are typically characterized radiographically by a fracture in the superior cortex of the femoral neck.[102] These fractures have a high likelihood of displacement with continued stress. Displaced femoral neck stress fractures are associated with serious complications, including osteonecrosis, nonunion, and varus deformity.[102,103] For these reasons, most authors recommend urgent surgical internal fixation of the femoral neck for tension-sided femoral neck stress fractures and displaced femoral neck fractures.[8,23,39,102] In addition to treatment of the fracture, any dietary or hormonal issues and the correction of training errors must be addressed to assist with healing and to prevent recurrence.[8]

Pubic rami

These injuries, which tend to occur in the inferior pubic ramus, represent a very small percentage of the stress fractures experienced by athletes.[106] According to one study, pelvic stress fractures accounted for 6% of all stress fractures in runners.[100] They are most common among long-distance runners and joggers, especially women.[13,106,107]

Clinical features Pain in the inguinal, perineal, or adductor region that is exacerbated by activity and relieved by rest is the presenting complaint.[42,100,106,107] On physical examination, patients often have an antalgic gait and severe tenderness to palpation over the affected pubic ramus.[4,13,100,107] A positive standing sign (frank pain or an inability to stand unsupported on the affected leg) is highly suggestive of a pubic ramus stress fracture.[107]

Diagnosis Radiographic findings such as periosteal new bone and sclerosis may not appear to be positive for 2 to 3 weeks after the onset of symptoms. If plain radiographs are nondiagnostic, a bone scan or MRI may be obtained.[106] Bone scintigraphy and MRI are both positive early during the course of this condition.

Treatment The treatment of pubic rami stress fractures is nonoperative, and it consists of activity modification (i.e., the cessation of running for 4 to 6 weeks followed by a gradual return to sports participation).[4,100,106] Most athletes show a response to this treatment within 1 to 3 months.[106,107] In addition to the treatment of the fracture, any dietary or hormonal issues and the correction of training errors must be addressed to assist with healing and to prevent recurrence.[8]

Sacrum

Sacral stress fractures typically present as low back and buttock pain in athletes, especially female distance runners[101,108,109] **(Figure 25.14)**. The most important risk factor is an increase in impact activity as a result of a more vigorous exercise program.[101,108]

Clinical features The pain, which usually begins insidiously without antecedent trauma, is activity related and progressive.[101,108,109] Physical examination usually reveals tenderness over the sacrum and the sacroiliac joint.[101,109] The neurologic examination is typically unremarkable, and the flexion, abduction, and external rotation (FABER) test may or may not be positive.[108,109]

Diagnosis Plain radiographs of the pelvis and spine are usually unremarkable, but they may reveal sclerosis as a result of endosteal callous formation.[101,109,110] Bone scintigraphy, which is very sensitive but lacks specificity, is the most common modality used for making the diagnosis.[110,111] On a bone scan, a sacral stress fracture appears as a focal round area of increased tracer uptake that is typically confined to the sacral alae.[108,109] Alternatively, MRI may be used to diagnose sacral stress fractures;

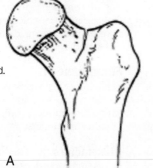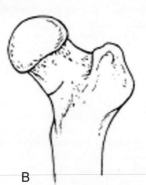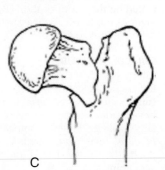

Figure 25.13 Fullerton and Snowdy[102] classification of femoral neck stress fractures. A, Tension type fracture. B, Compression type fracture. C, Displaced type fracture. (Redrawn from Canale ST: Campbell's Operative Orthopaedics, 10th ed. St. Louis, Mosby, 2003.)

A   B   C

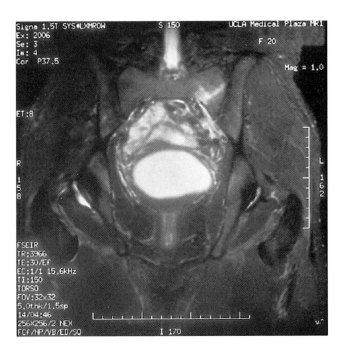

Figure 25.14 MRI of a stress fracture of the sacrum in a 20-year-old female distance runner with persistent low back pain and negative radiographic findings. (From DeLee JC, Drez D Jr, Miller MD [eds]: DeLee and Drez's Orthopaedic Sports Medicine: Principles and Practice, 2nd ed. Philadelphia, WB Saunders, 2003.)

it is slightly less sensitive than bone scintigraphy, but it has the advantages of ruling out other abnormalities and having a much smaller radiation load to the patient.[108,111] On MRI, a sacral stress fracture appears as an area of bone marrow edema, often with an adjacent sclerotic fracture line.[101,111]

Treatment The treatment of this injury involves a period of cessation from running and athletic activity (approximately 3 to 6 weeks) that is followed by a gradual return to activity.[101,108,109] Using this regimen, most athletes can return to their previous sporting activity, although it may take up to 6 months.[101,109] In addition to treatment of the fracture, any dietary or hormonal issues must also be addressed to assist with healing and to prevent recurrence.[8,101]

Gracilis syndrome

The gracilis syndrome comprises a fatigue avulsion fracture of traumatic origin that involves the bony origin of the gracilis muscle at the pubic symphysis.[112] The clinical picture is similar to that of osteitis pubis. Patients typically present with chronic groin, perineal, and medial thigh pain that is insidious in onset. The pain often radiates along the course of the gracilis muscle. On physical examination, focal tenderness is present over the pubic symphysis. Plain radiographs reveal a bony fragment at the inferior corner of the pubis adjacent to the symphysis. Histopathologic analysis suggests that the fragment results from an avulsion type of fatigue fracture, with the avulsion related to the directional pull of the gracilis muscle.[112] Nonoperative treatment is recommended, but, if it is ineffective, surgical removal of the free bony fragment has been shown to be successful.[112]

Osteoarthritis

Osteoarthritis of the hip is the end stage of many different disorders. Studies have shown that athletes may be at greater risk than

the general population for developing osteoarthritis of the hip. Vingard and colleagues[113] found that long-term sports exposure, especially for those involved in track and field and racket sports, places individuals at an increased risk for hip osteoarthrosis, particularly if this is associated with obesity and occupational weightlifting. Other studies have shown that soccer players are predisposed to hip osteoarthritis.[114,115] Symptoms of osteoarthritis of the hip include activity-related hip pain, joint stiffness, decreased range of motion, swelling, and crepitus. Plain radiographs reveal joint-space narrowing, osteophytes, subchondral sclerosis, and subchondral cysts. Initial treatment options are nonoperative modalities such as activity modification, range-of-motion exercises, assistive devices for ambulation, physical therapy, and NSAIDs. If these modalities fail, surgical options such as total hip arthroplasty are indicated.

Nerve compression syndromes
Ilioinguinal nerve

The ilioinguinal nerve arises from the ventral rami of the first lumbar nerve in the lumbar plexus with contributing filaments from the twelfth thoracic nerve.[116] The nerve passes through the psoas muscle, pierces the transversus abdominis near the ASIS, and continues through the internal and external abdominal obliques **(Figure 25.15)**. It provides motor innervation to the distal regions of the internal oblique and transversus abdominis muscles. The nerve then continues into the inguinal canal to provide sensory innervation to the medial thigh, the skin over the inguinal ligament, and the base of the penis and scrotum (or labia).[13,117]

Mechanism of injury and risk factors Abdominal muscle hypertrophy, pregnancy, and scar tissue from previous surgery (e.g., appendectomy, herniorrhaphy, or iliac crest bone grafting) predispose individuals to compression of the ilioinguinal nerve.[4,45] Among athletes, most cases of entrapment of the ilioinguinal nerve result from hypertrophy of the abdominal muscles as a result of excessive training.

Clinical features and diagnosis Patients with entrapment of the ilioinguinal nerve complain of burning or shooting iliac fossa pain that radiates to the groin, the proximal scrotum, the labia, and the upper medial thigh.[118] On physical examination, patients have altered sensation in the cutaneous distribution of the nerve and tenderness to palpation 2 to 3 cm medial and inferior to the ASIS.[2,118] In addition, hyperextension of the hip produces pain and hypoesthesia in the distribution of the nerve.[2] If a local nerve block medial to the ASIS alleviates the symptoms, the diagnosis is confirmed.[1,118]

Treatment The treatment is nonoperative, including ice, ultrasound, local steroid injections, NSAIDs, and altering the training program. If these modalities fail, operative exploration of the nerve may be indicated.[116]

Obturator nerve

The obturator nerve arises from the second to fourth ventral rami of the lumbar plexus. It exits the pelvis via the fibro-osseous obturator tunnel, where it splits into anterior and posterior divisions. The anterior division supplies motor innervation to the adductor longus, the adductor brevis, and the gracilis, and it supplies sensory innervation to the distal two thirds of the medial thigh.[117] The posterior division innervates the obturator externus and the superior portion of the adductor magnus, and it supplies sensory innervation to the articular capsule, the cruciate ligaments, and the synovium of the knee joint.[117,119]

Mechanism of injury and risk factors The obturator nerve can be compressed by pelvic fractures, hematomas, retroperitoneal

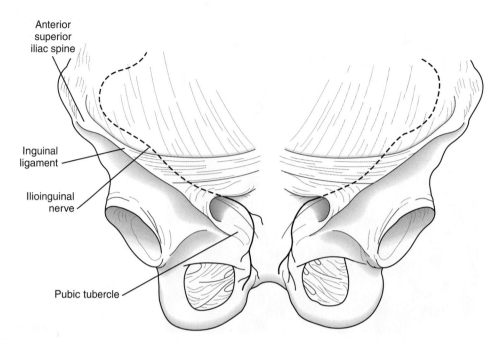

Figure 25.15 The course of the ilioinguinal nerve makes it susceptible to injury in athletes after pregnancy or as a result of excessive abdominal muscular training. (Redrawn from Stenchever MA, Droegmueller W: Comprehensive Gynecology, 4th ed. St. Louis, Mosby, 2001.)

masses, intrapelvic tumors, surgical trauma, or local inflammatory processes.[119,120] In athletes, it appears that the obturator nerve entrapment is the result of a fascial band at the distal end of the obturator canal.[119] This abnormality is common in skaters, Australian Rules football players, and soccer players as a result of adductor muscle development.[23,121]

Clinical features and diagnosis In the athlete, obturator nerve entrapment presents as exercise-induced medial thigh pain that begins insidiously.[119,121] The pain subsides with rest, but it resumes with activity. On physical examination, adductor muscle atrophy may be noted if there is an extrinsic source of compression. In addition, adductor weakness and paresthesias over the medial thigh may be present, especially after exercise.[120] Pain may be reproduced by hip external rotation and adduction in the standing patient.[120,121] Plain radiographs are unremarkable, but MRI may show atrophy of the adductor longus and brevis.[119] In cases that last for more than 3 months, EMG reliably shows a chronic denervation pattern in the adductor brevis and adductor longus muscles.[119,121] The injection of local anesthetic into the obturator nerve should reproduce the patient's weakness and relieve the pain associated with provocative maneuvers. This test is useful for confirming the diagnosis.

Treatment Nonoperative treatment including rest, physical therapy, adductor stretching and strengthening, NSAIDs, and local steroid injections has been shown to be beneficial only in early and mild cases.[119] Surgical intervention, which includes the release of the fascial bands overlying the adductor brevis and neurolysis of the obturator nerve, is required for the treatment of chronic entrapment.[119]

Lateral femoral cutaneous nerve: Meralgia paresthetica

The lateral femoral cutaneous nerve originates from the second and third ventral rami in the lumbar plexus. It exits the pelvis under the lateral attachment of the inguinal ligament, passing just medial to the ASIS. It supplies sensory innervation to the anterolateral thigh, and it has no motor function.[117]

Mechanism of injury and risk factors Entrapment of the lateral femoral cutaneous nerve, which is also known as *meralgia paresthetica,* has been reported after surgical procedures (including

iliac crest bone grafting, appendectomy, total abdominal hysterectomy, and pelvic osteotomy) in patients with diabetes mellitus, obese patients, patients who wear constrictive clothing (e.g., tight pants, pads, belts, or girdles), and seat-belted occupants of motor vehicles that are involved in accidents.[122,123] In athletes, often no identifiable cause is found.

Clinical features and diagnosis Patients present with pain or numbness in the anterolateral thigh, knee, and buttock with an absence of motor findings. Tinel's sign is usually present 1 cm medial and inferior to the ASIS. Radiographs and MRI are useful for ruling out other causes of pain and for evaluating intra-articular and intrapelvic sources of compression.[122] Nerve conduction studies, which show prolonged latency or decreased conduction velocity consistent with compression,[122,123] are the most useful tests for distinguishing meralgia paresthetica from lumbosacral radiculopathy.[122,123] A local nerve block should temporarily relieve patients' complaints, and thus it serves as a diagnostic confirmatory test and a predictor of benefit from surgical decompression[122,123] **(Figure 25.16).**

Treatment Nonoperative treatment consisting of the removal of the offending compressing agent, stretching, heat, physical therapy, local steroid injections, and NSAIDs is usually effective.[122,123] Williams and Trzil[123] showed that nonoperative treatment was effective in 91% of 277 patients with meralgia paresthetica. If nonoperative treatment measures fail, surgical treatment is indicated. Excellent results have been shown after neurectomy of the lateral femoral cutaneous nerve, with relief of symptoms in 23 of 24 (96%) patients.[123] In another study, surgical neurolysis also led to good or excellent results in 25 of 26 (96%) patients.[122]

Iliohypogastric nerve

The iliohypogastric nerve originates from the first ventral rami in the lumbar plexus. It supplies motor innervation to the transversus abdominis and the internal oblique muscles. The nerve perforates the transversus abdominis muscle and divides between the transversus abdominis muscle and the internal oblique muscle into two branches. The iliac branch pierces the internal and external oblique muscles and provides sensory innervation to the skin over the iliac crest. The hypogastric

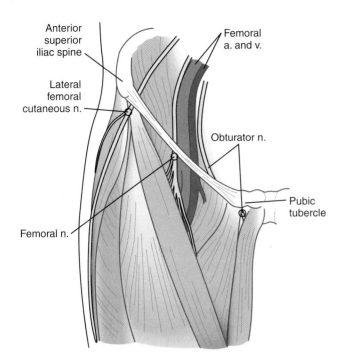

Figure 25.16 The courses of the lateral femoral cutaneous, femoral, and obturator nerves. *Circles* show typical regions for nerve blockade. a., artery; n., nerve; v., vein. (Redrawn from Miller RD: Miller's Anesthesia, 6th ed. Philadelphia, Churchill Livingstone, 2005.)

branch pierces the internal oblique muscle and the aponeurosis of the external oblique muscle just superior to the deep inguinal ring, and it provides sensory innervation to the skin of the hypogastric region.[117]

Tears in the external oblique aponeurosis at the site of emergence of small neurovascular bundles containing the terminal hypogastric branches of the iliohypogastric nerve may cause groin pain in the athlete. Ziprin and colleagues[124] described this condition in 23 athletes (most of whom were rugby or soccer players) who presented with groin pain that was intensified by sudden movements, such as kicking and coughing. On examination, focal tenderness to palpation was present just superior to the deep inguinal ring. Plain radiographs, ultrasound, bone scintigraphy, and MRI were all unremarkable. Nonoperative treatment failed in all 23 athletes, who thereafter underwent surgical exploration and repair of the tear(s) in the external oblique aponeurosis with neurectomy of the branches of the iliohypogastric nerve. This procedure lead to good or excellent results in 87% of the athletes, with the average return to sporting activities occurring in 11 weeks.[124]

Sciatic nerve: Piriformis syndrome
The sciatic nerve receives branches from the fourth and fifth lumbar nerve roots as well as the first and second sacral nerve roots. It exits the pelvis through the greater sciatic foramen below the piriformis muscle and above the short external rotators of the hip, and it descends down the posterior thigh, where it divides into the tibial and common peroneal nerves.[117]

Mechanism of injury and risk factors The piriformis syndrome is the result of the compression of the sciatic nerve at the greater sciatic notch. It is usually caused by an abnormal condition of the piriformis muscle, such as hypertrophy, adhesions, inflammation, spasm (often as a result of overuse, trauma, or prolonged sitting), or anatomic variation[22,125-127] **(Figure 25.17).**

Clinical features Piriformis syndrome is a cause of buttock, groin, and posterior thigh pain as well as sciatica; it therefore must be distinguished from lumbosacral causes of sciatica.[126] One study reported that 68% of 239 patients with chronic sciatica of unknown origin ultimately were diagnosed with piriformis syndrome.[125] The symptoms typically are exacerbated by prolonged sitting or lying supine, and they are relieved by walking.[23,125,126] Numbness is rare, but paresthesias, when present, typically involve all five toes (multiple dermatomes), unlike that seen among patients with lumbosacral radiculopathy.[125] Physical examination occasionally reveals tenderness and the reproduction of symptoms with palpation of the piriformis muscle.[126,128] Sciatic notch or greater trochanteric tenderness is usually present.[125] Straight-leg testing is usually negative, unlike that seen among patients with lumbosacral radiculopathy.[125] In the supine position, the patient may keep the affected leg slightly elevated and externally rotated (positive piriformis sign).[126,128] The patient may also have a positive Freiburg sign, which is characterized as the reproduction of the pain on passive internal rotation of the hip with the thigh in extension.[126,128] Finally, a positive Pace sign (pain on resisted abduction and external rotation of the flexed hip) may be elicited.[126,128]

Diagnosis Imaging studies are important for diagnosis and for ruling out other potential sources of the symptoms, such as lumbar disc herniation and lumbar spinal stenosis. Plain radiographs are typically unremarkable. MRI combined with magnetic resonance neurography is 93% specific and 64% sensitive for the diagnosis if piriformis muscle asymmetry (atrophy or hypertrophy) is found in association with sciatic nerve hyperintensity.[125] MRI may also reveal anatomic variations responsible for the syndrome.[127] Electromyography findings may support the diagnosis, but a negative study does not exclude the diagnosis because the electromyography findings depend on the duration of the symptomatology.[126]

Treatment The initial treatment of piriformis syndrome is nonoperative measures such as NSAIDs, piriformis stretching, massage, ultrasound, and local anesthetic or corticosteroid injections.[22,126] If nonoperative modalities fail, surgical treatment may be considered. Surgery consists of the sectioning of the piriformis muscle at the tendinous insertion or piriformis muscle resection,

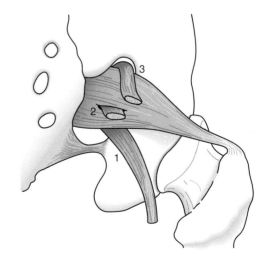

Figure 25.17 The sciatic nerve may traverse under (1), through (2), or over (3) the piriformis muscle as the nerve passes through the sciatic notch. (Redrawn from Frontera WR, Silver JK: Essentials of Physical Medicine and Rehabilitation, 1st ed. Philadelphia, Hanley and Belfus, 2002.)

the release of the fibrovascular bands that compress the sciatic nerve, and neuroplasty of the sciatic nerve.[125,126,128]

Sciatic nerve: Hamstring syndrome

Mechanism of injury and risk factors The hamstring syndrome is the result of compression of the sciatic nerve by tight tendinous structures of the lateral insertion area of the hamstring muscles (namely the long head of the biceps femoris and the semitendinosus muscles) to the ischial tuberosity.[129] The hamstring syndrome is commonly seen among athletes, especially sprinters and hurdlers.[129]

Clinical features This condition is a common cause of lower gluteal pain, with radiation down the posterior thigh to the popliteal space[129]; therefore, like the piriformis syndrome, it must be distinguished from lumbosacral causes of sciatica. The symptoms are exacerbated while sitting, stretching, sprinting, kicking, or hurdling, but they are seldom present while running slowly or lying supine.[129] There is frequently a history of recurrent hamstring tears.[129] In most patients, physical examination reveals local tenderness around the ischial tuberosity; it is frequently possible to palpate the tautness of the hamstring muscles.[129] The tenderness in hamstring syndrome is over the ischial tuberosity, which is more distal to the tenderness in the piriformis syndrome, typically over the piriformis muscle.[129] Neurologic examination is typically normal, and straight-leg raises only occasionally cause pain.[129]

Diagnosis Plain radiographs are typically unremarkable. CT or MRI may be necessary to rule out spinal stenosis or lumbar disc herniation.[129] Electromyography findings and nerve conduction velocity measurements are typically unremarkable.[129]

Treatment Nonoperative measures (rest, NSAIDs, and physical therapy) are usually unsuccessful, and, if so, operative treatment is recommended. Surgery consists of exploration of the sciatic nerve, the sectioning of taut tendinous structures of the hamstring muscle near the site of origin, and neuroplasty of the sciatic nerve.[129] Puranen and Orava[129] reported good results in 52 of 59 (88%) patients who were treated with this procedure.

Pudendal nerve

The pudendal nerve originates from the second through the fourth sacral nerves in the sacral plexus. It exits the pelvis through the greater sciatic foramen, crosses over the ischial spine, and then reenters the pelvis through the lesser sciatic foramen. The pudendal nerve provides motor innervation to the anal sphincters and the urethral sphincter; it also provides cutaneous sensory innervation to the perineum, the penis, the scrotum, the labia majora, and the clitoris.[117]

Neuropathic symptoms in the distribution of the pudendal nerve are extremely common among male bicyclists.[130] The probable cause of pudendal neuropathy in bicyclists is the compression of a branch of the pudendal nerve between the pubic symphysis and the bicycle seat.[131] Treatment involves temporary rest, changing the bicycle seat so that it does not tilt upward, changing to a different seat, or wearing padded bicycle pants.[130,131]

Other authors have attributed chronic perineal pain to the entrapment of the pudendal nerve between the sacrotuberous and sacrospinous ligaments, which are juxtaposed by an abnormally shaped and positioned ischial spine.[132] Because many of the patients in that study were involved in sports with hip flexion activities, the authors hypothesized that vigorous athletics leads to the hypertrophy of muscles of the pelvic floor, which then initiates the remodeling of the ischial spine.[132]

Lumbosacral causes

Lumbosacral causes of groin pain include radiculopathy from disc herniation, lumbar spinal stenosis, lumbar Scheuermann's disease, spondylosis, spondylolisthesis, or discogenic pain.[10,63] A full explanation of the cause, diagnostic workup, and treatment of these conditions is found in Chapter 24. A careful sports-specific history and physical examination and a thorough radiographic workup, including plain radiographs, CT, and/or MRI, should enable the clinician to differentiate these conditions from other causes of groin pain.[10]

Causes in pediatric patients

Additional discussion of these topics may be found in Chapter 31.

Osteoid osteoma

Osteoid osteoma is a benign tumor of adolescents and young adults that frequently affects the femoral neck. Therefore, it may present as a groin pain syndrome in young athletes, especially males.[22,133,134] The classic presentation includes well-localized, dull, aching pain, most noticeably at night; the pain is typically relieved by NSAIDs.[133,134] The physical examination is usually unremarkable. Plain radiographs may be normal, or they may reveal a radiolucent nidus that is surrounded by an area of reactive sclerosis.[133,134] Bone scintigraphy is extremely sensitive for detecting osteoid osteoma, and it shows focal increased uptake in the area of the lesion.[133,134] CT scanning is the definitive study for the diagnosis of osteoid osteoma, and it is useful for providing the accurate location and size of the lesion, especially in preparation for surgical treatment.[133,134] CT scanning shows the typical central lucent nidus and surrounding sclerosis[133] **(Figure 25.18).** MRI findings are variable and nonspecific, and they frequently lead to the incorrect diagnosis.[134] Treatment options include nonoperative management that consists of NSAIDs and observational treatment (because some authors suggest that the lesions will spontaneously regress), surgical excision, or radiofrequency ablation.[133,134]

Slipped capital femoral epiphysis

Slipped capital femoral epiphysis (SCFE) is the most common hip disorder among adolescents, with an incidence of approximately 2 per 100,000.[135] Therefore, this diagnosis must be considered in any adolescent with hip pain.[40] SCFE results from a mechanical shearing failure of the proximal femoral physis,[136] which in turn produces a posterior slippage of the proximal femoral epiphysis and concomitant extension and external rotation of the femoral neck and shaft. Risk factors include obesity and endocrinopathies.[137] SCFE is more common among males and blacks than in the general pediatric population, and it usually presents when patients are between 10 and 15 years of age.[42,136] Approximately 20% to 30% of SCFE cases are bilateral.[136]

Patients present with pain in the groin, thigh, or knee that is exacerbated by physical activity.[136] For this reason, any adolescent athlete presenting with knee pain should have a thorough hip examination. Physical examination may reveal a limp or external rotation gait and limited internal rotation of the hip.[135] With an acute slip, the hip often lies in a position of extension, adduction, and external rotation. Range of motion of the hip exacerbates pain. With a chronic slip, there is limited passive flexion, and the hip tends to rotate externally upon terminal flexion. Plain radiographs, including anteroposterior and frog-lateral views of both hips, are crucial for making the diagnosis of SCFE. Early radiographic findings include widening and blurring of the proximal femoral physis. As the amount of slip increases, a positive Klein line is identified as a line along the anterosuperior portion of the femoral neck that fails to intersect the anterolateral corner of the capital femoral epiphysis[135] **(Figure 25.19).**

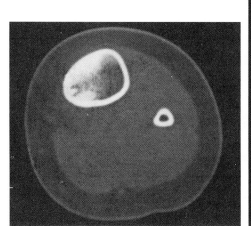

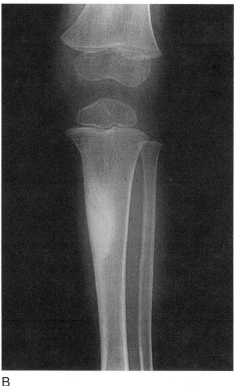

A   B

Figure 25.18   Osteoid osteoma. *A*, A computed tomography scan showing a small hypodense area with a central round density, the nidus *(arrow)*, which is surrounded by a large sclerotic zone. *B*, The large osteosclerotic area of the left tibial shaft that involves the greater part of the medullary canal. (From Grainger RG, Allison DJ, Dixon AK: Diagnostic Radiology: A Textbook of Medical Imaging, 4th ed. New York, Churchill Livingstone, 2001.)

Treatment typically consists of in situ fixation with one cannulated transphyseal screw placed perpendicular to the physis into the center of the femoral head.[136] Reduction of the slip before fixation is controversial, and it is associated with a significantly ($P < 0.001$) greater risk of osteonecrosis.[136] After pinning, patients are restricted from athletic activity until the growth plate is completely fused. Thereafter, the hardware is removed, and then the patient should wait an additional 2 to 3 months to allow bony healing across the pin site before the resumption of full athletic activity.[135]

Legg-Calvé-Perthes disease

Legg-Calvé-Perthes disease is a disorder of the capital femoral epiphysis in young children that is thought to be the result of a disruption of the blood supply of the growing femoral head. It most commonly occurs in children who are between 4 and 8 years old, but has been reported in children from 2 years of age to the late teenage years.[138,139] It is four to five times more common among males than females.[139] Patients typically present with a history of an intermittent, mildly symptomatic limp. Pain, when present, is usually related to activity and localized to the groin or referred to the anteromedial thigh or knee.[138] For this reason, any athlete who is less than 12 years old who presents with knee pain should have a thorough hip examination. Physical examination findings include limited hip range of motion, especially internal rotation and abduction.[138] Plain radiographs, including anteroposterior and frog-lateral views of both hips **(Figure 25.20),** are crucial for making the diagnosis.[138] Diagnosis typically warrants referral to a pediatric orthopedic surgeon for management and follow-up. In terms of athletics, if head involvement is more than 50%, most orthopedic surgeons will restrict high-impact athletic activity until the disease is well into the healing phase.[140]

Osteonecrosis of the femoral head

Osteonecrosis is bone death as a result of circulatory interruption. It most commonly occurs in the femoral head, in which case it presents as nonspecific groin or hip pain. This condition can occur in athletes, and it therefore must be considered in the differential diagnosis of pelvic pain in the athlete, especially in the presence of risk factors.[39] These risk factors include trauma (e.g., femoral neck fracture, hip dislocation, or hip subluxation), systemic corticosteroid use, alcohol abuse, sickle cell anemia, caisson disease, and a variety of hypercoagulable states. The physical examination is often unremarkable. Plain radiographs may show characteristic signs, including subchondral osteopenia, mottled sclerosis, subchondral collapse, and secondary degenerative changes, depending on the stage of the condition. Early in the course of the disease, plain radiographs may be unremarkable. MRI, which is very sensitive and specific for osteonecrosis, should be obtained if plain radiographs are normal and osteonecrosis is suspected on the basis of risk factors. Treatment depends on the stage of the disease and includes core decompression (with or without bone graft) during the early (precollapse) stages and total hip arthroplasty during the later (postcollapse) stages.

NONMUSCULOSKELETAL CAUSES

Pelvic floor dysfunction

Pelvic floor dysfunction is a poorly understood cause of pelvic pain that can be a serious impairment to the female athlete. The pelvic floor is a group of muscles that includes the coccygeus, the levator ani, the obturator internus, the adductor magnus, the piriformis, and the oblique abdominals.[141] These muscles act in coordination with musculoskeletal structures such as the hip joint, the lumbar spine, the sacroiliac joint, and the pubic symphysis as well as visceral structures such as the bladder, the vagina, the uterus, the ovaries, and the colon. A lack of balance and coordination among these numerous structures can cause pain, especially with voiding, defecation, intercourse, or menstruation.[141] The pain occurs in the region of the vagina, the rectum, the lower abdomen, the pubic symphysis, and the posterior pelvis.[141]

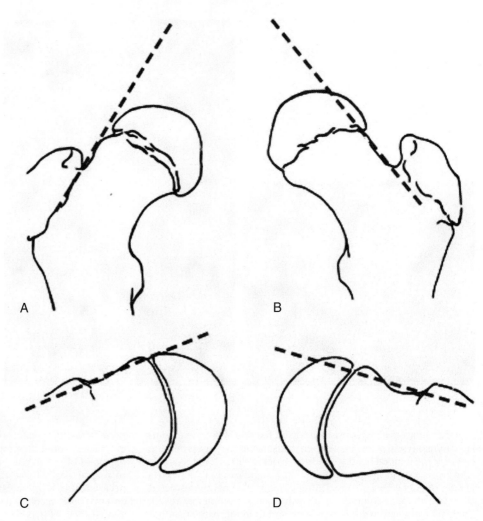

Figure 25.19 Slipped capital femoral epiphysis, anteroposterior view. A line superimposed on the superior femoral neck normally intersects part of the head (B and D are normal). With a slipped epiphysis, the line does not intersect the femoral head (A and C). Occasionally, the frog-leg view (C and D) is needed to show the slip. (Redrawn from Behrman RE, Kleigman R, Jenson HB: Nelson Textbook of Pediatrics, 17th ed. Philadelphia, WB Saunders, 2004.)

Pelvic floor dysfunction and pain can be the result of a primary muscle imbalance in the pelvic floor musculature or an increase in muscle tone in response to musculoskeletal abnormalities (e.g., hip osteoarthritis or local trauma) or visceral abnormalities (e.g., an ovarian cyst).[141] Evaluation for this dysfunction includes a manual examination of the pelvic floor and focal musculoskeletal and neurologic examinations.[141] Surface electromyography measurements are helpful for determining resting muscle activity. Treatment consists of physical therapy to address specific muscle imbalances; techniques such as myofascial release, postural education, biofeedback, and range-of-motion and strengthening exercises are used.[141]

Genitourinary causes

Although they are beyond the scope of this review, there are numerous urologic disorders that may present as groin pain in the athlete. Epididymitis is a clinical syndrome of pain, swelling, and inflammation in the epididymis that can present with testicular pain and swelling and, frequently, dysuria and urethral discharge.[2,24,142] Chronic prostatitis can present with pain, which most commonly localizes to the perineum, the suprapubic area, the penis, the testes, or the groin.[143] In addition, symptoms such as frequency, urgency, hesitancy, dysuria, and purulent discharge are also present.[143] A digital rectal examination of the prostate assists with the diagnosis and

should be included in the clinical evaluation of chronic groin pain.[2,24,143] The key for the sports medicine physician is to be aware that these conditions can cause groin pain in the athlete so that appropriate diagnosis and/or referral can be made.

General surgical cause: Inguinal hernia

Inguinal hernias are very common, and every athlete suffering from groin pain should be carefully examined to exclude this diagnosis. An inguinal hernia is located above and medial to the pubic tubercle.[13] The most common type of hernia is a direct inguinal hernia that, on physical examination, appears as a diffuse bulge at the internal ring, in the medial part of the inguinal canal.[13] An indirect inguinal hernia is congenital in origin, and it is caused by a failure of the processus vaginalis to close. Therefore, it appears at the external ring. Inguinal hernias result from weakness or a tear in the posterior wall of the inguinal canal. Patients with inguinal hernias typically present with groin pain and, often, a palpable mass.[20] The pain often radiates into the proximal thigh or the scrotum in males.[13] Activities that increase intra-abdominal pressure, such as Valsalva maneuvers and weight lifting, can cause or exacerbate the hernia. A careful physical examination to detect the presence of a hernia is essential. Maneuvers to increase intra-abdominal pressure, such as coughing or tensing the abdominal musculature, may produce a cough impulse or make the mass

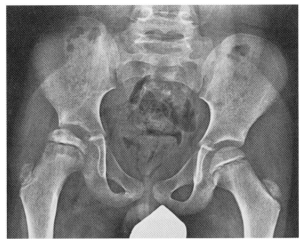

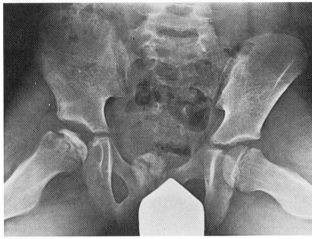

Figure 25.20 Legg-Calvé-Perthes disease, frontal *(A)* and frog-leg *(B)* views. Sclerosis and flattening of the right femoral head epiphysis are present, and the epiphysis and metaphysis show cystic changes. (From Johnson GA: Atlas of Emergency Radiology, 1st ed. Philadelphia, WB Saunders, 2001.)

more prominent.[13,20] Plain radiographs, if obtained, are unremarkable. Although MRI is not needed for diagnosis, it will show the inguinal hernia as an area of high signal on T1-weighted images within the inguinal canal.[10] The treatment of inguinal hernias is surgical herniorrhaphy via open or laparoscopic techniques.

PHYSICAL THERAPY: CORE STRENGTHENING

A discussion of groin and pelvic pain in the athlete would be incomplete without mentioning the role of preventive measures. Hip strength may be important for the prevention of groin injury, lower extremity injury, and lower back pain in athletes.[7,144] Tyler and colleagues[7] showed that adductor strengthening can decrease the incidence of adductor strains in professional hockey players. Nadler and colleagues[144] showed that there was a significant ($P = 0.04$) difference in the side-to-side symmetry of hip extensor strength in female athletes who reported lower extremity injury or back pain as compared with those who did not. Leetun and colleagues[145] reported that athletes who experienced an injury showed lower core stability measures than those who did not; these strength differences were most significant for hip abduction ($P = 0.04$) and external rotation ($P < 0.001$). Therefore, the concept of core strengthening has been proposed as a method to

condition athletes with the hope of preventing lower-extremity, groin, and back injuries.[144,145]

Anatomically, the core is defined as the musculature that surrounds the lumbopelvic region and that includes the abdominals anteriorly, the paraspinals and the gluteals posteriorly, the pelvic floor and the hip girdle musculature inferiorly, the hip abductors and the external rotators laterally, and the diaphragm superiorly.[146] These muscles act synergistically to maintain functional stability in the lumbopelvic region. Conceptually, the core is the anatomic and functional centerpiece and the powerhouse of the body; all motions are generated from the core and are translated to the extremities.[146]

The main emphasis of core strengthening is focused on muscular stabilization of the abdominal, paraspinal, and gluteal muscles to provide better stability and control for sporting activity. A typical core-strengthening program has recently been published.[146] Currently, core stability and its role in injury prevention is becoming increasingly popular as experience authenticates its benefits. Additional studies are needed to determine the role of core strengthening (if any) in the prevention of groin injuries in the athlete. In addition, studies will also be needed to establish sport- and gender-specific optimal training regimens.

CONCLUSION

The outcome of the treatment of hip and pelvic pain in athletes depends on a correct diagnosis. For athletes, correct diagnosis and effective treatment lead to less time missed from competition and earlier return to play. However, the diagnosis of pelvic pain can be problematic because of its many possible causes and the fact that symptoms are often vague and diffuse. In addition, many patients are found to have multiple causes of pelvic pain. Ekberg and colleagues[2] showed that more than 90% of patients with long-standing groin pain were found to have multiple diagnoses when examined by a multidisciplinary team of physicians. This fact underscores the importance of a multidisciplinary approach and of knowledge of the vast array of conditions that may cause pelvic pain in the athlete.

REFERENCES

1. Renstrom P, Peterson L: Groin injuries in athletes. Br J Sports Med 1980;14(1): 30-36.
2. Ekberg O, Persson NH, Abrahamsson PA, et al: Longstanding groin pain in athletes. A multidisciplinary approach. Sports Med 1988;6(1):56-61.
3. Lovell G: The diagnosis of chronic groin pain in athletes: a review of 189 cases. Aust J Sci Med Sport 1995;27(3):76-79.
4. Morelli V, Smith V: Groin injuries in athletes. Am Fam Physician 2001;64(8): 1405-1414.
5. Garrett WE Jr., Safran MR, Seaber AV, et al: Biomechanical comparison of stimulated and nonstimulated skeletal muscle pulled to failure. Am J Sports Med 1987;15(5):448-454.
6. Merrifield HH, Cowan RF: Groin strain injuries in ice hockey. J Sports Med 1973;1(2):41-42.
7. Tyler TF, Nicholas SJ, Campbell RJ, et al: The effectiveness of a preseason exercise program to prevent adductor muscle strains in professional ice hockey players. Am J Sports Med 2002;30(5):680-683.
8. Lynch SA, Renstrom PA: Groin injuries in sport: treatment strategies. Sports Med 1999;28(2):137-144.
9. Swain R, Snodgrass S: Managing groin pain: even when the cause is not obvious. Phys Sportsmed 1995;23(11):56-66.
10. Karlsson J, Jerre R: The use of radiography, magnetic resonance imaging, and ultrasound in the diagnosis of hip, pelvis, and groin injuries. Sports Med Arthrosc Rev 1997;5(4):268.
11. De Paulis F, Cacchio A, Michelini O, et al: Sports injuries in the pelvis and hip: diagnostic imaging. Eur J Radiol 1998;27(Suppl 1):S49-S59.
12. Fricker PA: Management of groin pain in athletes. Br J Sports Med 1997;31(2): 97-100.
13. Lacroix VJ: A complete approach to groin pain. Phys Sportsmed 2000;28(1):66-86.

14. Garrett WE Jr: Muscle strain injuries. Am J Sports Med 1996;24(6 Suppl):S2-S8.
15. Scopp JM, Moorman CT. III: Acute athletic trauma to the hip and pelvis. Orthop Clin North Am 2002;33(3):555-563.
16. Glazer JL, Hosey RG: Soft-tissue injuries of the lower extremity. Prim Care 2004;31(4):1005-1024.
17. Hughes C IV, Hasselman CT, Best TM, et al: Incomplete, intrasubstance strain injuries of the rectus femoris muscle. Am J Sports Med 1995;23(4):500-506.
18. Morelli V, Weaver V: Groin injuries and groin pain in athletes: part 1. Prim Care 2005;32(1):163-183.
19. Brown TD, Brunet ME: Adult thigh. In DeLee JC, Drez D Jr, Miller MD (eds): DeLee & Drez's Orthopaedic Sports Medicine: Principles and Practice, 2nd ed. Philadelphia, WB Saunders, 2003, pp 1481-1523.
20. Gilmore J: Groin pain in the soccer athlete: fact, fiction, and treatment. Clin Sports Med 1998;17(4):787-793.
21. Mozes M, Papa MZ, Zweig A, et al: Iliopsoas injury in soccer players. Br J Sports Med 1985;19(3):168-170.
22. Boyd KT, Peirce NS, Batt ME: Common hip injuries in sport. Sports Med 1997;24(4):273-288.
23. Anderson K, Strickland SM, Warren R: Hip and groin injuries in athletes. Am J Sports Med 2001;29(4):521-523.
24. Karlsson J, Sward L, Kalebo P, et al: Chronic groin injuries in athletes. Recommendations for treatment and rehabilitation. Sports Med 1994;17(2): 141-148.
25. Martens MA, Hansen L, Mulier JC: Adductor tendinitis and musculus rectus abdominis tendopathy. Am J Sports Med 1987;15(4):353-356.
26. Pomeranz SJ, Heidt RS Jr: MR imaging in the prognostication of hamstring injury. Work in progress. Radiology 1993;189(3):897-900.
27. Weinstein RN, Kraushaar BS, Fulkerson JP: Adductor tendinosis in a professional hockey player. Orthopedics 1998;21(7):809-810.
28. Akermark C, Johansson C: Tenotomy of the adductor longus tendon in the treatment of chronic groin pain in athletes. Am J Sports Med 1992;20(6):640-643.
29. Verrall GM, Slavotinek JP, Barnes PG, et al: Diagnostic and prognostic value of clinical findings in 83 athletes with posterior thigh injury: comparison of clinical findings with magnetic resonance imaging documentation of hamstring muscle strain. Am J Sports Med 2003;31(6):969-973.
30. Woods C, Hawkins RD, Maltby S, et al: The Football Association Medical Research Programme: an audit of injuries in professional football—analysis of hamstring injuries. Br J Sports Med 2004;38(1):36-41.
31. Dadebo B, White J, George KP: A survey of flexibility training protocols and hamstring strains in professional football clubs in England. Br J Sports Med 2004;38(4):388-394.
32. Gabbe BJ, Finch CF, Bennell KL, et al: Risk factors for hamstring injuries in community level Australian football. Br J Sports Med 2005;39(2):106-110.
33. Seward H, Orchard J, Hazard H, et al: Football injuries in Australia at the elite level. Med J Aust 1993;159(5):298-301.
34. Orava S, Kujala UM: Rupture of the ischial origin of the hamstring muscles. Am J Sports Med 1995;23(6):702-705.
35. Kujala UM, Orava S, Karpakka J, et al: Ischial tuberosity apophysitis and avulsion among athletes. Int J Sports Med 1997;18(2):149-155.
36. Worrell TW: Factors associated with hamstring injuries. An approach to treatment and preventative measures. Sports Med 1994;17(5):338-345.
37. Clanton TO, Coupe KJ: Hamstring strains in athletes: diagnosis and treatment. J Am Acad Orthop Surg 1998;6(4):237-248.
38. Askling C, Karlsson J, Thorstensson A: Hamstring injury occurrence in elite soccer players after preseason strength training with eccentric overload. Scand J Med Sci Sports 2003;13(4):244-250.
39. Nuccion SL, Hunter DM, Finerman GAM: Hip and pelvis. Section A: Hip and pelvis: adult. In DeLee JC, Drez D Jr, Miller MD (eds): DeLee & Drez's Orthopaedic Sports Medicine: Principles and Practice, 2nd ed. Philadelphia, WB Saunders, 2003, pp 1443-1463.
40. Waters PM, Millis MB: Hip and pelvic injuries in the young athlete. Clin Sports Med 1988;7(3):513-526.
41. Metzmaker JN, Pappas AM: Avulsion fractures of the pelvis. Am J Sports Med 1985;13(5):349-358.
42. Roos HP: Hip pain in sport. Sports Med Arthrosc Rev 1997;5(4):292-300.
43. Sallay PI, Friedman RL, Coogan PG, et al: Hamstring muscle injuries among water skiers. Functional outcome and prevention. Am J Sports Med 1996;24(2):130-136.
44. Schlonsky J, Olix ML: Functional disability following avulsion fracture of the ischial epiphysis. Report of two cases. J Bone Joint Surg Tm 1972;54A(3):641-644.
45. LeBlanc KE, LeBlanc KA: Groin pain in athletes. Hernia 2003;7(2):68-71.
46. Scudese VA: Traumatic anterior hip redislocation. A case report. Clin Orthop Relat Res 1972;88:60-63.
47. Byrd JWT: Labral lesions: an elusive source of hip pain case reports and literature review. Arthroscopy 1996;12(5):603-612.
48. Narvani AA, Tsiridis E, Tai CC, et al: Acetabular labrum and its tears. Br J Sports Med 2003;37(3):207-211.
49. Hase T, Ueo T: Acetabular labral tear: arthroscopic diagnosis and treatment. Arthroscopy 1999;15(2):138-141.
50. Fitzgerald RH Jr: Acetabular labrum tears. Diagnosis and treatment. Clin Orthop Relat Res 1995;311:60-68.
51. Dorrell JH, Catterall A: The torn acetabular labrum. J Bone Joint Surg 1986;68B(3):400-403.
52. Farjo LA, Glick JM, Sampson TG: Hip arthroscopy for acetabular labral tears. Arthroscopy 1999;15(2):132-137.
53. Ikeda T, Awaya G, Suzuki S, et al: Torn acetabular labrum in young patients. Arthroscopic diagnosis and management. J Bone Joint Surg Br 1988;70B:13-16.
54. Suzuki S, Awaya G, Okada Y, et al: Arthroscopic diagnosis of ruptured acetabular labrum. Acta Orthop Scand 1986;57(6):513-515.
55. Mitchell B, McCrory P, Brukner P, et al: Hip joint pathology: clinical presentation and correlation between magnetic resonance arthrography, ultrasound, and arthroscopic findings in 25 consecutive cases. Clin J Sport Med 2003;13(3):152-156.
56. Cotten A, Boutry N, Demondion X, et al: Acetabular labrum: MRI in asymptomatic volunteers. J Comput Assist Tomogr 1998;22(1):1-7.
57. Czerny C, Hofmann S, Neuhold A, et al: Lesions of the acetabular labrum: accuracy of MR imaging and MR arthrography in detection and staging. Radiology 1996;200(1):225-230.
58. Edwards DJ, Lomas D, Villar RN: Diagnosis of the painful hip by magnetic resonance imaging and arthroscopy. J Bone Joint Surg Br 1995;77B(3):374-376.
59. Czerny C, Hofmann S, Urban M, et al: MR arthrography of the adult acetabular capsular-labral complex: correlation with surgery and anatomy. AJR Am J Roentgenol 1999;173(2):345-349.
60. Mintz DN, Hooper T, Connell D, et al: Magnetic resonance imaging of the hip: detection of labral and chondral abnormalities using noncontrast imaging. Arthroscopy 2005;21(4):385-393.
61. Byrd JWT, Jones KS: Diagnostic accuracy of clinical assessment, magnetic resonance imaging, magnetic resonance arthrography, and intra-articular injection in hip arthroscopy patients. Am J Sports Med 2004;32(7):1668-1674.
62. Frost A, Bauer M: Skier's hip—a new clinical entity? Proximal femur fractures sustained in cross-country skiing. J Orthop Trauma 1991;5(1):47-50.
63. Hackney RG: The sports hernia: a cause of chronic groin pain. Br J Sports Med 1993;27(1):58-62.
64. Orchard JW, Read JW, Neophyton J, et al: Groin pain associated with ultrasound finding of inguinal canal posterior wall deficiency in Australian Rules footballers. Br J Sports Med 1998;32(2):134-139.
65. Larson CM, Lohnes JH: Surgical management of athletic pubalgia. Oper Tech Sports Med 2002;10(4):228-232.
66. Malycha P, Lovell G: Inguinal surgery in athletes with chronic groin pain: the "sportsman's" hernia. Aust N Z J Surg 1992;62(2):123-125.
67. Meyers WC, Foley DP, Garrett WE, et al: Management of severe lower abdominal or inguinal pain in high-performance athletes. Am J Sports Med 2000;28(1):2-8.
68. Van Der Donckt K, Steenbrugge F, Van Den Abbeele K, et al: Bassini's hernial repair and adductor longus tenotomy in the treatment of chronic groin pain in athletes. Acta Orthop Belg 2003;69(1):35-41.
69. Polglase AL, Frydman GM, Farmer KC: Inguinal surgery for debilitating chronic groin pain in athletes. Med J Aust 1991;155(10):674-677.
70. Schuricht A, Haut E, Wetzler M: Surgical options in the treatment of sports hernia. Oper Tech Sports Med 2002;10(4):224-227.
71. Simonet WT, Saylor H. III, Sim L: Abdominal wall muscle tears in hockey players. Int J Sports Med 1995;16(2):126-128.
72. Taylor DC, Meyers WC, Moylan JA, et al: Abdominal musculature abnormalities as a cause of groin pain in athletes. Inguinal hernias and pubalgia. Am J Sports Med 1991;19(3):239-242.
73. Kluin J, den Hoed PT, van Linschoten R, et al: Endoscopic evaluation and treatment of groin pain in the athlete. Am J Sports Med 2004;32(4):944-949.
74. Joesting DR: Diagnosis and treatment of sportsman's hernia. Curr Sports Med Rep 2002;1(2):121-124.
75. Ingoldby CJH: Laparoscopic and conventional repair of groin disruption in sportsmen. Br J Surg 1997;84(2):213-215.
76. Ekberg O, Sjoberg S, Westlin N: Sports-related groin pain: evaluation with MR imaging. Eur Radiol 1996;6(1):52-55.
77. Kesek P, Ekberg O, Westlin N: Herniographic findings in athletes with unclear groin pain. Acta Radiol 2002;43(6):603-608.
78. Ekberg O: Complications after herniography in adults. AJR Am J Roentgenol 1983;140(3):491-495.
79. Hamlin JA, Kahn AM: Herniography: a review of 333 herniograms. Am Surg 1998;64(10):965-969.
80. Sutcliffe JR, Taylor OM, Ambrose NS, et al: The use, value and safety of herniography. Clin Radiol 1999;54(7):468-472.
81. Azurin DJ, Go LS, Schuricht A, et al: Endoscopic preperitoneal herniorrhaphy in professional athletes with groin pain. J Laparoendosc Adv Surg Tech A 1997;7(1):7-12.
82. Srinivasan A, Schuricht A: Long-term follow-up of laparoscopic preperitoneal hernia repair in professional athletes. J Laparoendosc Adv Surg Tech A 2002;12(2):101-106.
83. Irshad K, Feldman LS, Lavoie C, et al: Operative management of "hockey groin syndrome": 12 years of experience in National Hockey League players. Surgery 2001;130(4):759-766.

84. Lacroix VJ, Kinnear DG, Mulder DS, et al: Lower abdominal pain syndrome in national hockey league players: a report of 11 cases. Clin J Sport Med 1998;8(1):5-9.

85. Fricker PA, Taunton JE, Ammann W: Osteitis pubis in athletes. Infection, inflammation or injury? Sports Med 1991;12(4):266-279.

86. Vitanzo PC Jr, McShane JM: Osteitis pubis: solving a perplexing problem. Phys Sportsmed 1996;29(7):33-48.

87. Holt MA, Keene JS, Graf BK, et al: Treatment of osteitis pubis in athletes. Results of corticosteroid injections. Am J Sports Med 1995;23(5):601-606.

88. Williams JGP: Limitation of hip joint movement as a factor in traumatic osteitis pubis. Br J Sports Med 1978;12(3):129-133.

89. Grace JN, Sim FH, Shives TC, et al: Wedge resection of the symphysis pubis for the treatment of osteitis pubis. J Bone Joint Surg Am 1989;71A:358-364.

90. Walheim G, Olerud S, Ribbe T: Mobility of the pubic symphysis: measurements by an electromechanical method. Acta Orthop Scand 1984;55:203-208.

91. Tuite MJ, DeSmet AA: MRI of selected sports injuries: muscle tears, groin pain, and osteochondritis dissecans. Semin Ultrasound CT MRI 1994;15(5):318-340.

92. Olerud S, Grevsten S: Chronic pubic symphysiolysis. A case report. J Bone Joint Surg Am 1974;56A(4):799-782.

93. Johnston CAM, Wiley JP, Lindsay DM, et al: Iliopsoas bursitis and tendinitis. A review. Sports Med 1998;25(4):271-283.

94. Jacobson T, Allen WC: Surgical correction of the snapping iliopsoas tendon. Am J Sports Med 1990;18(5):470-474.

95. Zoltan DJ, Clancy WG Jr, Keene JS: A new operative approach to snapping hip and refractory trochanteric bursitis in athletes. Am J Sports Med 1986;14:201-204.

96. Brignall CG, Stainsby GD: The snapping hip. Treatment by Z-plasty. J Bone Joint Surg Br 1991;73B(2):253-254.

97. Janzen DL, Partridge E, Logan PM, et al: The snapping hip: clinical and imaging findings in transient subluxation of the iliopsoas tendon. Can Assoc Radiol J 1996;47(3):202-208.

98. Taylor GR, Clarke NMP: Surgical release of the 'snapping iliopsoas tendon'. J Bone Joint Surg Br 1995;77B(6):881-883.

99. Brukner P, Khan K: Lateral, medial, and posterior knee pain. In Brukner P, Kahn K (eds): Clinical Sports Medicine, 2nd ed. Sydney, Australia, McGraw-Hill, 2001, pp 494-507.

100. McBryde AM Jr: Stress fractures in runners. Clin Sports Med 1985;4(4):737-752.

101. Johnson AW, Weiss CB Jr, Stento K, et al: Stress fractures of the sacrum. An atypical cause of low back pain in the female athlete. Am J Sports Med 2001;29(4):498-508.

102. Fullerton LR Jr, Snowdy HA: Femoral neck stress fractures. Am J Sports Med 1988;16(4):365-377.

103. Johansson C, Ekenman I, Tornkvist H, et al: Stress fractures of the femoral neck in athletes. The consequence of a delay in diagnosis. Am J Sports Med 1990;18(5):524-528.

104. Shin AY, Morin WD, Gorman JD, et al: The superiority of magnetic resonance imaging in differentiating the cause of hip pain in endurance athletes. Am J Sports Med 1996;24(2):168-176.

105. Devas MB: Stress fractures of the femoral neck. J Bone Joint Surg Br 1965;47B(4):728-738.

106. Pavlov H, Nelson TL, Warren RF, et al: Stress fractures of the pubic ramus. A report of twelve cases. J Bone Joint Surg Am 1982;64A(7):1020-1025.

107. Noakes TD, Smith JA, Lindenberg G, et al: Pelvic stress fractures in long distance runners. Am J Sports Med 1985;13(2):120-123.

108. Atwell EA, Jackson DW: Stress fractures of the sacrum in runners. Two case reports. Am J Sports Med 1991;19(5):531-533.

109. McFarland EG, Giangarra C: Sacral stress fractures in athletes. Clin Orthop Relat Res 1996;329:240-243.

110. Cooper KL, Beabout JW, Swee RG: Insufficiency fractures of the sacrum. Radiology 1985;156(1):15-20.

111. Featherstone T: Magnetic resonance imaging in the diagnosis of sacral stress fracture. Br J Sports Med 1999;33(4):276-277.

112. Wiley JJ: Traumatic osteitis pubis: the gracilis syndrome. Am J Sports Med 1983;11:360-363.

113. Vingard E, Alfredsson L, Goldie I, et al: Sports and osteoarthrosis of the hip. An epidemiologic study. Am J Sports Med 1993;21(2):195-200.

114. Klunder KB, Rud B, Hansen J: Osteoarthritis of the hip and knee joint in retired football players. Acta Orthop Scand 1980;51(6):925-927.

115. Lindberg H, Roos H, Gardsell P: Prevalence of coxarthrosis in former soccer players. 286 players compared with matched controls. Acta Orthop Scand 1993;64(2):165-167.

116. Starling JR, Harms BA, Schroeder ME, et al: Diagnosis and treatment of genitofemoral and ilioinguinal entrapment neuralgia. Surgery 1987;102(4):581-586.

117. Sandring S, Collins P, Wigley C: Nervous system. In Sandring S, Ellis H, Healy JC, et al (eds): Gray's Anatomy: The Anatomical Basis of Clinical Practice, 39th ed. New York, Elsevier, 2005, pp 43-67.

118. Knockaert DC, D'Heygere FG, Bobbaers HJ: Ilioinguinal nerve entrapment: a little-known cause of iliac fossa pain. Postgrad Med J 1989;65(767):632-635.

119. Bradshaw C, McCrory P, Bell S, et al: Obturator nerve entrapment. A cause of groin pain in athletes. Am J Sports Med 1997;25(3):402-408.

120. Bradshaw C, McCrory P: Obturator nerve entrapment. Clin J Sport Med 1997;7(3):217-219.

121. Brukner P, Bradshaw C, McCrory P: Obturator neuropathy: a cause of exercise-related groin pain. Phys Sportsmed 1999;27(5):62-73.

122. Nahabedian MY, Dellon AL: Meralgia paresthetica: etiology, diagnosis, and outcome of surgical decompression. Ann Plast Surg 1995;35(6):590-594.

123. Williams PH, Trzil KP: Management of meralgia paresthetica. J Neurosurg 1991;74(1):76-80.

124. Ziprin P, Williams P, Foster ME: External oblique aponeurosis nerve entrapment as a cause of groin pain in the athlete. Br J Surg 1999;86(4):566-568.

125. Filler AG, Haynes J, Jordan SE, et al: Sciatica of nondisc origin and piriformis syndrome: diagnosis by magnetic resonance neurography and interventional magnetic resonance imaging with outcome study of resulting treatment. J Neurosurg Spine 2005;2(2):99-115.

126. Rodrigue T, Hardy RW: Diagnosis and treatment of piriformis syndrome. Neurosurg Clin N Am 2001;12(2):311-319.

127. Lee EY, Margherita AJ, Gierada DS, et al: MRI of piriformis syndrome. AJR Am J Roentgenol 2004;183(1):63-64.

128. Foster MR: Piriformis syndrome. Orthopedics 2002;25(8):821-825.

129. Puranen J, Orava S: The hamstring syndrome. A new diagnosis of gluteal sciatic pain. Am J Sports Med 1988;16(5):517-521.

130. Weiss BD: Clinical syndromes associated with bicycle seats. Clin Sports Med 1994;13(1):175-186.

131. Goodson JD: Pudendal neuritis from biking [letter]. N Engl J Med 1981;304(6):365.

132. Antolak SJ Jr, Hough DM, Pawlina W, et al: Anatomical basis of chronic pelvic pain syndrome: the ischial spine and pudendal nerve entrapment. Med Hypotheses 2002;59(3):349-353.

133. Ahlfeld SK, Makley JT, Derosa GP, et al: Osteoid osteoma of the femoral neck in the young athlete. Am J Sports Med 1990;18(3):271-276.

134. Greenspan A: Benign bone-forming lesions: osteoma, osteoid osteoma, and osteoblastoma. Clinical, imaging, pathologic, and differential considerations. Skeletal Radiol 1993;22(7):485-500.

135. Kehl DK: Slipped capital femoral epiphysis. In Morrissy RT, Weinstein SL (eds): Lovell and Winter's Pediatric Orthopaedics, 5th ed. Philadelphia, Lippincott Williams & Wilkins, 2001, pp 999-1033.

136. Carney BT, Weinstein SL, Noble J: Long-term follow-up of slipped capital femoral epiphysis. J Bone Joint Surg Am 1991;73A(5):667-674.

137. Loder RT, Richards BS, Shapiro PS, et al: Acute slipped capital femoral epiphysis: the importance of physeal stability. J Bone Joint Surg Am 1993;75A(8):1134-1140.

138. Weinstein SL: Legg-Calvé-Perthes syndrome. In Morrissy RT, Weinstein SL (eds): Lovell and Winter's Pediatric Orthopaedics, 6th ed. Philadelphia, Lippincott Williams & Wilkins, 2006, pp 1039-1083.

139. Wynne-Davies R, Gormley J: The aetiology of Perthes' disease. Genetic, epidemiological and growth factors in 310 Edinburgh and Glasgow patients. J Bone Joint Surg Br 1978;60B(1):6-14.

140. Millis MB, Kocher M: Hip and pelvis. Section B: Hip and pelvic injuries in the young athlete. In DeLee JC, Drez D Jr, Miller MD (eds): DeLee & Drez's Orthopaedic Sports Medicine: Principles and Practice, 2nd ed. Philadelphia, WB Saunders, 2003, pp 1463-1479.

141. Prather H: Pelvis and sacral dysfunction in sports and exercise. Phys Med Rehabil Clin N Am 2000;11(4):805-836.

142. Berger RE, Lee JC: Sexually transmitted diseases: the classic diseases. In Walsh PC, Retik AB, Vanghan ED Jr, et al (eds): Campbell's Urology, 8th ed. Philadelphia, WB Saunders, 2002, pp 671-691.

143. Nickel JC: Prostatitis and related conditions. In Walsh PC, Retik AB, Vanghan ED Jr, et al (eds): Campbell's Urology, 8th ed. Philadelphia, WB Saunders, 2002, pp 603-630.

144. Nadler SF, Malanga GA, DePrince M, et al: The relationship between lower extremity injury, low back pain, and hip muscle strength in male and female collegiate athletes. Clin J Sports Med 2000;10(2):89-97.

145. Leetun DT, Ireland ML, Willson JD, et al: Core stability measures as risk factors for lower extremity injury in athletes. Med Sci Sports Exerc 2004;36(6):926-934.

146. Bliss LS, Teeple P: Core stability: the centerpiece of any training program. Curr Sports Med Rep 2005;4(3):179-183.

Knee Injuries

Andrew T. McDonald, MD, and Lyndon B. Gross, MD, PhD

KEY POINTS

· Anterior cruciate ligament tears are usually the result of a noncontact, twisting, or landing mechanism on a planted leg.

· Meniscal tears in the younger population often require surgical repair, whereas degenerative meniscal tears in an older population often improve with rehabilitation.

· Multiligamentous knee injuries should be referred to an orthopedic surgeon who is skilled in the treatment of such conditions.

· Patellofemoral pain must be evaluated in the context of finding anatomic and functional factors that may be contributing to the pain.

· Injury to the popliteus muscle is commonly missed by both examination and magnetic resonance imaging, but it can be easily identified with the use of special tests such as the Garrick test and the shoe removal test.

INTRODUCTION

The knee joint is the largest joint in the human body, and it is made up of three independent articulations: the patellofemoral articulation, the medial tibiofemoral articulation, and the lateral tibiofemoral articulation. Injury of the proximal tibiofibular articulation may also present as knee complaints, and it will be discussed in this chapter. Knee pain is one of the most common complaints reported in sports medicine clinics. A survey of National Collegiate Athletic Association member institutions reported a knee injury rate of 1 per every 1000 athlete encounters (with an athlete encounter being either a practice or a game).[1] Because the knee is a weight-bearing joint, injury to the knee has a significant impact on participation in all sports as well as on activities of daily living. Knee injuries can be broadly classified into acute and chronic injuries. Each type of injury has special considerations regarding predisposing risk factors and mechanisms of injury. This chapter will also discuss specific considerations involving the knee of a pediatric athlete.

MECHANISM OF INJURY

Because of the potentially serious acute and chronic morbidity of knee injuries, several studies have attempted to elucidate the extrinsic and intrinsic factors that lead to knee injuries. Extrinsic factors include shoe wear, training surface conditions, and training regimen; intrinsic factors include ligamentous laxity, decreased muscle flexibility, muscle weakness, and foot shape.

The majority of studies of acute knee injuries have concentrated on athletes participating in soccer and American football.[2] One extrinsic factor that has been studied in American football players is shoe type. During the 1970s, Torg and Quedenfeld[3] found a decreased number of knee and ankle injuries among high school football athletes using a "soccer style" shoe that had an increased number of cleats that were wider and shorter than those traditionally used. In response to these findings and the subsequent measurement of torque forces, the National High School Athletic Federation and the National Collegiate Athletic Association implemented regulations for cleat size and length.[2]

The National Football League performed a study comparing athletic injuries on natural grass and artificial turf during the 1980 through 1989 seasons and found that artificial turf accounted for an additional 36 knee injuries; however, only 11% of injuries were anterior cruciate ligament (ACL) injuries that necessitated surgery.[3]

Runners often develop overuse injuries as a result of wearing the improper shoe for their respective foot type or from failing to change to newer shoes as the mid sole of the older shoe loses its ability to absorb force. Chronic injuries may develop as a result of training on hard surfaces, running on uneven surfaces such as hills or sand, or running on the same banked edge of a road or track.

Overuse injuries tend to occur within the first few weeks of starting or significantly increasing the intensity of a training regimen. Injuries may also occur as athletes make the transition from high school to the collegiate level and the intensity of training increases. Athletes should be cautioned to gradually increase the level and duration of their training activities.

Benign hypermobility syndrome and its associated generalized ligamentous laxity have been associated with several overuse injuries, including patellofemoral pain syndrome. By contrast, several studies have shown that benign hypermobility syndrome has no relationship with ligamentous laxity in football players or with the incidence of knee ligament injuries.[2]

Weakness of the core (abdominal, paraspinous, and buttock) musculature can lead to an instability that may necessitate increased recruitment and loading of the knee. Quadriceps weakness is frequently implicated in knee overuse injuries, and it is also a sequelae of acute knee effusions. Decreased flexibility of hip flexors, hamstrings, iliotibial bands (ITBs), and calf muscles may increase the knee load and precipitate overuse injury. Atypical foot shape, pes planus, and pes cavus may predispose an athlete to knee injuries.

ACUTE KNEE INJURIES

The majority of acute knee injuries tend to be ligamentous and meniscal tears, osteochondral fractures, and patellar dislocations. Many cases of ligamentous injury to the knee occur when the foot is fixed to the ground as part of a closed kinetic chain. A force applied to the knee, either internally or externally, may exceed the elastic limits of the supporting knee ligaments.[2]

Ligamentous injury
Anterior cruciate ligament injury
The ACL is the primary restraint of anterior translation of the tibia on the femur and a secondary restraint of tibial rotation.[4] It arises from the posteromedial aspect of the intercondylar notch of the lateral femoral condyle, and it attaches directly in front of the intercondylar eminence of the tibia and just medial to the anterior horn of the lateral meniscus. The direction of putting one's hands in the front pockets serves as a simple mnemonic for the orientation of the ACL of the respective knee.

Clinical presentation Athletes typically present with the sudden onset of knee pain, often after a low-energy, noncontact mechanism such as a sudden change in direction while running, hyperflexion or hyperextension, or while initiating or landing a jump

(Figure 26.1). A "pop" may be heard at the time of injury.[2] These athletes may initially be unable to bear weight without assistance. Knee swelling commonly occurs within the first several hours. After an acute ACL injury, athletes will be unable to return to play that same day, although they may attempt to return to sport days or weeks later. An associated meniscal tear has been reported in up to 90% of acute ACL tears.[2] The lateral meniscus is more commonly injured in conjunction with acute ACL tears. Patients who present in a delayed fashion will commonly complain of a recurrent sensation of instability or giving way.

Diagnosis The most reliable examination can be performed shortly after the injury occurs and before the development of an effusion. Examination by means of the Lachman test can establish whether there is an ACL injury. The anterior drawer test is less accurate.[5] Both tests may be falsely negative in patients who are in significant pain and are unable to relax their hamstring musculature. A positive pivot shift is pathognomonic for ACL deficiency, but it is often only noted in the anesthetized patient who is no longer guarding.[6] Plain radiographs may show a bony avulsion of the anterior tibial intercondylar eminence, especially among children between the ages of 8 and 14 years. Alternatively, a lateral capsular bony avulsion (Segond fracture) may rarely be seen lateral to the tibia at the level of the joint; this is highly suggestive of an associated ACL rupture **(Figure 26.2).** Magnetic resonance imaging (MRI) is indicated to confirm the diagnosis of an ACL tear and to evaluate for concomitant injuries such as meniscal tears and osteochondral lesions **(Figure 26.3).**

Treatment The initial management of the suspected injury includes rest, ice, and compression to decrease swelling and crutches as necessary for weight bearing. The use of a knee immobilizer is not routinely indicated, and it may complicate

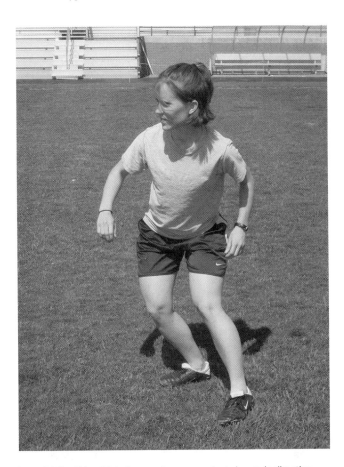

Figure 26.1 This athlete has made a noncontact change in direction as a possible mechanism for anterior cruciate ligament injury.

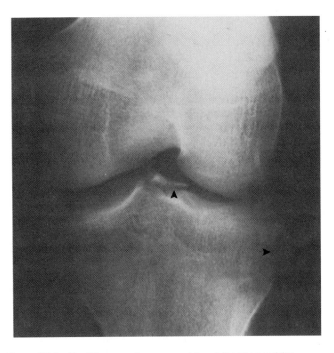

Figure 26.2 The *thin arrow* shows an avulsion of the intercondylar eminence. The *thicker arrow* shows the avulsion of the lateral capsule (Segond fracture). Both fracture patterns are indicative of an anterior cruciate ligament tear. (From DeLee JC, Drez D Jr, Miller MD [eds]: DeLee & Drez's Orthopedic Sports Medicine: Principles and Practice, 2nd ed. Philadelphia, WB Saunders, 2003.)

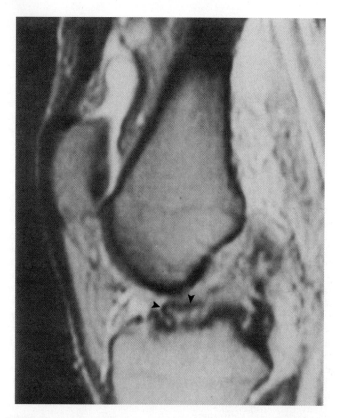

Figure 26.3 The *arrows* show the remnants of the anterior cruciate ligament, which has torn from its origin in the intercondylar notch. (From DeLee JC, Drez D Jr, Miller MD [eds]: DeLee & Drez's Orthopedic Sports Medicine: Principles and Practice, 2nd ed. Philadelphia, WB Saunders, 2003.)

rehabilitation efforts. Although there is no evidence that ACL reconstruction decreases the risk of developing osteoarthritis or that it is necessary for a return to activities of daily living, referral to an orthopedic surgeon should be considered for athletes or active individuals who wish to return to high-demand sports that require cutting or pivoting skills. Individuals who complain of recurrent instability or subluxation should either be referred for ACL reconstruction or fitted for a derotational brace. Immediate orthopedic consultation is not necessary for an uncomplicated ACL tear because reconstruction is typically delayed until 3 to 6 weeks after the injury in an effort to avoid the arthrofibrosis associated with performing surgery before the resolution of an acute hemarthrosis. Presurgical physical therapy to normalize the range of motion and to strengthen the quadriceps may provide a better postoperative outcome.

Return to play The ultimate return-to-play decision is made at the discretion of the physician in consultation with the athlete, but sports participation typically occurs no sooner than 6 to 9 months from the time of the surgery. The team physician should confirm that the range of motion has normalized and that the strength is similar to that of the uninjured side during a pre-participation evaluation. The athlete should be able to complete a progression of sport-specific agility drills without pain or instability before a return to competition.

Controversies Perhaps no greater controversy exists regarding the management of knee injuries than whether a bone–patella–bone autograft, a hamstring autograft, or a cadaveric allograft in the surgical reconstruction yields improved operative results. This debate is beyond the scope of this chapter.

Posterior cruciate ligament injury

The posterior cruciate ligament (PCL) has a broad femoral origin at the posterolateral aspect of the medial condyle, and it inserts posteriorly in a sulcus below the articular surface of the tibia.[2] It functions as the primary restraint of posterior translation and as a secondary restraint of external rotation of the tibia.[7] Injuries tend to be isolated to the PCL; however, when associated injuries do occur, it is the posterolateral corner structures (PLCS) of the knee (the lateral collateral ligament, the popliteus, the popliteofibular ligament, and the arcuate ligament) that are involved. Injury to the PLCS will increase the posterior laxity of the knee.[7]

Clinical presentation The athlete often presents with the acute onset of knee pain after either a hyperextension injury, a posteriorly directed trauma to the anterior aspect of the proximal tibia, or a hyperflexion injury with the ankle plantarflexed[8] **(Figure 26.4).** A fall onto a flexed knee with the ankle dorsiflexed often causes the force to be transmitted through the patella and distal femur, thus protecting the PCL.[2] Patients with combined PCL/PLCS injury are more likely to complain of knee instability with ambulation.

Diagnosis Knee effusion and tenderness to palpation may be most prominent in the popliteal fossa. Hyperextension of the knee may be noted as compared with the uninjured leg. Flexion of the knee to 90 degrees may elicit posterior sag of the tibia on the femur (Godfrey test). It is important to recognize the posterior sag of the tibia and not use this as a starting point for a Lachman's or anterior drawer test, thus yielding a false-positive test for ACL injury. Excessive posterior translation and a soft end point are

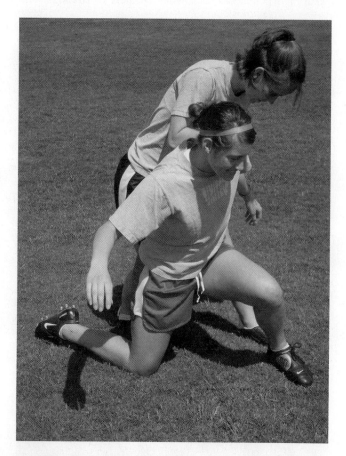

Figure 26.4 This athlete has her right knee in a hyperflexed position with the ankle in plantarflexion, which is a possible mechanism for posterior cruciate ligament injury.

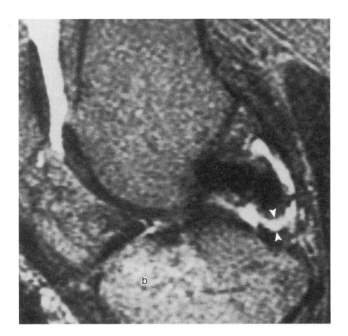

Figure 26.5 The *arrows* note the tear of the posterior cruciate ligament from its base. The defect has been replaced with hemorrhage. (From DeLee JC, Drez D Jr, Miller MD [eds]: DeLee & Drez's Orthopedic Sports Medicine: Principles and Practice, 2nd ed. Philadelphia, WB Saunders, 2003.)

noted on a posterior drawer test. More than 10 mm of translation with the tibial plateau displaced posterior to the condyles constitutes a grade III injury, and it is indicative of a complete tear of the PCL; PLCS injury should be highly suspected in these cases.[2] Plain radiographs may reveal an associated bony avulsion from the proximal tibia. In all suspected PCL injuries, the integrity of the PLCS should also be assessed with the dial test at 30 and 90 degrees of flexion with the patient in the supine/prone position (see Chapter 13). Excessive external rotation of the tibia as compared with the contralateral side is indicative of associated injury to the PLCS. MRI has greater than 95% sensitivity for detecting PCL tears, and it also helps to determine the precise location and degree of the tear[9] **(Figure 26.5).**

Treatment The initial treatment of grade I and II injuries consists of placing the patient in a hinged knee brace and beginning early quadriceps strengthening. With partial tears, range of motion can be advanced as tolerated, and rehabilitation should focus on maintaining quadriceps function.

The initial treatment of isolated grade III injuries consists of knee immobilization in extension for 2 to 4 weeks because of the high risk of occult injuries to the PLCS.[10] Ice and compression stockings are used to minimize swelling. Crutches should be used until the patient is able to ambulate without a limp. Range-of-motion and quadriceps-strengthening exercises may begin after immobilization. Patients often need 3 months of rehabilitation before they are able to perform a sports-specific agility drill progression without pain or instability. Isolated acute PCL injuries (including grade III) tend to do well with conservative treatment, with 60% of athletes able to return to preinjury levels of competition[11] (LOE: D).

Controversies There is debate among the orthopedic community regarding which (if any) PCL injuries should be repaired or reconstructed. It has been difficult to identify prognostic factors to predict outcomes; however, more evidence is showing that chronic PCL injuries will have a variable progression toward articular

degeneration.[12] Avulsion fractures, associated PLCS injury, and grade III injury have been advocated as indications for early primary repair or reconstruction by some orthopedic surgeons.[2] Because these indications are controversial, early referral to a physician who has experience with PCL injuries is recommended.

Medial collateral ligament injury

The medial collateral ligament (MCL) originates from the medial femoral epicondyle just anterior to the adductor tubercle and inserts on the anteromedial tibia approximately 5 to 7 cm below the joint line.[13] It is composed of a superficial and deep layer, the latter of which has fibers that attach to the medial meniscus. Up to 12% of knee injuries that occur in athletes are MCL injuries.[14]

Clinical presentation Athletes generally present with the acute onset of medial knee pain after either a valgus force on a partially flexed knee or an external rotational force on the tibia in relation to the femur[13] **(Figure 26.6).** The athlete may complain of a "pop" in the medial knee. Complaints of acute swelling or instability are uncommon in isolated MCL sprains. Sensations of locking or catching may occur with associated medial meniscal tears, which can occur in up to 5% of MCL injuries.[2]

Diagnosis Soft-tissue swelling is located over the medial aspect of the knee, and tenderness is noted along or adjacent to the medial joint line. Valgus stress testing in full extension and at 30 degrees of flexion should be performed for comparison with the unaffected side. Knee flexion to 30 degrees helps isolate the MCL. Pain in the location of the MCL during valgus stress testing but with minimal laxity is considered a grade I sprain. Laxity with 5 to 10 mm of joint

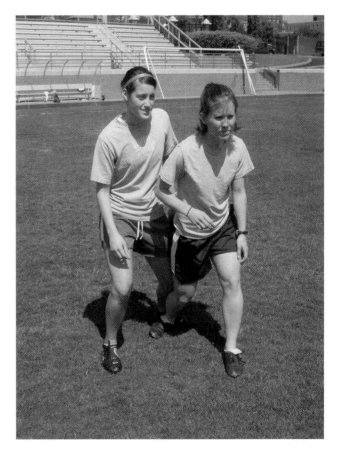

Figure 26.6 This athlete on the right is experiencing a valgus stress to the right knee. This is a possible mechanism for medial collateral ligament injury.

space opening but a firm end point is considered a grade II sprain. When there is a soft end point or no end point on valgus loading, it is considered a grade III sprain, and this is indicative of a complete tear of the ligament. If there is joint laxity with the knee locked in extension during valgus testing, there is a strong likelihood of an accompanying injury to the ACL, the posterior oblique ligament, or the posteromedial capsule.[13] Plain radiographs may detect an avulsion fracture or a calcification of the MCL from a previous injury (Pellegrini-Stieda lesion) **(Figure 26.7).** Among pediatric patients, valgus stress views may help detect a physeal injury.[2] On MRI, a grade I MCL sprain normally has edema around the ligament as opposed to displacement of the ligament fibers, which is seen in a grade II sprain. Grade III tears reveal a complete loss of continuity of the ligament.[15] MRI may also detect a concurrent bone contusion or other ligamentous or meniscal injuries.

Treatment Treatment of grade I and II sprains begins with ice and a compression wrap to decrease local swelling. The inability to tolerate weight bearing may initially require crutches. An MCL stabilizing brace may help with a sensation of instability during the rehabilitation process of grade II sprains.[16] Physical therapy to emphasize pain-free range of motion and quadriceps setting and eventual straight leg raising and hamstring isometrics may begin immediately with a grade I sprain and within a week for a grade II sprain.[13] Return to play is allowed after the completion of a functional training program; when the athlete has minimal or no pain, a full range of motion, and quadriceps and hamstring strength equal to 90% of the uninvolved limb; and when he or she can complete a sport-specific agility drill progression without pain or instability.[17] There are no current guidelines regarding return to play in a collateral stabilization brace. Many athletes will wear a brace for several weeks after an MCL injury to provide additional support against valgus stresses; however, the metal struts in the brace may not be allowed in certain sports.

Controversy Significant controversy continues to exist with regard to the surgical versus the conservative treatment of grade III tears, and orthopedic referral is indicated. Recent studies have shown

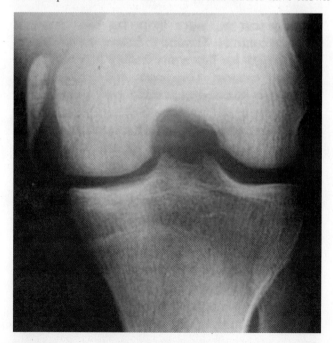

Figure 26.7 The radiograph demonstrates the classic Pellegrini—Stieda lesion, which is indicative of the avulsion fracture of the medial collateral ligament from the medial femoral condyle.

that, without associated injuries, conservative treatment is effective.[18] Current indications for the surgical repair of an isolated grade III MCL tear include functional instability despite adequate rehabilitation or an avulsion of the tibial insertion.[13]

Lateral collateral ligament and posterolateral corner structures injury

The components of the posterolateral corner of the knee act synergistically to resist varus stresses, external tibial rotation, and, to a lesser extent, posterior tibial translation.[13] The posterolateral corner can be divided into three layers. The first layer consists of the ITB and the biceps femoris tendon. The ITB has attachments on the lateral femoral condyle, and it inserts into Gerdy's tubercle on the anterolateral tibia. The biceps femoris tendon lies posterior to the ITB, and it inserts on the fibular head. The second layer consists of the patellar retinaculum and the lateral patellofemoral ligament. The third layer consists of the lateral collateral ligament (LCL), the popliteus muscle and tendon, the popliteofibular ligament, the arcuate ligament, and the lateral capsular fibers.[19] The LCL is the primary static restraint to varus forces of the knee. It originates on the lateral femoral condyle, and it inserts into the fibular head. Isolated injury to the LCL is relatively rare; it is frequently injured along with other PLCS.

Clinical presentation Athletes often present with the acute onset of lateral knee pain after a blow to the anteromedial knee while it is in full extension. Other mechanisms include hyperextension of the knee or excessive external tibial rotation. The knee may feel unstable in full extension, and the athlete may complain of buckling into hyperextension.[13] Complaints of numbness or tingling in the lateral leg or weakness with ankle dorsiflexion may indicate an associated injury of the common peroneal nerve.

Diagnosis Pain and localized soft-tissue swelling may be noted over the lateral femoral condyle, the breadth of the LCL, or the fibular head. Varus stress testing is performed in full extension and with the knee flexed to 30 degrees. Grade I injuries produce mild pain but minimal joint laxity with varus stressing in flexion. Grade II injuries produce 5 to 10 mm of joint space opening with a firm end point. Grade III injuries have greater than 10 mm of opening with a soft end point. Grade III tears indicate a complete LCL tear and are highly associated with injury to other PLCS or cruciate ligaments. Lateral joint line opening in full extension indicates a multiple ligament injury.[13] Performing Lachman's test and posterior drawer testing should evaluate the integrity of the ACL and PCL, respectively. The PLCS should be evaluated using the dial test, as discussed in the preceding section about PCL injuries. A neurologic examination is especially important as a result of the complication of common peroneal nerve injury with PLCS injuries. The avulsion of the biceps femoris from the proximal fibula is possible with a severe injury. MRI is helpful for confirming the degree and location of the LCL injury and for identifying associated injuries.

Treatment The initial management of grade I and II injuries is similar to that of MCL injuries. Orthopedic referral is recommended for grade III injuries and associated injuries to the posterolateral corner because early surgical repair or reconstruction has become the standard of care.[20]

Multiligamentous injuries

All acute knees injuries that involve the complete disruption of two or more ligaments should be classified as a multiple-ligament injury.

Clinical presentation

Many of these injuries are low-energy knee dislocations that sponta-neously reduce before medical evaluation. The multiple-ligament injured knee should be considered an orthopedic emergency as a result of the high incidence of vascular injury; the failure to recognize the full extent of these injuries can prove to be disastrous.

Treatment

The treatment of these injuries is beyond the scope of this chapter, but the initial assessment includes a through and expedient phys-ical examination, with particular attention paid to the neurovascu-lar examination. This should be followed by an immediate referral to an orthopedic surgeon who has experience with multiligamen-tous injuries.

Meniscal injuries

The medial and lateral menisci are C-shaped, fibrocartilaginous disks that help with load transmission between the femoral and tibial condyles. Traumatic tears in the periphery of the meniscus generally occur among athletes who are younger than 30 years of age.[2] Athletes who are more than 30 years of age typically suffer degenerative tears, which will be discussed later in this chapter. The medial meniscus is more commonly torn than the lateral meniscus in all sports, except for wrestling.[21]

Clinical presentation

The athlete with an injury to either meniscus will often present with the acute onset of sharp pain after a twisting or hyperflexion movement. A "pop" may be heard. Knee swelling may develop if the meniscus is torn from its vascular supply at the periphery of the anterior and posterior horns of the meniscus. The patient may describe a "locking" sensation of the knee with an inability to fully extend the knee.

Diagnosis

Physical examination may reveal an effusion. Joint line tenderness, especially along the respective posterior joint line, is commonly present. A block to passive extension may occur if there is a large, displaced, "bucket-handle" tear. The flexion McMurray test is pos-itive if a painful, palpable click is felt over the respective joint line.[6] In comparing physical examination findings to arthroscopic surgi-cal findings, a positive McMurray test is associated with a 66% prob-ability of a meniscal injury,[22] and an Apley compression test may support the diagnosis. Plain radiographs should be obtained to evaluate for a fracture or an osteochondral loose body. MRI of the knee will show a linear increased signal within the injured meniscus that extends to the articular surface (grade III signal change)[23] **(Figure 26.8).** The visualization of a grade III signal change in two or more images has 90% and 94% sensitivity for medial and lateral meniscal tears, respectively.[24] MRI may also show associated osteochondral injuries or a lateral meniscal vari-ant such as a discoid lateral meniscus, which may have predis-posed the athlete to a meniscal injury.[2]

Treatment

Initial treatment consists of protection from full weight bearing, nonsteroidal anti-inflammatory drugs (NSAIDs), progressive range-of-motion exercises, and isometric quadriceps strengthening as tolerated. Orthopedic referral should be made if the patient has locking or frequent catching, persistent symptoms after 3 months, or a desire for a prompt return to sports participation. If the patient presents with a locked knee or a knee that has a mechanical block to full extension, the orthopedic consult should occur within 24 hours.

Orthopedic considerations include arthroscopic partial menis-cectomy or primary repair of the meniscus in select cases.

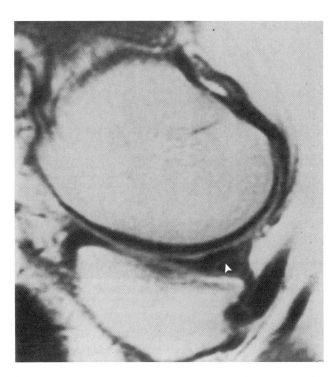

Figure 26.8 The *arrow* notes a grade III signal change on the lower surface of the posterior horn of the medial meniscus. (From DeLee JC, Drez D Jr, Miller MD [eds]: DeLee & Drez's Orthopedic Sports Medicine: Principles and Practice, 2nd ed. Philadelphia, WB Saunders, 2003.)

A primary repair is an attempt to maintain the chondroprotective role of the meniscus because contact stress between the femur and the tibia is increased by up to 45% after a partial meniscectomy.[25]

Return-to-play decisions after aggressive rehabilitation require a full, painless range of motion, quadriceps strength at 90% of that of the contralateral side, and the successful completion of a sport-specific agility progression. For the management of meniscal tears among athletes who are more than 40 years of age, please refer to the section about degenerative meniscal tears later in this chapter.

Patellar dislocation

The patella may dislocate from the patellofemoral joint. Dislocations almost always occur laterally.

Clinical presentation

The athlete presents with an acute onset of knee pain often after a sudden cutting movement or a sudden contraction of the quadriceps during deceleration. Significant knee swelling develops within the first few hours after injury. The patella typically reduces spontaneously as soon as the knee is straightened. The athlete may not recall the dislocation, thereby making the diagnosis more difficult. Patients with an old patellar dislocation may complain of a recurrent feeling of the patella subluxing or "going out" during activities.

Diagnosis

A knee effusion is evident on examination. Tenderness is often noted over the medial retinaculum and the lateral femoral condyle. The patella may show increased laxity with lateral or medial glide as compared with the unaffected leg. The athlete will have signif-icant apprehension and pain as the patella is pushed laterally during apprehension testing. Plain radiographs, including sunrise views, should be obtained to evaluate for an associated osteochon-dral fracture. MRI may be needed to rule out ligamentous or menis-cal injury if the diagnosis is questionable.

Treatment

The initial treatment is rest, ice, and compression to decrease swelling. If the knee is initially immobilized in full extension for 1 to 2 weeks, early isometric quadriceps exercises should be initiated to maintain quadriceps strength. Early range-of-motion exercises should begin when pain and swelling have decreased.[2] Resistance exercises of the quadriceps are not initiated until a full range of motion is achieved. A sport-specific return-to-play agility progression may begin when there is a pain-free range of motion, minimal or no swelling, and strength that is approximately 90% of that of the contralateral leg. Athletes will often return to sports in a patellar stabilization brace to minimize the risk of repeat dislocation. Orthopedic referral is indicated for recurrent dislocation events. Surgical options include proximal realignment (repair or reconstruction of the medial patellofemoral ligament) or distal realignment (medial translation of the tibial tubercle to correct an abnormal quadriceps angle).[2]

Disruption of the extensor mechanism of the knee

Certain injuries (e.g., quadriceps tendon rupture, patellar tendon rupture, and tibial tubercle avulsion) share a common trait as a disruption of the extensor mechanism. Quadriceps tendon rupture tends to occur among athletes who are more than 40 years of age, and it is three times more frequent than patellar tendon rupture.[26] Rupture of the patellar tendon is most common at the inferior pole of the patella. During knee flexion from 0 to 45 degrees, the quadriceps tendon has a mechanical advantage, and it is less susceptible to injury; however, during knee flexion beyond 45 degrees, the patellar tendon has a mechanical advantage, and it is less susceptible to injury.[27]

Clinical presentation

Athletes present after a sudden, forceful contraction of the quadriceps during vertical or horizontal deceleration or from a direct trauma to the anterior knee. A "pop" may be heard. Patients with a history of tendinitis may be predisposed to tendon rupture.

Diagnosis

Patients are often unable to passively extend the knee or to perform a straight-leg raise. An athlete with a partial quadriceps tendon injury that does not extend to the retinaculum may be able to extend against gravity with an associated extensor lag. There is tenderness over the injured tendon. A palpable defect in the quadriceps or the patellar tendon may be felt. Plain radiographs may reveal a tibial tubercle avulsion fracture that is primarily seen in the pediatric population.[2] Radiographs may also reveal patella alta in patellar tendon rupture and patella baja in quadriceps tendon rupture.

Treatment

The initial treatment is knee immobilization in extension. Immediate orthopedic referral is warranted for complete tendon rupture. Partial tendon ruptures may need surgical repair, especially in high-grade injuries. Because these repairs are most successful within 14 days, consultation with orthopedics within 72 hours is recommended for partial tears of the quadriceps or patellar tendons.

Patella fracture

Patella fractures are classified either by fracture pattern (transverse, vertical, comminuted) or location (lower pole, middle, or upper pole).

Clinical presentation

Athletes present with acute knee pain over the patella and an inability to fully straighten the leg after a direct blow to the patella. Patellar fractures are most commonly transverse, and they are often best seen on the lateral view of radiographs. The rarer vertical fracture may only be seen on sunrise views.

Diagnosis

Athletes have soft-tissue swelling and tenderness over the patella. They are often unable to hold the leg straight against gravity, which is similar to what occurs during other disruptions of the extensor mechanism. Plain radiographs confirm the diagnosis; however, caution is warranted to prevent the misdiagnosis of an incidental bipartite patella as a fracture (see the section on multipartite patella later in this chapter).

Treatment

Nondisplaced fractures are treated nonoperatively with bracing or casting in extension for 6 weeks followed by progressive range-of-motion exercises. Displaced fractures are those with 3 mm of cortical disruption or 2 mm of articular step off, and they are treated with open reduction and internal fixation.[2]

Proximal tibiofibular joint dislocation

Dislocation of the proximal tibiofibular joint is a very uncommon knee injury, and it is often missed on initial evaluation if it is not specifically considered. The dislocation is anterolateral in 90% of cases. Posteromedial dislocation is also seen in athletes, whereas superior dislocation is more commonly associated with displaced tibia fractures or congenital knee dislocation.[28]

Clinical presentation

In cases of anterolateral dislocation, the athlete classically complains of anterolateral knee pain after falling on a flexed, adducted leg with the ankle inverted. A posteromedial dislocation is often caused by direct trauma to the flexed knee. Patients may complain of numbness or tingling over the lateral leg and the dorsum of the foot if the common peroneal nerve is concurrently injured.

Diagnosis

The fibular head is prominent, tender to palpation, and excessively mobile. Anteroposterior plain radiographs will usually reveal a laterally displaced fibular head with a widening of the proximal interosseous space as compared with radiographs of the uninjured leg.

Treatment

Closed reduction can be performed after associated fracture is excluded. A period of immobilization may be indicated, and this may be followed by hamstring stretching exercises. Orthopedic referral is indicated for recurrent dislocations or for an associated injury to the common peroneal nerve.

CHRONIC KNEE INJURIES

The majority of chronic knee injuries tend to be overuse injuries with an insidious onset of pain. It is crucial for the history and physical examination to elucidate the extrinsic and intrinsic factors that predisposed the athlete to the injury to properly tailor treatment.

Patellofemoral pain syndrome

Patellofemoral pain syndrome (PFPS) is the most common and complex of all knee overuse injuries. It refers to anterior knee pain that originates from the patellofemoral joint and its supporting soft-tissue structures. It is also commonly referred to as *anterior knee pain, kneecap pain, retropatellar pain syndrome,* and *chondromalacia patella*. Intuitively, it is felt to manifest from overload stress of the patellar facets as they articulate with the trochlear groove of the femoral condyles. Cartilage effects range from symptomatic painful foci with no obvious arthroscopic changes to overt chondromalacia (thinning, fibrillation, fissuring, and denuding of the cartilage).[29] The source of pain in PFPS is unclear because there is no enervation of articular cartilage.[30] Pain may arise from excessive force transmission to underlying bone as a result of deficiencies in the load-bearing integrity of injured cartilage or, alternatively, from the nociceptive stimulation of adjacent structures, such as the peripatellar retinaculum or the extensor mechanism.[31]

Clinical presentation

Athletes present with the insidious onset of pain over the anterior knee, which is occasionally specific to the retropatellar region. Symptoms are commonly bilateral, and they are more common in adolescents and young adults. There may be a history of increased eccentric loading of the quadriceps (e.g., running). Pain is exacerbated by the loading of the patellofemoral joint (e.g., climbing stairs, squatting, or prolonged sitting). Pain (especially when arising) during a period of prolonged sitting (e.g., during a foreign film festival) is called a *positive theater sign*. Locking, catching, and swelling are uncommon; however, the knee may occasionally give out as a result of the pain-induced reflex inhibition of the quadriceps. Obtaining a history of intrinsic or extrinsic factors that may be contributing to knee pain is a crucial component of the evaluation of PFPS.

Diagnosis

The diagnosis is often made by history alone, and physical examination should focus on identifying the intrinsic biomechanical factors that predispose the athlete to PFPS. Visual inspection may reveal anatomic factors such as excessive valgus or varus deformity, femoral anteversion, external tibial torsion, patellar malposition, excessive lateral insertion of the patellar tendon (increased quadriceps angle), pes cavus, or pes planus. The knee will have a full range of motion; however, the evaluation of knee extension in a seated position may demonstrate excessive lateral tracking of the patella. This is called *J tracking* because the course of the patella resembles an upside-down letter J. Functional factors that may contribute to PFPS include hamstring tightness (determined by the measurement of the popliteal angle), ITB tightness (positive Ober's test), rectus femoris tightness (positive Ely test and positive Thomas' test), vastus medialis obliques atrophy, and a tight lateral retinaculum (decreased lateral patellar glide). Palpation of the femoral condyles and the patellar facets may elicit pain. Retropatellar pain with compression of the articular patellofemoral surfaces during quadriceps contraction is considered a positive Clarke sign. A direct, rocking pressure of the patella also elicits pain (positive grind test). Plain radiographs are not initially warranted, but they should be obtained if the athlete fails to respond to treatment. Abnormalities of patellar alignment within the trochlear groove may be noted on sunrise or merchant views. A multipartite patella may cause a diagnostic dilemma in patients with anterior knee pain because this is often an incidental finding (see the section on multipartite patella later in this chapter).

Treatment

Relative rest from offending activities such as squatting, excessive stair climbing, and hill running is often beneficial; however, it is important to prevent complete inactivity and subsequent deconditioning. A primary focus of therapy is correction of biomechanical factors that led to the overloading of the patellofemoral joint. Correctable extrinsic factors such as footwear, training surfaces, and training regimen should be addressed. Physical therapy may address core muscle and vastus medialis oblique weakness as well as hip flexor, ITB, calf, and hamstring tightness as identified on examination. McConnell taping techniques and lateral retinaculum mobility may facilitate proper patellar tracking.[31] Custom foot orthotics may be necessary to address pes planus, and ice massage after exercise may be useful for symptom control. NSAID therapy is not helpful for articular cartilage repair, but acetaminophen or NSAIDs can be given for short courses of acute pain control when requested.[32] Patellar support braces may be useful for decreasing the amount of patellar mobility. An alternative rationale for the benefit of patellar braces is the improved joint temperature and proprioceptive stimulation of the knee.[33] Crossley and colleagues[34] performed a systematic review of the literature for the treatment of patellofemoral pain, and they found a paucity of trials studying physical interventions such as physiotherapy, taping, bracing, and foot orthoses. The 16 studies that were identified did not meet criteria for a randomized, controlled trial, and they varied with regard to patient selection, intervention, and outcome measures, thus preventing a meta-analysis. There was some evidence to suggest that eccentric exercises were better than other forms of quadriceps strengthening. The review also supported the use of custom foot orthoses for females with varus of the rear of the foot.[34]

Athletes who fail to respond to nonoperative management after 12 months may be referred to an orthopedic surgeon for consideration for lateral retinacular release or tibial tuberosity transfer, although evidence to support these surgical treatments is sparse.

Multipartite patella (bipartite patella)

A multipartite patella occurs during a failed fusion of a secondary ossification center of the patella, and it is usually seen as a vertical lucency on a plain radiograph separating the patella into two components (bipartite patella). It occurs in 0.2% of the population.[2] Multipartite patella may be confused with an acute patella fracture; however, the bipartite patella variant can typically be distinguished from fracture by its minimal separation and smooth borders.[2] The majority of the time this multipartite variation is unilateral; it is more common among males by a ratio of 9:1.[35] The synchondrosis of the bipartite patella may become painful after trauma or with repetitive overuse of the knee.

Clinical presentation

Symptomatic athletes will present with the insidious onset of anterior knee pain. Like PFPS, it may be worsened with prolonged sitting or squatting. Athletes will also complain with kneeling or other activities that put direct pressure on the patella. They may temporally relate a direct blow to the kneecap with the onset of pain.

Diagnosis

Symptomatic athletes have point tenderness over the kneecap, usually in the area of the multipartite patella. Plain radiographs confirm the diagnosis **(Figure 26.9)**. Technetium bone scanning may assist with the diagnosis of an acute synchondrosis disruption from other causes of anterior knee pain.

Treatment

Initial treatment includes a short period of immobilization and progressive range-of-motion exercises before quadriceps strengthening and stretching exercises. NSAIDs may treat pain symptoms. Orthopedic referral for the consideration of lateral retinacular release or the excision of the ossicle fragments is recommended when conservative management fails.

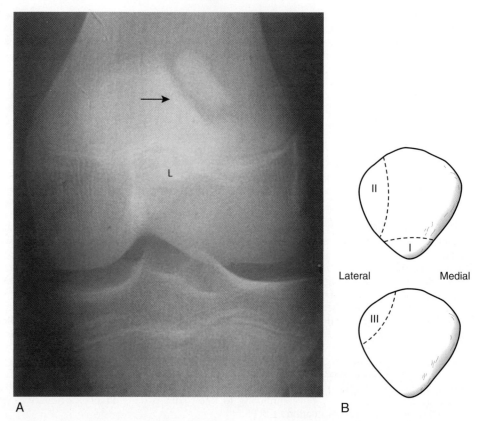

Figure 26.9 *A,* A bipartite patella with a separated superolateral compartment in a left knee (L). *B,* The classification of multipartite patella. Nonunion of the inferior pole (type I), lateral margin (type II), and superolateral quadrant (type III) occur in 5%, 20%, and 75% of cases, respectively. (From DeLee JC, Drez D Jr, Miller MD [eds]: DeLee & Drez's Orthopedic Sports Medicine: Principles and Practice, 2nd ed. Philadelphia, WB Saunders, 2003.)

Iliotibial band (ITB) friction syndrome

The ITB serves to abduct the leg and to help stabilize the pelvis in the single-leg stance. ITB friction syndrome often develops either from repetitive overload of the distal fibers of the ITB at its insertion on the Gerdy tubercle of the tibia or from excessive friction of the ITB as it glides over the lateral femoral epicondyle. ITB tightness, pes cavus, and/or gluteal weakness typically predispose an individual to ITB friction syndrome.

Clinical presentation

Athletes present with an insidious pain onset over the posterolateral knee that is often exacerbated by running on hills or banked surfaces. If there is a history of running on banked surfaces (e.g., a sloped track or a shoreline), pain is typically felt in the uphill leg.[30] Pain often escalates with attempts to continue running.

Diagnosis

The athlete has tenderness to palpation along the distal ITB that is often greatest at the lateral femoral epicondyle and, to a lesser extent, over the Gerdy tubercle. A positive Ober's test indicates ITB tightness, and pain is elicited with adduction overpressure. The Noble compression test is often positive.

Treatment

Activity modification to avoid the offending activity is the initial treatment. Alternative training such as elliptical training or deep water running should be advocated. Physical therapy should focus on aggressive ITB stretching and improving strength of the core (gluteal) and knee musculature. Ice massage, oral analgesics, and therapy modalities such as ultrasound and iontophoresis may help decrease pain symptoms. In refractory cases, corticosteroid injection of the ITB bursa may decrease pain and allow for a more effective rehabilitation strengthening program (see Chapter 48). A graduated return to running and the initial avoidance of vertical and horizontal grades may help prevent a recurrence of symptoms. Orthopedic referral is warranted for consideration of ITB lengthening in patients who fail to respond to months of conservative management.

Degenerative meniscal tears

Degenerative tears of both the medial and lateral menisci typically occur among patients who are more than 40 years of age.[32] With aging, there is a decrease in the elasticity, vascularity, and water content in the meniscus, and this is felt to predispose an individual to injury.

Clinical presentation

Athletes present with the insidious onset of knee pain. They often have no recollection of when the tear may have occurred. They may have a history of excessive running or frequent squatting. Although pain may be exacerbated by activities that load the tibiofemoral joints, there is usually no history of locking or catching, and swelling typically only occurs with high-impact activities like running or squatting.[30]

Diagnosis

Range of motion is often normal, and any effusion is minimal. There is typically tenderness to palpation along the respective joint line. Flexion McMurray testing and Apley testing often elicit pain, but they do not cause a catching or palpable click. Weight-bearing plain radiographs may suggest a decrease in joint space or reveal associated osteoarthritis. MRI or arthroscopy will confirm the diagnosis.

Treatment

Initial treatment is the avoidance of knee-loading activities, physical therapy to address associated flexibility and strength deficits, and judicious pain management.[36] Most athletes with degenerative meniscus tears will improve with nonoperative management. Orthopedic referral for arthroscopy with meniscal debridement should be considered for patients for whom conservative management fails. There is ongoing research in an attempt to regenerate meniscal tissue.[37]

Patellar tendinopathy (jumper's knee)

A chronic overuse injury to the patellar tendon is felt to be the result of the repeated loading of the extensor mechanism of the knee. It is more prevalent in sports involving some form of jumping, and it is thus commonly referred to as "jumper's knee."[38] It also commonly occurs among those who participate in activities that do not require jumping. Like many overuse tendon injuries, it has previously been described as a tendinitis; however, histopathologic studies have shown that the underlying pathology is tendon degeneration as opposed to tendon inflammation.[39] Intrinsic factors that may contribute to the development of patellar tendinopathy include patella alta and abnormal patellar laxity. Decreased quadriceps and hamstring flexibility were prospectively found to be predisposing factors for patellar tendinopathy[41] (LOE: D).

Clinical presentation

Athletes present with an insidious onset of a dull ache over the anterior knee during or after activity. It may be worsened by an increase in the intensity of training. Untreated, the pain usually worsens to become a constant ache at rest, and it may disturb sleep. Prolonged periods of sitting, climbing, or descending stairs may aggravate the pain[42] (LOE: D).

Diagnosis

Patients have a full range of motion, and the pain may lessen with the knee flexed. There is tenderness to palpation primarily over the inferior pole of the patella, but it may traverse the entire length of the patellar tendon. Pain may worsen with resisted knee extension, during jumping maneuvers, or during performance of a squat on a 30-degree decline. Athletes with prolonged symptoms may develop quadriceps wasting (specifically of the vastus medialis obliques). Although it is often unnecessary to confirm the diagnosis, MRI may reveal an increase in size and a focal increase in signal within the patellar tendon[43] **(Figure 26.10).** MRI has a 78% sensitivity and an 86% specificity for detecting patellar tendinopathy, but MRI appearance does not seem to correlate with clinical outcome.[42]

Treatment

Nonoperative treatment is advocated initially; however, it is important to tell the athlete that healing may take from 4 to 6 months and that conservative treatment may fail as a result of a too rapid a progression through rehabilitation. Relative rest from offending activities and ice massage to decrease pain is performed initially. Therapy to address quadriceps, hamstring, or calf inflexibility and to address quadriceps and core muscle weakness is initiated. Eccentric strengthening programs have been beneficial for this and for other tendinopathies.[44] Preliminary research into the use of eccentric decline squat strengthening has been advocated to treat chronic patellar tendinopathy.[40] A recent study found that eccentric training among volleyball players did not improve symptoms; however, these athletes continued to compete during their rehabilitation[45] (LOE: B). Ultrasound and electrical stimulation may be used to alleviate pain. Although there does not appear to be an inflammatory component to the patellar tendinopathy, NSAIDs have been used frequently to control pain, and they may benefit the tendinopathy via alternative mechanisms such as the accelerated formation of cross-linked collagen fibers.[42] Corticosteroid injection of the patellar tendon should be avoided because of its effects on tendon atrophy and the potential for tendon rupture.[46]

The failure of 6 months of conservative management warrants orthopedic referral to consider surgical intervention. Possible surgical options include arthroscopic excision and the debridement of degenerated areas, the repair of macroscopic defects, the drilling of the inferior pole of the patella, or percutaneous longitudinal tenotomy.[38] Evaluation of all surgical outcomes shows a best-case estimated success rate of 75% to 85%, with several athletes unable to return to their previous level of competition.[47]

Infrapatellar fat pad syndrome (Hoffa syndrome)

Infrapatellar fat pad syndrome involves hypertrophy and inflammation of the infrapatellar fat pad that is believed to be the result of repetitive trauma of the infrapatellar fat pad during activities that require repetitive knee extension.

Clinical features

Patients often report the insidious onset of pain that is deep and inferior to the inferior pole of the patella and that is exacerbated by knee extension. The condition may be associated with other chronic knee conditions such as patellar tendinopathy or trauma to the infrapatellar fat pad during arthroscopy or from intramedullary nail impingement.[48] Examination reveals swelling on either side of the patellar tendon. There is tenderness to palpation of the fat pad deep to the patellar tendon. A positive bounce test involves pain elicited during passive extension of the knee as pressure is applied on the fat pad.

Diagnosis

The injection of local anesthetic into the fat pad often alleviates symptoms and confirms the diagnosis. Plain radiographs are usually normal. MRI will show signal abnormality within the fat pad, but it is often not necessary for diagnosis.

Treatment

Initial treatment is nonoperative and consists of rest, ice massage, NSAIDs, and a rehabilitation program that avoids terminal extension. Injection with corticosteroids is avoided because of the potential for fat pad necrosis. For patients who do not respond to conservative management, arthroscopic surgical excision of the infrapatellar fat pad has shown positive results.[49]

Medial plica band syndrome

The mediopatellar plica runs from the medial lining of the suprapatellar pouch distally to the synovium over the infrapatellar fat pad, and it is palpable in most athletes. It is a well-vascularized, thin, pliable fold of the synovium.[2] Overuse of the patellofemoral joint or direct blunt trauma may cause the plica band to become thick and edematous. This enlarged plica can often become impinged during knee motion and cause pain, thus leading to medial plica band syndrome.

Clinical presentation

Athletes present with the insidious onset of nonspecific anterior knee pain. They may be able to recall a temporally related blunt trauma to the knee. Many athletes complain of a snapping or pinching sensation during a certain range of knee flexion.[2] There is typically no history of locking, catching, or swelling; however, pain may cause a reflex that causes the quadriceps musculature to give way.

Diagnosis

Physical examination reveals point tenderness with palpation or friction rub of the thickened plica. A palpable snap may be elicited

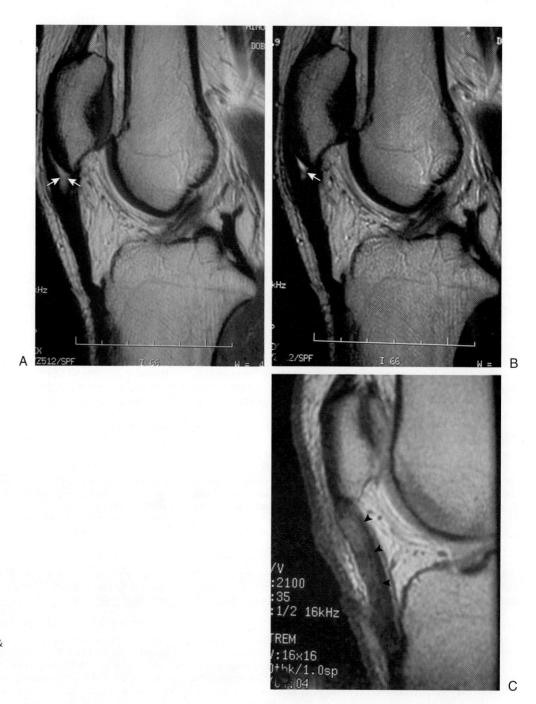

Figure 26.10 *A*, Thickening and increased signal is noted. *B*, Fluid signal is noted within the area of abnormal signal, which suggests a focal intrasubstance tear. *C*, Diffuse thickening and abnormal signal throughout the tendon. (From DeLee JC, Drez D Jr, Miller MD [eds]: DeLee & Drez's Orthopedic Sports Medicine: Principles and Practice, 2nd ed. Philadelphia, WB Saunders, 2003.)

during knee flexion from 40 to 60 degrees.[2] Medial retinacular tenderness after patellar subluxation may be confused with medial plica band syndrome. However, the patient with medial plica syndrome will have no patellar apprehension. Plain radiographs and MRI cannot make the diagnosis of a symptomatic plica. An injection of 1% lidocaine into the thickened plica band that alleviates the tenderness and pain with range of motion may confirm the diagnosis.

Treatment

The initial treatment is nonoperative, and it includes the avoidance of aggravating activities and ice massage. NSAIDs may help relieve pain. Physical therapy should address quadriceps and hamstring flexibility as well as strength deficits. Intra-articular steroid injection is not necessary; however, corticosteroid injection into the plica band may be considered. Failure to respond to 3 months of conservative therapy warrants orthopedic referral for arthroscopic plica excision, with reported success rates of more than 80%.[50]

Pes anserine bursitis

Inflammation of the bursa beneath the pes anserine tendon (the common insertion of the sartorius, the gracilis, and the semitendinosis muscles) occurs via overuse of the medial knee.

Clinical presentation

Athletes present with a vague and insidious onset of medial knee pain at the pes anserine insertion on the proximal tibial metaphysis approximately 2 cm below the medial joint line.

Diagnosis

Physical examination reveals point tenderness and perhaps localized swelling over the pes anserine insertion. Pain may radiate posteriorly, and tenderness may be found along the semitendinosis and gracilis tendons. Examination should focus on excluding other causes of medial knee pain, such as tibial plateau stress fracture, MCL injury, or meniscal injury. Plain radiographs can be obtained to exclude a bony lesion or a tibial plateau fracture.

Treatment

Initial treatment includes relative rest, local ice massage, and NSAIDs to control pain. Physical therapy should focus on hamstring and hip adductor flexibility and progressive strengthening as symptoms abate. A corticosteroid injection into the pes anserine bursa may decrease pain to help facilitate rehabilitation (see Chapter 48). Training errors and gait pattern should be addressed before a graduated progression back to sports participation.

Popliteus tendinopathy

The popliteus tendon is a static and dynamic stabilizer of the posterolateral knee. It has its origin on the posteromedial border of the proximal tibia, and it inserts primarily on the lateral femoral condyle as well as onto the lateral meniscus and the fibula. Its primary action is to internally rotate the tibia during open-chain movements. Popliteus tendinopathy has been associated with downhill running and other deceleration activities because it serves to aid the quadriceps with the prevention of the excessive anterior translation of the femur on the tibia.[51] Overuse or fatigue of the quadriceps places excessive stress on the secondary restraints, such as the popliteus muscle.

Clinical presentation

Patients may present with the insidious onset of pain over the posterolateral knee. There is frequently a history of cross-country or downhill running that further exacerbates symptoms. Occasionally, the pain will develop after an acute injury.

Diagnosis

Popliteus injury may be suspected with tenderness over the proximal aspect of the popliteus tendon with the patient in the prone position. There may be pain with resisted external rotation of the lower leg with the hip and knee flexed to 90 degrees (positive Garrick test)[52] **(Figure 26.11A).** A "shoe removal maneuver" in which the athlete internally rotates the injured lower leg to push off the contralateral shoe at the heel may also produce pain[53] (Figure 26.11B). Tenderness over the posterolateral knee may raise suspicion of a strain of the biceps femoris tendon or of injury to the lateral meniscus, which should be considered in the differential diagnosis. MRI may show edema within the muscle at the musculotendinous junction. An isolated acute rupture of the popliteus tendon was found in 2 of 2412 knee MRI studies.[54]

Treatment

General rehabilitation guidelines for muscular tendinopathy that incorporate relative rest, NSAIDs for pain, and ice are often the

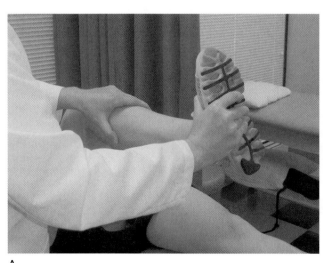

A

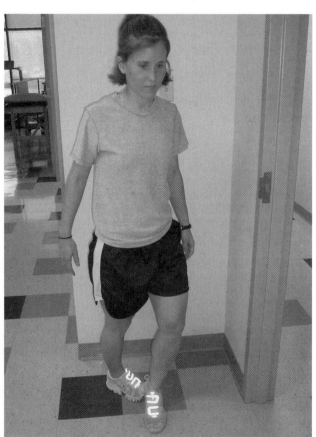

B

Figure 26.11 *A,* Active tibial external rotation against resistance (Garrick test). *B,* The shoe removal test. The back leg (being used to remove the contralateral shoe) is the leg that is under evaluation for popliteus tendon injury.

initial treatment modalities. Physical therapy should emphasize eccentric strengthening of the quadriceps muscles. Corticosteroid injection into the popliteus tendon over the point of maximal tenderness may help alleviate pain and allow for continued rehabilitation; however, care must be taken to avoid injury to the common peroneal nerve. Graduated return to activity is determined by symptoms.

Popliteal cyst (Baker cyst)

Popliteal cysts are the most common synovial-lined cyst in the body, and they are located behind the medial femoral condyle between the medial head of the gastrocnemius and the semimembranosus tendon. It is often an incidental finding on examination or imaging. In younger athletes, these may be associated with knee inflammation as a result of meniscal or ligamentous injuries.

Clinical presentation

Athletes present with an aching pain in the posterior knee and a feeling of fullness in the popliteal fossa. If the cyst communicates with the joint, there may be a history of a variably sized mass. If the cyst is large, it may restrict range of motion in the knee.

Diagnosis

The examination of the knee may reveal a discrete, cystic mass in the medial side of the popliteal fossa. If the mass is pulsatile, a popliteal artery aneurysm should be suspected. The cyst may transilluminate with light. If there is any question about the diagnosis, MRI can confirm a popliteal cyst and exclude other soft-tissue masses. The examination should exclude other knee injuries that may predispose the patient to a knee effusion.

Treatment

The initial treatment is relative rest from knee-loading activities, ice, and NSAIDs. External compression with a knee sleeve may decrease swelling, but it may also increase pain initially. Underlying knee pathology (classically a meniscus tear) should be addressed. Aspiration of the cyst is usually not recommended because the fluid is often too viscous for easy withdrawal, and surrounding neurovascular structures can be injured by blind attempts. Orthopedic referral is recommended for the consideration of open or arthroscopic-assisted cyst excision in refractory cases.

SPECIAL CONSIDERATIONS IN THE PEDIATRIC AND ADOLESCENT ATHLETE

Pediatric and adolescent athletes often suffer from unique injuries. As a result of differences between the mature (adult) and immature (child or adolescent) skeleton, younger athletes are at risk for osteochondral injuries (osteochondritis dissecans), apophysitis of the knee (Osgood–Schlatter disease and Sinding–Larsen–Johansson disease), and growth-plate fractures of the knee. A detailed discussion of the evaluation and treatment of these disorders can be found in Chapter 31A.

CONCLUSION

Multiple structures in the knee may be injured either acutely or with chronic overuse. A detailed history of the mechanism of injury and determination of risk factors for overuse injuries, combined with a detailed examination, will aid in the accurate diagnosis of knee injuries. This will allow either focused treatment of the injury or appropriate recognition of those conditions requiring consultation with an orthopedic surgeon versed in the surgical treatment of sports injuries.

REFERENCES

1. Arendt E, Dick R: Knee injury patterns among men and women in collegiate basketball and soccer. NCAA data and review of literature. Am J Sports Med 1995;23: 694-701.
2. In DeLee JC, Drez D Jr, Miller MD (eds): DeLee and Drez's Orthopaedic Sports Medicine: Principles and Practice, 2nd ed. Philadelphia, WB Saunders, 2003.
3. Torg J, Quedenfeld T: Effect of shoe type and cleat length on incidence and severity of knee injuries among high school football players. Res Q 1971;42:203-211.
4. Powell JW, Schootman M: A multivariate analysis of selected playing surfaces in the National Football League: 1980 to 1989. An epidemiologic study of knee injuries. Am J Sports Med 1992;20:686-694.
5. Koon D, Bassett F: Anterior cruciate ligament rupture. South Med J 2004;97(8): 755-756.
6. Donaldson WF, Warren RF, Wickiewicz T: A comparison of acute anterior cruciate ligament examinations: initial versus examination under anesthesia. Am J Sports Med 1995;13:5-10.
7. Magee DJ: Knee. In Magee DJ: Orthopedic Physical Assessment. Philadelphia, WB Saunders, 2002, p 661-763.
8. Grood ES, Stowers SF, Noyes FR: Limits of movement in the human knee: effect of sectioning the posterior cruciate ligament and posterolateral structures. J Bone Joint Surg Am 1988;70:88-97.
9. DeLee JC, Drez D Jr, Miller MD (eds): DeLee & Drez's Orthopedic Sports Medicine: Principles and Practice, 2nd ed. Philadelphia, WB Saunders, 2003.
10. Polly DW Jr, Callaghan JJ, Sikes RA, et al: The accuracy of selective magnetic resonance imaging compared with the findings of arthroscopy of the knee. J Bone Joint Surg Am 1988;70:192-198.
11. Shelbourne KD, Davis TJ, Patel DV: The natural history of acute, isolated, nonoperatively treated posterior cruciate ligament injuries: a prospective study. Am J Sports Med 1999;27:276-283.
12. Keller PM, Shelbourne KD, McCarroll JR, Rettig AC: Nonoperatively treated isolated posterior cruciate ligament injuries. Am J Sports Med 1993;21:132-136.
13. Quarles JD, Hosey RG: Medial and lateral collateral injuries: prognosis and treatment. Prim Care 2004;31:957-975.
14. Jensen JE, Conn RR, Hazelrigg G, Hewett JE: Systematic evaluation of acute knee injuries. Clin Sports Med 1985;4(2):295-312.
15. Stoller D, Cannon W, Anderson L: The knee. In Stoller D (ed): Magnetic Resonance Imaging in Orthopaedics and Sports Medicine, 2nd ed. Lippincott-Raven, Philadelphia, 1997, pp 203-442.
16. Paluska SA, McKeag DB: Knee braces: current evidence and clinical recommendations for their use. Am Fam Phys 2000;61(2):411-424.
17. Reider B: Medial collateral ligament injuries in athletes. Sports Med 1996;21(2):147-156.
18. Indelicato P, Hermansdorfer J, Huegel M: Nonoperative management of complete tears of the medial collateral ligament of the knee in intercollegiate football players. Clin Orthop 1990;256:174-177.
19. Seebacher JR, Inglis AE, Marshall JL, Warren RF: The structure of the posterolateral aspect of the knee. J Bone Joint Surg Am 1982;64(4):536-541.
20. LaPrade RF, Wentorf F: Diagnosis and treatment of posterolateral knee injuries. Clin Orthop 2002;402:110-121.
21. Baker BE, Peckham AC, Pupparo F, Sanborn JC: Review of meniscal injury and associated sports. Am J Sports Med 1985;13:1-4. (LOE: D).
22. Jackson JL, O'Malley PG, Kroenke K: Evaluation of acute knee pain in primary care. Ann Intern Med 2003;139:575-588. (LOE: D).
23. Crues JV 3rd, Mink J, Levy TL: Meniscal tears of the knee: accuracy of MR imaging. Radiology 1987;164:445-448.
24. DeSmet AA, Norris MA, Yandow DR, et al: MR diagnosis of meniscal tears of the knee: importance of high signal in the meniscus that extends to the surface. Am J Roentgenol 1993;161:101-107.
25. Baratz ME, Fu FH, Mengato R: Meniscal tears: the effect of meniscectomy and of repair on intraarticular contact areas and stress in the human knee. A preliminary report. Am J Sports Med 1986;16:1-5.
26. Ilan DI, Tejwani N, Keschner M, Leibman M: Quadriceps tendon rupture. J Am Acad Orthop Surg 2003;11(3):192-200.
27. Klimkiewicz JJ: Soft tissue knee injuries (tendon and bursae). In O'Connor FG, Sallis RE, Wilder RP, et al (eds): Sports Medicine: Just the Facts. McGraw-Hill, 2005, pp 359-365.
28. Safran M, Fu F: Uncommon causes of knee pain in the athletes. Orthop 1995;26:547-559.
29. Theut PC, Fulkerson JP: Anterior knee pain and patellar subluxation in the adult. In DeLee JC, Drez D Jr, Miller MD (eds): DeLee and Drez's Orthopaedic Sports Medicine: Principles and Practice, 2nd ed. Philadelphia, WB Saunders, 2003, pp 1799-1815.

30. Adams WB: Treatment options in overuse injuries of the knee: patellofemoral syndrome, iliotibial band syndrome, and degenerative meniscal tears. Curr Sports Med Rep 2004;3:256-260.

31. McConnell J: The management of chondromalacia patellae: a long term solution. Aust J Physiother 1986;32:215-223.

32. Bernstein J, Ahn J, Almekinders LC, et al: Analgesia in Sports Medicine, A Special Report to the Physician and Sportsmedicine. Minneapolis, MN, McGraw-Hill, 2003, pp 1-36.

33. Fredericson M, Powers CM: Practical management of patellofemoral pain. Clin J Sports Med 2002;12:36-38.

34. Crossley K, Bennell K, Green S, et al: A systematic review of physical interventions for patellofemoral pain syndrome. Clin J Sports Med 2001;11:103-110.

35. Iossifidis A, Brueton RN: Painful bipartite patella following injury. Injury 1995;26:175-176.

36. Bernstein J: Meniscal tears of the knee: diagnosis and individualized treatment syndrome. Phys Sportsmed 2000;28:83-90.

37. Huard J, Li Y, Peng H, Fu FH: Gene therapy and tissue engineering for sports medicine. J Gene Med 2003;5(2):93-108.

38. Cook JL, Khan KM, Harcourt PR, et al: A cross sectional study of 100 athletes with jumper's knee managed conservatively and surgically. Br J Sports Med 1997;31:332-336.

39. Khan KM, Cook JL, Taunton JE, et al: Overuse tendinosis, not tendinitis part I: a new paradigm for a difficult clinical problem. Phys Sportsmed 2000;28:38-48.

40. Purdam CR, Jonsson P, Alfredson H, et al: A pilot study of the eccentric decline squat in the management of painful chronic patellar tendinopathy. Br J Sports Med 2004;38(4):441-445.

41. Witvrouw E, Bellemans J, Lysens R, et al: Intrinsic risk factors for the development of patellar tendinitis in an athletic population, a two-year prospective study. Am J Sports Med 2001;29:190-195. (LOE: D).

42. Warden SJ, Brukner P: Patellar tendinopathy. Clin Sports Med 2003;22:743-759. (LOE: D).

43. McLoughlin RF, Raber EL, Vellet AD, et al: Patellar tendinitis: MR imaging features, with suggested pathogenesis and proposed classification. Radiology 1995;197:843-848.

44. Alfredson H, Pietila T, Jonsson P, et al: Heavy-load eccentric calf muscle training for the treatment of chronic Achilles tendinosis. Am J Sports Med 1998;26:360-366.

45. Visnes H, Hoksrud A, Cook J, et al: No effect of eccentric training on jumper's knee in volleyball players during the competitive season: a randomized clinical trial. Clin J Sports Med 2005;15(4):227-234. (LOE: B).

46. Nirschl RP: Elbow tendinosis/tennis elbow. Clin Sports Med 1992;11:851-870.

47. Coleman BD, Khan KM, Maffulli N, et al: Studies of surgical outcome after patellar tendinopathy: clinical significance of methodological deficiencies and guidelines for future studies. Scand J Med Sci Sports 2000;10:2-11.

48. Duri ZA, Aichroth PM, Dowd G: The fat pad: clinical observations. Am J Knee Surg 1996;9(2):55-66. (LOE: D).

49. Ogilvie-Harris DJ, Giddens J: Hoffa's disease: arthroscopic resection of the infrapatellar fat pad. Arthroscop. 1994;10(2):184-187. (LOE: D).

50. Johnson DP, Eastwood DM, Witherow PJ: Symptomatic synovial plicae of the knee. J Bone Joint Surg Am 1993;75:1485-1496. (LOE: B).

51. Petsche TS, Selesnick FH: Popliteus tendinitis: tips for diagnosis and management. Phys Sportsmed 2002;30(8):27-31.

52. Garrick JG, Webb DR. In Sports Injuries: Diagnosis and Management. Philadelphia, WB Saunders, 1999, Chapter 9-L (Popliteus tendonitis), pp 326-327.

53. Radhakrishna M, Macdonald P, Davidson M, et al: Isolated popliteus injury in a professional football player. Clin J Sports Med 2004;14(6):365-367.

54. Brown TR, Quinn SF, Wensel JP: Diagnosis of popliteus injuries with MR imaging. Skeletal Radiol 1995;24:511-514.

27 CHAPTER

Lower Leg Injuries

Greg Dammann, MD, and MAJ Duane R. Hennion, MD

KEY POINTS

- Women are up to 12 times more likely to develop a lower extremity stress fracture than men.
- Patients with stress fractures typically present with bone pain that is insidious in onset, that increases with activity, that is well localized, and that worsens over time.
- Medial tibial stress syndrome accounts for about 13% of all running injuries.
- The typical medial tibial stress syndrome pain initially occurs with exertion, and it may be relieved with continued running (i.e., if the athlete is able to run through the pain). The pain may also recur toward the end of the workout or after the cessation of running.
- The hallmark of chronic exertional compartment syndrome is pain that occurs at a predictable point during a run and that subsides gradually over 10-20 minutes with rest.

INTRODUCTION

As the number of recreational athletes involved in running and jumping sports has increased, so has the number of patients who present with lower leg pain. A thorough understanding of common lower leg injuries will aid the physician with diagnosing, treating, and expediting the return to play. In this chapter, we will discuss stress fractures of the tibia and fibula, medial tibial stress syndrome, exertional compartment syndrome in the lower leg, popliteal artery entrapment syndrome, and lower extremity nerve entrapments.

STRESS FRACTURES OF THE TIBIA AND FIBULA

Stress fractures of the tibia and fibula are overuse injuries that are caused by repetitive loading forces that result in bony microtrauma and finally biomechanical failure of the bony cortex. Runners are the athletes that are the most likely to suffer from stress fractures, with the tibia being the most frequent site of involvement.[1,2] The incidence of stress fractures in runners has been estimated to vary from 4% to 15%.[2,3] Female runners have been shown to have 12 times the risk of developing stress fractures than males.[4] Most stress fractures occur on the posteromedial (compression) side of the tibia, but they may also infrequently involve the mid-anterior region of the tibia or the distal fibula.[5] The specific sport or activity may affect the site of the stress fracture. Runners often develop fractures of the mid to distal third of the tibia, whereas basketball and volleyball players are prone to proximal tibial stress fractures.[6]

Mechanism of injury

A stress fracture develops when the human body's ability to adapt to repetitive stress is exceeded. Repetitive cyclic loading of the tibia triggers a physiologic bone remodeling. There is an initial increase in bone resorption by osteoclasts in response to the compressive forces, thereby causing increased bone porosity and a weakened cortex. This is followed by the production and deposition of new bone by osteoblasts. The resultant cortical hypertrophy is the appropriate bony functional adaptation response: the overall strengthening of the tibia. With adequate rest, the bone has time to repair and to adapt to the increased stress. If the tibia is continually stressed without an adequate rest period, an imbalance in bone remodeling occurs, with osteoblastic activity lagging behind osteoclastic activity. This results in an overall weakened bony cortex and, most likely, a resultant stress fracture.[7]

Risk factors

The causes underlying stress fracture development are multifactorial. Risk factors for stress fracture include female gender, increasing age, non-black race, and narrow tibial width.[8] Patients with eating disorders, who participate in sports that emphasize "leanness," who have a history of stress fractures, who are military recruits, and who are females with menstrual irregularities are at higher risk for developing stress fractures.[9] Special attention should be paid to the female athlete with menstrual irregularities, and this should include a high index of suspicion for the "female athlete triad" (disordered eating, amenorrhea, and osteoporosis). Because bony metabolism is affected by lower estrogen levels, women with irregular menses are predisposed to stress fractures.[10] Poor fitness level, an abrupt change in training, running on hard surfaces, poor athletic footwear, limb-length discrepancy, bone density, excessive pronation, and muscle fatigue have all been investigated as associated risk factors.[10-14] Although there are many associations, no causative factors have been identified.[10]

Clinical features

Patients with a stress fracture typically present with well-localized bony pain that occurs near the end of activity and that is relieved with rest. As the condition progresses, the pain becomes sharp and penetrating. It is easily exacerbated by any impact activity, and it may persist after the cessation of activity or at rest. The pain associated with a tibial stress fracture is localized to the fracture site, and it is typically more proximal than that of medial tibial stress syndrome (MTSS).[15,16] Patients may relate a history of an abrupt change in training habits to include increased intensity, duration, or frequency. Fibular stress fractures should be considered in those patients describing lateral leg or ankle pain.

Physical examination is remarkable for localized point tenderness along the tibia, with maximal tenderness at the fracture site. There can be associated erythema, swelling, or a palpable callus at the site of the fracture, depending on the duration of the injury. Jumping up and down or jogging in place in the examination room can often reproduce the characteristic pain. Applying a bending or twisting force to the leg can produce pain at the location of the fracture. Vibration with either a tuning fork or ultrasound applied to the fracture site may elicit pain and aid in the diagnosis of stress fracture. Severe pain when vibration is applied directly over the point of maximal tenderness is suggestive of a fracture. The vibratory stress test should not be relied on as conclusive evidence of stress fracture because the sensitivity and specificity have been reported as 75% and 67%, respectively.[17] Pain with compression of the tibiofibular syndesmosis may indicate a distal fibular stress fracture.[18] Neurovascular examination of the extremity should be normal.

Diagnosis

Early radiographs are often normal during the first few weeks after symptom onset. Faint periosteal reactions, a cortical lucency or cortical thickening, sclerosis, callus formation, and a fracture plane are radiographic abnormalities that are suggestive of stress fracture. Stress fractures of the tibia are typically transverse through the cortex, although longitudinal stress fractures have been reported.[19,20] Particular attention should be paid to the anterior cortical surface of the tibia for the presence of the "dreaded black line," which is indicative of the delayed healing or nonunion of an anterior cortex tibial stress fracture. The sensitivity of radiographs is only 15% to 35% initially, and it may take 2 to 12 weeks before the radiographic changes of stress fracture are evident.[21] Negative radiographs should not rule out the diagnosis of stress fracture if clinical suspicion is high **(Figure 27.1 and Box 27.1)**.

A triple-phase technetium bone scan is highly sensitive for stress fracture, and it is usually positive 3 to 5 days after the onset of pain. The scintigraphic pattern for stress fracture is a characteristic focal uptake in the area of the fracture that is often evident on all phases of the scan. Bone scan can differentiate MTSS from stress fracture. All three phases typically have positive findings for stress fracture in a localized area, which is in contrast with the diffuse reaction that is seen only on the delayed images (third phase) for MTSS. Bone scanning is highly sensitive for stress fractures in the patient with well-localized symptoms, and a negative scan virtually excludes the diagnosis of stress fracture. However, the specificity of a bone scan is low. It is important to note that the delayed images for stress fracture can remain positive for months, even after the resolution of symptoms and the patient's return to activity. Up to 50% of positive findings on bone scanning occur at asymptomatic sites that correspond with painless accelerated bone remodeling or bone strain.[22]

Magnetic resonance imaging (MRI) is slowly becoming the preferred study for the evaluation of stress fractures. Although it was initially felt to be an expensive imaging study that is no better than a bone scan, it has proven to be a sensitive tool for the detection of

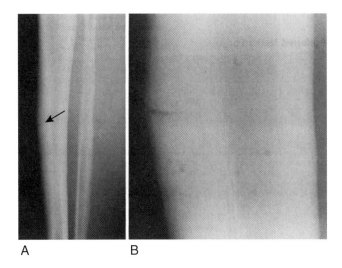

Figure 27.1 *A* and *B*, The "dreaded black line" of the anterior tibial cortex. (From DeLee JC, Drez D Jr, Miller MD [eds]: DeLee & Drez's Orthopaedic Sports Medicine: Principles and Practice, 2nd ed. Philadelphia, WB Saunders, 2003.)

stress fracture that avoids the use of radiation altogether at a comparable expense. MRI has been shown to be as sensitive as bone scanning for stress fracture but also to be more specific.[23,24] MRI can differentiate between MTSS and stress fracture, and it is additionally useful for differentiating bone injury from ligament or cartilage injury. An MRI is recommended to differentiate MTSS from a longitudinal stress fracture on a bone scan because both of these conditions will demonstrate diffuse tracer uptake along the posterior medial tibia.[25-27]

Treatment

The primary management of tibial and fibular stress fractures is rest and protection from further injury. The vast majority of stress fractures will heal with nonsurgical management. All running should cease. Patients are allowed to bear weight for daily activities if they can ambulate without discomfort; otherwise crutches should be used to decrease impact stress on the tibia until the pain has resolved. Casting or bracing is rarely necessary, although the use of a pneumatic leg brace has been shown to speed return to activity.[28] Ice massage and nonsteroidal anti-inflammatory medications (NSAIDS) are useful for analgesia. After the initial 1- to 2-week period of relative rest, aerobic conditioning may be maintained with low-impact cardiovascular activities including stationary biking, swimming, or water aerobics as long as participation in these activities does not result in bony pain. A stretching and flexibility program should be maintained. Predisposing factors such as nutritional, hormonal, or biomechanical abnormalities should be addressed. Menstrual irregularities should specifically be evaluated among female athletes. A gradually progressive training regimen

---

Box 27.1: Differential Diagnosis for Stress Fracture

Exertional compartment syndrome

Medial tibial stress fracture

Tendinitis

Bone tumor

Osteomyelitis

and appropriate footwear should be reviewed with the athlete to prevent recurrence. The diagnosis and treatment of stress fractures is discussed in more detail in Chapter 32.

Most stress fractures heal within 4 to 6 weeks, with a return to full sports participation in an additional 4 to 6 weeks. Rates of delayed union or nonunion have been reported to be as high as 10% in those individuals who are not compliant with the sufficient avoidance of impact activities.[2] Close follow up is an integral part of stress-fracture management. For those patients whose pain is not relieved after an initial 2- to 4-week period of relative rest, 3 to 12 weeks of immobilization with a cast or brace may be warranted.[29]

Stress fractures of the anterior cortex require special attention and account for about 5% of all tibial stress fractures. These fractures are at risk for delayed union or nonunion as a result of the decreased vascularity of the anterior tibial cortex and the constant tension from the pull of the posterior compartment muscles.[30] Suggested management is a short leg non–weight-bearing cast for 6 to 8 weeks followed by a walking cast for up to 6 months, with strict monitoring for evidence of healing through physical examination and imaging. Consultation with a physician experienced in the management of high-risk stress fractures is highly recommended for anterior cortex fractures, longitudinal stress fractures, and proximal tibial stress fractures that have failed nonsurgical management with immobilization. Intramedullary fixation or bone grafting may be required to allow healing.

Return to play

The patient may begin a gradual return to training when impact activities can be performed without pain after a minimum rest period of 2 to 4 weeks and when there is radiographic and clinical evidence of fracture healing. The patient should follow a gradual, slowly progressive training program, increasing distance in 10% increments each week. Pain should guide training progression. If at any point upon the resumption of activity the athlete experiences pain, he or she should cease the offending activity and seek medical consultation. By 12 weeks, most uncomplicated stress fractures are sufficiently healed to resume full training.

MEDIAL TIBIAL STRESS SYNDROME

MTSS was first defined as "a symptom complex seen in athletes who complain of exercise induced pain along the posterior medial border of the tibia."[31] It is the most prevalent of the lower-extremity overuse injuries, and it is often incorporated into the broad category of "shin splints," an ambiguous entity that does not clearly define location or cause. Runners are the athletes who are most frequently encountered with MTSS, which accounts for between 13.2% and 17.3% of all running injuries.[32] Two military studies have demonstrated the incidence to vary from 4.0% to 6.4%, and the only civilian prospective study demonstrated a higher incidence of 13%.[13-35] Athletes involved in jumping sports such as basketball, tennis, and volleyball are also prone to the development of MTSS.[36]

Mechanism of injury

MTSS is a tibial stress reaction that develops in response to repetitive loading forces on the lower extremity and the overuse of the muscles of the posterior compartment. The traction forces transmitted through the posterior compartment muscles result in a traction periostitis at the muscle origins with overuse. Physiologic bone remodeling is the adaptive response to activities that cause repetitive stress or insult to the periosteum. Initially, increased osteoclastic activity is triggered in response to the compressive

and traction forces of overuse, thereby causing increased bone porosity and a weakened cortex. This is followed by the production of new bone by osteoblasts to resist the compressive and traction forces.[37,38] Periosteal thickening and cortical hypertrophy occur, with the result being the appropriate functional adaptation response and an overall strengthened tibia. With adequate rest, the periosteum has time to adapt to the increased stress. If the tibia is continually stressed without an adequate rest period, an imbalance in bone turnover can occur with bone production lagging behind, which may result in a stress fracture. MTSS is one point along the continuum of the progression of skeletal injury as proposed by Matin.[39] Using triple-phase technetium bone scans, he described a five-stage progression of skeletal injury that begins with minimal periosteal reaction and continues through a complete full-thickness stress fracture. Fredericson and colleagues[40] proposed a similar grading system using MRI.

MTSS is a traction periostitis that results from the sheering stresses of the muscles in the posterior compartment on the posterior medial border of the tibia. The soleus muscle, the flexor digitorum longus muscle, and the deep crural fascia all originate along the medial aspect of the tibia. The sheering forces from the soleus muscle biomechanically appear to be the major cause of MTSS, with contributions from the flexor digitorum longus and the crural fascia. The tibialis posterior muscle originates from the lateral aspect of the tibia, so it is not considered to play a significant role in causing MTSS[38] **(Figure 27.2).**

Risk factors

Risk factors for MTSS can be classified as biomechanical or activity related. Activity-related risk factors include abrupt changes in training, running on hard surfaces, inadequate arch support, and poor athletic footwear. The degree of baseline conditioning is also a factor because an unconditioned athlete who begins an aggressive training program is more likely to develop MTSS as compared with a conditioned athlete.[34,41]

Excessive pronation of the foot in combination with repetitive impact activity is a well-described risk factor for the development of MTSS.[42-44] Muscle–tendon inflexibility, pes planus, subtalar joint mobility, and a greater Achilles tendon angle have all been implicated in the development of MTSS.[45] The risk of developing MTSS is multifactorial, but it is often the result of a combination of extrinsic (activity-related) and intrinsic (biomechanical) factors.

Clinical features

Patients with MTSS characteristically present with a gradually progressive pain along the middle to the distal posterior medial border of the tibia. Initially, the pain may be present only at the beginning of activity, and it may resolve quickly with continued exertion; in other words, the patient may describe an ability to "run through the pain." The pain is typically relieved by rest and exacerbated by activity. As the syndrome progresses, the patient's discomfort may intensify from a recurrent dull ache to a persistent sharp pain that is present both with exertion and at rest; athletic performance may eventually become impaired. A sudden increase in the frequency, intensity, or duration of athletic activity or significant changes in footwear, terrain, or running surface are key historic features that predispose an individual to the development of MTSS. Fifty percent of patients complain of bilateral lower extremity symptoms.[46]

Physical examination demonstrates tenderness to palpation along the posterior medial border of the tibial shaft. The tenderness is typically not well localized, and it involves the middle to distal third of the tibia. Mild edema coinciding with the area of tenderness may be present. The area of tenderness is more diffuse without specific point tenderness as is seen with a stress fracture. The patient's symptoms may often be reproduced with resisted

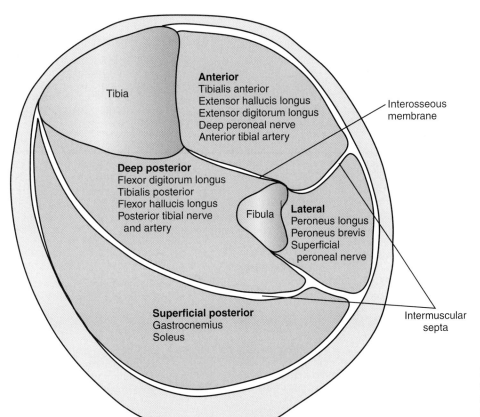

Figure 27.2 A diagram of the compartments of the lower extremity. (From Hamilton: Emergency Medicine: An Approach to Clinical Problem Solving, 2nd ed. Philadelphia, WB Saunders, 2003.)

plantarflexion or dorsiflexion of the foot. Neurovascular examination of the extremity should be normal. It is important to evaluate the patient for predisposing biomechanical deficiencies as part of a complete examination for MTSS.

Diagnosis

Lower-extremity radiographs should be obtained to rule out a stress fracture. Although radiographs are often normal for patients with MTSS, they may reveal signs of a stress reaction, such as cortical hypertrophy or longitudinal periosteal new bone formation with scalloping along the distal posterior medial tibial border.

For those patients whose symptoms do not resolve with rest or for athletes for whom a break in training is unacceptable, a triple-phase technetium bone scan should be performed to differentiate between MTSS and stress fracture. The typical findings that are indicative of periostitis include a diffuse longitudinal uptake pattern along the distal third or more of the length of the tibial periosteum in the delayed images.[42] The areas of tracer uptake correlate with periostitis of the soleus muscle, the flexor digitorum longus muscle, and the crural fascia origins on the tibia[47] **(Figure 27.3).**

MRIs are also useful for the evaluation and differentiation of MTSS and stress fractures. The appearance of MTSS on MRI has been described to include periosteal fluid and abnormal marrow signal intensity.[48] Caution should be used in the interpretation of both MRI and bone scans for the evaluation of MTSS because these studies may be normal early during the course of the condition **(Box 27.2).**

Treatment/prevention

The primary management of MTSS is rest. A 2- to 3-week period of rest or decreased training intensity may be curative.[49,50]

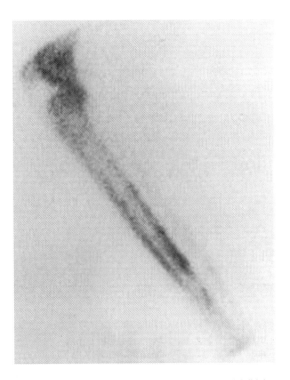

Figure 27.3 A technetium bone scan demonstrating medial tibial stress syndrome. (From Deutsch AL, Coel MN, Mink JH: Clin Sports Med 1997;16:280. In Rakel: Textbook of Family Practice, 6th ed. Philadelphia, WB Saunders, 2002.)

Box 27.2: Differential Diagnosis for Medial Tibial Stress Syndrome

Exertional compartment syndrome

Stress fracture

Tendinitis

Aerobic conditioning may be maintained with low-impact cardiovascular activities including stationary biking, swimming, and water aerobics without compromising the rate of recovery.[49,51] These activities should be performed in a manner that limits compression or traction stress on the tibia. Ice may be used acutely to reduce swelling and inflammation. NSAIDS are appropriate for analgesia. Stretching programs for the gastrocnemius, soleus, and hamstrings may be helpful for cases in which these muscles are excessively tight. Physical therapy modalities including ultrasound, iontophoresis, electrical stimulation, localized massage, and bracing may be useful adjuncts for the treatment of MTSS.[52,53] Biomechanical abnormalities (specifically excessive pronation) should be corrected with the use of orthotics and motion control footwear. A compressive sleeve may provide symptomatic relief with the premise that the uniform compression stabilizes the muscles and decreases the tension and sheer forces applied to the periosteum.

Surgical treatment should be reserved for patients with intractable MTSS for whom nonoperative modalities have failed. The failure of nonoperative treatment has been described as "at least 2 periods of rest and resumption of activity with recurrence of symptoms," and a period of relative rest can vary from 2 weeks up to 4 months.[46,54] In the rare instances in which surgery is required, a posterior medial fasciotomy involving the release of the superficial posterior compartment near its insertion to the medial border of the tibia can be performed.[43] Some authors recommend that the removal of a strip of periosteum along the medial tibial border be performed in addition to the fasciotomy.[46,55]

After the acute pain of MTSS subsides, the prevention of future recurrence becomes paramount. Prevention begins with correcting training errors and identifying biomechanical deficiencies. Flexibility of the gastronemius and soleus should be emphasized, as should the aggressive strengthening of the foot intrinsics, the dorsiflexors, the plantarflexors, the invertors, the evertors, and the gluteals[56] **(Figure 27.4).**

Biomechanical abnormalities must be identified and corrected before the patient returns to training, or else he or she will likely experience recurrent symptoms. The athlete should adhere to a gradual, progressive training program. He or she should be advised to choose a well-fitted, shock-absorbing shoe and to begin the initial running programs on compliant surfaces. To aid in the prevention of recurrence, warmup and cool-down stretching programs should be implemented (LOE: B).

Return to play

The best chance for avoiding symptom recurrence comes with a return to sports participation after a period of relative rest that is followed by strengthening, the correction of biomechanical factors, and then the completion of a gradual, progressive training program. Relative rest periods may vary from a minimum of 2 weeks to up to 4 months for severe MTSS. A gradual, slowly progressive training program should increase the exercise distance by no more than 10% each week. If symptoms return, the patient should cease activity for at least 2 weeks before resuming training at a lower intensity.

EXERTIONAL COMPARTMENT SYNDROME IN THE LOWER LEG

Chronic exertional compartment syndrome (CECS) is defined as a reversible ischemia that results from a noncompliant myofascial

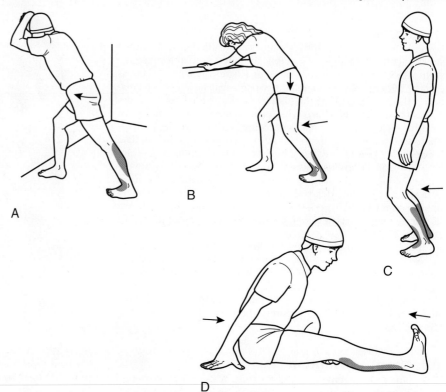

Figure 27.4 *A, B, C,* and *D,* Stretches for the muscles in the gastrocnemius and soleus area. *Shaded areas* indicate the areas that are the most likely to feel the stretch. (From Anderson B, Burke ER: Clin Sports Med 1991;10:63-86. In DeLee JC, Drez D Jr, Miller MD [eds]: DeLee & Drez's Orthopaedic Sports Medicine: Principles and Practice, 2nd ed. Philadelphia, WB Saunders, 2003.)

compartment that is unresponsive to the expansion of muscle volume that occurs with exercise. CECS is most commonly seen in the lower leg.

Mechanism of injury

This injury is typically seen in runners; however, any athlete can develop CECS. The true prevalence of this injury is unknown. The literature describes CECS as classically occurring in athletes who are less than 40 years of age who participate in running programs. Males and females are equally affected. About 50% to 70% of patients will have bilateral involvement, with one side being somewhat worse.[57] During exercise, muscles increase in volume. If the myofascial compartment does not allow for sufficient expansion to accommodate this increased volume, the compartment pressure increases. This increased myofascial compartment pressure can compromise blood flow, especially during exercise. When tissue perfusion is not adequate to meet the metabolic demands, the result is traversing neurologic and muscular ischemia, pain, and the impairment of muscular function.[58]

There are four main compartments in the leg. Each compartment is covered by a tight fascia, with structural support provided by the tibia and the fibula (see **Table 27.1** and Figure 27.2).

The anterior compartment is most commonly affected in patients with CECS (45%), followed by the deep posterior compartment (40%), the lateral compartment (10%), and the superficial posterior compartment (5%).[57]

Risk factors

Three classic risk factors have been identified that may contribute to an increase in the intracompartmental pressure seen during exercise[59]:

1. Decreased elasticity and increased thickness of the fascial sheath
2. Increased volume of skeletal muscle with exertion resulting from blood flow and edema caused by impaired tibial venous drainage
3. Muscle hypertrophy as a response to training

It has also been proposed that myofiber damage as a result of eccentric exercise causes a release of protein-bound ions and a subsequent increase in osmotic pressure within the compartment. The increase in osmotic pressure increases capillary relaxation pressure, thus decreasing the blood flow.

Table 27.1 Leg Compartments and Their Corresponding Muscles, Arteries, and Nerves

Compartment	Muscles	Artery	Nerve
Anterior	Extensor hallucis longus, tibialis anterior extensor, digitorum longus	Anterior tibial	Deep peroneal
Lateral	Peroneus longus, peroneus brevis	Perineal	Superficial peroneal
Deep posterior	Tibialis posterior,* flexor hallucis longus, flexor digitorum longus	Posterior tibial	Tibial nerve
Superficial posterior	Gastrocnemius, soleus plantaris		Sural nerve

*Some authors advocate a separate fifth compartment for the tibialis posterior because it is surrounded by its own fascia.[58]

It has been noted that the development of symptoms may be more common at the beginning of the running season as a result of muscle hypertrophy, which decreases the volume in the compartment. Recently, the role of creatine has been implicated as a risk for developing CECS because of the rapid increases in muscle size caused by fluid retention that are seen when patients take the substance.[56]

Clinical features

The classic presentation of patients with CECS is recurrent exertional leg pain that occurs at a well-defined and reproducible point of activity and that increases if the training activity persists. Typically, runners will be able to identify the distance or time required for the onset of their symptoms. Patients may also complain of altered running style after the onset of pain. For example, a runner may complain that the foot seems to be slapping the ground. The quality of the pain is described as a tight, cramplike, or squeezing ache over a specific compartment of the leg. The pain will typically decrease or dissipate after 10-20 minutes of rest; however, in extreme cases such as acute-on-chronic exertional compartment syndrome, the pain may persist even at rest. Patients occasionally report paresthesia in the leg and the dorsum of the foot during exercise, which may indicate the involvement of the nerve traversing the compartment. In addition, the patient may complain of muscle weakness or a sense of ankle instability.[60]

The physical examination of a patient with CECS is usually unremarkable, with a normal gait and a normal lower extremity examination unless the patient has recently exercised. Therefore, performing the physical examination after the patient has exercised strenuously enough to reproduce symptoms is recommended. After the reproduction of symptoms, the patient should be assessed for tenderness, tightness, and swelling over the involved compartment. Focal muscle herniation may be present through fascial defects; this commonly occurs where the superficial peroneal nerve exits the fascia. Another key aspect of the physical examination is testing muscle strength in the affected compartment **(Table 27.2)**.

Diagnosis

Although the history may be suggestive of CECS, no physical examination finding can firmly establish the diagnosis.[61] In addition to a physical examination, diagnostic testing including radiographs, bone scans, and MRI may assist with distinguishing between CECS and other possible lower-leg conditions.[62] Radiographs are typically normal in cases of CECS. Bone scanning can be done to eliminate MTSS and stress fracture from the differential diagnosis. When the physical examination suggests a vascular cause such as popliteal artery entrapment, MRI or magnetic resonance angiography is recommended. Electromyogram testing should be done to rule out nerve entrapment **(Box 27.3 and Table 27.3)**.

Table 27.2 Preliminary Diagnosis of Chronic Exertional Compartment Syndrome

Compartment	Weakness	Sensory Deficit
Anterior	Toe extension, foot dorsiflexion	Numbness in first web space
Lateral	Ankle eversion	Anterolateral aspect of the leg
Deep posterior	Toe flexion, foot inversion	Plantar aspect of the foot
Superficial posterior	Plantar flexion	Dorsolateral foot

Box 27.3: Differential Diagnosis of Exertional Leg Pain

Tendon injury

Medial tibial stress syndrome

Tibial stress fracture

Fibular stress fracture

Chronic exertional compartment syndrome

Peroneal nerve entrapment

Saphenous nerve entrapment

Sural nerve entrapment

Popliteal artery entrapment

Neurogenic claudication

Effort-induced venous thrombosis

Exertional rhabdomyolysis

Osteoid osteoma

The hallmark diagnostic tool for confirming CECS is the measurement of intracompartmental pressures (see Chapter 46 for a detailed discussion of how to perform the test). Generally accepted criteria for the diagnosis of CECS are described by Pedowitz and colleagues.[63] One or more of the following pressure criteria must be met in addition to a history and physical examination that are consistent with the diagnosis of CECS: (1) pre-exercise pressure of greater than 15 mm Hg; (2) 1 minute postexercise pressure of greater than 30 mm Hg; or (3) 5 minutes postexercise pressure of greater than 20 mm Hg (LOE: B).[63] Recent interest has focused on the use of noninvasive tests such as triple-phase bone scanning, MRI, near-infrared spectroscopy, and technetium-99m methoxyisobutyl isonitrile perfusion imaging for the diagnosis of CECS. The dynamic bone scan may support the diagnosis on the basis of specific tracer uptake patterns. The characteristic appearance is that of decreased radionuclide concentration in the vicinity of the area of increased pressure, with increased soft-tissue concentration both superior to and inferior to the abnormality. The area of decreased uptake is believed to be the result of the increased pressure and decreased blood flow to the region (LOE: E).[64] With MRI, exercise changes are characterized by swelling within a compartment, which manifests as intramuscular diffuse high signal intensity on T2-weighted images. Failure of the edematous muscle to return to the baseline normal appearance by 25 minutes after the completion of exercise is diagnostic.[65] Near-infrared spectroscopy measures the tissue deoxygenation of skeletal muscle by elevated intramuscular pressure during exercise (LOE: C).[66] Technetium-99m methoxyisobutyl isonitrile perfusion measures the ability of peripheral muscles to uptake intravenously injected radiopharmaceuticals.[67]

Treatment

The treatment of CECS can include both nonsurgical and surgical interventions. Nonsurgical interventions include addressing any

Table 27.3 Pedowitz Criteria for Chronic Exertional Compartment Syndrome

Timing of Test	Pressure
Before exercise	>15 mm Hg
1 minute postexercise	>30 mm Hg
5 minutes postexercise	>20 mm Hg

extrinsic or intrinsic contributing factors. Extrinsic factors such as training surface, shoe design, and training intensity can be modified as part of a treatment plan. Intrinsic factors such as muscle imbalance, flexibility, and limb alignment can be treated with stretching, strengthening, and orthoses. However, it is difficult or impossible to modify all of these factors, and even after addressing all possible contributing factors, athletes routinely remain symptomatic unless they refrain from symptom-producing activities (LOE: C).[68] Although the ischemia of CECS is generally considered reversible, the chronic and repetitive recurrence of elevated pressures can induce irreversible injury to the muscles and nerves within the involved compartment. Abnormal muscle and fascial biopsies taken at the time of fasciotomy have been described.[69] In addition, in athletes with chronic exertional ischemia, the risk of progression exists from reversible deficits to irreversible acute compartment syndrome.[70] Athletes who do not desire fasciotomy should be advised that continued symptoms or attempts to perform through the pain can result in acute compartment syndrome. Surgical intervention that involves fasciotomy is indicated if the athlete is unwilling to decrease the level of activity or if he or she experiences severe symptoms.

Return to play

After a patient presents with CECS, it is difficult to modify all risk factors that may have contributed to the symptoms. Athletes routinely remain symptomatic unless they abstain from symptom-producing activities. However, after fasciotomy, most athletes are able to return to full sports participation by 8 to 12 weeks, when symmetric strength has returned. Numerous researchers have reported rates of 80% to 100% good to excellent results.[71-73] Generally, athletes are able to return to sports participation without pain or with greatly diminished symptoms.

POPLITEAL ARTERY ENTRAPMENT SYNDROME

The diagnosis of popliteal artery entrapment syndrome (PAES) should be included in the differential diagnosis of the running athlete with exertional calf and upper-leg pain.

Mechanism of injury

This syndrome has classically been attributed to a congenitally abnormal relationship between the popliteal artery and the medial head of the gastrocnemius that causes intermittent arterial occlusion and subsequent claudication during exertion. However, a "functional" popliteal artery entrapment has been described in which no anatomic abnormalities are noted in the popliteal fossa, and entrapment has been attributed to compression from the soleus and plantaris muscles as well as to the hypertrophy of the gastrocnemius.[74]

Risk factors

PAES typically occurs during high-intensity exercises that require repetitive dorsiflexion and plantar flexion such as football, basketball, soccer, and running. This uncommon condition typically presents in young exercisers, most commonly males less than 30 years of age who complain of unilateral calf pain with exercise. Popliteal artery entrapment is bilateral in 25% to 40% of cases.[75]

Clinical features

The clinical presentation of PAES involves pain and claudication, which are related to the degree of entrapment of the popliteal artery.[76] Symptoms include calf pain and coolness and/or paresthesias of the foot that occur with exertion and that are relieved with rest. The pain is classically described as a deep ache or cramping. Physical examination at rest is often normal, and usually an exercise challenge is often required to reproduce symptoms. Popliteal, posterior tibial, and dorsalis pedis pulses should be examined before and after exercise to determine whether a reduction in pulse volume between limbs exist. The pulses should be examined with the ankle in passive dorsiflexion or active plantar flexion with the knee in extension because these positions place tension on the gastrocnemius, thereby leading to extrinsic compression of the popliteal artery.[77]

Diagnosis

Radiographs and bone scans often produce negative results in cases of PAES, but they should be done to rule out other causes of leg pain. When PAES is suspected, MRI and magnetic resonance angiography are recommended as screening tests because a decreased flow with provocation is suggestive of PAES.[78] If MRI or magnetic resonance angiography is positive for PAES, arteriography is the gold standard for the confirmation of the diagnosis.[79]

Treatment

PAES can be managed with nonoperative and operative interventions. However, nonoperative treatment involves the avoidance of the exacerbating activities. Surgery is the preferred treatment option because PAES typically recurs with activity; it may lead to long-term arterial damage if left untreated.[80]

LOWER EXTREMITY NERVE ENTRAPMENTS

Nerve entrapments and compression are less frequent causes of exertional leg pain. This diagnosis should be entertained in any athlete who is suspected of having exertional compartment syndrome but who has normal intracompartmental pressures. The common peroneal, superficial peroneal, and saphenous nerves are the most common nerves that are at risk for entrapment in the lower extremity.[81]

Mechanism of injury

The common peroneal nerve leaves the popliteal fossa and winds forward around the lateral aspect of the neck of the fibula. Then, in the lateral compartment, it divides into the superficial peroneal nerve, the deep peroneal nerve, and the lateral sural cutaneous nerve. The deep peroneal nerve enters the anterior compartment, innervates all the muscles, divides into the medial and lateral branches just proximal to the ankle, and then enters the foot deep to the inferior extensor retinaculum. Its medial branch supplies sensation to the first web space. The superficial nerve innervates the lateral leg compartment and then emerges from the lateral leg compartment by penetrating the crural fascia approximately 10 to 12 cm proximal to the tip of the lateral malleolus. Trauma is a primary cause of all three forms of entrapment.[82] Superficial peroneal nerve entrapment is often observed in dancers and athletes who are involved in bodybuilding, horse racing, running, soccer, and tennis. Common peroneal nerve entrapment is usually associated with repetitive exercises involving inversion and eversion, such as running and cycling. It can also be caused by external compressive sources (e.g., tight plaster casts and anterior cruciate ligament braces) as well as internal compressive sources (e.g., osteophytes and proximal tibiofibular joint ganglion cysts). Knee surgery is also a documented cause of both common peroneal and saphenous nerve entrapments.[79] The saphenous nerve is most vulnerable at the medial knee, where it pierces the fascia and emerges from the distal subsartorial canal. Causes of saph-enous neuritis include entrapment at the adductor canal, pes anserine bursitis, contusion, and postsurgical injury **(Figures 27.5 and 27.6)**.

Clinical presentation

The typical presentation of nerve entrapment consists of pain that is brought about by activity.[83] With entrapment of the common peroneal nerve, the athlete may report neuropathic symptoms that extend into the dorsum of the foot and the toe web spaces. The athlete may complain of foot drop or recurrent ankle sprains. On physical examination, there may be weakness with dorsiflexion. Superficial peroneal nerve entrapment often presents with burning, superficial pain with alterations in sensation over the sinus tarsi or the dorsolateral foot that are associated with activity and relieved by rest.[83] Examination may reveal percussion tenderness, a fascial defect in 60% of patients, or muscular herniation at the exit site. Deep peroneal nerve entrapment often presents with deep aching dorsal mid foot pain and paresthesias that extend into the first web space. Percussion along the course of the deep peroneal nerve may help to localize the entrapment. The athlete with saphenous nerve entrapment will complain of pain and numbness in the area of the medial knee and/or calf. There should be no motor deficits.

Diagnosis

Electrodiagnostic studies should be done to determine to location of the lesion. However, these may need to be done after exercise for exertional symptoms.[84]

Treatment

For common peroneal nerve entrapment, neuromodulatory medications and transcutaneous electrical neural stimulation (TENS) may be used for pain relief. Biomechanical interventions may be used to reduce neural tension, dorsiflexion support may be implemented, and a change in running style to avoid excessive varus/recurvatum knee movements may be required.[87] Nonoperative options include the use of NSAIDS in combination with relative rest, physical therapy for the strengthening of muscles in cases of associated weakness or recurrent ankle sprains, and the elimination of predisposing or triggering factors. Aids such as braces can be used to avoid recurrent ankle sprains. In-shoe orthotic devices may by helpful in certain instances, such as for the correction of a biomechanical malalignment in gait for patients with severe flatfoot or cavus foot. At times, the injection of steroids plus lidocaine near the site of involvement in the lower leg can reduce symptoms, and it can also serve as a diagnostic tool for confirming the zone of nerve compression. The use of antineuritic medications (e.g., gabapentin) can also be helpful for reducing and at times eliminating symptoms, particularly in cases that are associated with complex regional pain syndrome. In these cases, combination treatment with medication, physical therapy, and local and sympathetic nerve blocks may be required. Surgical decompression may be indicated for cases that are refractory to nonoperative options. This can include the release of the superficial peroneal nerve at the lateral leg for surgical decompression with partial or full fasciotomy. Some authors have also advocated fasciectomy in select cases. Neurolysis is generally not indicated because it has not been shown to improve outcome.

In 1997, Styf and Morberg[85] reported that 80% of their patients were free from symptoms or satisfied with their results after decompression of the superficial peroneal nerve. Three of 14 patients had local fasciectomy as well.[85]

Deep peroneal nerve entrapment has been successfully treated with several modalities. Nonsurgical care most importantly involves patient education to eliminate the predisposing factors.

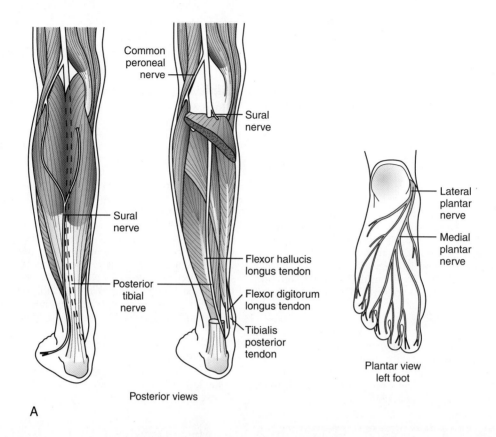

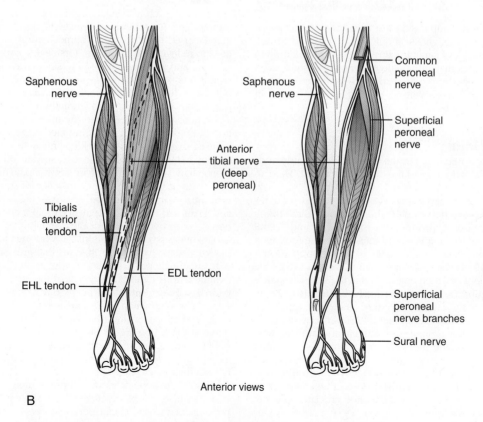

Figure 27.5 The anatomy of the lower extremity nerves. (From Shurman DH: Anesthesiology 1976;44:348.)

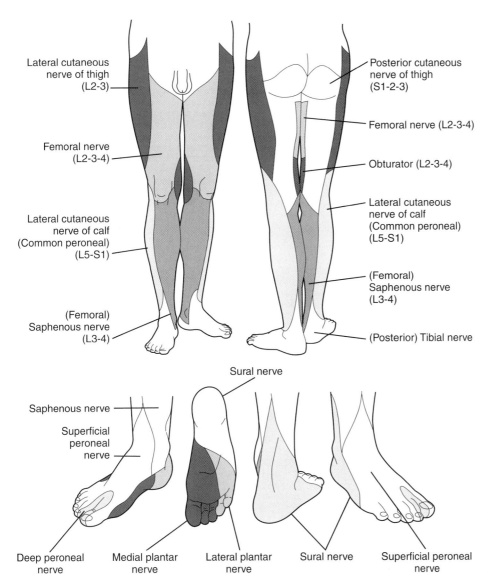

Lateral cutaneous nerve of thigh (L2-3)

Posterior cutaneous nerve of thigh (S1-2-3)

Femoral nerve (L2-3-4)

Femoral nerve (L2-3-4)

Obturator (L2-3-4)

Lateral cutaneous nerve of calf (Common peroneal) (L5-S1)

Lateral cutaneous nerve of calf (Common peroneal) (L5-S1)

(Femoral) Saphenous nerve (L3-4)

(Femoral) Saphenous nerve (L3-4)

(Posterior) Tibial nerve

Sural nerve

Saphenous nerve

Superficial peroneal nerve

Deep peroneal nerve

Medial plantar nerve

Lateral plantar nerve

Sural nerve

Superficial peroneal nerve

Figure 27.6 The cutaneous distribution of nerves to the lower extremity. (From Bridenbaugh PO: The lower extremity: somatic blockade. In Cousins M, Bridenbaugh PO [eds]: Neural Blockade in Clinical Anesthesia and Management of Pain, 2nd ed. Philadelphia, JB Lippincott, 1988, p 425.)

For example, padding of the tongue of the shoe, the elimination of shoes with laces, the use of alternative methods for lacing, and the avoidance of high-heeled shoes may be sufficient to resolve symptoms. Physical therapy is useful for strengthening the peroneal muscles for cases that are associated with weakness and for individuals with chronic ankle instability; the use of these modalities may also improve symptoms. In-shoe orthotic devices are helpful in certain instances, such as for the correction of a biomechanical malalignment in gait (e.g., for patients with severe flatfoot or cavus foot). The use of NSAIDS and antineuritic medications may be helpful as an adjunct to other treatment modalities. The injection of steroids plus lidocaine near the site of involvement can reduce symptoms in some individuals. In addition, consideration should be given to a metabolic workup to rule out thyroid dysfunction and diabetes in select individuals. Further workup may be necessary to rule out lumbar radiculopathy. Surgical options can be considered after symptoms are deemed refractory to nonoperative measures. Options include the surgical release of the deep peroneal nerve in primary and idiopathic cases to the excision of the nerve in cases of direct nerve injury as a result of previous surgery or direct trauma or in revision cases. Surgical decompression of the nerve can provide the immediate improvement of symptoms. In 1990, Dellon[84] reported about the surgical release of the deep peroneal nerve in 20 patients. With a mean follow-up time of more than 2 years, he reported excellent results in 60% of patients, good results in 20% of patients, and no improvement in 20% of patients.[84] The most common presenting symptom is a vague pain on the dorsum of the foot with occasional associated numbness or weakness. Treatment options are aimed at eliminating underlying causes of entrapment. Surgical release or excision is reserved for refractory cases.

CONCLUSION

Leg pain is among the most common complaints in running athletes. Although the differential diagnosis for exertional leg pain is relatively small, several diagnoses are complicated to accurately identify (e.g., exertional compartment syndrome and nerve entrapment). Careful attention to the details of the patients' complaints and their temporal relationship to exercise will assist the physician in coming to the proper diagnosis.

REFERENCES

1. Matheson GO, Clement DB, McKenzie DC, et al: Stress fractures in athletes: a study of 320 cases. Am J Sports Med 1987;15:46.
2. Hulkko A, Orava S: Stress fractures in athletes. Int J Sports Med 1987;8:221.
3. Matheson GO, Clement DB, McKenzie DC, et al: Scintigraphic uptake of 99m Tc at non-painful sites in athletes with stress fractures: the concept of bone strain. Sports Med 1987;4:65-75.
4. Geary SP, Kelly MA: The Leg. In Scuderi GR (ed): Sports Medicine: Principles of Primary Care. St. Louis, Mosby, 1997, p 379.
5. Andrish JT, Bergfeld JA, Walheim J: A prospective study on the management of shin splints. J Bone Joint Surg Am 1974;56:1697-1700.
6. Verma RB, Sherman O: Athletic stress fractures, part II: the lower body. Part III. The upper body—with a section on the female athlete. Am J Orthop 2001;30:848-860.
7. Matin P: Basic principles of nuclear medicine techniques for detection and evaluation of trauma and sports medicine injuries. Semin Nucl Med 1988;18:90.
8. Glorioso JG, Wilckens JH: Exertional leg pain. In O'Connor FG, Wilder RP (eds): Textbook of Running Medicine. New York, McGraw-Hill, 2001, pp 181-197.
9. Edwards PH, Wright ML, Hartman JF: A practical approach for the differential diagnosis of chronic leg pain in the athlete. Am J Sports Med 2005;33:1244.
10. Bennell K, Matheson G, Meeuwisse W, Brukner P: Risk factors for stress fractures. Sports Med 1999;28:91-122.
11. Monteleone GP: Stress fractures in the athlete. Orthop Clin North Am 1995;26:423.
12. Ekenman I, Tsai-Felländer L, Westblad P, et al: A study of intrinsic factors in patients with stress fractures of the tibia. Foot Ankle Int 1996;17:477-482.
13. Kaufman KR, Brodine SK, Shaffer RA, et al: The effect of foot structure and range of motion on musculoskeletal overuse injuries. Am J Sports Med 1999;27:585-593.
14. Bennell KL, Brukner PD: Epidemiology and site specificity of stress fractures. Clin Sports Med 1997;16:179-196.
15. Hershman EB, Mailly T: Stress fractures. Clin Sports Med 1990;9:183-214.
16. Jones DC, James SL: Overuse injuries of the lower extremity: shin splints, iliotibial band friction syndrome, and exertional compartment syndromes. Clin Sports Med 1987;6:273-290.
17. Lesho EP: Can tuning forks replace bone scans for identification of tibial stress fractures? Mil Med 1997;162:802-803.
18. Pell RF, Khanuja HS, Cooley GR: Leg pain in the running athlete. J Am Acad Orthop Surg 2004;12:400.
19. Clayer M, Krishnan J, Lee WK, et al: Longitudinal stress fractures of the tibia. Clin Radiol 1992;46(6):401-404.
20. Miniaci A, McLaren AC, Haddad RG: Longitudinal stress fractures of the tibia. Can Assoc Radiol J 1988;39(3):221-223.
21. Lassus J, Tulikoura I, Konttinen YT, et al: Bone stress injuries of the lower extremity: a review. Acta Orthop Scand 2002;73:359-368.
22. Brukner P, Bennell K, Matheson G: Diagnosis of stress fractures. Stress Fractures. Victoria, Australia, Blackwell Science, 1999, p 83.
23. Gaeta M, Minutoli F, Scribano E, et al: CT and MR imaging findings in athletes with early tibial stress injuries: comparison with bone scintigraphy findings and emphasis on cortical abnormalities. Radiology 2005;235:553.
24. Fredericson M, Bergman AG, Hoffman KL, Dillingham MS: Tibial stress reaction in runners: correlation of clinical symptoms and scintigraphy with a new magnetic resonance imaging grading system. Am J Sports Med 1995;23:472.
25. Brukner P: Exercise-related lower leg pain: bone. Med Sci Sports Exerc 2000;32(Suppl 3):S15-S26.
26. Fredericson M, Wun C: Differential diagnosis of leg pain in the athlete. J Am Podiatr Med Assoc 2003;93:321-324.
27. Verma RB, Sherman O: Athletic stress fractures, part I: history, epidemiology, physiology, risk factors, radiography, diagnosis, and treatment. Am J Orthop 2001;30:798-806.
28. Swenson EJ Jr, DeHaven KE, Sebastianelli WJ, et al: The effect of a pneumatic leg brace on return to play in athletes with tibial stress fractures. Am J Sports Med 1997;25:322-328.
29. Gillespie WJ, Grant I: Interventions for preventing and treating stress fractures and stress reactions of bone of the lower limbs in young adults. Cochrane Database Syst Rev 2000;2:CD000450.
30. Boden BP, Osbahr DC: High-risk stress fractures: evaluation and treatment. J Am Acad Orthop Surg 2000;8:344-353.
31. Mubarak S, Gould R, Lee Y: The medial tibial stress syndrome. Am J Sports Med 1988;10:201-205.
32. Yates B, White S: The incidence and risk factors in the development of medial tibial stress syndrome among naval recruits. Am J Sports Med 2004;32(3):772-780.
33. Almeida S, Trone D, Leone D, Shaffer R, et al: Gender differences in musculoskeletal injury rates: a function of symptom reporting? Med Sci Sports Exerc 1999;31: 1807-1812.
34. Andrish JT, Bergfeld JA, Walheim J: A prospective study on the management of shin splints. J Bone Joint Surg Am 1974;56:1697-1700.

35. Bennett JE, Reinking MF, Pluemer B, et al: Factors contributing to the development of medial tibial stress syndrome in high school runners. J Orthop Sports Phys Ther 2001;31:504-510.
36. Edwards PH, Wright ML, Hartman JF: A practical approach for the differential diagnosis of chronic leg pain in the athlete. Am J Sports Med 2005;33(8):1242.
37. Anderson MW, Greenspan A: Stress fractures. Radiology 1996;199:1-12.
38. Beck B, Osternig L: Medial tibial stress syndrome: the location of muscles in the leg and relation to symptoms. J Bone Joint Surg Am 1994;76:1057-1061.
39. Matin P: Basic Principles of nuclear medicine techniques for detection and evaluation of trauma and sports medicine injuries. Semin Nucl Med 1988;18:90.
40. Fredericson M, Bergman AG, Hoffman KL, et al: Tibial stress reaction in runners: Correlation of clinical symptoms and scintigraphy with a new magnetic resonance imaging grading system. Am J Sports Med 1995;23:472.
41. Detmer DE: Chronic leg pain. Am J Sports Med 1980;8:141.
42. Michael RH, Holder LE: The soleus syndrome: a cause of medial tibial stress (shin splints). Am J Sports Med 1985;13:87.
43. Mubarak SJ, Gould RN, LeeYF, et al: The medial tibial stress syndrome: a cause of shin splints. Am J Sports Med 1982;10:201.
44. Holder LE, Michael RH: The specific scintigraphic pattern of "shin splints in the lower leg": concise communication. J Nucl Med 1984;25:865.
45. Viitasalo JT, Kvist M: Some biomechanical aspects of the foot and ankle in athletes with and without shin splints. Am J Sports Med 1983;11:125.
46. Detmer DE: Chronic shin splints. Classification and management of medial tibial stress syndrome. Sports Med 1986;3:436.
47. Rupani MD, Molder LE, Espinola DA: The three-phase of radionuclide bone imaging in sports medicine. Radiology 1985;156:187-196.
48. Anderson MW, Ugalde V, Batt M, et al: Shin splints: MR appearance in a preliminary study. Radiology 1997;204:177-180.
49. Moore MP: Shin splints: diagnosis, management, prevention. Postgrad Med 1988;83:202.
50. Touliopolous S, Hershman EB: Lower leg pain: diagnosis and treatment of compartment syndromes and other pain syndromes of the leg. Sports Med 1999;27:193-204.
51. Kortebein PM, Kaufman KR, Basford JR, et al: Medial tibial stress syndrome. Med Sci Sports Exerc 2000;32(Suppl 3):S27-S33.
52. Beck BR: Tibial stress injuries: an aetiological review for the purposes of guiding management. Sports Med 1998;26:265-279.
53. Gillespie WJ, Grant I: Interventions for preventing and treating stress fractures and stress reactions of bone of the lower limbs in young adults. Cochrane Database Syst Rev 2000;2:CD000450.
54. Pell RF, Khanuja HS, Cooley GR: Leg pain in the running athlete. J Am Acad Orthop Surg 2004;12:396-404.
55. Yates B, Allen MJ, Barnes MR: Outcome of surgical treatment of medial tibial stress syndrome. J Bone Joint Surg Am 2003;85:1974-1980.
56. Glorioso JG, Wilckens JH: Exertional leg pain. In O'Connor FG, Wilder RP (eds): Textbook of Running Medicine. New York, McGraw-Hill, 2001, pp 181-197.
57. Edwards P, Myerson M:Exertional compartment syndrome of the leg: steps for expedient return to activity. Phys Sportsmed 1996;24(4).
58. Davey JR, Rorabeck CH, Fowler PJ: The tibialis posterior muscle compartment an unrecognized cause of exertional compartment syndrome. Am J Sports Med 1984;12:391.
59. McDermott AGP, Marble AE, Yabsley RH, et al: Monitoring dynamic anterior compartment pressures during exercise—a new technique using the STIC catheter. Am J Sports Med 1982;10:83.
60. Martens MA, Backaert M, Vermaut G, et al: Chronic leg pain in athletes due to recurrent compartment syndrome. Am J Sports Med 1984;12:148.
61. Styf J, Korner LM: Chronic anterior compartment syndrome of the leg: results of treatment by fasciotomy. J Bone Joint Surg Am 1986;68(9):1338-1347.
62. Blackman PG: A review of chronic exertional compartment syndrome in the lower leg. Med Sci Sport Exerc 2000;32(2):S4-S10.
63. Pedowitz RA, Hargens AR, Mubarak SJ, et al: Modified criteria for the objective diagnosis of chronic compartment syndrome of the leg. Am J Sports Med 1990;18:35.
64. Samuelson DR, Cram RL: The three-phase bone scan and exercise induced lower-leg pain. The tibial stress test. Clin Nucl Med 1996;21(2):89-93.
65. Kaplan P, Helms C, Dussault R: Musculoskeletal MRI. Philadelphia,, WB Saunders, 2001.
66. Breit G, Gross J, Watenpaugh O, et al: Near infrared spectroscopy for monitoring of tissue oxygenation of exercising muscle in a chronic compartment syndrome model. J Bone Joint Surg 1997;79:838-843.
67. Ownes S, Edwards P, Miles K, et al: Chronic compartment syndrome affecting the lower limb: MIBI perfusion imaging as an alternative to pressure monitoring: two case reports. Br J Sports Med 1999;33(1):49-51.
68. Detmer DE, Sharpe K, Sufit RL, et al: Chronic compartment syndrome: diagnosis, management, and outcomes. Am J Sports Med 1985;13:162.
69. Rorabeck CH, Fowler PJ, Nott L: The results of fasciotomy in management of chronic exertional compartment syndrome. Am J Sports Med 1988;16:224-227.

70. Rorabeck CH, Bourne RB, Fowler PJ: The surgical treatment of exertional compartment syndrome in athletes. J Bone Joint Surg Am 1983;65:1245-1251.

71. Martens MA, Backaert M, Vermaut G, et al: Chronic leg pain in athletes due to a recurrent compartment syndrome. Am J Sports Med 1984;12:148.

72. Stager A, Clement D: Popliteal artery entrapment syndrome. Sports Med 1999;28(1):61-70.

73. Rignault DP, Pailler JL, Lunel F: The functional popliteal artery entrapment syndrome. Int Angiol 1985;4(3):341-343.

74. Edwards PH, Wright ML, Hartman JF: A practical approach for the differential diagnosis of chronic leg pain in athletes. Am J Sports Med 2005;33(8):1241-1249.

75. Baltopoulos P, Filippou DK, Sigala F: Popliteal artery entrapment syndrome. Anatomic or functional syndrome? Clin J Sport Med 2004;14:8-12.

76. Lambert AW, Wilkins DC: Popliteal artery entrapment syndrome? Br J Surg 1999;86:1365-1370.

77. Stager A, Clement D: Popliteal artery entrapment syndrome. Sports Med 1999;28:61-70.

78. Baltopoulos P, Filippou DK, Sigala F: Popliteal artery entrapment syndrome. Anatomic or functional syndrome? Clin J Sport Med 2004;14:8-12.

79. Schon LC: Nerve entrapment, neuropathy, and nerve dysfunction in athletes. Orthop Clin North Am 1994;25(1):47-58.

80. McClusky L, Webb L: Compression and entrapment neuropathies of the lower extremity. Clin Podiatr Med Surg 1999;16:96.

81. Schon L, Baxter D: Neuropathies of the foot and ankle in athletes. Clin Sports Med 1990;9:489.

82. McCrory P, Bell S, Bradshaw C: Nerve entrapments of lower leg, ankle and foot in sport. Sports Med 2002;32:371-391.

83. Leach R, Purnell M, Saito A: Peroneal nerve entrapment in runners. Am J Sports Med 1989;17:287.

84. Dellon AL: Deep peroneal nerve entrapment on the dorsum of the foot. Foot Ankle 1990;11(2):73-80.

85. Styf J, Morberg P: The superficial peroneal tunnel syndrome. Results of treatment by decompression. J Bone Joint Surg Br 1997;79(5):801.

Ankle Fractures

Shawn F. Kane, MD

KEY POINTS

- The Ottawa ankle rules and the Buffalo modification of the Ottawa rules should be judiciously applied to adult patients with ankle trauma to decrease the total number of ankle radiographs obtained.
- The most important step in ankle fracture management is identifying stable verses unstable fractures. Stable fractures will have only one break in the supporting ankle "ring," whereas unstable fractures will have at least two.
- The entire length of the fibula must be palpated when examining a patient with a suspected ankle fracture to rule out a Maisonneuve fracture.
- Understanding the mechanism of injury will allow the practitioner to initially focus his or her examination on a certain injury pattern to improve diagnostic accuracy and treatment.
- Damage to the physeal plate in pediatric patients can result in growth arrest and abnormal limb length. Pediatric patients typically do not sprain their ankles; rather, they sustain Salter–Harris I fractures of the growth plate.

INTRODUCTION

The ankle is the key focal point in the transmission of forces from the foot–ground interface up to the rest of the appendicular and axial skeleton.[1] Because of its weight-bearing function and the construction of the articulation, the ankle is the most commonly injured joint among competitive and recreational athletes. The one thing that all ankle injuries—whether sprains or fractures—have in common is they result from an abnormal movement of the talus within the mortise.[2] More than 75% to 85% of ankle injuries are straightforward ligamentous injuries (i.e., sprains), which are easily diagnosed and treated. The remaining injuries consist of the simple, easily managed fractures, the more complex fractures that require operative intervention, and the subtle fractures that, if missed, can result in long-term disability.[3,4]

The key to the successful management of ankle fractures is distinguishing between those that are stable and those that are unstable. Stable fractures can usually be conservatively managed by primary care physicians alone or in consultation with an orthopedic surgeon. Unstable fractures almost always require operative

reduction and fixation, and they should be referred to an orthopedic surgeon for management. Understanding the mechanism of injury will allow the practitioner to initially focus his or her examination on a certain injury pattern to improve diagnostic accuracy and treatment.

EPIDEMIOLOGY

The exact incidence of ankle fractures in the general population is unknown, but it is thought to be increasing as a result of increasing longevity. Medicare data reveal that ankle fractures are the fourth most common fracture among the elderly and that women between 75 and 84 years of age had the highest age-specific incidence.[5] Among patients who are less than 50 years of age, ankle fractures are more common among men than women; however, after the age of 50, ankle fractures become more common among women. Falls from a height to the ground, sports and recreational activities, and work-related activities are the leading causes of ankle fractures in the general population. Football, soccer, basketball, snowboarding, and in-line skating are some of the physical activities that involve an increased incidence of ankle fractures.[6]

ANATOMY AND BIOMECHANICS

Understanding the anatomy and biomechanics of a joint is essential to the evaluation and treatment of injuries involving that joint. There are actually two joints that are vital to the structure and function of the ankle: the talocrural joint and the subtalar joint. The subtalar joint is commonly considered part of the foot, and it will be discussed in Chapter 29.

The talocrural joint is made up of the articulating surfaces of the distal tibia and fibula, which form a boxlike frame or "mortise" over the talar dome. The inferior surface of the distal tibia is articular and concave, and it is referred to as the *tibial plafond*, which means "ceiling." The talus is covered almost completely by articular cartilage, and it is interposed between the tibial plafond and the calcaneous. The stability of the ankle is increased by the static stabilization provided by the ligamentous structures and the dynamic stabilization provided by the numerous muscles that cross the joint **(Figure 28.1)**. The ankle is typically divided into medial, lateral, and syndesmotic complexes; this helps with the understanding of the mechanism of injury and of the commonly

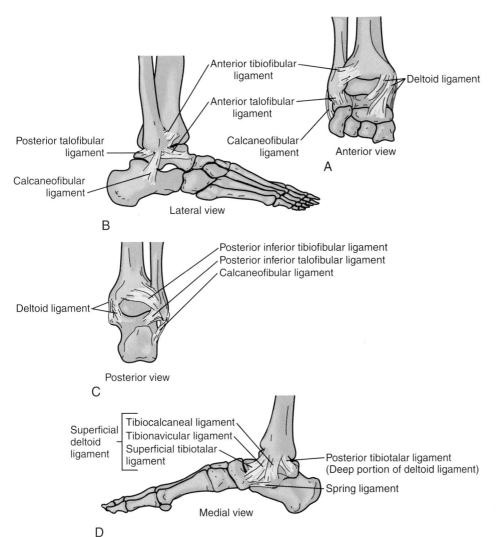

Figure 28.1   Bony and ligamentous anatomy of the ankle. *A*, Anterior view. *B*, Lateral view. *C*, Posterior view. *D*, Medial view. (From Pommering TL, Kluchursky L, Hall SL: Prim Care Clin Office Pract 2005:32;133-161.)

injured structures, and it also helps physicians better devise a treatment plan[7] **(Table 28.1).**

In a neutral position, 90% of the force load is transmitted through the tibial plafond, with the remaining load being borne by the lateral talofibular articulation.[8] The ankle is commonly thought of as a simple hinge joint with movement only in the sagittal (up and down) plane. Biomechanical studies have demonstrated that motion around the talocrural joint is actually very complex, with motion in the sagittal plane resulting in motion in both the axial and coronal planes. Both the talus and the plafond are wider anteriorly than posteriorly, which allows for increased bony contact and stability when the ankle is dorsiflexed. The plantar flexed ankle has the least amount of bony stability, and it is therefore more vulnerable to injury. The talus both slides and rotates under the plafond when it is moved in the sagittal plane. Dorsiflexion causes the talus to externally rotate and to cause posterolateral translation, external rotation, and minimal vertical motion of the fibula. Plantar flexion results in an internal rotation of the talus relative to the tibia. In summary, fractures to the medial malleolus typically result from eversion and abduction forces that cause the lateral displacement of the joint, and lateral malleolar fractures typically result from the medial displacement caused by inversion and adduction forces.

Table 28.1   Medial, Lateral, and Syndesmotic Complexes

Medial Complex	*Lateral Complex*	*Syndesmotic Complex*
Medial malleolus (distal tibia)	Lateral malleolus (distal fibula)	Anterior and posterior inferior tibia—fibular ligament
Medial facet of talus	Lateral facet of talus	Transverse tibiofibular ligament
Deltoid ligament:	Lateral ligaments	Tibia—fibular syndesmosis (interosseous membrane)
Posterior tibiotalar ligament	Anterior talofibular ligament	
Tibiocalcaneal ligament	Calcaneofibular ligament	
Tibionavicular ligament	Posterior talofibular ligament	
Anterior tibiotalar ligament		

The bones and ligaments of the ankle should be thought of as a ring that allows the talus to move through its normal, full range of motion under physiologic loading.[9] Stable injuries are those that involve damage to one side of the ring. With stable injuries, the normal motion of the talus remains intact. With unstable injuries, more than one injury to the ring results in nonphysiologic movement of the talus and decreased joint surface contact. Stable fractures can be managed with conservative casting, whereas unstable fractures generally require operative intervention to restore stability and motion.[8,9]

CLASSIFICATION

Classification systems were developed to provide diagnostic information and prognostic guidance for clinical decision making **(Table 28.2).** There are three main classification systems for ankle fractures: Lauge—Hansen, Danis—Weber, and AO, all of which attempt to accurately assess the extent of soft-tissue damage on the basis of radiographic fracture evidence. The Danis—Weber system is based on the level of the fibular fracture: inferior to the mortise, at the mortise, or superior to the mortise. The AO system is a comprehensive modification of the Danis—Weber system that is based on the presence of additional medial and posterior injuries. The Lauge—Hansen system was a landmark advancement in the classification of ankle fractures, and it remains the only system that attempts to correlate injury mechanism with observed fracture patterns (and vice versa).[10] It is a two-part system: the first part denotes the position of the foot at the time of injury and the direction of the deforming force, and the second part predicts the severity of the ankle injury on the basis of damage to other associated structures.

In clinical practice, none of these systems turns out to be ideal. There is poor intraobserver and interobserver reliability and reproducibility among them, and they have proven to be of limited prognostic value. However, familiarity with these systems will allow the practitioner to understand the mechanism of injury, and it will allow the referring physician to quickly convey the seriousness of the injury in simple terms.[7]

Table 28.2 Ankle Fracture Classification Systems

Fracture Classification	Type	Location of Fracture	Associated Injuries
Danis—Weber	A	Below ankle mortise and tibiofibular articulation	Syndesmosis likely intact
	B	At level of mortise and tibiofibular articulation	Syndesmosis likely intact
	C	Above level of mortise and tibiofibular articulation	Syndesmosis likely disrupted (positive squeeze test)
Lauge—Hansen	Supination/adduction	Transverse fracture of lateral malleolus	Stage 1: Tear of lateral ligaments.
			Stage 2: Fracture of medial malleolus
	Supination/external rotation	Avulsion fracture of the lateral malleolus	Stage 1: Rupture of anterior tibia—fibular ligament
			Stage 2: Spiral or oblique fracture of the lateral malleolus
			Stage 3: Posterior tibial fracture
			Stage 4: Fracture of medial malleolus or torn deltoid ligament
	Pronation/abduction	Medial malleolus	Stage 1: Torn deltoid ligament
			Stage 2: Syndesmotic disruption and posterior tibial fracture
			Stage 3: Oblique fracture of the fibula above mortise
	Pronation/external rotation	Medial malleolus	Stage 1: Torn deltoid ligament
			Stage 2: Syndesmotic disruption
			Stage 3: Spiral fracture of the fibula above mortise
			Stage 4: Posterior tibial fracture
	Pronation/dorsiflexion	Medial malleolus	Stage 1: Fracture of the anterior margin of the tibia
			Stage 2: Supramalleolar fracture of the fibula
			Stage 3: Transverse fracture of the posterior tibial surface
AO	A	Fibula at or below the plafond	Intact or possible medial and posterior avulsions
	B	Fibula at plafond extending proximally	Tibia—fibula ligaments torn; possible medial and lateral avulsions
	C	Fibula above plafond	Syndesmosis always torn, deltoid ligament torn

RADIOGRAPHIC IMAGING

Numerous imaging modalities—from plain radiography to computed tomography scanning to magnetic resonance imaging (MRI) to nuclear medicine—are available to aid in the diagnosis of injuries around the ankle. An appropriate physical examination and a thorough differential diagnosis will ensure that the studies obtained are both medically and financially appropriate. Plain radiographs are the most common imaging modality used for diagnosing injuries around the ankle, and they will be the primary focus of this section. The other, more advanced modalities will be discussed as required for the evaluation and diagnosis of specific injuries.

The standard radiographic evaluation of the ankle consists of three views: anteroposterior, mortise, and lateral. In the present era of cost-conscious medicine, numerous studies have evaluated whether two views (anteroposterior and lateral or lateral and mortise) were as effective for identifying fractures as the traditional three views. Two views successfully identify some fractures, but the classic, three-view combination detects significantly more fractures, and it is considered the gold standard for identifying ankle fractures[11] **(Figure 28.2).**

Does every ankle injury require radiographs? There are an estimated 6 million ankle radiographs performed annually in the United States and Canada at a cost of approximately $300 million dollars. Only 15% of the radiographs demonstrate a fracture, so, to save money, resources, and time in the emergency department and to improve overall patient care, Stiell and colleagues at the University of Ottawa in the early 1990s developed the Ottawa ankle rules **(Table 28.3).**[11] Numerous studies have been done on the application of the Ottawa ankle rules in many settings, and each has validated and reinforced their high sensitivity and negative predicative value. The Ottawa ankle rules can decrease the number of ankle radiographs by up to 30%.[13] In 1998, Leddy and colleagues recommended the Buffalo modification to the Ottawa ankle rules (i.e., pain to palpation over the crests or mid portions of the malleoli away from the ligamentous attachments) (see Table 28.3).[13] They found that this modification significantly increased the specificity of diagnosing malleolar fractures (59% from 42%) without decreasing the sensitivity and that it decreased the need for ankle radiographs by 54%[14] **(Figure 28.3).** Neither of these rules replace sound clinical judgment; rather, they augment the history and physical examination, and they help the clinician to determine the appropriateness of ankle radiographs. The application of these rules is not as clear-cut when they are applied to the immature skeleton with open epiphysial plates. The application of these rules for pediatric fractures will be discussed later in this chapter.

ADULT FRACTURES

The first step in successfully managing ankle injuries is to determine whether the fracture is stable or unstable. Stable fractures, which will be discussed first, have only one break in the ring, and they can be managed conservatively by most primary care physicians **(Figure 28.4).** All stable adult ankle fractures are isolated to either the medial, lateral, or posterior malleolus, and, by definition,

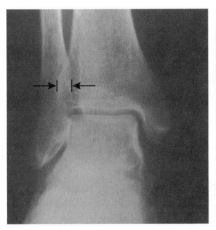

A

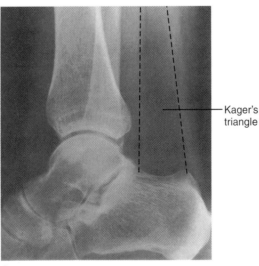

C

Kager's triangle

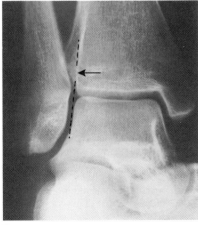

B

Figure 28.2 Radiograph demonstrating a normal anteroposterior, mortise, and lateral view of the ankle. (From Magee DJ: Orthopedic Physical Assessment, 4th ed. Philadelphia, WB Saunders, 2002, p 823.)

Table 28.3 Ottawa Ankle Rules and the Buffalo Modification

The Ottawa Ankle Rules	The Buffalo Modification
Patient has pain over either malleolus AND Patient has tenderness to palpation over the inferior and posterior poles of either malleolus (including the distal 6 cm) AND Patient unable to bear weight (four steps taken independently) at the time of injury and at the time of evaluation	Same as the Ottawa ankle rules, except the area of malleolar tenderness to palpation is moved to over the crests or the mid portions of the malleoli, away from the ligamentous attachments

they have no appreciable injury to any other structure in the ankle (i.e., the second break in the ring).

Isolated medical or lateral malleolar fractures
Mechanism of injury
These injuries usually result from a significant inversion (lateral malleolus), eversion (medial malleolus), or a combination of supination and external rotation (posterior malleolus). Isolated fractures of the lateral malleolus are the most common fractures of the ankle, with isolated medial or posterior fractures being less common and requiring a more thorough evaluation to not miss any associated injuries.

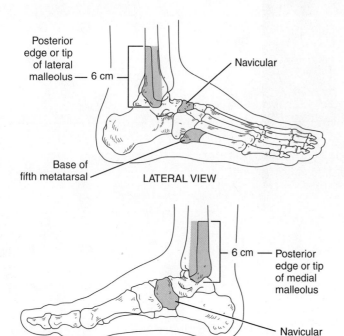

Figure 28.3 Graphic representation of the Ottawa ankle rules and the Buffalo modification. Tenderness over the shaded areas requires evaluation with an ankle series. (From Magee DJ: Orthopedic Physical Assessment, 4th ed. Philadelphia, WB Saunders, 2002, p 822.)

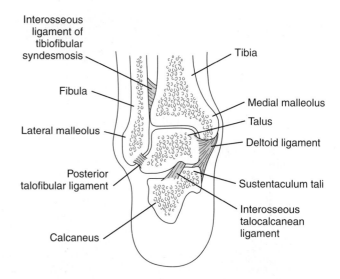

Figure 28.4 Coronal section through the ankle demonstrating the "ring" that helps identify stable versus unstable fractures. (From Magee DJ: Orthopedic Physical Assessment, 4th ed. Philadelphia, WB Saunders, 2002, p 767.)

Risk factors
No risk factors for this injury have been identified.

Clinical features
The area of maximal tenderness and a history of the events surrounding the injury are usually good aids for determining which ankle structures are injured. The absence or presence of swelling is not a reliable indicator of injury severity. The amount of swelling is usually related more to the amount of elapsed time between injury and presentation than to the severity of injury. Examination soon after injury usually provides the best information because swelling has not set in to obscure physical findings. Isolated malleolar fractures are at times challenging to distinguish from severe sprains. Any time that a patient has tenderness on both the medial and lateral side of the ankle, there must be a high index of suspicion for an unstable ankle. At the same time, the clinician cannot solely focus all of his or her attention on the ankle. Because of the possibility of proximal fractures, the full length of both the tibia and the fibula must be palpated in patients with an acute ankle injury.

Diagnosis
Isolated malleolar fractures are routinely diagnosed on plain radiographs **(Figure 28.5)**. The fracture pattern can aid in the determination of the mechanism of injury, and it can also be helpful for categorizing the fracture as stable. Nondisplaced fractures may only be seen on one x-ray view. An avulsion or distraction force on the ankle will result in transverse fractures of the malleoli, whereas torsion of the talar dome with subsequent impact on the malleoli can cause oblique fractures.[9] A vertical fracture in either malleoli increases the probability of another injury that can create an unstable ankle and thus warrants a thorough search. Stability of the ankle can be assessed by analyzing the displacement of various bones of the ankle on plain radiographs. Typically, the medial clear space, the tibiofibular clear space, the tibiofibular overlap, the talar tilt, and the talocrural angle are evaluated to determine stability. The most reliable criteria for instability is lateral talar displacement relative to the tibia, which is demonstrated by the medial clear space being larger than the superior clear space[8] **(Figure 28.6)**.

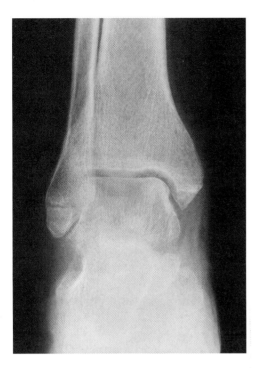

Figure 28.5   Stable, nondisplaced transverse fracture through the lateral malleolus. Note the fracture line. (From Eiff MP, Hatch RL, Calmbach WL [eds]: Fracture Management for Primary Care, 2nd ed. Philadelphia, WB Saunders, 1998, p 290.)

Treatment

Treatment of suspected ankle fractures ideally begins on the side of the field or as soon as possible after the injury has occurred. Ankle injuries, suspected fractures, and sprains are all initially treated in the same way. The athlete will usually have to be removed from the contest and examined. If it is evident that the athlete will not return to competition, then the injured ankle should be iced, compressed, and elevated to try to reduce the impact of swelling. The patient may require crutches for ambulation immediately after the injury. If a fracture is suspected, then standard radiographs should be obtained at the earliest possible convenience. Before or after the radiographs are performed, the ankle should be placed in a bulky posterior (bulky jones) or a U-and-L–type splint.

Small, nondisplaced avulsion fractures of either the lateral or medial malleolus are best treated with early mobilization (i.e., functional treatment) that is similar to that of an ankle sprain. Randomized controlled trials have shown that the functional treatment of these fractures is equally as effective whether functional braces, elastic bandages, air-casts, or hard casts are used.[15]

Minimally displaced fractures of the malleoli can be treated with immobilization in either a cast or a fracture boot for at least 4 to 6 weeks. The foot must be immobilized in a neutral position to minimize the risk of Achilles tendon shortening. Compliance with the fracture boot is a concern, and proper patient selection is vital to achieving a successful outcome. The amount of displacement that is acceptable to be managed nonoperatively has changed through the years. Currently, less than 3 mm of displacement of the lateral malleolus and less than 2 mm of displacement with less than 25% articular surface involvement are manageable nonoperatively.[7,8] Immediate orthopedic evaluation is required if there is an open fracture, a dislocation with or without fracture that cannot be

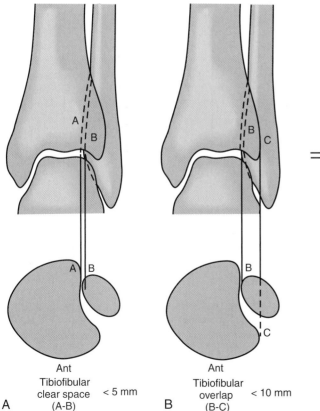

A
Ant
Tibiofibular
clear space   < 5 mm
(A-B)

B
Ant
Tibiofibular
overlap   < 10 mm
(B-C)

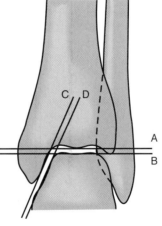

Medial clear space (CD) > superior clear space (AB) consistent with lateral talar displacement

C

Figure 28.6   Graphic representation of radiographic findings associated with an unstable ankle fracture. *A*, Tibiofibular clear space of less than 5 mm is normal. *B*, Tibiofibular overlap of greater than 10 mm is normal. *C*, Medial and superior clear spaces are normal. The medial clear space being greater than the superior clear space is a very good indicator of a displaced ankle fracture. (From Griend RV, Michelson JD, Bone LB: J Bone Joint Surg Am 1996;78[11]:1772-1783.)

reduced, or evidence of persistent distal vascular compromise after reduction or splinting.

Patients should be seen 2 weeks after immobilization to check on the condition of the cast and compliance. At 4 weeks, if there is radiographic evidence of fracture union and the site is nontender to palpation, then the patient may begin gradual weight bearing and ankle rehabilitation. If there is no evidence of healing or the site is still tender to palpation, then the weight bearing and rehabilitation should be delayed at least another 2 weeks. If at 6 weeks the fracture is still not clinically healed and the patient is in a cast, the cast should be removed, and a fracture boot should be used for help with walking and so that rehabilitation to decrease the amount of stiffness and atrophy can begin. After immobilization, rehabilitation should begin with range of motion and then progress to strength training. After the patient has a normal, pain-free range of motion and at least 85% strength as compared with the uninjured side, he or she may begin returning to physical activity. When the patient is back to 100% strength and when he or she can execute sport-specific motions, then he or she may return to competition. Diligent effort during rehabilitation should help patients resume physical activity as soon as is practical **(Table 28.4).**

Malleolar stress fractures

Stress fractures are a partial or complete bone fracture that results from the repeated application of a stress lower than the stress required to fracture the bone in a single loading. Medial and lateral malleolar stress fractures occur infrequently, with fibular stress fractures occurring more commonly. Epidemiologic studies often do not distinguish between proximal, middle, and distal (lateral malleolar) stress fractures, thereby making the exact incidence of lateral malleolar stress fractures hard to discern. Distal fibular stress fractures (within 4 to 7 cm of the tip of the lateral malleolus) occur more frequently than proximal or middle stress fractures.[16] Medial malleolar stress fractures were not identified until 1975, and they account for 0.6% to 4% of all stress fractures.[15] Medial malleolar stress fractures occur almost entirely among athletes (runners) and, most commonly, in the skeletally immature.

Lateral malleolar stress fractures are caused by a combination of muscular forces and axial loading. Young male athletes tend to sustain stress fractures that are 5 to 6 cm proximal to the tip, whereas middle-aged females sustain the fracture 3 to 4 cm from the proximal tip. Medial malleolar fractures arise from abnormal weight transmission and torsional forces. Characteristically, these fractures present with a vertical to oblique fracture line that arises from the junction of the medial malleolus and the tibial plafond.[16]

Mechanism of injury
The failure of bone to adequately adapt to a mechanical load experienced during physical activity is the cause of this injury. Over time, this lack of adaptation leads to the spectrum of overuse injuries, which, if not cared for, can lead to a stress fracture.

Risk factors
Risk factors for this condition are listed in **Table 28.5.**

Clinical features
A history of increased or recently changed physical activity precedes the development of symptoms. Pain, which is the primary symptom, is usually aggravated with activity and relieved with rest. It is initially hard to localize, but, as the injury progresses, it localizes to the malleolar area, and it is associated with stiffness and swelling. Patients tend to have the symptoms for a couple of days to several months before presentation.

Physical examination usually reveals a normal range of motion and strength. Localized tenderness to palpation over the

Table 28.4 Management Guidelines for Isolated Stable Medial and Lateral Malleolar Fractures

Acute Treatment	
Splint type and position	Stirrup or posterior splint with ankle in neutral position
Initial follow-up visit	3 to 5 days for definitive casting
Patient instructions	No weight bearing until definitive casting; icing and elevation to minimize swelling
Definitive Treatment	
Cast or splint type and position	Short-leg walking cast, walking cast fracture boot with ankle in neutral position
Length of immobilization	Malleolar: 4 to 6 weeks
	Distal fibular: 6 to 8 weeks
	Immobilization continued for up to 8 weeks if no evidence of radiographic healing
Healing time	6 to 8 weeks and possibly several months for complete radiographic healing
Follow-up interval	Malleolar: 4 weeks to check radiographic healing
	Distal fibular: every 2 to 4 weeks
	Every 2 weeks after discontinuing immobilization to assess status of ankle rehabilitation
Repeat x-ray interval	Malleolar: at 4 weeks to check radiographic healing
	Distal fibular: at 7 to 10 days to check positioning
	Every 2 weeks if no healing at 4 weeks
Patient instructions	Range of motion, calf stretching. and strengthening after immobilization; full dorsiflexion and peroneal muscle strength are emphasized
Indications for referral	Unstable fractures; bimalleolar and trimalleolar fractures; posterior malleolar fractures with >25% articular involvement and >2 mm displacement; symptomatic nonunion

affected malleoli is common, as is some focal pitting edema and doughy skin.[17]

Diagnosis
Up to 70% of initial radiographs are normal, and they may not show any evidence of injury for 2 to 4 weeks after symptoms begin. Radionuclide bone scanning and MRI are the best imaging modalities to aid in the diagnosis of a stress fracture. Radionuclide scanning demonstrates increased uptake that correlates with increased bone activity. Bone scans are very sensitive, but they have a low specificity, and they can yield a false-positive rate of approximately 14%. In addition, precise anatomic location is difficult. MRI has replaced bone scanning in most areas as a result of its precise anatomic locating, its ability to differentiate between stress reactions and fractures, and its decreased radiation exposure.[15]

Treatment
The extent of the fracture, seasonal timing, and the caliber of the athlete will aid in making the decision about whether to manage

Table 28.5 Risk Factors for Stress Fractures

Extrinsic (Avoidable) Risk Factors	Intrinsic (Biomechanical or Unavoidable) Risk Factors
Poor training regimen	History of previous stress fracture
Running on hard or uneven surfaces	Leg-length discrepancies
Poor footwear	Tibial torsion
Inadequate nutrition	Pes cavus/planus
Long distances (>20 miles per week)	Narrow tibial cross section
	Increased hip rotation
Smoking	Forefoot varus
Alcohol	Subtalar varus
Inhaled corticosteroid use	Tibial varum
Low level of aerobic fitness	Female gender
Menstrual irregularities (no menses in 6 or more months of the previous year)	Increased age
	Energy imbalance

Adapted from Sherbondy PS, Sebastianelli WJ: Clin Sports Med 2006;25:129-137; Wilder RP, Sethi S: Clin Sports Med 2004;23:55-81; Wall J, Feller JF: Clin Sports Med 2006;25;781-802; Rauh MJ, Macera CA, Trone DW, et al: Med Sci Sports Exerc 2006;38(9):1571-1577.

the patient operatively or nonoperatively. All distal fibular and most medial malleolar stress fractures can be managed nonoperatively. Typical treatment involves modified rest, limited weight bearing for limping patients, and symptom-limited cross training for 3 to 8 weeks followed by a gradual return to increased levels of activity. Complete rest should be avoided. Pneumatic ankle braces, fracture boots, casts, taping, and strict activity modification all have similar results, and they all have a role in treatment, depending on the individual patient.[17] Surgical intervention for radiographically detectable or displaced stress fractures in highly competitive in-season athletes is an acceptable treatment, without any significant complications.[18] The primary reason for operative intervention is to return the athlete to competition as soon as 24 days after surgery.

After the first stress fracture is treated, the next step is to identify and treat as many of the risk factors associated with stress fractures to try and prevent a recurrence. Even with aggressive prevention and treatment, a history of a previous stress fracture increases the risk of recurrence by to 2 to 3.5 times. Because of the complex nature of these risk factors, a multidisciplinary team approach will be most beneficial for the athlete.[19]

Unstable ankle fractures

Unstable fractures involve two breaks in the ring, and they may require consultation with an orthopedic surgeon for proper treatment. The initial treatment is basically the same as it is for stable ankle fractures. The force required to cause an unstable fracture is usually more significant than the force that causes a stable fracture. Patients will usually be in a significant amount of pain and unable to ambulate, and they will have an ankle that appears to be abnormal. A key step in evaluating a severely injured ankle is ensuring that there has been no vascular compromise by palpating either the posterior tibial or dorsalis pedis pulses and by checking distal capillary refill. An ankle fracture with distal vascular compromise is a medical emergency that requires immediate attention. If there is no evidence of vascular compromise, the ankle should be splinted, elevated, and iced; crutches should be used for ambulation, and radiographs should be obtained as soon as is practical. It has been estimated that more than 65% of unstable ankle fractures can be managed with closed reduction to achieve satisfactory results.

Even with these acceptable results, closed reduction is generally reserved for patients with severe medical conditions that preclude their undergoing a surgical procedure.

The definitive treatment of these fractures requires consultation and operative intervention by an orthopedic surgeon. If there is no vascular compromise, it is acceptable to obtain orthopedic consultation 24 to 72 hours after the injury. Open fractures and injuries with persistent neurovascular injury should be referred immediately to an orthopedic surgeon for treatment. The timing of the surgery is variable, with the amount of soft-tissue swelling, soft-tissue compromise and associated injuries being the main factors in the decision. Early surgical intervention commonly results in wound complications, osteomyelitis, and other issues as compared with delayed surgery. As a result, most operative interventions are done somewhere in the window of 7 to 10 days after the injury.[20] The exact technique will depend on what the surgeon finds interoperatively. The techniques used are numerous and beyond the scope of this chapter, but the general concept is to restore joint integrity and to maintain as much of the articular cartilage as possible to help minimize the long-term morbidity.

Rehabilitation and return to play are usually a little longer for operatively managed unstable fractures than for stable fractures. Patients with operatively reduced ankles usually should not bear weight for 6 to 8 weeks. Placing the patient in a functional brace or cast immobilization is based on a combination of surgeon preference and patient selection. There is evidence to support functional bracing in conjunction with active and passive ankle physical therapy. Patients who are functionally braced have demonstrated higher subjective and objective outcomes as compared with those who are casted.[21,22] At this time, if there is evidence of bone healing, transition to a fracture boot for the next 4 to 6 weeks should occur, with a gradually decreased dependence on crutches for ambulation. After the removal of all braces or casts, the patient will have to begin a vigorous rehabilitation program to regain the range of motion and strength that were lost as a result of the injury. At this point, the rehabilitation criteria are the same as they are for an unstable fracture; it just takes longer to get to this point.

Bimalleolar and bimalleolar equivalent fractures

Bimalleolar and bimalleolar equivalent fractures consist of either a fracture of the lateral and medial malleolus or a lateral malleolar fracture with complete disruption of the deltoid ligament (Figure 28.7). Injuries to the deltoid ligament are estimated to occur in 10% to 36% of ankle fractures.[23] Missing an injury to the deltoid ligament and treating only the radiographically evident lateral malleolus fracture may potentially lead to complications and a less-than-satisfactory outcome.

Mechanism of injury
A pronation abduction force typically causes these fracture patterns.

Risk factors
No risk factors for this condition have been identified.

Clinical features
The main clinical feature of this type of fracture is tenderness to palpation over both malleoli or significant tenderness of the medial ankle ligaments in the presence of a lateral malleolar fracture. The fracture pattern will help with the identification of the mechanism that caused the injury, and it will also increase the suspicion for a possible deltoid ligament injury. Inversion injuries are associated with a vertical fracture of the medial malleolus and a transverse

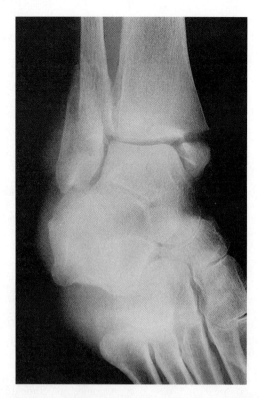

Figure 28.7 An unstable bimalleolar fracture that will most likely require open reduction. Note the presence of both tibia and fibula fractures. (From Eiff MP, Hatch RL, Calmbach WL [eds]: Fracture Management for Primary Care, 2nd ed. Philadelphia, WB Saunders, 1998, p 296.)

fracture of the lateral malleolus. Eversion injuries usually have a transverse fracture of the medial malleolus and a spiral/vertical fracture of the lateral malleolus. A spiral fibular fracture that is 2 to 3 inches proximal to the mortise or a fibular fracture at the joint line should prompt a thorough evaluation of the medial structures of the ankle.[1]

Diagnosis

Tenderness to palpation over the medial side of the ankle along with evidence of a talar shift (>4 mm of medial clear space widening) on radiographs is diagnostic for a complete deltoid ligament disruption. The diagnostic challenge is when there is tenderness medially but no evidence of talar shift on the radiographs. Gravity stress views (anteroposterior radiograph taken with the leg horizontal, medial side up, without ankle support) may be beneficial for helping to correctly identify the fracture. An increased talar tilt (>15%) or a talar shirt (>2 mm) as compared with the uninjured ankle occurs only when the superficial and deep divisions of the deltoid ligament are disrupted; this is pathognomonic for a bimalleolar equivalent fracture.[8] This simple, easy-to-obtain radiograph is not difficult to interpret, and it has proven to be less problematic than MRI or ultrasound for the proper diagnosis of deltoid ligament injuries in the presence of lateral malleolar fractures.[24]

Treatment

These injuries should be treated like the other unstable ankle fractures, and patients should be referred to an orthopedic surgeon for definitive treatment. Bimalleolar fractures are typically treated with open reduction and internal fixation. Closed reduction can provide satisfactory results in up to 65% of cases, but it is usually reserved for patients with severe medical contraindications to surgery. Surgery involves the reduction and plating of the lateral malleolus followed by the reduction and fixation of the medial malleolus.

The current treatment of choice for bimalleolar equivalent fractures is the repair of the lateral component without the repair of the deltoid ligament. Surgical repair of the deltoid has not resulted in significant improvements in outcome, and it may lead to worse long-term results. Medial exploration should be undertaken only if the talus does not reduce anatomically beneath the plafond, in which case exploration to remove the incarcerated deltoid ligament is warranted.[25]

As with the other unstable, operatively reduced ankles, the ankle should be immobilized in the neutral position. The choice of protected weight bearing and early motion versus no weight bearing and no motion is based on surgeon and physical therapist preference because studies have not demonstrated one being better than the other.

Trimalleolar fractures

A trimalleolar fracture includes the addition of a fracture to the posterior tibial plafond component or of the posterior malleolus to the bimalleolar fracture **(Figure 28.8)**.

Mechanism of injury

A high-energy rotatory supination external rotation mechanism can lead to this injury.

Risk factors

Skateboarding is one of the primary risk factors for this type of injury.

Clinical features

A lateral avulsion fracture results from the pull of the posterior-inferior tibiofibular, which is also attached inferiorly to the distal fibular fragment. Less frequently, the impaction of the externally

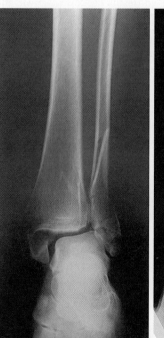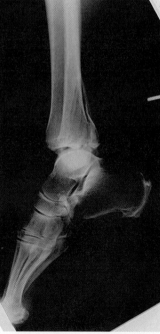

Figure 28.8 Anteroposterior and lateral views of a trimalleolar fracture, which is by definition an unstable fracture that will require open reduction. Note the medial and lateral fractures on the anteroposterior view and the posterior malleolar fracture on the lateral view. (From Eiff MP, Hatch RL, Calmbach WL [eds]: Fracture Management for Primary Care, 2nd ed. Philadelphia, WB Saunders, 1998, pp 288-306, 296.)

rotating talus on the posterior lip of the tibia may result in a trimalleolar fracture.

Diagnosis

Typically, plain radiographs are all that is required to diagnose this fracture. Computed tomography scanning may also be useful for further defining the degree of damage and location of fragments.

Treatment

Open reduction is required for these fractures, and it is very similar to the treatment of bimalleolar fractures. Typically, the posterior malleolus portion of the fracture reduces spontaneously after treatment of the fibular fracture.[8]

Syndesmotic rupture of high-grade syndesmotic injury

Complete syndesmotic rupture is a unique subset of ankle injuries that is thought to occur in between 1% and 10% ankle sprains. The fracture is typically fibular and at or above the level of the plafond. However, the rupture of the syndesmotic ligament results in mortise widening and a very unstable ankle. The syndesmotic ligament complex consists of the anterior and posterior inferior tibiofibular ligaments, the transverse tibiofibular ligament, and, more proximally, the interosseus membrane **(Figure 28.9)**. The syndesmotic ligaments provide a strong restraint to external rotational forces, and they are injured when the talus is abducted or externally rotated in the mortise.[26]

Mechanism of injury

This injury typically occurs during an abrupt change in direction with internal rotation of the leg while the ankle undergoes forced pronation/external rotation, pronation/abduction, or supination/external rotation.

Risk factors

Syndesmotic injuries are more common among athletes who participate in contact sports that involve cutting or pivoting maneuvers. These sports include football, rugby, basketball, lacrosse, and soccer. However, syndesmotic injuries may occur in other athletes and in nonathletes as well.

Clinical features

The identification of an unstable syndesmosis is primarily based on the mechanism of injury and the associated fracture pattern. Clinically, patients with these fractures usually have supramalleolar edema, pain with passive dorsiflexion, a positive squeeze test (manual medial–lateral compression across the syndesmosis), pain during the external rotation stress test, and pain during the tibiotalar shuck (cotton) test[27] **(Figure 28.10).**

Diagnosis

The physical examination and history may be suggestive of this injury, although acutely the physical examination may not be that reliable as a result of pain. Radiographic findings provide additional clues regarding the identification of this injury. A tibiofibular clear space of less than 5 mm and a widening of the medial clear space of more than 4 mm are strong indicators of a syndesmotic injury.[7] Plain radiographs are not always sensitive enough to aid in the diagnosis of syndesmotic injuries. For cases in which there is a high index of suspicion, either graded stress plain radiography or MRI can be used to diagnose injury to the syndesmotic complex.[28] Old syndesmotic injuries can be identified by visualizing calcifications in the area of the interosseus membrane.

Treatment

Initially, high-grade syndesmotic injuries should be treated like all other unstable ankle injuries and then referred to an orthopedic surgeon for definitive treatment. The key to managing patients with a suspected syndesmotic injury is close follow-up, a high

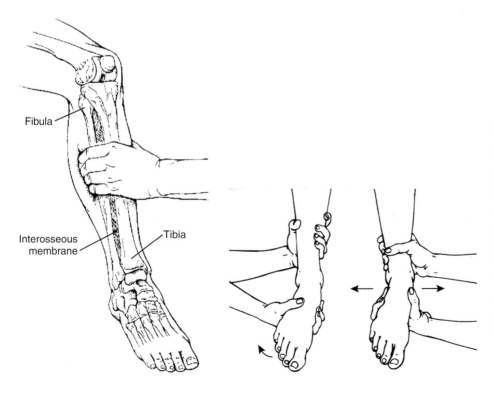

Figure 28.9 Graphic representation of the squeeze (A), external rotation (B), and cotton tests (C). The squeeze test is performed by grabbing the leg proximally and squeezing. Pain distally is a positive test. The external rotation test is performed by stabilizing the lower leg with one hand and externally rotating the ankle with the other. Pain in the syndesmotic area is a positive test. The cotton test is performed by stabilizing the leg with one had and providing alternate medial and lateral force on the talus with the other. Pain in the syndesmosis or a feeling of looseness as compared with the noninjured side is positive for a probable syndesmotic injury. (From Stephenson K, Saltzman CL, Brotzman SB. Foot and ankle injuries. In Brotzman SB, Wilk KE [eds]: Clinical Orthopedic Rehabilitation, 2nd ed. Philadelphia, Mosby, 2003, p 377.)

Fibula

Interosseous membrane

Tibia

Anterior view   Posterior view

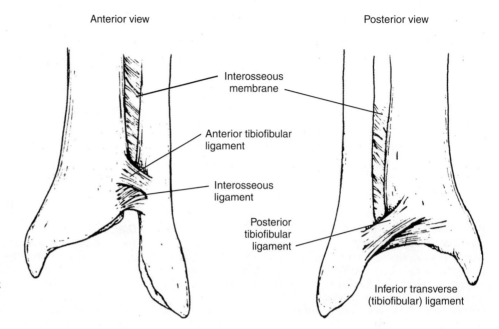

Interosseous membrane

Anterior tibiofibular ligament

Interosseous ligament

Posterior tibiofibular ligament

Inferior transverse (tibiofibular) ligament

Figure 28.10 The components of the distal lower extremity syndesmosis. (From Stephenson K, Saltzman CL, Brotzman SB. Foot and ankle injuries. In Brotzman SB, Wilk KE [eds]: Clinical Orthopedic Rehabilitation, 2nd ed. Philadelphia, Mosby, 2003, p 377.)

index of suspicion, and a low referral threshold because the outcome of these injuries is much better if they are operatively treated early. The exact operative repair will be based on the fracture pattern, but it usually involves, at a minimum, a syndesmotic screw to allow those structures to heal.

Maisonneuve fracture

The Maisonneuve fracture, which was first described in 1840 by a French surgeon, is a specific type of unstable ankle fracture that is characterized by a proximal fibular fracture with the associated failure of the deltoid ligament, the medial malleolus, and/or the tibiofibular syndesmosis.[29] Although it is an uncommon fracture that accounts for approximately 5% of all operatively treated ankle fractures, the Maisonneuve fracture is considered one of the most unstable ankle fractures. The impaction of the talus on the fibula acts as a wedge that disrupts the anterior tibiofibular and interosseous ligaments. This rotational force exits the fibula at the site of the fibular fracture[29] **(Figure 28.11)**. Increased injury forces result in more proximal fibular fractures.

Mechanism of injury

A severe pronation/external rotation of the ankle can lead to this type of fracture.

Risk factors

No risk factors for this type of injury have been identified.

Clinical features

This fracture presents like other medial or syndesmotic ankle injuries, with the patient complaining of pain around the ankle. Patients usually do not complain of pain in their proximal fibula until it is palpated during the examination.

Diagnosis

The diagnosis of the Maisonneuve fracture may be easily overlooked; studies have demonstrated that 14% to 45% of these fractures are missed on initial presentation. The entire fibula must be palpated, and, if there is any suspicion, full-leg radiographs must be obtained. Proximal fibular tenderness with a positive "squeeze" test are consistent with the diagnosis, even in the absence of obvious radiographic findings.

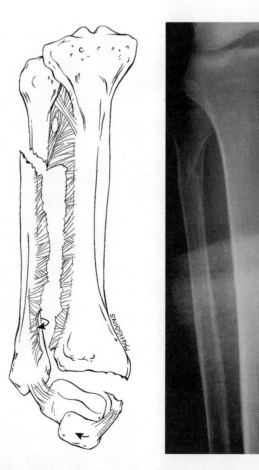

Figure 28.11 A drawing and radiograph of a Maisonneuve fracture. (From Eiff MP, Hatch RL, Calmbach WL [eds]: Fracture Management for Primary Care, 2nd ed. Philadelphia, WB Saunders, 1998, pp 288-306.)

Treatment

In the absence of an open fracture, the patient should be placed on crutches, put in a bulky dressing, and referred to and seen by an orthopedic surgeon in approximately 72 hours for internal fixation. Anatomic restoration of the mortise and the correction of any fibular shortening are the most important factors for determining a positive outcome. The extent and the specific damage to the syndesmosis and the medial ankle structures will dictate how they are repaired. There is usually no need to repair the proximal fibular injury, because it is enclosed in considerable muscle tissue, and there is a substantial risk of damage to the peroneal nerve when dissecting to the fracture.

Patients should not bear weight, and their injuries should be immobilized in a cast for 6 to 8 weeks. At this point, they should have the syndesmotic screws removed, and they can then begin aggressive physical therapy. If there is no evidence of healing, the syndesmotic screws can be left in for 3 to 4 months, but they should be removed before weight bearing and rehabilitation because they may limit dorsiflexion and promote stiffness and pain.

Ankle dislocations

Dislocations of the ankle typically occur in the presence of a fracture as a result of the mechanical efficiency of the mortise and the fact that bones are mechanically weaker than ligaments. A pure dislocation or a dislocation without a fracture is quite rare.

Mechanism of injury

Dislocations of the ankle are the result of high-energy trauma, which produces a combination of plantar flexion and either forced inversion or eversion of the foot. Probably the most common circumstances that surround an ankle dislocation are a plantarflexed ankle meeting an unyielding inversion force, like that seen when a baseball or softball player slides into a base that does not break away.[30] These injuries can either be open or closed, depending on the status of the overlying skin.

Risk factors

No risk factor have been identified.

Clinical features

Dislocations are usually described by the dislocated position of the talus with respect to the mortise versus the normal anatomic alignment. Ankle dislocations almost always occur in conjunction with some type of fracture. Pure dislocations of the ankle (i.e., those not accompanied by fractures) do occur, although at a significantly lower rate than fractures with dislocations.[31]

Diagnosis

The diagnosis of ankle dislocations is usually primarily clinical, and it is based on the appearance of the ankle and the position of the talus. Radiographs are very helpful for identifying the exact fracture pattern associated with the dislocation.

Treatment

The acute management of ankle dislocations requires the immediate evaluation of two things: the distal neurovascular status and the skin condition. If there is acute compromise of the distal circulation as determined by a nonpalpable dorsalis pedis or a posterior tibialis pulse, if there are significant neurologic deficits, or if the dislocated bones are stretching the overlying skin taught (commonly referred to as "tenting"), then the situation is a medical emergency. The ankle must be reduced to return blood flow to the extremity and to save the overlying skin from pressure necrosis, which will drastically complicate this injury. The general concept of reducing a dislocated ankle is to reverse the force that caused the injury; this can usually be accomplished with distal traction in combination

with a force opposite from the current location of the talus. If there is no vascular compromise and the skin is not overly stretched, then the dislocated ankle can be splinted in place, and the patient can be transported to definitive care. After the reduction of the dislocation, definitive treatment depends on whether the dislocation is associated with an unstable or a stable fracture or any open wounds. Because these injuries are uncommon, no "standard" treatment protocol exists; rehabilitation will be guided by associated injuries and individual response to treatment.[30]

Tibial plafond (pilon) fractures

These are relatively uncommon fractures that constitute approximately 1% of lower-extremity fractures and 7% to 10% of tibial fractures.[32]

Mechanism of injury

Plafond fractures can be categorized as either high- or low-energy fractures. The high-energy fractures are typically the result of a significant axial load, whereas torsion is usually the mechanism behind a low-energy fracture. High-energy fractures tend to have significant comminution and damage to the articular cartilage and a worse outcome as compared with the low-energy fractures.[33]

Risk factors

Participation in adventure sports (e.g., parachuting, hang gliding) or high-speed motor sports is associated with the high-energy fractures, whereas skiing and rollerblading are associated with the low-energy fractures.

Clinical features

The patient is typically in a significant amount of pain, and he or she will have a markedly swollen and deformed ankle. Low-energy fractures may have a less dramatic appearance than high-energy ones, so, on the basis of the mechanism of injury, a high index of suspicion must be maintained. The worse the initial soft-tissue injury, the poorer the overall outcome. In addition, 20% to 25% of pilon fractures may be open, which is not unexpected when considering the energy involved in this type of injury.

Diagnosis

The diagnosis is usually straightforward given the presence of a deformed ankle in combination with a history of significant trauma. The neurovascular status of the extremity and the overall condition of the patient must be immediately addressed. Anteroposterior, lateral, and oblique radiographs will confirm the diagnosis, and a computed tomography scan will probably be indicated to fully assess the damage and to help with surgical planning. Because the most common mechanism of injury is a significant axial load, strong consideration should be given to obtaining lumbosacral radiographs to rule out occult injury to the spine. Although compartment syndrome is rare with these fractures, vigilance on the part of the physician is required to ensure that it does not develop.

Treatment

Orthopedic consultation will definitely be required to treat this injury, and it should be obtained as soon as it is clinically warranted. Surgical treatments for a pilon fracture should not be conducted until the full extent of the soft-tissue damage is known. A delay of up to 10 to 14 days is justified to allow the soft-tissue damage to declare itself and to allow for late reduction while minimizing further tissue damage.[34] Low-energy fractures with little or no soft-tissue compromise respond well to operative internal fixation. Because of the significant amount of damage, external fixation with limited internal fixation usually provides the best outcome for high-energy fractures. Prognosis for a patient with a plafond fracture is guarded until 1 year has passed since the injury.

The best potential for good long-term results comes with the perfect anatomic reconstruction of the joint surface and with a patient who is motivated to participate in his or her own rehabilitation.[7,35]

PEDIATRIC FRACTURES

The skeletal system of a child significantly differs from that of an adult. These differences create unique patterns of injury and special treatment requirements for pediatric fractures. The long bones of children have many discrete areas, with the physis, the epiphysis, and the metaphysis being the most important with regard to fractures around the ankle. The physis or growth plate is the areas where bones grow longitudinally by undergoing endochondral ossification.[36] Bones may have proximal and distal physes, and each may contribute differently to overall bone growth. For example, the proximal ends of the tibia and the fibula contribute 55% of overall growth, with the distal end providing the other 45%.[37] Damage to the physis is reported to account for 15% to 30% of skeletal injuries in children. When unrecognized and improperly treated, up to 15% of these injuries can lead to physeal arrest; however, proper treatment of these injuries reduces the incidence of physeal arrest to 1% to 2%.[38] The epiphysis is the area between the physis and the adjacent joint, and the metaphysis is the area between the physis and the mid shaft. The physis is the weak part of the bone; it is two- to five-times weaker than the surrounding ligamentous structures, and it is susceptible to shearing, bending, and tension stresses **(Figure 28.12).** Chapter 31 contains a more complete overview of pediatric and adolescent injuries.

Foot and ankle problems in the young athlete are the second most common reason for a visit to a physician.[38] In contrast with adults, ligamentous injuries to the ankle are rare among children because the ligaments are stronger than the growing bone. Children are more likely to suffer a fracture than a sprain, and any skeletally immature patient with a significant injury should have radiographs done to evaluate for the possibility of a fracture.[39] The physis (or growth plate) is the weakest link in the bone—tendon—muscle chain, and it is the most commonly injured structure in the ankle of a child with open growth plates. Fracture of the distal tibia and the fibular physis is second in frequency only to fractures of the distal radius physis. Physeal ankle fractures usually occur in children who are between 9 and 14 years of age (average age: 12 years), and there is a 2:1 male predominance.[9,39]

Dias and Tachdjian developed a pediatric ankle fracture classification system that was modified from the adult Lauge–Hansen

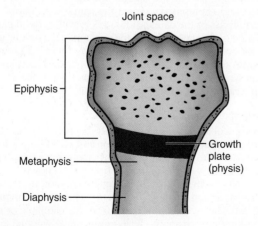

Joint space

Epiphysis

Metaphysis

Diaphysis

Growth plate (physis)

Figure 28.12 The anatomy of a long bone, with the different anatomic areas identified. (From Grover G: Orthopedic injuries and growing pain. In Berkowitz CD [ed]: Pediatrics: A Primary Care Approach, 2nd ed. Philadelphia, WB Saunders, 2000, p 372.)

system **(Figure 28.13).** However, this system has its limitations because children are notoriously unable to recall the position of the foot and the force applied to the ankle at the moment of injury.[38] The Salter–Harris (SH) physeal fracture classification system **(Table 28.6)** is based on the location of the fracture line and the fragment in relation to the physis. **(Figure 28.14).** Knowledge of this system is helpful for describing fractures in the area of the physis.

The Ottawa ankle rules have a sensitivity of only 83% and a specificity of only 50% for patients with an open physis; therefore, these rules should not be applied to children.[39,40]

Pediatric isolated fibula fractures
Mechanism of injury
This injury usually results from an inversion/supination injury.

Risk factors
Slower running speed, decreased dorsiflexion strength, and less balance in males have been identified as risk factors for inversion injuries.[39]

Clinical features
An SH I fracture of the distal fibula is the childhood equivalent of the lateral ankle sprain in an adult. This condition is primarily diagnosed clinically on the basis of localized tenderness and swelling over the lateral malleolus.

Diagnosis
Radiographs of SH I or II fractures tend to be normal, or they may demonstrate only minimal displacement, thereby making the radiographic diagnosis difficult. As a rule of thumb, bilateral x-rays should be obtained for all pediatric patients to allow for comparison with the noninjured leg. The radiographs and the clinical examination tend to be more obvious and dramatic in fractures that are SH III or greater, and bilateral x-rays are usually not required. Computed tomography scanning and MRI may be needed to fully define the extent of complex fractures.[38]

Treatment
The initial and on-field management of a suspected ankle fracture in children is the same as it is for an adult (Rest Ice Compression Elevation).

Nondisplaced SH type I and II fractures can be managed by experienced primary care physicians. Nondisplaced or minimally displaced, less than 2 mm, SH I and II fractures are best treated with a short-leg walking cast for 3 to 4 weeks.[9] These patients have a low likelihood of growth arrest as long as the fracture remains nondisplaced.

Patients with displaced SH II or greater fractures of the distal fibula should be referred to an orthopedic surgeon due to the high association of these fractures with tibial physeal injuries that may require internal fixation. These injuries have a higher risk of growth arrest.

All other fractures around the ankle in children should be managed (or, at a minimum, comanaged) by an orthopedic surgeon because of the involvement of the growth plate and the potential for operative management that may be required to ensure the best outcome. Postfracture rehabilitation for children is the same as it is for adults, but it tends to move at a more rapid pace. Rehabilitation after immobilization should be limited by symptoms in children.

Pediatric tibial fractures
Mechanism of injury
This injury usually results from an eversion/pronation injury.

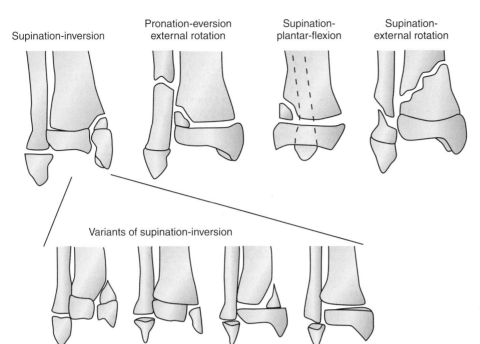

Supination-inversion

Pronation-eversion external rotation

Supination-plantar-flexion

Supination-external rotation

Variants of supination-inversion

Figure 28.13 The Dias–Tachdjian ankle fracture classification system for skeletally immature patients. (From Chambers HG: Orthop Clin North Am 2003;34[3]:445-459.)

Risk factors

No risk factors for this injury have been identified.

Clinical features

Nondisplaced SH I and II fractures of the tibia are often mistakenly treated as sprains, and then patients return for follow up because of continued pain and swelling. As with the fibular fractures, tenderness and swelling should provide clues to the diagnosis.

Diagnosis

The diagnosis is similar to that of fibular fractures, although bilateral comparison films may be needed.

Treatment

SH I fractures usually respond to treatment with immobilization in a short-leg walking cast for 4 weeks. SH II fractures can be treated in the same way, although another option is a long-leg (above the

knee) cast with 30 degrees of knee flexion for 3 weeks followed by a short-leg walking cast for another 3 to 4 weeks.

Displaced (>2 mm) SH type II and all type III, IV, and V fractures require operative intervention by an orthopedic surgeon. Patients with these fractures should not bear weight, and their fractures should be placed in a bulky compression dressing until the surgeon can be consulted.

Patients with displaced SH II or greater fractures should receive follow-up radiographs every 6 months for 2 years or until Park–Harris growth arrest lines parallel to the physis appear. These lines represent transient calcification of the physeal plate during injury repair; if growth is normal, they are parallel to the physis. Angulated or tented lines are a sign of damage to the physeal plate and of the potential for growth arrest.

Juvenile tillaux fractures

An avulsion fracture of the lateral epiphysis by the anteroinferior tibiofibular ligament is the most common SH III fracture of the distal tibia **(Figure 28.15)**. These fractures typically occur in teenagers close to the end of their growth as a result of the fact that the distal tibial physis closes in a medial-to-lateral fashion.[9,37] A Tillaux

Table 28.6 Salter–Harris Physeal Fracture Classification System

Type I	A shear or slide injury; the epiphysis separates ever so slightly from the metaphysis, with the periosteal attachments surrounding the physis remaining intact; frequently seen in infants and toddlers.
Type II	The fracture line extends from the physis proximally through the metaphysis; the most common Salter–Harris fracture; most commonly occurs in children who are more than 8 years of age.
Type III	The fracture line extends from the physis distally through the epiphysis; an intra-articular fracture.
Type IV	The fracture line originates on the articular surface and travels proximally through the epiphysis, the physis, and the metaphysis.
Type V	A profound compressive force that crushes the physis; the rarest Salter–Harris fracture.

A mnemonic to aid in remembering the location of a Salter–Harris fracture is based on the name SALTR: S, slide injury; A, above physis; L, lower (distal) to the physis; T, through the physis; and R, ruined (physis severely crushed).

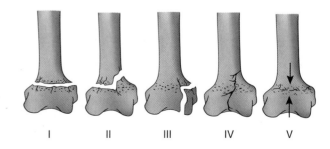

I   II   III   IV   V

Figure 28.14 The Salter–Harris classification of fractures. The *arrows* point to the physis. (From Grover G: Orthopedic injuries and growing pain. In Berkowitz CD [ed]: Pediatrics: A Primary Care Approach, 2nd ed. Philadelphia, WB Saunders, 2000, p 374.)

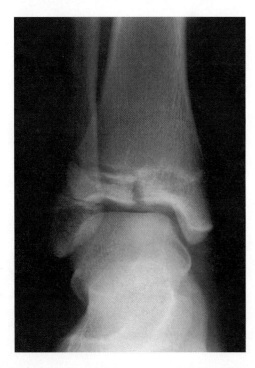

Figure 28.15 A radiograph demonstrating a juvenile tillaux fracture. Note the lateral Tillaux fragment. (From Ankle fractures. In Eiff MP, Hatch RL, Calmbach WL [eds]: Fracture Management for Primary Care, 2nd ed. Philadelphia, WB Saunders, 1998, p 303.)

fracture may be minimally displaced (i.e., <2 mm) and therefore amenable to closed reduction in a long-leg cast. Tillaux fractures that do not meet this criterion will require open reduction with either Kirschner wires or cortical screws.

CONCLUSION

Injuries to the ankle are very common, and most of them are straightforward, easily managed sprains or fractures. Improperly diagnosed and treated ankle injuries can lead to significant morbidity for the patient. Identifying stable and unstable fractures is an important first step in determining the appropriate treatment. The Ottawa and Buffalo ankle rules can be used to help identify which adult patients need radiographs but should not be applied to children and adolescents. Patients with open physeal plates require special attention to minimize the chance of permanent injury to the growth plate.

REFERENCES

1. Birrer RB: Chapter 53: Ankle injuries. Birrer RB, O'Connor FG (eds): Sports Medicine for the Primary Care Physician, 3rd ed. Boca Raton, Florida, CRC Press, 2004.
2. Hintermann B, Regazzoni P, Lampert C, et al: Arthroscopic findings in acute fractures of the ankle. J Bone Joint Surg (Br) 2000;82-B(3):345-351.
3. Wexler RK: The injured ankle. Am Fam Physician 1998;57(3):474-485.
4. Judd JB, Kim DH: Foot fractures frequently misdiagnosed as ankle sprain. Am Fam Physician 2002;66(5):785-794.
5. Ashman ES, Abell BE: Tibial and ankle fractures. O'Connor FG, Sallis RE, Wilder RP, St. Pierre P (eds): Sports Medicine: Just the Facts. New York, McGraw-Hill, 2005.
6. Windhagen H, Wulker N, Hurschler C: Ankle fractures. Curr Opin Orthop 1999;10:218-223.
7. Griend RV, Michelson JD, Bone LB: Fractures of the ankle and the distal part of the tibia. J Bone Joint Surg Am 1996;78-A(11):1772-1783.
8. Michelson JD: Ankle fractures resulting from rotational injuries. J Am Acad Orthop Surg 2003;11(6):403-412.
9. Ankle fractures. Eiff MP, Hatch RL, Calmbach WL (eds): Fracture Management For Primary Care, 2nd ed. Philadelphia, WB Saunders, 1998, pp 288-306.
10. Michelson J, Solocoff D, Waldman B, et al: Ankle fractures: the Lauge-Hansen classification revisited. Clin Orthop 1997;345:198-205.
11. Brandser EA, Kerbaum KS, Dorfman DD, et al: Contribution of individual projections alone and in combination for radiographic detection of ankle fractures. Am J Roentgenol 2000;174:1691-1698.
12. Stiell IG, McKnight RD, Greenberg GH, et al. Implementation of the Ottawa Ankle Rules. JAMA 1994;271:827-832.
13. Nugent PJ: Ottawa ankle rules accurately assess injuries and reduce reliance on radiographs. J Fam Pract 2004;53(10):785-788.
14. Leddy JJ, Smolinski RJ, Lawrence J, et al: Prospective evaluation of the Ottawa ankle rules in a university sports medicine center. Am J Sports Med 1998;26:158-165.
15. Wykes PR, Eccles B, Thannavan B, Barrie JL: Improvement in the treatment of stable ankle fractures: an audit based approach. J Injury 2004;35:799-804.
16. Sherbondy PS, Sebastianelli WJ: Stress fractures of the medial malleolus and distal fibula. Clin Sports Med 2006;25:129-137.
17. Wilder RP, Sethi S: Overuse injuries: tendinopathies, stress fractures, compartment syndrome and shin splints. Clin Sports Med 2004;23:55-81.
18. Wall J, Feller JF: Imaging of stress fractures in runners. Clin Sports Med 2006;25:781-802.
19. Rauh MJ, Macera CA, Trone DW, et al: Epidemiology of stress fracture and lower extremity overuse injury in female recruits. Med Sci Sports Exerc 2006;38(9):1571-1577.
20. Tull F, Borrelli J: Soft-tissue injury associated with closed fractures: evaluation and management. J Am Acad Orthop Surg 2003;11:431-438.
21. Egol KA, Dolan R, Koval KJ: Functional outcome of surgery for fractures of the ankle: a prospective, randomized comparison of management in a cast or a functional brace. J Bone Joint Surg (Br) 2000;82-B(2):246-249.
22. Lehtonen H, Jarvinen TLN, Honkonen S, et al: Use of a cast compared with a functional ankle brace after operative treatment of an ankle fracture: a prospective randomized study. J Bone Joint Surg 2003;85-A(2):205-211.
23. Campbell SE: MRI of sports injuries of the ankle. Clin Sports Med 2006;25:727-762.
24. Michelson JD, Varner KE, Checcone M: Diagnosing deltoid injury in ankle fractures: the gravity stress view. Clin Orthop Relat Res 2001;387:178-182.
25. Stromsoe K, Hoqevold HE, Skjeldal S, Alho A: The repair of a ruptured deltoid ligament is not necessary in ankle fractures. J Bone Joint Surg (Br) 1995;77-B:920-921.
26. Candal-Couto JJ, Burrow D, Bromage S, Briggs PJ: Instability of the tibio-fibular syndesmosis: have we been pulling in the wrong direction? J Injury 2004;35:814-818.
27. Stephenson K, Saltzman CK, Brotzman SB: Foot and ankle injuries. In Brotzman SB, Wilk KE (eds): Clinical Orthopedic Rehabilitation, 2nd ed. Philadelphia, Mosby, 2003, pp 371-439.
28. Uys HD, Rijke AM: Clinical association of acute lateral ankle sprain with syndesmotic involvement. Am J Sports Med 2002;30:816-822.
29. Sproule JA, Khalid M, O'Sullivan M, et al: Outcome after surgery for Maisonneuve fracture of the fibula. J Injury 2004;35:791-798.
30. Tranovich M: Ankle dislocation with fracture. Phys Sportsmed 2003;31(5):42-44.
31. Rivera F, Bertone C, De Martino M, et al: Pure dislocation of the ankle: three case reports and literature review. Clin Orthop 2001;382:179-184.
32. Germann CA, Perron AD, Sweeney TW, et al: Orthopedic pitfall in the ED: tibial plafond fractures. J Emerg Med 2005;23:357-362.
33. Thoradson DB: Detecting and treating common foot and ankle fractures: part 1: the ankle and hindfoot. Phys Sportsmed 1996;24(9):29-36.
34. Pinzur MS: Pitfalls in the treatment of fractures of the ankle and talus. Clin Orthop Relat Res 2001;391:17-25.
35. Watson TJ, Moed BR, Karges DE, et al: Pilon fractures: treatment protocol based on severity of soft tissue injury. Clin Orthop Relat Res 2000;375:78-90.
36. Bassewitz HL, Shapiro MS: Persistent pain after ankle sprain: targeting the causes. Phys Sportsmed 1997;25(12):58-65.
37. Christoph RA: Musculoskeletal disorders in children. Tintinalli JE, Ruiz E, Krome RL (eds): Emergency Medicine: A Comprehensive Study Guide, 4th ed. New York, McGraw-Hill, 1978, pp 674-686.
38. Perron AD, Brady WJ: Evaluation and management of the high-risk orthopedic emergency. Emerg Med Clin North Am 2003;21:159-204.
39. Soprano JV: Musculoskeletal injuries in the pediatric and adolescent athlete. Curr Sports Med Rep 2005;4(6):329-334.
40. Teebaggy AK: Leg and ankle. In Steinberg GC, Atkins CM, Baran DT, Ramamurti CP (eds): Ramamurti's Orthopedics in Primary Care, 2nd ed. Baltimore, Lippincott Williams & Wilkins, 1992.

CHAPTER 29

Foot Fractures

LTC Kevin deWeber, MD, FAAFP

KEY POINTS

- Because of the tenuous blood supply and/or critical weight-bearing nature of many foot bones, the rate of nonunion of several foot fractures is very high. Attention to anatomic reduction, adequate immobilization, and close follow-up can optimize the rate of healing.
- Early recognition of hindfoot and midfoot fractures is critical, and computed tomography scanning has an important role in accurate evaluation and management planning. Accurate anatomic alignment and reduction are of paramount importance to minimize chronic pain and abnormal gait.
- The careful examination of seemingly isolated fractures of the foot is necessary to rule out concomitant tarsometatarsal (Lisfranc) sprains or fracture dislocations, which can lead to more disability than the original fracture. The early recognition of these midfoot injuries and accurate assessment with computed tomography scanning or magnetic resonance imaging are important for proper management and optimal healing.
- Most of the recommended treatments of foot fractures are based on case series or case reports. Only calcaneal fractures and avulsion fractures of the fifth metatarsal have treatment recommendations that are supported by clinical trials.
- Careful neurovascular examination of the sole if the foot is necessary for the evaluation of sustentaculum tali calcaneal fractures and to rule out damage to the adjacent posterior tibial artery and nerve.

INTRODUCTION

In addition to the significant forces of gravity during normal ambulation, the relatively small bones and articulations of the foot must absorb tremendous forces during acceleration, deceleration, and collisions that can occur in sporting activities, some of which may result in fractures. Foot fractures can lead to disproportionately long periods of sport disability because treating them often requires significant periods of limited weight bearing that are followed by proper rehabilitation and reconditioning. Furthermore, foot fractures have relatively high incidences of posttraumatic degenerative arthritis, especially when joint surfaces are involved. This propensity for arthritis can be lessened by (but not eliminated by) prompt diagnosis, careful reduction, and proper treatment. Painful posttraumatic arthritis has put an early end to many a promising season and countless sports careers.

The bones of the foot are commonly described in three anatomic sections: the hindfoot, the midfoot, and the forefoot. The hindfoot is comprised of the talus and the calcaneus. The midfoot includes the navicular, three cuneiforms (medial, middle, and lateral), and the cuboid. The forefoot is composed of the five metatarsals, 14 phalanges, and two sesamoids, which lie within the volar capsule of the first metatarsophalangeal joint. The junction between the midfoot and the forefoot is called the *Lisfranc joint*, and it is comprised of the articulations between the five metatarsals and the cuboid and cuneiforms. Nonfracture injuries to this joint can be just as disabling as broken bones.

The fractures discussed in this chapter are those that are known to occur in sporting activities. Many other fractures of the foot may occur (e.g., fractures of the body of the calcaneus and injuries to the body/neck of the talus), but these are not discussed here because they usually result only from high-energy trauma (e.g., motor vehicle accidents, industrial falls). The reader is referred to current fracture texts for detailed discussions of these non–sports-related injuries.

OSTEOCHONDRAL FRACTURES OF THE TALAR BODY

These injuries are commonly missed because they are often accompanied by the more obvious ankle sprains or fractures. However, if they are not treated, they can slowly lead to subtalar arthritis and possibly the need for ankle fusion.

Mechanism of injury
Shearing forces created by ankle inversion episodes are the most common cause of osteochondral talar fractures.

Risk factors
There are no stated risk factors for this condition.

Clinical features
Patients initially have symptoms that are more specific to the concomitant ankle sprain or fracture. Athletes commonly present

6 to 8 weeks after such an injury complaining of persistent pain that may be vague and occasionally with a history of the ankle catching or locking (as a result of a loose osteochondral fragment). There may be tenderness to palpation over the dome of the talus and a swelling of the ankle joint, but the examination is often normal.

Diagnosis

Large osteochondral fragments may be visible with standard ankle x-rays, but smaller ones will not be. Bone scintigraphy has been shown to be 99% sensitive but only 76% specific for talar osteochondral lesions (LOE: D).[1,2] If osteochondral lesions of the talus are in the differential diagnosis, magnetic resonance imaging (MRI) should be strongly considered, because it is more specific, and it allows for the classification of the lesion (LOE: D).[3] Stage I lesions are characterized by intact but contused cartilage and subchondral trabecular bone compression, and they are not visible on plain films. Stage II lesions have incomplete separation of the cartilage from the underlying bone. Stage III lesions are osteochondral fragments that have no underlying attachments but that remain in their beds. Stage IV lesions are detached from their beds and act as loose bodies within the joint. See **Figure 29.1** for the classification of these lesions.

Treatment

Asymptomatic lesions discovered incidentally do not require treatment (LOE: D).[4-6] Stage II and symptomatic stage I lesions should be treated initially with short-leg cast immobilization for 6 weeks (LOE: D).[6] Stage III lesions can be managed with up to 6 months of conservative management (LOE: D)[5] or with arthroscopic debridement of the cartilage and debridement of the subchondral bone to stimulate the formation of a fibrocartilaginous scar (LOE: D).[6] Arthroscopic evaluation should also be done if stage I or II lesions fail to heal with conservative management, at which time treatment options include continued conservative treatment for stage I lesions, drilling of the overlying cartilage for stage II lesions, and debridement of stage III lesions. Most authors recommend the arthroscopic debridement of stage IV lesions, with debridement of the fragment bed down to bleeding subchondral bone if it is not already covered by a fibrocartilaginous scar (LOE: D)[7,8] **(Figure 29.2).**

FRACTURES OF THE LATERAL PROCESS OF THE TALUS

A fracture of the lateral process of the talus has been called *snowboarder's fracture* as a result of its frequent association with this sport. In many cases, it presents as an ankle sprain that just has not healed after several weeks. Early recognition and treatment can reduce the risk of nonunion and the need for fragment excision.

Mechanism of injury

Although commonly thought to result from the dorsiflexion and inversion of the ankle joint, a recent study in cadavers showed that forceful dorsiflexion with eversion was much more likely to produce this fracture than inversion.[9]

Risk factors

Sports that subject the ankles to forceful eversion are the primary risk factors for this relatively uncommon fracture.

Clinical features

Patients usually have swelling and ecchymosis localized to the lateral aspect of the ankle, with point tenderness just anterior and inferior to the lateral malleolus. Because of this, the injury can easily be overlooked and/or misdiagnosed as a lateral ankle sprain.

Diagnosis

This fracture should be in the differential diagnosis of chronic lateral ankle pain after a sprain. It is usually visible on the mortise view x-ray of the ankle **(Figure 29.3).** Computed tomography (CT) scanning is helpful for further defining the degree of articular involvement and the fragment size (LOE: D).[10] The lateral process of the talus articulates with the fibula superiorly and with the calcaneus inferiorly **(Figure 29.4).** The importance of these articulations has led to a classification of these fractures into the following categories: simple nonarticular chip fractures, larger fractures involving the talofibular or talocalcaneal articulations, and comminuted fractures involving both articulations.[3]

Treatment

Nondisplaced, nonarticular fractures can be treated with cast immobilization for about 6 weeks, with the first 4 weeks involving no weight bearing.[3] The management of fractures that are either displaced by more than 2 mm and/or that involve fragments that are more than 1 cm in diameter is controversial, but the literature favors surgical treatment with open reduction and internal fixation (ORIF) because it involves better outcomes (LOE: D).[11,12] Most authors recommend primary surgical excision for comminuted fractures to avoid the development of arthritic changes at the subtalar joint (LOE: E).

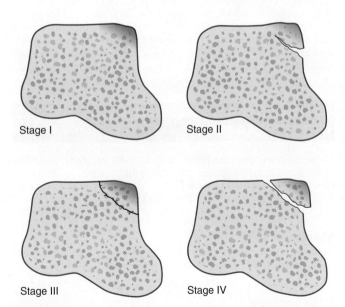

Stage I

Stage II

Stage III

Stage IV

Figure 29.1 The Berndt and Harty classification system of osteochondral lesions. Stage I: subchondral trabecular compression lesion. Stage II: incomplete separation of the osteochondral fragment. Stage III: osteochondral fragment that has a detached base but that remains positioned within the fracture bed. Stage IV: fragment displaced and loose within the ankle joint.

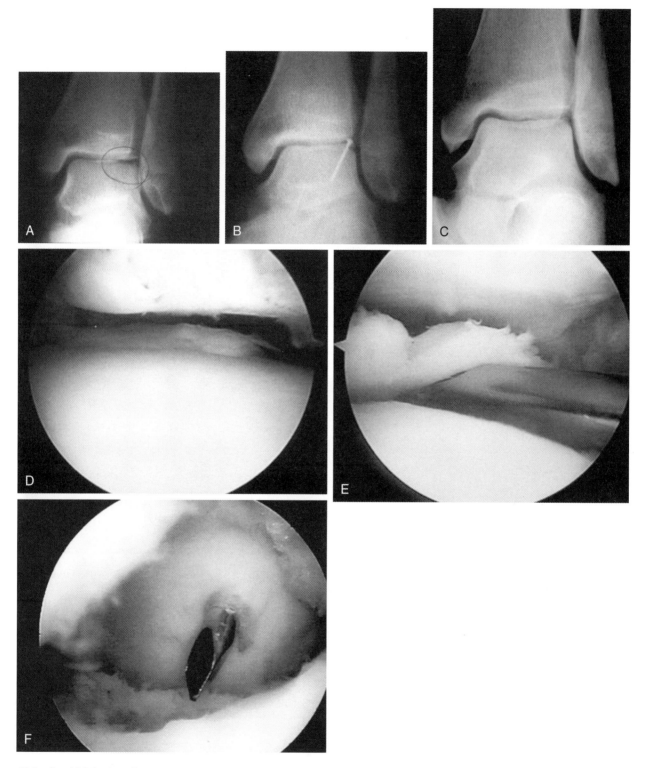

Figure 29.2   *A* and *B,* Talar dome fracture repaired with 1.5-mm mini fragment screw. *C,* Displaced osteochondral fracture at the lateral aspect of the shoulder of the talus, seen better as a step off *(D)* on initial arthroscopic evaluation. The large, unstable fragment *(E)* was excised, and the defect was treated with drilling *(F)*. (From Browner L: Skeletal Trauma: Basic Science, Management, and Reconstruction, 3rd ed. Philadelphia, Saunders, 2003.)

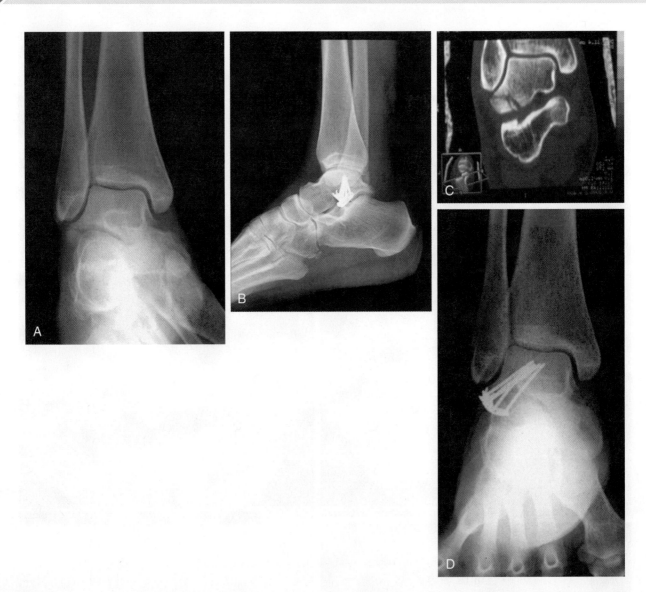

Figure 29.3 Isolated lateral talar process fracture on plain films (A and B), computed tomography (C), and after internal fixation (D). (From Browner L: Skeletal Trauma: Basic Science, Management, and Reconstruction, 3rd ed. Philadelphia, Saunders, 2003.)

FRACTURES OF THE LATERAL TUBERCLE OF THE POSTERIOR PROCESS OF THE TALUS AND OS TRIGONUM SYNDROME

The posterior talar process is composed of two tubercles (medial and lateral) that are separated by a groove for the tendon of the flexor hallucis longus (see Figure 29.4). Fractures of the entire posterior process or of the medial tubercle are rare, and they are not discussed in this text. About 6% of ankles have a separate accessory ossicle called the os trigonum just posterior to the lateral tubercle. About 60% of persons with an os trigonum will have them bilaterally. The synostosis between the accessory ossicle and its tubercle is susceptible to acute and chronic injury.[13]

Mechanism of injury
Fractures of the lateral tubercle of the posterior process are well described in the literature. This injury has been reported in football and rugby players, presumably as a result of repetitive forceful equinus positioning of the foot during kicking. It can also occur with inversion injuries of the ankle.

Risk factors
Factors that predispose athletes to posterior talar process fractures include activities that lead to repetitive forceful equinus positioning of the ankle (e.g., kicking sports) and toeing in ballet.

Clinical features
Patients are most likely to present with symptoms similar to those of lateral ankle sprains, with pain being more posteriorly located than it is with the average sprain. There will usually be tenderness to palpation on the posterolateral aspect of the ankle, and movement of the ankle and subtalar joints will be painful. Actively moving the great toe may also cause pain as a result of the proximity of the flexor hallucis longus tendon to the fracture site. A useful provocative maneuver is forceful plantar flexion of the ankle; pain suggests an injury to the posterior process of the talus or to the surrounding structures.

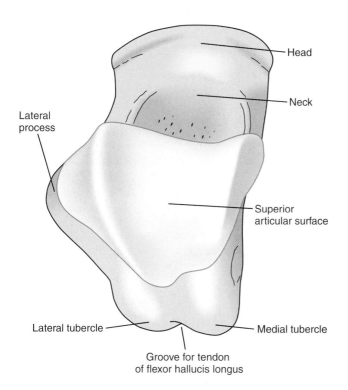

Figure 29.4 Anatomy of the talus, superior view.

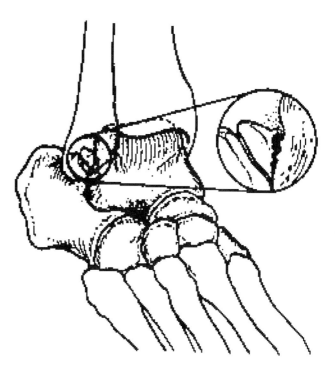

Figure 29.5 Fracture of the lateral tubercle of the posterior talar process. (Redrawn from Amis JA, Gangl PM: J Musculoskel Med 1987;68. In DeLee JC, Drez D Jr, Miller MD [eds]: DeLee & Drez's Orthopaedic Sports Medicine: Principles and Practice, 2nd ed. Philadelphia, WB Saunders, 2003.)

Diagnosis

A lateral x-ray of the ankle best demonstrates the lateral tubercle. Comparison x-rays with the contralateral foot may be helpful for patients with an os trigonum because of the significant rate of bilaterality. A lateral process fracture can usually be distinguished from an os trigonum by its fracture line, which has a rough, irregular surface, as opposed to that of an os trigonum, which appears to be more smooth and rounded **(Figure 29.5)**. However, at times, the distinction is not clear; in these cases, a bone scan or MRI should be considered. Acute injury will cause increased uptake in that area on a bone scan (LOE: D).[14] However, this imaging modality is nonspecific, because the area can have increased uptake, even in asymptomatic athletes (LOE: D).[15] MRI is useful for distinguishing fractures from bone bruises, acute fractures, synostosis injury, and soft-tissue causes of pain in the so-called "posterior impingement syndrome" (LOE: D).[16,17]

Treatment

Acute, nondisplaced fractures of the lateral tubercle of the posterior process of the talus should be treated initially with a short-leg cast or compressive dressing with protection from weight bearing for 4 to 6 weeks. X-rays should be repeated periodically until evidence of healing is seen (LOE: D).[3,18] Conservative treatment should be continued for up to 3 months in the case of a symptomatic os trigonum. If the fracture site remains symptomatic, excision of the symptomatic fragment or the os trigonum usually eliminates the pain (LOE: D).[14,19-21]

FRACTURES OF THE CALCANEUS

Significant force is usually required to fracture the calcaneus. Calcaneal fractures are broadly categorized as those that involve the posterior facet and those that do not. The posterior facet is the largest articular facet of the calcaneus, and it lies on its superior

surface, articulating with the talus **(Figure 29.6)**. Fractures through this very thick part of the calcaneus usually result from motor vehicle accidents and major falls, and they are not discussed in this text. Fractures that may occur in sporting activities are those that involve the anterior process, the body (not involving an articular facet), and, less commonly, the sustentaculum tali.[22]

FRACTURES OF THE ANTERIOR PROCESS OF THE CALCANEUS

Mechanism of injury

Injury to this anterior "beak" of the calcaneus usually results from the forced inversion of the ankle **(Figure 29.7)**.

Risk factors

No risk factors for this injury have been identified.

Clinical features

Patients often present with symptoms and a physical examination that is consistent with a lateral ankle sprain, and this fracture may be missed if radiographs are not ordered and examined carefully. Patients will have pain in the anterolateral aspect of the hindfoot and tenderness to palpation in the area of the sinus tarsi. Swelling and ecchymosis may also be present locally.

Diagnosis

The oblique view of the foot is the x-ray view most likely to identify an anterior process fracture, although lateral and anteroposterior (AP) views are important. The anterior process has articular surfaces with the cuboid bone anteriorly, so an intra-articular

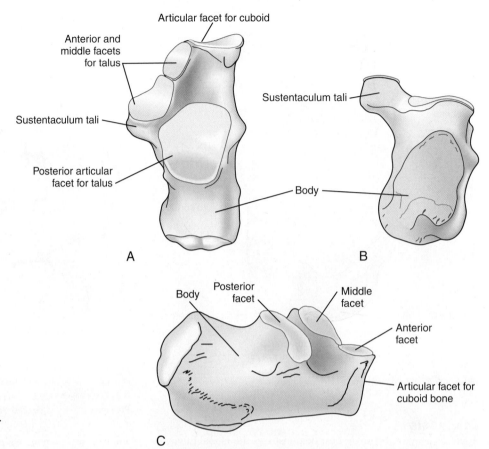

Figure 29.6 Anatomy of the right calcaneus. *A*, Superior view. *B*, Posterior view. *C*, Lateral view.

fracture may be present. Abnormalities on plain films may be subtle, so bone scanning, CT scanning, or MRI may also be beneficial for determining the presence of a fracture, the extent of articular involvement with the calcaneocuboid joint, and the degree of displacement **(Figure 29.8).**

Treatment
Nondisplaced anterior calcaneal process fractures involving less than about 25% of the calcaneocuboid joint are typically treated symptomatically with a short-leg walking cast or a removable fracture boot for 4 to 6 weeks, with partial weight bearing. For larger fragments, ORIF should be considered (LOE: D).[22]

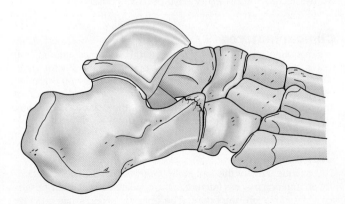

Figure 29.7 Fracture of the anterior process of the calcaneus.

CALCANEAL BODY FRACTURES

Mechanism of injury
Fractures of the calcaneal body in areas other than through the posterior facet usually result from a forceful injury or a motor vehicle accident.

Risk factors
Men are four to five times more likely than women to fracture the calcaneus.[23]

Clinical features
Patients will be unable to bear weight on the affected foot. Examination will reveal diffuse swelling and possibly ecchymosis in the hindfoot that extends onto the midfoot and ankle.

Diagnosis
AP, lateral, and oblique x-rays will usually reveal the fracture line, but the involvement of the subtalar joint cannot reliably be determined without CT scanning, so this should be performed (LOE: D).[24] Note that, in fractures of the body of the calcaneus, the incidence of other injury to the lower extremity or back is significant, so a careful examination of these areas should also be performed.

Treatment
The treatment of nonarticular calcaneal body fractures is primarily nonsurgical, initially with ice, elevation, and a compressive

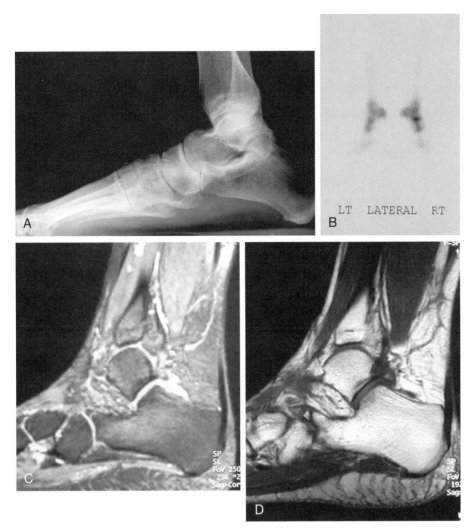

Figure 29.8 Fracture of the anterior process of the calcaneus. Note the difficulty of seeing a fracture line on plain films (A). In this patient, a bone scan (B) was positive, which led to magnetic resonance imaging (C and D) to further characterize the fracture. (From Browner L: Skeletal Trauma: Basic Science, Management, and Reconstruction, 3rd ed. Philadelphia, Saunders, 2003.)

soft-tissue dressing to minimize swelling and pain. Patients can progress to non–weight-bearing range-of-motion exercises when symptoms improve. When the swelling resolves, these patients may be placed in a removable fracture boot, and they may be limited to touchdown-only weight bearing for about 4 to 6 weeks. These patients may then progress to partial weight bearing followed by full weight bearing as tolerated. Surgical treatment should be considered when there is severe disruption of the calcaneal arch, including a widening of the calcaneus or a loss of calcaneal height (LOE: D).[22]

FRACTURES OF THE SUSTENTACULUM TALI

Mechanism of injury
Isolated fractures of the sustentaculum tali are rare, but they can occur as a result of axial compression on an inverted ankle.

Risk factors
No risk factors for this injury have been determined.

Clinical features
There may be isolated swelling in the medial hindfoot, with tenderness concentrated inferior to the medial malleolus. Resisted

motion of the flexor hallucis longus tendon may be painful because it passes under the sustentaculum and presses on the fracture site.

Diagnosis
Lateral, axial, and oblique x-rays are indicated. If plain films are normal but a fracture is suspected, CT scanning is sensitive for detecting even nondisplaced fractures. Careful examination of the distal foot is required to assess for injury to the posterior tibial artery and nerve that course just medial and superior to the sustentaculum. Compromise of the artery can lead to prolonged capillary refill in the sole of the foot, and injury to the nerve will cause paresthesia, numbness, and/or decreased sensation in the sole.

Treatment
Nondisplaced fractures are treated with non–weight-bearing immobilization in a short-leg cast for about 6 weeks. The patient can then be transitioned to a removable fracture boot and progressed to weight bearing as tolerated. Displaced fractures should be reduced. Closed reduction is difficult, but it can be attempted under regional or general anesthesia by placing the ankle in inversion and plantar flexion and applying digital pressure over the sustentaculum. If this is not successful or if the reduction is not maintained, ORIF should be performed.[22]

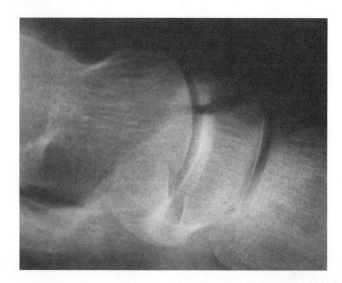

Figure 29.9 Avulsion fracture of the navicular. (From Browner L: Skeletal Trauma: Basic Science, Management, and Reconstruction, 3rd ed. Philadelphia, Saunders, 2003.)

ACUTE FRACTURES OF THE NAVICULAR

Fractures of the navicular can be the result of either acute injuries or chronic stress, but only the former type will be discussed in this chapter. The navicular bone forms the keystone of the medial arch of the foot. The talonavicular joint provides most of the foot's supination and pronation, and it works in conjunction with the subtalar joint during inversion and eversion. Its tenuous blood supply can also sometimes lead to inadequate fracture healing.

Mechanism of injury

Acute fractures of the navicular can occur among players of various sporting activities or as a result of major trauma that occurs during motor vehicle accidents or falls. Avulsion fractures, which account for about 50% of navicular fractures, result from twisting type trauma **(Figure 29.9)**. They can occur dorsomedially from the pull of the superficial deltoid ligament or plantarmedially from the pull of the posterior tibial tendon or the spring ligament. Fractures of the body usually result from more significant trauma **(Figure 29.10)**.

Risk factors

No risk factors for this condition have been identified.

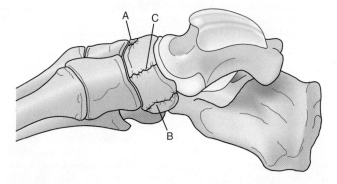

Figure 29.10 Fractures of the navicular. A, Dorsomedial avulsion fracture. B, Plantar–medial avulsion fracture. C, Nondisplaced body fracture.

Clinical features

The medial two thirds of the navicular is palpable in the medial aspect of the dorsum of the midfoot. Fractures will cause local tenderness to palpation, ecchymosis, and/or local edema, and patients will have pain with weight bearing. Because navicular injuries are frequently associated with other injuries, the careful examination of surrounding areas is important.

Diagnosis

AP, lateral, medial oblique, and lateral oblique x-rays of the foot are indicated, and they will reveal most of these fractures; however, CT scanning is indicated if operative repair is being considered. CT scanning allows for better visualization of the talonavicular joint, and it can characterize other associated injuries. An accessory navicular bone (the os tibiale externum) is present in about 25% of persons, so the careful examination of x-rays is indicated to distinguish this from acute fractures. Comparison x-rays are useful because this accessory bone is bilateral about 90% of the time[22,25] **(Figure 29.11)**. Radiographs should be done while the patient is bearing weight to rule out associated ligamentous instability (see section on tarsometatarsal joint injuries later in this chapter).

Treatment

The talonavicular articulation works with the subtalar joint during inversion and eversion of the hindfoot, and it is essential during pronation (cushioning heel strike) and supination (strengthening push off). Therefore, restoring the anatomy is important for resuming normal gait mechanics. Any fracture that is displaced by 2 mm

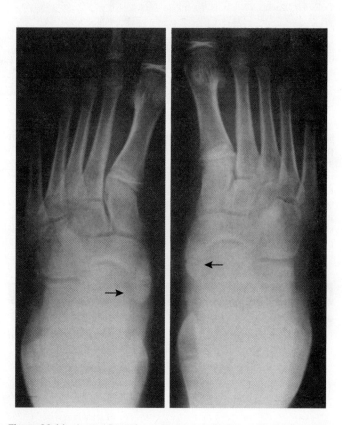

Figure 29.11 Large bilateral accessory navicular bones (os tibiale externum). (From DeLee JC, Drez D Jr, Miller MD [eds]: DeLee & Drez's Orthopaedic Sports Medicine: Principles and Practice, 2nd ed. Philadelphia, WB Saunders, 2003.)

or more requires open reduction and internal fixation (LOE: D).[26,27] Isolated, nondisplaced fractures can be treated with a non–weight-bearing short-leg cast for 6 to 8 weeks (LOE: D).[26] Repeat weight-bearing x-rays should be done out of plaster 10 to 14 days after the initial injury to evaluate for any instability, which, if present, should prompt surgical intervention. Progression to protected weight bearing in a walking cast may begin when the foot is nontender to palpation and when no pain is elicited by the manipulation of the foot.[22]

CUBOID FRACTURES

Isolated cuboid injuries occur, but this bone is more commonly injured in conjunction with a tarsometatarsal joint injury (described later) or with an injury to the talonavicular complex.

Mechanism of injury
Cuboid fractures can occur from a direct blow, but they more commonly occur when the foot is forced into a position of plantar-flexion and abduction, thus creating a compression fracture along the lateral column of the foot that is called the "nutcracker fracture" **(Figure 29.12).**

Risk factors
No risk factors for this injury have been described.

Clinical features
Cuboid injuries can present with findings that range from subtle swelling, ecchymosis, and tenderness to palpation over the dorso-lateral midfoot to severe distortion of the anatomy.[22] Keep in mind that the two columns of the foot—the lateral column, which is composed of the third and fourth metatarsals and the cuboid; and the medial column, which is composed of the first through third metatarsals, the cuneiforms, and the navicular—act in concert to maintain foot stability. If, for example, the lateral column is injured by a compression injury, as it is with a cuboid nutcracker fracture, the medial column should be examined carefully for a distraction injury, such as a fracture, a ligament injury, or both (see Figure 29.12).

Diagnosis
Routine x-rays of the foot can be helpful, especially the medial oblique view, which best assesses the cuboid articulations. Weight-bearing views are important to assess for ligamentous instability. If x-rays suggest a cuboid injury, a CT scan is recommended to further delineate the injury. Cuboid fractures are usually classified as nondisplaced, unstable, or crush fractures for the purposes of management.[22]

Treatment
There is a paucity of literature regarding the treatment of cuboid injuries. For isolated cuboid fractures in which there is less than 2 mm of displacement and no significant loss of bone length from compressive injury, current treatment is a well-molded non–weight-bearing cast for 4 to 6 weeks. Weight-bearing x-rays should be taken after 2 weeks to assess for occult injuries as the swelling subsides. Progressive weight bearing can begin when the fracture is nontender, using a fracture boot or short-leg cast. Fractures involving any adjacent joint instability, a loss of body length, or more than 2 mm of displacement or joint surface disruption should undergo ORIF (LOE: D).[26,28,29]

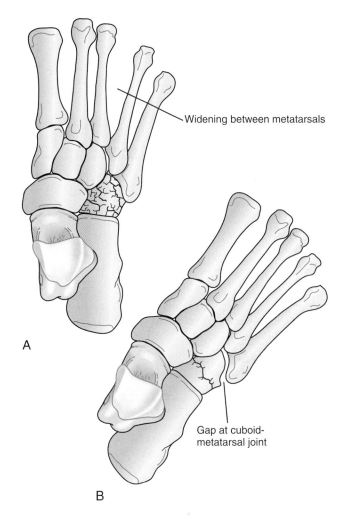

Figure 29.12 Examples of fractures of the cuboid. *A,* "Nutcracker" fracture caused by compression in the lateral column of the foot. *B,* Nondisplaced fracture associated with fourth and fifth tarsometatarsal joint disruption.

OS PERONEUM FRACTURES

The os peroneum is a sesamoid bone within the peroneus longus tendon, where the tendon passes over the cuboid. It is present in 5% to 26% of individuals, and about 25% of the sesamoids are bipartite or multipartite.[30] The bone can be injured either with an intact tendon or in conjunction with tendon rupture **(Figure 29.13).**

Mechanism of injury
The os peroneum can be fractured by a direct blow or by forces that place tensile loads on its tendon, such as an inversion-type sprain injury.

Risk factors
Athletes with chronic lateral ankle instability from past sprains may rely more on the peroneal muscles, which provide dynamic lateral ankle stability. This over reliance on the peroneals can lead to stress on the os peroneum, which can result in a fracture.

Clinical features
Athletes may hear a pop during the injury, and they will complain of pain over the lateral foot, especially during push off.

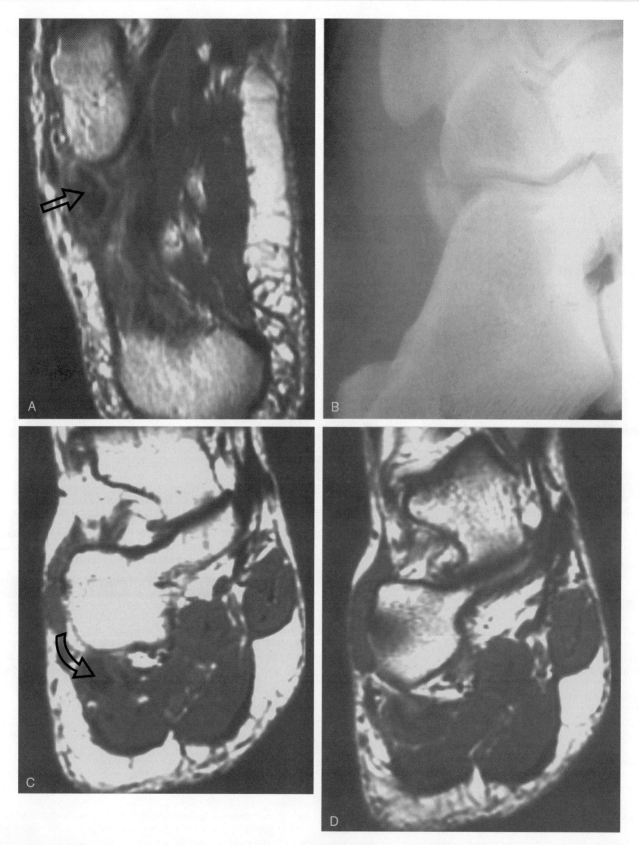

Figure 29.13 *A*, A T1-weighted axial magnetic resonance image shows a fracture of the os peroneum (linear gray signal) *(arrow)* traversing the normally black signal of the os peroneum. *B*, An oblique radiograph of the foot shows elongation and a transversely oriented fracture of the os peroneum, which suggests a peroneus longus tendon tear. *C* and *D*, Coronal T1-weighted images show a flattening of the os peroneum with a transversely oriented fracture *(curved arrow)* and attenuation of the peroneus longus tendon. (From DeLee JC, Drez D Jr, Miller MD [eds]: DeLee & Drez's Orthopaedic Sports Medicine: Principles and Practice, 2nd ed. Philadelphia, WB Saunders, 2003.)

Examination may reveal localized tenderness and swelling over the peroneal tendon where it courses over the cuboid. There may be pain with resisted plantar flexion of the first metatarsal or with forced passive dorsiflexion of the first ray because the peroneus longus tendon inserts partially on the volar surface on the first metatarsal base. Resisted eversion may also be painful.

Diagnosis

AP, lateral, and oblique x-rays may show a fracture of the os peroneum. A bipartite os peroneum or a nondisplaced fracture should have 2 mm or less separation of the fragments. The separation of fragments by 6 mm or more is consistent with a fracture and a tendon rupture (LOE: D).[31] The usefulness of bone scintigraphy is unknown. MRI may be useful to delineate coexistent tendon pathology (LOE: E).[32]

Treatment

Acute nondisplaced os peroneum fractures with an intact peroneus longus tendon can be treated with a non–weight-bearing cast or a removable fracture boot for 6 weeks. When the fracture is nontender to palpation and x-rays show healing, rehabilitation with motion, strengthening, and proprioceptive exercises may begin (LOE: E). If conservative treatment for 3 months is not successful for alleviating pain, surgical excision of the fragments from the intact tendon should be performed (LOE: D).[33] Rupture of the tendon associated with acute os peroneum fracture should be treated with ORIF or with the excision of the fragments and tendon repair (LOE: E).[34]

TARSOMETATARSAL JOINT INJURIES

The tarsometatarsal (TMT) joints include the three metatarsocuneiform joints medially and the two metatarsocuboid joints laterally (Figure 29.14). Collectively, they are referred to as the *Lisfranc joint*, after the 19th-century French surgeon who briefly served in Napoleon's army and who first described the complex midfoot injuries that happened when a cavalry soldier fell from his horse with his forefoot trapped in the stirrup.

The semirigid TMT articulations comprise the important transverse arch of the foot, which protects the neurovascular structures

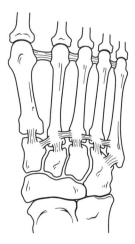

Figure 29.14 The Lisfranc articulation with its ligamentous attachments. Note the recessed second tarsometatarsal joint and the Lisfranc ligament in place of the first–second intermetatarsal ligament. (From DeLee JC, Drez D Jr, Miller MD [eds]: DeLee & Drez's Orthopaedic Sports Medicine: Principles and Practice, 2nd ed. Philadelphia, WB Saunders, 2003.)

of the plantar aspect of the foot. It also comprises the distal portion of the longitudinal arch and creates a lever arm that allows for the transfer of weight smoothly from the hindfoot to the forefoot during walking. The disruption and improper healing of these important joints can cause long-term pain and disability, and it can preclude athletic participation at previous levels.

Mechanism of injury

There are several variables that can serve as mechanisms of injury to the TMT joints in athletics. Jumping athletes may land on the foot with the ankle in full plantarflexion, which causes the transmission of large axial forces through the foot. This can disrupt the relatively weak dorsal TMT ligaments or fracture the base of the second metatarsal, which is the only metatarsal base that is more proximally inset (keystoned) as compared with the others. In a football pileup, if the dorsiflexed foot of an athlete lying on the ground is fallen on by a large lineman, the axial forces may also disrupt the articulations and collapse the midfoot. These injuries sometimes occur when the planted forefoot is stepped on by a large athlete, which creates a twisting injury of the midfoot as the foot and the rest of the body continue moving while the forefoot is trapped. A similar mechanism of action occurs in equestrian or biking sports when the athlete falls off the mount but the forefoot remains trapped in a stirrup or pedal clip.[35]

Risk factors

Risk factors are those sports with the potential to trap the forefoot while the hindfoot continues to move or those that subject the foot to high axial forces. Such sports include football, biking, or equestrian sports.

Clinical features

Lisfranc joint injuries range from clinically subtle sprains to multiple fracture–dislocations. Midfoot pain is the chief complaint. Athletes with mild injury may have dorsal midfoot swelling or ecchymosis and tenderness to palpation in one or several of the TMT articulations. Careful physical examination and maintaining a high index of suspicion for these injuries remain paramount for timely diagnosis and early treatment, which are important for preventing long-term disability. Each TMT joint should be assessed for pain or instability by a dorsally directed stress of the metatarsal heads. Passive pronation, supination, abduction, and adduction of the entire forefoot (with the hindfoot stabilized) can elicit pain in injured TMT joints. Checking sensation in the first dorsal web space and palpating for diminished dorsalis pedis arterial pulse are important because this artery and the deep peroneal nerve course over the second TMT joint and may be damaged in Lisfranc injuries. Compartment syndrome may also occur if the first intermetatarsal branch of the dorsalis pedis artery is injured, so the clinician should maintain a high index of suspicion for this complication.

Diagnosis

AP, lateral, and oblique x-rays may be sufficient to diagnose TMT injuries and to assist with treatment. Stress views are widely advocated to detect subtle ligamentous instability, although they have not been proven to be effective clinically. Dorsal stress views may be done by obtaining an AP x-ray while the patient bears weight on the affected foot. Abduction stress views are done by exerting lateral pressure on the distal medial forefoot against a stationary fulcrum located at the level of the anterior calcaneal process on the lateral foot. Patients with severe pain may require anesthesia with a regional ankle block to allow these maneuvers.

Fractures of the metatarsal bases, the cuneiforms, the cuboid, and the navicular may occur in various combinations in these injuries. Careful examination of the films is necessary to also detect subtle findings that may indicate ligamentous instability and the need for aggressive treatment. On the AP view, the space between the first and second metatarsal bases should not be 2 mm more than that of the uninjured side (LOE: D).[36,37] The medial border of the first metatarsal should be in line with the medial border of the first cuneiform, and the same alignment should be present between the medial borders of the second metatarsal and the second cuneiform. The lateral base of the third metatarsal should also be aligned with the lateral border of the lateral cuneiform (LOE: E).[38] A small avulsion fracture at the base of the second metatarsal (fleck sign) may also be a sign of ligamentous instability (LOE: E)[39] **(Figure 29.15).** The lateral view should be examined for any dorsal step offs at the TMT joints, which indicate instability. Flattening of the longitudinal arch on lateral weight-bearing views as compared with the unaffected side has been correlated with greater injury severity (LOE: D).[40] On the oblique view, the medial border of the fourth metatarsal should line up with the medial border of the cuboid, and the medial border of the third metatarsal should be continuous with the medial border of the lateral cuneiform.

CT and MRI may be more sensitive for detecting midfoot fractures and instability, according to recent prospective studies of patients with acute "foot sprains." In a study of 75 patients, CT and MRI detected 79% more metatarsal fractures than plain radiography. MRI detected 315% more tarsal fractures than x-rays and 35% more tarsal fractures than CT. MRI and CT both diagnosed 82% more Lisfranc joint malalignments than stress x-rays. The study also found that stress views did not increase the diagnostic yield of plain films. A similar study of 49 patients showed similar results.[41,42] These studies suggest that MRI may be the best imaging modality but that it is followed closely by CT for clinically suspected midfoot sprains (LOE: B).

On the basis of the results of imaging and examination, injuries may be generally classified as stable (grade I and II sprains, in which ligaments are only partially torn) or unstable (grade III sprains, which are characterized by complete ligament tears, with or without fractures).

Treatment

There is mounting evidence that treatment results are directly related to the quality of the anatomic reduction obtained, not only for fractures but just as importantly for ligamentous joint instability. Injuries with displaced fractures, articular diastasis, or loss of normal foot arches are considered unstable and require reduction by ORIF (LOE: D).[43-46] There is limited evidence that athletes with subtle injuries that are characterized by the widening of the first–second intermetatarsal space by 2 to 5 mm as compared with the uninjured side may be treated successfully with casting, as described later in this chapter (LOE: D).[37,40]

Grades I and II sprains, which are manifested by midfoot pain with weight bearing, pain with manipulation of the TMT joints, but no fractures or instability on imaging may be treated symptomatically. After several days of edema-control treatment, patients who cannot bear weight without pain can be placed in a well-molded, non–weight-bearing cast for 3 weeks, followed by progressive weight bearing in a short-leg cast or fracture boot with an arch support insert (LOE: D).[47,48] Aggressive rehabilitation exercises should begin at this time. When there is no pain with weight bearing, these patients can progress to shoes with a semirigid foot orthosis and low-impact cross-training. Progress should be based on the amount of pain and swelling with activity.

Because of the serious complications of improperly (and even properly) treated Lisfranc injuries, any clinical suspicion of a Lisfranc-type injury should result in prompt referral to a provider with experience in treating them.

Return to play

Athletes should be counseled that the length of time until return to play may be prolonged relative to common ankle sprains and that it varies with the severity of injury. Patients with mild sprains with no instability may resume sports participation in a few weeks.

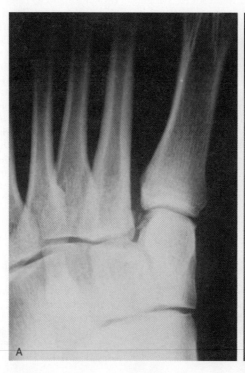 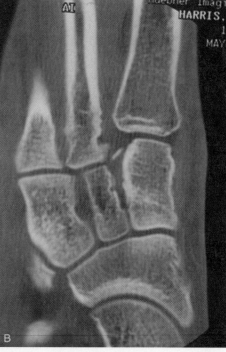

Figure 29.15 A diastasis and occasionally a bone fragment between the first and second metatarsal bases suggest injury to the Lisfranc joint. *A*, A Lisfranc injury as seen on a routine standing radiograph. *B*, A Lisfranc injury as seen on a computed tomography scan. (From DeLee JC, Drez D Jr, Miller MD [eds]: DeLee & Drez's Orthopaedic Sports Medicine: Principles and Practice, 2nd ed. Philadelphia, WB Saunders, 2003.)

Athletes with subtle instability treated with casting took an average of 4 months to return to full participation in two case series (LOE: D).[40,47] Those with severe injuries can take up to 2 years to fully recover,[44] and some may not be able to return to their previous level of activity.

FRACTURES OF THE FIRST METATARSAL

The first metatarsal is shorter, thicker, and more mobile than the other metatarsals. Therefore, only significant trauma results in fractures, and open fractures are common.

Mechanism of injury
Athletic injuries may result from a twisting mechanism when the forefoot is fixed to the ground.

Risk factors
There are no stated risk factors for this condition.

Clinical features
Athletes will present with localized pain in the forefoot and difficulty bearing weight. Swelling will usually be present dorsally, and there will be point tenderness to palpation over the medial forefoot and possibly deformity.

Diagnosis
If the injury is isolated, standard non–weight-bearing AP, lateral, and oblique views of the foot are adequate for diagnosing metatarsal fractures **(Figure 29.16)**. If fractures are present in proximal metatarsals, careful physical examination and stress radiographs may be indicated to assess for Lisfranc joint injury. The amount of fracture angulation in any plane should be assessed radiographically, and rotation can be assessed on examination. Open fractures should be obvious on examination, and attention should be given in all injuries to skin tenting or symptoms of compartment syndrome.

Treatment
There is very little literature on which to base the treatment of first metatarsal fractures; most management is based on anecdotal

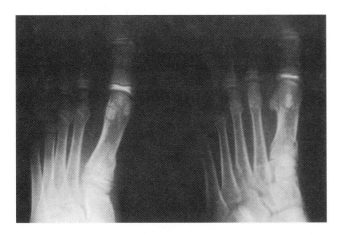

Figure 29.16 Fracture of the first metatarsal shaft sustained in a football player when his foot was stepped on during a game. (From DeLee JC, Drez D Jr, Miller MD [eds]: DeLee & Drez's Orthopaedic Sports Medicine: Principles and Practice, 2nd ed. Philadelphia, WB Saunders, 2003.)

evidence. Indications for surgical treatment with ORIF include significant fracture displacement in any plane, multiple fractures, intra-articular injury, open wounds, compartment syndrome, and the presence of skin that is at risk for pressure necrosis. Unreduced displacement of the first metatarsal can result in abnormal weight-bearing distribution with ambulation and difficulty with shoe wear.

Nondisplaced, uncomplicated fractures may be treated in a short-leg cast for about 4 weeks, with gradual progression to weight bearing as tolerated. Consideration may also be given to treatment with a controlled ankle motion walker boot for some patients. The athlete is then transitioned as soon as it will be tolerated to a well-cushioned shoe and to participation in a rehabilitation program (LOE: E).

FRACTURES OF THE SECOND, THIRD, AND FOURTH METATARSALS

These metatarsals are fractured more frequently than the first metatarsal as a result of their smaller diameters and their relative lack of mobility. However, there is a paucity of literature available regarding their evaluation and treatment.

Mechanism of injury
The mechanism of injury for central metatarsal fractures is similar to that of the first metatarsal, with direct blows and twisting injuries being the most common.

Risk factors
There are no known risk factors for this condition.

Clinical features
Athletes will complain of difficulty bearing weight and localized forefoot pain. If fractures are proximal and associated with a Lisfranc joint complex injury, pain may be more proximal and diffuse. There is usually point tenderness and swelling over the affected metatarsal(s); ecchymosis, crepitus, and deformity may be present with severe fractures.

Diagnosis
Standard non–weight-bearing AP, lateral, and oblique views are adequate for diagnosis **(Figure 29.17)**. Additional imaging, such as CT or MRI, can be considered if a Lisfranc joint injury is suspected. The amount of angulation, displacement, rotation, and involvement of joint surfaces should be assessed because these may determine treatment.

Treatment
The same general indications for the operative treatment of the first metatarsal apply to the central metatarsals, but the latter are more forgiving of mild displacement than is the first metatarsal. Multiple metatarsal head fractures should be treated with ORIF. Proximal fractures associated with Lisfranc joint complex injury should be treated as indicated for the Lisfranc injury. For isolated metatarsal fractures, commonly quoted criteria for operative treatment are 10 degrees or more of angulation in the dorsal/plantar plane or more than 3 to 4 mm of displacement in any plane.[49] However, as little as 2 mm of elevation or shortening of a metatarsal can lead to metatarsalgia or plantar keratoses, so consideration for tolerating less displacement should be made (LOE: E).

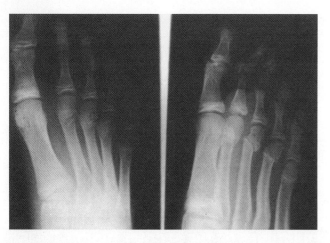

Figure 29.17 Fractures of the lateral four metatarsal necks resulting from a baseball player catching his foot on a base while sliding. (From DeLee JC, Drez D Jr, Miller MD [eds]: DeLee & Drez's Orthopaedic Sports Medicine: Principles and Practice, 2nd ed. Philadelphia, WB Saunders, 2003.)

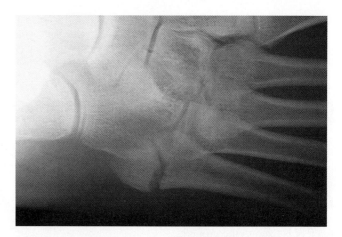

Figure 29.18 Avulsion fracture of the fifth metatarsal base. (From DeLee JC, Drez D Jr, Miller MD [eds]: DeLee & Drez's Orthopaedic Sports Medicine: Principles and Practice, 2nd ed. Philadelphia, WB Saunders, 2003.)

The initial treatment of uncomplicated, isolated central metatarsal fractures should include the reduction of displaced fractures by hanging the toes in finger traps and using the weight of the leg for traction. Casting is then done, with radiographs in plaster to assess the adequacy of the reduction. ORIF should be done if reduction is not maintained adequately. A short-leg walking cast or even a padded, hard-soled shoe (with weight bearing as tolerated) can be used for closed nondisplaced or minimally displaced fractures. These usually heal in 4 to 6 weeks.[50]

ACUTE FIFTH METATARSAL FRACTURES

The fifth is the most commonly fractured of the metatarsals. Types of injuries seen include avulsion fractures of the base, proximal metaphyseal–diaphyseal junction fractures (Jones fractures), and diaphyseal fractures. Stress fractures of the proximal 1.5 cm of the diaphysis will be discussed in Chapter 32.

Mechanism of injury
Most injuries to the fifth metatarsal are the result of sporting activities. Avulsion fractures of the base are the most common, and they usually occur in conjunction with an inversion ankle injury. Jones fractures are usually caused by forceful adduction of the forefoot. Distal spiral fractures of the diaphysis typically result from axial forces with a rotational component when dancers roll into or out of a fully plantarflexed foot position. Some fractures may occur after direct blows to the lateral forefoot.

Risk factors
Dancers (more than other athletes) seem particularly prone to acute fractures of the distal diaphyseal shaft of the fifth metatarsal.[51] Jones fractures typically occur among soccer, football, and basketball players, but they occur among players of many sports. Those who have lateral ankle instability are probably more prone to avulsion fractures of the base.

Clinical features
Athletes typically complain of sudden pain in the lateral forefoot after an inversion injury or a difficult landing. They will have localized tenderness over the fracture site. If there are prodromal

symptoms in the same area, a stress fracture should be considered, and treatment may be different.

Diagnosis
Standard AP, lateral, and oblique x-rays of the foot are adequate for the diagnosis of fifth metatarsal fractures **(Figures 29.18 and 29.19).** If stress fractures are suspected, additional imaging techniques may be needed. Attention to the location and type of fracture is necessary to determine treatment, especially among elite athletes.

Treatment
Avulsion fractures of the fifth metatarsal base can be treated conservatively. One study showed that treatment with a bulky dressing verses a walking short-leg cast resulted in radiographic and clinical healing in 100% of patients, but those who were treated with just the bulky dressing returned to normal activity 13 days sooner (33 versus 46 days) than those treated with casting (LOE: B).[52]

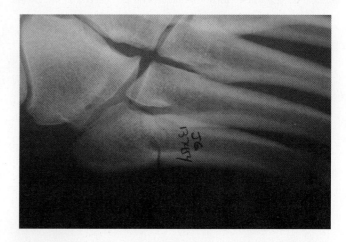

Figure 29.19 Acute Jones fracture at the diaphyseal–metaphyseal junction of the fifth metatarsal. (From DeLee JC, Drez D Jr, Miller MD [eds]: DeLee & Drez's Orthopaedic Sports Medicine: Principles and Practice, 2nd ed. Philadelphia, WB Saunders, 2003.)

Jones fractures can be treated successfully with a non–weight-bearing short-leg cast for about 6 weeks or with intramedullary screw fixation. Both methods result in high rates of healing, but the trend among athletes is surgical treatment. There is limited evidence that surgical treatment returns athletes to play faster than nonsurgical treatment: athletes miss about 6 to 8 weeks with surgical treatment as compared with about 12 weeks for nonsurgical treatment (LOE: D).[53-55] Surgical treatment among American collegiate football players was also recently shown to result in a lower rate of nonunion (7%) than that seen among those treated who were conservatively (20%) (LOE: D).[56]

Distal diaphyseal fractures can be treated symptomatically with elastic wrap, bulky dressings, hard-soled shoes (even for those with displaced fractures), or walking casts for those who need additional support. Surgical treatment does not seem to afford any advantage. In one large series, dancers returned to walking after about 6 weeks and to professional dancing after approximately 19 weeks (LOE: D).[51]

SESAMOID FRACTURES

The hallucal sesamoids are two 9- to 15-mm oval bones that are located just proximal to the volar aspect of each first metatarsal head within the substance of the collateral ligament of the metatarsophalangeal (MTP) joint and the flexor hallucis brevis tendons. They act to cushion impact to the first metatarsal head and to give a mechanical advantage to the toe flexors.

Mechanism of injury

The hallucal sesamoids are susceptible to acute injury from a direct blow or from a hard jump landing, especially among dancers.

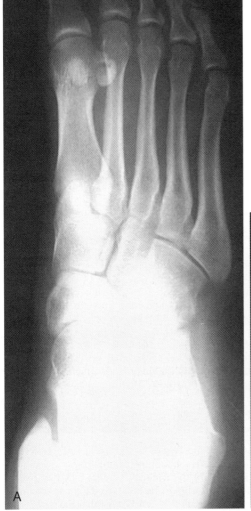
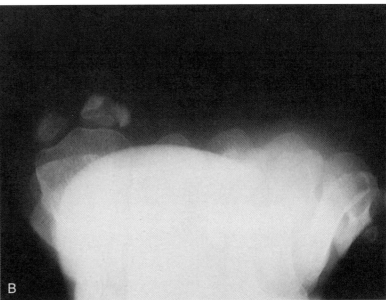

Figure 29.20   Fracture of the fibular sesamoid seen on oblique (A) and tangential (B) views. (From Browner L: Skeletal Trauma: Basic Science, Management, and Reconstruction, 3rd ed. Philadelphia, Saunders, 2003.)

Risk factors

Risk factors for sesamoid fractures include inadequate padding at the first MTP joint.

Clinical features

Athletes with an acute sesamoid fracture will usually give a history of a difficult landing or of a direct blow to the first MTP area and complain of pain during ambulation, especially during the push-off phase. Physical findings can include painful and restricted motion at the MTP joint, pain on direct palpation to the plantar aspect of the first MTP joint area, swelling in the first MTP joint, and decreased strength in plantar flexion or dorsiflexion.

Diagnosis

AP, lateral, oblique, and tangential sesamoid view x-rays should be done, but they may miss sesamoid abnormalities **(Figure 29.20)**. Furthermore, 8% to 31% of sesamoids can be bipartite, and even the acute fracture of a bipartite sesamoid may produce symptoms that are similar to those of a fractured unified sesamoid.[57] Therefore, if radiographs are negative but the area of the sesamoids is tender, bone scanning may be useful for determining whether a sesamoid injury has occurred (LOE: E).[58,59]

Treatment

Treatment for nondisplaced acute sesamoid fractures is usually successful with a short-leg walking cast with a toe plate for about 6 weeks, followed by placement in a wood-soled shoe with a pad placed proximal to the sesamoids for an additional 4 to 6 weeks (LOE: D).[60-62] Surgical excision or bone grafting of the fractured sesamoid may be considered if the fragments are displaced (LOE: E).[63,64]

FRACTURES OF THE TOES

Toe fractures are the most common acute bony injuries of the forefoot. Fortunately, their treatment is straightforward, and recovery is usually full and relatively rapid. Great toe fractures should be approached more cautiously and perhaps treated more aggressively than lesser toe factures because the great toe bears more weight than the lesser toes, and it may not heal as well with the same conservative measures, thereby resulting in chronic pain.

Mechanism of injury

Fractures of the toes can occur as a result of a direct blow (e.g., a collision with an object, such as a ball or another player) or from crush injuries (e.g., when an athlete's foot is stepped on).

Risk factors

Kicking athletes are at the most risk for collisions of the foot with objects, and ballet dancers may sustain diaphyseal fractures of the phalanges as a result of repetitive axial loading. Inadequate shoe wear may also predispose an individual to injury.

Clinical features

The fractured toes may display swelling, ecchymosis, tenderness to palpation, and deformity. Careful examination is needed to assess the amount of clinical angulation and the rotation of the toes because this is more predictive of future problems than is the appearance of the radiographs (LOE: E).

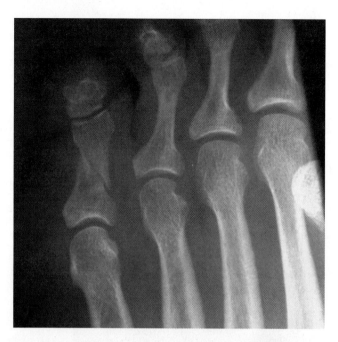

Figure 29.21 Nondisplaced fracture of the fifth proximal phalanx sustained from stubbing the toe; often called the "night walker's fracture." (From Browner L: Skeletal Trauma: Basic Science, Management, and Reconstruction, 3rd ed. Philadelphia, Saunders, 2003.)

Diagnosis

Standard AP, lateral, and oblique x-rays are sufficient for identifying fractured phalanges.

Treatment

The treatment of nondisplaced fractures **(Figure 29.21)** is successful with hard-soled shoes and protected weight bearing, as tolerated. Buddy taping of the injured toe to its adjacent toe may decrease pain by providing stabilization. Any fractures with displacement or angulation must be reduced, usually by gravity traction. After reduction, the fractured toe may then be buddy taped with a piece of soft, absorbent material between the two toes to prevent maceration. Weight bearing and return to activity are advanced as tolerated.

In addition, great toe fractures may require immobilization in a splint to maintain reduction. The restoration of axial alignment and rotation is important to avoid deformity that could result in abnormal pressure on a digital prominence. Intra-articular fractures of the great toe may also require surgical intervention to ensure optimal outcome **(Figure 29.22)**.

Surgical reduction should be considered for fractures of either the great toe or the lesser toes that display persistent clinical deformity or intra-articular discontinuity after attempts at reduction (LOE: E).

CONCLUSION

Fractures of the foot are common and are a source of potential disability to athletes. They require careful physical examination and judicious choice of the optimal imaging modality for proper diagnosis. Special care should be taken to diagnose fractures that predispose many to long-term disability or that have high rates of nonunion. Achieving anatomic alignment is paramount in nearly all of these fractures because this is often what determines the speed of healing and the risk for chronic disability.

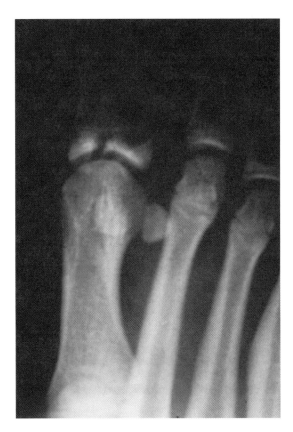

Figure 29.22 Intra-articular fracture of the first proximal phalanx. (From DeLee JC, Drez D Jr, Miller MD [eds]: DeLee & Drez's Orthopaedic Sports Medicine: Principles and Practice, 2nd ed. Philadelphia, WB Saunders, 2003.)

REFERENCES

1. Urman M, Amman W, Sisler J, et al: The role of bone scintigraphy in the evaluation of talar dome fractures. J Nucl Med 1991;32:2241-2244.
2. Loomer R, Risher C, Lloyd-Smith R, et al: Osteochondral lesions of the talus. Am J Sports Med 1993;21(1):13-19.
3. Heckman JD: Fractures of the talus. In Bucholz RW, Heckman JD (eds): Rockwood and Green's Fractures in Adults, 5th ed. Philadelphia, Lippincott Williams & Wilkins, 2002, pp 2094-2132.
4. Alexander AH, Lichtman DM: Surgical treatment of transchondral talar-dome fractures (osteochondritis dissecans): long-term follow-up. J Bone Joint Surg 1979;62A(4):646-652.
5. Canale ST, Bending RH: Osteochondral lesions of the talus. J Bone Joint Surg 1980;62A(1):97-102.
6. Pettine KA, Morrey BF: Osteochondral fractures of the talus: a long-term follow-up. J Bone Joint Surg 1987;69B(1):89-92.
7. Parisien JS: Arthroscopic treatment of osteochondral lesions of the talus. Am J Sports Med 1986;14(3):211-217.
8. VanBuecken K, Barrack RL, Alexander AH, et al: Arthroscopic treatment of transchondral talar dome fractures. Am J Sports Med 1989;17(3):350-356.
9. Funk JR, Srinivasan SC, Crandall JR: Snowboarder's talus fractures experimentally produced by eversion and dorsiflexion. Am J Sports Med 2003;31(6):921-928.
10. Ebraeim NA, Skie MC, Podeszwa DA, et al: Evaluation of process fractures of the talus using computed tomography. J Orthop Trauma 1994;8(4):332-337.
11. Mukherjee SK, Pringle RM, Baxter AD: Fracture of the lateral process of the talus: a report of thirteen cases. J Bone Joint Surg 1974;56B(2):263-273.
12. Valderrabano V, Perren T, Ryf C, et al: Snowboarder's talus fracture: treatment outcome of 20 cases after 3.5 years. Am J Sports Med 2005;33(6):871-880.
13. DiGiovanni CW, Benirschke SK, Hansen ST Jr: Foot injuries. In Browner BD, Jupiter JB, Levine AM, et al (eds): Skeletal Trauma: Basic Science, Management, and Reconstruction, 3rd ed. Philadelphia, WB Saunders, 2003, pp 2375-2492.
14. Veazey BL, Heckman JD, Galindo MJ, et al: Excision of ununited fractures of the posterior process of the talus: a treatment for chronic posterior ankle pain. Foot Ankle 1992;13(8):453-457.
15. Sopov V, Liberson A, Groshar D: Bone scintigraphic findings of os trigonum: a prospective study of 100 soldiers on active duty. Foot Ankle Int 2000;21(10):822-824.
16. Larciprete M, Guidice G, Balocco P, et al: Ankle impingement syndrome. Radiol Med (Torino) 2000;99(6):415-419.
17. Peace KA, Hillier JC, Hulme A, et al: MRI features of posterior ankle impingement syndrome in ballet dancers: a review of 25 cases. Clin Radiol 2004;59(11):1025-1033.
18. Mouhsine E, Djahangiri A, Garofalo R: Fracture of the non fused os trigonum, a rare cause of hindfoot pain. A case report and review of the literature. Chir Organi Mov 2004;89(2):171-175.
19. Wredmark T, Carlstedt CA, Bauer H, et al: Os trigonum syndrome: a clinical entity in ballet dancers. Foot Ankle 1991;11(6):404-406.
20. Ihle CL, Cochran RM: Fracture of the fused os trigonum. Am J Sports Med 1982;10(1):47-50.
21. Abramowitz Y, Wollstein R, Barzilay Y, et al: Outcome of resection of a symptomatic os trigonum. J Bone Joint Surg Am 2003;85A(6):1051-1057.
22. Fitzgibbons TC, McMullen ST, Mormino MA: Fractures and dislocations of the calcaneus. In Bucholz RW, Heckman JD (eds): Rockwood and Green's Fractures in Adults, 5th ed. Philadelphia, Lippincott Williams & Wilkins, 2002, pp 2131-2179.
23. Rammelt S, Zwipp H: Calcaneus fractures: facts, controversies and recent developments. Injury 2004;35(5):443-461.
24. Miric A, Patterson BM: Pathoanatomy of intra-articular fractures of the calcaneus. J Bone Joint Surg Am 1998;80(2):207-212.
25. Early JS: Fractures and dislocations of the midfoot and forefoot. In Bucholz RW, Heckman JD (eds): Rockwood and Green's Fractures in Adults, 5th ed. Philadelphia, Lippincott Williams & Wilkins, 2002, pp 2180-2245.
26. Miller C, Winter W, Bucknell A, et al: Injuries to the midtarsal joint and lesser tarsal bones. J Am Acad Orthop Surg 1998;6(4):249-258.
27. Sangeorzan BJ, Benirschke SK, Mosca V, et al: Displaced intra-articular fractures of the tarsal navicular. J Bone Joint Surg 1989;71A(10):1504-1510.
28. Main BJ, Jowett RL: Injuries to the midtarsal joint. J Bone Joint Surg Br 1975;57(1):89-97.
29. Sangeorzan BJ, Mayo K, Hansen S: Intraarticular fractures of the foot: talus and lesser tarsals. Clin Orthop Relat Res 1993;292:41-135.
30. Mann RA, Casillas MM, Coughlin MJ: The foot and ankle tendons. In Garrett WE, Speer KP, Kirkendall DT (eds): Principles and Practice of Orthopedic Sports Medicine. Philadelphia, Lippincott Williams & Wilkins, 2000, pp 979-1010.
31. Brigido MK, Fessell DP, Jacobson JA, et al: Radiography and US of os peroneum fractures and associated peroneal tendon injuries: initial experience. Radiology 2005;237(1):235-241.
32. Sobel M, Bohne WH, Markisz JA: Cadaver correlation of peroneal tendon changes with magnetic resonance imaging. Foot Ankle 1991;11(6):384-388.
33. Peterson D, Stinson W: Excision of the fractured os peroneum: a report of five patients and review of the literature. Foot Ankle 1992;13(5):277-281.
34. Patterson MJ, Cox WK: Peroneus longus tendon rupture as a cause of chronic lateral ankle pain. Clin Orthop Relat Res 1999;(365):163-166.
35. Bowman M: Athletic injuries of the midfoot and hindfoot. In Garrett WE, Speer KP, Kirkendall DT (eds): Principles and Practice of Orthopedic Sports Medicine. Philadelphia, Lippincott Williams & Wilkins, 2000, pp 893-943.
36. Myerson M: The diagnosis and treatment of injuries to the Lisfranc joint complex. Orthop Clin North Am 1989;20(4):655-664.
37. Shapiro MS, Wascher DC, Finerman GA: Rupture of Lisfranc's ligament in athletes. Am J Sports Med 1994;22(5):687-691.
38. Foster SC, Foster RR: Lisfranc's tarsometatarsal fracture dislocation. Radiology 1976;120:79-83.
39. Brown DD, Gumbs RV: Lisfranc fracture-dislocations: report of two cases. J Natl Med Assoc 1991;83(4):366-369.
40. Faciszewski T, Burks RT, Manaster BJ: Subtle injuries of the Lisfranc joint. J Bone Joint Surg Am 1990;72(10):1519-1522.
41. Preidler KW, Peicha G, Lajtai G, et al: Conventional radiography, CT, and MR imaging in patients with hyperflexion injuries of the foot: diagnostic accuracy in the detection of bony and ligamentous changes. Am J Roentgenol 1999;173(6):1673-1677.
42. Peicha G, Preidler KW, Lajtai G, et al: Diagnostic value of conventional roentgen image, computerized and magnetic resonance tomography in acute sprains of the foot. A prospective clinical study. Unfallchirurg 2001;104(12):1134-1139.
43. Myerson MS, Fisher RT, Burgess AR, et al: Fracture dislocations of the tarsometatarsal joints: end results correlated with pathology and treatment. Foot Ankle 1986;6(5):225-242.
44. Kuo RS, Tejwani NC, Digiovanni CW, et al: Outcome after open reduction and internal fixation of Lisfranc joint injuries. J Bone Joint Surg Am 2000;82-A(11):1609-1618.
45. Arntz CT, Veith RG, Hansen ST Jr: Fractures and fracture-dislocations of the tarsometatarsal joint. J Bone Joint Surg Am 1988;70(2):173-178.
46. Arntz CT, Hansen ST Jr: Dislocations and fracture dislocations of the tarsometatarsal joints. Orthop Clin North Am 1987;18(1):105-114.
47. Curtis MJ, Myerson M, Szura B: Tarsometatarsal joint injuries in the athlete. Am J Sports Med 1993;21(4):497-502.
48. Meyer SA, Callaghan JJ, Albright J, et al: Midfoot sprains in collegiate football players. Am J Sports Med 1994;22(3):392-401.

49. Shereff M: Fractures of the forefoot. Instr Course Lect 1990;39:133-140.

50. Alelpuz E, Carsi V, Alcantara P, et al: Fractures of the central metatarsal. Foot Ankle Int 1996;17(4):200-203.

51. O'Malley MJ, Hamilton WG, Munyak J: Fractures of the distal shaft of the fifth metatarsal. "Dancer's fracture." Am J Sports Med 1996;24(2):240-243.

52. Wiener B, Linder J, Giattini J: Treatment of fractures of the fifth metatarsal: a prospective study. Foot Ankle Int 1997;18(5):267-269.

53. Konkel KF, Menger AG, Retzlaff SA: Nonoperative treatment of fifth metatarsal fractures in an orthopaedic suburban primate multispeciality practice. Foot Ankle Int 2005;26(9):704-707.

54. Portland G, Kelikian A, Kodros S: Acute surgical management of Jones' fractures. Foot Ankle Int 2003;24(11):829-833.

55. Wright RW, Fischer DA, Shively RA, et al: Refracture of proximal fifth metatarsal (Jones) fracture after intramedullary screw fixation in athletes. Am J Sports Med 2000;28(5):732-736.

56. Low K, Noblin JD, Browne JE, et al: Jones fractures in the elite football player. J Surg Orthop Adv 2004;13(3):156-160.

57. Coughlin MJ: Conditions of the forefoot. In DeLee JC, Drez D Jr, Miller MD (eds): DeLee & Drez's Orthopaedic Sports Medicine, 2nd. Philadelphia, WB Saunders, 2003, pp 2483-2587.

58. Beidert R, Hintermann B: Stress fractures of the medial great toe sesamoids in athletes. Foot Ankle Int 2003;24(2):137-141.

59. Beidert R: Which investigations are required in stress fracture of the great toe sesamoids? Arch Orthop Trauma Surg 1993;112(2):94-95.

60. Mouhsine E, Leyvraz PF, Borens O, et al: Acute fractures of medial and lateral great toe sesamoids in an athlete. Knee Surg Sports Traumatol Arthrosc 2004;12(5):463-464.

61. Mittlmeier T, Haar P: Sesamoid and toe fractures. Injury 2004;35(suppl 2):SB87-SB97.

62. Hobart MH: Fracture of sesamoid bones of the foot. J Bone Joint Surg 1929;11:298-302.

63. Richardson EG: Injuries to the hallucal sesamoids in the athlete. Foot Ankle 1987;7(4):229-244.

64. Anderson R, McBryde A: Autogenous bone grafting of hallux sesamoid nonunions. Foot Ankle Int 1997;18(5):293-296.

CHAPTER **30**

Foot and Ankle Soft-Tissue Injuries

Ahmed A. Radwan, MD; Peter H. Seidenberg, MD, FAAFP; and Greg Dammann, MD

KEY POINTS

- Tenderness over the medial ankle, especially with an acute presentation (less than 24 hours from injury), mandates careful attention to rule out other associated injuries.

- Partial or complete rupture of the posterior tibialis tendon as a result of trauma has distinct pain at the navicular tuberosity in approximately 50% of cases. Overuse injuries with tendon degeneration present with pain just distal to the medial malleolus

- Achilles tendinosis and insertional Achilles enthesopathy are two separate entities and should be treated as such. An eccentric exercise program has a 90% or more improvement rate in cases of chronic Achilles tendinosis but less than 50% success for patients with insertional enthesopathy.

- Anterolateral ankle impingement is caused by an impingement of a distal fascicle of the anterior inferior tibiofibular ligament or a meniscoid lesion of the anterior lateral ankle against the talar dome in ankle dorsiflexion. By contrast, anterior ankle impingement is caused by a bony impingement of the anterior tibial osteophytes on the talar neck.

INTRODUCTION

Foot and ankle injuries are the most common injuries sustained by athletes and seen by sports medicine physicians. Studies of sports-related injuries in running and jumping sports have suggested an incidence of injury of 10% to 15% for the ankle and of 3% to 15% for the foot.[1]

Ankle sprains are the most common injuries in sports, with a high prevalence among participants in basketball, soccer, cross-country, dance, and ballet.[1] Each year, an estimated 1 million people present to physicians with acute ankle injuries.[2] At least 40% of ankle sprains have the potential to cause chronic problems as a result of inadequate rehabilitation and the missed diagnosis of concomitant insults.[3] Injury is either the result of extremes of functional motion beyond normal limits or forced motion in a plane that is unintended for joint function. A schematic drawing of the ankle ligaments is shown in **Figure 30.1.**

ANKLE SPRAINS

Lateral ankle sprain

The lateral ligaments are the most commonly injured, accounting for 85% of ankle sprains. The anterior talofibular ligament is considered the weakest lateral ankle ligament, with isolated testing of the individual ligaments demonstrating that it is the first to fail, followed by the calcaneofibular ligament (LOE: B).[4-7]

Mechanism of injury

Landing on an inverted and plantarflexed ankle is the mechanism of injury for lateral ankle sprain. With plantar flexion, the wider anterior part of the talus rotates downward, bringing the narrower, less stabilizing posterior portion into the tibiofemoral mortis. Furthermore, with plantarflexion, the anterior talofibular ligament becomes taut and longitudinally oriented, thereby acting as a collateral ligament or the lateral static stabilizer of the ankle against an inversion force. By contrast, dorsiflexion causes the calcaneofibular ligament to become taut and longitudinally oriented, but it also moves the wider anterior part of the talus into the mortise, thus giving the ankle more bony support. Hence, isolated injury to the calcaneofibular ligament is uncommon **(Figure 30.2).**

Depending on the force, the ligament will partially or completely tear. Typically, the ligaments will tear in the mid substance, although occasionally an avulsion of the tip of the lateral malleolus will occur. A large fragment of lateral malleolus may fracture if the bones are brittle (e.g., in older individuals or those with metabolic disorders). If the inversion force continues, the talus is pushed under the short medial malleolus, thereby opening up the lateral side of the ankle and causing more extensive damage to the lateral ligaments. It may even cause compression injury to the medial malleolus and result in a fracture that typically extends from the lateral margin of the medial malleolus vertically up the shaft of the tibia.

Clinical features

Pain, swelling, and the inability to bear weight comfortably are the presenting symptoms. Careful palpation over individual ligaments will help isolate the ligaments that are injured. The anterior drawer test assesses the integrity of the anterior talofibular ligament. This test may be falsely negative within 48 hours of injury as a result of pain and guarding; it is most sensitive when it is

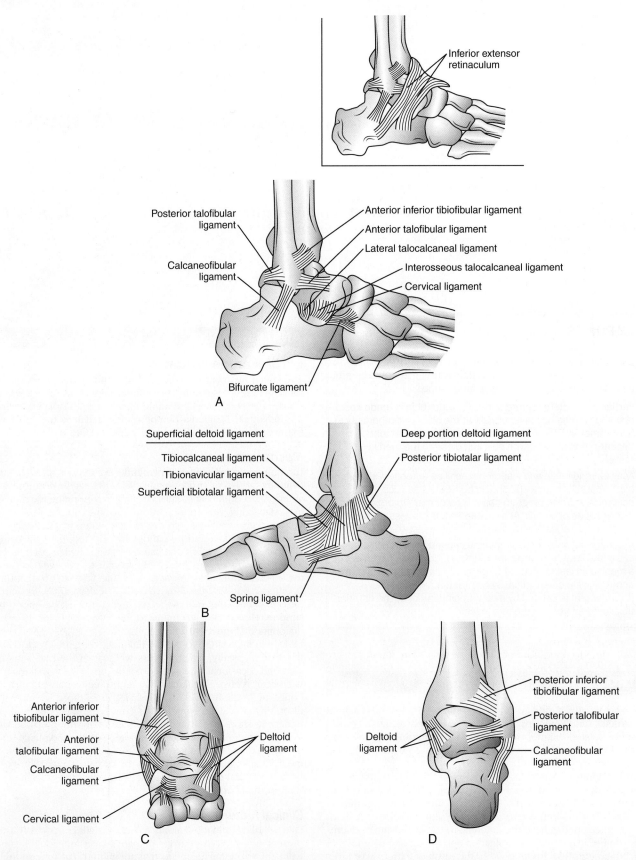

Figure 30.1 Compendium of the foot and ankle ligaments. *A*, Lateral view of the foot and ankle. *B*, Medial view of the foot and ankle. *C*, Anterior view of the ankle and hindfoot. *D*, Posterior view of the ankle and hindfoot. (From DeLee JC, Drez D Jr, Miller MD [eds]: DeLee and Drez's Orthopedic Sports Medicine: Principles and Practice, 2nd ed. Philadelphia, WB Saunders, 2002.)

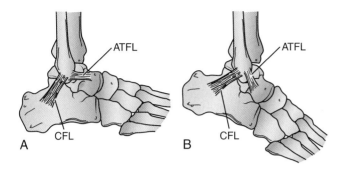

Figure 30.2 *A,* In the dorsiflexed position, the ankle is relatively stable: The wide anterior talus stabilizes the ankle joint and the calcaneofibular ligament (CFL) is oriented longitudinally. *B,* In plantar flexion, the ankle is less stable because the narrower posterior talus is engaged in the tibiofibular plaford and the weaker anterior talofibular ligament (ATFL) assures a longitudinal, stabilizing position. (From DeLee JC, Drez D Jr, Miller MD [eds]: DeLee and Drez's Orthopedic Sports Medicine: Principles and Practice, 2nd ed. Philadelphia, WB Saunders, 2002.)

performed 4 to 5 days after injury (LOE: B).[8,9] The talar tilt (inversion stress), when performed with the ankle in plantarflexion, can also be used to assess the anterior talofibular ligament. When performed with the ankle in neutral flexion, it is used to assess the integrity of the calcaneofibular ligament.

Diagnosis
The diagnosis of lateral ankle sprain is a clinical diagnosis. Careful examination should help with the assessment of the grade of ligament injury; the need for imaging is explained below.

Grades of ligamentous injury Ligament injuries, as suggested by the American Medical Association, are graded on the basis of stretch, partial tear, or complete rupture of the ligament[10]:

- Grade I: Mild, minor tearing of the ligament fibers and no demonstrable increase in translation on examination.
- Grade II: Moderate, partial tearing of the ligament without complete disruption and with slight to moderate increased translation on examination.
- Grade III: Severe, complete tearing of the ligament, with a marked increase in translation on examination.

Imaging
The Ottawa ankle rules are used to determine when radiographic studies are indicated for the adult patient with ankle trauma (LOE: B).[11] For a more complete discussion of the Ottawa ankle rules, see Chapter 28, Ankle Fractures, and Chapter 31A, Treatment of Common Pediatric and Adolescent Injuries. Stress radiographs can help document lateral ligamentous ankle injuries, but they are not required to make the diagnosis of an acute ankle sprain. Talar tilt stress radiographs and anterior drawer stress radiographs are primarily used to document mechanical instability as a cause of chronic lateral ankle instability.[12]

Magnetic resonance imaging (MRI) is not required for acute ankle sprains. However, MRI should be considered for patients who present with chronic ankle pain or persistent ankle symptoms 6 weeks after injury and appropriate rehabilitation.[12]

Treatment
The management of all lateral sprains is conservative, with protection, rest, ice, compression, and elevation (PRICE) followed by a functional ankle rehabilitation protocol (as outlined in the next section). Recovery time varies with the grade of the injury.

Grade I takes from 1 to 3, whereas grade II usually requires 2 to 4 weeks.

For a grade III sprain, a fracture boot or a short-leg cast is often used for the first 5 to 7 days, with crutches being used until full weight bearing is tolerated. Often this immobilization eliminates the need for crutches and allows the patient to do weight-bearing activities of daily living comfortably.[13] Functional treatment with early mobilization is the currently the favored rehabilitative method. By minimizing immobilization, the recovery period may be shortened (LOE: B).[14] A semirigid pneumatic or lace-up ankle brace is used throughout the rehabilitation period. Return to play can occur after 5 to 8 weeks with optimal rehabilitation.

Functional treatment has the same outcomes as primary surgical repair. If conservative, nonoperative management fails, the athlete can still be treated effectively with delayed reconstruction (LOE: B).[8,15]

Initial management (PRICEMM)
Pain and swelling are the immediate tissue response to an injury. Initial management aims at controlling those body responses to limit the extent of damage and to protect the ankle from further reinjury.

Protection Removable devices facilitate rehabilitation and cryotherapy. An air-filled or gel-filled ankle brace that restricts inversion–eversion and allows limited plantarflexion–dorsiflexion or a simple plaster posterior splint can be used for immobilization. Circumferential casting generally is not recommended.[16]

Rest The athlete should refrain from any activity that exacerbates the pain. An initial period of complete rest may be required. The use of two properly fitted crutches may be considered during the immediate period after injury until the patient is able to achieve pain-free weight bearing.[13]

If the main complaint is pain with the regular exercise program of the athlete (e.g., running at a certain distance and pace), relative rest may be advised by decreasing duration and intensity to a pain-free limit with a gradual functional progression.

Ice Different methods of cryotherapy can be used: crushed ice in a plastic bag, commercially available cold applications, or foot and ankle immersion in water at a temperature of approximately 12.7°C (55°F). Ice should be used immediately after the injury for approximately 20 minutes, this should be repeated every 2 to 3 hours for the first 48 hours or until edema and inflammation have stabilized. Heat should not be applied to an acutely injured ankle joint because it encourages swelling and inflammation through hyperemia. While cold therapy is being used, exercises should be initiated to maintain the range of motion and to assist with lymphatic drainage.[13]

Compression Because increased swelling is directly associated with a loss of range of motion in the ankle joint, the initial goals are to prevent swelling and maintain range of motion. To milk edema fluid away from the injured tissues, the ankle should be wrapped with an elastic bandage. The bandaging should start just proximal to the toes and extend above the level of maximal calf circumference. A U-shaped felt pad applied around the lateral malleolus further helps compress an area that is prone to increased swelling.[13]

Elevation The injured extremity should be elevated 15 to 25 cm (6 to 10 inches) above the level of the heart to facilitate venous and lymphatic drainage until the swelling has begun to resolve.[16]

Medications Nonsteroidal anti-inflammatory drugs (NSAIDs), cyclo-oxygenase-2 inhibitors, acetaminophen, and/or other analgesics are commonly employed. Generally, NSAIDs are preferable to narcotics for pain relief.

Modalities Ultrasound, ice massage, electrical stimulation, and iontophoresis may assist with pain control. No definitive evidence suggests that these modalities speed or improve ligamentous healing.

Functional rehabilitation

Functional rehabilitation begins on the day of injury and continues until pain-free gait and activity are attained. Prolonged immobilization and avoidance of weight bearing are common treatment errors that should be avoided (LOE: A).[17,18] Functional stresses stimulate the incorporation of stronger replacement collagen and help to correctly orient the repaired collagen fibers.[18] A prerequisite to the institution of functional rehabilitation is ankle joint stability. Because grade I and II sprains are considered stable, functional rehabilitation can begin immediately.[13] The four components of the program are range-of-motion rehabilitation, progressive muscle-strengthening exercises, proprioceptive training, and activity-specific training.

Range of motion must be regained before functional rehabilitation is initiated. Regardless of weight-bearing capacity, Achilles tendon stretching should be instituted within 48 to 72 hours after the ankle injury because of the tendency of the surrounding muscular tissues to contract after trauma.[13] Achilles tendon stretching can be done without weight bearing using a towel to pull the toes and foot toward the face and with weight bearing by standing with the heel on the floor and bending at the knees. Perform pain-free stretches for 15 to 30 seconds, complete five repetitions, and repeat the process three to five times a day. Moving the ankle in multiple planes of motion by drawing the letters of the alphabet with the foot four to five times a day may also be helpful.[13]

Progression to the strengthening phase begins after range of motion is attained and swelling and pain are controlled. The strengthening of weakened muscles (especially the peroneals with a lateral injury) is essential to rapid recovery and important for preventing reinjury (LOE: B).[18,19]

Strengthening begins with isometric exercises performed against an immovable object in each of the four directions of ankle movement: plantarflexion, dorsiflexion, eversion, and inversion. The patient then progresses to dynamic resistive exercises using ankle weights, resistance bands, or elastic tubing. Strengthening exercises should only be done in positions that do not cause pain. Resistance for the isometric exercises can be provided by an immovable object (wall or floor) or the contralateral foot. For each exercise, hold the position for 5 seconds, do 10 repetitions, and repeat the process three times a day. The contralateral foot, rubber tubing, or weights can provide resistance for isotonic exercises. For each exercise, hold the concentric component for 1 second and the eccentric component for 4 seconds; this should be performed slowly and under control. Do three sets of 10 repetitions, and repeat the process two times a day (LOE: B).[20]

For toe curls and marble pickups, place the foot on a towel and then curl the toes, moving the towel toward the body. Use the toes to pick up marbles or other small objects. Perform two sets of ten repetitions, and repeat the process two times a day.

Strengthening can also occur from using the body as resistance through weight bearing. For toe raises, heel walks, and toe walks, perform three sets of ten repetitions; repeat the process two times a day, and progress walking as tolerated.[13]

As the patient achieves full weight bearing without pain, proprioceptive training is initiated for the recovery of balance and postural control. Inadequate proprioceptive rehabilitation is one of the most common treatment errors when working with lateral ankle sprains, and it may predispose the patient to repeat injury. Various devices are used in concert with a series of progressive drills to return patients to a high functional level.

The simplest device for proprioceptive training is the wobble board. It is a small discoid platform that is attached to a hemispheric base. With the patient sitting, have him or her rotate the board clockwise and then counterclockwise using one foot and then both feet. With the patient in the standing position, instruct him or her to rotate the board using one leg and then both legs. Have the patient do five to ten repetitions and repeat the exercises two times a day. Advance to different heights, add resistance, and have the patient train with the eyes closed (LOE: B).[21]

Another method to try is having the patient walk on different surfaces. Have him or her walk in normal, heel-to-toe fashion over various surfaces. Progress from hard, flat floors to uneven surfaces, and have the patient walk 50 feet two times a day. Walking exercises can be performed with the eyes open or closed and with or without resistance.[13]

Training for return to activity

When the previous ambulation is no longer limited by pain, the patient may progress to a regimen of 50% walking and 50% jogging. When this can be done without pain, jogging eventually progresses to forward, backward, and pattern running. Circles and figure eights are commonly employed for pattern running. These routines are the final phase of ankle joint rehabilitation.

The completion of the program is essential for the recovery of ankle stability. A patient who will be returning to sports participation may require additional athletic therapy. This sport-specific component of the rehabilitation process should be supervised by a certified athletic trainer or a sports physical therapist who is familiar with the physical demands of the athlete's specific sport and position. Using taping or bracing with subsequent weaning may be recommended during the early period of activity-specific training.[13]

Medial ankle sprain

Deltoid (medial) ligament tears are not as common and routine as injuries to the lateral ankle. The force required to tear the deltoid ligament is much greater than that required to injure the relatively weaker lateral structures. These increased forces can also cause injuries that require operative intervention, such as Maisonneuve fracture, severe syndesmosis injury, distal fibular fracture, and avulsion fracture of the medial malleolus.

Mechanism of injury

Medial ankle injuries can occur during eversion. A common example is a basketball player landing awkwardly on the ankle after a dunk.

Diagnosis

Pain and swelling are the presenting symptoms. Deltoid ligament injuries display tenderness to palpation over the deltoid ligament and/or laxity on eversion stress testing (reverse talar tilt).[22] Tenderness over the medial ankle, especially with an acute presentation (<24 hours from injury), mandates careful attention to rule out other associated injuries as described previously. Isolated deltoid sprains (without other associated injuries) can be treated in a way that is similar to inversion sprains, with the exception that rehabilitation tends to be more prolonged.

Treatment

The treatment of grade I and II medial ankle sprains is functional ankle rehabilitation as previously described. The treatment of grade III injury requires initial non—weight-bearing immobilization using a fracture boot or a short-leg cast. After the acute pain and swelling remit (usually within 48 hours), weight bearing to tolerance is encouraged. Immobilization (typically for 3 to 5 weeks) is continued until swelling, tenderness, and instability have resolved. A comprehensive ankle rehabilitation program is used along with a semirigid pneumatic orthosis for up to 6 months from the date of injury (LOE: B).[23,24]

Syndesmotic sprain (high ankle sprain)

Syndesmotic injury accounts for 1% to 11% of all ankle sprains, with higher incidence among players of contact sports. Unlike the lateral sprain, this injury is associated with little swelling and less chance of recurrence.

Mechanism of injury

The mechanism of syndesmosis sprain is typically ankle external rotation with hyperdorsiflexion (i.e., being tackled or twisted down by the ankle).[8]

Clinical features

Patients typically have tenderness over the anterior inferior tibiofibular ligament and proximally along the interosseous membrane.

Diagnosis

The external rotation stress test and the squeeze test are used to assess the injury. When the squeeze test is performed closer to the knee and pain is still elicited in the syndesmosis, this indicates a more severe injury that will take longer to heal and that should make the examiner suspicious of a Maisonneuve fracture.[22]

Treatment

Grade I high ankle sprains are managed with the functional ankle rehabilitation protocol. Immobilization with a long, semirigid pneumatic stirrup brace that extends to just below the knee can be beneficial. Protected weight bearing may be necessary for up to 3 weeks. Grade II syndesmosis injuries are also managed nonoperatively. Weight bearing is restricted longer than with a grade I injury, with 3 to 6 weeks of no weight bearing currently being recommended. Grade III sprains have radiographic evidence of syndesmosis widening. With or without fracture, Grade III syndesmotic sprains are treated surgically (LOE: B).[22,25] For further discussion of high-grade syndesmotic injury, see Chapter 28, Ankle Fractures.

Sinus tarsi syndrome and subtalar joint sprains

Sinus tarsi syndrome is a condition that is characterized by persistent pain in the lateral ankle area and by instability of the rear foot. There is usually a history of severe or recurrent inversion sprains. The sinus tarsi is a funnel-shaped cavity located between the anterosuperior surface of the calcaneus and the inferior aspect of the neck of the talus. It opens laterally anterior to the lateral malleolus, and it terminates medially with a small opening posterior to the sustentaculum tali. The ligamentous structures within the tarsal canal include the inferior attachment of the extensor retinaculum of the foot, the interosseous talocalcaneal ligament, and the cervical ligament (see Figure 30.1).

Mechanism of injury

The tarsal canal ligaments maintain alignment between the talus and calcaneus, and they limit inversion. With inversion trauma, the ligaments are usually injured in the following order: anterior talofibular ligament, calcaneofibular ligament, cervical ligament, and interosseous talocalcaneal ligament. The more severe the injury incurred, the more of these ligaments are injured. Thus, tarsal canal ligament injury does not occur as an isolated lesion; rather,

it will also involve the rupture of the calcaneofibular ligament and/or the anterior talofibular ligament.[26]

Other causative factors include hypertrophy of the synovial membrane as a result of a pinching and compressive situation from lateral ankle sprains, ganglion cysts, entrapment of the superficial peroneal nerve, and exostosis associated with degenerative joint disease (LOE: E).[27]

Clinical features

Patients present with pain over the lateral sinus tarsi opening that is aggravated by weight-bearing activity and improved with rest. A perception of instability of the rear foot over uneven surfaces is a common complaint. Physical examination reveals tenderness to the palpation of the sinus tarsi, with worsening on foot inversion and eversion. Laxity and instability of the ankle and foot joints may be present as well.

Diagnosis

The diagnosis of sinus tarsi syndrome is usually made clinically, and it is confirmed by symptomatic relief after an injection of 2 to 3 mL of local anesthetic into the tarsal canal (see Chapter 48, Therapeutic and Diagnostic Injections and Aspirations, for more details about sinus tarsi injections). Radiographs can help rule out associated pathology (e.g., arthritis, fracture, and instability). MRI can best demonstrate changes in the sinus tarsi that result from inflammation or scar tissue from previous injury. Ankle arthroscopy may also be beneficial for direct visualization (LOE: B).[28]

Treatment

Conservative treatment has been quite successful. It includes NSAIDs, stable shoes, immobilization, ankle sleeves, and over-the-counter orthoses. Resistant cases have been treated with a course of oral steroids, a series of steroid injections, physical therapy, or custom orthoses. Sinus tarsectomy should be considered if conservative treatment is not effective (LOE: B).[29]

Bifurcate ligament sprains

Bifurcate ligament sprains are reported in 18.6% of ankle inversion injuries.[30]

Mechanism of injury

Because the bifurcate ligament is taut with plantarflexion and inversion, injury to it usually occurs with violent dorsiflexion, forceful plantarflexion, or direct trauma. This mechanism can also avulse the anterior process of the calcaneus.

Clinical features

Patients present with lateral midfoot pain and swelling, usually after an ankle injury.

Diagnosis

A bifurcate sprain is often mistaken for a lateral ankle sprain because of the proximity to the lateral malleolus. In contrast with anterior talofibular ligament injury, the point of maximal tenderness in bifurcate sprains is found midway on a line that connects the tuberosity of the fifth metatarsal and the distal tip of the lateral malleolus. Pain may be elicited at this site with simultaneous forefoot supination and plantar flexion (Figure 30.3).

Treatment

Acute injuries are treated with PRICEMM (as described previously for lateral ankle sprains), which is followed by gentle range-of-motion exercises. Weight bearing should be protected with taping, a splint, a removable walking cast, or a functional ankle brace for 6 to 8 weeks after injury.[8]

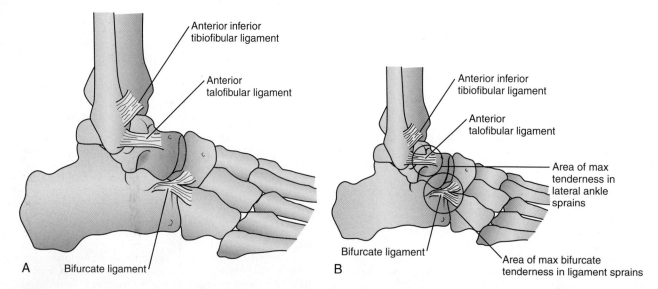

Figure 30.3 *A*, A schematic drawing demonstrating the bifurcate ligament. *B*, Bifurcate ligament sprains present with maximal tenderness to palpation midway between the distal fibula and the fifth metatarsal base. This is distinct from the area of maximal tenderness in lateral ankle sprains surrounding the anterior talofibular ligament. (From DeLee JC, Drez D Jr, Miller MD [eds]: DeLee and Drez's Orthopedic Sports Medicine: Principles and Practice, 2nd ed. Philadelphia, WB Saunders, 2002.)

ANKLE IMPINGEMENT SYNDROMES

Chronic anterolateral ankle impingement

Chronic anterolateral ankle impingement after inversion ankle injury is a well-recognized entity.

Mechanism of injury

Pain results from the impingement of a distal fascicle of the anterior inferior tibiofibular ligament or a meniscoid lesion of the anterior lateral ankle against the talar dome during ankle dorsiflexion.

Clinical features

Patients will describe multiple inversion injuries, and they will have pain at the anterior aspect of the lateral malleolus and an intermittent catching sensation.

Diagnosis

Tenderness is felt by the patient over the lateral gutter and anterolateral talus. A standing impingement test is performed by asking the patient to dorsiflex the ankle maximally while keeping the heel in contact with the ground. The angle formed by the back of the leg and the floor is measured with a goniometer. A difference between the sides of 5 degrees or more suggests impingement (LOE: B).[31]

Treatment

An aggressive 6-week course of physical therapy and bracing to eliminate subtle instability is the first step in treatment. Oral anti-inflammatories and cortisone injection may also be used (see Chapter 48, Therapeutic and Diagnostic Injections and Aspirations). Patients for whom conservative management is ineffective are treated with ankle arthroscopy and the debridement of the anterolateral meniscoid lesion, if one is present.[32]

Anterior ankle impingement

By contrast, anterior ankle impingement is caused by a bony impingement of anterior tibial osteophytes on the talar neck rather than soft-tissue impingement. It is thought to result from multiple episodes of dorsiflexion,[33] typically among football players and dancers.[34]

Clinical features

Patients complain of anterior ankle pain with a feeling of blocking on dorsiflexion. As the impingement develops, the patient complains of ankle stiffness and a loss of takeoff speed.

Diagnosis

On examination, there is restricted and painful dorsiflexion and occasionally palpable soft-tissue swelling.[31] A plain lateral x-ray showing less than 60 degrees between osteophytes and the talar neck will confirm the diagnosis.

Treatment

Most patients respond to conservative management with standard ankle rehabilitation. In resistant cases, arthroscopic resection of the osseous spurs has excellent results (LOE: B).[31]

Posterior soft-tissue impingement

Posterior soft-tissue impingement results from the compression of the posterior ankle soft tissues against the posterior tibia when the ankle is in plantar flexion. Several bony processes can produce this compression against the tibia, including the posterior process of the calcaneus, the posterolateral process of the talus, or an os trigonum (os trigonum syndrome[23]).

Mechanism of injury

The syndrome usually arises insidiously in predisposed athletes participating in activities that require repetitive forced plantarflexion. Ballet dancers are especially prone to this injury.

Clinical features

Patients complain of posterior ankle pain that is exacerbated by plantarflexion or dorsiflexion.

Diagnosis

On examination, there is posterior tenderness anterior to and not involving the Achilles tendon that is exacerbated by plantarflexion or dorsiflexion.[35] Occasionally, there is palpable soft-tissue thickening. Lateral radiography may show an ossicle or a small avulsion. MRI may identify hypertrophic lesions or soft-tissue edema.

Treatment
Conservative treatment includes physical therapy, NSAIDs, injection, and bracing. Patients for whom conservative treatment is ineffective may benefit from surgical debridement.[36]

PLANTAR FASCIITIS

Plantar fasciitis is the most common cause of heel pain among adults. The plantar fascia is a thickened fibrous aponeurosis that originates from the medial tubercle of the calcaneus and that runs forward to form the longitudinal foot arch. The function of the plantar fascia is to provide static support of the longitudinal arch and dynamic shock absorption.

Mechanism of injury
The underlying pathology of plantar fasciitis is collagen degeneration caused by repetitive microtears that overcome the body's ability to repair itself.[37] It is important to remember that, despite the -itis suffix, there is little to no acute inflammation associated with plantar fasciitis.

Patients with flat feet or high arches are at increased risk for developing planter fasciitis. Flatfoot deformity will place an increased strain on the origin of the plantar fascia at the calcaneus as the plantar fascia attempts to maintain a stable arch during the propulsive phase of the gait. With the pes cavus deformity, excessive strain results from the inability of the foot to pronate to adapt itself to the ground. Other structural risk factors may include overpronation, leg-length discrepancy, lateral tibial torsion, and femoral anteversion. Functional risk factors include inflexibility and weakness in the gastrocnemius, the soleus, the Achilles tendon, and the intrinsic foot muscles.[37]

Clinical features
Patients complain of heel pain when taking the first few steps in the morning or when arising after prolonged sitting. The symptoms typically lessen as walking continues. The point of maximal tenderness is at the medial tubercle at the plantar aspect of the calcaneus. Tenderness along the proximal plantar fascia may be present as well. The pain may be exacerbated by passive dorsiflexion of the toes or by having the patient stand on the tips of the toes.

Diagnosis
The diagnosis is usually made clinically. Radiographs are only necessary if another abnormality (e.g., fracture, tumor, or rheumatoid arthritis) is suspected. Heel spurs are often visualized on the plantar aspect of the anterior calcaneus on lateral radiographs. Although patients may become fixated on removal or other treatments for these "heel spurs", physicians should reassure them that heel spurs are present in 15% to 25% of the asymptomatic general population and that many patients with severe plantar fasciitis pain have no spurs on x-ray. Clearly then, plantar-plane calcaneal spurs do not cause plantar fascia pain, and their removal is not necessary for pain relief (LOE: B).[38]

The differential diagnosis of plantar fasciitis is broad. It may include calcaneal stress fracture, bursitis of the plantar heel, and tarsal tunnel syndrome. Entrapment of the posterior tibial, medial plantar, or lateral plantar nerve can cause symptoms that mimic those of plantar fasciitis.

Treatment
Successful treatment depends on a correct understanding of the underlying pathogenesis of plantar fasciitis. As previously mentioned, collagen degradation in the plantar fascia typically begins as an effect of chronic overuse injury. This injury is most commonly the result of a tight and/or weak Achilles/gastrocnemius/soleus muscle tendon unit. If the gastrocnemius/soleus muscles are insufficiently flexible or unable to absorb the force of recurrent ground impact, the plantar fascia will be injured, and the process of plantar fasciosis begins (see Chapter 6, Victim or Culprit: A Pathoanatomic Approach to the Correct Diagnosis, for further discussion). First-line treatments for plantar fasciitis include correcting the intrinsic and extrinsic risk factors associated with this injury. This usually requires relative rest (running at 30% to 50% of the previous level), ice and ice massage (especially after activities), and the correction of biomechanical factors with new, appropriate footwear (first line), a stretching and strengthening program (first line), and, finally, orthotics, if necessary (second line). **Table 30.1** reviews common therapies for plantar fasciitis.

Frequently used stretching techniques for improving gastrocnemius/soleus flexibility include wall stretches and curb or stair stretches **(Figure 30.4)**. Dynamic stretches such as towel stretching and rolling the foot arch over a 15-oz–sized can or a tennis ball are also useful. Strengthening exercises for the intrinsic foot muscles improve longitudinal arch support and provide dynamic shock absorption. A simple, low-cost exercise program is outlined in **Figure 30.5** and Box 30.2. Patients should be warned at the outset that the processes that resulted in their plantar fasciitis pain took months and years to develop. Correcting these forces through stretching, strengthening, and even orthotics will reliably improve symptoms, but only over a time course of weeks to months.

Orthotics and night splints can be used if the patient does not improve with 4 to 6 weeks of stretching and strengthening. Corticosteroid injection is usually a second- or third-line treatment because it does nothing to address the underlying forces and that factors that resulted in the pain and because of the potential risks, including rupture of the plantar fascia and fat pad atrophy (LOE B).[39] Surgery is uncommon, and it is only indicated for a few patients for whom the prolonged use of conservative measures (>6 to 12 months) has failed.

INSERTIONAL ACHILLES PAIN

Insertional Achilles pain includes retrocalcaneal bursitis, adventitial Achilles bursitis, insertional Achilles enthesopathy, and Haglund's deformity.

Pain in the area of the calcaneal insertion of the Achilles is occasionally difficult to diagnose accurately, and it is also often difficult to treat. Four distinct anatomic structures can each be the source of pain in this region. Hence, a precise and accurate diagnosis is paramount because the first step in proper treatment is correctly identifying the offending tissue(s) **(Figure 30.6)**. Identifying the offending tissue or tissues can typically be done with a careful physical examination. However, MRI may also provide definitive evidence of which tissues are involved.

Each of these different entities will briefly be described. However, the clinician should be aware that cases of insertional Achilles pain will commonly involve more than a single entity.

Retrocalcaneal bursitis
Mechanism of injury
Retrocalcaneal bursitis is an overuse injury that is aggravated by pressure and that commonly occurs among athletes wearing overly tight-fitting shoes. In some cases, retrocalcaneal bursitis

Table 30.1 Common Treatments for Plantar Fasciitis

Stretching the Gastrocnemius and Soleus Muscles

See Figure 30.4

A must for prolonged symptom relief

Strengthening the Calf and Foot Intrinsics

Can use barefoot walking, heel raises, or towel drag exercises (see Figure 30.6)

A must for prolonged symptom relief because strong muscles help absorb the forces that would otherwise reinjure the healing plantar fascia

Ice

Simply cannot have too much of this good thing

Use of ice four times daily for a minimum of 15 minutes each time is preferred

Has been shown in studies and clinical practice to be better than nonsteroidal anti-inflammatory drugs for pain control, with no side effects

Orthotics and Night Splints

Second-line interventions for those patients for whom previous treatments are ineffective

Off-the-shelf orthoses used for first-time sufferers, custom orthotics for those with recurring problems

Night splints proven in multiple studies to be very helpful for morning pain

Commercially made night splints have fallen dramatically in price over the past few years and are now quite affordable

Nonsteroidal Anti-inflammatory Drugs

Used for pain control only

Best used only for short courses (<2 weeks)

Steroid Injection

Used for pain control only

Third-line therapy

Insert the needle through the lateral heel (not the plantar heel); do not inject into the fat pad (see Chapter 48, Therapeutic and Diagnostic Injections and Aspirations, for a review of the technique)

Extracorporeal Shockwave Lithotripsy

A modality that is in search of an orthopedic indication

Studies done so far only in recalcitrant, recurrent fasciitis; results unimpressive

Surgery

Last resort

Try conservative treatment for 6 to 18 months before surgical referral

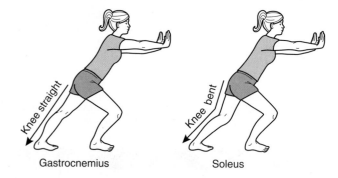

Figure 30.4 Heel cord stretching. Stretching the gastrocnemius and soleus is a therapeutic key in the treatment of many types of heel pain. **Box 30.1** illustrates the recommended routine.

Box 30.1: Heel Cord Stretching

1. Stretching the heel cord involves stretching two separate muscles: the gastrocnemius and the soleus. Both muscles should be stretched individually for best results. Place the leg to be stretched behind the other leg, and lean forward against a wall, keeping the back knee straight.
2. Continue to lean forward, keeping the knee straight and the heel on the ground, until the pull is felt in the upper calf (gastrocnemius).
3. Hold this position for a full 30 seconds. Muscle begins to lengthen after 20 seconds of stretching, so the final 10 seconds are the most essential.
4. Next, lean forward again, but bend the knee of the back leg, still keeping the heel on the ground. It is often helpful to visualize yourself trying to kneel while keeping your heel on the ground.
5. Continue to kneel and lean until a pull is felt in the lower calf (soleus).
6. Hold this position for a full 30 seconds.
7. Repeat these exercises with the opposite leg.
8. Stretch each leg three times during each stretching session.
9. To improve heel cord flexibility, three stretching sessions per day are recommended. To maintain flexibility, one session per day is adequate.

---

may be caused by bursal impingement between the Achilles tendon and an excessively prominent posterior–superior aspect of the calcaneus (Haglund's deformity).[40]

Clinical features

The athlete will complain of posterior heel pain that worsens when first beginning an activity. Some individuals also may report obvious swelling (e.g., pump bump, which is presumably named after an association with high-heeled shoes or pumps).[40]

Diagnosis

Tenderness specific to retrocalcaneal bursitis is isolated best by palpating just anterior to both the medial and lateral edges of the distal Achilles tendon. This is in contrast with Achilles enthesopathy, which is notable for tenderness where the Achilles tendon inserts into the calcaneus. Lateral radiographs of the calcaneus may reveal a Haglund's deformity, which is described later in this chapter.

Treatment

Changing footwear may be the most important form of treatment. The use of an open-backed shoe may relieve pressure on the affected region. NSAIDs and ice can be used during the acute phase. Stretching and strengthening of the Achilles tendon may help relieve impingement on the subtendinous bursa. Although steroid injection is possible, it should be performed only by experienced providers because the Achilles tendon will be exposed to steroids and placed at risk for rupture (even with properly placed injections) given the appositional proximity of the Achilles tendon and the retrocalcaneal bursa. Immobilization in a walking boot or short-leg walking cast can be helpful for recalcitrant cases. The surgical removal of the inflamed bursa is required only rarely, but it may be necessary if the condition is complicated by Haglund's deformity.[40]

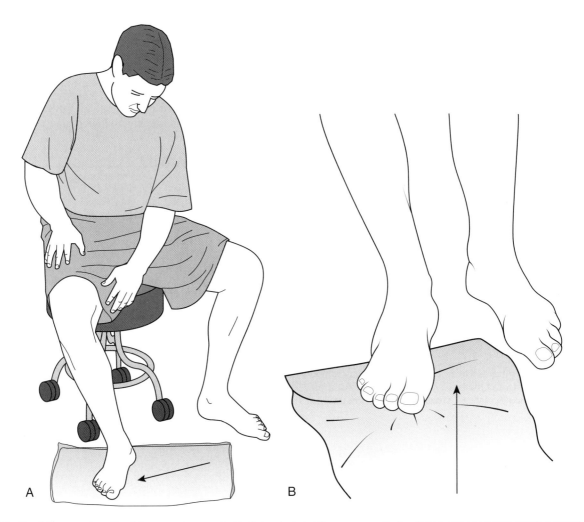

Figure 30.5 Towel drag exercises. Towel drag exercises are decidedly low-tech, but they are very effective for strengthening ankle and foot muscles. *A*, Towel drag (side to side). *B*, Towel crunch (front to back) **(Box 30.2).**

Box 30.2: Towel Drag Exercises

- Start with the towel spread to its maximum length, but folded to a width of 4 to 6 inches.
- Place the towel medial to the bare foot on wood, tile, or another smooth surface.
- Keeping the heel on the ground, drag the towel from a medial to a lateral position until the entire towel is bunched lateral to the foot (see Figure 30.5*A*).
- Refold the towel, and place it lateral to the foot.
- Keep the heel on the ground while using the toes to drag the towel from a lateral to a medial position until the entire towel is bunched medial to foot.
- Refold towel, and place it anterior to the foot.
- Lift the heel off of the ground, and use the toes to curl the towel back toward the heel until the entire towel is bunched under the arch of the foot (see Figure 30.5*B*).
- Perform the same three towel drags with the opposite foot.
- Repeat each set of drags 10 times with each foot once or twice daily.
- A can of soup can be placed on top of the towel and dragged with the towel for added resistance.

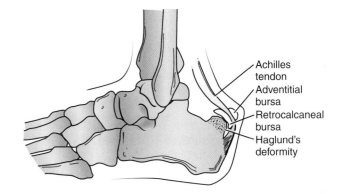

Figure 30.6 The insertional fibers of the Achilles tendon, the adventitial bursa, the retrocalcaneal bursa, and Haglund's deformity (a bony abnormality of the posterior calcaneus). Any or all of these structures can contribute to insertional Achilles pain. (From DeLee JC, Drez D Jr, Miller MD [eds]: DeLee and Drez's Orthopedic Sports Medicine: Principles and Practice, 2nd ed. Philadelphia, WB Saunders, 2002.)

Adventitial Achilles bursitis

Isolated adventitial Achilles bursitis is uncommon among athletes. It occurs most commonly in women with ill-fitting footwear. Its mechanism of injury and clinical presentation are very similar to those of retrocalcaneal bursitis; however, the tenderness in adventitial Achilles bursitis is more posteriorly superficial than in retrocalcaneal bursitis. Treatment focuses on relieving pressure. A U-shaped Achilles pad can be very helpful for cases in which open-backed shoes cannot be worn. Steroid injection is even more complicated than in retrocalcaneal bursitis because the risk of Achilles rupture with a deep injection is compounded by the risk of catastrophic skin necrosis if the injection is too superficial.

Athletes with retrocalcaneal and/or adventitial bursitis can return to play when pain subsides and strength and agility (post-immobilization) have returned to normal. Because both bursitises are primarily the result of inflammation, after this has resolved and the offending pressure has been relieved, the athlete can return to sports with relative rapidity.

Insertional Achilles enthesopathy

Achilles enthesopathy is a tendinosis-like injury that involves the Achilles tendon as it inserts into the calcaneus. It is generally considered to be a syndrome of overuse, and it is often concomitant with retrocalcaneal bursitis and Haglund's disease. Achilles enthesopathy is the most common source of pain in insertional Achilles pain and the second most common Achilles disorder after noninsertional or true Achilles tendinosis, which is discussed in the next section.[41,42]

Mechanism of injury

Jumping activities, direct trauma, ill-fitting shoes, calcaneal varus, and abnormal foot biomechanics have been proposed to precipitate pain and injury of the Achilles tendon insertion.

Diagnosis

Examination may reveal pain with passive dorsiflexion and resisted plantarflexion. Tenderness may be elicited with direct palpation over the Achilles tendon insertion.

Treatment

The treatment of insertional tendinopathy can be difficult and prolonged. Initial treatment options include open-backed shoes (to reduce pressure on the area), heel lifts, or orthoses to correct excessive calcaneal valgus. An Achilles stretching program should be implemented, and the athlete should rest from all offending activities for at least 2 to 4 weeks. Second-line therapy includes immobilization in a walking boot or a short-leg walking cast for 4 to 6 weeks. While immobilized, the athlete may maintain cardiovascular fitness by using an exercise bike. An eccentric loading program can be implemented for insertional Achilles tendinopathy. However, the reported response rate is 32% as opposed to the more than 90% rate of response to eccentric loading in true Achilles tendinosis (LOE: B).[43] Still, the conservative treatment of insertional Achilles tendinopathy with the use of rest, ice, modification in training, heel lifts, and orthoses produces an 85% to 95% success rate (LOE: D).[44]

Patients who do not benefit from two trials of immobilization (or one round of immobilization if they have a pronounced Haglund's deformity) should be referred for surgical evaluation. The principles of surgery include the debridement of the calcific or diseased portion of the Achilles insertion, the excision of the retrocalcaneal bursa, and the resection of the superior prominence. Surgical debridement of the Achilles tendon can necessitate tendon transfer from the flexor hallucis longus.

Return to play

Recovery from Achilles enthesopathy can be prolonged, especially given the frequent need for prolonged immobilization (either as a nonoperative treatment and/or for postsurgical recovery). The return of a normal range of motion and near-normal concentric and eccentric muscle strength is essential to a successful return to play. The time required for healing and rehabilitation is seldom less than 6 weeks and often more than 6 months.

Haglund's deformity

Haglund's deformity is a prominence of the posterior–superior portion of the os calcis. It predisposes patients to and complicates cases of insertional Achilles pain. Although Haglund's deformity may be suspected on physical examination, lateral radiographs of the foot are required for a definitive diagnosis. Multiple criteria for diagnosing a Haglund's deformity have been described; see Chapter 17, Radiographic Lines and Angles, for a more complete discussion. The presence of a Haglund's deformity does not mean that the athlete will be recalcitrant to conservative treatment, so surgical excision is not first-line or default treatment. However, Haglund's deformity does make an athlete less likely to heal with conservative measures, so surgical referral may be hastened.

ACHILLES TENDINOSIS

True Achilles tendinosis is a degenerative, noninflammatory process that involves the distal, "narrow neck" region of the Achilles tendon.[41,42] One large study by Kvist evaluated the epidemiology of Achilles tendon injuries. According to the study, which involved 698 patients, 66% had tendinopathy of the main body of the Achilles, 23% had Achilles tendon insertional problems, 8% had injury at the myotendinous junction, and 3% had a complete tendon rupture (LOE: D).[45] Eighty-nine percent of those injured in this study were men, and running was the main sport reported in these patients. In another study of 470 patients, Paavola and colleagues[46] found that 41% of patients who had Achilles tendinopathy developed symptoms in the contralateral leg during an 8-year follow-up period (LOE: D).

Risk factors

Overuse, an increase in mileage, an increase in hill running, poor calf and hamstring flexibility, and/or strength may predispose an athlete to the development of this condition.

Mechanism of injury

The pathogenesis of chronic tendinosis is not well understood. However, recent work by Alfredson[47] suggests that pain from Achilles tendinosis may be mediated by glutamate and associated with the neovascularization of the injured Achilles tendon.

Clinical features

The athlete may give a history of a recent change in shoes and/or training level. The patient will complain of an activity-related pain that is localized to the tendon approximately 3 to 4 cm above its insertion into the calcaneus.

Diagnosis

Tenderness, swelling, and possibly crepitus are found in the tendon neck 3 to 4 cm above the calcaneus. In chronic cases, a fusiform, tender swelling of the tendon may be palpated. Inflexibility of hamstring and of the gastrocnemius and soleus muscles as well as functional overpronation may be found concomitantly. Imaging is rarely needed for diagnosis, but, when it is needed, musculoskeletal ultrasound is being used more frequently for the evaluation of Achilles tendon disorders. It has several advantages over MRI: it is ready assessable, it has a quick scan time, and it is better tolerated by patients. However, musculoskeletal ultrasound is operator dependent, with a long learning curve. Ultrasound is accurate for the diagnosis of full-thickness tears of the Achilles tendon. Paavola and colleagues[48] correctly diagnosed 25 out of 26 full-thickness tears before surgery, and Hartgerink and colleagues[49] showed that ultrasound can be effective for the differentiation of full-thickness tears versus partial-thickness tears or tendinopathy, with a sensitivity and specificity of 100% and 83%, respectively, and an accuracy of 92% (LOE: D). Despite the ability of ultrasound to detect structural abnormalities of the Achilles tendon accurately, only a moderate correlation exists between the ultrasound appearance and clinical assessment of chronic Achilles tendinopathy.[50] MRI is also an excellent imaging modality for the Achilles tendon because of its excellent soft-tissue contrast characteristics. Karjalainen and colleagues[51] examined Achilles tendons with MRI and documented the overall sensitivity of MRI for the detection of abnormalities in cases of a painful Achilles tendon to be 94% with a specificity of 81% and an overall accuracy of 89% (LOE: D).[51]

Treatment

Initial treatment options include relative rest from offending activity and modification to decrease mileage and avoid hill running. Orthotics to correct hyperpronation can be helpful, and so can aggressive Achilles stretching.

If the previously described initial treatment has failed or if the patient has had pain for more than 6 weeks at the time of presentation,* the preferred treatment is an eccentric exercise program, which has been proven to be successful in more than 90% of cases of chronic tendinosis. Initially using body weight for resistance, the patient stands at the edge of the a step with the ankle in a neutral position. The patient then lowers the heel to maximum dorsiflexion in a controlled fashion **(Figure 30.7).** No concentric component is allowed; the patient should use the contralateral leg and knee to return to the start position. The patient is instructed to do three sets of 15 repetitions with the knee flexed (soleus) and three sets of 15 repetitions with the knee extended (gastrocnemius). The exercises are repeated twice daily. The patient should be warned to expect increased pain during the initial 10 to 14 days of exercises. When the pain begins to subside (after 2 to 3 weeks), resistance is increased by adding weights to a backpack or by performing the exercises using a squat bar or leg sled (LOE: B).[52] The exercises are performed for 10 to 12 weeks. Typically, no additional exercise (e.g., running or biking) is allowed during the first 6 weeks. During the second 6 weeks, the patient may gradually progress from biking to fitness jogging. By 12 weeks of the program, athletes are ready to begin sport-specific drills and a relatively rapid return to play.

Local injections of corticosteroids are not recommended as a result of the risk of delayed tendon rupture. Surgical debridement is reserved for patients for whom prolonged conservative measures are not effective.[41] For cases of tendon rupture, surgical referral is warranted.

ACHILLES RUPTURE

Achilles tendon ruptures are increasingly frequent, mainly because of the greater participation in recreational sports by the general

*Eccentric exercises are not routinely used before 6 weeks because it is clinically difficult to distinguish a partial Achilles rupture from tendinitis in this time frame.

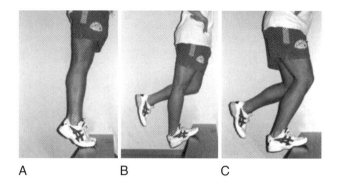

Figure 30.7 *A,* Begin in an upright body position with all weight on the forefoot and the ankle joint in plantar flexion. *B,* Lower the heel slowly, eccentrically loading the calf and keeping the knee straight. *C,* The exercise is also done with the knee bent to eccentrically load the soleus. In both exercises, the patient returns to the starting position by stepping back up with the opposite leg. (From Alfredson H, Pietilä T, Jonsson P, et al: Am J Sports Med 1998;26:360-366.)

population that alternates exercise with inactivity.[53] Achilles tendon rupture is predominantly a male disease. Studies of Achilles tendon rupture have revealed a male-to-female ratio ranging from 2:1 to 12:1, which is thought to reflect the greater number of men who are involved in sports.

Risk factors

Epidemiologic data from Nillius and colleagues[54] showed an incidence curve with two peaks: a large peak during middle age and a smaller peak between the ages of 70 and 79 years. A review by Arndt[55] showed that 57% of 1823 Achilles tendon ruptures were left sided, probably as a result of the greater prevalence of right-side–dominant individuals who push off with the left lower limb (LOE: D).[55] The exact reason why the Achilles tendon ruptures is not known. Degeneration of the tendon can result from several factors, including physiologic alterations in the tendon, chronic overloading with microtrauma, pharmacologic treatment, and association with other systemic diseases. Kannus and Jozsa[56] compared the histopathology of 397 Achilles tendon ruptures with 220 control tendons. They found characteristic histopathologic degenerative changes in most (97%) of the ruptured tendons. However, most patients had no symptoms before the rupture (LOE: D).[56] Nine of the 176 patients who presented to a clinic in Sweden with rupture of the Achilles tendon between 1990 and 1995 had previous symptoms, whereas the other 95% did not have symptoms (LOE: D).[57] Certain medications also place the Achilles tendon at risk for rupture; during the last decade, local and systemic corticosteroids and fluoroquinolones such as ciprofloxacin have been implicated in the rupture of the Achilles tendon.

Clinical features

In most cases, the history of Achilles tendon rupture is typical and does not pose diagnostic problems. The patient will report feeling a "pop" or "snap" in the calf and feeling that he or she has been struck or kicked in the posterior aspect of the distal part of the leg. The immediate pain resolves quickly, and the patient will often walk into the office with a level of pain and swelling that can be surprisingly minimal. Persistent weakness, poor balance, and altered gait are common complaints.

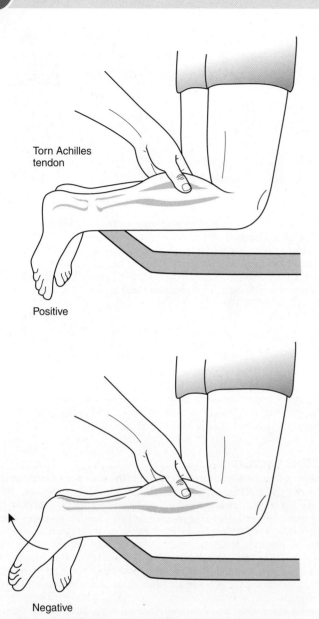

Torn Achilles tendon

Positive

Negative

Figure 30.8 Thompson's test is a reliable clinical test to identify the presence of a complete tear in the Achilles tendon. When the Achilles tendon is torn, a positive test is elicited by squeezing the calf and seeing no plantarflexion of the foot. A negative test occurs when the calf is squeezed and plantarflexion occurs in the foot. (From Frontera WR, Silver JK: Essentials of Physical Medicine and Rehabilitation. Philadelphia, Hanley and Belfus, 2002.)

Diagnosis

The diagnosis of Achilles tendon rupture is clinical. Within 2 to 3 days after the injury, a gap can be palpated that is 2 to 7 cm proximal to the insertion of the Achilles tendon on the calcaneus. Later the gap is often filled with hematoma and fibrous tissue; swelling, edema, and bruising may make palpation more difficult (LOE: C).[58] The calf squeeze test, which is also known as the *Thompson test*, is a reliable predictor of Achilles rupture **(Figure 30.8)**. With the patient prone on the examining table and the ankles clear of the table, the examiner squeezes the calf from side to side. Squeezing the calf deforms the soleus muscle and causes the overlying Achilles tendon to bow away from the tibia if

the tendon is intact.[59] If there is plantarflexion of the foot, the test is negative, and the Achilles tendon has not sustained a complete rupture. If plantarflexion is absent, the test indicates a complete rupture. Although clinical examination is generally sufficient for a diagnosis of acute Achilles tendon rupture, longstanding or partial ruptures may produce ambiguous clinical findings, and these may need to be confirmed by MRI or ultrasound imaging.

Treatment

The goals of the management of Achilles tendon rupture are to minimize the morbidity of the injury, to optimize a rapid return to full function, and to prevent complications. Despite the development and study of several treatment methods and procedures during the last decade, there is no consensus regarding the best way to deal with Achilles tendon rupture. Treatment options can be broadly divided into surgical and nonsurgical. The most common nonsurgical treatment has been immobilization in a below-knee plaster cast in a gravity equines position for 4 weeks and then in a more neutral position for another 4 weeks. The nonsurgical management option is best for those patients who are elderly and/or inactive, who have poor skin integrity, and who have wound healing problems. Advantages of nonsurgical treatment include no wound complications, decreased hospital costs, and no exposure to anesthesia. Disadvantages of nonsurgical repair include a higher incidence of rerupture (up to 40%) and a more difficult repair in the cases of rerupture. The surgical management of Achilles rupture is recommended to those who are young, healthy, and more active. There are a variety of surgical techniques for the repair of the ruptured Achilles tendon, including the traditional open repair and a newer percutaneous repair. Advantages of operative treatment include a lower rerupture rate (0% to 5%), a higher percentage of patients who return to sports, and a greater return of strength, endurance, and power. The main disadvantage of operative management is wound complication. Cetti and colleagues[60] compared the results of 111 patients who underwent either nonsurgical management in a cast versus operative treatment involving simple end-to-end sutures followed by cast immobilization. They reported that the surgical management resulted in better outcomes and increased patient satisfaction (LOE: D).[60]

PERONEAL TENDON PATHOLOGY

Peroneal tendon injury is a relatively common entity that may be associated with ankle inversion injury. The tendons of the peroneus brevis and longus muscles pass behind the lateral malleolus to turn anteriorly toward their respective insertions at the base of the fifth metatarsal and the base of the first metatarsal. The tendons are retained within the peroneal groove by the superior peroneal retinaculum.

Mechanism of injury

The condition may be related to chronic lateral instability, or it may result from a sudden, forceful, passive ankle dorsiflexion with the foot in slight inversion that results in a sudden, strong reflex contraction of the peroneals, which serve as the dynamic lateral stabilizers of the ankle.[23] Injury may result in tenosynovitis or tendinosis. Severe acute injury may cause elevation of the superior peroneal retinaculum off of the lateral border of the fibula with concomitant subluxation, dislocation, or dissection of the tendons; tear of the superior peroneal retinaculum; or fracture of the posterolateral margin of the fibula.

Clinical features

Patients will complain of pain, swelling in the lateral ankle region, a sense of instability, or an audible painful snapping during activity.

Diagnosis

Tenosynovitis or tendinosis presents with fullness and tenderness along the tendons as well as pain with passive inversion or with active resisted eversion. Usually a partial tear within the tendon presents with more localized tenderness, normal strength, and pain with resisted eversion.[23]

Patients with subluxation of the peroneal tendons complain of snapping or popping in the region of the lateral malleolus. Pain with resisted eversion may be present. During active eversion and dorsiflexion, the prominent tendons can be palpated or seen as they subluxate laterally (pop out) in the fibular groove. If frank peroneal tendon dislocation is occurring, active dorsiflexion and eversion cause the tendons to displace outside of the fibular groove, and they become palpable over or even anterior to the lateral malleolus.[23]

Rupture of the peroneal tendons often presents with diffuse tenderness and fullness along the peroneal tendon sheath. The patient may have weakness with eversion, but he or she may not have significant pain after the acute phase of the inflammatory reaction has subsided.

Peroneal disease is best imaged with MRI. The modality is used to confirm tenosynovitis, partial or complete peroneal tendon rupture, peroneal tendon subluxation or dislocation, integrity of the superior peroneal retinaculum, the competency of lateral ankle ligaments, and the internal derangement of the ankle and subtalar joints.[23]

Treatment

The conservative treatment of tenosynovitis and tendinosis is functional ankle rehabilitation with emphasis on peroneal tendons exercises. The conservative treatment of subluxation with immobilization in mild plantarflexion and inversion for 4 to 6 weeks has a 50% to 60% success rate, and the stability of the peroneal tendons is then verified clinically. An ankle rehabilitation program is instituted with an emphasis on peroneal strength and proprioception.[61] A felt pad may be taped over the tendons temporarily if the athlete with subluxation wishes to complete his or her season. Primary surgical repair is recommended for athletes with subluxations, frank dislocations, partial or complete tendon tears, and for those patients who do not want to risk the chance of failure (LOE: C).[62]

POSTERIOR TIBIALIS INJURY

Posterior tibialis tendinitis is uncommon among young athletes overall, but it can be seen relatively frequently among dancers, ice skaters, and middle-aged and older athletes.

Mechanism of injury

Sports that require rapid changes in direction (e.g., basketball, tennis, soccer, and ice hockey) place increased stress across the tendon. Sudden impact forces on the foot and ankle may cause the tendon to rupture. However, a tendon weakened from overuse and repetitive trauma provides the substrate for that injury to occur. Simply put, a ruptured tendon was not strong enough to stand up to an athlete's chosen frequency, intensity, and volume of training.[63,64]

The tendon of the tibialis posterior passes within in its own synovial sheath posterior to the medial malleolus and restrained by the flexor retinaculum. It then turns anteriorly and divides into three distinct components proximal to the navicular tuberosity. The anterior component inserts primarily into the navicular tuberosity. The middle component continues distally, inserting into the cuneiforms, the cuboid, and the medial three metatarsal

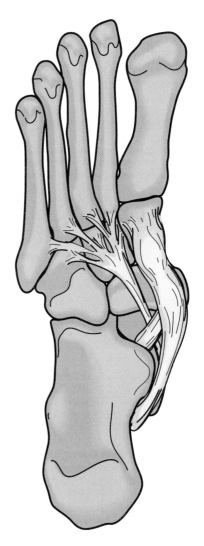

Figure 30.9 The tibialis posterior tendon inserts into the medial tuberosity of the navicular (one main slip) and continues through the second slip into the plantar surface of foot, where it arborizes and inserts into all three cuneiforms, the cuboid, and the bases of the first, second, third, fourth, and fifth metatarsals. (Redrawn from Canale ST: Campbell's Operative Orthopedics, 10th ed. Philadelphia, Mosby, 2003.)

bases. The posterior component inserts as a band on the spring ligament. All three components provide the function of supporting the medial longitudinal arch[65,66] **(Figure 30.9).**

Clinical features

Patients present with diffuse swelling, tenderness, and warmth at the medial ankle and along the course of the tendon. They generally complain of a gradual loss of the medial longitudinal arch, and they may have excessive medial heel wear of the shoes.[67]

There is tenderness to palpation along the course of the tendon. Holding the foot in an everted position and instructing the patient to invert against resistance can demonstrate muscle weakness. Toe raises are difficult, and there is often delay in or a lack of heel varus with toe raising on the affected side when viewed from behind. If partial or complete rupture has occurred, a distinct defect will be felt; more often, no tendon will be available for palpation.[68]

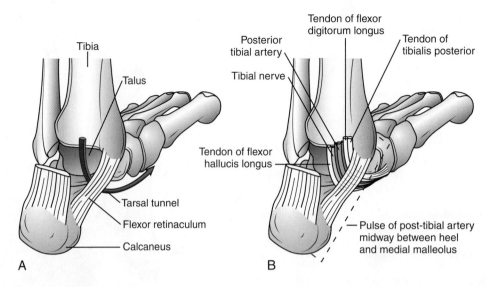

Figure 30.10 Tarsal canal anatomy and contents.

Diagnosis

It is vitally important to determine the exact location of the patient's pain and tenderness. Partial or complete rupture of the tendon as a result of trauma involves distinct pain at the navicular tuberosity in approximately 50% of cases. Overuse injuries with tendon degeneration present with pain just distal to the medial malleolus. MRI is highly sensitive and specific for the detection of a rupture (LOE: B).[67]

The plantar calcaneonavicular or spring ligament runs from the anteromedial aspect of the calcaneus to the medial pole of the navicular.[23] It serves as the major support for the medial arch and head of the talus. Injury is usually a resulting complication of a prior rupture of the posterior tibial tendon with an acquired flatfoot. MRI confirms the diagnosis.

Treatment

Treatment is ideally dependent on the stage of the deformity, the presenting symptoms, and the severity of the pain. The disorder is disabling, and, therefore, treatment should be implemented rapidly and aggressively to avoid further progression.[69] During the early stages, conservative methods such as NSAIDs, ultrasound, taping, muscle strengthening, and rigid orthoses can be used to control excessive pronation, to reduce tendon strain, and to allow the muscle to function more efficiently.

Immobilization with the foot in inversion for several weeks to months may be needed. If the patient is unresponsive after approximately 8 weeks of conservative treatment, then he or she is considered a surgical candidate. In cases of tenosynovitis, a synovectomy may be performed. Alternatively, in cases of severe tendinopathy or tendon rupture, a reconstruction may be required.[65,66,68,69]

TARSAL TUNNEL SYNDROME

Tarsal tunnel syndrome is an entrapment neuropathy of the tibial nerve or one of its branches either inside the tarsal tunnel or just distal to tunnel. The tarsal tunnel is a space behind the medial malleolus that is covered by the flexor retinaculum. In addition to the tibial nerve, the tendons of the flexor hallucis longus muscle, the flexor digitorum longus muscle, the tibialis posterior muscle, and the posterior tibial artery also pass through the tarsal tunnel **(Figures 30.10 and 30.11).**

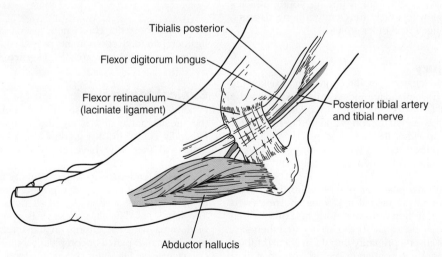

Figure 30.11 Contents of the tarsal tunnel. (From Canale ST: Campbell's Operative Orthopedics, 10th ed. Philadelphia, Mosby, 2003.)

Mechanism of injury

Causes of tarsal tunnel syndrome include chronic ankle sprains, fractures, dislocations, posttraumatic fibrosis, ganglions, tendon sheath tumors, repetitive stress, pes planus, and hyperpronation. Excessive stretch of the medial plantar nerve in joggers can cause tarsal tunnel syndrome, a condition that is often referred to as "jogger's foot."[23] Any condition that may cause peripheral neuropathy will also predispose an individual to this condition; this list includes alcoholism, diabetes, and thyroid disorders. Radiculopathy to the L4, L5, and S1 regions can produce pain in the tarsal tunnel area. People going from high heels to flat shoes on the weekend may also develop this pain syndrome.[70]

Clinical features

Patients present with heel pain and a tingling sensation around the plantar and medial aspect of the heel. Symptoms are often exacerbated by weight bearing and ambulation, but they may persist at rest.

Diagnosis

Palpation of the course of the posterior tibial nerve may cause patients to experience an uncomfortable burning pain that radiates proximally or distally (Tinel's sign). Nerve conduction velocity studies and electromyographic tests can confirm the diagnosis of tarsal tunnel syndrome.[23]

Treatment

Treatment is initially conservative, with rest, NSAIDs, and casting. The correction of foot biomechanics with arch supports and heel wedges is also helpful. Corticosteroid injection into the tarsal tunnel can provide long-term or even permanent relief from symptoms by reducing both the inflammation and the pain associated with nerve entrapments. For persistent symptoms, surgery is indicated (LOE: B).[71]

FLEXOR HALLICUS LONGUS TENDINOPATHY

Injury to the flexor hallucis longus occurs during activities that require repetitive extreme dorsiflexion, such as ballet. The flexor hallucis longus passes through the tarsal tunnel behind the medial malleolus and inserts into the plantar surface of the base of the distal phalanx of the greater hallux.

Mechanism of injury

Chronic inflammation and hypertrophy may result as dancers repetitively go from a flatfoot stance to en pointe position (extreme plantarflexion). Eventually, the inflamed tendon gets compressed in plantarflexion over the posterior talar tubercle (LOE: B).[72] In advanced cases, the tendon can actually lock in demi pointe (forefoot in plantarflexion) and become unable to release in plié (forefoot in neutral/dorsiflexion).[73]

Risk factors

Wearing shoes that are too big and that require the athlete to "toe grip" is associated with an increased risk of injury.

Clinical features

Flexor hallucis longus tendinitis will usually present in the young athlete as pain with forefoot weight bearing over the posteromedial aspect of the calcaneus around the sustentaculum tali.

Diagnosis

On examination, pain may be aggravated with resisted great toe flexion or passive stretch into full dorsiflexion. Passive flexion or extension of the interphalangeal joint may produce a snap posterior to the medial malleolus. It is not typically associated with other injuries, but it is commonly misdiagnosed as Achilles or posterior tibial tendinitis.

Treatment

Conservative treatment includes decreased activity, physical therapy, and NSAIDs. For persistent symptoms, surgical management is advised for the release of the tendon sheath. After surgery, athletes usually go back to their previous levels of dancing (LOE: C).[43]

ANTERIOR TIBIALIS TENDINOPATHY

The anterior tibialis tendon accounts for 80% of the dorsiflexion power of the ankle. It passes medially over the anterior ankle joint and runs to insert into the medial and plantar aspects of the medial cuneiform and the base of the first metatarsal. Anterior tibialis tendinitis is a chronic problem that is most commonly seen in runners.

Mechanism of injury

A common cause of tendon irritation is tight footwear laces, a condition that is commonly seen among beginning skaters and that is often referred to as "lace bite." The tendon is rarely injured acutely except in the elderly, in whom it can rupture either mid substance or at its insertion.

Clinical features

The athlete presents with pain, swelling, and stiffness in the anterior ankle that are aggravated by running.

Diagnosis

Localized tenderness, swelling, and, occasionally, crepitus along the tendon are present. Foot drop is common, and resisted dorsiflexion will be weak or tender.

Treatment

Treatment includes rest, gel pads, tibialis anterior stretching, strengthening, and icing. Casting may be required in advanced or unresponsive cases of tendinopathy. Rupture or avulsion injuries are treated surgically.[74]

HALLUX VALGUS (BUNION DEFORMITY)

Hallux valgus results from the lateral deviation of the hallux with respect to the first metatarsal.

Mechanism of injury

Hallux valgus is caused by a combination of familial predisposition, the presence of pes planus, and improper shoe wear. With increasing lateral deviation of the hallux, the metatarsophalangeal (MTP) joint becomes incongruent, the sesamoids subluxate laterally, the hallux pronates, and the medial aspect of the first metatarsal head becomes more prominent as weight bearing shifts from the first to the second metatarsal head.

Clinical features

The athlete will usually present with a red, enlarged, painful area (bunion) on the medial aspect of the first metatarsal head. The enlarged first metatarsal head may compress the second ray, and, in severe cases, a second toe deformity may occur. A painful keratosis can also form under the second metatarsal head.[40]

Treatment

Symptomatic treatment to relieve pressure on the big toe includes the use of a wider athletic shoe; a silicone pad can be placed over the bunion to alleviate direct pressure on the medial prominence. Achilles stretching is helpful in cases of Achilles tightness, and a simple toe spacer between the first and second toes can decrease second ray compression. In cases of pes planus associated with hallux valgus, a medial longitudinal arch support with a Morton's extension under the first MTP joint may also alleviate symptoms.[40] The definitive treatment for bunions is surgical. However, a randomized controlled trial (nonblinded) of surgery, orthotics, or watchful waiting (control) showed no difference in health-related quality of life scores between the three groups after 1 year. Surgery patients reported less subjective pain and disability, but they also reported five times the number of days missed from work as a result of surgery and a lengthy recovery time.[45]

TURF TOE

Turf toe is a hyperextension injury to the first tarsometatarsal joint that results in sprain of the plantar plate and the joint capsule. The plantar plate is the ligamentous attachment of the sesamoids and the flexor hallucis brevis to the base of the proximal phalanx.

Mechanism of injury

Forced dorsiflexion results in tearing of the plantar plate and the collateral ligaments. Severe injury may cause fracture of the sesamoids, dorsal dislocation, or articular injury of the first MTP joint. The risk of this injury increases when athletes are playing on old artificial turf that has hardened over time.[40]

Clinical features

The injured athlete presents with a red, swollen, stiff first MTP joint. There may also be a history of injuries to this region. Typically, the joint is tender on the plantar side, although dorsal tenderness can also occur. Players may have a limp and be unable to run or jump because of pain.

Diagnosis

The severity of injury is graded from I to III.[75] Grade I injury is a stretch or minor tearing of the capsuloligamentous complex with localized plantar tenderness and minimal swelling. The athlete is usually able to continue playing. Grade II injury is a partial tear with more tenderness, moderate swelling, ecchymosis, and a mild limp. Symptoms worsen over 24 hours. Grade III injury is a complete tear of the capsule off of the metatarsal head, severe plantar and dorsal tenderness, swelling and ecchymosis, severe loss of motion, and no ability to bear weight medially. Radiographs of the foot are obtained to assess joint congruity and to rule out fracture of the sesamoids or the articular surface.[40]

Treatment

Conservative treatment (i.e., PRICEMM, NSAIDs, and a rigid orthotic with a toe plate) can proceed if displacement of the sesamoids on x-ray is less than 2 mm. A fracture boot may be used if the patient is unable to bear weight comfortably. Physical therapy is instituted when the foot is comfortable for passive range of motion and progressive resistance exercise (LOE: B).[76]

Patients with grade I sprains are allowed to return to sports participation as soon as their symptoms allow, which is usually immediately. Patients with grade II sprains will require 3 to 14 days of rest from athletic training. Those with grade III sprains will require crutches for a few days to as long as 6 weeks. Early return to sports training after turf toe injury can result in long-term complications such as impaired push off, hallux rigidus, persistent symptoms, and chronic pain. Shoe modifications that incorporate a stiffer sole or an orthotic with a rigid forefoot section are recommended for the prevention of reinjury (LOE: B).[77]

INTERDIGITAL NEUROMA (MORTON'S NEUROMA)

Interdigital neuroma is a common cause of forefoot pain that is frequently reported among runners and dancers.

Mechanism of injury

This lesion is caused by entrapment neuropathy of the plantar nerve between the metatarsal heads, most commonly between the third and fourth toes.

Clinical features

Patients present with the numbness and tingling of the toes as well as aching and burning in the distal forefoot. The pain usually radiates from the metatarsal heads to the third and fourth toes, and it is exacerbated by walking on hard surfaces or wearing tight or high-heeled shoes.

Diagnosis

There is tenderness in the plantar web space between the metatarsal heads. Squeezing the forefoot with one hand while carefully palpating the involved interspace with the thumb and index finger of the other hand will cause marked discomfort. Rarely, the neuroma itself can be palpated as it subluxes out from between the metatarsal heads. This compressive examination may also produce a painful audible click that is known as *Mulder's sign*[78] **(Figure 30.12).**

Treatment

Treatment involves the modification of shoe wear with the use of stiff shoes, orthotic inserts, and metatarsal pads while avoiding high heels. Good footwear with a wide toe box is essential. The injection of corticosteroids with local anesthetic may give lasting or permanent relief (LOE: B).[79] One to two injections can be tried, but multiple injections should be avoided because corticosteroids may cause atrophy of the plantar fat pad. Additionally, surgical treatment is minimally invasive and quite successful.[79]

FREIBERG'S INFARCTION

Freiberg's disease is an osteochondrosis with a congenital, traumatic, or vascular cause. It is most common in the second metatarsal head. The typical patient is a female adolescent between 11 and 17 years of age. The female-to-male ratio is 5:1.

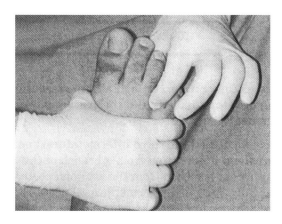

Figure 30.12   The technique to use to elicit Mulder's sign/click. (From Frontera WR, Silver JK: Essentials of Physical Medicine and Rehabilitation. Philadelphia, Hanley and Belfus, 2002.)

Mechanism of injury

An unknown injury leads to osteonecrosis and the eventual collapse and deformity of a lesser metatarsal head.

Clinical features

Patients most frequently present with second MTP joint pain, although metatarsals two through five may be affected, and the pain worsens with activity. Examination shows tenderness on the affected MTP joint, swelling, a limited range of motion, and, occasionally, a plantar callosity under the second metatarsal head.[40,80]

Radiographs may show rarefaction of the metatarsal subchondral bone at the site of the subchondral fracture, flattening and collapse of the dorsal aspect of the metatarsal head, narrowing of the joint space, and loose bodies during later stages.

Treatment

Conservative treatment includes rest, the use of a metatarsal pad, the avoidance of high-impact activities, the use of a walking boot, and the use of crutches until the gait is pain free. Gradual return to activity is allowed as symptoms decrease. Surgery is not recommended during the acute stage, which may persist for 6 months to 2 years. Patients typically return to full activity without surgical intervention, despite the affected metatarsal's persistently abnormal x-ray appearance. However, surgery may be indicated later as a result of persistent pain, deformity, and disability. Surgery involves the debridement of the joint and the removal of metatarsal head osteophytes with reshaping of the head.[80]

CONCLUSION

Soft-tissue injuries to the ankle and foot are common and involve many different structures. Accurately identifying the injured tissue, determining and correcting offending forces, and providing evidence-based treatment are essential to expedite recovery. An adequate rehabilitation program is an essential component for all lower-extremity injuries.

REFERENCES

1. Garrick JG, Requa RK: The epidemiology of foot and ankle injuries in sports. Clin Sports Med 1988;7:29-36.
2. Perlman M, Leveille D, DeLeonibus J, et al: Inversion lateral ankle trauma: differential diagnosis, review of the literature, and prospective study. J Foot Surg 1987;26:95-135.
3. Safran MR, Benedetti RS, Bartolozzi AR, et al: Lateral ankle sprains. Sci Sports Exerc 1999;31(7 suppl):S429-S437.
4. Bulucu C, Thomas KA, Halvorson TL, Cook SD: Biomechanical evaluation of the anterior drawer test: The contribution of the lateral ankle ligaments. Foot Ankle Int 1991;11:389-393.
5. Cass JR, Morrey BF, Chao EYS: Three-dimensional kinematics of ankle instability following serial sectioning of lateral collateral ligaments. Foot Ankle Int 1984;5:142-149.
6. Attarian DE, Mccracken HJ, Devito DP: Biomechanical characteristics of human ankle ligaments. Foot Ankle Int 1985;6:54-58.
7. Dias LS: The lateral ankle sprain: An experimental study. J Trauma 1979;19:266-269.
8. Thomas HT, McKeag DB: Ankle sprains: expedient assessment and management. Phys Sportsmed 1998;26(10).
9. Van Dijk CN, Lim LS, Bossuyt PM, et al: Physical examination is sufficient for the diagnosis of sprained ankles. J Bone Joint Surg (Br) 1996;78(6):958-962.
10. American Medical Association: Standard Nomenclature of Athletic Injuries. Chicago, American Medical Association, 1966.
11. Stiell IG, McKnight RD, Greenberg GH, et al: Implementation of the Ottawa ankle rules. JAMA 1994;271:827-832.
12. Hockenbury T, Sammarco GJ: Evaluation and treatment of ankle sprains. Phys Sportsmed 2001;29(2).
13. Wolfe MW, Uhl TL, Mattacola CG, McCluskey LC: Management of ankle sprains. Am Fam Physician 2001;63:93-104.
14. Eiff MP, Smith AT, Smith GE: Early mobilization versus immobilization in the treatment of lateral ankle sprains. Am J Sports Med 1994;22(1):83-88.
15. Cass JR, Morrey BF, Katoh Y, Chao EY: Ankle instability: comparison of primary repair and delayed reconstruction after long-term follow-up study. Clin Orthop Relat Res 1985;(198):110-117.
16. Wexler RK: The injured ankle. Am Fam Physician 1998;57:474-480.
17. Dettori JR, Pearson BD, Basmania CJ, Lednar WM: Early ankle mobilization. Part I: The immediate effect on acute, lateral ankle sprains (a randomized clinical trial). Mil Med 1994;159:15-20.
18. Karlsson J, Lundin O, Lind K, Styf J: Early mobilization versus immobilization after ankle ligament stabilization. Scand J Med Sci Sports 1999;9:299-303.
19. Hartsell HD, Spaulding SJ: Eccentric/concentric ratios at selected velocities. Br J Sports Med 1999;33:255-258.
20. Hartsell HD: Eccentric/concentric ratios at selected velocities for the invertor and evertor muscles of the chronically unstable ankle. Br J Sports Med 1999;33(4):255-258.
21. Bahr R, Lian O, Bahr IA: A twofold reduction in the incidence of acute ankle sprains in volleyball after the introduction of an injury prevention program: a prospective cohort study. Scand J Med Sci Sports 1997;7(3):172-177.
22. Smith AH, Bach BR Jr: High ankle sprains. Phys Sportsmed 2004;32(12).
23. Keene JS: Ankle and foot. In DeLee JC, Drez D Jr, Miller MD (eds): DeLee and Drez's Orthopaedic Sports Medicine: Principles and Practice, 2nd ed. Philadelphia, WB Saunders, 2003, pp 2323-2388.
24. Harper MC: The deltoid ligament. An evaluation of need for surgical repair. Clin Orthop 1988;226:156-168.
25. Jackson R, Wills RE, Jackson R: Rupture of deltoid ligament without involvement of the lateral ligament. Am J Sports Med 1988;16:541-543.
26. Liberatore R: Sinus tarsi syndrome or ligament injury? J Am Podiatr Med Assoc 1987;77(11):623.
27. Giorgini RJ, Bernard RL: Sinus tarsi syndrome in a patient with talipes equinovarus. J Am Podiatr Med Assoc 1990;80(4):218-222.
28. Frey C, DiGiovanni C, Feder KS: Arthroscopic evaluation of the subtalar joint: does sinus tarsi syndrome exist? Foot Ankle Int 1999;20(3):185-191.
29. Kuwada GT: Long-term retrospective analysis of the treatment of sinus tarsi syndrome. J Foot Ankle Surg 1994;33(1):28-29.
30. Broström L: Sprained ankles: III. Clinical observations in recent ligament ruptures. Acta Chir Scand 1965;130:560-569.
31. Tol JL, Verheyen CPPM, Van Dijk CN: Arthroscopic treatment of anterior impingement in the ankle. J Bone Joint Surg Br 2001;83:9-13.
32. Bassewitz HL, Shapiro MS: Persistent pain after ankle sprain: targeting the causes. Phys Sportsmed 1997;25(12).
33. Vincelette P, Laurin CA, Levesque HP: The footballer's ankle and foot. Can Med Assoc J 1972;107:872-874.
34. Stetson WB, Ferkel RD: Ankle arthroscopy: indications and results. J Am Acad Orthop Surg 1996;4:24-34.
35. Karasick D, Schweitzer ME: The os trigonum syndrome: imaging features. AJR Am J Roentgenol 1996;166:125-129.
36. Kirchner JS, Musgrave AL, Musgrave DS: Chronic pain continues after ankle sprain resolution. Biomech 2005. Available at http://www.biomech.com/showarticle;html?articleID=173500601
37. Singh D, Angel J, Bentley G, Trevino SG: Plantar fasciitis. BMJ 1997;315:172-175.

38. Cornwall MW, McPoil TG: Plantar fasciitis: etiology and treatment. J Orthop Sports Phys Ther 1999;29(12):756-760.

39. Sellman JR: Plantar fascia rupture associated with corticosteroid injection. Foot Ankle Int 1994;15:376-381.

40. Hockenbury RT: Forefoot problems in the athlete. Med Sci Sports Exerc 1999;31(7 Suppl):S448-S458.

41. Williams SK, Brage M: Heel pain-plantar fasciitis and Achilles enthesopathy. Clin Sports Med 2004;23:123-144.

42. Schepsis AA, Jones H, Haas AL: Achilles tendon disorders in athletes. Am J Sports Med 2002;30:287-305.

43. Koleitis GJ, Micheli LJ, Klein JD: Release of the flexor hallucis longus tendon in ballet dancers. J Bone Joint Surg Am 1996;78A:1386-1390.

44. Myerson MS, McGarvey W: Disorders of the Achilles tendon insertion and Achilles tendonitis. Instr Course Lect 1999;48:211-218.

45. Torkki M, Malmivaara A, Seitsale S, et al: Surgery vs orthosis vs watchful waiting for hallux valgus. A randomized controlled trial. JAMA 2001;285:2474-2480.

46. Paavola M, Kannus P, Paakkala t, et al: Long-term prognosis of patients with Achilles tendinopathy. An observational 8-year follow-up study. Am J Sports Med 2000;28:634-642.

47. Alfredson H: Conservative management of Achilles tendinopathy: new ideas. Foot Ankle Clin 2005;10(2):321-329.

48. Paavola M, Paakkala T, Kannus P, et al: Ultrasonography in the differential diagnosis of Achilles tendon injuries and related disorders. A comparison between pre-operative ultrasonography and surgical findings. Acta Radiol 1998;39(6):612-619.

49. Hartgerink P, Fessell DP, Jacobsen JA, et al: Full-versus partial thickness Achilles tendon tears: sonographic accuracy and characterization in 26 cases with surgical correlation. Radiology 2001;220(2):406-412.

50. Khan KM, Forster BB, Robinson J, et al: Are ultrasound and magnetic resonance imaging of value in assessment of Achilles tendon disorders? A two year prospective study. Br J Sports Med 2003;37:149-153.

51. Karjalainen PT, Soila K, Aronen HJ, et al: MR imaging of overuse injuries of the Achilles tendon. AJR Am J Roentgenol 2000;175:251-260.

52. Alfredson H, Pietila T, Jonsson P, Lorentzon R, et al: Heavy-load eccentric calf muscle training for the treatment of chronic Achilles tendinosis. Am J Sports Med 1998;26(3):360-366.

53. Maffulli N, Kader D: Tendinopathy of tendo achillis. J Bone Joint Surg Br 2002;84:1-8.

54. Nilius Sa, Nilsson Be, Westlin ND: The incidence of Achilles tendon rupture. Acta Orthop Scand 1976;47:118-121.

55. Arndt KH: Achilles tendon rupture. Zentralbl Chir 1976;101:360-364.

56. Kannus P, Jozsa L: Histopathological changes preceding spontaneous rupture of a tendon. A controlled study of 891 patients. J Bone Joint Surg Am 1991;73:1507-1525.

57. Maffulli N: Rupture of the Achilles tendon. J Bone Joint Surg Am 1999;81:1019-1036.

58. Maffulli N: The clinical diagnosis of subcutaneous tear of the Achilles tendon. A prospective study in 174 patients. Am J Sports Med 1998;26:266-270.

59. Scott BS, al Chalabi A: How the Simmonds-Thompson test works. J Bone Joint Surg Br 1992;74:314-315.

60. Cetti R, Christensen SE, Ejsted R, et al: Operative versus nonoperative treatment of Achilles tendon rupture. A prospective randomized study and review of the literature. Am J Sports Med 1993;21(6):791-799.

61. Keene JS, Lange RH: Diagnostic dilemmas in foot and ankle injuries. JAMA 1986;256(2):247-251.

62. McLennan JG: Treatment of acute and chronic luxations of the peroneal tendons. Am J Sports Med 1980;8(6):432-436.

63. Myerson M: Current Therapy in Foot and Ankle Surgery. In Myerson M (ed): Posterior tibial tendon insufficiency. St Louis, BC Decker, 1993.

64. Smerdelj M, Madjarevic M, Oremus K: Overuse injury syndromes of the calf and foot. Arh Hig Rada Toksikol 2001;52(4):451-464.

65. Hutchinson HB, O'Rourke EM: Tibialis posterior tendon dysfunction and peroneal tendon subluxation. Clin Podiatr Med Surg 1995;12(4):703-723.

66. Roukis TS, Hurless JS, Page JC: Functional significance of torsion of the tendon of tibialis posterior. J Am Podiatr Med Assoc 1996;86(4):156-163.

67. Lim PS, Schweitzer ME, Deely DM, et al: Posterior tibial tendon dysfunction: secondary MR signs. Foot Ankle Int 1997;18(10):658-663.

68. Mann RA, Thompson FM: Rupture of the posterior tibial tendon causing flat foot. J Bone Joint Surg Am 1985;67A(4):556-561.

69. Johnson KA: Surgery of the Foot and Ankle. New York, Raven Press, 1989.

70. Glazer JL, Hoser RJ: Soft-tissue injuries of the lower extreinity. Prim Care 2004;31(4):1005-1024.

71. Baili DS, Kelikian AS.: Tarsal tunnel syndrome: diagnosis, surgical technique, and functional outcome. Foot Ankle Int 1998;19(2):65-72.

72. Hamilton WG, Geppert MJ, Thompson FM: Pain in the posterior aspect of the ankle in dancers. J Bone Joint Surg 1996;78A:1491-1500.

73. Khan K, Brown J, Way S, et al: Overuse injuries in classical ballet. Sports Med 1995;19:341-357.

74. Omey ML, Micheli LJ: Foot and ankle problems in the young athlete. Med Sci Sports Exerc 1999;31(7 Suppl):S470-S486.

75. Clanton TO, Ford JJ: Turf toe injury. Clin Sports Med 1984;13:731-741.

76. Clanton TO, Butler JE, Eggert A: Injuries to the metatarsophalangeal joints in athletes. Foot Ankle 1986;7(3):162-176.

77. Rodeo SA, O'Brian S, Warren RF, et al: Turf-toe: an analysis of metatarsophalangeal joint sprains in professional football players. Am J Sports Med 1990;18(3):280-285.

78. Mulder JD: The causative mechanism in Morton's metatarsalgia. J Bone Joint Surg Br 1951;33-B:94-95.

79. Greenfield J, Rea J Jr, Ilfeld FW: Morton's interdigital neuroma. Indications for treatment by local injections versus surgery. Clin Orthop Relat Res 1984;(185):142-144.

80. Binek R, Levinsohn EM, Bersani F, Rubenstein H: Freiberg disease complicating unrelated trauma. Orthopedics 1988;11(5):753-757.

CHAPTER 31

Pediatric and Adolescent Injuries

Part A   TREATMENT OF COMMON PEDIATRIC AND ADOLESCENT CONDITIONS

Mark B. Stephens, MD, MS

KEY POINTS

- Back pain in children and adolescents is not normal; look for the underlying cause.
- Pain on internal rotation and limited internal rotation of the hip or preferential external rotation of the hip indicates hip joint pathology; look for the underlying cause.
- Routine screening for scoliosis is not recommended.
- Consider osteochondritis dissecans in pediatric patients presenting with a knee effusion.
- Pitch count limits prevent overuse injuries of the upper extremity in young throwing athletes.

INTRODUCTION

It is estimated that 30 million American youth participate in some sort of sporting activity[1]; this equates to roughly half of all children between the ages of 5 and 18 years.[2] More than a third of these young participants sustain an injury at some point in their experience that is significant enough to be evaluated by a medical professional. The peak injury rate occurs in children between the ages of 5 and 14, who account for more than 750,000 annual visits to the emergency department for sports-related injuries.[3] However, the absolute number of injuries is much higher because many young athletes do not seek medical attention. Therefore, sports-related injuries are something that all physicians who care for adolescents or children will encounter commonly in their practices.

In general, pediatric and adolescent sports injuries can be divided into two broad categories: traumatic injuries and overuse injuries. Traumatic injuries occur when kinetic forces across a bone or joint exceed local tissue stability. Fractures are the prime example of traumatic sports injuries. Alternatively, overuse injuries occur when repetitive movements about a particular musculotendinous unit or joint result in tissue microtrauma, tissue fatigue, and, finally, tissue injury.

Children are susceptible to predictable types of sports injuries for several reasons. First, children have a greater body surface area to body mass ratio. This places relatively greater kinetic forces across certain joints, and it places young athletes at increased risk for fracture. Second, children are less coordinated and have less developed motor skills than adolescents or adults, thus making them susceptible to injury as a result of miscoordination during sports activity. Third, the biomechanical properties of cartilage and bone in children differ significantly from that of adults. Growing cartilage and the areas in which tendons insert into bone (apophyses) **(Table 31A.1)** are particularly susceptible to stress and injury.[4] Finally, a relatively recent phenomenon is that children are specializing in certain sports at increasingly younger ages.[5] Many youth play on challenge or elite teams that travel. A common by-product of such specialization is overtraining with resultant overuse injury.

Given these underlying principles, the location and types of athletic injuries sustained by children and adolescent are quite predictable.[1] There are three primary anatomic zones of injury in young athletes.[6] The first zone is the epiphyseal plate. Known more commonly as the "growth plate," this is the cartilaginous zone where bone growth occurs. The epiphyseal plate is mechanically the weakest area of growing bone. It is weaker than surrounding ligament, muscle, or tendon. Injuries to the growth plate are more common among young boys, with a peak incidence in individuals who are between the ages of 14 and 16 years.[4] Most growth plate injuries are traumatic in nature, and they occur primarily as the result of a fall. Fractures of the growth plate are most commonly classified according to the taxonomy of Salter–Harris **(Figure 31A.1 and Table 31A.2).**

The second zone that is commonly injured in this group of patients is the joint surface. The growing tissues of the articular surface are particularly vulnerable to injury at the ankle, knee, and elbow.[7] This contributes to the pathophysiology of osteochondritis dissecans at these sites.

The third zone of injury is the apophyseal insertion site. The apophysis is the anatomic junction where tendon inserts into bone. Repetitive traction on the tissues of the apophysis (such as occurs with repetitive throwing, running, or jumping) results in local inflammation and tissue damage. Calcaneal apophysitis (Sever's

Table 31A.1 Definitions

Child	An individual between the ages of 2 and 11 years, before the onset of secondary sexual characteristics
Adolescent	An individual between the ages of 12 and 21 years, from the onset of secondary sexual characteristics to formal adulthood
Youth	A term used to describe both children and adolescents
Sprain	An injury to a ligament
Strain	An injury to a muscle
Contusion	A local hemorrhage into soft tissue or muscle
Apophysis	The site of insertion of a tendon into a bone

Table 31A.2 Salter–Harris Classification

Type I	The physeal plate is widened, and there is separation of the epiphysis.
Type II	The fracture passes through a section of the metaphysis and extends obliquely through the epiphysis.
Type III	An intra-articular fracture extends through the epiphysis and across the epiphyseal plate to the periphery.
Type IV	The fracture is through the metaphysis, the physis, and the epiphysis.
Type V	There is a crush injury to the growth plate.

disease) and tibial tubercle apophysitis (Osgood–Schlatter disease) are prime examples of this.

The most commonly injured parts of the body among young athletes are the lower extremities (knee, foot, and ankle) followed by the upper extremities (elbow, shoulder, forearm, wrist, and hand) and the head and neck region.[8] Young children more commonly sustain injuries of the head and upper extremities, whereas adolescents typically injure the lower extremities. Sprains, strains, and contusions are the most common types of injuries, and these are followed by more serious enthesopathies and, finally, fractures.

As with all medical conditions, a careful history is essential when evaluating pediatric and adolescent sports injuries.[9] As previously noted, sports injuries among young athletes typically fall into two patterns: acute (traumatic) and repetitive (overuse). For all acute injuries, it is important to determine the specific mechanism of injury (Did you twist or fall? Was your foot planted?). Note the exact location of the patient's pain. Ask if there are any associated signs or symptoms (Did you hear a pop? Did the joint give way? Did the joint lock? Is there any swelling?). If swelling is present, it is important to note whether the swelling occurred immediately at the time of injury or if fluid gradually accumulated over time. For overuse injuries, it is important to inquire when during the activity pain occurs (e.g., the throwing phase, the cocking phase, the follow-through phase). Note any alleviating or exacerbating factors (e.g., jumping, running). Ask the patient

to describe his or her training regimen, and note whether any acute change in this pattern has occurred. Also, it is important to inquire about the types and locations of previous sports injuries. Finally, explore the young athlete's equipment and environment (e.g., shoes, terrain). It is also important to determine what type of protective equipment, if any, the athlete was using at the time of the injury.

With these basic principles in mind, this chapter reviews the most common sports injuries of children and adolescents.

DISORDERS OF THE LOWER EXTREMITY

Ankle sprains

Ankle sprains are the most common acute sports injury among children and adolescents, accounting for 10% to 30% of all sports-related injuries.[10] A majority of ankle sprains (85%) are the result of an inversion injury. It should be emphasized that young children typically injure the distal fibular physis (Salter–Harris I fracture) rather than injuring the ligamentous structures of the lateral ankle.[10] This has important clinical implications because the treatment for bony Salter–Harris fractures is quite different from that of routine ligamentous sprains. Older children and adolescents typically injure the ligaments and soft tissues surrounding the ankle and respond well to traditional "adult" therapies for ankle sprains.

Mechanism of injury

During an inversion injury, the athlete typically rolls his or her foot inward upon landing during jumping activities. There may or may not be an audible pop at the time of injury. Basketball, soccer, football, dance, volleyball, and gymnastics are the activities that are most commonly associated with ankle sprains. The most commonly injured structure is the anterior talofibular ligament followed by the calcaneofibular ligament and the posterior talofibular ligament. Athletes who have sustained prior ankle sprains are at risk for recurrent injury.[4]

Clinical features

Swelling is the most common clinical sign associated with ankle sprains. Pain with weight bearing is also common and merits radiographic imaging. Physical examination should include an assessment of distal pulses and sensation. Physical examination should also include an assessment of the point of maximal tenderness. Patients who are tender at the medial or lateral malleolus, the fifth metatarsal, or the talus should have x-rays performed. It is important to note that the Ottawa ankle rules should not be applied to skeletally immature athletes.[11]

The integrity of the anterior talofibular ligament is assessed by the anterior drawer test. To perform this test, the examiner cups the heel of the athlete's affected foot with the ankle held at 5 degrees of plantar flexion; the heel is then pulled forward.

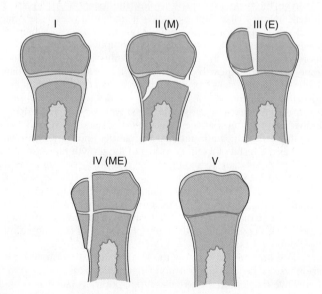

Figure 31A.1 Salter–Harris fracture classification.

A positive test occurs when there is a discrepancy in laxity of the affected joint as compared with the contralateral side.

A second test to evaluate the soft-tissue integrity of the ankle is the talar tilt. This is performed by grasping the forefoot of the affected ankle and firmly adducting the heel. This maneuver tests for the integrity of the calcaneofibular ligament. As with the anterior drawer test, a positive talar tilt test is indicated when there is a discrepancy in laxity as compared with the contralateral side.

A final diagnostic maneuver to use to evaluate ankle sprains is the squeeze test. This is performed by squeezing the sagittal midshank. This maneuver is used to evaluate for potential syndesmotic injury (commonly referred to as a *high ankle sprain*) or proximal fibular fracture. A positive squeeze test is indicated by the presence of significant pain at the site of injury (either the syndesmosis or the proximal fibula).

Finally, it is always important to rule out a Maisonneuve fracture when evaluating ankle injuries. This type of fracture occurs when kinetic forces are transmitted cephalad along the interosseous membrane and result in the fracture of the proximal fibular head. Palpation of the fibular head is, therefore, an important adjunct to the physical examination of the injured ankle. If the patient is tender at the fibular head, x-rays of the tibia and fibula should be obtained.

Diagnosis

The diagnosis of ankle sprains is primarily clinical and made on the basis of the history, the mechanism of injury, and the clinical examination. Radiographs should be obtained when there is appropriate point tenderness on examination or when the patient is unable to bear weight.

Normal radiographs do not exclude a fracture. Many foot and ankle fractures are difficult to visualize on routine x-rays. Growth plate fractures are especially common among younger children, who often will have normal x-rays. Skeletally immature children who are tender over a growth plate should be diagnosed with a growth plate fracture and treated as such. Adolescents who are skeletally mature, who have ligamentous tenderness, and who have no indication for x-rays or who have normal x-rays should be treated initially as having a sprain and told to return if their symptoms do not quickly resolve. Children and adolescents with open growth plates and diffuse, poorly localized tenderness should be treated conservatively and have close follow-up until symptoms and examination clearly point to the underlying process.

Treatment

Treatment of ankle sprains in children and adolescents consists primarily of ice, compression, elevation, and early rehabilitation. The injury should be iced acutely for the initial 24 to 48 hours. Compression and elevation of the affected extremity help to alleviate swelling. This initial period should be followed by rehabilitation that consists of progressive weight bearing and kinesthetic training. The use of support bracing has been shown to speed recovery in acute ankle sprains.[12] A systematic review of the literature supports functional rehabilitation for the treatment of acute ankle sprains as the most effective means of returning skeletally mature athletes to competition[13] (LOE: B). Patients should have pain-free range of motion, and they should be able to complete functional testing (e.g., running, cutting, performing figure-of-eight drills) before returning to competition.[10] Patients with mild ankle sprains can typically return to competition within 1 to 2 weeks, whereas individuals with more severe ankle sprains may take up to 3 to 8 weeks to fully heal.[14] Patients who have persistent symptoms 6 to 8 weeks after their injuries should be reevaluated by a physician and have further radiographic imaging performed. There should never be a temptation to rush a young athlete back into competition; to do so risks reinjury and further complications.

Sever's disease (calcaneal apophysitis)
Mechanism of injury
Sever's disease is a traction apophysitis at the point where the Achilles' tendon inserts on the calcaneus.[15] This condition (rather than "disease") typically presents during the period of rapid musculoskeletal growth that usually occurs between the ages of 8 and 13 years for girls and between the ages of 12 and 15 years for boys. Kinetic forces from the pull of the Achilles tendon on the unossified calcaneal insertion site result in microtrauma of the apophysis and nearby epiphyseal growth plate during the period of rapid growth[16]; this results in the clinical symptomatology.

Clinical features
Patients with calcaneal apophysitis typically complain of chronic, aching heel pain that is exacerbated by running, walking, or jumping activities.[10] Hard playing surfaces and/or poor-quality footwear exacerbate these symptoms. Biomechanically, these children often have difficulty putting full pressure on the affected heel. As a result, to reduce pain, they will subconsciously foreshorten the Achilles tendon by walking on their toes. Some children will present without pain but may have a history of a limp or of heel pain that is exacerbated by physical activity.

Diagnosis
The diagnosis of Sever's disease is made primarily on the basis of a consistent history and supported by physical examination that reveals point tenderness at the growth plate, just inferior to where the Achilles inserts on the calcaneus. The main body of the calcaneus is not tender in patients with Sever's disease. A decreased range of dorsiflexion of the ankle is common as well. Radiographs are nonspecific, often showing fragmentation, irregular ossification, or sclerosis at the calcaneal apophysis (**Figure 31A.2**). These radiographic findings are not considered pathologic, and they can often be demonstrated on the unaffected side.[3] The differential diagnosis of Sever's disease includes calcaneal stress fracture, osteomyelitis, and calcaneal bone cysts.

Treatment
The treatment of Sever's disease is based on relative rest of the affected area. Heel cord stretching is essential to promote symptom relief. Patients should be instructed to perform three sets of heel cord stretches, holding each exercise for 20 minutes three times daily. This should take approximately 20 minutes per session (see Chapter 30, Box 30.1 and Figure 30.5 for a detailed discussion of heel cord stretching). After pain subsides, patients should begin muscle-strengthening exercises that focus on the gastrocnemius–soleus complex. Strengthening of this muscle group increases the ability to absorb force and lessens the chance of symptom recurrence with return to play. Children should begin with bilateral heel raises using only their body weight and progress

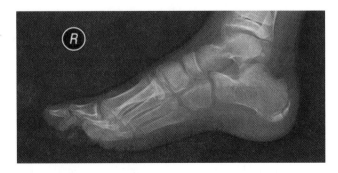

Figure 31A.2 Sever's disease. Nonspecific changes of fragmentation, irregular ossification, and bony sclerosis at the calcaneus of a skeletally immature patient. (Photo courtesy of Dr. Ulrich A. Rassner.)

slowly to single-leg exercises with added weight as their individual strength, balance, and symptoms allow.

In addition to stretching and strengthening, the use of heel cup inserts, properly fitting footwear, ice massage, and the judicious use of anti-inflammatory medications are helpful adjuncts for the treatment of Sever's disease. Parents and patients should not use anti-inflammatory medications to mask pain during sporting activities or to speed return to play; patients should only return to full sports activity when they are pain free. Inappropriate attempts to speed return to play result in symptom recurrence and further slow recovery times.

Using these principles of treatment, most athletes can expect to return to competition in 2 to 4 weeks. Athletes who experience persistent pain should continue to ice and stretch, and they should be restricted from competition until they are pain free. Although this condition is self-limited, some cases may take up to 12 to 18 months to completely heal. Although it is extremely uncommon, particularly recalcitrant cases may require a 2-week trial of immobilization in a short-leg walking cast. Difficult cases or cases in which the child is unable to return to play within 4 to 6 weeks merit consultation with a musculoskeletal specialist.

ANTERIOR KNEE PAIN

Anterior knee pain is another condition that is very common among young athletes.[17] This section covers anterior knee pain syndrome, Osgood-Schlatter disease, and Sinding–Larsen–Johansson disease.

Anterior knee pain syndrome
Mechanism
Historically, multiple terms have appeared in the literature to describe anterior knee pain in athletes, including *chondromalacia patella, retropatellar pain syndrome, runner's knee,* and *patellofemoral pain syndrome.* The currently preferred nomenclature is *anterior knee pain syndrome.* Anterior knee pain syndrome is the most common cause of adolescent knee pain.[16] Anterior knee pain syndrome results from a combination of biomechanical factors, overuse, and muscular dysfunction in the adolescent athlete. In adolescents, a relative imbalance of quadriceps strength coupled with kinetic forces at the hip, knee, and ankle results in the relative misalignment of the patella within the patellofemoral groove; this misarticulation creates the clinical pain syndrome.[18] Anterior knee pain syndrome is typically not a problem among younger children because of their lower body masses and correspondingly lower forces on the patellofemoral joints.

Clinical features
Patients with anterior knee pain syndrome present with chronic, dull, aching anterior knee pain that is often hard to localize. Pain is often pronounced when patients stand after a prolonged period of sitting (i.e., "movie-goers sign"). Pain is typically worse when going down stairs and with downhill running or walking. Patients often complain of a sensation of the muscle "giving way."

Diagnosis
It is important to examine the hip and knee and to observe gait in all patients who present with anterior knee pain. The hip examination is normal in patients with anterior knee pain syndrome, and the patient's gait is also normal when he or she is ambulating on a flat surface. The patient may exhibit antalgia or compensation when asked to descend stairs. Physical examination of the knee commonly reveals patellar inhibition; this is noted when the examiner occludes the superior pole of the patella and compresses it against the patellofemoral groove with the patient in the supine position

with the knee fully extended. A positive test occurs when the patient is asked to maximally contract the quadriceps, and there is a marked inhibition of contraction of the quadriceps and/or pain. Patients with anterior knee pain syndrome may also have tenderness to palpation of the articular surface of the superolateral (or, less commonly, the superomedial) aspect of the patella. These patients often exhibit a weak vastus medialis complex and tight hamstrings. The remainder of the knee examination reveals a full range of motion and no evidence of ligamentous or meniscal injury. X-rays (anteroposterior, lateral, and sunrise views) are normal in patients with anterior knee pain syndrome. X-rays are routinely obtained to rule out incidental bony or osteochondral pathology.

Treatment
The treatment of anterior knee pain syndrome is conservative. Activity modification is important to reduce overload or the overuse of the patellofemoral complex. Historically, rehabilitation has focused on quadriceps strengthening and hamstring stretching exercises. With regard to quadriceps exercises, strengthening the vastus medialis may be particularly useful because it is responsible for the terminal 5 to 10 degrees of knee extension. Controversy exists, however, regarding the practicality of individual muscle strengthening as opposed to global quadriceps strengthening. Additionally, a recent systematic review of the literature indicates equal functional outcomes in patients with a dedicated exercise rehabilitation program and in those without exercise rehabilitation (SOR: C).[19] It is also important to consider intrinsic factors (i.e., strength, flexibility, and alignment) and extrinsic factors (i.e., training program, equipment, and running surface) that contribute to anterior knee pain. Chapter 26, Knee Injuries, further discusses individual risk factors for anterior knee pain.

Nonsteroidal anti-inflammatory medications are useful only for short-term pain control in patients with anterior knee pain syndrome (SOR: B).[20] Bracing is controversial, but it has been shown to neither reduce the incidence of anterior knee pain nor speed return to activity.[21] Anecdotally, athletes may prefer to brace for comfort. Athletes may return to competition when their pain improves. The recurrence of anterior knee pain is common, so young athletes should be encouraged to continue with their strengthening, stretching, and rehabilitative regimen even when they are symptom free.

Osgood–Schlatter disease (tibial apophysitis)
Mechanism
Originally described in 1903, Osgood–Schlatter disease is another form of traction apophysitis (similar to Sever's disease)[4]. With this condition, there is an imbalance of forces where the patellar tendon inserts on the anterior tibial tubercle. This results in local tissue microtrauma, swelling of the tibial tubercle, and pain. Patients with increased external tibial torsion are particularly predisposed to the mechanical forces that result in the clinical symptoms of tibial apophysitis.[22]

Clinical features
Historically, males are more commonly affected than females—although increased and younger participation of women in sports has narrowed this gap. As with Sever's disease, patients with Osgood–Schlatter disease present during the period of rapid musculoskeletal growth between the ages of 8 and 15 years. Pain is localized to the tibial tubercle and increased during activities with forced extension of the knee such as running or jumping. Patients will complain of pain when kneeling, and they often exhibit a decrease in knee flexion. Pain is relieved by rest. In 80% of cases, the pain is unilateral. Patients who have intermittent symptoms (as opposed to those with persistent symptoms) typically have a longer time to complete resolution.

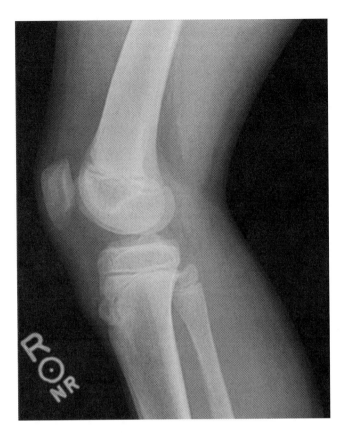

Figure 31A.3 Osgood–Schlatter disease. Note the irregular ossification of the tibial tubercle.

Diagnosis

On physical examination, patients with Osgood–Schlatter disease are point tender to palpation at the anterior tibial tubercle. There is often visible swelling of the tubercle as well. The remainder of the knee examination is structurally unremarkable. Patients may present with a limp, depending on the level of disease activity. When radiographs are obtained, they typically demonstrate some fragmentation of the tibial tubercle[16] **(Figure 31A.3).**

Treatment

Treatment of Osgood–Schlatter disease can be very frustrating. Although it is a self-limited condition, the complete resolution of symptoms may take up to 2 years. A systematic review of the literature reveals that Osgood–Schlatter disease is best treated conservatively (LOE: B).[23] Treatment is based on rest and activity modification. Ice massage, balanced strengthening and stretching of the hamstrings and quadriceps, and anti-inflammatory medications are helpful adjuncts. Strapping or taping of the patellar tendon may help to reduce pain for some patients. Kneepads are useful for athletes who wish to continue participating in sports in which there is potential for the knees coming in contact with the playing surface (e.g., volleyball). Despite these therapies, some patients will still have pain. Casting has been advocated as a potential treatment for these patients, but evidence to support its routine use is lacking. Surgery is rarely needed, and it is typically reserved for persistent pain in skeletally mature patients.[24] An athlete's return to competition is limited only by his or her level of pain. Continued activity will not structurally damage the affected knee, but an athlete should never be forced to "play through" the pain because avulsions of the tibial apophysis, while rare, have occurred. Typically, the most difficult aspect of the management of tibial apophysitis is communicating with coaches and parents about the benign—yet potentially lengthy—natural history of this condition.[3]

Sinding–Larsen–Johansson disease

Sinding–Larsen–Johansson disease is another form of traction apophysitis that is localized to the inferior pole of the patella. This condition results from forces of the patellar ligament on the inferior pole of the patella. It is analogous to Sever's disease and Osgood–Schlatter disease. Patients present with activity-related pain and swelling of the inferior pole of the patella. On examination, patients are tender at the inferior pole of the patella with an otherwise structurally normal knee. Radiographs may reveal elongation and/or fragmentation of the inferior pole of the patella. This condition is also self-limited, and pain typically abates as the skeleton matures. Treatment is conservative and similar to the other traction apophyses. Strapping or taping of the patellar tendon may also help to alleviate symptoms. The principles for return to competition are similar to the other conditions as well.

Osteochondritis dissecans
Mechanism

Osteochondritis dissecans (OCD) is a musculoskeletal lesion wherein a segment of subchondral bone and its associated articular cartilage have separated from surrounding bone. The condition results from a combination of factors including trauma, genetics, and/or local bony ischemia.[25] Three quarters of cases involve the knee (most typically the lateral aspect of the medial femoral condyle). The other most common sites for OCD lesions are the elbow and the talus.

Clinical features

Males are more commonly affected than females. Patients with osteochondritis dissecans of the knee typically present with vague complaints of knee pain that is worsened with activity; they may or may not report a history of trauma. In general, there are two subsets of patients who present with OCD lesions of the knee. In the first group, there is a clear history of trauma that correlates with symptoms and a loss of function. The second and more common subset of patients presents with the insidious waxing of symptoms and a loss of function.

Patients will usually complain of pain with activity and relative stiffness after periods of rest. Swelling is common among patients with OCD lesions **(Figure 31A.4).** This is important because patients with anterior knee pain syndrome, Osgood–Schlatter disease, and Sinding–Larsen–Johansson disease typically do not have an effusion. Patients may also complain of mechanical (foreign body) symptoms within the joint, such as locking or the muscle giving way. Patients are sometimes unable to fully extend the knee. The presence of an effusion in combination with a subtle restriction in the range of motion is the most important clinical clue that should lead a physician to suspect underlying OCD.[26]

Diagnosis

Although the diagnosis of OCD is based on radiography, there are important signs on physical examination that should not be overlooked. In a compensatory effort to alleviate pain, patients may externally rotate the tibia and alter their gait accordingly. Patients who present with a limp may already have a relatively advanced subchondral lesion. On physical examination, Wilson's sign is used to detect lesions of the medial femoral condyle. This test is performed by having the patient sit on the edge of the examination table. The knee is placed in 90 degrees of flexion, and the tibia is then internally rotated as the knee is slowly extended.

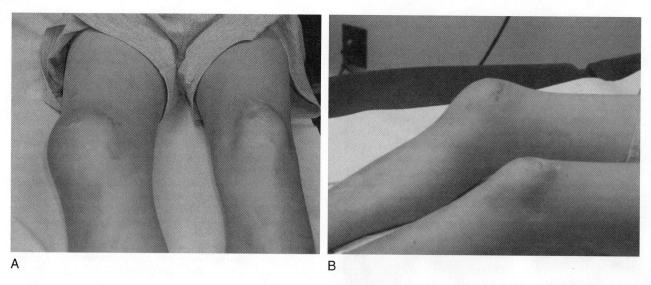

A   B

Figure 31A.4 *A* and *B*, The knees of an 11-year-old boy with osteochondritis dissecans of the right knee. Notice the effusion and the lack of full extension in the right knee.

Pain resulting from the impingement of the lateral aspect of the medial femoral condyle against the tibia constitutes a positive test.

Radiographs are central to the diagnosis and management of OCD. Plain films should include posteroanterior, lateral, and tunnel views. When plain films indicate the presence of an osteochondral lesion **(Figure 31A.5),** advanced imaging is used to stage the disease[27] **(Table 31A.3).** Magnetic resonance imaging (MRI) is currently the modality of choice **(Figure 31A.6).** Staging is important to determine the clinical stability of osteochondral lesions and the need for surgical intervention. Typically, stage 1 and 2 lesions can be managed conservatively, whereas stage 3 and 4 lesions require surgery. Arthroscopy is the gold standard for defining osteochondral injuries,[25] particularly if there is confusion regarding the extent of the injury on the basis of MRI alone.

Treatment

The treatment of OCD lesions in children and adolescents differs from their treatment in adults. Most OCD lesions in the pediatric population can be managed conservatively. Patients who have nondisplaced lesions and who are skeletally immature should be treated conservatively.[25] Sports activity should be suspended for a minimum of 6 to 8 weeks. Conservative treatment specifically entails gentle range-of-motion activity, protected weight bearing, and strengthening of the quadriceps complex. The goal of protected weight bearing is to unload the affected extremity. The use of dedicated physical therapy is quite helpful in this setting. Patients who continue to have symptoms despite conservative therapy, patients with mechanical symptoms that are consistent with a loose body, and all patients with stage 3 or 4 lesions should be referred for arthroscopic exploration and debridement (SOR: C).[28]

TRAUMATIC KNEE INJURIES

Traumatic knee injuries are rare among young children. As athletes age, however, they are susceptible to the same patterns of injuries as adults. The most commonly injured structures of the knee in young athletes are the menisci, the anterior cruciate ligament, and the medial collateral ligament. The principles of the diagnosis and treatment of traumatic knee injuries for children are largely the same as for adults, as discussed in Chapter 27, Lower Leg Injuries.

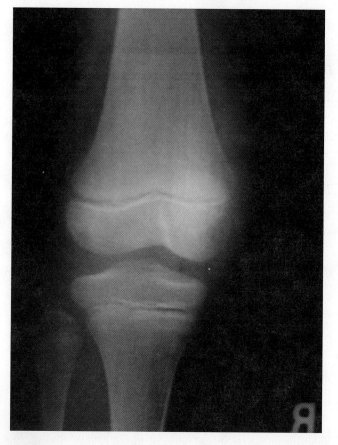

Figure 31A.5 An anteroposterior x-ray demonstrating osteochondritis dissecans of the lateral femoral condyle.

Disorders of the hip

Table 31A.3 Magnetic Resonance Imaging Staging of Osteochondritis Dissecans[27,53]

Stage 1	Low-intensity signal change that is consistent with injury to the articular cartilage; normal subchondral bone
Stage 2	High-intensity signal change that is consistent with articular cartilage compromise; subchondral fragment stable
Stage 3	High-intensity signal consistent with articular cartilage compromise; subchondral fragment dissociated from subchondral bone but partially attached
Stage 4	Frank loose body

DISORDERS OF THE HIP

Slipped capital femoral epiphysis

Mechanism

Slipped capital femoral epiphysis (SCFE) **(Figure 31A.7)** is the most common musculoskeletal disorder of the hip among adolescents.[29] It occurs when a shear force across the proximal femoral epiphysis is sufficient to cause a posteromedial displacement of the epiphysis with respect to the metaphysis. In addition to these biomechanical forces, there is also a genetic predisposition to SCFE. The condition is also more common among patients with hypothyroidism, panhypopituitarism, and renal osteodystrophy, raising the possibility of an endocrine contribution to the disease as well.

Clinical features

Obese males between 8 and 15 years of age are at the highest risk for SCFE. The condition is more common among black children than white or Hispanic children. In 30% to 50% of cases, the condition is bilateral.[30] The incidence of SCFE is roughly 2 per 100,000. Patients typically present with vague and chronic hip,

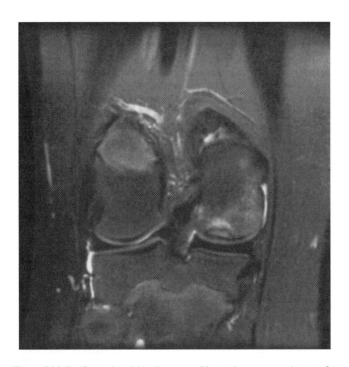

Figure 31A.6 Osteochondritis dissecans. Magnetic resonance image of the knee. Note the defect of the lateral aspect of the medial femoral condyle. (Photo courtesy of Dr. Ulrich A. Rassner.)

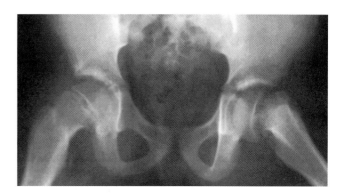

Figure 31A.7 Slipped capital femoral epiphysis. Note the slippage of the left femoral head relative to the femoral shaft. (Photo courtesy of Dr. Ulrich A. Rassner.)

groin, or medial knee pain. In one series, nearly 25% of patients with SCFE initially presented with knee pain.[31] For this reason, all young patients presenting with knee pain should also undergo a thorough examination of the hip. There may or may not be a history of antecedent trauma. Patients often present with a noticeable limp with the affected extremity held in a posture of flexion, abduction, and external rotation.

Diagnosis

Obese adolescents who present with a history of hip, groin, or medial knee pain of weeks' to months' duration should be considered to have SCFE until proven otherwise. Depending on the degree of slippage, the affected SCFE joint is considered to be either stable or unstable. Patients with stable SCFE present with a mildly antalgic gait and manifest the telltale sign of pain at the limit of passive internal rotation of the hip. Extreme passive external rotation is also often painful.

As the slip progresses, pain increases, the limp becomes more pronounced, and the affected extremity is forced into the characteristic position of external rotation, abduction, and flexion. When the patient is unable to bear weight, the joint is considered to be unstable. Susceptible patients presenting in severe pain with the extremity held in external rotation with a clinical history that is consistent with SCFE should not bear weight until radiographs can be obtained to either confirm or exclude the diagnosis. Unnecessary manipulation of the hip should be avoided until radiographs are obtained to prevent iatrogenic transformation of a stable SCFE into an unstable SCFE.

Anteroposterior, lateral, and frog-leg hip views of the affected and unaffected hips should be obtained. Radiographs of the affected extremity define the degree of slippage. Early during the course of the disease, radiographs may be normal. As the slip progresses, a step off is noted at the anterior epiphyseal–metaphyseal junction. *Klein's line* refers to a straight line drawn along the superior surface of the femoral neck on an anteroposterior film **(Figure 31A.8).** In the normal state, this line runs through the superior pole of the femoral head. In early SCFE, Klein's line is even with the superior pole of the femoral head. As the slip progresses, the femoral head falls below Klein's line.

Treatment

SCFE lesions should be managed in consultation with an orthopedic surgeon. The definitive treatment for SCFE is orthopedic pinning.[32] Both stable and unstable SCFE lesions can be fixed with a single in situ pin. In cases of stable SCFE, consultation should occur within 36 hours; unstable cases should be evaluated within 24 hours. In either case, the patient must not bear weight

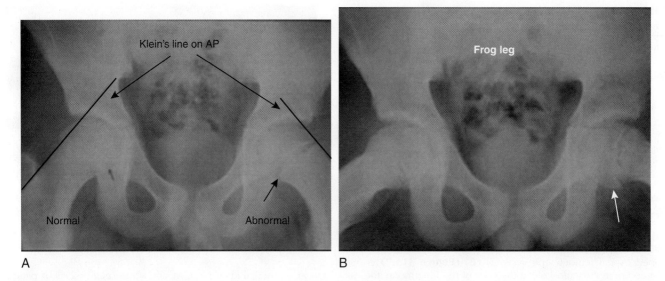

Figure 31A.8 Anteroposterior pelvis *(A)* and frog-leg *(B)* images demonstrating slipped capital femoral epiphysis of the left hip. *A,* Klein's line barely intersects the left femoral head on the anteroposterior view. *B,* The frog-leg view demonstrates the classic "ice cream falling off the cone" appearance of the left hip.

until he or she is evaluated by an orthopedist. Delays in diagnosis and treatment increase the risk for avascular necrosis, arthritic degeneration, and the potential need for hip replacement.[33]

Legg–Calvé–Perthes disease (osteochondrosis of the capital femoral epiphysis)
Mechanism
Legg–Calve–Perthes disease (LCPD) is a temporary condition in which the femoral head of young patients loses its vascular supply. The result is short-term femoral osteonecrosis and subsequent bony regeneration. The exact cause and mechanism are unknown. The condition is self-limiting because, with gradual revascularization, the femoral head resorbs, reorganizes, and heals.

Clinical features
LCPD typically presents in males who are between 4 and 10 years of age. There is a 4:1 male-to-female predilection,[34,35] and 80% of cases are unilateral. Patients present with an intermittent limp and pain of the groin or medial thigh caused by local joint irritation that is associated with the avascular changes of the femoral head. Pain often radiates to the knee, and it is worsened with motion and relieved with rest. Age is a key feature because patients who present after the age of 8 years have a poorer prognosis than those who present earlier. Females also typically have a poorer prognosis than males.[35] The primary long-term complication of LCPD is premature arthritis and degeneration of the hip.

Four stages of LCPD have been defined radiographically. In stage 1, there is an interruption of the blood supply to the femoral head. Growth around the capital femoral epiphysis ceases, and this is manifested as a physically smaller femoral head and a widening of the articular space on the affected side. This phase lasts for several months or up to a year. During stage 2, there is an initiation of healing as the blood supply returns and bony regeneration starts. Stage 2 reveals subchondral fractures within the epiphysis of the femoral head; this stage can last from 1 to 3 years. Stage 3 shows evidence of bone resorption as the femoral head continues to remodel; this stage also lasts from 1 to 3 years.

Stage 4 shows evidence of reossification with new bone formation and healing.

Diagnosis
On physical examination, patients often have limited active internal rotation and abduction of the hip. They may also have pain at the limits of passive internal rotation. Patients will often present with a limp. The key to diagnosis is clinical suspicion and appropriate radiographic evaluation. If clinical suspicion indicates, bone scans can be helpful for establishing avascular change in patients with normal early plain films.

Treatment
Treatment of LCPD can be surgical or nonsurgical, but most patients respond well to nonsurgical treatments. Patients who present with LCPD at less than 8 years of age do particularly well with conservative therapy. Specifically, this consists of a combination of bracing, orthotics, no weight bearing, and staged exercise rehabilitation. These patients should be managed in consultation with a musculoskeletal specialist. Patients who present after 8 years of age or with significant radiographic change show improved outcomes with surgical intervention and should be managed in consultation with an orthopedic specialist (LOE: C).[36]

DISEASES OF THE SPINE

Spondylolysis
Mechanism
The term *spondylolysis* refers to a stress fracture of the pars interarticularis of the vertebral body.[37] It is a relatively common cause of back pain in the adolescent athlete, but the true mechanism of injury is not known. Shear forces across the facet joint and the pars interarticularis occur with excess loading and repetitive flexion and extension of the back, and this results in a stress fracture of the pars[37] **(Figure 31A.9).** Excessive lordosis (associated with hyperextension of the back in sports such as gymnastics), excessive loading (associated with weight lifting or repetitive landing sports), and heredity also play roles in the pathophysiology of spondylolysis.[4]

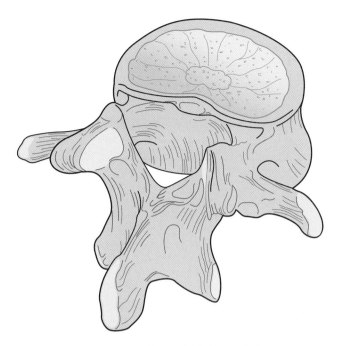

Figure 31A.9 Stress fractures in spondylolysis occur in the pars interarticularis. This drawing depicts bilateral spondylolytic fractures that would predispose an individual to spondylolisthesis. (Redrawn from Canale ST: Campbell's Operative Orthopaedics, 10th ed. Philadelphia, Mosby, 2002.)

For a discussion of the diagnosis and treatment of spondylolysis, see Part B of this chapter.

Spondylolisthesis

A bilateral pars interarticularis defect with a complete fracture and associated slippage of one vertebra across another is referred to as *spondylolisthesis.* The exact cause is not known, but the mechanism is felt to be the result of a repetitive overload of the posterior spinal elements leading to bilateral fractures of the pars interarticularis. Weight lifters are at particular risk. Patients present with signs and symptoms similar to those seen with spondylolysis, although radicular symptoms are more common with spondylolisthesis. The principles of the diagnosis and management of spondylolisthesis are similar to those of spondylolysis[38] **(Figure 31A.10).**

Lateral plain films are used to grade the degree of slippage in patients with spondylolisthesis. Grading is defined as the degree of translation of one vertebral segment relative to the adjacent segment. Grade I is defined as a slippage of 0% to 25%; grade II is a slippage of 25% to 50%; grade III slippage is 50% to 75%; grade IV slippage is 75% to 100%, and grade V slippage is slippage of more than 100%.[39] MRI is helpful to evaluate for spinal cord or nerve root compression in patients with focal neurologic symptoms (see Figure 24.17).

Patients with grade I and II slippage can be managed conservatively with activity modification, physical therapy, and bracing. The principles for return to activity are the same as for spondylolysis. Patients with greater degrees of slippage are candidates for potential surgical intervention and should be referred accordingly.

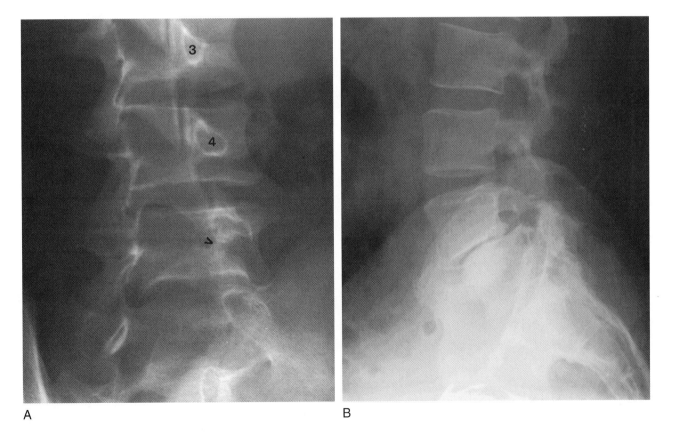

A

B

Figure 31A.10 *A,* A defect in the pars interarticularis of L5 *(arrowhead)* is seen on the oblique radiograph. The normal bony continuity of the pars (the "neck of the Scottie dog") of L3 and L4 can also be appreciated. *B,* The pars interarticularis defect of spondylolysis. Note the "Scottie dog" collar. (*A,* From DeLee JC, Drez D Jr, Miller MD [eds]: DeLee & Drez's Orthopedic Sports Medicine: Principles and Practice, 2nd ed. Philadelphia, WB Saunders, 2003. *B,* Photo courtesy of Dr. Ulrich A. Rassner.)

Scoliosis

Scoliosis can be divided into several forms: infantile (<3 years of age), juvenile (3 to 10 years of age), and adolescent (10 years of age through skeletal maturity).[40] Idiopathic adolescent scoliosis is the form that will be encountered most commonly by primary care physicians. Although the exact pathophysiology is not known, it is clear that genetics play a central role in the development of scoliosis. The prevalence of idiopathic scoliosis in the general adolescent population is 2% to 4%. Higher rates are noted among swimmers, gymnasts, and dancers.[39]

Clinical features

Most cases of scoliosis are incidentally noted. Although patients with scoliosis can present with back pain, scoliosis itself is not a primary cause of low back pain. Previous recommendations called for routine population screening to detect scoliosis in adolescents. The most recent US Preventive Services Task Force Guidelines, however, recommend against routine screening for scoliosis (LOE: A).[41]

Diagnosis

On physical examination, most patients have thoracic scoliotic curves that deviate to the right. The Adams forward bend test is an office test that can be used to assess for scoliosis. To perform this test, the patient is asked to bend forward at the hips with the arms extended slightly forward. The examiner stands behind the patient and looks for an asymmetry of the thoracic cage ("rib hump") that manifests as thoracic rotational deformity with forward flexion of the spine.

Radiographs also play a central role in the management of idiopathic adolescent scoliosis. Films should be obtained to determine the degree of curvature as well as the level of skeletal maturity. The degree of curvature is calculated using the Cobb angle on a standard posteroanterior film. This angle is calculated by determining the intersection of two lines drawn perpendicular to the superior and inferior most vertebrae of the scoliotic curve **(Figure 31A.11)**; the angle formed by the intersection of these two lines is the Cobb angle. The degree of skeletal maturity is determined by assessing the amount of bony fusion of the iliac crest. The iliac apophysis ossifies in a predictable fashion from lateral to medial. The level of ossification correlates well with skeletal maturity.

Treatment

The treatment of patients with idiopathic adolescent scoliosis is based on both the degree of curvature and the level of skeletal maturity.[40] Skeletally immature patients with curves of less than 20 degrees can be managed by observation and serial examinations. Skeletally immature patients with curves between 20 and 30 degrees should be considered for bracing. Skeletally immature patients with curves of greater than 30 degrees should be referred to an orthopedic surgeon for potential surgical intervention. At present, there is no evidence that specific exercise either worsens or reduces the degree of curvature. Similarly, there is no evidence that spinal manipulation alters the degree of curvature.[39] Scoliosis itself does not preclude an athlete from participation. Patients with severe curves, however, will require activity modification during phases of active treatment or bracing.

DISORDERS OF THE UPPER EXTREMITY

Little Leaguer's elbow (medial epicondylar apophysitis/avulsion and osteochondritis dissecans)

The term *Little Leaguer's elbow* generically refers to elbow pain in young throwing athletes.[42] Young overhead athletes typically have

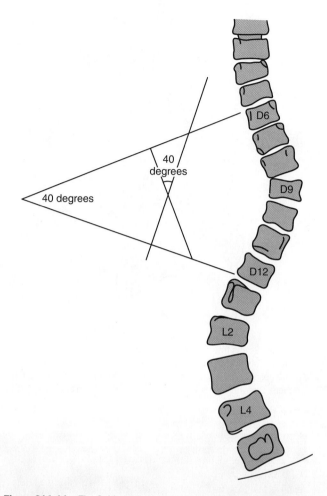

Figure 31A.11 The Cobb angle can be measured by the angle formed from the intersection of the two vertebral lines or by the angle of intersection of their perpendiculars. (From Grainger et al: Diagnostic Radiology: A Textbook of Medical Imaging. Philadelphia, Churchill Livingstone, 2001.)

relatively poor mechanics and poor core strength, and they are prone to throwing more with enthusiasm rather than with technique. This in combination with early sports specialization can predispose young throwers to injury. During the cocking phase of the overhead throw, valgus forces are placed on the medial elbow structures (the medial collateral ligament and the humeral epicondyle). There is compensatory compression of the lateral elbow structures (particularly the capitellum) at the same time. This excess tension, valgus strain, and lateral compressive force results in osteochondral change at the capitellum (see earlier section on OCD) and apophyseal changes at the medial epicondyle. If medial forces exceed apophyseal tissue load capacity, an avulsion fracture is the result **(Figure 31A.12)**. See Chapter 20, Elbow Injuries, for descriptions of the features and treatment of these injuries.

For Little Leaguer's elbow and Little Leaguer's shoulder, prevention is important. Youths who throw too much, too soon, and too fast are particularly at risk. Young throwing athletes should not be allowed to overpitch. Strong evidence suggests that programs to limit pitch count among young throwers are effective for reducing overuse syndromes. In particular, a pitch count of between 300 and 600 pitches per season (50 to 75 pitches per outing) has been associated with the lowest incidence of medial epicondylar apophysitis.[43]

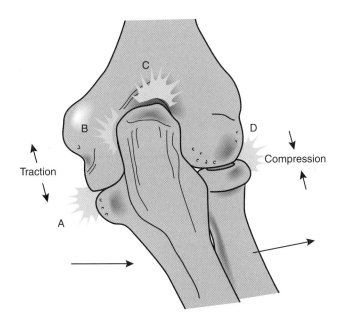

Medial   Lateral

Figure 31A.12 During the throwing motion, the medial elbow structures experience traction forces while the lateral structures undergo compressive loading. Sites A through D are typical sites of injury. (From DeLee JC, Drez D Jr, Miller MD [eds]: DeLee & Drez's Orthopedic Sports Medicine: Principles and Practice, 2nd ed. Philadelphia, WB Saunders, 2003.)

Supracondylar humeral fractures
Mechanism
Supracondylar fractures of the humerus in children merit special mention because of the unique neurovascular structure of the elbow and the potential for adverse long-term sequelae associated with this type of fracture. Supracondylar humeral fractures occur most commonly among children around 7 years of age. They account for more than 70% of elbow fractures in children.[44] In 98% of cases, the injury is the result of an extension mechanism, typically when the patient falls on an outstretched hand. In 2% of cases, the fracture is the result of a flexion injury.

The diagnosis of a supracondylar humeral fracture is one not to be missed. Chronic complications from supracondylar fractures include cubitus varus, median or radial nerve injury, and Volkmann's ischemic contracture. A further discussion of condylar fractures and supracondylar fractures can be found in Chapter 20, Elbow Injuries.

Clinical features
Patients typically present with pain and swelling of the affected extremity. Patients will often favor the affected extremity, holding it in flexion against the torso. It is particularly important to perform a careful neurovascular examination to document the presence of distal pulses and to ensure the integrity of distal median and ulnar nerve function. It is also very important that the evaluating physician look carefully for potential signs of child abuse in all young patients who present with supracondylar fractures.

Diagnosis
Anteroposterior and lateral plain films should be obtained when a fracture is suspected. Patients can be splinted in 30 degrees of flexion for comfort[45] while awaiting radiographs. It is helpful to obtain films of the contralateral extremity, because radiographic findings can be subtle. A useful anatomic landmark

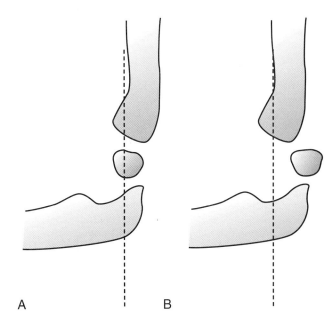

A   B

Figure 31A.13 *A*, A line drawn down the anterior surface of the humerus on a lateral film should transect the middle of the capitellum. *B*, With an extension supracondylar fracture, the line passes more anteriorly. (Redrawn from Marx et al: Rosen's Emergency Medicine: Concepts and Clinical Practice, 6th ed. Philadelphia, Mosby, 2005.)

in supracondylar fractures is the anterior humeral line. On the lateral radiograph, a line is dropped from the anterior humeral cortex through the capitellum; this line should pass through the middle third of the capitellum[45] **(Figure 31A.13)**. Another useful radiographic sign is the fat pad or "ship's sail" sign that occurs with subtle or occult elbow fractures **(Figure 31A.14)**. Interruption of the intra-articular space around the elbow results in a hemarthrosis

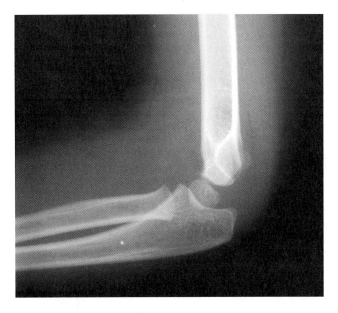

Figure 31A.14 The "sail sign." An increased anterior fat pad on lateral elbow radiographs indicates a fracture, even if no fracture is apparent on x-rays. The appearance of any posterior fat pad lucency is also abnormal. This x-ray demonstrates an obvious supracondylar fracture with both an anterior sail sign and a posterior fat pad being visible. (From Marx et al: Rosen's Emergency Medicine: Concepts and Clinical Practice, 6th ed. Philadelphia, Mosby, 2005.)

that is apparent radiographically as the pathognomonic fat pad. The fat pad sign can be either anterior or posterior, and it is associated with fractures of the radial head as well as the humerus. The posterior fat pad is typically associated with supracondylar fractures.

Supracondylar fractures are graded on the basis of the level of displacement. Type I fractures are nondisplaced, and a posterior fat pad sign is often present. Type II fractures are moderately displaced, but the posterior cortex is intact. Type III fractures are completely displaced in either the posteromedial or posterolateral planes.[46]

Treatment

The goal of the treatment of supracondylar humeral fractures is always anatomic reduction with the preservation of function. Type I fractures can be managed by immobilization in a long-arm splint for 3 weeks. Repeat x-rays and close follow-up are required to ensure that the fracture does not displace to a type II fracture. Because of their high-risk nature, it is preferable to manage type I fractures in conjunction with orthopedic surgery. After 3 weeks in a long-arm splint and x-rays that verify no fracture displacement, patients with type I fractures can begin range-of-motion activity if the patient is pain free. Type II and III supracondylar fractures require reduction and fixation and mandate orthopedic referral. Full return to activity after type II and III supracondylar fractures may take up to 1 full year.

Rotator cuff impingement/swimmer's shoulder
Mechanism

The muscles of the rotator cuff (the supraspinatus, the infraspinatus, the teres minor, and the subscapularis) form a common tendon (the rotator cuff) that helps to situate the head of the humerus within the glenoid fossa to provide stability. However, the shoulder joint sacrifices stability to increase mobility, thereby allowing for the precise positioning of the hand in space. This lack of stability predisposes the shoulder joint to sporting injury, particularly with repetitive overhead motion. This is particularly true among young athletes who have more inherent laxity than older patients. Injuries to the rotator cuff typically occur among older adolescents who participate in overhead sports activities. For example, it is estimated that competitive swimmers who swim up to 7000 m per day will perform more than 750,000 shoulder rotations per year.[47] Thus, it is easy to imagine how the soft-tissue structures of the shoulder are subject to considerable tensile overload, impingement, and instability. Despite this, tears of the rotator cuff are extremely rare among young athletes. The anatomy of the shoulder is reviewed in Chapter 9, Physical Examination of the Shoulder.

Clinical features

Patients with rotator cuff impingement typically present with the complaints of night pain, a sore shoulder, or a "dead arm." Symptoms often have been present for weeks to months before presentation.[4] The pain is often vague, but it is located anteriorly or laterally and exacerbated with overhead activity.

Diagnosis

The diagnosis of impingement is based on the clinical history and specific signs found during the physical examination. The previously described Neer's, Hawkins', and empty beer can tests (see Chapter 9, Physical Examination of the Shoulder) are used to determine the affected anatomic structures. However, it is important to note that rotator cuff injuries among young patients are typically the result of instability or laxity rather than degeneration or arthritis.

It is important to query young athletes about a history of prior shoulder dislocations and to test for glenohumeral instability by using the crank test or the load-shift test or looking for the sulcus sign (see Chapter 9, Physical Examination of the Shoulder). Plain films of the shoulder, including anteroposterior, outlet, and axillary views, may be obtained to assess underlying bony integrity. If necessary, MRI is the diagnostic imaging modality of choice to evaluate rotator cuff integrity.[16]

Treatment

The treatment of rotator cuff impingement centers on activity modification and shoulder rehabilitation. Shoulder rehabilitation exercises (see Chapter 21, Part A, Soft-Tissue Shoulder Injuries) are specifically designed to balance the shoulder musculature and strengthen the rotator cuff. Because the rotator cuff is the primary dynamic stabilizer of the shoulder, these exercises lead to improved glenohumeral stability and allow for pain-free overhead movement. If no improvement is noted after 6 to 12 weeks, an MRI should be obtained[46] and referral to a sports medicine specialist considered. It is imperative that athletes with a history of rotator cuff problems or glenohumeral instability continue to perform these exercises even while they are pain free to prevent the recurrence of symptoms.

The diagnosis and treatment of shoulder pain in the young athlete is also discussed in Chapter 21, Part A, Soft-Tissue Shoulder Injuries.

PREVENTION OF INJURY IN YOUNG ATHLETES

Sports and athletics are inextricable components of modern American society. The push to participate and the pressure to succeed undoubtedly contribute to many otherwise preventable injuries. With this in mind, there are several principles that should govern participation in youth sports[48,49]:

- Children should always participate in athletics at a level that is commensurate with their skills and abilities.
- Organized sporting activities should always have adequate supervision.
- Organized sporting activities should always provide participants with the proper protective equipment.
- Training programs for young athletes should always proceed at the proper intensity.
- Early recognition and treatment can prevent numerous overuse injuries, and the proper use of protective athletic equipment can prevent numerous traumatic injuries.

CONCLUSION

Children have a unique musculoskeletal system and experience a different set of sports-related injuries than adults. Because an open growth plate is typically the weakest link in the musculotendinous kinetic chain, children and adolescents are at high risk for growth plate injury, many of which can be serious. An understanding of the unique risk factors of young athletes coupled with knowledge of the wide array of injuries that can occur in pediatric athletes will help the sports medicine physician better care for this young and vulnerable population.

REFERENCES

1. Adirim T, Cheng T: Overview of injuries in the young athlete. Sports Med 2003;33(1):75.
2. Kann L, Kinchen SA, Williams B, et al: Youth risk behavioral surveillance–United States, 1999. MMWR CDC Surveill Summ 2000;49(5):1-32.

3. Stanitski C: Primary care of the injured athlete. Part 2: Pediatric and adolescent sports injuries. Clin Sports Med 1997;16(4).

4. Bernhardt D, Landry G: Sports injuries in young athletes. Adv Pediatr 1995;42:465-500.

5. Hawkins D, Metheny J: Overuse injuries in youth sports: biomechanical considerations. Med Sci Sports Exerc 2001;33(10):1701-1707.

6. Gill T IV, Micheli L: The immature athlete: common injuries and overuse syndromes of the elbow and wrist. Clin Sports Med 1996;15(2):401-423.

7. DiFiori J: Overuse injuries in children and adolescents. Phys Sportsmed 1999;27(1):95-99.

8. Conn J, Annest J, Gilcrist J: Sports and recreation related injury episodes in the US population, 1997–1999. Inj Prev 2003;9:117-123.

9. Robinson J: Diagnostic workup of sports injuries. Can Fam Physician 1993;39:1754-1758.

10. Chambers H: Ankle and foot disorders in skeletally immature athletes. Orthop Clin North Am 2003;34:45-459.

11. Steill I, et al: Decision rules for the use of radiography in acute ankle injuries. Refinement and prospective validation. JAMA 1993;269(9):1127-1132.

12. Beynnon BD, Renstrom PA, Haugh L, et al: A prospective, randomized clinical investigation of the treatment of first-time ankle sprains. Am J Sports Med 2006;34(9):1401-1412.

13. Kerkoffs G, et al: Immobilisation and functional treatment for acute lateral injuries in adults. Cochrane Database Syst Rev 2002;3:CD003762.

14. Patel D, Greydanus D, Luckstead E Sr: The college athlete. Pediatr Clin North Am 2005;52:25-60.

15. Hendrix C: Calcaneal apophysitis (Sever disease). Clin Podiatr Med Surg North Am 2005;22(1):55-62.

16. Ryu R, Fan R: Adolescent and pediatric sports injuries. Pediatr Clin North Am 1998;45(6):1601-1635.

17. Roach J: Knee disorders and injuries in adolescents. Adolesc Med 1998;9(3):589-597.

18. Juhn M: Patellofemoral pain syndrome: a review and guidelines for treatment. Am Fam Physician 1999;60:2012-2022.

19. Heinties E, et al: Exercise therapy for patellofemoral pain syndrome. Cochrane Database Syst Rev 2003;4:CD003472.

20. Heinties E, et al: Pharmacotherapy for patellofemoral pain syndrome. Cochrane Database Syst Rev 2004;3:CD003470.

21. Cutbill J, et al: Anterior knee pain: a review. Clin J Sports Med 1997;7:40-45.

22. Gigante A, et al: Increased external tibial torsion in Osgood-Schlatter disease. Acta Orthop Scand 2003;74(4):431-436.

23. Bloom O, Mackler L: Clinical inquiries. What is the best treatment for Osgood-Schlatter disease? J Fam Pract 2004;53(2):153-156.

24. Flowers M, Bhadreshwar D: Tibial tuberosity excision for symptomatic Osgood-Schlatter disease. J Pediatr Orthop 1995;15:292-297.

25. Bruce E, Hamby T, Jones D: Sports-related osteochondral injuries: clinical presentation, diagnosis and treatment. Prim Care 2005;32(1):253-276.

26. Hixon A, Gibbs L: Osteochondritis dissecans: a diagnosis not to miss. Am Fam Physician 2000;61:151-158.

27. Loredo R, Sanders T: Imaging of osteochondral injuries. Clin Sports Med 2001;20(2):249-278.

28. Kocher M, et al: Management of osteochondritis dissecans of the knee: current concepts. Am J Sports Med 2006;34(7):1181-1191.

29. Manoff E, Banffy M, Winell J: Relationship between body mass index and slipped capital femoral epiphysis. J Pediatr Orthop 2005;25(6):744-746.

30. Lavallee M, Cox Cohoon K, Elek K: Fractures and Dislocations. In American Academy of Physicians (ed): Home Study Self-Assessment Program, Volume 273. Leawood, KS, American Academy of Family Physicians, 2002.

31. Matava M, et al: Knee pain as the initial symptom of slipped capital femoral epiphysis: an analysis of initial presentation and treatment. J Pediatr Orthop 1999;19(4):455-460.

32. Guzzanti V, Falciglia F, Stanitski C: Slipped capital femoral epiphysis in skeletally immature patients. J Bone Joint Surg Br 2004;86(5):731-736.

33. Loder R: Slipped capital femoral epiphysis. Am Fam Physician 1998;57(9):2135-2150.

34. Boyd K, Peirce N, Batt M: Common hip injuries in sport. Sports Med 1997;24(4):273-288.

35. Horn B, Moseley C: Current concepts in the management of pediatric hip disease. Curr Opin Rheumatol 1992;4(2):184-192.

36. Herring J, Kim H, Browne R: Legg-Calve-Perthes disease. Part II: Prospective multicenter study of the effect of treatment on outcomes. J Bone Joint Surg Am 2004;86-A(10):2121-2134.

37. Micheli L, Curtis C: Stress, fractures in the spine and sacrum. Clin Sports Med 2006;25(1):75-88.

38. Herman M, Pizzutillo P, Cavalier R: Spondylolysis and spondylolisthesis in the child and adolescent athlete. Orthop Clin North Am 2003;34(3):461-467, vii.

39. Baker R, Patel D: Lower back pain in the athlete: common conditions and treatment. Prim Care 2005;32(1):201-229.

40. Reamy B, Slakey J: Adolescent idiopathic scoliosis: review and current concepts. Am Fam Physician 2001;64:111-116.

41. U.S. Preventive Services Task Force: Screening for idiopathic scoliosis in adolescents. Available at http://www.ahrq.gov/clinic/uspstf/uspsaisc.htm. Accessed July 10, 2007.

42. Gerbino P: Elbow disorders in throwing athletes. Orthop Clin North Am 2003;34(3):417-426.

43. Lyman S, et al: Effect of pitch type, pitch count and pitching mechanics on risk of elbow and shoulder pain in youth baseball pitchers. Am J Sports Med 2002;30(4):463-468.

44. de las Heras J, et al: Supracondylar fractures of the humerus in children. Clin Orthop Relat Res 2005;432:57-64.

45. Lins R, Simovitch R, Waters P: Pediatric elbow trauma. Orthop Clin North Am 1999;30(1):119-132.

46. Wilkins K: Fractures and dislocations of the elbow region. In Rockwood C, Wilkins K, King R (eds): Fractures in Children. Philadelphia, Lippincott-Raven, 1996, pp 363-375.

47. Chen F et al: Shoulder and elbow injuries in the skeletally immature athlete. J Am Acad Orthop Surg 2005;13:172-185.

48. American Academy of Pediatrics: Intensive training and sports specialization in young athletes. Pediatrics 2000;106(1):154-157.

49. Current comment from the American College of Sports Medicine. August 1993–"The prevention of sport injuries of children and adolescents." Med Sci Sports Exerc 1993;28(5):S1-S7.

Part B SPONDYLOLYSIS: A PRACTICAL APPROACH TO AN ADOLESCENT ENIGMA

Francis G. O'Connor, MD, MPH; Pierre A. d'Hemecourt, MD; and Melissa Nebzydoski, DO

KEY POINTS

- Spondylolysis is a controversial and complex disorder that presents many diagnostic and management challenges to the physician.
- Spondylolysis should be suspected and must be ruled out of the differential diagnosis in any young athlete with extension-related low back pain.
- Oblique x-rays should not be used to diagnose spondylolysis because they expose the patient to increased levels of radiation and will only detect one third of pars interarticularis fractures. Instead, posteroanterior and lateral x-rays plus single photon emission computed tomography scanning should be used as the initial imaging modalities in the spondylolysis workup.
- Fine-cut computed tomography is a useful secondary imaging modality for antatomic diagnosis and risk stratification.
- Athletes with proven spondylolysis who continue to have pain after 4 months of treatment should undergo repeat computed tomography scanning to evaluate healing and to guide further therapy.

INTRODUCTION

Spondylolysis is among the most controversial, complex, and challenging disorders that confront the sports clinician. Strategies for management range from benign neglect to prolonged bracing and electrical bone stimulators and, eventually, to surgical intervention. Although the literature suggests that the natural history of this disorder may be favorable, questions remain regarding the impact of this ailment on the early termination of sports participation as well as its possible role in degenerative lumbar disease in later years. This chapter represents the authors' preferred strategy for attempting to sequence and orchestrate the complex roles of imaging, activity modification, bracing, and physical therapy in the diagnosis and management of the athlete with active spondylolysis. The cornerstone philosophy of this algorithm remains the belief that spondylolysis represents a fracture and thus warrants all attempts to facilitate fracture healing.

DIAGNOSIS

Spondylolysis is a clinical diagnosis that is suggested by a history of extension-related low back pain. The diagnosis is especially common in athletes who are involved in high-risk sports activities, including football blocking, military press, tennis serving, baseball pitching, gymnastics back walkover, and the butterfly swim stroke. Athletes typically have low back pain that is aggravated by extension with occasional radiation to the buttocks and associated hamstring tightness. The single-leg hyperextension (i.e., the stork test,

see Figure 24.10) assists with the confirmation of a clinical diagnosis of an active spondylolysis lesion.

The role and timing of imaging in the diagnosis of spondylolysis is controversial. Traditionally, spondylolysis has been diagnosed by the clinician using a five-view radiographic series of the lumbar spine that includes anteroposterior, lateral, spot, and oblique views. Studies have shown, however, that the vast majority of spondylolysis defects can be ascertained without the additional radiation incurred by adding oblique sequences. Congeni and colleagues explained that anteroposterior, lateral, spot, and bilateral oblique views can be useful for evaluating spondylolisthesis but that especially oblique radiographs are not as sensitive for detecting spondylolysis and expose the patient to the same surface radiation as a computed tomography (CT) scan.[1] Further evidence also suggests that an oblique view cannot always be considered reliable. A study done by Saifuddin and colleagues demonstrated that only 32% of pars defects will appear within 15 degrees of the 45-degree angle of the oblique view.[2]

Single photon emission computed tomography (SPECT) represents a radiographic imaging modality that can provide additional information to the clinician regarding the metabolic activity of the spondylolytic lesion. In a study done by Bellah and colleagues, it was found that SPECT bone scans are considered more sensitive but less specific than planar bone scans as a result of the anatomic overlap that occurs in planar images.[3] SPECT should still be used if plain radiographs are negative when there is high suspicion for spondylolysis. Lesions that are identified as "hot" imply a stress reaction with an active fracture site. Alternatively, "cold" lesions suggest chronic or terminal defects, which tend to be asymptomatic. Differentiating between "hot" and "cold" lesions is important because it can affect both the protocol and goals of treatment.

Reverse gantry CT scanning, when performed with fine-cut sequences, is of great use to the clinician who is managing spondylolysis. Not only does this modality clearly and more specifically identify the anatomic location of the lesion, but it assists with risk stratifying the fracture for the management protocol. CT can also assist in identifying other etiologies of low back pain where the SPECT is positive, such as an osteoid osteoma. In a study done by Congeni and colleagues, lesions were classified as acute fractures, subacute or healing fractures, or terminal, nonunion fractures on CT scan.[1] This classification allows more aggressive treatment with activity restriction and bracing for fractures that are acute and subacute because they appear to have a better opportunity for bony healing. When treating spondylolysis, repeat CT scanning can also be considered after 4 months of treatment if there is no clinical improvement.

Magnetic resonance imaging (MRI) is not routinely used in the diagnosis of spondylolysis. However, MRI may be useful in those cases where prior imaging is found to be inconclusive or in which neurologic symptoms are present. When ordering an MRI to evaluate spondylolysis, it is important to involve a neuroradiologist to ensure that appropriate axial images are taken of not only the intervertebral discs but also of the pars interarticularis. MRI can be helpful for diagnosing early or prespondylitic lesions by showing high signal intensity on T2-weighted, fat-saturated images that appear as bone marrow edema. A retrospective study done by Ulmer and colleagues demonstrated that 40% of patients diagnosed with spondylolysis had reactive marrow change within the pedicles.[4]

Authors' preferred diagnostic strategy

In a young athlete who presents to the clinic with a 2- to 3-week history of extension-related low back pain, we currently order plain films (anteroposterior, lateral, and lumbar spot views) and a SPECT bone scan on the first clinic visit. These images allow us to diagnose the condition and to proceed with advanced imaging to properly risk stratify the lesion for management **(Figure 31B.1)**.

MANAGEMENT

If there is a high suspicion for spondylolysis in a young athlete on the basis of the history and physical examination findings, treatment is initiated at the first visit while a further diagnostic workup is ordered. Treatment (just as diagnosis) remains a controversial area and requires individualization. Early options include activity modification, a lumbar corset, or the initiation of a bracing protocol. Activity modification and physical therapy are initiated at the first visit; these and other treatment modalities will now be discussed in further detail.

Bracing

The role of bracing is controversial, with recommendations ranging from a simple off-the-shelf corset to a customized thoracolumbar-sacral orthosis. In the treatment described by Congeni and McClearly, a brace is prescribed for those individuals with either an acute reaction or an acute fracture on SPECT, whereas a corset may be used in a subacute fracture or a "cold" lesion on SPECT.[5] It is the authors' practice that after the diagnosis of spondylolysis is finalized a Boston overlap brace should be the treatment of choice for all acute and subacute fractures (see Figure 31B.1). Stress responses and chronic fractures may be initially treated with a lumbar corset brace. The brace is fitted at 0 degrees of extension, worn for 23 to 24 hours a day, and only removed to bathe. This has been previously described in a study done by d'Hemecourt and colleagues.[6]

The first phase of brace treatment for spondylolysis involves fitting the Boston overlap brace and allowing several weeks for adjustment. Patients are counseled to carry on their normal daily activities but to avoid sports or other strenuous activities. In general, a stress reaction will be temporarily braced for 4 to 6 weeks, whereas an acute fracture will require bracing for 4 months. If a chronic fracture is diagnosed by a cold bone scan or an MRI without T2 signal intensity, the patient is only braced if symptoms are present or until symptoms resolve. In the event of a subacute fracture, with only mild uptake on bone scan, the bracing is variable, depending on symptoms and the age of the patient. In the adolescent who is experiencing a growth spurt, the brace may be used for the full duration of 4 months. Eighty percent of patients treated using this approach by d'Hemecourt and colleagues achieved good to excellent results.[7]

The patient is reevaluated after 4 to 6 weeks of brace treatment. At this time, the authors allow the athlete to return to modified play wearing the brace if he or she is pain free and comfortable in the brace. In addition to continued brace treatment, patients are instructed to continue physical therapy and home exercises that can improve and maintain flexibility, strength, and aerobic fitness. It is important to remember that the brace will inhibit

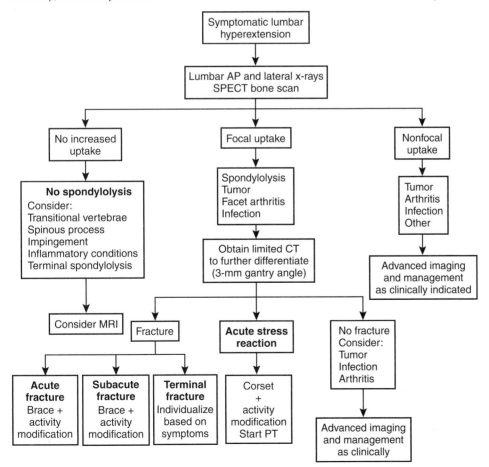

Figure 31B.1 Diagnostic imaging for the management of spondylolysis in a young athlete. AP, anterior posterior; PT, physical therapy; SPECT, single photon emission computed tomography.

Table 31B.1   Modified Boston Brace Protocol for Acute Spondylolysis in the Young Athlete

Week	Time in Brace	Activity/Rehabilitation Exercises
1 to 4	23 hours per day	Activities of daily living; no sports
5 to 8	23 hours per day	Gradual progression of core stabilization and flexibility with sport-specific drills and gradual sport participation
9 to 12	23.5 hours per day	Can be out of brace for selected rehabilitation exercises; sport participation allowed in brace if pain free
13 to 16	Wean from brace; increase time out of brace by 6 hours per week	Continue general conditioning; progressive trunk stabilization
17+	Soft lumbosacral corset during activity	Return to running program; transition back to sport-specific skills, practice, and play

some sports, such as a back walkover in gymnastics, but gymnasts may be able to start some bar and floor work. Other athletes, such as soccer players, can play while wearing the brace. It should be emphasized that the return to sports at this time is gradual and not sudden. The braces may be trimmed a few centimeters along the inferior and lateral borders to allow for better lateral motion.

Patients may slowly begin weaning from the brace during the fourth month. The weaning process takes place over 4 weeks, with the time out of the brace being increased by 6 hours each week, starting with the elimination of night wear. The use of a soft lumbosacral corset may afford added protection and comfort during the transition back to full activity.

Table **31B.1** summarizes the authors' recommendations for managing bracewear in the athlete with spondylolysis.

Physical therapy

During the initial phase of treatment, the authors start physical therapy that focuses on antilordotic (abdominal) strengthening and peripelvic flexibility. If the patient is pain free, the authors also allow cycling and freestyle swimming with no brace during this initial phase. Physical therapy is done out of the brace only if the athlete is demonstrates proficiency with the exercise protocol. At the 4- to 6-week visit, the athlete is progressed to phase 2 of the treatment if he or she reports being pain free during routine activities in the brace and having no pain on lumbar extension and stork testing.

The second phase of physical therapy is a continuation of phase 1 with the addition of neutral core stabilization exercises and extensor muscle strengthening but without allowing for lumbar hyperextension. Some examples include bridges and balance ball exercises. Initially, spine stabilization exercises are done in the brace, whereas limited range-of-motion exercises are attempted out of the brace. During the third month, neutral spine aerobic exercise can be done out of the brace. During phase 2, the patient may slowly return to sports as long as he or she remains pain free and continues to use the brace. Sport-specific drills are added before the actual return to play.

Bone stimulator

If the athlete continues to have pain at the 4-month mark, a CT scan should be repeated. If the patient is symptomatic and there is a nonunion on CT scan, the authors recommend the consideration of bone stimulation; options include pulsed ultrasound and electrical stimulation. Electrical stimulation is generally continued for 4 months at which time a CT scan is repeated, and the fracture is then reassessed for healing. Currently, however, there are no evidence-based indications or protocols for bone stimulation in the treatment of spondylolysis. The second author's institution is

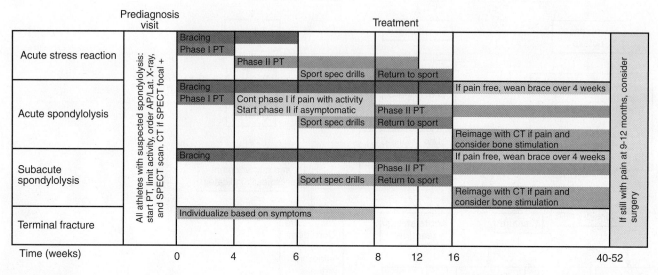

Figure 31B.2   Putting it all together: An overview of spondylolysis treatment. AP/Lat, anterior-posterior and lateral radiographs; PT, physical therapy; SPECT, single photon emission computed tomography.

currently engaged in ongoing research to ascertain the use and sequencing of bone stimulation for the treatment of this disorder.

Surgery

If the patient remains symptomatic and has a persistent nonunion at 9 to 12 months or if progression is made to spondylolisthesis grade III or IV, surgical posterolateral in situ fusion at L5 is recommended. A return to sports participation after surgery is allowed after there is demonstrated union and when the athlete is pain free and manifests a full range of motion.

Advanced imaging

If patients progress smoothly through rehabilitation without pain or other limitations, there is no need for follow-up radiographs or other studies to confirm healing. A follow-up bone scan/SPECT scan is not as useful clinically because the scan may remain positive well after the patient has recovered. However, if there is residual pain or other limitations, a CT scan may be helpful to assess the degree of healing. Persistent pain at 4 months merits patient reevaluation and a search for a possible comorbid diagnosis. If healed, the patient can be weaned from the brace, and another source of the patient's low back pain should be considered. If the interval CT demonstrates no healing, electrical stimulation with continued bracing should be considered.

CONCLUSION

Spondylolysis remains a complex and controversial disorder that confronts both the athlete and the sports clinician. Many diagnostic and treatment strategies are presented in the literature; the authors have presented a strategy that has been found to be successful for the treatment of many athletes with this condition. The sequencing of patient visits is demonstrated in **Figure 31B.2.** Ongoing research will hopefully improve the diagnosis and management of this disorder.

REFERENCES

1. Congeni J, McCulloch J, Swanson K: Lumbar spondylolysis: a study of natural progression in athletes. Am J Sports Med 1997;25:248-253.
2. Saifuddin A, White J, Tucker S, Taylor BA: Orientation of lumbar pars defects: implications for radiological detection and surgical management. J Bone Joint Surg 1998;80:208-211.
3. Bellah RD, Summerville DA, Treves ST, Micheli LJ: Low-back pain in adolescent athletes: detection of stress injury to the pars interarticularis with SPECT. Radiology 1991;180:509-512.
4. Ulmer JL, Elster AD, Mathews VP, Allen AM: Lumbar spondylolysis: reactive marrow changes seen in adjacent pedicles on MR images. Am J Roetgenol 1995;164:429-433.
5. McCleary MD, Congeni JA: Current concepts in the diagnosis and treatment of spondylolysis in young athletes. Curr Sports Med Rep 2007;6:62-66.
6. d'Hemecourt PA, Zurakowski D, Kriemler S, Micheli LJ: Spondylolysis: returning the athlete to sports participation with brace treatment. Orthopedics 2002;25:653-657.
7. d'Hemecourt PA, Gerbino PG, Micheli LJ: Back injuries in the young athlete. Clin Sports Med 2000;19:663-669.

Stress Fractures

MAJ Christopher M. Prior, DO, FAAFP,
and CPT Jessica A. Pesce, MS, PT

KEY POINTS

- Stress fractures are common injuries, accounting for up to 10% of diagnoses in primary care sports medicine clinics (LOE: B).[2]
- As a result of hormonal and anatomic factors, women are up to 12 times more likely than men to suffer a stress fracture (LOE: A).[1]
- Track and field athletes account for a large proportion of stress fracture injuries: half of all stress fracture injuries among male athletes will occur in track and field athletes, and two thirds of all female stress fractures are diagnosed in female track athletes (LOE: A).
- Initial imaging for suspected stress fractures includes plain films plus either magnetic resonance imaging or bone scan imaging. The choice between bone scan and MRI is largely made on the basis of cost and availability.
- Critical stress fractures are fractures with delayed healing or high potential for complications. These fractures should be aggressively identified, and patients with these injuries must be referred for early orthopedic intervention (LOE: varies on the basis of the specific fracture).
- Noncritical stress fractures are best managed by activity modification until the athlete is pain free for at least 2 weeks. After this, a gradual return to activity is allowed on the basis of clinical symptomatology (LOE: varies on the basis of the specific fracture).

INTRODUCTION

Overuse injuries involving both soft tissues and bones are extremely common among athletes. The cause of overuse injuries is usually multifactorial, and almost all overuse injures are preventable. An overuse injury involving bone is referred to as a *stress fracture*, and most of these fractures occur in the lower extremities.[1] In 2002, Matheson and colleagues[2] reported an incidence of stress fractures in sports medicine clinics that approached 10%.

TYPES OF STRESS FRACTURES AND THE PATHOPHYSIOLOGY OF BONY STRESS INJURY

There are two types of stress fractures: fatigue and insufficiency. A fatigue fracture involves a normal bone that is abnormally loaded, whereas an insufficiency fracture involves an abnormal bone that fails under normal stresses. These types of fractures are not mutually exclusive, and both involve a disruption of bone homeostasis.

A greater understanding of bone homeostasis is explained by Wolff's law, which relies on the increased reabsorption of bone by osteoclasts when bone is stressed. The osteoclastic activity stimulates osteoblasts to rebuild damaged bone. When the osteoclasts are more active than the osteoblasts, the bone is theoretically weaker and more vulnerable to fracture. Sufficient recovery time will result in stronger bone. Alternatively, insufficient recovery will result in accumulative microdamage, a loss of bone integrity, and stress fractures (Table 32.1).

CAUSES OF STRESS FRACTURES

The causes of stress fractures can be broken down into both intrinsic and extrinsic factors. Previous injury, misalignment, and low bone density are common intrinsic factors. The previous injury may be a stress fracture or perhaps any injury to the opposite leg that places greater stresses on the previously uninjured leg. An athlete with a history of stress fracture is 60% more likely to suffer another stress fracture.[3] Poor technique, poor training, and inadequate rehabilitation may contribute to recurrent injury. Improper alignment of the foot, ankle, or knee may accelerate the accumulated microtrauma that leads to stress fractures. For example, pes planus or cavus can put enormous stress on the metatarsals, which are then unable to properly dissipate forces as they would in a properly aligned, normal foot.

There are many causes of decreased bone density that are of great concern for female athletes; some of these can also be found in male athletes. Inadequate caloric intake or excessive expenditure can lead to a decreased bone density. Lower estrogen levels may increase calcium excretion, thereby decreasing bone density and accelerating remodeling. Relatively increased progesterone levels may have a similar effect. Contraceptives containing only progesterone can produce a relatively decreased estrogen level, which also predisposes athletes to a lower bone density and a

Table 32.1 Risk Factors for Stress Fracture

Intrinsic	Extrinsic
Poor alignment	Playing surfaces
Low bone density	Protective equipment
Previous injury	Training equipment

greater risk of stress fractures. Traditional oral contraceptive pills may provide enough estrogen to regulate menstrual cycles, but they will not correct the caloric deficit that sometimes causes the menstrual irregularities. Diets that are simply deficient in calcium will also increase the risk of stress fractures.[4] Thus, menstrual status is an imprecise marker for nutritional adequacy because an athlete may still be nutritionally deficient without exhibiting any correlating menstrual changes. Overall, females are 12 times more likely than males to suffer a stress fracture.[1]

Intrinsic factors that are somewhat controversial include improper muscle strength, balance, and inflexibility. It is well known that eccentric muscle contraction can function as an active shock absorber to lessen the repetitive microtrauma load on bone. Weak and fatigued muscles do not effectively dissipate these mechanical stresses, thus leaving bones vulnerable to stress fractures. Less well defined is the concept of muscular balance: when a muscle group is overpowered by its antagonist muscle group, a relative weakness may occur that can result in mechanical overload. Flexibility is often discussed as a risk factor for stress factors and overuse injuries. Although the precise interaction of flexibility and overuse injuries (including stress fractures) is much discussed, it is little studied and even less understood.

Protective equipment, playing surfaces, and training methods are examples of extrinsic causes of stress fractures. The weight of protective and training equipment can place excessive stresses on bone. Gradually increasing the amount of equipment carried, mileage, duration, and intensity can help decrease the incidence of overuse injuries and stress fractures. Another important consideration is the sport or the specific type of athletic activity. Track and field sports account for 50% of stress fractures among males and for 64% of these injuries among females in the general population.[5]

The most common site of lower-extremity stress fractures is the tibia. In children, these fractures are usually in the anterior proximal third of the tibia, whereas in adults they are usually at the junction of the middle and distal third.[6] Metatarsal fractures represent 25% of stress fractures, and these usually involve the distal second and third metatarsals.[7] Navicular stress fractures are the most common stress injuries of the tarsal bones[8] **(Box 32.1)**.

CLINICAL PRESENTATION OF STRESS FRACTURES (BOX 32.2)

Complaints that increase suspicion of a stress fracture include dull, bony, aching pain that worsens with activity or with the loading of the affected bone. Occasionally patients may recall a specific time when they felt a snap or another sensation of initial injury, although this is less common. Typically the pain initially occurs only during extended activity, and it then progresses to being present with any activity and finally to being persistent even at rest or at night. Bony tenderness to palpation is usually present, although stress fractures can develop in areas that are relatively inaccessible to direct palpation. Stress fractures in certain locations may present with atypical symptoms. For example, femoral neck stress fractures can present with groin pain or knee pain. Other physical examination techniques such as the fulcrum test (the bone is bowed by the examiner to reproduce symptoms)

Box 32.1: Common Predisposing Factors for Stress Fracture Injury

- Menstrual irregularities
- Smoking
- Eating disorders
- Irregular running surfaces
- Decreased bone density
- Lack of recovery time
- Sudden increase in training schedule
- Inappropriate footwear
- Malalignment
- Female gender
- Poor conditioning
- Running and jumping exercises

---

and the hop test (the patient is instructed to repeatedly hop on the affected leg to see if activity increases symptoms) are nonspecific and should be used judiciously. Both the fulcrum and the hop test could, at least in theory, "complete" an injury by converting a stress fracture to a frank fracture.

Focal pain that is aggravated by palpation, percussion, vibration, or ultrasound has a low sensitivity (<50%) but a high specificity for stress fracture injury. Boam and colleagues[9] and Romani and colleagues[10] demonstrated the limited accuracy of ultrasound to diagnose stress fractures. However, ultrasound and tuning fork testing are still commonly used in clinical settings as a result of their ease of use and their wide availability.

IMAGING CONSIDERATIONS IN STRESS FRACTURES

Early radiographs are often normal during the first few weeks after symptom onset **(Figure 32.1)**. Faint periosteal reactions and sclerosis are the earliest abnormalities of stress fractures, with cortical lucency or cortical thickening (or stress reaction) appearing later and callus formation trailing behind **(Figure 32.2)**. Radiographic fracture planes are less commonly seen in stress injuries. Stress fractures of the long bones (i.e., the tibia, the fibula, the metatarsals, and the femur) are typically transverse in orientation, although rare longitudinal fractures have been reported. During the first weeks of symptoms, the sensitivity of radiographs is often less than 20% because it may take 2 weeks to 3 months for stress fractures to become radiographically apparent. Therefore, negative radiographs should never eliminate the diagnosis of stress fracture if any clinical suspicion suggests the possibility of this type of injury.

Box 32.2: Symptoms of Stress Fracture Injury

- Dull ache
- No trauma
- Pain with or worsened with activity
- Night pain
- Gradual onset

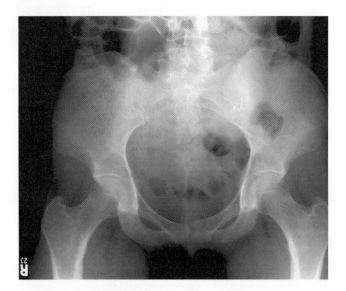

Figure 32.1 Hip radiographs of a young runner with right hip pain. These were originally read as normal. (Courtesy of Dr. York.)

A triple-phase technetium bone scan is highly sensitive for stress fracture, and it is usually positive 3 to 5 days after the onset of pain **(Figure 32.3).** The scintigraphic pattern for stress fracture is a characteristic focal uptake in the area of the fracture that is often evident during all phases of the scan. Bone scanning can differentiate medial tibial stress syndrome (MTSS) from stress fracture. All three phases typically involve positive findings for stress fracture in a localized area; this is in contrast with the diffuse reaction that is seen solely on the delayed images (third phase) for MTSS.

Triple-phase bone scanning is 84% to 100% sensitive; however, it is not very specific. A triple-phase bone scan can be diagnostic

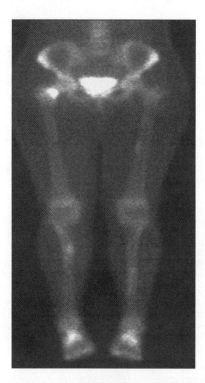

Figure 32.3 A bone scan of the same young runner shown in Figure 32.1 that shows increased uptake in the right femoral neck. (Courtesy of Dr. York.)

within 3 days of the onset of symptoms. Increased signal during the first phase (flow) will demonstrate acute soft-tissue inflammation. Increased uptake during the second phases (pool phases) indicates the increased capillary permeability of bone and soft tissue. Diffuse uptake only during the first two phases is

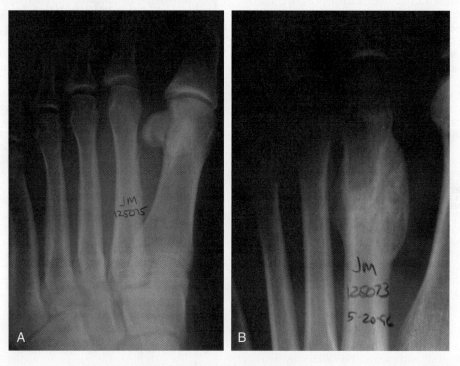

Figure 32.2 Classic metatarsal stress fracture. *A,* The initial film shows a minor crack in the diaphyseal cortex. *B,* Later radiograph shows the exuberant callus formation characteristic of healing stress fractures. (From DeLee JC, Drez D Jr, Miller D [eds]: DeLee & Drez's Orthopaedic Sports Medicine: Principles and Practice, 2nd ed. Philadelphia, WB Saunders, 2003.)

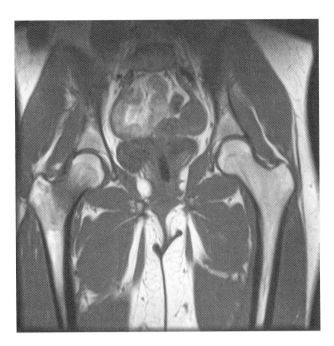

Figure 32.4 Magnetic resonance image showing marrow edema and the disruption of cortical bone. (Courtesy of Dr. York.)

Box 32.3: Some Potential Treatment Options for Stress Fractures

- Non—weight-bearing cast
- Orthotics
- Stretching and strengthening
- CAM Walker
- Calcitonin
- Parathyroid hormone
- Pneumatic brace
- Nonsteroidal anti-inflammatory drugs
- Bone stimulator
- Relative rest
- Ice massage
- Compression

---

characteristic of soft-tissue injuries without bony involvement. Increased focal uptake during all three phases indicates the bony involvement that is seen with a stress fracture, osteomyelitis, bony infarct, bony dysplasia, and osteoid osteoma. Bone scanning is highly sensitive for stress fractures in the patient with well-localized symptoms, and a negative scan virtually excludes the diagnosis of stress fracture. However, the specificity of a bone scan is low. Bone scans can remain positive for stress fracture for up to 12 months after symptom resolution and return to normal activity. Additionally, clinical judgment is a prerequisite to interpreting bone scan results because 50% of positive bone scan findings occur at asymptomatic sites that correspond histologically to areas of accelerated bone remodeling or bone strain.[9] A positive bone scan can remain positive for up to 1 year after diagnosis and treatment; therefore, it is not a good modality to evaluate for healing. Clinical judgment and findings on physical examination are the best indicators of healing.

Limited magnetic resonance imaging (MRI) can be as sensitive as a triple-phase bone scan without the radiation exposure, and, in some settings, it may even be cheaper than a bone scan **(Figure 32.4)**. MRI is also vastly more specific than bone scanning.

MRI can distinguish between bone stress (MTSS), stress fracture, and soft-tissue injury in adjacent locations. Also, because the prognosis and treatment of certain stress fractures is determined by the exact location of the fracture, MRI can be very useful for determining the exact location of the stress fracture, thereby increasing the likelihood of proper grading and treatment. **Table 32.2** illustrates the MRI and bone scan grading criteria for long-bone stress fractures.

Treatment

The main treatment of stress fractures is removal from the overloading forces. Relative rest continues until the patient is pain free. Bruckner and colleagues[11] found that rest only (without immobilization or restrictions on weight bearing) increased the risk of delayed union and nonunion. Casting, taping, partial weight bearing, and bracing are all techniques for unloading the weakened bone. Pain-free cross training will help the patient to maintain cardiovascular fitness and positive outlook. Ice massage and anti-inflammatory medications are modalities that decrease discomfort, whereas a gradual return to training, directed stretching and strengthening programs, and bone stimulators are other modalities that have been used to hasten the healing process **(Box 32.3)**.

In 2000, Gillespie and Grant[12] discovered that pneumatic braces speed recovery when they are used to treat and rehabilitate tibial stress fractures. In 1999, Finestone and colleagues[13] proved that the incidence of lower-extremity stress fractures was reduced

---

Table 32.2 Grading of Tibial or Long Bone Stress Fractures by Bone Scan or MRI Appearance[14]

Grade	Bone Scan	Magnetic Resonance Imaging
I	Small ill-defined cortical area of increased activity	Periosteal edema Mild to moderate on T2 Marrow edema normal
II	Better-defined cortical area of increased activity	Periosteal edema Moderate to severe on T2 Marrow edema on T2 images
III	Wide fusiform cortical—medullary area of highly increased activity	Periosteal edema Moderate to severe on T2 Marrow edema on T1 and T2 images
IV	Transcortical area of increased activity	Periosteal edema Moderate to severe on T2; marrow edema on T1 and T2 images Fracture line clearly visible

Box 32.4: Critical Fractures

- Anterior cortex of the tibia
- Medial malleolus
- Talus
- Navicular
- Fifth metatarsal
- Sesamoids
- Femoral neck

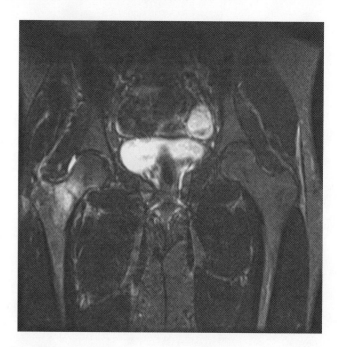

Figure 32.5 Magnetic resonance image of a compression side femoral neck stress fracture.

with the use of orthoses. The same authors also discovered that soft biomechanical orthoses, although they were better than no orthoses at all, were not as affective as semirigid orthoses.[13]

Drinkwater and colleagues[14] found that calcitonin–salmon improved the bone density of the spine and proximal femurs of young amenorrheic athletes. Cummings and Cummings[15] found improvements in bone density among athletes who took estrogen replacements. Biphosphonates are not currently recommended for females of childbearing age. Dietary advice includes 1200 to 1500 mg of calcium and 400 to 800 U of vitamin D **(Box 32.4).**

Critical stress fractures have an increased risk of nonunion. Particularly concerning areas include the anterior cortex of the tibia, the medial malleolus, the talus, the navicular, the fifth metatarsal, the sesamoids, and the femoral neck. These lesions have to be followed closely, and they should most likely be followed by an orthopedic surgeon.

Stress fractures of the anterior cortex of the tibia take up to a year to heal. These stress fractures must be monitored for both clinical and radiographic evidence of healing. There is little evidence to suggest that casting or avoiding aggravating events is the best treatment. Rettig and colleagues[16] suggested that the subcutaneous location of the anterior tibia may cause the relative hypovascularity of the anterior tibial cortex, which is a predisposing condition for delayed union.

Runners are vulnerable to stress fractures of the medial malleolus. These fractures are usually vertical through the tibial plafond. Stress fractures of the medial malleolus present with tenderness and an ankle effusion as well as discomfort with activity. Nondisplaced or minimally displaced fractures usually respond to immobilization in a pneumatic brace, whereas displaced or nonunion fractures should be treated operatively.

Stress fractures of the talus that usually involve the body of the talus can be found in runners and jumpers. Stress fractures involving the lateral process are easily confused with sinus tarsi syndrome. Although intervention may not be very comfortable, the prognosis is poor if intervention is delayed. These injures should be casted and not allowed to bear weight, and they should be followed closely.

Similarly, runners, jumpers, hurdlers, and basketball players with an insidious onset of medial arch pain on the dorsum may have a navicular stress fracture. Increased discomfort in the region of the navicular bone (i.e., the "N spot") after running or jumping is suggestive of a stress fracture. The middle third is the area that is the most at risk. Pain usually radiates to the arch or the dorsum of the foot. There is little use for radiographs, but computed tomography and bone scanning are highly diagnostic. Treatment usually involves a prolonged period of non–weight-bearing immobilization. Patients will generally recover without surgery if their treatment includes strict non–weight bearing.

Sesamoid stress fractures are prone to nonunion, and they may require extended periods of non–weight bearing. Symptoms usually include mild swelling and tenderness at the sesamoid bones. X-rays may show a stress fracture; however, a bone scan can be used to confirm clinical suspicion. Casting with reduced

dorsiflexion is the first-line treatment. Bone grafting and excision are potential surgical treatments, and this should be followed by a gradual increase in activity. There is little evidence of the effectiveness of bone stimulators.

Proximal fifth metatarsal stress fractures are usually treated with 6 weeks of a short-leg non–weight-bearing cast. Most patients cannot tolerate prolonged immobilization; therefore, internal fixation with a medullary compression screw may be used. Occasionally bone grafting and open reduction may be necessary. Regardless, early intervention improves the prognosis.

Although they are relatively uncommon, femoral neck stress fractures have a high morbidity. Patients usually complain of pain radiating to the groin and a decreased range of motion; they may have knee or night pain without tenderness on palpation. These fractures are classified as distraction or compression fractures. Distraction-type fractures involve the superior margin of the femoral neck, and they tend to occur more frequently in the mature athlete. Immediate orthopedic referral is recommended because these injuries are prone to fracture and displacement. These patients should bear no weight until being evaluated by an orthopedic surgeon. After definitive treatment, patients should remain non–weight bearing or partial weight bearing until pain-free passive range of motion returns with radiographic or MRI evidence of healing. Open reduction and internal fixation are indicated if there is a widening of the distractive type fracture.

Compression fractures are found along the inferior medial border of the femoral neck, and they are more common among younger athletes **(Figure 32.5).** These fractures are at risk for nonunion and avascular necrosis. Primary treatment is generally nonsurgical, and it involves complete rest until the pain-free passive range of motion is restored, followed by a gradual, careful increase in activity level.

Noncritical stress fractures

Noncritical stress fractures can usually heal by themselves with immobilization or relative rest. Typical areas include the medial

Table 32.3 Stress Fracture Rehabilitation Program, Darnall Army Community Hospital Sports Medicine

	Day 1	Day 2	Day 3	Day 4	Day 5	Day 6	Day 7
Week 1	Walk 5 minutes	Walk 10 minutes	Walk 10 minutes	Walk 20 minutes	Walk 20 minutes	Walk 30 minutes	Walk 30 minutes
Week 2	Walk 20 minutes Jog 5 minutes Walk 10 minutes	Walk 20 minutes Jog 5 minutes Walk 10 minutes	Walk 15 minutes Jog 10 minutes Walk 15 minutes	Walk 15 minutes Jog 10 minutes Walk 15 minutes	Walk 10 minutes Jog 15 minutes Walk 10 minutes	Walk 10 minutes Jog 15 minutes Walk 10 minutes	Jog 40 minutes
Week 3	Jog 20 minutes Sprint 5 minutes	Jog 20 minutes Sprint 5 minutes	Jog 20 minutes Sprint 10 minutes	Jog 20 minutes Sprint 10 minutes	Jog 15 minutes Sprint 20 minutes	Jog 15 minutes Sprint 20 minutes	Jog 10 minutes Sprint 30 minutes
Week 4	Gradually increase functional activities						
Week 5	Resume full activities						
Week 6	Resume full activities (noncontact)						

A sample "return to running" regimen for an uncomplicated lower-extremity stress fracture. We typically begin the week 1 activities after 2 weeks of the patient being pain free at rest and after a week or two of nonimpact aerobics, (e.g., bike riding, elliptical training). Each progression should be pain free. If pain returns, weight-bearing activities should be stopped until the patient is free of pain, and then the regimen should be started again at a slower pace. The final week involves the wearing of protective gear.

tibia, the fibula, and the second, third, and fourth metatarsals. Physicians, coaches, and athletes must identify and alter modifiable factors that may predispose their bodies to stress fractures.

The tibia shaft is the most common site of stress fractures, especially among those patients with a cavus foot or excessive subtalar pronation. Stress fractures of the anterior medial cortex of the tibia are the most feared; many times they will require internal fixation.

Metatarsal stress fractures are commonly found in distance runners and ballet dancers. The second metatarsal is the most common, and this is followed by the third, the first, the fourth, and finally the fifth metatarsals. Fifth metatarsal stress fractures are sometimes confused with Jones fractures. However, it is important to remember that stress fractures of the fifth metatarsal shaft are classified as critical fractures and should be promptly referred to orthopedics for consideration of surgical management because they are prone to nonunion.

CONCLUSION

Stress fractures are extremely common among participants in running sports and among those whose occupations involve repetitive motions. Attention to the modifiable causes of stress fractures can reduce the incidence and morbidity of these overuse injuries. Imaging modalities are commonly used to confirm clinical suspicion, and a few of these can be used to monitor healing when clinically indicated. Treatment involves reducing aggravating activities, altering modifiable causes, and gradually returning to activity after a period of pain-free rest **(Table 32.3).** Some stress fractures are considered critical, and they may require surgery for healing to occur. In general, the earlier a proper diagnosis is reached and treatment begins, the better the long-term prognosis will be.

REFERENCES

1. Hulkko A, Orava S: Stress fractures in athletes. Int J Sports Med 1987;8(3):221-226.
2. Matheson GO, Clement DB, McKenzie DC, et al: Stress fractures in athletes: a study of 320 cases. Am J Sports Med 1987;15(1):46-58.
3. Couture CJ, Karlson A: Tibial stress injuries: decisive diagnosis and treatment of stress injuries. Phys Sportsmed 2002;30(6):29-36.
4. Myburgh KH, Hutchins J, Fataar AB, et al: Low bone density is an etiologic factor for stress fractures in athletes. Ann Intern Med 1990;113(10):754-759.
5. Sanderlin BW, Raspa RF: Common stress fractures. Am Fam Physician 2003;68(8):1527-1532.
6. Coady CM, Micheli LJ: Stress fractures in the pediatric athlete. Clin Sports Med 1997;16:225-238.
7. Monteleone GP Jr: Stress fractures in the athlete. Orthop Clin North Am 1995;26:423-432.
8. Bennell KL, Bruckner PD: Epidemiology and site specificity of stress fracture. Clin Sports Med 1997;16:179-196.
9. Boam WD, Miser WF, Yuill SC, et al: Comparision of ultrasound examination with bore scintiscan in the diagnosis of stress fractures. J Am Board Fam Pract 1996;9:414-417.
10. Romani WA, Perrin DH, Dussault RG, et al: Identification of tibial stress fractures using therapeutic continuous ultrasound. J Orthop Sports Phys Ther 2000;30:444-452.
11. Bruckner P, Bradshaw C, Bennell K: Managing common stress fractures: let risk level guide treatment. Phys Sportsmed 1998;26(8):39-47.
12. Gillespie WJ, Grant I: Interventions for preventing and treating stress fractures and stress reaction of bone of the lower limbs in young adults. Cochrane Database Syst Rev 2000;(2):CD000450.
13. Finestone A, Giladi M, Elad H: Prevention of stress fractures using custom biomechanical shoe orthoses. Clin Orthop 1999;(360):182-190.
14. Drinkwater BL, Healy NL, Rencken ML, et al: Effectiveness of nasal calcitonin in preventing bone loss in amenorrheic women, abstracted. J Bone Miner Res b 1993;8(suppl 1):S264.
15. Cummings DC, Cummings CE: Estrogen replacement therapy and female athletes: current issues. Sports Med 2001;31(15):1025-1031.
16. Rettig AC, Shelburne KD, McCarroll JR, et al: The natural history and treatment of delayed union and nonunion stress fractures of the anterior cortex of the anterior tibia. Am J Sports Med 1988;16(3):250-255.
17. Zwas ST, Elkanovitch R, Frank G: Interpretation and classification of bone scintigraphic findings in stress fractures. J Nucl Med 1987;28(4):452-457.

SECTION 4

Rehabilitation

CHAPTER 33

Principles of Sports Rehabilitation

Jennifer Reed, MD, FAAPMR,
and Jimmy D. Bowen, MD, FAAPMR, CSCS

KEY POINTS

- The rehabilitation framework can be organized around four principles: (1) the type of injury that is present; (2) the presentation of the injury; (3) the complete and accurate diagnosis of the injury; and (4) the treatment plan of the injury and the athlete's return to play.
- Injury type can be categorized as either macrotrauma or microtrauma. Acute injuries are generally the result of macrotrauma, whereas chronic injuries are typically the result of microtrauma.
- Goals of the acute rehabilitative stage include the control of inflammation and pain, protecting the injured tissue from further damage, maintaining general strength and cardiovascular fitness, and regaining/maintaining range of motion through joint activation.
- During the recovery stage, emphasis is placed on restoration of function by addressing tissue overload and functional biomechanical deficit complexes.
- An advancing program of isometric, concentric, eccentric, and plyometric strength should be undertaken. Recovering strength is essential because muscle weakness is a common finding among athletes with both acute injuries and more chronic overuse problems.
- The major goals of a well-constructed rehabilitation plan are to reduce the risk of reinjury and to reduce the risk of subsequent injuries along the kinetic chain.

INTRODUCTION

Musculoskeletal overuse and injury cause impairment through the partial or complete loss of anatomic form and physiologic function. The goal of sports rehabilitation is to prevent or reverse the impairments realized from an injury. Sports rehabilitation (or "pre-habilitation") arguably begins before injury or surgery. Without argument, rehabilitation must begin immediately after injury or surgery with the goal of the restoration of optimal form, function, and sport-specific activity.

FRAMEWORK FOR SPORTS REHABILITATION

Rehabilitation protocols in sports medicine are numerous and vary in their content. If a hundred different sports medicine physicians were polled regarding the best protocol for the rehabilitation of a specific injury type, one would likely get a hundred different responses. In reality, one size does not fit all patients. Each patient's rehabilitation should ideally be tailored to his or her unique needs and athletic demands. Therefore, rather than attempting to apply rigid protocols to different patients with the same injury, it is much more useful to think about rehabilitation conceptually.

A rehabilitation framework can be organized around four principles: (1) the discovery of the type of injury that is present; (2) the determination of the method of presentation of the injury; (3) the complete and accurate diagnosis of the injury; and (4) the plan of treatment of the injury and of the return to play of the athlete.[1]

During the course of daily practice as one applies this framework to individual patients, it is also useful to keep the concept of the kinetic chain in mind. As described by Steindler,[2] the kinetic chain is a "combination of several successively arranged joints working together to successfully complete a desired motor task of the body." Kibler[3] expounds on this concept by stating the following:

> ...individual body segments and joints, collectively called *links*, must move in certain specific sequences to allow efficient accomplishment of the task. The sequencing of the links is called the *kinetic chain* of an athletic activity. Each kinetic chain has its own sequence, but the basic organization includes proximal to distal sequencing, a proximal base of support or stability, and successive activation of each segment of the link and each successive link. The net result is generation of force and energy in each link, summation of the developed force and energy through each of the links, and efficient transfer of the force and energy to the terminal link.

For example, the kinetic chain involved in propelling the ball in jai alai (**Figure 33.1**) is as follows: ground > plant leg > hip/trunk > shoulder > elbow > wrist > hand.

A breakdown in force generated at any link or the inefficient transfer of force from one link to the next will result in an increased load on the next link in the chain as it tries to compensate for the weak link. The end result may be injury in the distal link. For example, if the jai alai player in Figure 33.1 has underlying

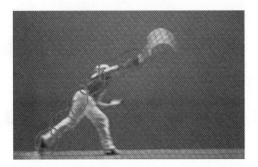

Figure 33.1 Kinetic chain: jai alai player.

inflexibility in his hip or trunk rotation that interferes with the efficient transfer of force to the next link (the shoulder), he most likely will present with complaints of shoulder pain, rather than describing hip tightness (see Chapter 6 for a more complete discussion and application of the kinetic chain process).

Injury type

Injury type can be categorized as either macrotrauma or microtrauma. Macrotrauma injuries are readily identified events (e.g., an anterior cruciate ligament tear). The tissue is essentially normal before the event, and it becomes abruptly abnormal after the event. Microtrauma injuries are more insidious. Over time, as a result of repetitive insult to a tissue, the integrity of the tissue is altered. Cellular repair mechanisms are disrupted, and the cells cannot produce the proper matrix required for healing. Examples include Achilles tendinitis and lateral epicondylitis.[1,4,5]

Method of injury presentation

The method of injury presentation may be acute, chronic, or an acute exacerbation of a chronic injury.[1] Acute injuries are generally the result of macrotrauma, whereas chronic injuries are typically the result of microtrauma. Acute exacerbations of chronic injuries may occur as the result of incomplete rehabilitation. It is important to note that the resolution of symptoms does not necessarily equate with normal function. For example, a subacromial injection may resolve the shoulder pain of an overhead athlete with rotator cuff impingement. However, if the athlete returns to play before addressing the biomechanical factors that contributed to the injury (i.e., poor scapular control), symptoms are likely to return at the original site or elsewhere along the kinetic chain (often in the same limb).[5,6]

Complete and accurate diagnosis

To formulate an effective and thorough rehabilitation plan, it is useful to render a complete and accurate diagnosis by identifying and addressing the following clinical, anatomic, and mechanical complexes[5,7]:

1. *Clinical symptoms complex:* pain, swelling, and decreased range of motion
2. *Tissue injury complex:* the tissue that has been injured
3. *Tissue overload complex:* tissues that have been stressed or overloaded and that are contributing to or exacerbating the injury
4. *Functional biomechanical deficit complex:* physiologic and mechanical alterations such as strength imbalances or inflexibilities that affect the proper mechanics of athletic activity
5. *Subclinical adaptation complex:* substitution patterns that an athlete develops to compensate for the injury in an effort to maintain performance

Table 33.1 Complete Diagnosis of Plantar Fasciitis

Clinical symptom complex	Point tenderness over the plantar fascia insertion onto the calcaneus; symptoms worse in the morning and after running
Tissue overload complex	Plantar fascia and gastrocnemius
Tissue injury complex	Plantar fascia
Functional biomechanical deficit complex	Gastrocnemius inflexibility and weakness; decreased ankle dorsiflexion
Subclinical adaptation complex	Running on toes; decreased stride length; decreased stance phase on the affected side

Table 33.1 demonstrates the application of this concept to a patient with plantar fasciitis.

Plan of treatment for the injury and return to play of the athlete

When organizing a treatment plan for an athlete, it is helpful to consider rehabilitation in terms of the acute, recovery, and functional stages.

ACUTE STAGE OF REHABILITATION

During the acute stage of rehabilitation **(Table 33.2)**, attention is focused on the clinical symptoms complex and the tissue injury complex. Goals include the control of inflammation and pain, protecting the injured tissue from further damage, maintaining general strength and cardiovascular fitness, and regaining/maintaining range of motion though joint activation. Criteria for advancing to the next phase of rehabilitation include adequate tissue healing, near-normal range of motion, pain control, and tolerance for strengthening. Functional rehabilitation cannot be initiated until analgesia is effective and the control of inflammation is

Table 33.2 Acute Stage of Rehabilitation

Focus of Treatment	Clinical Symptom Complex/Tissue Injury Complex
Tools	Relative rest and/or immobilization Physical modalities Medications Manual therapy Initial exercise Surgery
Goals	Control inflammation and pain Protect injured tissue from further damage Maintain general strength and cardiovascular fitness Maintain/regain range of motion
Criteria for advancing to the next rehabilitation phase	Pain control Adequate tissue healing Near-normal range of motion Tolerance for strengthening

Modified from Kibler WB, Herring SL, Press JP (eds): Functional Rehabilitation of Sports and Musculoskeletal Injuries. Gaithersburg, MD, Aspen Publishers, 1998.

accomplished.[8] Biologic impairments and the physiologic losses that occur after injury begin immediately and may become substantial in a matter of days. The sooner the injured athlete can transition from the acute phase to the recovery phase, the better. Symptom relief does not mean that functional capacity has been restored. It is important to remember that the resolution of pain indicates that it is time to transition to the next phase of rehabilitation rather than for a premature return to training or competition.

RECOVERY STAGE OF REHABILITATION

During the recovery stage **(Table 33.3)**, treatment emphasis is placed on the restoration of function by addressing the tissue overload complex and the functional biomechanical deficit complex. Goals include regaining local flexibility and strength, correcting biomechanical deficits, and maintaining fitness. The recovery phase may be the longest stage of the rehabilitation process. To advance to the next phase of rehabilitation, the athlete should be free from pain; exhibiting a normal range of motion, complete tissue healing, and restored flexibility; and demonstrating strength of 75% or greater as compared with the uninjured side.

Early during this phase, the recovery of joint range of motion and the restoration of flexibility receive priority. Full range of motion and joint flexibility will prepare the injured area for more dynamic training and sport-specific activity. Stretching exercises should be done after adequate warm-up. The combination of warm-up followed by stretching is more effective for improving joint range of motion than either used in isolation.[9-11] The proposed benefits of improved flexibility are a reduction in risk of injury or reinjury, pain reduction, and improved athletic performance. "However, a lack of definitive research makes it difficult to make recommendations regarding an effective flexibility program."[12] If stretching is considered to be effective, the debate then becomes what type of stretching to use. Do you begin with static stretches or ballistic stretching? Do proprioceptive neuromuscular facilitation techniques (also know as *contract–relax*) provide a more effective method for the restoration of flexibility? Or do dynamic range of motion and eccentric flexibility training provide additional benefits? The bottom line seems to be that after weighing economy of time, the need for intervention from the facilitator, injury protection, and the proposed improvement of athletic performance, the most commonly used

program is static stretching.[12] The greatest benefits seem to be achieved when this type of stretching is used in combination with warm-up activity and as a prelude to strengthening. However, there is much controversy with regard to this topic. Definitive research will be helpful for defining the recommendations associated with flexibility training.

Recovering strength is also essential because muscle weakness is a common finding in athletes with acute injuries and overuse problems. Here again it is important that functional strengthening continue even when the symptoms of the injury have abated. It is not unusual to have strength deficits proximal to the injury site (e.g., hip abductors after knee injury) and even contralateral to the injury site.[13] An advancing program of isometric, concentric, eccentric, and plyometric strengthening programs should be undertaken, culminating in local and kinetically associated muscles exhibiting increased aerobic muscle endurance and anaerobic power. Progressive resistance training during the recovery phase, as described by Kraemer,[14] optimally consists of 60% to 80% of the 1-repitition maximum with 3-5 sets of 8-12 repetitions each being performed 3-4 days per week. Generally during this period of rehabilitation, as the injured athlete gains strength, exercise intensity is maintained while the load increases. Strength conditioning recommendations during rehabilitation have many important variables: the selection of muscle groups, the sequence of the exercises, the combination of routines with and without equipment, and the appropriate rest activity.[14]

FUNCTIONAL STAGE OF REHABILITATION

During the final stage of rehabilitation **(Table 33.4)**, attention remains focused on any residual biomechanical deficits as well as on the subclinical adaptation complex. Goals include the normalization of movement patterns, strength balance, improved joint neuromuscular control, and return to athletic competition. This stage of rehabilitation ideally continues as an ongoing program to reduce the risk of future reinjury.[1,4,15] The criteria for return to play include normal sports mechanics, normal strength/flexibility and range of motion, good general fitness, and the demonstration of sport-specific skills.

The major goals of a well-constructed rehabilitation plan are to reduce the risk of reinjury and to reduce the risk of subsequent injuries along the kinetic chain. Consider the development of a rehabilitation plan for a female basketball player after a lateral ankle sprain. During the latter stages of the functional phase of her rehabilitation, the physician may elect to introduce a series of plyometric jumping exercises not only to reintroduce the

Table 33.3 Recovery Stage of Rehabilitation

Focus of Treatment	Tissue Overload Complex/Functional Biomechanical Deficit Complex
Tools	Manual therapy Flexibility Proprioception/neuromuscular control training Specific, progressive exercise
Goals	Restoration of function Regain local flexibility and strength Address biomechanical deficits away from the site of injury Maintain general fitness
Criteria for advancing to the next rehabilitation phase	Pain free Complete tissue healing Normal range of motion Good flexibility 75% or greater strength as compared with uninjured side

Modified from Kibler WB, Herring SL, Press JP (eds): Functional Rehabilitation of Sports and Musculoskeletal Injuries. Gaithersburg, MD, Aspen Publishers, 1998.

Table 33.4 Functional Stage of Rehabilitation

Focus of Treatment	Functional Biomechanical Deficit Complex/Subclinical Adaptation Complex
Tools	Power and endurance exercise (e.g., plyometrics) Sport-specific functional progression Technique/skills instruction
Goals	Normalize movement patterns Return to athletic competition Reduce the risk of reinjury
Criteria for advancing to the next rehabilitation phase	Normal strength and strength balance Normal sports mechanics Demonstration of sport-specific skills

Modified from Kibler WB, Herring SL, Press JP (eds): Functional Rehabilitation of Sports and Musculoskeletal Injuries. Gaithersburg, MD, Aspen Publishers, 1998.

necessary sport-specific skills needed to challenge her ankle but also as a means of possible protection from injury elsewhere in the kinetic chain. The knee (specifically the anterior cruciate ligament) is a particularly vulnerable proximal link in the lower extremity of the female athlete. In women, neuromuscular differences appear to modify the ability to dissipate landing forces as compared with what is seen in men. Irmischer and colleagues[16] observed a significant reduction in ground reaction forces during landing among women completing a 9-week, plyometric-based jumping program as compared with controls. This study demonstrates the successful use of a plyometric training program to alter landing strategies in females, which may result in a reduced risk of knee injury while landing.[16]

KINESIOLOGY BASICS OF SPORTS REHABILITATION

A basic understanding of rehabilitation kinesiology helps the sports medicine physician to plan an appropriate rehabilitation program and to coordinate that plan with other members of the rehabilitation team (i.e., physical therapists, athletic trainers).

Types of muscle action
Concentric contraction
Concentric contraction occurs when the total length of the muscle shortens as tension is produced. For example, the upward phase of a biceps curl is a concentric contraction.

Eccentric contraction
Eccentric contraction occurs when the total length of the muscle increases as tension is produced. For example, the lowering phase of a biceps curl constitutes an eccentric contraction. Muscles are capable of generating greater forces under eccentric conditions than under either isometric or concentric contractions.[17-19] Large tensile forces are generated during sudden eccentric contractions (e.g., a linebacker coming to a rapid stop at the line of scrimmage generates large eccentric quadriceps forces).

Traditional rehabilitation programs have often omitted eccentric training. Although there are no definitive studies to support eccentric training as an absolute prerequisite before returning to athletic play,[19] research is emerging to support its use, particularly for the rehabilitation of microtrauma/overuse injuries. For example, Roos and colleagues[20] designed a prospective randomized clinical trial to test the hypothesis that eccentric calf muscle exercises reduce pain and improve function in patients with Achilles tendinopathy. At 12 weeks, members of the group who performed eccentric exercises reported significantly less pain, and more patients in that group returned to sports participation after 12 weeks.[20]

Isometric contraction
Isometric contraction occurs when muscle length remains relatively constant as tension is produced. For example, during a biceps curl, holding the dumbbell in a constant/static position rather than actively raising or lowering it is an example of isometric contraction.[21,22] Although the forces generated during isometric contractions are potentially greater than during concentric contractions, muscles are seldom injured during this type of contraction. Isometric exercises are often used during the early phases of rehabilitating a musculotendinous injury because the intensity of contraction and the muscle length at which it contracts can be controlled.[19]

Closed kinetic chain
During a closed kinetic chain exercise, the terminal joint is stationary, thus prohibiting free motion.[2] A lower-extremity example

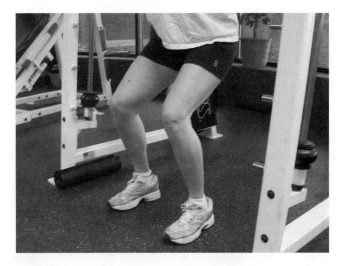

Figure 33.2 Closed kinetic chain: two-leg squat.

would be leg squats **(Figure 33.2)**, and an upper-extremity example would be pushups.[23] Closed kinetic chain exercises have several advantages over open-chain exercises. Rather than having muscle groups work in isolation, closed-chain exercises allow for the simultaneous activation of antagonistic muscle groups (e.g., the quads and the hamstrings during leg squats), thus promoting increased joint stability and a simulation of functional movement patterns.[24] Lower-extremity closed kinetic chain exercises have often been touted as a more functional type of exercise for the rehabilitation of the lower extremity because sport-related activities are performed with the feet in fixed positions.

For example, in the setting of rehabilitation after anterior cruciate ligament reconstruction, Bynum and colleagues[25] performed a randomized prospective trial comparing open and closed kinetic chain rehabilitation. "The closed kinetic chain group had lower mean KT-1000 arthrometer side-to-side differences, less patellofemoral pain, was generally more satisfied with the end result, and more often thought they returned to normal daily activities and sports sooner than expected." The authors thus concluded that closed kinetic chain exercises do offer some important advantages over open kinetic chain exercises during rehabilitation after anterior cruciate ligament reconstruction.[25]

Open kinetic chain
During an open-chain kinetic exercise, the terminal link is allowed to move freely through space. Muscle groups may act in isolation with this type of exercise. For example, during an open-chain lower-extremity exercise such as knee extension, the quadriceps predominates **(Figure 33.3)**.

Both open and closed kinetic chain exercises have a role in rehabilitation. For example, rehabilitation for an overhead-throwing athlete (e.g., a baseball player) after the repair of a superior labral tear may involve closed-chain exercises to develop scapular control early during the postoperative phase, when shoulder range of motion is protected. As rehabilitation progresses toward the functional phase, open-chain exercises will be added to more closely simulate the throwing motion.

Plyometrics
Plyometric exercises emphasize explosive motions **(Figure 33.4)**. This type of exercise takes advantage of the elastic properties of connective tissue coupled with the force generated by muscle itself. A rapid prestretch (eccentric load) is followed immediately

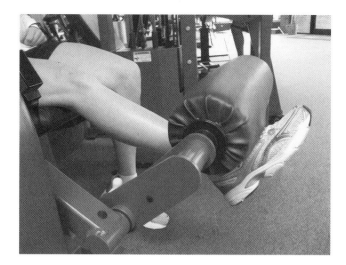

Figure 33.3 Open kinetic chain: single-leg extension.

by a forceful concentric contraction.[17,18] For example, high jumpers first lower their bodies toward the ground, placing a pre-stretch on the leg muscles; this is followed by the forceful contraction of the same muscles, which propels the athlete over the bar.[19] Plyometric exercises are introduced during the functional phase of rehabilitation and are among the most sport-specific exercises performed during this stage.

Proprioception

A complete rehabilitation program must not overlook the neuromuscular control that is necessary for joint control. The repair of static and dynamic constraints and the strengthening of muscles do not necessarily prepare the joint of an athlete for the sudden positional changes seen in the athletic arena. Therefore, the rehabilitative process must address the structure that contributes to the awareness of posture, movement, changes in equilibrium, and the knowledge of position, weight, and the resistance of objects related to the body.[26] The joint capsule receptors, the ligament receptors, the muscle, and the tendon receptors must be appreciated and

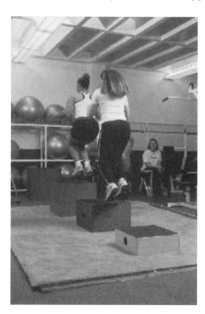

Figure 33.4 Plyometrics: box jumps.

progressively and systematically assessed and trained before an effective return to sport-specific activities. The use of taping and orthotics and their benefits for joint proprioception should also be considered.[27] (See Chapter 38 for a discussion of bracing and Chapter 37 for a discussion and primer on athletic taping.)

PSYCHOLOGIC ASPECTS OF REHABILITATION

Addressing the active patient's emotional needs is just as important as the physical recovery. An athlete may be depressed about the current injury and apprehensive about future injuries. Recognizing the psychologic and emotional needs of the injured athlete during each phase of rehabilitation will go a long way toward enhancing recovery and ensuring the enthusiastic participation of the patient.[28] Framing the rehabilitation plan in a positive way by instructing the athlete regarding what he or she *can* do (not just what he or she *cannot* do) is integral to facilitating a successful outcome.

CONCLUSION

Sports rehabilitation is a dynamic program of exercise, guided evaluation and instruction, and psychologic support that is designed to prevent or reverse the deleterious functional and physiologic effects of injury. The goals of rehabilitation are best appreciated in general conceptual terms as opposed to rigid protocols. Understanding the phases of sports rehabilitation and the goals of each phase will help sports physicians to individualize programs to meet the needs of each specific athlete.

REFERENCES

1. Kibler WB: A framework for sports medicine. Phys Med Rehabil Clin North Am 1994;5:1.
2. Steindler A: Kinesiology of the Human Body Under Normal and Pathologic Conditions. Springfield, IL, Charles C. Thomas, 1955.
3. Kibler WB: Determining the extent of the functional deficit. In Kibler WB, Herring SL, Press JM (eds): Functional Rehabilitation of Sports and Musculoskeletal Injuries. Gaithersburg, MD, Aspen Publishers, 1998, pp 16-19.
4. Kibler WB, Herring SA: Formulating a rehabilitation program. In Griffin LY (ed): Rehabilitation of the Injured Knee, 2nd ed. St. Louis, Mosby, 1995.
5. Herring SA, Kibler WB: A framework for rehabilitation. In Kibler WB, Herring SL, Press JM (eds): Functional Rehabilitation of Sports and Musculoskeletal Injuries. Gaithersburg, MD, Aspen Publishers, 1998, pp 1-8.
6. Lysens, et al: The predictability of sports injuries. Sports Med 1984;1:6.
7. Herring SA: Rehabilitation of Muscle Injuries. Medicine and Science in Sports and Exercise, vol 22. Williams & Wilkins, 1990.
8. Frontera WR: Exercise and musculoskeletal rehabilitation. Phys Sportsmed 2003;31(12).
9. Schwellnus M: Flexibility and joint range of motion. In Frontera WR (ed): Rehabilitation of Sports Injuries: Scientific Basis. Malden, MA, Blackwell Science, 2003, pp 232-257.
10. Murphy DR: A critical look at static stretching: are we doing our patients harm? Chiropractic Sports Med 1994;8:59-70.
11. Kuland DN, Tottossy M: Warm-up, strength and power. Orthop Clin North Am 1983;14:427-448.
12. Nelson RT, Brandy WD: An update on flexibility. Strength Condition J 2005;27(1):10-16.
13. Urbach D, Awiszus F: Impaired ability of voluntary quadriceps activation bilaterally interferes with functional testing after knee injures: a twitch interpolation study. Int J Sports Med 2002;23(4):231-236.
14. Kraemer WJ: Strength training basics: designing workouts to meet patients' goals. Phys Sportsmed 2003;31(8):39-45.
15. Kibler WB, Chandler TJ, Pace BK: Principles of rehabilitation after chronic tendon injuries. Clin Sports Med 1992;11(3):661-671.
16. Irmischer BS, Harris C, Pfeiffer RP, et al: Effects of a knee ligament injury prevention exercise program on impact forces in women. J Strength Cond Res 2004;18(4):703-707.

17. Komi PV (ed): Strength and Power in Sport. London, Blackwell Scientific Publications, 1992.
18. McArdle WD, Katch FI, Katch VL. Exercise Physiology: Energy, Nutrition and Human Performance, 3rd ed. Philadelphia, Lea & Febiger, 1991.
19. Young JL, Press JM: The physiologic basis of sports rehabilitation. In Kibler WB, Herring SL, Press JM (eds): Functional Rehabilitation of Sports and Musculoskeletal Injuries. Gaithersburg, MD, Aspen Publishers, 1998, pp 9-16.
20. Roos EM, Engstrom M, Lagerquist A, Soderberg B: Clinical improvement after 6 weeks of eccentric exercise in patients with mid-portion Achilles tendinopathy—a randomized trial with 1-year follow-up. Scand J Med Sci Sports 2004;14(5):286-295.
21. Kinesiology: A Scientific Basis of Human Motion, 7th ed. Philadelphia, WB Saunders, 1982.
22. Hunter GR: Muscle physiology. In Baechle TR (ed): Essentials of Strength Training and Conditioning, 2nd ed. Champaign, IL, Human Kinetics, 2000, pp 3-15.
23. Hillman S: Principles and techniques of open kinetic chain rehabilitation: the upper extremity. J Sports Rehabil 1994;3:319-330.
24. Draganich LF, Jaeger RJ, Fralj AR: Coactivation of the hamstrings and quadriceps during extension of the knee. J Bone Joint Surg Am 1989;71:1075-1081.
25. Bynum EB, Barrack RL, Alexander AH: Open versus closed chain kinetic exercises after anterior cruciate ligament reconstruction. A prospective randomized study. Am J Sports Med 1995;23(4):401-406.
26. Harrelson GL, Leaver-Dunn D: Introduction to rehabilitation. In Andrews, Harrelson, Wilk (eds): Physical Rehabilitation of the Injured Athlete, 2nd ed. Philadelphia, WB Saunders, 1998, pp 175-217.
27. Grossman T, Serenelli K, Mistry D: Taping and bracing. In O'Connor F, Sallis R, Wilder R, St. Pierre P (eds): Sports Medicine: Just the Facts. McGraw-Hill, pp 442-445.
28. Brewer BW, Andersen MB, Van Raalte JL: Psychological aspects of sports injury rehabilitation: toward a biopsychosocial approach. In Mostofsky DI, Zaichkowsky LD (eds): Medical and Psychological Aspects of Sport and Exercise. Morgantown WV, Fitness Information Technology, 2002, pp 41-54.

CHAPTER 34

Practical Application of Osteopathic Manipulation in Sports Medicine

Lori A. Boyajian-O'Neill, DO, and Dennis A. Cardone, DO

KEY POINTS

- The body has an inherent ability to heal and maintain or acquire health. Physicians seek to facilitate this inherent propensity for health through a variety of interventions, including pharmacologic, surgical, biopsychosocial, and manual therapies.
- Manual therapeutic techniques are applied to restore or improve function by targeting barriers to normal function. There are many specific techniques, including those that are applied to soft tissue and others that are applied to joints.
- Structure and function are inextricably connected; that which affects one conversely affects the other.
- "Normal" joint biomechanics vary within and among athletes even in the same sports or positions. Training alters biomechanics and neuromuscular patterns to achieve a desired level of performance. When there is injury, there is an alteration of structure and function and, thus, performance.
- Acute trauma, overuse injury, or abnormal anatomy that leads to abnormal biomechanics in one area will eventually adversely affect structure and function at distant sites if there is no intervention (i.e., prehabilitation or rehabilitation).
- Neuromusculoskeletal integrity is developed and maintained through training that optimizes function and performance. Muscle-activating patterns, which are established through training and interrupted by injury, may be reestablished through rehabilitation that includes strengthening, proprioception, and range of motion.

INTRODUCTION

What is osteopathic medicine?

Andrew Taylor Still, MD, who founded osteopathic medicine in 1874, was one of the first sports medicine physicians in the United States. At the American School of Osteopathy in Kirksville, Missouri, he advocated exercise as being inextricably tied to health. An anatomist by avocation, Dr. Still observed the connection between structure (anatomy) and function (physiology) in normal and pathologic states and promoted three principles of osteopathic medicine: (1) the body is a unit; (2) structure and function are reciprocally interrelated; and (3) the body is self-healing. These tenets are the basis of osteopathic medical education and osteopathic sports medicine practice. In founding osteopathic medicine, Dr. Still put into practice his philosophy that structure and function are interconnected and thus that they affect the work and capabilities of the body (performance).

The American Osteopathic Association describes osteopathic medicine as a "complete system of medical care with a philosophy that combines the needs of the patient with current practice of medicine, surgery and obstetrics and emphasizes the interrelationship between structure and function and has an appreciation of the body's ability to heal itself."[1] The concept of body unity means that the human being is a dynamic unit of function. Athletes use their bodies to the extreme to maximize function and achieve performance. Osteopathic sports medicine physicians apply the tenets of osteopathic medicine to assist athletes with preparing for sport, optimizing performance, and recovering from injury with the philosophy that the athlete's structure and function are interrelated.

Osteopathic sports medicine physicians use osteopathic manipulative techniques or manual techniques to improve physiologic function and/or to support homeostasis that has been altered by somatic dysfunction. The term *somatic dysfunction* is used in osteopathic medicine, and the American Osteopathic Association defines it as "impaired or altered function of related components of the somatic (body framework) system: skeletal, arthrodial and myofascial structures, and related vascular, lymphatic and neural elements."[1] In osteopathic sports medicine, somatic dysfunction is treated using osteopathic manipulative techniques, pharmacotherapeutics, modalities, and surgery. Osteopathic manipulative techniques encompass a variety of techniques, including soft-tissue mobilization and manipulative techniques. This chapter focuses on the approach and application of osteopathic principles and practices to the rehabilitation of athletes, with an emphasis on osteopathic manipulation techniques.

What is osteopathic sports medicine?

Osteopathic medicine is deeply rooted in the care of the athlete, whether he or she is a competitor on the playing field or a working or "industrial" athlete. Forrest "Phog" Allen, DO, won 771 basketball games at Kansas University, and he was well known to use manual medicine techniques in the treatment of his players. The American Osteopathic Academy of Sports Medicine defines sports medicine as the branch of the healing arts profession that uses a holistic, comprehensive approach to the prevention, diagnosis, and management of sports- and exercise-related injuries, disorders, dysfunctions, and disease processes.[2]

REHABILITATION PRINCIPLES OF OSTEOPATHIC SPORTS MEDICINE

When structure is altered (e.g., as the result of an injury), function (or performance) is affected. Think of the athlete with a sprained ankle: ligaments (structure) are damaged, and function (performance) is adversely affected. Correspondingly, when function is altered, structure is affected. Think of a golfer who develops a new swing that causes stress at the shoulder; this may lead to acromioclavicular joint sprain, acromial spur, or other structural abnormalities. Alteration in structure or function may lead to compensatory changes through kinetic linkage, and it may cause somatic dysfunction not only locally but also at distant sites. An understanding of the kinetic chain is critical to understanding performance and osteopathic musculoskeletal pathology (somatic dysfunction).

The body is a unit, and forces that affect one area will predictably evoke a series of responses in other areas of the body, including the soft tissue, the bones, and the joints. The kinetic chain requires constant feedback mechanisms to maintain homeostasis whether at rest or in dynamic states of motion. Breakdowns of the kinetic chain occur when neuromusculoskeletal systems do not function in concert. These breakdowns often occur as a result of poor muscle activation patterns that may be the result of inexperience, deconditioning, injury, or preexisting anatomic abnormalities (e.g., leg-length discrepancy, rotoscoliosis). Any interruption in the normal biomechanics of the kinetic chain predisposes the athlete to injury. Athletes demonstrate the kinetic chain of events during any sports maneuver. For example, a volleyball player who spikes a ball must first get into a crouched or "ready" position; explosively jump; hyperextend the lumbar spine; and severely hyperextend, abduct, and externally rotate the shoulder as he or she gets ready to strike the ball. Dynamic stabilizers keep the body balanced and aligned to complete this task. In a pathologic state, the kinetic chain is affected, and sports maneuvers or performance may be adversely affected, thus leading to injury. For example, a dysfunction of the quadriceps femoris muscle could limit jumping ability. Lumbosacral dysfunction might limit back extension. Both of these injuries, which are remote from the shoulder, could interrupt normal kinetic chain biomechanics and cause effects that are detrimental to the shoulder complex. Another example is a baseball pitcher with shoulder pain who may compensate by altering his or her delivery during the acceleration phase, thus leading to elbow pain. Understanding the kinetic chain is essential to understanding the interrelatedness of structure and function, especially during rehabilitation. The reestablishment of proprioception and neuromusculoskeletal abilities to preinjury levels is a challenge that is recognized by osteopathic sports medicine physicians and a primary goal of kinetic chain rehabilitation.

The kinetic chain links one structure and function to another, and a dysfunction in any area of the kinetic chain will cause compensatory changes in the chain. If the precipitating factors are not corrected, gross trauma may occur. Recognition that the problem may not be at the obvious site of injury but rather the result of a dysfunction occurring at another part of the kinetic chain is important when developing a treatment plan.

If rehabilitation is focused only on the obvious area of injury with disregard to the entire kinetic chain, then unusual and uncompensated stress may result in further injury.

Predictable patterns of fascial rotation have been described that influence or are influenced by spinal curves and that may be altered when there is somatic dysfunction of the kinetic chain. Zink and Lawson[3] described predictable fascial motion preferences at transitional regions of the body as "common compensatory patterns." These transitional areas are the occipitoatlantal junction, the cervicothoracic junction, the thoracolumbar junction, and the lumbosacral junction.[3]

Over time, the body will adapt to stress, and compensatory patterns will result. These patterns may be caused by a structural source or a functional stress. For the highly trained athlete, compensatory patterns are the result of years of training. The development of this complex of muscles—including the development and refinement of the neurologic feedback mechanisms (proprioception)—is important to the performance of the player. Symmetry is not typically the desired goal. Rather, asymmetry is the goal, and it is the result of countless hours performing a sport-specific maneuver and the development of highly complex muscle activation patterns. Think of the right-handed tennis player with relatively overdeveloped (hypertrophied) musculature of the right forearm, shoulder complex, thorax, and back. Dysfunction affecting the massive right latissimus dorsi muscle, which extends from the iliac crest to the thoracolumbar fascia to the humerus, could interrupt the kinetic chain, thereby affecting the serve of this tennis player. However, when treating this patient, it would be a mistake to assume or attempt to make the left and right latissimus muscles equal in strength or flexibility.

During rehabilitation, the osteopathic sports medicine physician recognizes the somewhat predictable patterns of compensation to more effectively render an exercise/rehabilitation prescription that will address somatic dysfunction throughout the kinetic chain.

The osteopathic structural examination

Osteopathic sports medicine physicians receive extensive training in recognizing injury patterns. The foundation of the evaluation of the injured athlete is the comprehensive medical and injury history and physical examination. The physical examination includes a systems-based evaluation, a traditional orthopedic examination, and an osteopathic structural examination.

The osteopathic structural examination is the examination of a patient by an osteopathic physician with emphasis on the neuromusculoskeletal system, including palpatory diagnosis for somatic dysfunction and viscerosomatic/somatosomatic change within the context of total patient care. The examination is concerned with finding somatic dysfunction in all parts of the body, and it is performed with the patient in multiple positions to provide static and dynamic evaluation.[1] Components of the osteopathic structural examination are described in **Table 34.1**.

Somatic dysfunction and barriers

Osteopathic sports medicine physicians use the structural examination to recognize and treat somatic dysfunction using osteopathic manipulative techniques. The characteristics of somatic dysfunction can be described with the mnemonic *STAR*: *S*ensitivity changes, *T*issue texture abnormality, and *A*symmetry and alteration of the quality and quantity of *R*ange of motion. Another mnemonic for somatic dysfunction is *TART*: *T*issue texture abnormality, *A*symmetry, *R*estriction of motion, and *T*enderness, any one of which must be present for diagnosis **(Table 34.2)**.

Acute somatic dysfunction is the immediate or short-term impairment or altered function of related components of the

Table 34.1 Components of the Osteopathic Structural Examination

Structures Evaluated	Specific Evaluation
Pelvis and sacrum	Anterior superior iliac spine heights and distance from midline Sacral base motion
Lumbar and lower thoracic spine	Tissue texture changes Vertebral rotational motion Asymmetry Viscerosomatic reflexes Spinal curvature
Abdomen and abdominal diaphragm	Fascial restrictions Sternal motion Tender points
Respiratory motion and ribs	Rib motion Thoracic inlet
Upper thoracic and cervical spines	Tissue texture changes Vertebral motion Tender points Occipitoatlantal dysfunction Atlantoaxial dysfunction
Upper extremities	Shoulder height Carrying angle at elbow Orientation of forearms and wrists
Lower extremities	Iliac crest heights Q angles Fibular head motion Tibial tubercle inversion/eversion Medial malleoli heights Achilles tendon orientation Medial arches of the foot

somatic (body framework) system. Somatic dysfunction is characterized in its early stages by vasodilation, edema, tenderness, pain, and tissue contraction (e.g., an acute sprain). Somatic dysfunction is diagnosed by the history and by palpatory assessment for STAR/TART.[1]

Chronic somatic dysfunction is the long-term impairment or altered function of related components of the somatic (body framework) system. In contrast with acute somatic dysfunction, it is characterized by tenderness, itching, fibrosis, paresthesias, and tissue contraction. *Tissue texture abnormality* is a palpable change in tissue from skin to particular structures that represent any combination of the following signs: vasodilation, edema, flaccidity, hypertonicity, contracture, and fibrosis as well as the symptoms of itching, pain, tenderness, and paresthesias. Types of tissue texture abnormality include bogginess, thickening, stringiness, ropiness, firmness (hardening), increased or decreased temperature, and increased or decreased moisture.[1]

There are positional and motion aspects of somatic dysfunction that are best described using at least one of three parameters: (1) the position of a body part as determined by palpation and referenced to its adjacent defined structure; (2) the directions in which motion

Table 34.2 Features of Somatic Dysfunction

TART	STAR
Tissue texture changes	**S**ensitivity changes of tissues
Asymmetry	**T**issue texture abnormality
Restriction of motion	**A**symmetry
Tenderness	**R**ange-of-motion abnormalities

Table 34.3 Barriers

Physiologic	The end of the active range of motion
Anatomic	The end of the passive range of motion
Restrictive	The end of the range of motion that is less than normal

is freer; and (3) the directions in which motion is restricted.[1] The point at which motion is restricted, either normally or pathologically, is called a *barrier* (**Table 34.3**).

Schneider and Dvorak described physiologic and anatomic barriers to the normal range of motion in a joint and also pathologic barriers that can develop with injury.[4] *Anatomic barriers* refer to the limit of motion imposed by anatomic structure. Clinically, this is the limit of passive range of motion. A breach of anatomic barrier will result in dislocation and/or fracture. *Physiologic barriers* are the limits of active range of motion. Clinically, these barriers mark the beginning of passive range of motion, which ends at the anatomic barrier. The term *elastic barriers* refers to the range of motion between physiologic and anatomic barriers of motion in which passive ligamentous stretching occurs before tissue disruption. A breach of elastic barriers will result in tissue disruption, as is seen in sprains. The term *pathologic barriers* refers to the restriction of joint motion associated with pathologic change of tissues (e.g., the impingement caused by an osteophytic acromion, which limits shoulder flexion). *Restrictive barriers* are functional limits that abnormally diminish the normal physiologic range of motion. Restrictive barriers are very common and include "tight muscles" (e.g., tight hamstrings). Athletes commonly engage the restrictive barrier and, through stretching, seek to relieve or reset this barrier to increase their range of motion. When range of motion is normalized, the athlete will engage the physiologic barrier.

Facilitation and somatic dysfunction

Facilitation refers to the maintenance of a pool of neurons in a hyperexcited state or a state in which less afferent stimulation is required to elicit a neural impulse.[5] A sustained or inappropriate impulse can cause somatic dysfunction through continuous sensory input (e.g., from overstretched muscles, tendons, or ligaments). The resultant prolonged muscle contraction restricts the range of motion and can cause the activation of inflammatory mediators such as bradykinins, prostaglandins, and leukotrienes, which can cause local vasodilation and tissue texture changes (TART/STAR). Reflex activity can sustain the muscle contraction and also cause adjacent muscles to contract.

Viscerosomatic reflexes are observed when there is a reflexive neurologic response that results in recognized patterns of somatic or tissue changes. These reflexes involve localized visceral stimuli that produce patterns of response in segmentally related somatic structures. An example of a visceral somatic reflex is an abdominal wall muscle spasm that occurs as a result of appendicitis.

Somatosomatic reflexes are localized somatic stimuli that produce patterns of reflex response in segmentally related somatic structures. These may manifest as muscle spasms, tender points (Jones[6]), trigger points (Travell[7]), and tissue temperature or texture changes. Somatosomatic reflexes may represent underlying pathology that is causing sympathetic nervous system activation or hyperactivation, which result in the clinically apparent tissue texture changes.

Tender points and trigger points

Tender points are hypersensitive points in the myofascial, tendinous, and ligamentous tissues of the body that are approximately 1 cm in size and that do not have a pattern of pain radiation. Lawrence H. Jones, DO, FAAO, described tender points as a manifestation of somatic dysfunction and developed a system called *strain and counterstrain* to diagnose and treat somatic dysfunction related to tender points.[6] Counterstrain is discussed later in this chapter.

A *myofascial trigger point* is a small, hypersensitive site that, when stimulated consistently, produces a reflex mechanism that gives rise to referred pain and/or other consistent manifestations.[1] Myofascial trigger responses are consistent from person to person, and so patterns of trigger-point location and radiation have been mapped. These myofascial trigger points were most extensively and systematically documented by Janet Travell, MD, and David Simons, MD.[7]

OSTEOPATHIC APPROACH TO THE INJURED ATHLETE

History

A comprehensive history of the injury, including precipitating factors and the mechanism of injury, is critical to understanding the current injury and preventing future injury. Deconditioning, poor training, and abnormal biomechanics certainly can contribute, and they may be the primary cause of acute injury. In addition, factors such as poor nutrition and the use of supplements and performance-enhancing drugs (both banned and acceptable) can contribute to injury. Knowledge of these factors forms a basis for examination and investigation.

Sports medicine physicians must have an understanding of the physical demands and risks associated with specific sports and positions. An understanding of the level of competition (i.e., elite, collegiate, club, recreational, or school-based) is important for developing an approach to injury assessment, rehabilitation, and return to play. Athletes with poorly or incompletely rehabilitated injuries may be at a greater risk for the acute exacerbation of injury, chronic injury patterns, and compensatory changes that may cause injury at other, previously unaffected joints and soft tissues, as described previously. A detailed history is the basis for the comprehensive physical evaluation of the injured athlete.

Physical examination

A focused examination of the affected area as well as of areas of compensation is necessary for complete diagnosis. This would include what is traditionally thought of as an orthopedic evaluation in addition to the osteopathic structural examination. Osteopathic sports medicine physicians perform a structural examination that places emphasis on the neuromusculoskeletal system and that includes palpatory diagnosis for somatic dysfunction. Assessment for postural patterns, asymmetry, and functional kinetic chain abnormalities are also included in the examination. The examination is performed with the patient in multiple positions to provide both static and dynamic evaluation; an overview is provided in Table 34.1. The physical examination should include sport-specific maneuvers to gain information about abilities and disabilities. For example, a baseball pitcher with shoulder pain may have a primary somatic dysfunction of the ilium or thoracolumbar areas that affects the latissimus dorsi muscles, thereby causing an alteration of normal overhead throwing mechanics that leads to shoulder strain or injury.

This comprehensive assessment of the injured athlete provides the information that is needed to formulate a comprehensive, holistic approach to rehabilitation. Although osteopathic sports medicine physicians use a variety of methods to treat athletes, including nonpharmacologic, pharmacologic, and surgical methods, the remainder of this chapter will focus further discussion on the use of osteopathic manipulative techniques for the treatment of athletes.

Overview of osteopathic techniques

The manipulative techniques used by osteopathic sports medicine physicians to treat somatic dysfunctions can be described in various manners. One way is to segregate by mode of therapy (i.e., soft tissue, mobilization, or manipulative), and another is a classification based on the method of technique (direct or indirect) relative to the barrier engaged when performing the technique.

Direct techniques are those techniques in which the restrictive barrier is engaged as part of the treatment. There are many types of specific techniques under the umbrella of direct technique in which an impulse is applied across a joint. These have been developed to restore the symmetry of the movements that are associated with the vertebral or extremity joints. A well-known example of a direct technique is high-velocity/low-amplitude manipulation.

Indirect techniques are those techniques in which the restrictive barrier is not engaged as part of the treatment. Rather than engaging the barrier directly (direct technique), with indirect techniques, the treatment is focused on the "normal" direction of motion (i.e., into the direction of freedom) rather than the direction of restriction. These techniques enhance muscle relaxation, flexibility, and the circulation of body fluids. The focus is primarily on restoring physiologic movements to altered joint mechanics. Examples of such techniques include massage, myofascial release (stretching), strain and counterstrain, muscle energy, unwinding, and indirect functional techniques. Indirect techniques do not involve the application of impulse (quick force) across a joint. Rather, the joint is gently carried repeatedly and passively through the normal range of motion. The purpose is to increase the range of motion in a joint in which the normal motion has become restricted. One example of indirect techniques is facilitated positional release, which will be described later in this chapter.

Specific osteopathic manipulative techniques

The American Osteopathic Association describes more than 15 separate osteopathic manipulative techniques.[1] Included in this chapter are basic descriptions of a few of the most commonly used techniques and descriptions of the application of these techniques for the treatment of athletes.

Muscle energy

Muscle energy (ME) is a soft-tissue technique that refers to a system of treatment in which the patient voluntarily moves the body as specifically directed by the osteopathic physician. This directed patient action is from a precisely controlled position against a defined resistance.[1] Fred L. Mitchell, Sr, DO, first developed this method, which seeks to increase range of motion through the relaxation of antagonistic muscles.[1] The goal of ME techniques is to cause a neurophysiologic reflex that will lead to muscle relaxation. It is postulated that ME, when used directly on involved restrictions, activates the Golgi tendon organ, which relieves the muscle spasm.[8] Another theory is that engaging the affected muscle in an isometric contraction causes muscular fatigue and subsequent relaxation. Active and passive joint ranges of motion are assessed in all three planes, and barriers to normal or baseline motion are observed. For example, in the spine, these ranges of motion may be flexion–extension, rotation, and side bending. In the extremities, the assessment involves flexion–extension, pronation–supination, and abduction–adduction. Upon identification of a restrictive barrier, the joint is moved to the point of the restricted barrier (engaged), and the patient is asked to move the joint away from the barrier and toward the direction of ease of movement. The patient's force is countered by an equal opposing force by the physician, thereby causing isometric contraction of the muscle in spasm. This isometric contraction is 3 to 5 seconds in duration, and it is followed by the complete relaxation of the muscle for an additional 3 to 5 seconds;

Table 34.4   Steps of Muscle Energy Technique

1	The physician places the joint so that restrictive barriers are engaged in all planes.
2	The patient contracts muscles to move the joint away from the barrier and into the direction of ease of motion.
3	The physician applies an equal counterforce for isometric contraction.
4	The counterforce is applied for 3 to 5 seconds.
5	The patient relaxes, and the counterforce is removed.
6	The joint is passively moved to a new restrictive barrier.
7	Steps 1 through 6 are repeated 3 to 5 times until the desired range of motion is achieved.

Table 34.5   Indications and Contraindications for High-Velocity/Low-Amplitude Technique

Indications	Absolute Contraindications	Relative Contraindications
Decreased range of motion	Suspected or known fracture	Acute cervical strain
	Bone metastasis	Pregnancy
	Osteoporosis	Postoperative condition
	Unstable joints	Herniated nucleus pulposus
	Osteomyelitis	Coagulopathy
	Atlantoaxial (AA) instability	Vertebral artery ischemia

this increases the range of motion (elastic barrier) and resets the restricted barrier. The joint is then repositioned to the new barrier, and the process is repeated. The entire treatment outlined in **Table 34.4** is repeated until normal or baseline range of motion is reestablished, which usually takes 3 to 6 repetitions. Think of a contracted biceps muscle that restricts elbow extension. ME would be applied by first extending the elbow to engage the restricted barrier and then having the patient contract the biceps to flex the elbow against resistance (isometric) in the manner described previously. This would activate the Golgi tendon reflex, and the biceps would relax.

ME is very useful for precompetition warmup and for rehabilitation in which improved joint range of motion or muscle complex lengthening/stretching is desired. For example, the massive biceps femoris complex (hamstrings) can cause restriction to full knee extension and, when in a contracted or shortened state, be vulnerable to injury from a sudden and forceful knee extension. This somatic dysfunction of the hamstrings may render the athlete more susceptible to hamstring injury. This is typically as a result of immobilization of the knee in even slight flexion (after surgery or trauma) or simply as a result of repeated abnormal positioning. Think of the "weekend warrior" who sits at a desk with his or her hips and knees flexed for most of the week whose hamstrings are normally contracted and not conditioned for a weekend of sporting activity. Pregame ME can be applied to lengthen the hamstrings and increase knee extension, thereby decreasing the risk of hamstring injury or injury to associated parts of the kinetic chain.

High-velocity/low-amplitude technique

High-velocity/low-amplitude (HVLA) technique is a mobilization technique that employs a strong therapeutic impulse (high velocity) of brief duration that pushes the joint for a short distance (low amplitude) within its anatomic range of motion of a joint. HVLA is commonly known as "thrust technique." The goal of HVLA is to engage and thrust through a restrictive barrier in one or more planes of motion to elicit the release of that restriction (physiologic barrier). Thrusting techniques are used to increase motion, improve function, decrease pain, and modify somatovisceral reflexes.

HVLA is a passive technique and therefore the thrust is rendered completely by the physician, which can render the patient vulnerable to injury. HVLA is applied frequently to the cervical and lumbar spine, and so complications can arise in these areas as a result of operator error, anatomic anomaly, or preexisting conditions such as osteoporosis, an undiagnosed herniated disk, or fracture. Contraindications to consider when working with athletes include ligamentous laxity (acute sprains or chronic instability), suspected or diagnosed fractures, and atlantoaxial instability (often seen in Down syndrome and rheumatoid arthritis) **(Table 34.5)**. Although demonstrated to be very safe, major complications including vertebrobasilar injury and cauda equina syndrome have

been reported. However, the risk of serious injury is quite low and reportedly in the range of 1 in 400,000 to 1 in 1,000,000.[9]

HVLA can be applied to the axillary and appendicular joints as well as the spine. For example, athletes who engage in overhead motion and weight lifting often experience trigger or tender points related to the spasm of the muscles of the posterior shoulder complex. The levator scapulae and rhomboid muscles can be especially affected as a result of scapular motion and thoracic spinal movement. These muscles attach at the ribs and vertebra and so motion at the costovertebral joints and functional vertebral units (two vertebrae) can be affected by muscle contraction and spasm, thereby leading to somatic dysfunction. Restrictions of the motion of vertebral units and costovertebral joints may cause pain, maintain muscle spasm, and adversely affect performance. The release of these restrictions may restore normal or baseline functioning of the shoulder complex and relieve abnormal and potentially pathologic stresses. Mobilization techniques may be enhanced when they are preceded by myofascial or ME techniques to relax the muscles.

Myofascial release

Myofascial release (MFR), which was first described by Andrew Taylor Still and his early students, is a system of techniques that is directed at myofascial structures. Techniques can be described as either direct or indirect. Direct MFR techniques engage the restrictive barrier, and the tissue is then loaded with a constant force until tissue release/relaxation occurs.[1] An example of this would be the very common practice of stretching myofascial tissues during warm up or rehabilitation. Indirect MFR involves gliding the dysfunctional tissues along the path of least resistance (away from the barrier) until free movement is achieved.[1]

MFR is generally well tolerated, and most athletes have experienced some type of MFR during their careers (i.e., stretching). MFR is often used to stretch muscles before competition and during rehabilitation. Myofascial techniques can restore range of motion and decrease pain, thus allowing for the earlier return of function. The goals of myofascial treatment include the relaxation of contracted muscles; increased circulation to an area of ischemia (often accompanying muscle spasm); increased venous and lymphatic drainage; and the stimulation of stretch reflexes in hypotonic muscles.[8] Myofascial techniques are useful for interrupting the pain–muscle tension–pain cycle. Complications include increased pain, muscle spasm, and headaches (from cervical techniques).

Counterstrain

Counterstrain is a system of diagnosis and treatment that considers the dysfunction to be a continuing, inappropriate strain reflex that is inhibited by applying a position of mild strain in the direction exactly opposite that of the reflex.[1] The physiologic basis of counterstrain is based on the presumption that somatic dysfunction has a neuromuscular basis.

The goals of counterstrain are to "relieve spinal or other joint pain by passively putting the joint into its position of greatest comfort" and to "relieve pain by reducing the continuing inappropriate proprioceptive activity."[10] These goals are accomplished by specific, directed positioning around the point of tenderness, usually shortening the muscle in spasm by applying a strain to its antagonists; this interrupts the neurophysiologic reflex and relieves tension. Counterstrain is a very safe technique, and it is well tolerated by almost all athletes, including senior athletes in whom osteoporosis and osteoarthritis may be a concern. However, care should be taken when positioning the patient to minimize the development of conditions such as herniated disc, fracture (osteoporosis), or muscle spasm.

With counterstrain, the diagnosis is made by finding tender points or areas of somatic or viscerosomatic reflexes within ligaments, muscles, or joints. These reflex points are characterized by palpable and rather superficial tissue texture changes that compromise a tense, fibrotic area approximately 1 to 2 cm in size. Tenderness at this point is greater than would be expected for the applied pressure (usually to the degree that there is blanching of the nail bed). Typically, tender points are located near the bony attachments of tendons and ligaments or in the belly of the muscles.[6] There is some thought that these "Jones' tender points" may be related to "Travell's trigger points" and acupuncture points. However, trigger points radiate pain, which Jones' tender points do not, and acupuncture points are more superficial and not necessarily associated with myofascial, ligamentous, or tendinous structures.

Counterstrain is a passive technique that is based on positioning the area in a manner that shortens the involved muscle, thus ameliorating pain and dysfunction. When performing the technique, the physician places a finger pad over the tender point and, through joint positioning, relieves the intensity of pain at the tender point. Patients may report a decrease in pain, or the physician may note a change of tissue texture that reflects the release of the tender point. When pain is ameliorated to an acceptable degree (usually about 30%), the position is held for 90 seconds. This is the length of time that is usually required for the proprioceptive firing to decrease in frequency/amplitude and for the mechanoreceptors to reduce the stimulation of muscle contraction. At this point, the joint is slowly and deliberately moved into a neutral position by the physician without any patient effort. This lack of active patient effort during repositioning prevents the reinitiation of the inappropriate proprioceptive firing.

Because counterstrain is passive and gentle, it is ideal for senior athletes, athletes recovering from surgery, and disabled athletes. Contraindications include an inflammatory process at the site of the tender point, which may be evidence of an underlying pathogenic process.

Facilitated positional release

Facilitated positional release (FPR) is a system of indirect techniques developed by Stanley Schiowitz, DO, that is an enhancement of myofascial techniques.[1] FPR is performed by placing the affected region in a neutral position and adding a facilitating force of compression or torsion to the tissues to induce relaxation or release of the tissues. FPR is directed toward the normalization of hypertonic muscles, both superficial and deep.[8] The mechanism of FPR relates to the action of the muscle spindle gamma loop when the gain is suddenly decreased. As the spindles in the muscle become unloaded, there is a decline in the firing from the Ia fibers.[11] The muscle begins to relax and subsequently lengthens. Complications of FPR are postulated to include fracture (osteoporosis) and the

Table 34.6 Categories and Types of Manipulation

Mobilization	Soft Tissue	Joint Manipulation
Articulatory	Myofascial release	High-velocity/low-amplitude technique
Facilitated positional release	Muscle energy	
	Counterstrain	

aggravation of herniated discs, although no studies have investigated the incidence of complications.

FPR is performed with the use of three steps. First, the physician places the body region to be treated in neutral position (usually in the supine position). Second, compression, torsion, or a combination thereof is applied in an effort to decrease tissue tension, thus shortening the large muscle group; this position is held for 3 to 4 seconds. Finally, the treating position is released and the area is reassessed for somatic dysfunction.[12]

Articulatory techniques

Articulatory techniques are passive methods that are designed to increase joint range of motion. These techniques include direct and indirect methods. With articulatory techniques, which are also called *low-velocity/low- to moderate-amplitude techniques*, the involved joint is gently assessed for full range of motion in all planes, and barriers are assessed (anatomic barriers if normal, restrictive barriers if pathologic).[1] Restrictive barriers are engaged and gently moved through a series of maneuvers to increase range of motion. Low-velocity/low- to moderate-amplitude techniques are generally well tolerated by injured athletes because the techniques are passive and slow. Common indications include a decreased range of motion, especially among athletes who would benefit from a passive technique but who may not tolerate HVLA or who would not be able to participate in an active technique such as ME.

To perform articulatory manipulation, the affected joint and the position at which the surrounding tissue is least taut are determined. The joint and tissue are moved into the directions of ease in all planes. The position is slightly exaggerated to increase the relaxation of the affected myofascial elements. Traction and compression are the most common forces applied to decrease tissue tension. The force and motion will commonly mobilize the joint and release the tissue to the point that there may be a sudden release as reflected by a pop, a click, or another sound. When mobilization and release occur, the forces are relaxed, and the region is brought back to a neutral position for the reassessment of the dysfunction.

Articulatory techniques are very easily applied to appendicular and axial joints. An example of their use for the treatment of athletes is with the sacroiliac joint, which often develops somatic dysfunction among participants in jumping and collision sports. The sacroiliac joint is especially easily mobilized using the lower extremity as a lever to initiate motion at the joint with the athlete in the supine position. Also, athletes recovering from shoulder surgery tolerate this gentle, passive technique very well **(Table 34.6)**.

CONCLUSION

The osteopathic sports medicine physician combines the basic tenets of osteopathic medicine—the body is a unit; structure and function are reciprocally interrelated; and the body is self-healing—with the needs of the athlete often in unique clinical settings, including in the office, on the sidelines, in a medical tent, or in a rehabilitation facility. The understanding that structure and function are interrelated and that somatic dysfunction can be a consequence of sports participation provides a unique perspective with regard to injury and rehabilitation. The use of manual medicine techniques to treat somatic dysfunction in an effort to restore function and enhance performance is an important aspect of osteopathic sports medicine, and it enhances traditional approaches to injury management and rehabilitation. The approaches and techniques described in this chapter are purely introductory, and they will certainly be expanded on as osteopathic sports medicine and rehabilitation medicine evolve.

REFERENCES

1. The Glossary Review Committee of the Educational Council on Osteopathic Principles: Glossary of osteopathic terminology. In AOA Yearbook and Directory of Osteopathic Physicians. Chicago, American Osteopathic Association, 2006.
2. American Osteopathic Academy of Sports Medicine home page (Web site). Available at www.aoasm.org. Accessed December 12, 2006.
3. Zink J, Lawson W: An osteopathic structural examination and functional interpretation of the soma. Osteopathic Ann 1979;7(12):433-440.
4. Schneider W, Dvorak J: Manual Medicine Therapy. Stuttgart, Georg Thieme Verlag, 1988.
5. Ward R (ed): Foundations for Osteopathic Medicine, 2nd ed. Philadelphia, Lippincott Williams & Wilkins, 2003.
6. Jones LH: Tender points. In Jones LH (ed): Strain and Counterstrain. Newark, OH, The American Academy of Osteopathy, 1988, pp 28-29.
7. Simons DG, Travell JG: Myofascial Pain and Dysfunction: The Trigger Point Manual. Baltimore, MD, Lippincott Williams & Wilkins, 1992.
8. DiGiovanna E, Schiowitz S: An Osteopathic Approach to Diagnosis and Treatment, 3rd ed. Philadelphia, Lippincott Williams & Wilkins, 2005.
9. Stevinson C, Ernst E: Risks associated with spinal manipulation. Am J Med 2002;112(7):566-571.
10. Jones LH: Strain and Counterstrain. In Jones LH (ed): Strain and Counterstrain. Newark, OH, The American Academy of Osteopathy, 1988, p 11.
11. Carew T: The control of reflex action. In Kandel E, Schwartz J (eds): Principles of Neural Science, 2nd ed. New York, Elsevier, 1985.
12. Savarese R, Capobianco J: OMT Review: A Comprehensive Review in Osteopathic Medicine, 3rd ed. Privately published, 2003.

Core Stabilization

*Daniel L. Munton, MD; Geof D. Manzo, MS, ATC;
and Elizabeth J. Caschetta, MS, ATC*

KEY POINTS

- The core is comprised of groups of muscles that form the lumbo–pelvic–hip complex.
- Power is generated in the core and transferred distally to the extremities.
- Athletes must display appropriate core strength, stability, and dynamic control to produce efficient movements.
- A thorough evaluation of the core must take place to evaluate possible weak links along the kinetic chain.
- In overhead athletes, evaluation of the scapula is an integral part of the assessment of core strength and stability.

INTRODUCTION

Core strength and stability are important and often overlooked aspects of athletics. Historically, rehabilitation and reconditioning programs have concentrated on the extremities. However, all power is generated in the core and transferred distally to the extremities. Therefore, neglect of the core during assessment and rehabilitation can impede an athlete's future success. The purpose of this chapter is to explain the importance of core stability and its effect on the athlete.

CORE STRENGTH AND STABILITY DEFINED

The term *core* refers to the lumbo–pelvic–hip complex, where the center of gravity is located.[1,2] The muscles that make up this complex provide a stable base from which the extremities work. The term *core strength* refers to the strength and endurance of the muscles of the lumbo–pelvic–hip complex, whereas *stability* refers to the ability to use strength and endurance in a functional manner.[3,4] *Function* is defined as a multiplanar movement that involves acceleration, deceleration, and stabilization.[5,6] To be mechanically efficient, athletes must combine strength and stability training in their reconditioning programs. Core strength and stability together is called *functional strength*. Functional strength is the ability to produce concentric acceleration force, isometric stabilization force, and eccentric deceleration force in all three planes of movement during activity.[5,6]

The central nervous system plays an integral role in core stability. This system controls proprioception, which is the interpretation of sensory information and the response to position sense.[7] Receptors in the skin, joints, muscles, and tendons send information to the central nervous system, which, in turn, sends appropriate information back to the muscles to provide neuromuscular control.[7] In other words, core stability is the ability of the central nervous system to interpret the position of the body in space and to react accordingly. Appropriate muscle strength is needed to support the spine and to dynamically stabilize the body. With injury or a lack of training, proprioception can be altered, thus emphasizing the need for stabilization exercises.

CORE MUSCULATURE

The muscles that make up the core can be divided into three groups: the abdominal muscles (**Figure 35.1**), the hip muscles (**Figure 35.2**), and the spinal muscles (**Figure 35.3**). The origins, insertions, and actions of these muscles are described in **Tables 35.1, 35.2, and 35.3**. In the overhead athlete, the scapular stabilizers (**Figure 35.4**) are also considered an essential core group.

THE IMPORTANCE OF CORE STABILITY IN ATHLETICS

An athlete with a stable core will decrease the likelihood of injury as a result of his or her increased efficiency of movement (LOE: B).[1,2,4,7-10] When the lumbo–pelvic–hip complex is stable, the peripheral muscles require less forceful contractions to produce the same amount of power.[2,4,9] Adequate pelvic stability allows for the efficient transfer of power from the lower extremities to the upper extremities.[7] For example, the act of throwing requires the legs and trunk to initiate movement and to transfer forces up the arm to the ball.

Low back pain is a common complaint among both athletes and nonathletes.[1,8] Up to 30% of college football players will miss at least one game as a result of lumbar pain.[8] This pain is caused by the repeated mechanical irritation of the tissues that occupy the spine.[1,2] Repeated irritation occurs as a result of the instability of

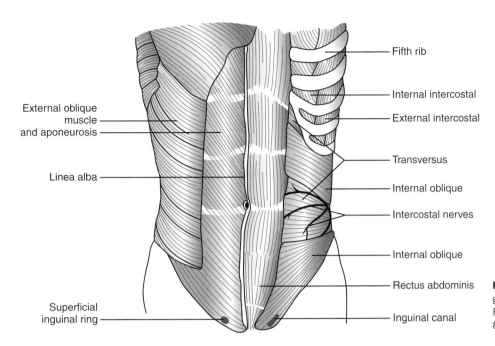

External oblique muscle and aponeurosis

Linea alba

Superficial inguinal ring

Fifth rib

Internal intercostal

External intercostal

Transversus

Internal oblique

Intercostal nerves

Internal oblique

Rectus abdominis

Inguinal canal

Figure 35.1 The abdominal core muscle group. (From Jenkins DB: Hollinshead's Functional Anatomy of the Limbs and Back, 8th ed. Philadelphia, WB Saunders, 2002.)

the spine and pelvis. Therefore, core stabilization must be incorporated into a low back pain rehabilitation program.[1,8]

The assessment of core stability

The assessment of the athlete must include all segments of the kinetic chain. Emphasis on one joint without attention to the cervical, thoracic, and lumbo–pelvic segments can lead to an incomplete picture of dysfunction. All links in the chain must have appropriate length/tension relationships for each progressive segment to be used efficiently.

The evaluation of the core must include the assessment of posture, flexibility, strength, endurance, and stabilization.[6] These

components of assessment go hand in hand with determining the appropriate function of the athlete. Optimal posture is the correct alignment of each segment. Flexibility is the appropriate length of a muscle, which has a direct relationship with posture. For example, a tight psoas muscle will anteriorly rotate the pelvis, which, in turn, will increase lumbar lordosis. In addition, a tight muscle can affect the strength of other muscles. For example, the gluteus maximus will have decreased neural drive if the hip flexors are tight. This is called *reciprocal inhibition*.[5,6] To make up for this decreased output, other muscles must compensate. Synergistic dominance will take place when synergists take over the role of the primary muscle.[5,6] An example would be the hamstring dominance of hip extension when the neural drive to the gluteus

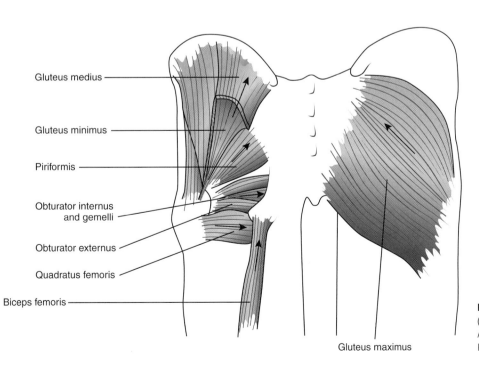

Gluteus medius

Gluteus minimus

Piriformis

Obturator internus and gemelli

Obturator externus

Quadratus femoris

Biceps femoris

Gluteus maximus

Figure 35.2 The hip core muscle group. (From Jenkins DB: Hollinshead's Functional Anatomy of the Limbs and Back, 8th ed. Philadelphia, WB Saunders, 2002.)

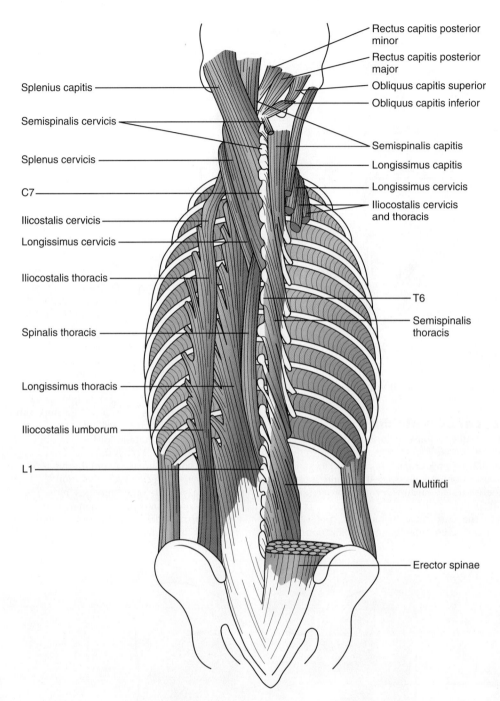

Splenius capitis

Semispinalis cervicis

Splenus cervicis

C7

Ilicostalis cervicis

Longissimus cervicis

Iliocostalis thoracis

Spinalis thoracis

Longissimus thoracis

Iliocostalis lumborum

L1

Rectus capitis posterior minor

Rectus capitis posterior major

Obliquus capitis superior

Obliquus capitis inferior

Semispinalis capitis

Longissimus capitis

Longissimus cervicis

Iliocostalis cervicis and thoracis

T6

Semispinalis thoracis

Multifidi

Erector spinae

Figure 35.3 The spinal core muscle group. (From Jenkins DB: Hollinshead's Functional Anatomy of the Limbs and Back, 8th ed. Philadelphia, WB Saunders, 2002.)

maximus is decreased. This compensation pattern leads to decreased efficiency and possible injury.

Range of motion and flexibility must be assessed at the lumbo–pelvic–hip complex. The athlete must have a full range of motion at the hip to function appropriately. If the hip opens up too early during the cocking phase of throwing, all distal segments will rotate prematurely, and this may place additional stress on the anterior shoulder (LOE: E).[11,12] Flexibility assessments at the hip should include the rectus femoris, the iliopsoas, the tensor fasciae latae, the hamstrings, and the piriformis.

Strength should be assessed for the hip extensors, the back extensors, the abdominals, and the obliques. This can be accomplished by manual muscle testing as described by Kendall and McCreary.[13] Other authors have advocated additional testing procedures that may be more functional. Bliss[4] recommends four tests for core stability: the prone bridge, the lateral bridge, torso flexor endurance, and torso extensor endurance. The athlete must hold each position with a neutral spine. Normative values in seconds are as follows: right lateral bridge, 83; left lateral bridge, 86; flexion, 34; and extension, 173 (LOE: E).[4] Norms for the prone bridge have yet to be calculated, but 60 seconds seems to be ideal. Dynamic lower-extremity stabilization tests may include a single-leg stance, an overhead squat, a single-leg squat, and a step down. Inadequate lower-extremity stabilization may cause a

Table 35.1   Abdominal Muscles of the Core

Muscle	Origin	Insertion	Action
Rectus abdominus	Pubic symphysis and pubic crest	Cartilage of the fifth to seventh ribs and the xiphoid process	Flexion of lumbar and compression of abdomen during defecation, urination, forced exhalation, and childbirth
External obliques	Inferior portion of the eighth rib	Iliac crest and the linea alba	Flexion of the lumbar vertebra when fired simultaneously; when fired unilaterally, lateral flexion and rotation
Internal obliques	Iliac crest, inquinal ligament, thoracalumbar fascia	Cartilage of the last three or four ribs and the linea alba	Flexion of the lumbar and compression of the abdomen when fired bilaterally; lateral flexion and rotation when fired unilaterally
Transverse abdominus	Iliac crest, inguinal ligament, lumbar fascia, cartilage of the inferior six ribs	Xiphoid process, linea alba, pubis	Compression of the abdomen

Table 35.2   Hip Muscles of the Core

Muscle	Origin	Insertion	Action
Tensor fascia lata	Iliac crest	Lesser trochanter of the femur	Flexes and laterally rotates the thigh; flexes the trunk at the hip joint
Gluteus maximus	Iliac crest, sacrum, coccyx	Iliotibial band, linea aspera of the femur	Extends the femur and laterally rotates the thigh
Gluteus medius and minimus	Ilium	Greater trochanter of the femur	Medially rotates the thigh; abduction
Piriformis	Anterior sacrum	Greater trochanter of the femur	Lateral rotation of the hip
Obturator externus	Inner surface of the obturator foramen, pubis, and ischium	Greater trochanter of the femur	Lateral rotation of the hip
Obturator internis	Outer surface of the obturator membrane	Greater trochanter of the femur	Lateral rotation of the hip
Superior gemellus	Ischial spine	Greater trochanter of the femur	Lateral rotation of the hip
Inferior gemellus	Ischial tuberosity	Greater trochanter of the femur	Hip stabilizer

Table 35.3   Back Muscles of the Core

Muscle	Origin	Insertion	Action
Quadratus laborum	Iliac crest, iliolumbar ligaments	Inferior border of the twelfth rib, transverse process of the first four lumbar vertebrae	Extends the lumbar region when fired bilaterally; laterally flexes the lumbar region when unilaterally fired; moves the twelfth rib inferiorly during forced exhalation
Serratus anterior	Superior eight or nine ribs	Vertebral border and the inferior angle of the scapula	Abducts and rotates the scapula upward; elevates the ribs when the scapula is stabilized
Trapezius	Nuchal line of the occipital bone and the spines of the seventh cervical and all twelve thoracic vertebra	Lateral third of the clavicle and the acromion process, medial margin of the acromion and the superior lip of spine of scapula, the tubercle at the apex of the spine of the scapula	Elevates, adducts, depresses, and upwardly rotates the scapula, along with help to extend the head
Erector spinae	Longitudinal axis of the back	Onto the ribs, upper vertebra, and head	Principal extensors of the vertebra
Multifidus	Sacrum, ilium, transverse processes of the lumbar, thoracic, and inferior four cervical vertebra	Spinous process of a more superior vertebra	Extends the vertebral column when fired bilaterally; when fired unilaterally, laterally flexes the vertebral column and rotates the head

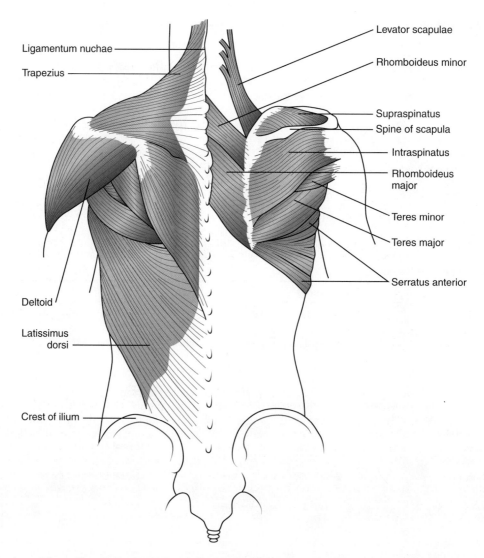

Ligamentum nuchae

Trapezius

Deltoid

Latissimus
dorsi

Crest of ilium

Levator scapulae

Rhomboideus minor

Supraspinatus

Spine of scapula

Intraspinatus

Rhomboideus
major

Teres minor

Teres major

Serratus anterior

Figure 35.4 The scapular stabilizers. (From Jenkins DB: Hollinshead's Functional Anatomy of the Limbs and Back, 8th ed. Philadelphia, WB Saunders, 2002.)

pitcher to rush through the delivery and to place increased loads on the shoulder or elbow (LOE: E).[12]

The scapula should be included in the core assessment of the overhead athlete. The scapula should be evaluated both statically and dynamically. Manual muscle testing can be undertaken, but it can be tedious. A scapular pinch test will decrease assessment time. The athlete should isometrically pinch the shoulder blades together and hold this position 15 to 20 seconds; burning in the periscapular area indicates weakness. Kibler[14] also advocates the lateral slide test. A measurement from the inferior angle of the scapula to its associated spinous process is taken with the arm at the side, with the hands on the hips, and with the arms abducted and internally rotated at 90 degrees. A positive test is a 1.5 cm or greater difference on one side as compared with the other.[14]

REHABILITATION AND RECONDITIONING

The rehabilitation and reconditioning program should be systematic and progressive.[3-6,14-17] Training begins with the most

challenging environment that an athlete can control.[6] Local muscles such as the transverse abdominus and the multifidus, however, must be activated before the global muscles of the lumbo–pelvic–hip complex. The progression is from muscle activation to dynamic stabilization.[3,4]

Tactile, auditory, and visual feedback may be necessary at first.[3,4,17] Cues can be eliminated as the athlete masters a specific task. For example, the transverse abdominus may need several cues to fire correctly. Many athletes have difficulty firing the transverse abdominus as a result of previous concentration on the other abdominal muscles for stabilization. When an athlete masters the active contraction of the transverse abdominus, cueing can be eliminated, and more dynamic movements can take place. Progression guidelines are as follows: simple to complex, stable to unstable, static to dynamic, and single plane to multiplane.[3-6,17]

Flexibility is an important aspect of the core stabilization program. Flexibility training in conjunction with stability training yields results. Appropriate length/tension relationships must be maintained throughout the kinetic chain for efficient movements to take place. All muscles of the lumbo–pelvic–hip complex must be flexible and strong.

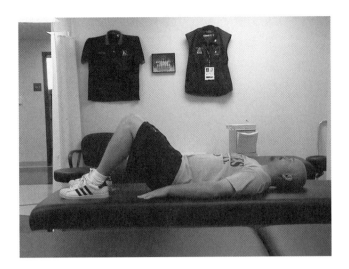

Figure 35.5 Pelvic tilt.

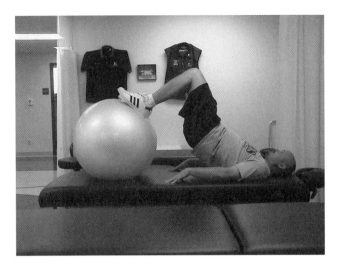

Figure 35.7 Bridge with hamstring curl on a physioball.

CORE STABILIZATION EXERCISES

Pelvic tilt progression

In a study using electromyography, the following series of exercises was found to activate the abdominal muscles significantly more than abdominal hallowing exercises (LOE: B).[18]

The athlete is supine with the feet flat on the table. He or she should be instructed to flatten the low back onto the table and then hold it there for 5 seconds. A good verbal cue for this exercise is to instruct the athlete to pull his or her belly button back toward the spine while flattening the back. Pulling the belly button back toward the spine without tilting the pelvis is an abdominal hollowing (drawing in) exercise only. Breathing should be normal while performing the pelvic tilt **(Figure 35.5)**.

When the athlete masters the pelvic tilt, he or she may be progressed to bridging exercises. The athlete performs the pelvic tilt and then lifts his or her hips off of the table and holds them up for 5 seconds **(Figure 35.6)**.

The final progression of the supine pelvic tilt is to have the athlete extend one lower extremity during the bridge. Lower extremities should alternate with each bridge. To make this exercise

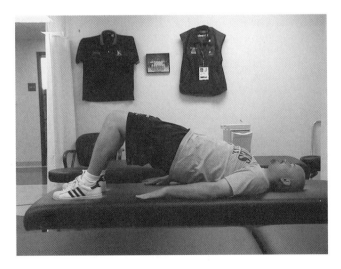

Figure 35.6 Bridge.

more difficult, the upper extremities can be alternated with the lower extremities.

Quadruped progression

The athlete is positioned on his or her hands and knees and instructed to draw in the abdominal muscles. The lower extremity on one side is then extended and held for up to 5 seconds, and the extremities should be alternated. A technique that can be used to aid in the proper performance of this exercise is to place a dowel across the back, in line with the spine. The dowel should not move. When this is mastered, the dowel can be placed perpendicular to the spine, and it must then be held in a level position.

The next progression is to extend both the upper and lower extremities on the same side and hold.

The final progression of the quadruped exercise involves the athlete extending the opposite upper and lower extremities at the same time. A dowel can be used for this exercise as well.

Physioball exercises
Seated physioball

The athlete is seated on the physioball and raises one lower extremity off the ground. This exercise can be advanced by alternating the opposite upper and lower extremities.

Bridging

The athlete is supine with the feet on the ball. The abdominals are drawn in, and the athlete lifts his or her hips off of the ground. Another way to perform a bridge on the physioball is to have the athlete seated on the ball and then to walk his or her legs out away from the ball. The hips should be level and must not sag. To make the bridge more difficult, one lower extremity can be extended.

Crunch

A simple crunch can be performed on the physioball. The athlete starts in a supine position with the back supported on the ball. A crunch is then performed. A medicine ball can be added to provide resistance.

Wall squat

The physioball is placed between the athlete and the wall. The athlete draws in his or her abdominal muscles and then performs a

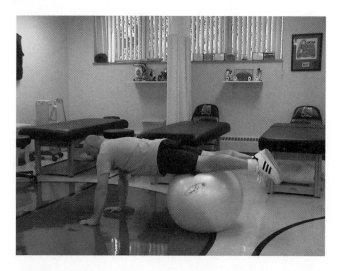

Figure 35.8 Walkouts.

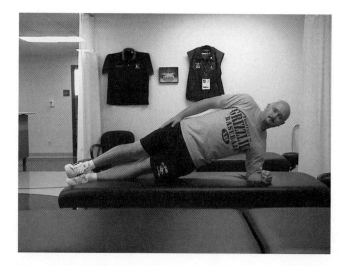

Figure 35.10 Side-lying plank.

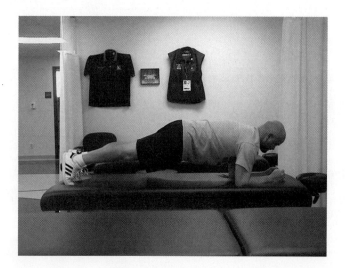

Figure 35.9 Prone plank.

squat to parallel. Moving the arms or adding a medicine ball can further challenge the core.

Hamstring curl

An additional progression to the bridge exercise is to add a hamstring curl. The athlete is supine with his or her feet on the physioball, and he or she then performs a bridge. At the completion of the bridge, the athlete performs a hamstring curl while holding the bridge **(Figure 35.7)**.

Push-ups

Wall push-ups and standard push-ups can be progressed by using a physioball. The athlete must draw in his or her abdominals before performing the push-up.

Walkouts

The athlete is prone on the physioball with his or her hands in contact with the ground. The athlete then walks forward while keeping the abdominals tight and the spine neutral. This exercise can be progressed from slow to fast **(Figure 35.8)**.

Gluteus medius exercises
Clamshell

The athlete is positioned on his or her side with the knees and hips bent. With the feet together, the athlete rotates his or her top knee up and back. The trunk should not rotate. To progress this exercise, the athlete extends his or her knee and performs a single-leg raise in abduction with slight extension.

Monster walk

A resistance band is placed around the athlete's ankles. The athlete assumes an athletic stance position and side shuffles a set distance.

Plank exercises
Prone plank

The athlete props up on his or her forearms and toes while in the prone position. The spine should be neutral, and this position is then held for 15 seconds. The athlete can progress to 30 seconds as stabilization improves **(Figure 35.9)**.

Side-lying plank

The athlete props up on his or her forearm in the side position while drawing in the abdominals. This position is held for 15 seconds and progressed to 30 seconds as stability improves **(Figure 35.10)**.

Medicine ball exercises
Crunches

Athletes can progress crunching exercises by using a medicine ball. Oblique crunches and trunk twisting maneuvers can be progressed using medicine balls as well.

Lunges

With the arms outstretched and holding the medicine ball, the athlete lunges forward and twists to the side of the lunging leg. The clinician should ensure proper form. The knees should be in line with the foot, and the knees should not go past the toes. The abdominals should be tight, and the spine should be neutral. **(Figure 35.11)**.

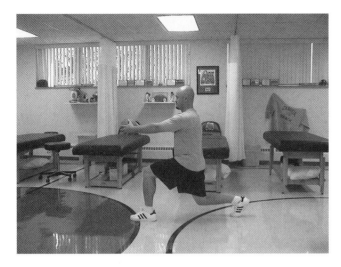

Figure 35.11   Lunge with medicine ball.

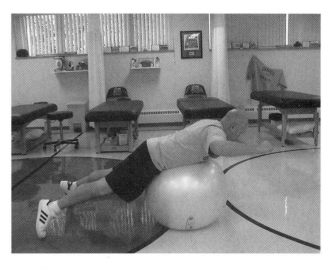

Figure 35.14   Physioball 90/90 external rotation.

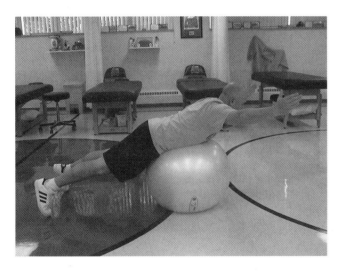

Figure 35.12   Physioball Y.

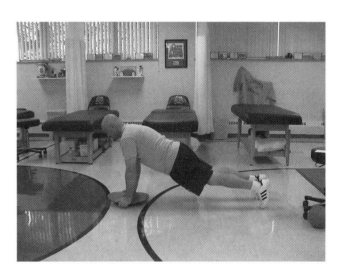

Figure 35.15   Push-up plus on a wobble board.

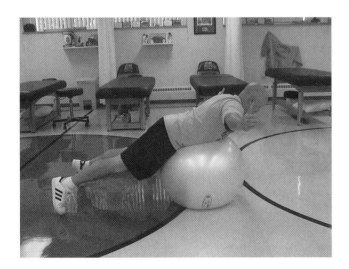

Figure 35.13   Physioball T.

Scapular stabilization exercises
Physioball Y

The athlete assumes a prone position on the physioball with the chest off of the ball. The shoulder blades are drawn back and down while the upper extremities are lifted up to form a "Y." The thumbs should be pointing upward **(Figure 35.12).**

Physioball T

The athlete is positioned in a similar fashion as he or she is to perform the physioball Y. The shoulder blades are pinched together while the upper extremities are horizontally abducted with the shoulder externally rotated. The upper extremities should not go beyond parallel with the ground because this places additional stress on the anterior shoulder **(Figure 35.13).**

Physioball 90/90 external rotation

The athlete is positioned prone on the ball as described previously. The elbows are bent at 90 degrees and then horizontally abducted to 90 degrees. The athlete then externally rotates to 90 degrees, lowers, and repeats **(Figure 35.14).**

Push-up "plus" on the wobble board

The athlete assumes a push-up position with his or her hands on the outer edge of the wobble board. The shoulder blades are protracted, and the spine is held in neutral. The athlete will hold this position for 15 seconds, and this is progressed to 30 seconds as stability improves **(Figure 35.15).**

CORE STABILITY AND THE OVERHEAD ATHLETE

The role of the scapula must not be overlooked when discussing core stability in the overhead athlete. The scapula attaches to the trunk via a suction-like mechanism that is provided by the serratus anterior and the subscapularis.[15] Three groups of muscles attach to the scapula.[14] The first group is made up of the trapezius, the rhomboids, the levator scapulae, and the serratus anterior. The second group includes the deltoid, the biceps, and the triceps. The rotator cuff makes up the final group.

The scapula serves three functions.[14,15] The first function is to maintain dynamic stability. The scapula must move along with the humerus in a coordinated manner to maintain the humeral head within the glenoid. The second function is to serve as a base for muscle attachment. These muscles serve as important force couples to maintain humeral head congruity. The lower trapezius and the serratus anterior are a pivotal force couple for acromial elevation.[14-16] The third function of the scapula is to provide proximal-to-distal energy transfer. The scapula is the link between the legs and the trunk to the arm and hand.

For the scapula to function correctly, the distal segments must be working correctly.[14] Hip and spine extension are necessary for full scapular retraction.[17,19] Kibler[14] describes scapular retraction as a "full tank of energy" that is necessary for efficient force production during throwing. In addition, the muscles that control scapular movement must be strong. The serratus anterior and the lower trapezius must upwardly rotate the scapula to elevate the acromion[14-16]; failure to do so may lead to impingement. The serratus anterior must also protract the scapula to keep up with a rapidly internally rotating and horizontally adducting humerus during the throwing motion. The inability of the scapula to keep up with the humerus may cause injury to the posterior rotator cuff and lead to instability (LOE: B).[15] The middle and lower trapezius eccentrically contract to control protraction because too much protraction can close off the subacromial space and lead to impingement.[14,15] When the scapula is functioning correctly, the rotator cuff has a stable base from which to work.

The rehabilitation and reconditioning of the overhead athlete should involve the mimicking of sport-specific movements.[6,15-17] This can be initiated early during the process. An overhead athlete with a rotator cuff injury can begin core strengthening before rotator cuff work. Scapular stabilization should be initiated as well (see Figures 35.12 through 35.15). The rotator cuff is dependent on a stable base, and this base must be developed before isolated rotator cuff exercise (LOE: E).[16,17] Closed kinetic chain exercises in low-range elevation can be initiated early as well to promote cocontraction of the rotator cuff. An athlete can do this in a standing position with an athletic stance to promote the proximal-to-distal transfer of energy.[16]

After an athlete has developed appropriate core stability; a full, pain-free range of motion; and strength and endurance peripherally, he or she may progress back to throwing. The overhead thrower should take part in an interval throwing program. Progression is from a short to a long toss and then finally off the mound. Other overhead athletes (i.e., tennis players) should follow a similar pattern of strengthening and sport-specific rehabilitation progression.

CONCLUSION

Athletes must display appropriate core strength, stability, and dynamic control of the lumbo–pelvic–hip complex produce efficient movements. A strong core is necessary for force absorption and transfer in a proximal-to-distal fashion. A thorough evaluation of the core must take place to determine possible weak links along the chain, and these "weak links" must be corrected for appropriate length/tension and force couple relationships to exist. An athlete with a strong, stable core will be able to transfer energy efficiently with more power and with less stress distally. This makes for a productive, successful athlete.

REFERENCES

1. Hodges PW: Core stability exercise in chronic low back pain. Orthop Clin North Am 2003;34:245-254.
2. Arnheim DD, Prentice WE. Principles of Athletic Training, 11th ed. St. Louis, Mosby, 2003.
3. Standaert CJ, Herring SA, Pratt TW: Rehabilitation of the athlete with low back pain. Curr Sports Med Rep 2004;3:35-40.
4. Bliss LS, Teeple P: Core stability: the centerpiece of any training program. Curr Sports Med Rep 2002;4:179-183.
5. Clark MA, Russell AM: Low Back Pain: A Functional Perspective. Thousand Oaks, CA, National Academy of Sports Medicine, 2002.
6. Clark MA: Rehabilitation: core competency underlies functional rehabilitation. Biomechanics 2000;7(2):67-73.
7. Houglum PA: Therapeutic exercise for athletic injuries. In Houglum PA (ed): Athletic Training Education Series. Champaign, IL, Human Kinetics, 2001, pp 496-562.
8. Eck JC, Riley LH: Return to play after lumbar spine conditions and surgeries. Clin Sports Med 2004;13(1):367-379.
9. Allen S: Core strengthening. Gatorade Sports Science Exchange Roundtable 2002;13(1):1-4.
10. Mandelbaum BR, Silvers HJ, Watanabe DS, et al: Effectiveness of a neuromuscular and proprioceptive training program in preventing anterior cruciate ligament injuries in female athletes. Am J Sports Med 2005;33(7):1003-1009.
11. Ceasrine V, Mundorff C: Preseason screening for the overhead-throwing athlete. NATA News 2004;17(2):41-47.
12. Cappel KR: How lower extremity biomechanics affects upper body pitching. Biomechanics 1996;3(4):22-26.
13. Kendall FB, McCreary EK: Muscle Testing and Function, 4th ed. Baltimore, Md, Williams & Watkins, 1993, pp 215-226, 284–293.
14. Kibler WB: The role of the scapula in athletic shoulder function. Am J Sports Med 1998;26(2):325-337.
15. Voight ML, Thompson BC: The role of the scapula in the rehabilitation of shoulder injuries. J Athl Train 2000;35(3):364-372.
16. Wilk KE, Andrews JR: Current concepts in the rehabilitation of overhead throwing athlete. Am J Sports Med 2002;30(1):136-151.
17. McMullen J, Uhl TL: Kinetic chain approach for shoulder rehabilitation. J Athl Train 2000;35(3):329-337.
18. Drysdale CL, Earl JE, Hertel J: Surface electromyographic activity of the abdominal muscles during pelvic tilt and abdominal hallowing exercises. J Athl Train 2004;39(1):32-36.
19. Walendzak D: Rehabilitation: lower extremity theory enhances shoulder rehabilitation. Biomechanics 1998;5(10):45-51.

CHAPTER 36

Physical Therapy Modalities

MAJ Guy R. Majkowski, PT, DSc, OCS, FAAOMPT,
and Norman W. Gill III, PT, DSC, Cert MPT, OCS, FAAOMPT

KEY POINTS

- Physical therapy modalities should be used as part of a multifaceted approach to rehabilitation.
- The proper selection of the modality depends on the stage of healing and the goal of treatment.
- Within the multimodal approach, modalities have a variable and proportional contribution that is based on the nature and extent of the injury, the body area, and the tissue healing timeline.
- Although there is reasonable underlying scientific evidence for most modalities, there is limited evidence for clinical efficacy as a result of the heterogeneity of samples, poor research designs and methodology, and the diverse parameters available for each modality.
- A lack of evidence is not evidence against using a particular modality.

INTRODUCTION

Physical therapy modalities play a vital role in a multimodal approach to rehabilitation, but they represent only a fraction of the total treatment options available to provide comprehensive management of the injured athlete **(Figure 36.1).** Although it is important that the clinician understand the general goals of each modality, it is more critical to know when to use a particular modality on the basis of the tissue healing timeline. Modalities typically serve as adjunctive treatments during the subacute or chronic phases, and they can serve as the primary treatment during the acute phase of injury. Physical therapy modalities encompass a wide range of therapeutic interventions that use various forms of energy to affect human tissue **(Figure 36.2).** Although alternative treatment options such as lasers, magnets, and ultraviolet lights are also referred to as "modalities," this chapter addresses those modalities that are most often employed as part of sports medicine rehabilitation (see Figure 36.2). Many modalities possess a broad, basic-science evidence base for their underlying principles or mechanisms[1-3]; however, there is much less evidence in the applied sciences to support their clinical use. Recent attempts to validate therapeutic efficacy are limited by poor methodology, a lack of homogenous study samples, and the clinical practice of using multiple simultaneous modalities.[1,3-27]

CRYOTHERAPY

Cryotherapy is the most commonly used modality in sports medicine. The immediate goal of cryotherapy after acute injury is purported to be the cooling of the involved tissues to control pain and to decrease blood flow to the area. The theory behind reducing blood flow to the area is to minimize the impact of secondary tissue hypoxia resulting from edema. Karunakara and colleagues determined that an ice bag applied to the forearm for a cycle of 20 minutes on, 10 minutes off, 10 minutes on, and 10 minutes off was able to reduce blood flow in the forearm/wrist (LOE: C).[28] However, the authors recommended that, if decreased blood flow was the goal of therapy, treatment times of up to an hour are indicated. Cryotherapy has additional physiologic effects that are listed in **Table 36.1.**

Despite its prominent role in the widely advocated treatment acronym *PRICE* (*P*rotection, *R*est, *I*ce, *C*ompression and *E*levation) for the early management of acute injuries, limited evidence exists to guide the clinician in recommending the best method for the application of cryotherapy. Debates continue regarding the best method of application; however, the evidence recommends crushed ice in a bag with a wet towel as being the most effective.[29,30] Zemke and colleagues compared ice massage to the use of an ice bag and found no difference between methods except that the ice massage reached its lowest temperature in approximately 18 minutes as compared with an ice bag, which reached its lowest temperature after approximately 28 minutes at mean depth of 1.7 cm (LOE: C).[31] The authors were unable to confirm that subcutaneous tissue variations effected the reduction in tissue temperature.[31] Enwemeka and colleagues found that during a 20-minute cold pack treatment, tissue temperatures at depths of more than 1 cm remained unchanged.[32] However, after removing the cold pack, the researchers found that the deeper tissues conducted heat to the superficial tissue, thereby resulting in a deep tissue (3 cm deep) temperature reduction up to 40 minutes after treatment (LOE: C).[32] Another research team investigated the effectiveness of commonly prescribed home treatments (a mixture of water and alcohol, gel packs, and frozen peas) as compared with an ice bag with a wet towel. Kanlayanaphotporn and colleagues validated the common practice of using an ice bag in a wet towel and also reported that a mixture of water and alcohol was superior to gel packs and frozen peas for reducing superficial skin temperatures to therapeutic levels (LOE: B).[29] Although basic scientific studies conducted on knee

MULTIMODAL APPROACH TO REHABILITATION

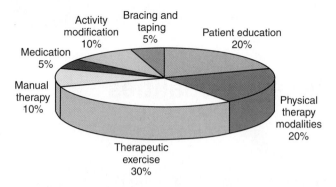

Figure 36.1 Typical percentage breakdown of the contribution of each therapeutic intervention to the comprehensive management of an injured athlete.

patients confirm that superficial cryotherapy with compression via a Cryocuff (Aircast, Inc, Summit, NJ) can reduce intra-articular knee temperatures up to 6°C after knee arthroscopy (LOE: C)[2] and after anterior cruciate ligament reconstruction (LOE: C),[33] current clinical studies have been unable to demonstrate patient-oriented evidence in the form of improved clinical outcomes (LOE: B).[34-36]

In general, cryotherapy is relatively safe. The literature describes the possible risks of frostbite and nerve damage as the only severe complications that can directly result from this modality; therefore, caution is required in its application.[37] These risks are minimized by careful screening for contraindications (see Table 36.1), supervising its application (i.e., frequently checking the area), reducing treatment duration to 20 minutes, and avoiding areas of superficial nerves (e.g., fibular head).

Ultimately, insufficient evidence exists to make strong conclusions as a result of a lack of randomized controlled trials, poor methodology, and a tendency to use ice with additional interventions[8,13,16,17] **(Table 36.2).**

Techniques and equipment
Ice
- Body area targeted: large body area such as the spine or the thighs; large joints such as the knee, shoulder, or ankle

- Advantages: conforms to surface contours, inexpensive, and widely available
- Temperatures: target tissue temperature—15 to 25°C
- Techniques:
  - Ice massage
  - Crushed ice in wet towel
  - Ice cubes in plastic bag
  - Frozen mixture of water and isopropyl alcohol (2:1 or 3:1 ratio)
- Typical progression of sensation after application: freezing, burning, aching, and numbness
- Special considerations: increased awareness of potential for superficial nerve injury (e.g., common peroneal nerve around fibular head); prevent injury by padding area or keeping ice off of the superficial nerve

Cold whirlpool bath
- Body area targeted: primarily used for extremities (typically the ankle, knee, wrist, and hand)
- Advantages: rapid circumferential cooling via convection; allows for range of motion and weight-bearing activities during treatment
- Disadvantages: costly equipment, requires daily tank cleaning, limited portability, and restricted to aforementioned body areas
- Temperatures: target water temperature at 10 to 15°C (50 to 60°F)
- Techniques: static cooling by submerging the extremity in water versus therapeutic exercise during immersion (range-of-motion or weight-bearing exercises); optional home treatment with the patient placing either the foot or hand into an ice water bucket and performing gentle exercises as instructed by the provider; duration of treatment should be 12 to 20 minutes or until numb
- Special consideration: increased awareness that digits cool more rapidly than larger joints

Gel packs
- Body area targeted: large body area such as the spine or the thighs; large joints such as the knee, shoulder, or ankle
- Advantages: more readily conforms to surface contours than ice cubes; reusable
- Temperatures: gel packs stored at −15 to −17°C (1 to 5°F); tissue temperature dropped 3.78°C for superficial tissue (skin) and 2.49°C for deep tissue (1-cm depth) after a 20-minute application (LOE: C)[32]
- Techniques: wet or dry cloth barrier placed between the gel pack and the skin; target treatment time of 20 minutes

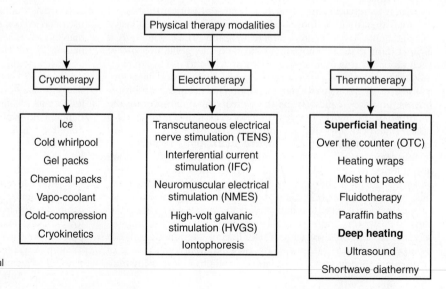

Figure 36.2 Subtypes of common modalities in physical therapy.

Table 36.1   Cryotherapy General Effects, Indications, and Contraindications

General Effects	Indications	Contraindications
Joint and soft-tissue stiffness	Pain	Circulatory or sensory impairments
Analgesic or sedative effect	Loss of joint motion	Cold hypersensitivity
Muscle relaxation	Muscle spasm	Cold uticaria (hives)
Reduced nerve conduction velocity	Acute inflammation	Cold-induced hemoglobinuria
Reduced motor power	Edema	Cryoglobinemia
Reduced muscle spasm		Communication impairments
Reduced blood flow		Raynaud's syndrome
Reduced metabolic tissue demand		
Reduced joint proprioception		

Chemical packs

- Advantages: portable without external cold source; conforms to body area
- Disadvantages: relatively expensive; one-time use; small size limits treatment area
- Special consideration: beware of the potential for the rupture of the pack and superficial skin burns

Vapocoolant sprays (e.g., fluoromethane spray)

- Body area targeted: used extensively on neck, shoulder girdle, and thigh muscles; two main uses are as a counterirritant while stretching (spray and stretch technique) and as treatment for myofascial trigger points (desensitization)
- Advantages: portable without external cold source; provides immediate analgesia
- Disadvantages: relatively expensive; transient effect
- Techniques: apply stretch to muscle; protect eyes/nose/mouth from spray; spray in parallel lines approximately 2 inches apart; hold applicator 12 to 18 inches from target area; increase stretch as tolerated
- Special consideration: use only on intact skin; avoid inhalation of spray; allow skin adequate recovery time

Cold-compression units

- Body area targeted: knee, shoulder, ankle, elbow, thigh, leg/calf, or forearm
- Advantage: most units are portable with ice water maintained in an insulated container during use; can provide 360-degree cooling of a joint; avoids melting ice
- Technique: joint/body part is secured in a pad/sleeve; ice water is forced into (or circulated through) a tube and into the pad/sleeve surrounding the joint or body part to provide simultaneous cooling and compression; can provide cooling from 30 minutes up to several hours (continuous circulation machines)

Table 36.2   Summary of Evidence for Cryotherapy

Body Region	Condition	Usefulness or Effect	Evidence	Reference
Knee	Joint proprioception	Decreased	C	Uchio et al, 2003[51]
Wrist	S/P CTR	Benefit	B	Hochberg 2001[52]
Knee	S/P arthroscopy	Benefit	B	Lessard et al, 1997[53]
Nonspecific	—	Benefit	SR	Swenson et al, 1996[37]
Knee	S/P ACLR	No Benefit	B	Konrath et al, 1996[54]
Knee	S/P ACLR	Benefit	B	Dervin et al, 1998[35]
Knee	S/P ACLR	No Benefit	B	Edwards et al, 1996[34]
Ankle	Soft-tissue injuries	Benefit	CR	Ogilvie-Harris and Gilbart, 1995[55]
Lumbar	LBP	ID	SR	French et al, 2006[13]
Elbow	DOMS	No benefit	B	Yackzan et al, 1984[56]
Elbow	DOMS	No benefit	C	Paddon-Jones et al, 1997[57]
	Soft-tissue injuries	Benefit	SR	Mac Auley, 2001[58]
	Acute soft-tissue injuries	ID	SR	Bleakley et al, 2006[8]
Forearm	Blood flow	Decreased	C	Karunakara et al, 1999[28]

Recommendation: The current evidence suggests the following: Protect the skin from frostbite by placing a cloth barrier between the ice and the patient. Protect superficial nerves by placing padding over the nerve or keeping ice off of these areas. Recommended crushed ice wrapped in a wet towel or a mixture of water and alcohol. The duration of treatment depends on the goal of treatment: pain control and deep tissue cooling = 20 minutes; reduce blood flow = alternating 10 minutes on and 10 minutes off for 1 hour.

Evidence ratings: A, double-blind study; B, clinical trial, >20 subjects; C, clinical trial, <20 subjects; D, series, ≥5 subjects; E, anecdotal case reports.

ACLR, anterior cruciate ligament reconstruction; CR, critical review; CTR, carpal tunnel release; DOMS, delayed-onset muscle soreness; ID, insufficient data; LBP, low back pain; S/P, status post; SR, systematic review.

Cryokinetics

- Body area targeted: ankle, knee, or shoulder
- Technique: numb the joint before exercise to allow progressive, active exercise of the target area; typically the area is numbed by ice massage or an ice bath; exercise continues until pain starts to return; reapply ice massage (usually 2 to 3 minutes) several times during the exercise session as needed

THERMOTHERAPY

Therapeutic heat is a commonly used modality in sports medicine as a result of its wide applicability and general ease of use. It is often well tolerated by patients, and it psychologically provides a degree of relaxation and comfort in addition to its physiologic benefits. Therapeutic heat is generally divided into superficial heat and deep heat modalities. The method of heat transfer and the length of time of application are the key factors for determining the depth of penetration. The general principle is that heat energy moves from areas of high concentration to areas of low concentration. Energy is transferred to body tissue for therapeutic heating in one of four ways:

1. Radiation: The environment is hotter than the body, and the heat is absorbed by the tissue; there is no contact (e.g., diathermy).
2. Conduction: Direct contact allows for the direct transfer down the energy gradient (e.g., hot packs).
3. Convection: There is direct contact, but the medium moves across the body (e.g., fluidotherapy/whirlpool).
4. Conversion: One form of energy, such as sound or electricity, is converted into heat (e.g., ultrasound).

Therapeutic heat is used primarily during the subacute phase of healing or when symptoms have become chronic; and it is contraindicated for patients with acute injuries. The overarching goals of heat application are the reduction of pain and increased circulation to promote healing. Some heating modalities are purely passive (e.g., hot packs, paraffin), whereas fluidotherapy is a more vigorous heat application, and it is often combined with therapeutic exercise during treatment. The size of the area to be treated often affects the choice of modality. For deep heat especially, ultrasound is limited to a very small, specific area, whereas diathermy can treat a broad area. Both have their advantages, depending on the clinical problem facing the clinician.

Evidence shows that superficial heating modalities can raise the skin temperature by 1 to 6°C and intramuscular temperatures by between 0.4 (LOE: D)[38] and 2.2°C (LOE: D).[39] The intramuscular temperature has been shown to remain elevated for at least 16 minutes after application.[38] It is thought that collagen fibers in heated tissues will have improved elasticity. Although some research indicates that this is the case, the overall effect appears to be small, and, therefore, it may be clinically irrelevant. For example, Robertson and colleagues found that shortwave diathermy increased tissue extensibility (without stretching) in ankle dorsiflexion motion by 1.8 degrees; this was in contrast with superficial heating (hydrocollator packs), which increased extensibility by 0.7 degrees, and no heat, which resulted in a −0.1-degree change (LOE: B).[40] Although the results of the shortwave diathermy treatment were statistically significant and demonstrated the scientific result of increased tissue extensibility, the 1.8-degree increase in motion is of questionable clinical significance. Similar conclusions were found by Funk and colleagues and Lin and colleagues, who studied moist heat packs with stretching for increasing hamstring length in the 90/90 position and knee flexion range of motion, respectively.[41,42] Funk and colleagues found a statistical difference after a 20-minute moist heat treatment, but the clinical effect was only a 2.6-degree increase in knee extension (LOE: B)[41]

Lin and colleagues found that the maximum benefit of moist heat appears to have a ceiling effect after 20 minutes, with a maximum increase of 6 to 7 degrees (LOE: B).[42] Cosgray and colleagues found that any benefit gained from their protocols for superficial heating lasted for less than 24 hours (LOE: B).[43] The physiologic effects of thermotherapy have been noted in other tissues, too. For example, increased nerve conduction velocity was found in the superficial radial sensory nerve after 20 minutes of fluidotherapy treatment (LOE: C).[44]

The general therapeutic effects of thermotherapy as well as its indications and contraindications are summarized in **Table 36.3.**

The clinical evidence to support superficial heat modalities is either insufficient or lacking data. By contrast, evidence for deep-heating modalities shows conflicting results regarding its efficacy. The Philadelphia Panel performed the most recent systematic review of the literature about physical therapy treatments for four major areas of the body: the knee, the shoulder, the neck, and the low back.[21-24] The conclusions of this review and of more recent studies are located in the following summary of evidence tables for each modality.

Techniques and equipment
Superficial heating modalities (penetration depth, approximately 1 cm)

Over-the-counter heat wraps
- Use an exothermic reaction of iron disks to transfer heat by conduction (e.g., ThermaCare heat wraps)
- Body areas targeted: back, neck, and shoulders
- Temperature: skin temperature rises of 1 to 6°C and intramuscular temperature rises of up to 1.5°C
- Techniques: applied directly onto the skin for up to 8 hours

Moist hot packs
- Heat transfer by conduction
- Most commonly used modality
- Body areas targeted: large body areas such as the spine or the thighs; large joints such as the shoulders and the knees
- Temperatures: hot packs heated in a hydrocollator at 71 to 79°C (150 to 170°F)
- Technique: prepare/drape area; wrap hot pack in 6 to 8 layers of dry towel (hot pack covers typically count as two layers); apply to target area
- Special considerations: do not let patient lie on hot pack

Fluidotherapy
- Heat transfer by convection
- Medium: small particles heated by forced hot air vigorously circulate around the body part
- Body areas targeted: hand/wrist and foot/ankle
- Also used for skin desensitization
- Temperatures: provides constant heat at 38.8 to 47.8°C (102 to 118°F)
- Technique: body part is washed and inserted into machine; range of motion during therapy is encouraged

Paraffin
- Heat transfer by conduction
- Medium: paraffin wax and mineral oil in a ratio of 1:7
- Body areas targeted: hand/wrist and foot/ankle
- Also aids in skin moisturizing and scar management
- Temperatures: 47.8°C (118 to 130°F)
- Technique: body part is washed, dipped in wax 7 to 10 times to add layers, covered with plastic bag, and wrapped in a towel for approximately 20 to 30 minutes

Table 36.3 Thermotherapy General Effects, Indications, and Contraindications

General Effects	Indications	Contraindications
Analgesic and/or sedative effect	Pain	Acute trauma
Promote muscle relaxation	Loss of joint motion	Acute inflammation
Removal of waste/debris	Contractures/adhesions	Hemorrhage
Increase in collagen extensibility	Muscle spasm	Edema
Increase in range of motion	Chronic inflammation	Infection
Increase in blood flow/vasodilatation	Myositis ossificans	Malignancy
Increase in oxygen	Tendinitis/bursitis	Communication impairments
Increase in cellular metabolism		Circulatory and/or sensory impairments
Decrease in muscle spasm		Hypersensitivity
		Skin breakdown

- Special considerations: do not use if the individual has open cuts, sores, or active infection in the area to be treated **(Table 36.4)**.

Deep-heating modalities (penetration depths, >1 cm)

Ultrasound
- Heat transfer by conversion
- Physics: sound waves formed by the vibration of a piezoelectric crystal are absorbed within the tissue
- Body area targeted: deeper tissue and smaller areas, typically the shoulder, neck, elbow, ankle, and knee

- Depth of penetration: 1 to 2 cm at 3 MHz and 4 to 6 cm at 1 MHz frequencies
- Power: 1.5 watts/cm^2 typically used
- Technique: The area is prepared and draped. Ultrasound gel (coupling agent) is applied to the sound head using small, slow, circular movements, and it is applied in an area not to exceed 4×4 inches. With continuous ultrasound, the sound head must be in motion at all times, or it will burn the tissue. Despite previously held beliefs that pulsed ultrasound does not provide a thermal effect, Gallo and colleagues found an equivalent thermal effect when comparing pulsed ultrasound (3 MHz, 1.0 watts/cm^2, 50% duty cycle, 10 minutes)

Table 36.4 Summary of Evidence for Superficial Heat

Body Region	Condition	Usefulness or Effect	Evidence	Reference
Neck	Pain	ID	CR	Wright and Sulka, 2001[1]
Neck	Acute and chronic	ND	SR	Philadelphia Panel, 2001[22]
Shoulder	Calcific tendinitis	ND	SR	Philadelphia Panel, 2001[21]
	Capsulitis	ID		
	Bursitis, tendinitis	ID		
	Nonspecific pain	ID		
Lumbar	LBP	Benefit	SR	French et al, 2006[13]
	Acute LBP	Benefit	B	Nuhr et al, 2004[59]
Lumbar	Acute LBP	ND	SR	Philadelphia Panel, 2001[24]
	Subacute LBP	ND		
	Chronic LBP	ID		
	Postsurgical LBP	ND		
Knee	PFS	ND	SR	Philadelphia Panel, 2001[23]
	Postsurgical	ND		
	OA	ND		
	Tendinitis	ND		
Hamstring	Flexibility	Benefit*	B	Cosgray et al, 2004[43]
	Flexibility	No benefit	B	Funk et al, 2001[41]
Quadriceps	DOMS	No benefit	B	Jayaraman et al, 2004[60]

Recommendation: Overall, there are insufficient or lacking clinical trials to establish a strong recommendation for or against superficial heat. Recent reviews indicate moderate evidence for a small, short-term decrease in pain and disability in acute and subacute patients with LBP, with an additional benefit observed from adding exercise.

*Range of motion gained during treatment returned to baseline in less than 24 to 48 hours.

Evidence ratings: A, double-blind study; B, clinical trial, >20 subjects; C, clinical trial, <20 subjects; D, series, ≥ 5 subjects; E, anecdotal case reports.

CR, critical review; DOMS, delayed-onset muscle soreness; ID, insufficient data; LBP, low back pain; ND, no data; OA, osteoarthritis; PFS, patellofemoral syndrome; SR, systematic review.

Table 36.5 Summary of Evidence for Ultrasound

Body Region	Condition	Usefulness	Evidence	Reference
Neck	Acute	ND	—	Philadelphia Panel, 2001[22]
	Chronic	No benefit	SR	
Shoulder	Calcific tendinitis	Benefit	A	Ebenbichler et al, 1999[61]
Shoulder	Calcific tendinitis	Benefit	SR	Philadelphia Panel, 2001[21]
	Capsulitis	No benefit	SR	
	Bursitis, tendinitis	No benefit	SR	
	Nonspecific pain	No benefit	SR	
Shoulder	Shoulder impingement	ID	B	Johansson et al, 2005[62]
Wrist	CTS	Benefit	SR	O'Conner et al, 2005[65]
	CTS	Benefit	B	Bakhtiary et al, 2004[63]
	CTS	Benefit	A	Ebenbichler et al, 1998[64]
Lumbar	Acute LBP	No benefit	SR	Philadelphia Panel, 2001[24]
	Subacute LBP	ND		
	Chronic LBP	No benefit		
	Postsurgical LBP	ND		
Hip	OA	No benefit	SR	Welch et al, 2005[65]
Quadriceps	DOMS	No benefit	B	Jayaraman et al, 2004[60]
Knee	PFS	No benefit	SR	Brosseau et al, 2005[9]
	OA	No benefit	SR	Welch et al, 2005[65]
Knee	PFS and OA	No benefit	SR	Philadelphia Panel, 2001[23]
	Postsurgical	ND		
	Tendinitis	ND		
Ankle	Ankle injuries	Limited	CR	Ogilvie-Harris and Gilbert, 1995[55]
	Acute ankle sprains	No benefit	SR	Van der Windt et al, 2005[66]
	Achilles tendinitis			
Foot	Plantar fasciitis	ND	SR	Crawford & Thomson, 2006[12]
General	Epicondylitis, tendinitis, tenosynovitis	No benefit	A	Klaiman et al, 1998[47]

Recommendation: Increasing numbers of clinical trials do not support the use of ultrasound for PFS, knee OA, LBP, chronic neck pain, or shoulder pathologies, with the exception of calcific tendinitis and CTS.

Evidence ratings: A, double-blind study; B, clinical trial, >20 subjects; C, clinical trial, <20 subjects; D, series, ≥5 subjects; E, anecdotal case reports. CR, critical review; CTS, carpal tunnel syndrome; DOMS, delayed-onset muscle soreness; ID, insufficient data; LBP, low back pain; ND, no data; OA, osteoarthritis; PFS, patellofemoral syndrome; SR, systematic review.

and continuous ultrasound (3 MHz, 0.5 watts/cm^2, 10 minutes).[45] Hence, practitioners should consider continuous movement of the sound head, regardless of the setting. Another clinical application of ultrasound is phonophoresis. Phonophoresis is therapeutic ultrasound with the addition of a medicated gel or conductive medium. Cagnie and colleagues concluded that pulsed ultrasound delivered a higher concentration of the medication when treating the knee as compared with continuous ultrasound.[46] Although in vivo studies have demonstrated drug penetration via phonophoresis, the clinical outcome studies have not demonstrated any additional benefit of adding medications to the ultrasound treatments (LOE: A, A).[47,48]

- Special considerations: do not use over eyes, testes, ovaries, heart, pregnant uterus, pacemaker/implanted stimulators, cemented joint implants, or epiphyseal plates in children **(Table 36.5)**.

Shortwave diathermy

- Heat transfer by nonionizing radiation
- Physics: electromagnetic energy in the radiofrequency spectrum is absorbed within the tissue
- Body areas treated: large body areas such as the spine, shoulders, arms, thighs, and hips

- Two main types of diathermy: capacitive (energy derived primarily from the electric field) and inductive (energy derived primarily from the magnetic field; provides the greatest thermal effect)
- Depth of penetration: capacitive, 1 cm; inductive, 3 cm
- Frequency: commonly 27.12 MHz
- Power: 80 to 120 watts
- Equipment: capacitive machines use plates, inductive machines use drums (most common) or cables
- Techniques: the body part to be treated is draped with a cloth towel to absorb moisture, and the plates or drums are placed near the treatment area. The distance between the device and the skin is specific to the treatment, and it is dependent on a number of factors: the type of device, the size of the device, and the amount of subcutaneous fat. Treatment time is 15 minutes.
- Special considerations: do not use over eyes, testes, ovaries, intrauterine device, pregnant uterus, pacemaker/implanted stimulators, metal objects, or epiphyseal plates in children; be cautious of moist skin, sweat, and blisters, which can focus or concentrate energy and cause burns **(Table 36.6)**

ELECTROTHERAPY

Electrotherapy is an increasingly popular modality in sports medicine. Electrotherapy is the application of low-level electrical

Table 36.6 Summary of Evidence for Shortwave Diathermy

Body Region	Condition	Usefulness or Effect	Evidence	Reference
Knee	Analgesic effect	No benefit	A	Laufer et al, 2005[67]
Neck	Analgesic effect	No benefit	B	Dziedzic et al, 2005[68]
Calf	Increased tissue extensibility	Benefit	B	Robertson et al, 2005[40]
Calf		Benefit	B	Peres et al, 2002[69]
Hamstring		Benefit	B	Draper et al, 2004[70]
Calf	Increased tissue temperature	Benefit	C	Draper et al, 1999[71]

Recommendation: Shortwave diathermy appears to have no benefit in the treatment of knee osteoarthritis. Limited evidence is available supporting the scientific foundation of shortwave diathermy and the short-term results of its use for increasing tissue temperature and extensibility. Well-designed controlled trials are lacking, thus preventing evidence-based recommendations for specific patient populations.
Evidence ratings: A, double-blind study; B, clinical trial, >20 subjects; C, clinical trial, <20 subjects; D, series, ≥5 subjects; E, anecdotal case reports.

current to the peripheral nervous and musculoskeletal systems. It has widespread applicability for the treatment of orthopedic conditions and varied indications, although its application in sports medicine is typically for pain control and muscle reeducation. This class of modalities has many advantages, including portability, ease of use, and noninvasive special applications for cutaneous wound and fracture healing **(Table 36.7).**

The immediate goals of electrotherapy are to improve muscle performance and control pain. Several mechanisms of action are proposed for each type of modality, and indications often depend on the stage of healing. After acute injury, transcutaneous electrical nerve stimulation (TENS) can be used to control pain, and neuromuscular electrical stimulation or interferential current can be used to address edema (pumping action through muscle contraction) and muscle spasm or to prevent disuse atrophy. In the case of painful inflammatory conditions, electrical currents can be used for the transdermal delivery of anti-inflammatory or pain-controlling medications by driving charged ions through the skin; this modality is known as *iontophoresis.* Electrical stimulation is a valuable modality after surgery or injury, and it is widely used to improve neuromuscular control and to provide biofeedback for muscles of the rotator cuff, the quadriceps, or the anterior tibialis. Electrical stimulation and interferential current are also applied with the goal of breaking the pain–spasm–pain cycle during the acute or subacute phases of healing. The tonic contraction of a muscle induces an ischemic event that further increases muscle tone. Electrical stimulation of the muscle is thought to improve blood flow to the muscle and to break the pain and spasm cycle.

There is sufficient evidence to support the theories behind the use of electrotherapy; however, it must be recognized that the clinical evidence is limited.[1,19,21-24] As with cryotherapy and thermotherapy, electrical modalities offer a wide range of parameters and available treatment options. Therefore, they present a challenge with regard to the methodologic design of studies. In addition, electrical modalities are typically used as adjunctive treatments, so other treatments occurring simultaneously may confound the ability to establish direct cause-and-effect relationships. Although it is difficult to make strong conclusions about the efficacy of electrical modalities alone, they appear to be a reasonable choice as an adjunctive therapy for the treatment of sports-related injuries.

Techniques and equipment
General

Types of stimulators
- Direct current
  - Iontophoresis
  - Muscle denervation

- Wound healing
- Alternating current
  - Pain control
  - Muscle reeducation
  - Edema management
  - Fracture healing

Common parameters
- Wave form
- Amplitude (intensity)
- Pulse width (duration)
- Pulse rate (frequency)

Transcutaneous electrical nerve stimulation
- Indication: pain control
- Theories: Gate theory proposes the inhibition of small C-fibers from the periphery as a result of the stimulation of larger-diameter afferents.[49] The competing theory is that TENS causes a release of endogenous opioids (endorphins); this is typically associated with higher-frequency settings.
- Wave form: typically biphasic
- Modes: TENS is usually delivered in three types of modes:
  Conventional (high-rate TENS)
  - Good after acute injury or immediately after surgical
  - Gate control action; avoids muscle contraction
  - High frequency (40 to 150 Hz)
  - Low intensity (minimally above threshold)
  - Current (10 to 30 mA)
  - Short pulse duration (usually <50 microseconds)
  - Pain relief only while on (30 to 60 minutes several times a day)
  Acupuncture-like
  - For trigger points and subacute pain
  - Elicits motor response
  - Low frequency (1 to 10 Hz)
  - Maximally tolerated intensity; treatment times are minimal
  - Pain relief tends to occur after the completion of the treatment rather than during treatment, but effects typically last longer than with conventional TENS
  High frequency or burst
  - Burst of 1 to 2 Hz
  - 100 Hz frequency in each burst
- Advantages: units are small and portable; patient easily trained in their use
- Disadvantages: units can range between $200 and $800
- Special considerations: accommodation to stimulus common over time and may result in the need to increase intensity;

Table 36.7 Electrotherapy General Effects, Indications, and Contraindications

General Effects	Indications	Contraindications
Analgesia	Pain	Sensory impairments
Gate control theory	Muscle spasm	Hypersensitivity
Endogenous pain control theory	Muscle re-education	Communication impairments
Reduced muscle spasm	Prevention of atrophy	Demand-type cardiac pacemaker
Promotion of muscle relaxation	Loss of motion	Cardiac arrhythmias
Increased blood flow via vasodilation	Stimulating denervated muscle	Use over a pregnant uterus (premature contractions)
Iontophoretic transdermal medication delivery	Edema	Use over the anterior neck (laryngospasms possible)
Strengthening	Wound healing	Use over the carotid sinus (vasovagal reflex)
Biofeedback	Fracture healing	

Table 36.8 Summary of Evidence for Transcutaneous Electrical Nerve Stimulation

Body Region	Condition	Usefulness or Effect	Evidence	Reference
Neck	MND	ID	SR	Kroeling et al, 2005[3]
Neck	Acute	No benefit	SR	Philadelphia Panel, 2001[22]
	Chronic	ID		
Shoulder	Calcific tendinitis	ND	SR	Philadelphia Panel, 2001[21]
	Capsulitis	ID		
	Bursitis, tendinitis	ID		
	Nonspecific pain	ID		
Forearm	Pain	Benefit*	B	Johnson et al, 2003[72]
Lumbar	Acute LBP	No benefit	SR	Philadelphia Panel, 2001[24]
	Subacute LBP	ND		
	Chronic LBP	No benefit	A	
	Postsurgical LBP	ND		
Lumbar	Nonspecific LBP	No benefit	B	Herman et al, 1994[73]
Knee	OA	Benefit	SR	Osiri et al, 2000[20]
Knee	OA	Benefit	A	Law et al, 2004[74]
Knee	PFS	ND		Philadelphia Panel, 2001[23]
	Postsurgical	No benefit	SR	
	OA	Benefit	SR	
	Tendinitis	ND		

Recommendation: Increasing numbers of clinical trials do not support the use of transcutaneous electrical nerve stimulation for acute or chronic LBP, acute neck pain, or postsurgical pain. Recent reviews indicate moderate evidence for transcutaneous electrical nerve stimulation for the treatment of knee OA. Additional well-designed controlled trials are needed that will determine more specific, evidence-based recommendations for treatment protocols and specific patient populations.

*Healthy subjects
Evidence ratings: A, double-blind study; B, clinical trial, >20 subjects; C, clinical trial, <20 subjects; D, series, ≥5 subjects; E, anecdotal case reports.
ID, insufficient data; LBP, low back pain; MND, mechanical neck disorder; ND, no data; OA, osteoarthritis; PFS, patellofemoral syndrome; SR, systematic review.

Table 36.9 Summary of Evidence for Interferential Current Stimulation

Body Region	Condition	Usefulness or Effect	Evidence	Reference
Elbow	DOMS	Benefit	D	Minder et al, 2002[75]
Shoulder	Shoulder pain	No benefit	B	Van der Heijden et al, 1999[76]
Lumbar	LBP	Benefit	B	Hurley et al, 2004[77]
Lumbar	LBP	Benefit	B	Hurley et al, 2001[78]
Lumbar	LBP	No benefit	B	Werners et al, 1999[79]
Forearm	Induced ischemic pain*	Benefit	B	Johnson and Tabasam, 2003[72]

Recommendation: There is insufficient evidence to formulate a recommendation. Hurley and colleagues[75] did not include a true control group, and they demonstrated that all groups improved with no significant difference at 6 and 12 months whether they received manual therapy, interferential current stimulation, or a combination of both. The prior study by Hurley and colleagues[76] suggests greater effectiveness with spinal nerve root electrode placement, but the absence of a control or placebo group prevents the determination of efficacy.

*Healthy subjects
Evidence ratings: A, double-blind study; B, clinical trial, >20 subjects; C, clinical trial, <20 subjects; D, series, ≥5 subjects; E, anecdotal case reports.
DOMS, delayed-onset muscle soreness; LBP, low back pain.

Table 36.10   Summary of Evidence for Neuromuscular Electrical Stimulation

Body Region	Condition	Usefulness or Effect	Evidence	Reference
Cervical	Acute and chronic pain	ID	SR	Philadelphia Panel, 2001[22]
Shoulder	Calcific tendinitis	ND	SR	Philadelphia Panel, 2001[21]
	Capsulitis, bursitis, tendinitis	ND		
	Nonspecific pain	ND		
Lumbar	Acute and subacute LBP	ND	SR	Philadelphia Panel, 2001[24]
	Postsurgical LBP	ND		
	Chronic LBP	ID		
Quadriceps	Strengthening*	Benefit	B	Parker et al, 2003[80]
Knee	S/P TKA	Benefit	D	Stevens et al, 2004[81]
Knee	S/P ACLR	Benefit	B	Fitzgerald et al, 2003[82]
Knee	PFS	ND	SR	Philadelphia Panel, 2001[83]
	Postsurgical	ID		
	Osteoarthritis	No benefit		
	Tendinitis	ND		

Recommendation: There are no data or insufficient evidence for most applications, with limited evidence of any benefit of this treatment for knee rehabilitation protocols.
*Healthy subjects
Evidence ratings: A, double-blind study; B, clinical trial, >20 subjects; C, clinical trial, <20 subjects; D, series, ≥5 subjects; E, anecdotal case reports.
ACLR, anterior cruciate ligament reconstruction; ID, insufficient data; LBP, low back pain; ND, no data; PFS, patellofemoral syndrome; S/P, status post; SR, systematic review; TKA, total knee arthroplasty.

skin irritation can occur from the electrodes (gel drying) or from the tape used to hold the electrodes in place **(Table 36.8)**

Interferential current stimulation
- Indications: pain control, muscle stimulation, and increased circulation
- Theory: Two AC signals at different medium frequencies are crossed, thus generating a perceived signal in the intersection (phase overlaps) that is thought to penetrate into the deeper tissue than the cutaneous stimulation found with TENS. Higher currents are better tolerated with interferential current.
- Special considerations: can use multiple pairs of electrodes (2, 3, or 4) to cover large regions; requires an electrical source; involves large-expense equipment; requires a provider for setup and adjustments **(Table 36.9)**

Neuromuscular electrical stimulation
- Indications: muscle re-education, prevention of disuse atrophy, and edema management
- Mechanism: electrical stimulation of the peripheral nerve causing strong muscle contraction
- Techniques: Basic application involves device selection, parameter selection, and electrode placement. The application of

different waveforms (e.g., Russian, monophasic, and biphasic) is routinely used. Pulse rate may affect patient comfort, and varying levels of intensity can be used, from submaximal to maximal tolerance. Larger electrodes are better tolerated; small electrodes may be used if trying to isolate a specific muscle.
- Advantage: can be combined with active therapeutic exercise to enhance muscle contraction
- Special considerations: will not help a denervated muscle; must have an intact peripheral nerve; console units may provide a better effect than portable, battery-powered units (LOE: C)[50] **(Table 36.10)**

High-volt galvanic stimulation (direct current)
- Indications: stimulate denervated muscle and aid in edema management
- Mechanism: A muscle denervated by an injured peripheral nerve can be stimulated to contract by the direct depolarization of the muscle, thus circumventing the regenerating nerve. For edema management, the polarity of the charges delivered is thought to affect ions in the interstitial fluid to reduce edema, and the pumping action of the muscles aids in the movement of fluids and lymph from the injured area.
- Techniques: A large dispersive pad is usually placed on a large surface area, such as the back or the opposite thigh, and the

Table 36.11   Summary of Evidence for High-Volt Galvanic Stimulation

Body Region	Condition	Usefulness or Effect	Level of Evidence	Reference
Neck	Chronic neck pain	ID	SR	Kroeling et al, 2005[3]
	Acute and subacute pain	ID		
	Occipital headaches	ID		
Wrist	CTD	Benefit	B	Stralka et al, 1998[83]
Ankle	Lateral epicondylitis	No benefit	B	Michlovitz et al, 1988[84]

Recommendation: There is insufficient evidence available to provide a clinical recommendation for or against the use of high-volt galvanic stimulation.
Evidence ratings: A, double-blind study; B, clinical trial, >20 subjects; C, clinical trial, <20 subjects; D, series, ≥5 subjects; E, anecdotal case reports.
CTD, cumulative trauma disorder; ID, insufficient data; SR, systematic review.

Table 36.12   Summary of Evidence for Iontophoresis

Body Region	Condition	Usefulness or Effect	Evidence	Reference
Neck	Whiplash (<2 months)	ID	SR	Kroeling et al, 2005[3]
Ankle	Achilles tendinitis	Benefit	A	Neeter et al, 2003[85]
Foot	Plantar fasciitis	Benefit*	A	Gudeman et al, 1997[86]
Elbow	Lateral epicondylitis	Benefit	A	Nirschl et al, 2003[87]
Elbow	Lateral epicondylitis	No benefit	A	Runeson et al, 2002[88]
Shoulder	Calcific tendinitis	No benefit	A	Leduc et al, 2003[89]
Temporomandibular joint	Temporomandibular disorders	Benefit	A	Schiffman et al, 1996[90]
Shoulder	Calcific tendinitis	No benefit	B	Perron et al, 1997[91]
Wrist	Carpal tunnel syndrome	Benefit†	B	Gokoglu et al, 2005[92]
Cervicothoracic	Myofascial trigger points	No benefit	A	Evans et al, 2001[93]

Recommendation: Limited evidence exists to suggest a beneficial role of iontophoresis for the treatment of acute Achilles tendinitis and temporomandibular joint disorders. Studies of other areas of the body have resulted in either conflicting evidence or insufficient evidence to make a recommendation for or against the use of this modality.

*Iontophoresis treatments provided enhanced short-term decreases in symptoms, but no difference was present at 1 month as compared with the ice, stretching, and strengthening group.
†This study identified a clinical benefit from iontophoresis, but it was not superior to corticosteroid injection at both 2 and 8 weeks.
Evidence ratings: A, double-blind study; B, clinical trial, >20 subjects; C, clinical trial, <20 subjects; D, series, ≥5 subjects; E, anecdotal case reports.
ID, insufficient data; SR, systematic review.

active electrodes are placed on the treatment site. Pulse rates may be adjusted to improve comfort, and voltage is gradually increased to patient tolerance. During the acute phase of edema management, intensity is kept at the submuscular contraction level. For denervated muscle, maximum tolerated intensities are recommended. Treatment times of 20 to 30 minutes are standard.

- Special considerations: tolerance may build within or between treatments, typically resulting in frequent voltage increases **(Table 36.11)**

Iontophoresis (direct current galvanic stimulation)

- Indications: reduce pain and inflammation
- Mechanism: A transcutaneous delivery of medication is provided. Charged ions in solution are placed under an electrode that delivers the same charge; the resultant repelling charge forces ions through the skin.
- Technique: Two electrodes are placed on skin (one with medication, one for electrical ground) with an initial current at 0.1 to 0.5 mA/cm^2 and gradually increased until the patient feels tingling. The maximum current applied is 4.0 mA/cm^2.
- Special considerations: electrical burns possible if current too high; thermal burns possible if electrodes not well adhered to skin; skin irritation if skin is not clean or if it is oily; occasional lightening seen among darker-skinned people with corticosteroid use (dexamethasone) **(Table 36.12)**

CONCLUSION

The use of modalities serves an important role in the rehabilitation of an injured athlete. The main modalities used in sports medicine consist of cryotherapy, thermotherapy (superficial and deep), and electrical therapies. The goals of each modality drive their application; however, other important factors must be considered, such as the tissue-healing timeframe, the body area to be treated, the size of the treatment area, the depth of target tissue, and coexisting conditions that may contraindicate certain treatment options. The evidence base for modalities is strong in the basic sciences but less robust regarding the clinical efficacy as a result of numerous methodologic challenges. It is important to highlight that modalities typically serve as adjunctive treatments; however, they can be the primary treatment during the acute phase of injury. When used in conjunction with other treatments, the prescription of modalities offers a range of therapeutic choices for the sports medicine practitioner who is looking to optimize healing and to facilitate the return of function of the athlete.

REFERENCES

1. Wright A, Sluka KA: Nonpharmacological treatments for musculoskeletal pain. Clin J Pain 2001;17(1):33-46.
2. Martin SS, Spindler KP, Tarter JW, et al: Does cryotherapy affect intraarticular temperature after knee arthroscopy? Clin Orthop Relat Res 2002;(400):184-189.
3. Kroeling P, Gross AR, Goldsmith CH: A Cochrane review of electrotherapy for mechanical neck disorders. Spine 2005;30(21):E641-E648.
4. Murphy K, Guiliani J, Freedman B: The diagnosis and treatment of lateral epicondylids. Curr Opin Orthop 2006;17:134-138.
5. O'Conner D, Marshall S, Massy-Westropp N: Non-surgical treatment (other than steroid injection) for carpal tunnel syndrome. Cochrane Database Syst Rev 2005;(1):CD003219.
6. Pelland L et al: Electrical stimulation for the treatment of rheumatoid arthritis. Cochrane Database Syst Rev 2005;(5):CD003687.
7. Aker PD et al: Conservative management of mechanical neck pain: systematic overview and meta-analysis. BMJ 1996;313(7068):1291-1296.
8. Bleakley C, McDonough S, MacAuley D: The use of ice in the treatment of acute soft-tissue injury: a systematic review of randomized controlled trials. Am J Sports Med 2004;32(1):251-261.
9. Brosseau L et al: Therapeutic ultrasound for treating patellofemoral pain syndrome. Cochrane Database Syst Rev 2001;(4):CD003375.
10. Cole C, Seto C, Gazewood J: Plantar fasciitis: evidence-based review of diagnosis and therapy. Am Fam Physician 2005;72(11):2237-2242.
11. Brosseau L et al: Thermotherapy for treatment of osteoarthritis. Cochrane Database Syst Rev 2003;(4):CD004522.
12. Crawford F, Thomson C: Interventions for treating plantar heel pain. Cochrane Database Syst Rev 2003;(3):CD000416.
13. French SD et al: A Cochrane review of superficial heat or cold for low back pain. Spine 2006;31(9):998-1006.
14. Goodyear-Smith F, Arroll B: What can family physicians offer patients with carpal tunnel syndrome other than surgery? A systematic review of nonsurgical management. Ann Fam Med 2004;2(3):267-273.
15. Green S, Buchbinder R, Hetrick S: Physiotherapy interventions for shoulder pain. Cochrane Database Syst Rev 2003;(2):CD004258.
16. Gross AR et al: Physical medicine modalities for mechanical neck disorders. Cochrane Database Syst Rev 2000;(2):CD000961.

17. Hubbard TJ, Aronson SL, Denegar CR: Does cryotherapy hasten return to participation? A systematic review. J Athl Train 2004;39(1):88-94.
18. Maher CG: Effective physical treatment for chronic low back pain. Orthop Clin North Am 2004;35(1):57-64.
19. Nyland J, Nolan MF: Therapeutic modality: rehabilitation of the injured athlete. Clin Sports Med 2004;23(2):299-313, vii.
20. Osiri M et al: Transcutaneous electrical nerve stimulation for knee osteoarthritis. Cochrane Database Syst Rev 2000;(4):CD002823.
21. Philadelphia Panel: Philadelphia Panel evidence-based clinical practice guidelines on selected rehabilitation interventions for shoulder pain. Phys Ther 2001;81(10):1719-1730.
22. Philadelphia Panel: Philadelphia Panel evidence-based clinical practice guidelines on selected rehabilitation interventions for neck pain. Phys Ther 2001;81(10):1701-1717.
23. Philadelphia Panel: Philadelphia Panel evidence-based clinical practice guidelines on selected rehabilitation interventions for knee pain. Phys Ther 2001;81(10):1675-1700.
24. Philadelphia Panel: Philadelphia Panel evidence-based clinical practice guidelines on selected rehabilitation interventions for low back pain. Phys Ther 2001;81(10):1641-1674.
25. Robinson V et al: Thermotherapy for treating rheumatoid arthritis. Cochrane Database Syst Rev 2002;(1):002826.
26. Speed CA: Therapeutic ultrasound in soft tissue lesions. Rheumatology (Oxford) 2001;40(12):1331-1336.
27. Verhagen AP et al: Conservative treatments for whiplash. Cochrane Database Syst Rev 2004;(1):003338.
28. Karunakara RG, Lephart SM, Pincivero DM: Changes in forearm blood flow during single and intermittent cold application. J Orthop Sports Phys Ther 1999;29(3):177-180.
29. Kanlayanaphotporn R, Janwantanakul P: Comparison of skin surface temperature during the application of various cryotherapy modalities. Arch Phys Med Rehabil 2005;86(7):1411-1415.
30. Belitsky RB, Odam SJ, Hubley-Kozey C: Evaluation of the effectiveness of wet ice, dry ice, and cryogenic packs in reducing skin temperature. Phys Ther 1987;67(7):1080-1084.
31. Zemke JE et al: Intramuscular temperature responses in the human leg to two forms of cryotherapy: ice massage and ice bag. J Orthop Sports Phys Ther 1998;27(4):301-307.
32. Enwemeka CS et al: Soft tissue thermodynamics before, during, and after cold pack therapy. Med Sci Sports Exerc 2002;34(1):45-50.
33. Glenn RE Jr et al: Cryotherapy decreases intraarticular temperature after ACL reconstruction. Clin Orthop Relat Res 2004;(421):268-272.
34. Edwards DJ, Rimmer M, Keene GC: The use of cold therapy in the postoperative management of patients undergoing arthroscopic anterior cruciate ligament reconstruction. Am J Sports Med 1996;24(2):193-195.
35. Dervin GF, Taylor DE, Keene GC: Effects of cold and compression dressings on early postoperative outcomes for the arthroscopic anterior cruciate ligament reconstruction patient. J Orthop Sports Phys Ther 1998;27(6):403-406.
36. Healy WL et al: Cold compressive dressing after total knee arthroplasty. Clin Orthop Relat Res 1994;(299):143-146.
37. Swenson C, Sward L, Karlsson J: Cryotherapy in sports medicine. Scand J Med Sci Sports 1996;6(4):193-200.
38. Sawyer PC et al: Effects of moist heat on hamstring flexibility and muscle temperature. J Strength Cond Res 2003;17(2):285-290.
39. Blankenship K, et al.: Temperature rise in deep muscle tissue during a three-hour therapeutic heat wrap application. Med Sci Sports Exerc 2003;35(5 Supplement 1):S108.
40. Robertson VJ, Ward AR, Jung P: The effect of heat on tissue extensibility: a comparison of deep and superficial heating. Arch Phys Med Rehabil 2005;86(4):819-825.
41. Funk D et al: Efficacy of moist heat pack application over static stretching on hamstring flexibility. J Strength Cond Res 2001;15(1):123-126.
42. Lin YH: Effects of thermal therapy in improving the passive range of knee motion: comparison of cold and superficial heat applications. Clin Rehabil 2003;17(6):618-623.
43. Cosgray NA et al: Effect of heat modalities on hamstring length: a comparison of pneumatherm, moist heat pack, and a control. J Orthop Sports Phys Ther 2004;34(7):377-384.
44. Kelly R et al: Effect of fluidotherapy on superficial radial nerve conduction and skin temperature. J Orthop Sports Phys Ther 2005;35(1):16-23.
45. Gallo JA et al: A comparison of human muscle temperature increases during 3-MHz continuous and pulsed ultrasound with equivalent temporal average intensities. J Orthop Sports Phys Ther 2004;34(7):395-401.
46. Cagnie B et al: Phonophoresis versus topical application of ketoprofen: comparison between tissue and plasma levels. Phys Ther 2003;83(8):707-712.
47. Klaiman MD et al: Phonophoresis versus ultrasound in the treatment of common musculoskeletal conditions. Med Sci Sports Exerc 1998;30(9):1349-1355.
48. Penderghest C, Kimura I, Gulick D: Double-blind clinical efficacy study of pulsed phonophoresis on perceived pain associated with symptomatic tendonitis. J Sport Rehabil 1998;7(1):9-19.
49. Melzack R, Wall PD: Pain mechanisms: a new theory. Science 1965;150(699):971-979.
50. Snyder-Mackler L et al: Electrical stimulation of the thigh muscles after reconstruction of the anterior cruciate ligament. Effects of electrically elicited contraction of the quadriceps femoris and hamstring muscles on gait and on strength of the thigh muscles. J Bone Joint Surg Am 1991;73(7):1025-1036.
51. Uchio Y et al: Cryotherapy influences joint laxity and position sense of the healthy knee joint. Arch Phys Med Rehabil 2003;84(1):131-135.
52. Hochberg J: A randomized prospective study to assess the efficacy of two cold-therapy treatments following carpal tunnel release. J Hand Ther 2001;14(3):208-215.
53. Lessard LA et al: The efficacy of cryotherapy following arthroscopic knee surgery. J Orthop Sports Phys Ther 1997;26(1):14-22.
54. Konrath GA et al: The use of cold therapy after anterior cruciate ligament reconstruction. A prospective, randomized study and literature review. Am J Sports Med 1996;24(5):629-633.
55. Ogilvie-Harris DJ, Gilbart M: Treatment modalities for soft tissue injuries of the ankle: a critical review. Clin J Sport Med 1995;5(3):175-186.
56. Yackzan L, Adams C, Francis KT: The effects of ice massage on delayed muscle soreness. Am J Sports Med 1984;12(2):159-165.
57. Paddon-Jones DJ, Quigley BM: Effect of cryotherapy on muscle soreness and strength following eccentric exercise. Int J Sports Med 1997;18(8):588-593.
58. Mac Auley DC: Ice therapy: how good is the evidence? Int J Sports Med 2001;22(5):379-384.
59. Nuhr M et al: Active warming during emergency transport relieves acute low back pain. Spine 2004;29(14):1499-1503.
60. Jayaraman RC et al: MRI evaluation of topical heat and static stretching as therapeutic modalities for the treatment of eccentric exercise-induced muscle damage. Eur J Appl Physiol 2004;93(1-2):30-38.
61. Ebenbichler GR et al: Ultrasound therapy for calcific tendinitis of the shoulder. N Engl J Med 1999;340(20):1533-1538.
62. Johansson KM, Adolfsson LE, Foldevi MO: Effects of acupuncture versus ultrasound in patients with impingement syndrome: randomized clinical trial. Phys Ther 2005;85(6):490-501.
63. Bakhtiary AH, Rashidy-Pour A: Ultrasound and laser therapy in the treatment of carpal tunnel syndrome. Aust J Physiother 2004;50(3):147-151.
64. Ebenbichler GR et al: Ultrasound treatment for treating the carpal tunnel syndrome: randomised "sham" controlled trial. BMJ 1998;316(7133):731-735.
65. Welch V et al: Therapeutic ultrasound for osteoarthritis of the knee. Cochrane Database Syst Rev 2001;(3):003132.
66. Van Der Windt DA et al: Ultrasound therapy for acute ankle sprains. Cochrane Database Syst Rev 2002;(1):001250.
67. Laufer Y et al: Effect of pulsed short-wave diathermy on pain and function of subjects with osteoarthritis of the knee: a placebo-controlled double-blind clinical trial. Clin Rehabil 2005;19(3):255-263.
68. Dziedzic K et al: Effectiveness of manual therapy or pulsed shortwave diathermy in addition to advice and exercise for neck disorders: a pragmatic randomized controlled trial in physical therapy clinics. Arthritis Rheum 2005;53(2):214-222.
69. Peres SE et al: Pulsed shortwave diathermy and prolonged long-duration stretching increase dorsiflexion range of motion more than identical stretching without diathermy. J Athl Train 2002;37(1):43-50.
70. Draper DO et al: Shortwave diathermy and prolonged stretching increase hamstring flexibility more than prolonged stretching alone. J Orthop Sports Phys Ther 2004;34(1):13-20.
71. Draper DO et al: Temperature change in human muscle during and after pulsed shortwave diathermy. J Orthop Sports Phys Ther 1999;29(1):13-18; discussion 19-22.
72. Johnson MI, Tabasam G: An investigation into the analgesic effects of interferential currents and transcutaneous electrical nerve stimulation on experimentally induced ischemic pain in otherwise pain-free volunteers. Phys Ther 2003;83(3):208-223.
73. Herman E et al: A randomized controlled trial of transcutaneous electrical nerve stimulation (CODETRON) to determine its benefits in a rehabilitation program for acute occupational low back pain. Spine 1994;19(5):561-568.
74. Law PP, Cheing GL: Optimal stimulation frequency of transcutaneous electrical nerve stimulation on people with knee osteoarthritis. J Rehabil Med 2004;36(5):220-225.
75. Minder PM: Interferential therapy: lack of effect upon experimentally induced delayed onset muscle soreness. Clin Physiol Funct Imaging 2002;22(5):339-347.
76. Van der Heijden GJ et al: No effect of bipolar interferential electrotherapy and pulsed ultrasound for soft tissue shoulder disorders: a randomised controlled trial. Ann Rheum Dis 1999;58(9):530-540.
77. Hurley DA et al: A randomized clinical trial of manipulative therapy and interferential therapy for acute low back pain. Spine 2004;29(20):2207-2216.
78. Hurley DA et al: Interferential therapy electrode placement technique in acute low back pain: a preliminary investigation. Arch Phys Med Rehabil 2001;82(4):485-493.
79. Werners R, Pynsent PB, Bulstrode CJ: Randomized trial comparing interferential therapy with motorized lumbar traction and massage in the management of low back pain in a primary care setting. Spine 1999;24(15):1579-1584.
80. Parker MG et al: Strength response in human femoris muscle during 2 neuromuscular electrical stimulation programs. J Orthop Sports Phys Ther 2003;33(12):719-726.

81. Stevens JE, Mizner RL, Snyder-Mackler L: Neuromuscular electrical stimulation for quadriceps muscle strengthening after bilateral total knee arthroplasty: a case series. J Orthop Sports Phys Ther 2004;34(1):21-29.

82. Fitzgerald GK, Piva SR, Irrgang JJ: A modified neuromuscular electrical stimulation protocol for quadriceps strength training following anterior cruciate ligament reconstruction. J Orthop Sports Phys Ther 2003;33(9):492-501.

83. Stralka SW, Jackson JA, Lewis AR: Treatment of hand and wrist pain. A randomized clinical trial of high voltage pulsed, direct current built into a wrist splint. AAOHN J 1998;46(5):233-236.

84. Michlovitz S, Smith W, Watkins M: Ice and high voltage pulsed stimulation in treatment of lateral ankle sprains. J Orthop Sports Phys Ther 1998;(9):301-304.

85. Neeter C et al: Iontophoresis with or without dexamethazone in the treatment of acute Achilles tendon pain. Scand J Med Sci Sports 2003;13(6):376-382.

86. Gudeman SD et al: Treatment of plantar fasciitis by iontophoresis of 0.4% dexamethasone. A randomized, double-blind, placebo-controlled study. Am J Sports Med 1997;25(3):312-316.

87. Nirschl RP et al: Iontophoretic administration of dexamethasone sodium phosphate for acute epicondylitis. A randomized, double-blinded, placebo-controlled study. Am J Sports Med 2003;31(2):189-195.

88. Runeson L, Haker E: Iontophoresis with cortisone in the treatment of lateral epicondylalgia (tennis elbow)—a double-blind study. Scand J Med Sci Sports 2002;12(3):136-142.

89. Leduc BE et al: Treatment of calcifying tendinitis of the shoulder by acetic acid iontophoresis: a double-blind randomized controlled trial. Arch Phys Med Rehabil 2003;84(10):1523-1527.

90. Schiffman EL, Braun BL, Lindgren BR: Temporomandibular joint iontophoresis: a double-blind randomized clinical trial. J Orofac Pain 1996;10(2):157-165.

91. Perron M, Malouin F: Acetic acid iontophoresis and ultrasound for the treatment of calcifying tendinitis of the shoulder: a randomized control trial. Arch Phys Med Rehabil 1997;78(4):379-384.

92. Gokoglu F et al: Evaluation of iontophoresis and local corticosteroid injection in the treatment of carpal tunnel syndrome. Am J Phys Med Rehabil 2005;84(2):92-96.

93. Evans T et al: The immediate effects of lidocaine iontophoresis on trigger-point pain. J Sports Rehabil 2001;10(4):287-297.

CHAPTER 37

Athletic Taping

Raymond D. Chronister, ATC, and Gregg Calhoon, ATC

KEY POINTS

- Athletic taping is used for joint support and to control joint motion. It can be used for prevention of injury or in response to injury.
- The cosmetic appearance of taping is less important than its function: Support the joint or region without causing complications or injury.
- Contact allergies to tape and tape adherent can occur. Offending substances should be discontinued.
- Blisters are caused by friction. Rolls or bubbles in the prewrap or tape can cause friction and should be avoided.

INTRODUCTION

Taping is used to support joints and to limit the motion of various body parts. Whether it is for prevention or as a response to an acute or chronic injury, athletes in any sport may use taping. Before doing any tape job, it is important to understand why it is being done. How much support is needed? What motion is being supported or prevented? What motion is still required? Often a lot of misguided emphasis is placed on doing a "pretty" tape job, but what is important is that the tape supports what it needs to and that it does not cause blisters. If the tape provides support without causing harm, then remember the old adage, "It all looks the same under a sock." This chapter describes some commonly used taping techniques, but remember that there any many ways that each can be done.

BASIC SUPPLIES

The athletic training kit and the training room should be stocked with these basic supplies.

Tape adherent

Tape adherent is used to help secure the prewrap or tape to the skin. This should be sprayed over the area to be taped and given a few seconds to dry. As it dries, it will become sticky. Some athletes may be allergic to the adhesive, so watch for signs of contact dermatitis. Common tape adherent products are Tuff-Skin and QDA.

Underwrap or prewrap

Underwrap or prewrap is commonly used as a barrier between the skin and tape, for unshaved ankles or other hairy body parts, or to decrease the irritation that comes with the daily removal of the tape. For optimal results, prewrap should not be used for ankle taping. When using underwrap or prewrap, all skin should be covered, and wrinkles in the prewrap material must be strictly avoided because these can cause blisters. Use as thin a layer of underwrap as possible.

Athletic tape

Athletic tapes comes in widths of $^{1}/_{2}$, 1, $1^{1}/_{2}$, and 2 inches. In general, $1^{1}/_{2}$-inch tape is the most commonly used size, because it can be easily split into smaller widths but can still be used as a substitute for 2-inch tape.

Elastikon

Elastikon is a flexible but very strong tape that is very difficult to tear). It comes in 1-inch, 2-inch, and 3-inch sizes.

Elastic stretch tape

Elastic stretch tape is a very flexible tape that is used where other tape may constrict a body part, such as around the thigh or calf. It comes in 1-inch, 2-inch, and 3-inch sizes, and it is also used to cover other tape applications.

Other supplies

Tape scissors and heel and lace pads are other common taping supplies.

BASIC TERMS

Anchors

Anchors are the first strips of tape to be laid down, and there are usually two of them. These are used as structural support to "anchor" the strips that are subsequently applied.

Stirrups

Stirrups are supporting strips for an ankle tape that pull the calcaneus either laterally (to support against inversion) or medially (to support against eversion). They should start and end at the proximal anchor strip.

Horseshoe

A *horseshoe* is made of supporting strips of ankle tape that run medially to laterally behind the ankle, starting and ending at the distal anchor strip. These are used to interlock with the stirrups to add strength.

Cover/seal

Covering or *sealing* with tape is done to overwrap all of the supporting strips, ensuring that no skin is exposed. Covering or sealing with tape minimizes possible friction points and also helps cross-tie all of the support strips for added strength.

Supporting strip

A *supporting strip* is a piece of tape that is applied to the skin for the primary function of motion support (i.e., not to anchor or seal).

POINTS TO REMEMBER

- Blisters are caused by friction. Rolls in the prewrap or wrinkles in the tape may be a source of friction in the active ankle and thus can lead to blistering.
- Practice tearing the tape. Many people try to tear the tape against the body part being taped, but this can cause the athlete pain if it is a swollen or tender area. The tape should be torn with two hands off of the body part **(Figure 37.1).** It is a good idea to take a roll of tape and practice tearing off 2-inch to 3-inch strips.
- Steady tension is important. The tape should be applied evenly so that neither edge is digging into the skin (a possible cause of blisters). Care also must be taken so that the proper amount of pressure is applied as the tape unrolls. If it is laid down too loosely, then it will not be effective; if it is too tight, it will restrict circulation to the extremity.
- The best technique for handling the tape roll is to grip with your thumb on the back surface of the tape and to place either your index or middle finger in the hole of the tape roll. This way, the tension of the tape coming off of the roll can be controlled by squeezing the roll between your thumb and finger. Tearing the tape will also be easier and quicker **(Figure 37.2).**
- When applying the tape, the roll should be held out about 3 or 4 inches from the patient's skin. This will make it easier to manipulate turns while maintaining the desired amount of tension **(Figure 37.3).**
- Remember that each body part that you tape is different. The tape will need to be angled in a way that causes it to lay evenly (i.e., no edges digging in). It is important for both strength of structure and blister prevention that the tape is laid flat against the skin. Continuous strips are generally not used (except for heel locks and spicas) because they will pinch and constrict the changing contours of the body. For the ankle, the strips around the lower leg must be angled to fit the conical shape of the leg (i.e., the leg narrows toward the ankle).

- As a general rule, the loose end of stretch tape that is used to cover an application should either be tucked under itself or sealed with a few strips of athletic tape to keep it from rolling up.

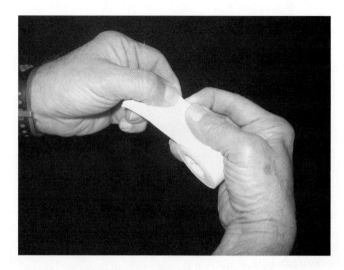

Figure 37.1 Tear athletic tape with two hands.

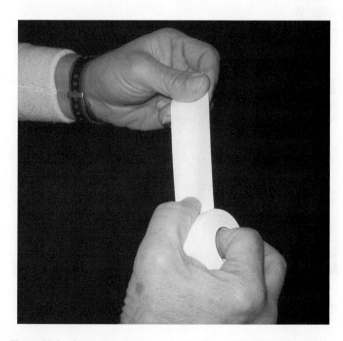

Figure 37.2 Control the tension of the tape by squeezing the roll between the thumb and the forefinger.

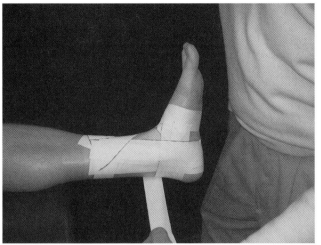
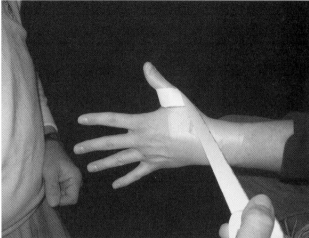

A   B

Figure 37.3 *A* and *B,* Hold the roll of tape about 3 to 4 inches away from the skin.

STANDARD ANKLE TAPING

Supplies
- $1^1/_2$-inch tape
- Tape adherent
- Possibly underwrap and heel and lace pads

Body position
The athlete should sit with his or her ankle hanging off of the table about halfway up the lower leg. The foot should be in a relatively talar/calcaneal neutral position, with 0 degrees of dorsiflexion. Remind the athlete to keep the foot in this position until the taping is complete. If the athlete changes the position of the foot during taping, it will cause wrinkles that may lead to blisters.

Procedure
(Note: Remember to consider whether you are supporting inversion or eversion because this will dictate the direction in which you pull the stirrups.)

1. Spray the ankle with Tuff-Skin.
2. Apply the heel and lace pads.
3. Cover the ankle with underwrap, if required. Remember to avoid rolls in the underwrap and to cover all of the skin with as thin a layer as possible **(Figure 37.4).**
4. Apply a circumferential anchor strip at the distal and proximal ends. If underwrap is used, each strip should overlap the edge of the underwrap onto the skin **(Figure 37.5).**
5. Apply the first stirrup. Start at the anchor (proximal), and pull the tape down under the calcaneus and up to the anchor on the other side. Use the malleolus as your guide **(Figure 37.6).** Remember to pull the stirrup laterally for inversion support and medially for eversion support.
6. Apply the first horseshoe strip. Start on the medial side at the distal anchor, and pull the horseshoe around behind the posterior ankle

to the other side, on the anchor again, using the malleolus as a guide. Cover the bottom third first **(Figure 37.7).**
7. Repeat steps 5 and 6 two more times. Each successive strip should overlap the previous strip by half **(Figure 37.8).**
8. Start the heel lock by placing a strip diagonally across the top of the ankle **(Figure 37.9A).** The tape should start at the styloid process on the base of the fifth metatarsal and run to the medial malleolus. The tape will then make the turn around the heel (Figure 37.9B) and back over to the lateral aspect of the heel; note that the tape is placed on the lateral heel posterior and inferior to the lateral malleolus (Figure 37.9C). The tape continues across the plantar surface of the foot and then comes up the medial side before it crosses back over the top of the ankle (Figure 37.9D). Running nearly exactly anterior to posterior, the strip continues directly over the lateral malleolus and then crosses behind the heel, coming around inferior to the medial malleolus. The tape will continue under the foot to the lateral side, where it will be torn off on the dorsal aspect of the foot (Figure 37.9E). When this procedure is performed correctly, the heel lock tape forms a cross (makes an "X") behind the ankle (Figure 37.9F) and on the anterior ankle/foot (Figure 37.9G).
9. The tape will then need to be sealed with circumferential strips from the top to the malleolus, with each previous strip overlain by half. The forefoot must be sealed as well **(Figure 37.10)** so that all skin is covered (except the very tip of the heel) as well as all of the previous strips (steps 5 through 8).

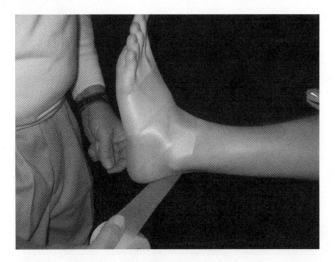

Figure 37.4   Cover the skin with a very thin layer of underwrap.

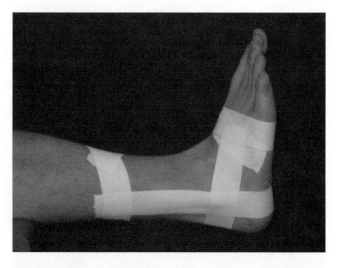

Figure 37.7   Apply the first horseshoe strip.

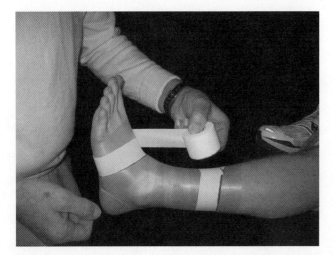

Figure 37.5   Apply the anchor strip at the distal and proximal ends.

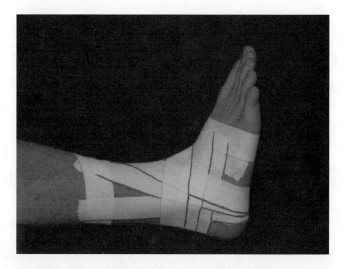

Figure 37.8   Apply a stirrup strip and a horseshoe strip twice more, with each strip overlapping the previous one by half.

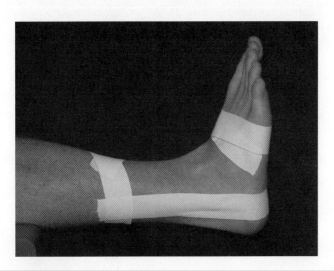

Figure 37.6   Apply the first stirrup.

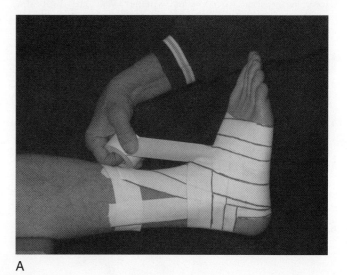

A

Figure 37.9   A through G, Heel-lock taping technique.

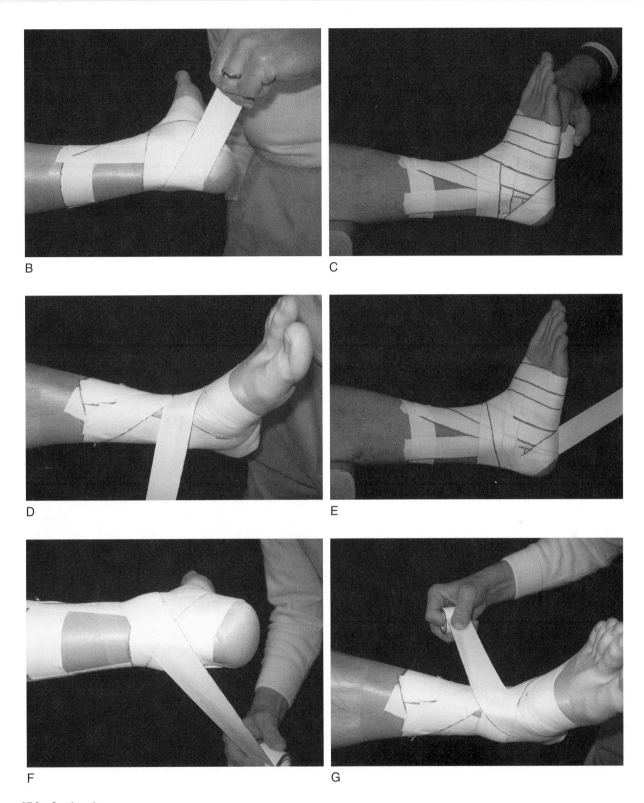

B

C

D

E

F

G

Figure 37.9 Continued

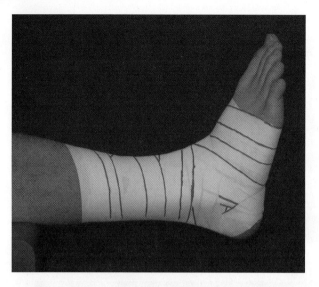

Figure 37.10 Seal the foot so that all previous strips are covered and so that all skin is covered, except for the very tip of the heel.

ARCH TAPING (X ARCH)

Supplies
- Tape adherent
- 1-inch athletic tape
- 2-inch stretch tape

Body position
The athlete should be sitting up with the leg extended off of the table, with about half of the lower leg hanging off. The foot should be in a neutral position with 0 degrees of dorsiflexion.

Procedure
1. Start with an anchor strip along the plantar aspect of the metatarsal heads from the first through the fifth metatarsals. The strip should not go around the top of the forefoot.
2. The first support strip starts at the head of the fifth metatarsal, runs on the lateral side of the foot around the back of the heel,

and then crosses under the arch to end at the starting point **(Figure 37.11).**

3. Continue with the successive strips, placed each strip next to the previous strip **(Figure 37.12A)** until you reach the first metatarsal head. This should create, when viewed from the bottom, a fan-like appearance that extends toward the toes, with an open teardrop shape left over the heel (Figure 37.12B).
4. The supporting strips should then be sealed in by cover strips that are parallel to the first anchor strip **(Figure 37.13A).** These are applied to cover the area from the metatarsal heads to the heel (Figure 37.13B). Remember, these need to be half strips (on the plantar aspect of the foot only) (Figures 37.13C and D) so that they do not restrict the spread of the metatarsals during weight bearing.
5. The entire application can then be covered by overwrapping it with stretch tape **(Figure 37.14).** Because stretch tape is elastic, the overwrap can be wrapped around the entire foot (including top of foot).

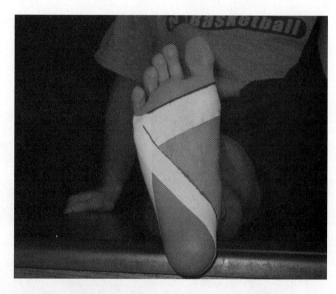

Figure 37.11 For an arch taping, start the first support strips at the head of the fifth metatarsal, continue along the lateral side of the foot, and cross the tape under the arch.

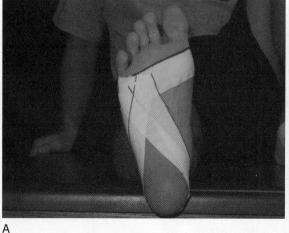
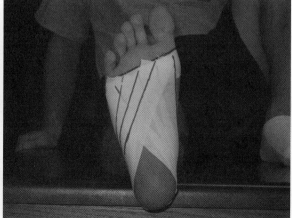

A   B

Figure 37.12 A and B, Place successive strips next to the previous ones to create a "fan" that extends toward the toes. Note that the open skin of the heel creates a teardrop shape.

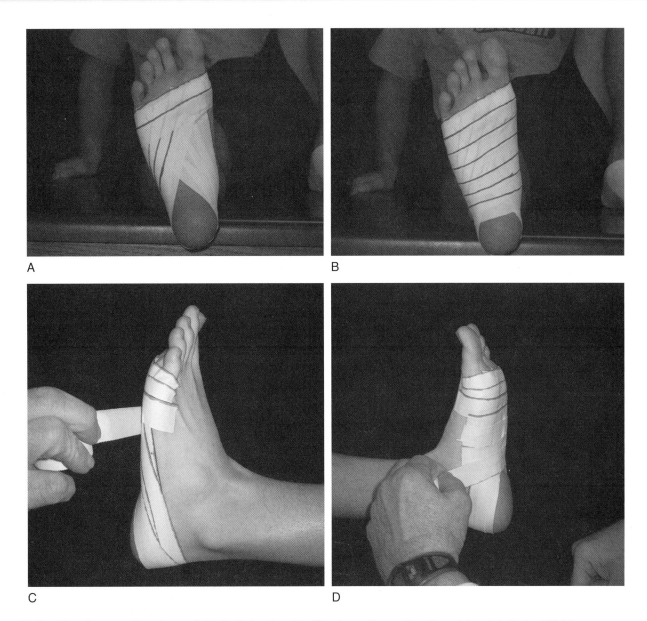

A   B

C   D

Figure 37.13 Place the supporting strips parallel to the first anchor strip *(A)*, and cover the area from the metatarsals to the heel *(B)*. Take care to not restrict the spread of the metatarsals *(C and D)*.

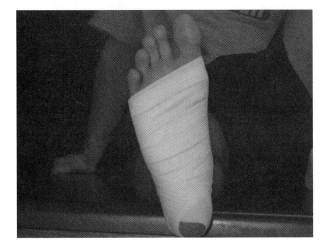

Figure 37.14 Finish the arch taping with a final overwrap of stretch tape.

TURF TOE TAPING

Supplies
- Tape adherent
- 1-inch athletic tape
- 2-inch stretch tape

Body position
The athlete should be sitting up with his or her leg extended off of the table and about half the lower leg hanging off. Their foot should be pulled back in a relatively neutral position.

Procedure
1. With 1-inch tape, place an anchor around the great toe (just proximal to the nail) and another anchor at the base of the arch just before the heel **(Figure 37.15).**

2. Place the first support strip from the inferior portion of the great toe straight to the bottom anchor **(Figure 37.16)**.
3. The next strip will be placed in the same manner, overlapping the first strip by half and pulling toward the medial part of the foot **(Figure 37.17)**. Steps 2 and 3 can be repeated if more support is needed.
4. The support strips should then be sealed with strips that halve each other from the metatarsal heads (don't forget the great toe!) toward the bottom anchor **(Figure 37.18A)**. Again, these are half strips that involve only the plantar aspect of the foot (Figure 37.18B).
5. The entire application and foot can then be covered in stretch tape **(Figure 37.19)**.

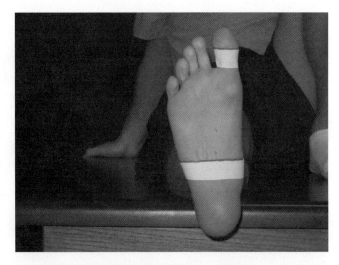

Figure 37.15 Anchor the great toe and the base of the arch.

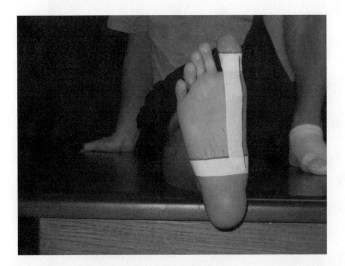

Figure 37.16 Place a support strip from the inferior portion of the great toe to the bottom anchor.

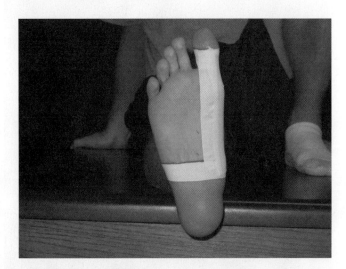

Figure 37.17 The next support strip will overlap the first by half.

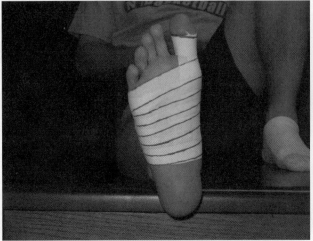

A

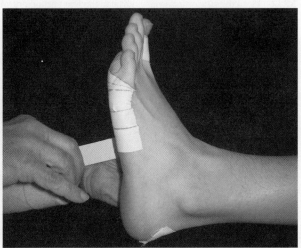

B

Figure 37.18 *A* and *B*, Seal the support strips with horizontal strips that overlap each other by half from the metatarsals to the bottom anchor.

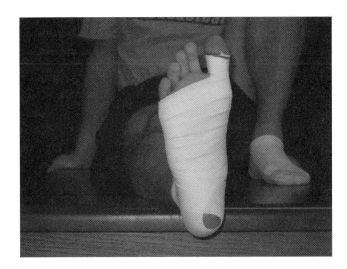

Figure 37.19   Finish the turf toe taping with a final overlay of stretch tape.

ACHILLES TAPING

Supplies
- Tape adherent
- 2-inch stretch tape
- 3-inch Elastikon
- Underwrap, if needed

Body position
The athlete should be sitting straight up with the leg extended off the table and about half of the lower leg hanging off. The foot should be relaxed and plantarflexed.

Procedure
1. Two anchor strips are placed using stretch tape. The distal anchor will go around the metatarsal heads, and the proximal anchor will go around the lower third of the leg at the level of the gastrocnemius–Achilles junction **(Figure 37.20).**
2. A strip of Elastikon should then be stretched along the bottom of the foot (from anchor to anchor) to be measured and cut to length. Each end should then be split down the middle for about 2 inches. The Elastikon should be stretched along the back of the ankle from the top to the bottom, with

the cut ends being stretched around to then be secured on the front of the anchor strips **(Figures 37.21A and B).** Another strip of Elastikon can be applied in this same manner over the previous strip to add more support, if desired.
3. The application should then be sealed and covered with stretch tape **(Figure 37.22A, B, and C).**

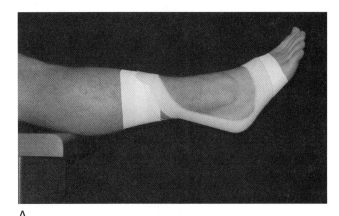

A

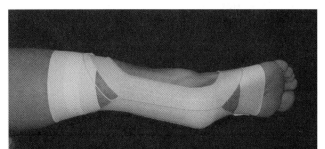

B

Figure 37.21   A and B, Apply the Elastikon along the bottom of the foot from anchor to anchor.

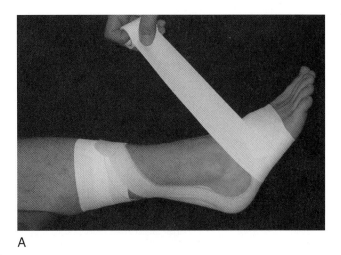

A

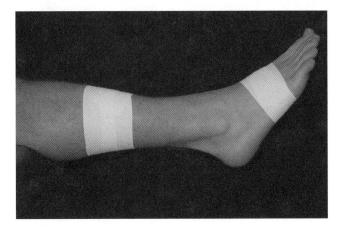

Figure 37.20   For an Achilles taping, place one anchor around the metatarsal heads and one around the lower third of the leg.

Figure 37.22   A, B, and C, Seal the Achilles tape application with stretch tape.

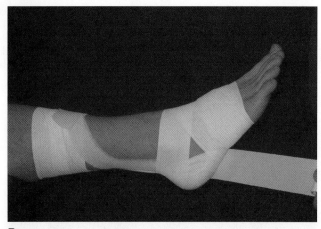

B

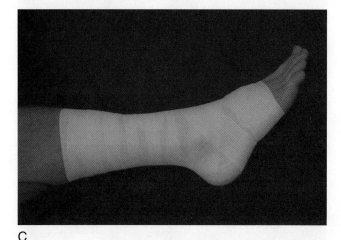

C

Figure 37.22 Continued

COLLATERAL SUPPORT TAPING OF THE KNEE

Supplies
- Tape adherent
- 2-inch stretch tape
- 2-inch athletic tape
- Possibly underwrap and 3-inch Elastikon

Body position
The athlete should stand on the taping table in a slight straddle stance with most of his or her weight on the back leg. A roll of tape can be placed under the heel of the front leg (the leg to be taped) to achieve the proper knee flexion **(Figure 37.23)**.

Procedure
1. Two anchor strips are placed using stretch tape. The distal anchor will go around the mid calf, and the proximal anchor will go around the proximal third of the thigh **(Figure 37.24)**.
2. The first support strip will run from the thigh anchor on the lateral side and then down, crossing over the lateral joint line and continuing diagonally in front of the knee, just below the kneecap, to secure to the calf anchor on the medial side of the leg **(Figure 37.25A and B)**.

3. The second strip will start on the medial side of the thigh anchor and come across the front of the thigh, just above the kneecap, crossing the previous strip at the lateral joint line and then continuing to secure to the calf anchor in the back **(Figure 39.26)**.
4. Steps 2 and 3 should be repeated with each strip halving the previous strip **(Figure 37.27)**.
5. Two strips should then be run vertically over the lateral joint line, and these strips should also halve each other. The top portion of these strips should be a little anterior on the thigh, and the distal portion will end at the anchor on the lateral side **(Figure 37.28)**.
6. Stretch tape should then cover the thigh and calf portion of the application, leaving a gap at the joint line **(Figure 37.29A and B)**.

(Note: This method can be used for medial collateral ligament support as well by applying tape as described but instead supporting the medial joint line of the knee.)

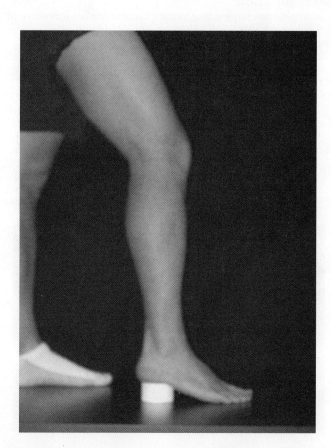

Figure 37.23 Achieve proper knee flexion by placing a roll of tape under the heel.

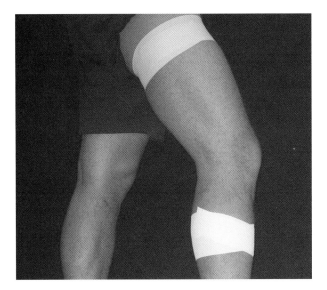

Figure 37.24   Place one anchor around the mid calf and one around the proximal third of the thigh.

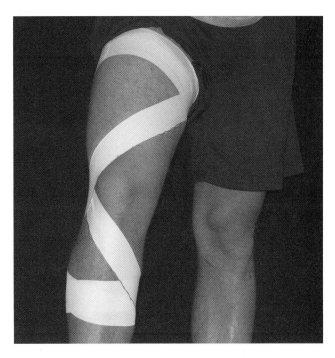

Figure 37.26   Apply the second support strip diagonally from the medial thigh anchor to just above the kneecap, and secure it to the calf anchor on the lateral side.

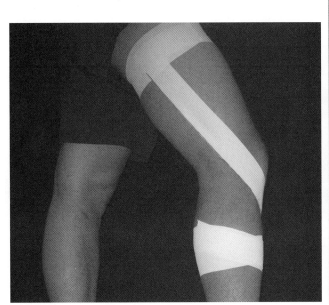

A

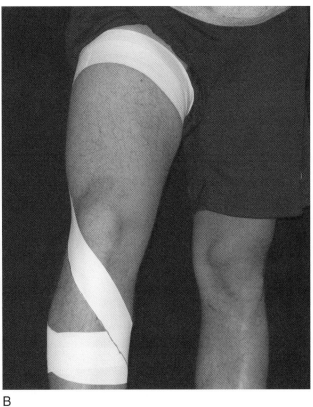

B

Figure 37.25   A and B, Apply the first support strip diagonally from the lateral thigh anchor to just below the kneecap, and secure it to the calf anchor on the medial side.

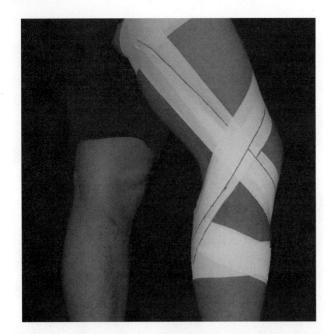

Figure 37.27 Each successive strip should overlap the previous strip by half.

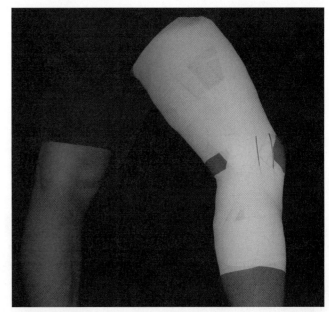

A

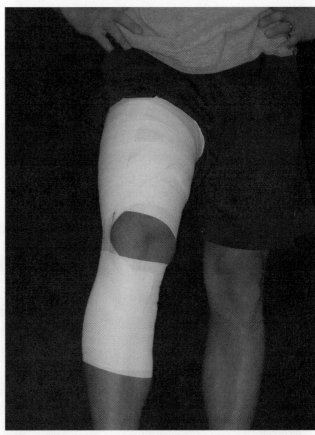

B

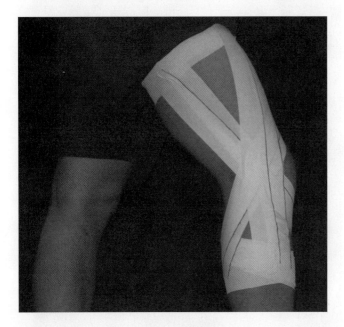

Figure 37.28 Run two overlapping vertical strips over the lateral joint.

Figure 37.29 *A* and *B*, Apply stretch tape over the calf and thigh, leaving a gap at the joint.

HYPEREXTENDED KNEE TAPING

Supplies
- Tape adherent
- 2-inch stretch tape
- 2-inch athletic tape
- Padding
- Possibly underwrap and 3-inch Elastikon

Body position
The athlete should stand on the taping table in a slight straddle stance with most of his or her weight on the back leg. A roll of tape should be placed under the heel of the front (affected) leg to achieve proper knee flexion (see Figure 37.23).

Procedure
1. Two anchor strips are placed using stretch tape. The distal anchor will go around the mid calf, and the proximal anchor will go around the proximal third of the thigh (see Figure 37.24).
2. Place some padding (e.g., Webril) in the popliteal area behind the knee to prevent irritation.
3. The first support strip should be placed on the lateral side of the thigh anchor, and it will run across the front of the thigh to the back of the knee, crossing the popliteal pad and continuing around anteriorly to finish on the calf anchor on the medial side **(Figure 37.30).**
4. The next strip will start on the medial side of the thigh anchor and run across the front of the thigh (crossing the previous strip) to the back of the knee, crossing the popliteal padding (and the previous strip) area and continuing around the front (again crossing the previous strip) to finish on the calf anchor

on the posterior lateral side **(Figure 37.31A and B).** These strips can be reinforced by duplication.
5. Stretch tape should then cover the thigh and calf portion of the application, crossing and covering the popliteal area but leaving the kneecap area open. **(Figure 37.32).**

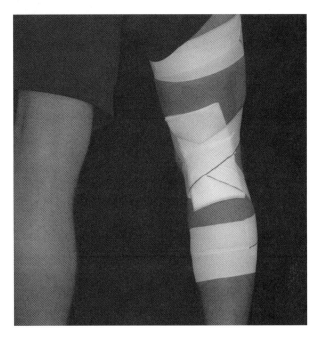

Figure 37.30 Apply the first support strip diagonally from the lateral thigh anchor across the front of the thigh to the back of the knee, and secure it to the calf anchor on the medial side.

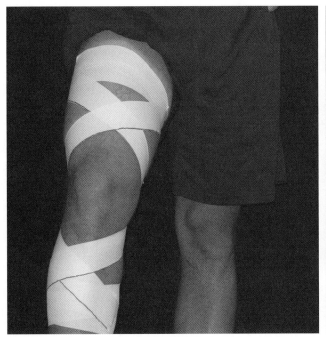

A

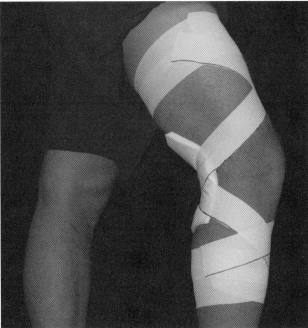

B

Figure 37.31 A and B, Apply the second support strip diagonally from the medial thigh anchor across the front of the thigh to the back of the knee, and secure it to the calf anchor on the posterior lateral side.

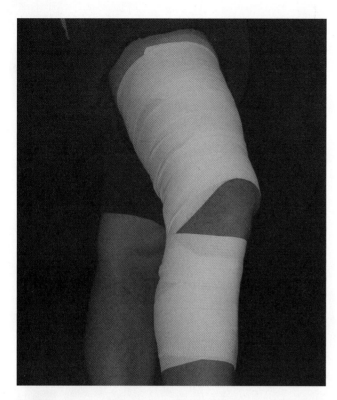

Figure 37.32 Apply stretch tape over the calf and thigh, leaving a gap at the kneecap.

THUMB SPICA TAPING

Supplies
- Tape adherent
- Prewrap
- 1-inch athletic tape
- Underwrap

Body position
The athlete should stand facing you with his or her hand pointed toward your chest. The athlete's thumb will be pointing up, and his or her hand will be open. The athlete should maintain neutral wrist alignment (no radial or ulnar deviation) during thumb spica taping.

Procedure
1. Underwrap is used to cover the palm of the hand, the thumb shaft, and the wrist **(Figure 37.33).**
2. The first strip is started on the palmar aspect over the pisiform. It will run vertically along the wrist and curve around the top of the thumb and around the metacarpophalangeal joint **(Figure 37.34A).** It will continue to circle the thumb and cross itself behind the thumb at the metacarpophalangeal joint (Figure 37.34B). It will then continue down the back side of the wrist to the starting point (Figure 37.34C).
3. The continuous strip will continue with each repetitive wrap overlapping the previous strip by about a third **(Figure 37.35A and B)** so that the portion around the thumb progresses distally (Figure 37.35C). Three overlapping strips typically provide enough support, but more strips may be added, depending on the particular injury.

4. The spica wrap can then be sealed with 1½-inch tape using circumferential strips and overlapping by half from the interphalangeal joint back down to the metacarpophalangeal joint of the thumb.

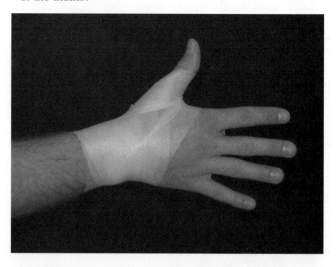

Figure 37.33 Cover the palm, the thumb shaft, and the wrist with underwrap.

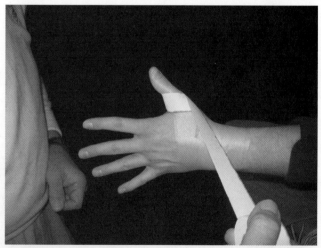

A

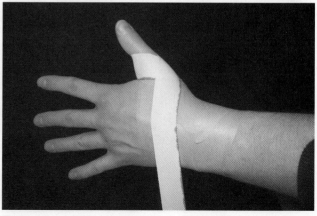

B

Figure 37.34 A, B, and C, Continue the tape down the back side of the wrist to the starting point.

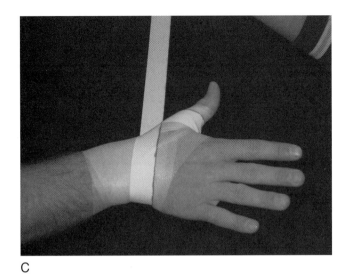

C

Figure 37.34 Continued

REGULAR WRIST TAPING

Supplies
- Tape adherent
- Prewrap
- 1-inch or 1½-inch athletic tape
- Underwrap

Body position
They athlete should be standing and facing you with his or her hand pointed toward your chest. The athlete's hand should be clinched in a fist.

Procedure
1. Underwrap is applied around the wrist from the base of the hand and then continued proximally for about 3 to 4 inches **(Figure 37.36)**.
2. The tape is applied in a circular motion around the wrist **(Figure 37.37)**, working distal to proximal. The taped portion should be about 3 inches in total length.

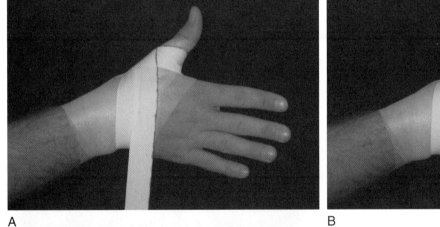

A

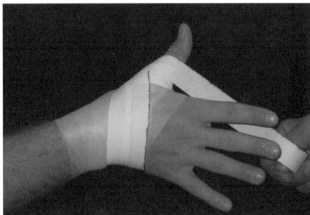

B

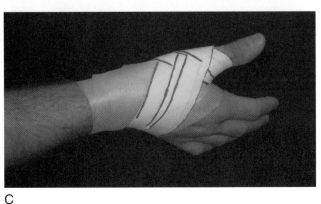

C

Figure 37.35 *A, B*, and *C*, Overlap each successive strip by a third.

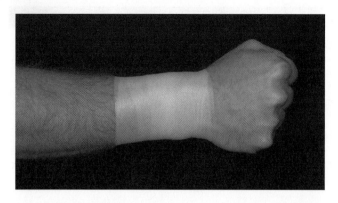

Figure 37.36 Apply the underwrap from the base of the hand, and continue in a proximal direction.

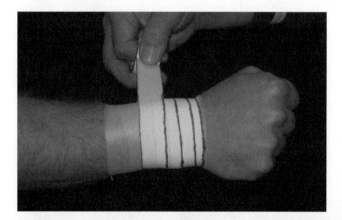

Figure 37.37 Continue to apply the tape from a distal to a proximal direction.

EXTRA SUPPORT WRIST TAPING

Supplies
- Tape adherent
- Prewrap
- 1-inch or 1½-inch athletic tape
- Underwrap

Body position
The athlete should stand facing you with his or her hand pointed toward your chest. The athlete's thumb will be pointing up, and his or her hand should be open.

Procedure
1. Underwrap is applied around the palm of the hand and the wrist. Anchor straps are placed proximal to the wrist and around the metacarpophalangeal joints **(Figure 37.38).**
2. Start the first strip over the dorsal aspect of the fourth metacarpal head, wrap between the thumb and the index finger in the web space, and then proceed ulnarly across the metacarpal heads. As you cross back to the dorsal hand, angle diagonally across the dorsal wrist, and end the first strip on the palmar and ulnar side of the proximal anchor **(Figure 37.39A).**
3. The second strip is the mirror image of the first, and it will start on the dorsal aspect at the second metacarpophalangeal joint, heading ulnarly, and wrapping around the fifth metacarpal head. Continue palmarly to the thumb and index finger web

space, wrap through the web space, and then begin to angle proximally, crossing over the first strip at the dorsal wrist joint line and ending on the proximal anchor at the radial aspect. The wrapping will start on the radial side of the palm (around the fourth metacarpal) and angle back and down to cross the previous strip at the anterior wrist (crossing over the pisiform). It will continue around the ulnar side and finish on the posterior wrist (Figure 37.39B).
4. Steps 2 and 3 should be duplicated, starting on the palmar aspect of the hand, and crossing each other over the palmar wrist **(Figure 37.40).** This step may also be repeated as desired for extra support.
5. Stretch tape will be used to seal the job **(Figure 37.41).**

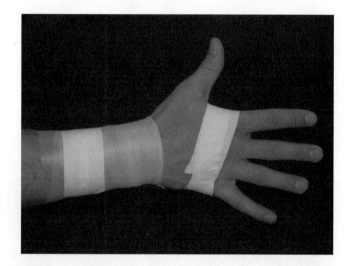

Figure 37.38 For extra support in a wrist taping, apply one anchor strap proximal to the wrist and a second anchor around the metacarpophalangeal joints.

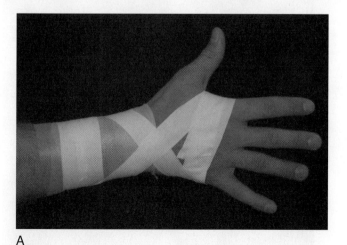

A

Figure 37.39 A and B, Apply a support strip as indicated in steps 2 and 3 of Extra Support Wrist Taping Section.

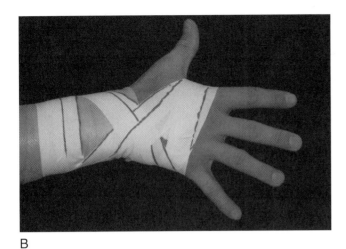

B

Figure 37.39 Continued

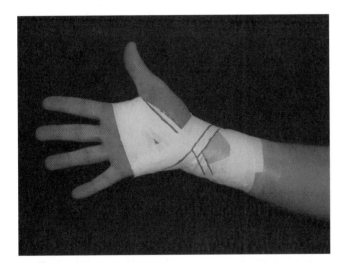

Figure 37.40 Duplicate the support strips on the palmar aspect of the hand, and cross each over the palmar wrist. Each successive strip should overlap the previous one by half.

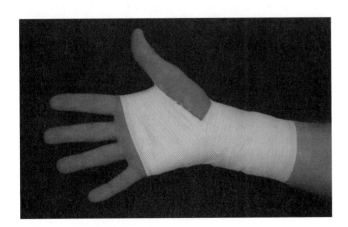

Figure 37.41 Use stretch tape to seal the application.

ELBOW HYPEREXTENSION TAPING

Supplies
- Tape adherent
- 2-inch stretch tape
- 1¹/₂- or 2-inch athletic tape
- Padding

Body position
The athlete should be standing in front of you with his or her arm extended with the palm up and with about 30 degrees of elbow flexion.

Procedure
1. Two anchor strips will be placed using stretch tape. The distal anchor will be placed at about the mid forearm. The proximal anchor will be placed below the deltoid tubercle **(Figure 37.42)**.
2. Padding should be placed in the cubital fossa to limit irritation.
3. The first strip should start at the posteromedial aspect of the arm, at the humeral anchor. It will run diagonally down to cross at the antecubital fossa, and it will then end on the posterior portion of the forearm anchor **(Figure 37.43*A* and *B*)**.
4. The next strip will start on the posterolateral part of the upper arm anchor. It will run diagonally down to cross the antecubital fossa (as well as the previous strip), and it will continue to and end at the posterior portion of the forearm anchor.
5. Steps 3 and 4 should be repeated **(Figure 37.44)**.
6. Stretch tape should be used to cover and seal the job. The cubital fossa should be covered, but the posterior elbow should remain uncovered **(Figure 37.45*A* and *B*)**.

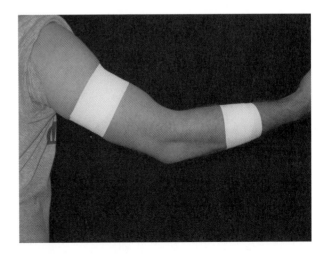

Figure 37.42 To tape a hyperextended elbow, place one anchor strip at the mid forearm and a second anchor strip below the deltoid tubercle.

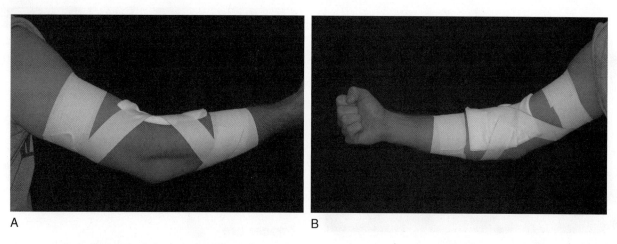

A

B

Figure 37.43 *A* and *B*, Run the first support strip diagonally from the posteromedial aspect of the deltoid anchor, cross the cubital fossa, and end on the posterior portion of the forearm anchor. Run the second support strip from the posterolateral aspect of the deltoid anchor, cross the cubital fossa, and end on the posterior portion of the forearm anchor.

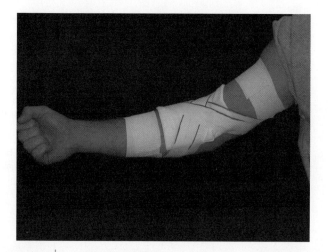

Figure 37.44 Continue applying the support strips until the elbow is secured.

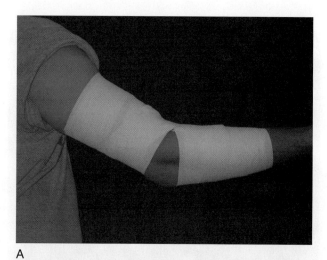

A

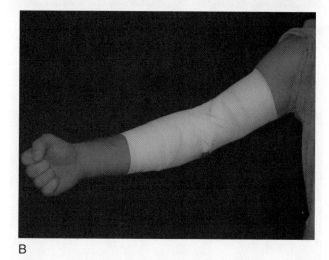

B

Figure 37.45 *A* and *B*, Use stretch tape to cover the application, making sure that the posterior elbow remains uncovered.

CONCLUSION

Remember that these are just some of the many techniques that can be used in athletic training. Not only are there other techniques, but there are also many different variations of each technique that may achieve the desired effect. Many comprehensive taping textbooks provide more information about this subject. However, in the end, you must always think about what you are trying to accomplish with each taping job. Taping should always have a purpose, and it should serve that purpose without posing an increased risk of injury to the athlete.

CHAPTER 38

Proper Indications and Uses of Orthopedic Braces

LTC Jeff C. Leggitt, MD,
and MAJ Christopher G. Jarvis, MD, FAAFP

KEY POINTS

- Orthotic devices (braces/orthoses) are not a substitute for a correct anatomic diagnosis and proper rehabilitation.
- Neutral wrist splints have been found to be more effective than "cock-up" wrist splints for the treatment of carpal tunnel syndrome. Wrist splints perform best when worn continuously rather than just at nighttime.
- The key to treating mallet finger is to maintain continuous splinting in slight extension for 4 to 6 weeks.
- Return to activity after a tibial stress fracture can be hastened with the use of a pneumatic long-leg stirrup brace.
- Semirigid ankle braces in combination with rehabilitative exercises prevents recurrent lateral ankle sprains.

INTRODUCTION

The use of braces for musculoskeletal injuries is widespread. The evidence for their use is far from definitive, however, and the majority of the evidence is either anecdotal or expert opinion. Despite the controversy and myth surrounding the use of braces, there is a role for bracing in many injuries. This chapter will discuss the most common devices and their proposed mechanism of action in relation to overuse and nonfracture traumatic injuries. A discussion of scientific merit will also be highlighted when available.

GENERAL CONSIDERATIONS IN BRACING

Defining the terms

The various terms used for braces are often inconsistent and confusing. The correct medical term for a brace is an *orthosis* (plural *orthoses*), which is Greek for "making straight." According to *Dorland's Medical Dictionary,* an *orthosis* is "an orthopedic appliance or apparatus used to support, align, prevent, or correct deformities or to improve the function of movable parts of the body."[1] The term *brace* can be used interchangeably with *orthosis.* The term *orthotic* is an adjective,

and it is used to describe an instrument or tool, such as an *orthotic device.*[1] Furthermore, *orthotics* is the field of knowledge that relates to orthoses and their use; it does not mean "many orthoses". Further adding to the confusion is the common practice of using the term *orthorics* as a synonym for orthotic shoe inserts. For simplicity, the term *braces* will be used preferentially throughout this chapter.

Types of braces

Braces can be prophylactic, to prevent or reduce injury; functional, to provide stability to injured tissue while allowing some level of participation; or rehabilitative, to provide protection and a controlled range of motion during the rehabilitative period. Some braces can perform all of these functions, and their application in a specific situation determines their functional classification. For example, an ankle stirrup brace could fit all three categories, even for the same patient. After a lateral ankle sprain, it would initially be a rehabilitative brace. As treatment progressed, it would become a functional brace. Finally, to prevent recurrent sprains, it could function as a prophylactic brace as the athlete returned to sports participation.

Regardless of the indication or the brace, no orthotic device is a substitute for a correct pathoanatomic diagnosis and proper rehabilitation.

The proposed mechanisms for braces are multifactorial. Some restrict motion, whereas others correct anatomic or biomechanical alignment. Some displace forces to other tissues (e.g., counterforce bracing), some provide cushioning to protect injured tissue from impact, some are thought to exert their effects by aiding in proprioception, and some perform all of these functions. In addition to these recognized mechanisms, there is probably a large placebo effect among patients with braces.[2]

Proper brace prescribing practices

Braces are not a "one size fits all" treatment, and education must accompany their use. It is incumbent on the prescriber to observe the patient applying the brace and to ensure correct brace positioning and function. Orthoses can cause discomfort, or they may slip during movement; this should be discovered in the examination room and not during competition or while the patient is on the job. The correct brace depends on many patient and disease factors, including (but not

Table 38.1 Condition and Brace Recommendations

Condition	Brace Recommendation
Lateral elbow pain (tennis elbow)	Counterforce brace as part of a rehabilitative program emphasizing eccentric strengthening
Carpal tunnel syndrome	Neutral wrist splint to avoid repetitive flexion; strengthening exercises
Mallet finger	Continuous splinting with any brace that allows slight extension; authors recommend the Oval-8 or a similar waterproof brace
Ulnar collateral ligament (skier's or gamekeeper's thumb)	Commercial thumb spica splint if compliance can be ensured and if a complete tear or avulsion fracture is ruled out
Medial or lateral collateral ligament tear	Hinged functional knee brace if the injury is isolated
Anterior or posterior cruciate ligament tear	Hinge-postshell brace to provide some stability early during the rehabilitative period or before surgery to decrease instability; treatment decisions should be made in concert with an orthopedic surgeon
Patellar femoral pain syndrome	Simple neoprene sleeve or a sleeve with a buttress as a part of a comprehensive rehabilitation protocol
Patellar tendinopathy	Patellar tendon strap along with quadriceps strengthening and stretching
Osteoarthritis	Unloader brace as a bridge to or substitute for surgery, particularly in patients with unicompartmental disease
Tibial stress fractures	Long-leg, pneumatic stirrup brace to hasten return to activity
Lateral ankle sprain	Either a stirrup or nonstirrup semirigid brace along with intensive strengthening and proprioceptive training to achieve secondary (and perhaps primary) prevention
Achilles tendinosis	Eccentric strengthening and possibly Achilles straps
Plantar fascia pain syndrome	Heel cups/pads, foot orthoses, or tension night splints in conjunction with regular stretching and strengthening

limited to) diagnosis, desired effect, compliance, cognition, dexterity, edema, and cost.[3] Some braces are to be used over clothing, whereas others are to be applied directly to the skin. The patient should demonstrate technical competence in applying the brace as well as a cognitive knowledge of the brace's uses and limitations. Fortunately almost all braces come with patient instructions, which should be read by both the provider and the patient.

It is impractical for any clinic to carry every brace for every condition. The physician is encouraged to become familiar with one or two braces for the most common conditions and stock and provide only these familiar braces. **Table 38.1** summarizes common conditions and their possible bracing solutions. **Box 38.1** provides resources for obtaining braces. Physicians may also consult with a certified orthotist, especially when dealing with complex or difficult bracing situations. Certified orthotists specialize in all braces, both off the shelf and custom made, and can be invaluable resources. In the case of upper extremity braces, an occupational therapist can also provide assistance. Occupational therapists are often trained in the fabrication of custom splints and braces for the upper extremity, and they know how to provide a range of conservative treatments for upper-extremity ailments.

Potential detrimental effects of bracing

Both providers and patients may wonder if a brace may cause muscular atrophy or inhibition. Unfortunately, there is no

definitive answer to this question. A recent review noted contradictory studies (LOE: meta-analysis).[4] This is most likely a result of the multitude of braces available and the multiple clinical variables related to their application. Another area of bracing concern is the possible predisposition to injury of another joint in the kinetic chain. There is evidence that ankle bracing leads to the transfer of load forces to other joints, but whether that leads to an increase in injuries is unknown (LOE: C).[5] Thus, although common sense dictates that braces should only be worn when necessary, every patient and situation is unique, and continued follow-up and clinical acumen should dictate the most prudent course.

DIAGNOSIS-SPECIFIC CONSIDERATIONS IN BRACING

Lateral elbow pain (tennis elbow)

The most common orthosis for lateral elbow pain is the counterforce brace **(Figure 38.1)**. The proposed mechanism for this brace is the dissipation of the forces away from the injured tissue to the surrounding noninjured area.[6] This type of brace can be both a rehabilitative and a functional orthosis. Bracing for lateral epicondyle pain has had mixed results. A study comparing physical therapy and bracing showed that physical therapy was superior with regard to pain control, whereas bracing increased daily activity level. The combination of the two was superior to either for the first 6 weeks only; however, by 6 months, there was no difference in any therapeutic arm (LOE: B).[7] A 2004 Cochrane review and a more recent systematic review and meta-analysis were inconclusive (LOE: A).[8,9]

A practical approach is to use a counterforce brace while having the patient participate in a rehabilitative program that includes progressive strengthening to include eccentric exercises. No one make or model of brace has been shown to be better than any other (LOE: E).[6] The brace should be snug but not compressive. In addition, the physician must be cognizant that if the brace causes an increase in pain, then the diagnosis of lateral epicondylitis may be incorrect. Pain that worsens with counterforce bracing is often seen in patients with nerve entrapments at the elbow.

Box 38.1: Popular Brace Resources

- Air Cast: www.aircast.com
- Berg: www.berg.com
- Bledsoe: www.bledsoebrace.com
- Cho-Pat: www.cho-pat.com
- Don-Joy: www.djortho.com
- 3-Point Products (Oval-8 finger splint): www.3pointproducts.com

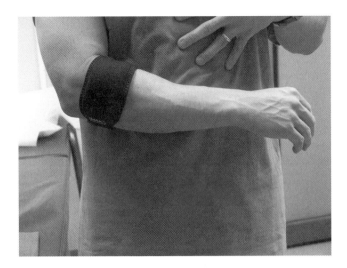

Figure 38.1   Lateral elbow counterforce brace.

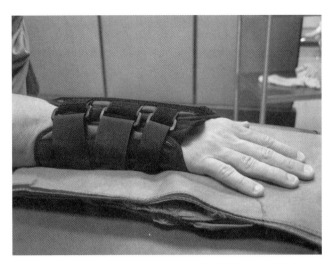

Figure 38.2   Neutral wrist splint for carpal tunnel syndrome.

Authors' recommendation: Prescribe a counterforce brace for lateral elbow pain as part of a comprehensive rehabilitative program.

Carpal tunnel syndrome: Median nerve entrapment at the wrist

The most common type of bracing for carpal tunnel syndrome is the wrist splint* **(Figure 38.2).** The wrist splint is a rehabilitative type of brace. The proposed mechanism is to limit flexion and thus avoid compressing the median nerve in the carpal tunnel. While *cock-up wrist splints* are commonly used to treat carpal tunnel syndrome, a recent study showed that neutral splinting was superior to cock-up splinting (20 degrees of extension) (LOE: A).[10]

Limited evidence indicates that bracing can improve symptoms during the first 2 to 3 weeks of use (LOE: A).[11] Although many prescribe only nighttime use, evidence shows that continuous wear is superior (LOE: A).[10] As compared with nighttime-only splinting, full-time use not only provided greater improvement of symptoms, but it also showed superior electrophysiologic measures (LOE: A).[12] Unfortunately, compliance may be lower with full-time wear, so nighttime-only prescription may be appropriate in certain cases.

Authors' recommendation: Prescribe a neutral wrist splint to a patient with carpal tunnel syndrome, and recommend its continuous use. Nighttime only use is acceptable. In addition, make an ergonomic assessment of the patient's environment to avoid repetitive flexion of the wrist.

Distal extensor tendon injury (mallet finger)

The purpose of a splint for mallet finger is to keep the ends of the distal extensor tendon approximated while the injury heals. A Cochrane review found that patient compliance with splinting (rather than the type of splint used) was the single most important factor in successful treatment outcome[13] **(Figure 38.3).** The same review showed that the use of surgical wires did not improve clinical outcomes.

The patient with a mallet finger must understand that the distal interphalangeal joint should never be allowed to flex at any time during treatment or else the splinting period restarts from the beginning.[14] The normal splinting time is 6 weeks (LOE: meta-analysis).[15] Support of the distal phalanx during splint changes must be demonstrated (LOE: E).[16] This is very difficult to do alone, and, if a reliable assistant is not available, the patient may need to come into the clinic for splint changes. Necrosis of the skin can occur if the distal interphalangeal joint is overextended during splinting. It is useful to remember that skin blanching indicates that there is too much extension. Skin maceration can also occur; letting the skin "breathe" for 10 to 20 minutes between splint changes minimizes this.

Authors' recommendation: Use a device such as the Oval-8 splint (see Figure 38.3*C*), which can get wet and be applied or changed by the patient. Regardless of the splint that is chosen, ensure that distal interphalangeal joint extension is maintained for a full 6 weeks.

Ulnar collateral ligament injury of the thumb (skier's or gamekeeper's thumb)

Similar to the treatment for mallet finger, a splint for skier's thumb is used to maintain approximation of the ulnar collateral ligament while healing occurs, usually 4 to 6 weeks. Stable ulnar collateral ligament injuries can be treated with a thumb spica cast or a splint. In this capacity, the orthosis functions as both a rehabilitative and functional brace. Commercial splints are available that provide an alternative to casting if compliance can be ensured **(Figure 38.4).** Immobilization should be for 4 to 6 weeks. Competition can continue with splinting if the athlete's sport and position allow for this accommodation. After 6 weeks of continuous splinting, most experts recommend dynamic splinting (i.e., splinting during activity) for another 6 weeks if the patient is continuing to participate in athletics (LOE: E).[17,18] The only readily available evidence-based recommendations for ulnar collateral ligament splinting are consensus opinions, which are summarized here.

Authors' recommendation: In stable injuries (i.e., incomplete tears without fracture), commercial thumb spica splinting can be used to treat the injury. The splint must be used for a minimum of 4 weeks and then continued for another 4 to 6 weeks during competition. If there is any suspicion of a complete tear with or without bony avulsion, the patient should be referred to an orthopedist because early surgical intervention is advocated as the best treatment (LOE: E).[19]

---

*The term splint is used here to denote a brace that is used to limit motion to protect an injured part.[1]

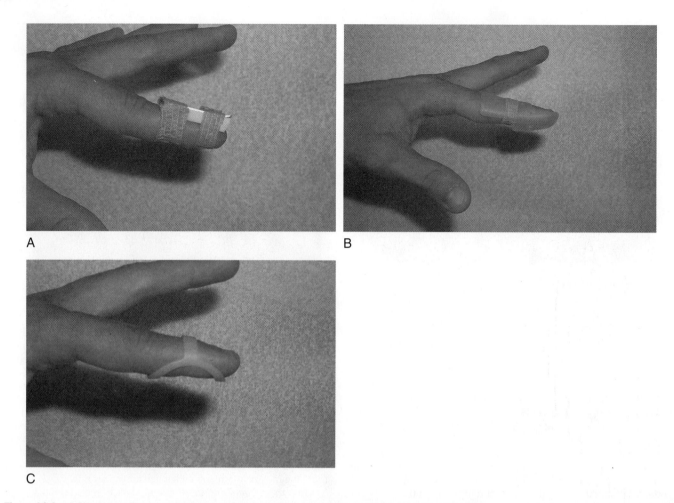

A

B

C

Figure 38.3   *A*, Aluminum splint for mallet finger. *B*, Stack splint for mallet finger. *C*, Oval-8 splint for mallet finger.

Traumatic ligamentous knee injuries

Braces for ligamentous knee injuries can be prophylactic, rehabilitative, or functional.[20] A common prophylactic knee brace attempts to protect the medial collateral ligament in response to a valgus knee stress, usually from a lateral blow, and to support the cruciate ligaments during rotational stresses by dissipating impact forces both above and below the joint[21] **(Figure 38.5).** An American Academy of Orthopedic Surgeons (AAOS) position

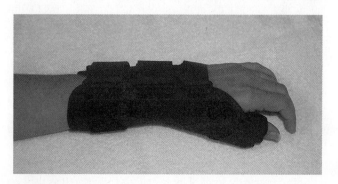

Figure 38.4   Thumb spica splint.

statement contends that there is evidence to suggest that prophylactic knee bracing provides limited protection to a lateral blow for the medial collateral ligament in football players but that there is insufficient evidence to suggest that any other ligaments, menisci, or cartilage are protected by these braces. Despite their claim of limited evidence for medial collateral ligament protection, the AAOS does not currently endorse the universal use of prophylactic knee braces in football or any other sport as a result of the lack of definitive evidence (LOE: E).[20] The American Academy of Pediatrics also states that there is currently insufficient evidence to recommend prophylactic knee bracing for pediatric athletes (LOE: E).[22]

Authors' recommendation: Do not use prophylactic knee braces to prevent ligamentous injury to the knees.

The hinge-postshell **(Figure 38.6)** and hinge-poststrap (Figure 38.5*B*) models are types of functional knee braces. These braces have medial and lateral vertical hinges and a variable stop to limit hyperextension, thereby providing protection to injured or postoperative tissues while allowing the athlete some level of participation during healing.[22,23] Some studies suggest that the hinge-postshell type also provides improved tibial displacement control, greater rigidity, enhanced durability, and better soft-tissue contact as compared with the hinge-poststrap type (LOE: E).[22,23] The AAOS states that functional knee braces offer limited functional

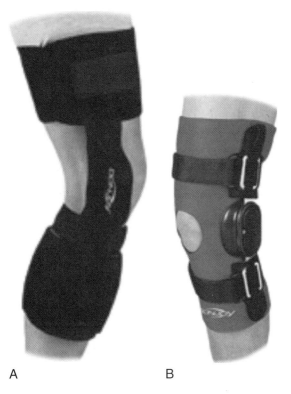

A   B

Figure 38.5 Prophylactic knee braces. *A*, With a unilateral-hinged bar, viewed from the side. *B*, With bilateral-hinged bars. (From Pulaska SA, McKeag DB: Am Fam Physician 2000;61:411-418, 423-424.)

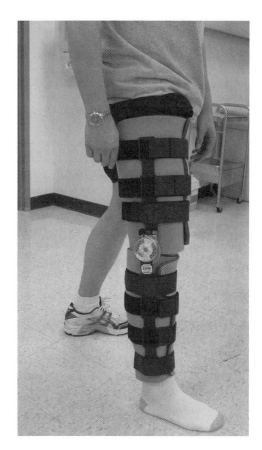

Figure 38.7 Postoperative or rehabilitative knee brace.

improvements for the anterior cruciate ligament (ACL)—deficient knee, but the braces have not been shown to protect against meniscal tears or articular cartilage wear. Furthermore, functional knee braces may be effective under low-force conditions, but likely do not restore the knee to normal stability under the high-force conditions of many sports. Indeed, braces may actually provide a false sense of security that may place the athlete at increased risk for further injury (LOE: E).[20] Specifically, bracing appears to significantly improve proprioception during limited somatosensory input tasks (e.g., balancing on one leg) but not significantly during functional tasks in post-ACL reconstruction patients (LOE: B).[24] Additionally, the use of a functional brace beyond the initial rehabilitative period does not appear to provide any added protection to a well-performed ligamentous reconstruction (LOE: C).[20] However, several authors continue to advocate the use of bracing for up to 12 months after ACL reconstruction to reduce postoperative strain (LOE: E).[22,23,25,26] Still, most agree that lower-extremity strengthening, flexibility, and athletic technique improvement are more important than the application of a functional brace for the long-term outcomes of ligamentous knee injuries (LOE: E).[22,23] Muscular fatigue has been implicated as a significant limitation for the use of functional knee braces during athletic activities. Functional bracing has also not been shown to be effective for chronic posterior cruciate ligament deficiency, but it can help during the acute postinjury setting (LOE: B).[27-29]

Rehabilitative knee braces attempt to protect knee ligaments and menisci from further injury during conservative management or after surgical treatment[21] **(Figure 38.7)**. Rehabilitative braces protect injured or reconstructed ligaments through controlled extension and flexion and by controlling varus and valgus stresses. Commonly, these braces allow adjustments to permit increasingly free range of motion during the rehabilitative period. Most authors

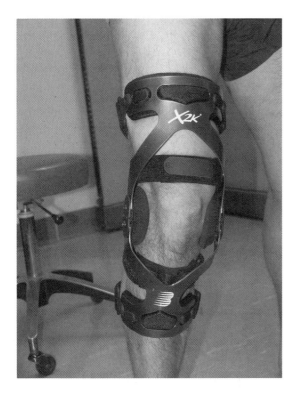

Figure 38.6 Hinge-postshell anterior cruciate ligament brace.

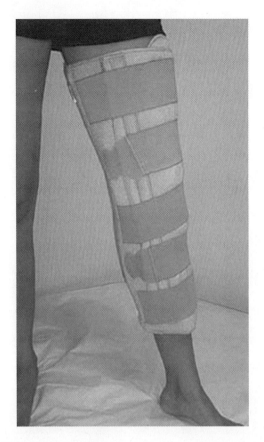

Figure 38.8 Knee immobilizer.

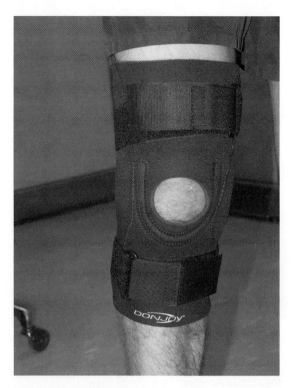

Figure 38.9 Simple hinged knee brace.

recommend using rehabilitative braces (as compared with a knee immobilizer) during the first week or two after an acute injury[21] **(Figure 38.8).** Knee immobilizers can result in recalcitrant stiffness, especially if the prescribed follow-up is not immediately obtained. Another benefit of the rehabilitative brace over the knee immobilizer is the adjustable straps, which allow for easy access for examinations and ice application. The AAOS states that there is a role for rehabilitative braces during the early post-surgical phase after ACL reconstruction.[20] Rehabilitative knee braces also may be used for pediatric patients with nondisplaced epiphyseal fractures in lieu of casting (LOE: E).[22]

Authors' recommendations for specific injuries
Medial collateral ligament injury
Depending on the severity and laxity of the injury, either a simple hinged knee brace or a functional postshell knee brace can be used during rehabilitation **(Figure 38.9).** The majority of isolated medical collateral ligament injuries heal well after 4 to 6 weeks. For athletes returning to play, we also recommend continued bracing with at least a hinged knee brace during the rest of the competitive season.

Lateral collateral ligament injury
Grade I injuries may only need basic initial treatment and rehabilitation, with return to activity occurring within a few weeks. Grade II injuries need a lateral stabilizing rehabilitative knee brace, and the return to activity may take several weeks. Grade III injuries should be managed in concert with a orthopedic surgeon.

Anterior cruciate ligament injury
Early orthopedic consultation should be sought with an ACL-deficient knee in active athletes who are involved in jumping, pivoting, or hard-cutting sports. Initial treatment depends on the severity of dysfunction. A rehabilitative brace can be used before surgery for athletes who experience recurrent subluxation or symptoms of instability during their preoperative therapy. At the discretion of the treating physician and athlete, this brace may be used after ACL surgery as well. Patients who are not involved in pivoting activities may benefit from conservative management, which would include bracing and rehabilitation (specifically hamstring strengthening).

Posterior cruciate ligament injury
A functional brace can be tried in conjunction with aggressive quadriceps strengthening. If the patient perceives improved stability, the brace may be worn during at-risk activities.

Unknown knee injuries
Other than bony fractures of the knee, there is usually no contraindication to limited weight bearing and passive range of motion. Indeed, both of these are helpful for preserving the health of articular cartilage in the knee joint. We discourage the regrettably common practice of treating all patients who present with knee pain and who have negative x-rays with a knee immobilizer. The only indications for knee immobilizers are patellar fracture, patellar dislocation, post-surgical immobilization, and a few other rare cases. Prolonged immobilization can be harmful to the patient and may unduly predispose him or her to other serious complications (e.g., deep venous thrombosis). Knee immobilization will result in limited range of motion, which can greatly complicate future examinations and cause delays in diagnosis and rehabilitation. Patients with knee pain and no evidence of fracture on x-ray may be given crutches to assist with weight bearing as tolerated. If bracing is desired, a hinged brace is far superior to an immobilizer for nearly all acute injuries.

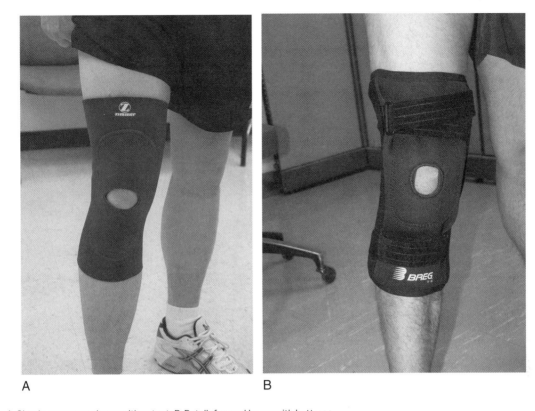

A   B

Figure 38.10   *A*, Simple neoprene sleeve with cutout. *B*, Patellofemoral brace with buttress.

Patellofemoral pain syndrome

All patellofemoral braces are functional braces **(Figure 38.10).**
Their proposed mechanisms of action are to maintain proper
patella alignment, typically with an emphasis on controlling lateral
displacement, and to improve malalignment-associated anterior
knee pain.[21,23] Proprioception may also be improved. Recent
Database of Abstracts of Reviews of Effectiveness and Cochrane
reviews have found contradictory results, and, as such, they have
failed to find enough evidence to recommend for or against the
use of patellofemoral braces for the treatment of patellofemoral
pain (LOE: A).[30-33] More high-quality studies are needed before
any definitive conclusions about their use can be drawn.

Authors' recommendation: Quadriceps strengthening and identifying the source of the individual patient's dysfunction are the
cornerstones of the treatment of patellofemoral pain. A simple neoprene sleeve, a fixed buttress brace, or a brace with an adjustable
strap buttress may be offered as a second-line therapy and as a part
of a comprehensive rehabilitation plan. If the patient perceives no
pain relief with bracing, then the brace should be discontinued.

Patellar tendinopathy

Patellar tendon straps are functional braces that are designed to
apply counterforce pressure on the patellar tendon, thereby distributing the forces to the surrounding tissue **(Figure 38.11).**
There are no evidence-based reviews to support the use of these
very simple and common braces. Anecdotally, patients regularly
espouse their positive effects, and most authors recommend a trial
of their use (LOE: E).[23]

Authors' recommendations: The first-line treatment for patellar tendinopathy is quadriceps strengthening and stretching.

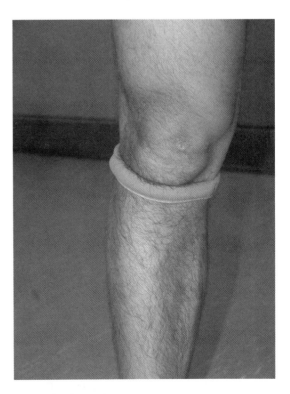

Figure 38.11   Patellar tendon strap.

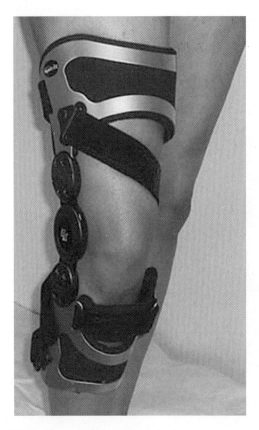

Figure 38.12 Unloader/offloader brace.

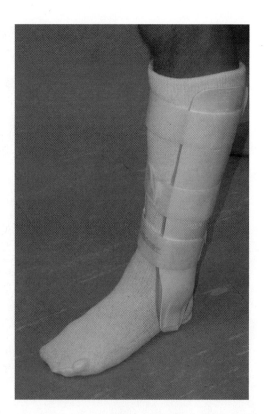

Figure 38.13 Long-leg pneumatic stirrup tibial stress fracture brace.

In conjunction with a comprehensive rehabilitation plan, patellar straps may be tried and continued if the patient finds them to be helpful.

Osteoarthritis

Unloader/offloader braces are designed to reduce the loading of a specific compartment or area of an osteoarthritic knee and thereby reduce its associated pain **(Figure 38.12)**. Specifically, the brace dissipates forces away from the injured articular surface to the opposite (and hopefully less injured) joint compartment. However, the increased forces transmitted to nonarthritic areas may be too uncomfortable for the patient to tolerate.[34] The AAOS states that unloader braces may provide significant pain reduction in some osteoarthritic knees (LOE: E).[20] This decreased level of pain may allow the arthritic patient to increase his or her level of physical/athletic activities, and this can lead to weight loss and muscular strengthening, both of which have been proven to be effective for osteoarthritis treatment (LOE: A).[35] A recent Cochrane review supported the AAOS views, stating that an unloader knee brace provided greater pain relief than a neoprene sleeve, which was better than medical therapy alone.[36] The unloader brace is also another option for those patients who do not desire surgery or who are poor candidates for it. Unloader braces are designed for use during short-term bouts of activity. Only rarely can patients wear an unloader brace for longer than 2 to 3 hours at a time.

Authors' recommendations: An unloader knee brace should be offered to patients with primarily unicompartmental articular damage, especially if they have an angular deformity. When used in conjunction with other conservative treatment options, unloader braces can help return the osteoarthritic athlete to episodic bouts of the activities that he or she enjoys.

Tibial stress fractures

There is some evidence that the use of pneumatic bracing may hasten the recovery of tibial stress fractures and aid in rehabilitation. The mechanism of action of these braces is proposed to be similar to that of counterforce braces in that stresses are directed away from the injured bone and dissipated to a larger area (LOE: B).[37] The brace that is widely advocated is a long stirrup-type brace that extends up to the proximal tibia (as opposed to the typical pneumatic ankle stirrup brace) **(Figure 38.13)**. Consensus from three small but very different trials showed a significantly quicker return to full activity among those patients wearing long stirrup braces (LOE: Cochrane review).[38] In the individual studies, braced patients returned to activity 20 to 45 days before nonbraced individuals. Although the study groups were very heterogeneous, the results are very encouraging and warrant further study. Providers should be mindful that stress-fracture healing still requires more than bracing. Activity modification, relative rest, and the correction of intrinsic and extrinsic risk factors are still critical to the successful treatment plan.

Authors' recommendation: Use long-leg pneumatic bracing as a part of the comprehensive treatment plan for patients with tibial stress fractures. The brace should be worn continuously for 4 to 6 weeks and then during activity for another 4 to 6 weeks.

Lateral ankle sprains

As stated previously, braces for the lateral ankle can be prophylactic, functional, or rehabilitative. The typically proposed mechanism for efficacy involves limiting the range of motion, especially inversion. Proprioception also appears to be improved, but only in those patients with previous injury (LOE: C).[4] The braces come in several different varieties **(Figure 38.14)**. General categories are rigid stirrup braces (pneumatic; Air-Cast) and gel stirrup braces

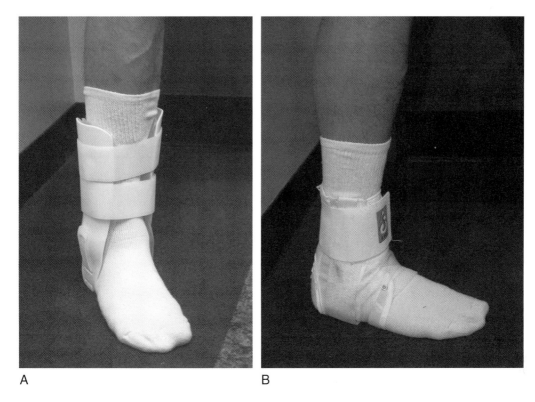

A   B

Figure 38.14 *A*, Stirrup-style ankle brace. *B*, Fabric-style ankle brace.

(most common); semirigid braces, which combine fabric and a rigid plastic support; lace-up braces with and without crossing straps; and elastic or fabric ankle sleeves.[39] A comparison of different braces has shown that the stirrup variety provides the most support and that all semirigid braces outperform soft braces. Elastic wrapping provides no benefit, except perhaps some edema control (LOE: B).[39] Taping initially performs as well as a stirrup-type brace, but the effect wanes after about 10 minutes as a result of loosening (LOE: B).[40,41] Any benefit from taping after 10 minutes of activity is probably the result of enhanced proprioception or placebo effect.[42] Although similar loosening occurs with other semirigid and lace-up braces, braces can be retightened after 10 minutes of activity, whereas taping cannot.

It is difficult to study the effect of ankle bracing as a result of the inconsistencies of braces and methodologies in different trials. Additionally, passive laboratory (in vitro) tests do not always approximate actual athletic participation. Still, systematic reviews and randomized controlled trials generally agree that recurrent lateral ankle sprain can be reduced with a combination of appropriate rehabilitation and a semirigid ankle orthosis (LOE: A).[42] In addition, there is some evidence that even primary injury may be prevented with the prophylactic use of a semirigid brace for high-risk activities like basketball or volleyball (LOE: A).[43] After an initial injury, bracing to prevent recurrent injury (secondary prevention) should be carried out for a minimum of 12 months because this is about the time it takes for a ligament to regain all of its normal strength and proprioceptive capabilities.[44] Many athletes may choose to use the brace permanently. It must be emphasized again that bracing is no substitute for proper rehabilitation. The best recurrent injury prevention results were achieved from a combination of intensive reconditioning (including proprioceptive rehabilitation and muscular strengthening) and brace use (LOE: B).[44] Interestingly, a recent study has shown that, for acute grade III lateral ankle injury, 1 week of treatment in a fracture boot **(Figure 38.15)** in combination with immediate range-of-motion exercises and as-tolerated strengthening exercises may be the best initial treatment (LOE: B).[4]

Authors' recommendation: For acute ankle sprains that can tolerate some weight bearing, use a stirrup-type ankle brace in combination with range-of-motion exercises and strengthening as tolerated. As range of motion and strength improve (usually after 1 week or so), transition to a nonstirrup brace, and begin proprioceptive retraining.. This brace can be continued throughout the remainder of the season, and, depending on the athlete, it may become a staple of his or her equipment for prevention. If the athlete cannot bear weight and a fracture has been ruled out, then he or she should be fitted for a fracture boot and given range of motion and isometric exercises for 1 week. After 1 week, he or she should return to the regular rehabilitation track as outlined previously.

Achilles tendinosis

There are several braces or orthotic devices advocated for the treatment of Achilles tendinosis. The first and probably the oldest is a simple heel lift **(Figure 38.16).** The proposed mechanism is to elevate the heel and decrease the tension on the tendon. Evidence to corroborate this assumption can be found in a study of 13 subjects in which decreased peak muscle activity in the gastrocnemius muscle was found with heel wedge use (LOE: C).[45] Unfortunately, in a blinded, randomized, prospective study of 33 subjects, more improvement was observed among patients who were treated with exercise and ultrasound as opposed to exercise and heel lift (LOE: A).[46] Still, many authors continue to advocate the use of heel lifts, especially for patients with acute Achilles conditions.[47] The verdict is not in yet, and clearly more study is needed.

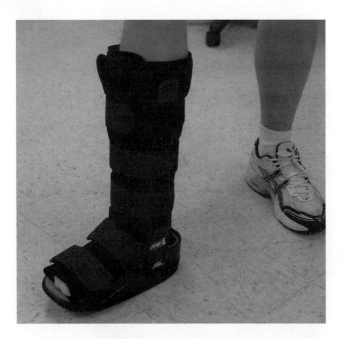

Figure 38.15 Fracture boot.

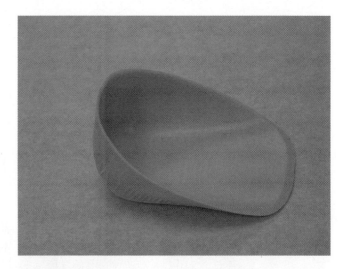

Figure 38.17 Heel cup.

Other authors recommend heel cups or foot orthoses, reportedly to restrict or accommodate calcaneal movement (LOE: E)[48] **(Figure 38.17)**. Still others advocate using an Achilles strap **(Figure 38.18)**, which applies the principles of counterforce bracing to Achilles disorders (LOE: E).[49] Again, only anecdotal evidence exists in support of these devices.

Authors' recommendation: The primary treatment of chronic Achilles tendinopathy is eccentric exercises. Heel lifts may actually shorten the tendon and tighten the cord, which may be counterproductive in the long run. Therefore, we do not routinely recommend them. We have had modest success with a counterforce Achilles strap. If there is a pes cavus or pes planus deformity with underpronation or overpronation, a full-foot orthosis may be helpful. However, the mainstay for Achilles tendinosis treatment is overload eccentric exercise[48] as described in Chapter 30, Foot and Ankle Soft-Tissue Injuries.

Plantar fascia pain

There are several types of orthoses available for plantar fascia pain. Heel pads and cups are usually used as first-line therapy, and purportedly work by either fixing the calcaneous and/or by providing extra cushion for the heel.[50] Custom-made foot orthoses are also advocated, supposedly by correcting biomechanical abnormalities. However, the less-expensive heel pads and cups and Achilles stretching performed better than the more expensive custom orthoses and stretching in a head-to-head trial (LOE: A).[51]

Another brace that is commonly employed is the tension night splint **(Figure 38.19)**. It works by keeping the plantar fascia stretched at night, thus avoiding the pain that occurs with the first steps in the morning. A Cochrane review found limited evidence to support the use of night splints to treat patients with pain that has lasted for more than 6 months. The same review indicates that patients treated with custom-made night splints improved but that patients treated with prefabricated night splints did not.[52] Many other plantar fascia braces exist, but no evidence exists to support their use.

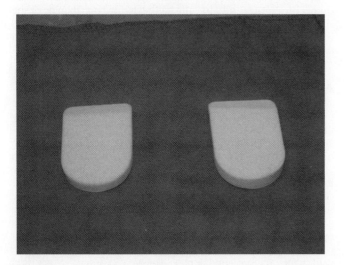

Figure 38.16 Heel wedges.

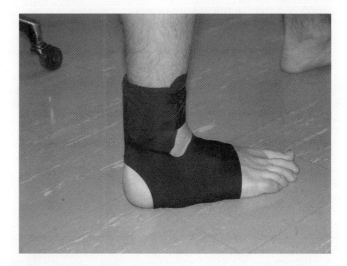

Figure 38.18 Achilles strap.

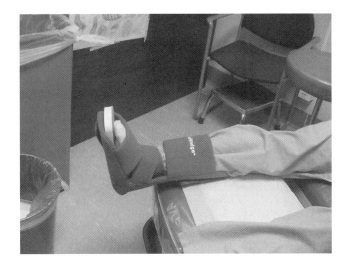

Figure 38.19 Prefabricated tension night splint.

Authors' recommendation: The mainstay of treatment for plantar fascia pain is frequent stretching of the plantar fascia and the Achilles tendon, along with the strengthening of the intrinsic muscles of the foot. Biomechanical abnormalities that may contribute to the pain syndrome can be treated with foot orthosis. In addition, training errors (including worn-out shoes) should be sought out and corrected. Night splints can be considered as second-line therapy for recalcitrant plantar fascial pain.

CONCLUSION

Braces are an integral part of treating musculoskeletal injuries and ailments. Proper bracing first requires proper pathoanatomic diagnosis, followed by a comprehensive treatment plan—with bracing being just a single aspect of the overall rehabilitation. Familiarity with some common braces and their indications will provide the physician with another tool in returning the athlete promptly and safely to the playing field.

REFERENCES

1. Dorland's Medical Dictionary online: Definition of "orthosis." Available at www.mercksource.com/pp/us/cns/cns_hl_dorlands.jspzQzpgzEzzSzppdocszSzuszSzcommonzSzdorlandszSzdorlandzSzdmd_o_07zPzhtm#12597938. Accessed December 28, 2005.
2. Segedy A: Effectiveness of bracing depends on application. BioMechanics (serial online), March 2004. Available at www.biomech.com/db_area/archives/2004/0403.braces.bio.shtml. Accessed December 29, 2005.
3. Aiello DD, George P: Orthotic options. Rehab Management (serial online), March 2003. Available at http://www.rehabpub.com/features/32003/2.asp. Accessed on December 30, 2005.
4. Arnold BL, Docherty CL: Bracing and rehabilitation—what's new. Clin Sports Med 2004;23:83-95.
5. Segedy A: Braces' joint effects spur research surge. BioMechanics (serial online), February 2005. Available at www.biomech.com/showArticle.jhtml?articleID=59302060. Accessed December 28, 2005.
6. Peters T, Baker CL: Lateral epicondylitis. Clin Sports Med 2001;20:549-563.
7. Struijs PAA, Kerkhoffs GMMJ, Assendelft WJJ, et al: Conservative treatment of lateral epicondylitis brace versus physical therapy or a combination of both—a randomized clinical trial. Am J Sports Med 2004;32:462-469.
8. Struijs PAA, Smidt N, Arola H, et al: Orthotic devices for the treatment of tennis elbow (Cochrane review). In The Cochrane Library, Issue 3. Chichester, UK: John Wiley & Sons, 2004. Available at http://www.mrw.interscience.wiley.com/cochrane/clsysrev/articles/CD001821/frame.html.
9. Bisset L, Paungmali A, Vicenzino B: A systematic review and meta-analysis of clinical trials on physical interventions for lateral epicondylalgia. Br J Sports Med 2005;39:411-422.
10. Goodyear-Smith F, Arroll B: What can family physicians offer patients with carpal tunnel syndrome other than surgery? A systematic review of nonsurgical management. Ann Fam Med 2004;2:267-273.
11. O'Connor D, Marshall S, Massy-Westropp N: Non-surgical treatment (other than steroid injection) for carpal tunnel syndrome (Cochrane review). In The Cochrane Library, Issue 3. Chichester, UK: John Wiley & Sons,, 2004. Available at http://www.mrw.interscience.wiley.com/cochrane/clsysrev/articles/CD003219/frame.html.
12. Viera AJ: Management of carpal tunnel syndrome. Am Fam Physician 2003;68:265-272, 279-280.
13. Handoll HHG, Vaghela MV: Interventions for treating mallet finger injuries. Cochrane Review (serial online). Available at www.cochrane.org/cochrane/revabstr/AB004574.htm. Accessed March 22, 2005.
14. Rettig AC: Closed tendon injuries of the hand and wrist in the athlete. Clin Sports Med 1992;11:77-99.
15. Leggit JC, Meko CJ: Acute common finger injuries: part I. Tendons and ligaments. Am Fam Physician 2006;73(5):810-816.
16. Wang QC, Johnson BA: Fingertip injuries. Am Fam Physician 2001;63:1961-1966.
17. Lee SJ, Montgomery K: Athletic hand injuries. Orthop Clin North Am 2002;33:139-146.
18. Bach AW: Finger joint injuries in active persons. Pointers for acute and late-phase management. Phys Sportsmed 1999;27:90.
19. Graham TJ, Mullen DJ: Athletic injuries of the adult hand. In DeLee JC, Drez D Jr, Miller MD (eds): DeLee & Drez's Orthopaedic Sports Medicine, 2nd ed. Philadelphia, WB Saunders 2003, pp 1408-1445.
20. American Academy of Orthopaedic Surgeons: The use of knee braces. Document number 1124. Published October 1997, revised December 2003. Available at www.aaos.org/wordhtml/papers/position/1124.htm. Accessed November 20, 2005.
21. Baker CL: Bracing and Taping for Prevention and Treatment of Injuries. The Hughston Clinic Sports Medicine Field Manual. Baltimore, Williams & Wilkins, 1996, pp 271-284.
22. Martin TJ: the Committee on Sports Medicine and Fitness. American Academy of Pediatrics: Technical report: knee brace use in the young athlete. Pediatrics 2001;108(2):503-507.
23. Pulaska SA, McKeag DB: Knee braces: current evidence and clinical recommendations for their use. Am Fam Physician 2000;61:411-418, 423-424.
24. Birmingham TB, Kramer JF, Kirkley A, Inglis JT: Knee bracing after ACL reconstruction: effects on postural control and proprioception. Med Sci Sports Exerc 2001;33(8):1253-1258.
25. Risberg MA, Holm I, Steen H, et al: The effect of knee bracing after anterior cruciate ligament reconstruction. A prospective, randomized study with two years' follow-up. Am J Sports Med 1999;27:76-83.
26. Kramer JF, Dubowitz T, Fowler P, Schachter C: Functional knee braces and dynamic performance: a review. Clin J Sports Med 1997;7:32-39.
27. Allen CR, Kaplan LD, Fluhme DJ, Harner CD: Posterior cruciate ligament injuries. Curr Opin Rheumatol 2002;14:142-149.
28. St Pierre P, Miller MD: Posterior cruciate ligament injuries. Clin Sports Med 1999;18:199-221.
29. Miller MD, Johnson DJ, Harner CD, Fu FH: Posterior cruciate ligament injuries. Orthop Rev 1993;22:1201-1210.
30. D'hondt NE, Struijs PA, Kerkhoffs GM, Verheul C: Orthotic devices for treating patellofemoral pain syndrome. Cochrane Database Syst Rev 2005;4. Available at http://www.mrw.interscience.wiley.com/cochrane/clsysrev/articles/CD002267/frame.html.
31. Arroll B, Ellis-Pegler E, Edwards A, Sutcliffe G: Patellofemoral pain syndrome: a critical review of the clinical trials on nonoperative therapy. Am J Sports Med 1997;25(2):207-212 and Database of Abstracts of Reviews of Effectiveness 2005, Volume 4.
32. Crossley K, Bennell K, Green S, McConnell J: A systematic review of physical interventions for patellofemoral pain syndrome. Clin J Sport Med 2001;11(2):103-110 and Database of Abstracts of Reviews of Effectiveness 2005, Volume 4.
33. Yeung EW, Yueng SS: Interventions for preventing lower limb soft-tissue injuries in runners. Cochrane Database Syst Rev 2005;4. Available at http://www.mrw.interscience.wiley.com/cochrane/clsysrev/articles/CD001256/frame.html.
34. Pruitt AL: Orthotic and brace use in the athlete with degenerative joint disease with angular deformity. Clin Sports Med 2005;24:93-99.
35. Manek NJ, Lane NE: Osteoarthritis: current concepts in diagnosis and management. Am Fam Physician 2000;61:1795-1804.
36. Brower RW, Jakma TS, Verhegan AP, Verhaar JA: Braces and orthosis for treating osteoarthritis of the knee. Cochrane Database Syst Rev 2005;4.
37. Whitelaw FP, Wetzler MJ, Levy AS, et al: A pneumatic leg brace for the treatment of tibial stress fractures. Clin Orthop Relat Res 1991;270:301-305.
38. Rome K, Handoll HHG, Ashford R: Interventions for preventing and treating stress fractures and stress reactions of bone of the lower limbs in young adults. Cochrane

Database Syst Rev 2005;4. Available at http://www.mrw.interscience.wiley.com/cochrane/clsysrev/articles/CD0000450/frame.html.

39. Boyce SH, Quigley MA, Campbell S: Management of ankle sprains: a randomised controlled trial of the treatment of inversion injuries using an elastic support bandage or an Aircast ankle brace. Br J Sports Med 2005;39:91-96.

40. Vaes PH, Duquet W, Handelberg F, et al: Influence of anklestrapping, taping, and nine braces: a stress roentgenologic comparison. J Sport Rehabil 1998;7:157-171.

41. Eils E, Demming C, Kollmeier G, et al: Comprehensive testing of 10 different ankle braces Evaluation of passive and rapidly induced stability in subjects with chronic ankle instability. Clin Biomech 2002;17:526-535.

42. Thacker SB, Stroup DF, Branche CM: The prevention of ankle sprains in sports. A systematic review of the literature. Am J Sports Med 1999;27:753-760.

43. Handoll HHG, Rowe BH, Quinn KM, et al: Interventions for preventing ankle ligament injuries. Cochrane Database Syst Rev 2005;4. Available at http://www.mrw.interscience.wiley.com/cochrane/clsysrev/articles/CD000018/frame.html.

44. Stasinopoulos D: Comparison of three preventive methods in order to reduce the incidence of ankle inversion sprains among female volleyball players. Br J Sports Med 2004;38:182-185.

45. Lee KH, Matteliano A, Medige J, et al: Electromyographic changes of leg muscles with heel lift: therapeutic implications. Arch Phys Med Rehabil 1987;68:298-301.

46. Lowdon A, Bader DL, Mowat AG: The effect of heel pads on the treatment of Achilles tendinitis: a double blind trial. Am J Sports Med 1984;12:431-435.

47. Keene JS: Section G: Tendon injuries of the foot and ankle. In DeLee JC, Drez D Jr, Miller MD (eds): DeLee and Drez's Orthopaedic Sports Medicine: Principles and Practice, 2nd ed. Philadelphia, WB Saunders, 2003, pp 2410-2445.

48. Wilson JJ, Best TM: Common overuse tendon problems: a review and recommendations for treatment. Am Fam Physician 2005;72:811-818.

49. Greene BL: Case report: Physical therapist management of fluoroquinolone-induced Achilles tendinopathy. Physical Therapy 2002:82 (serial online). Available at www.ptjournal.org/PTJournal/Dec2002/v82n12p1224.cfm. Accessed December 27, 2005.

50. Cole C, Seto C, Gazewood J: Plantar fasciitis: evidence-based review of diagnosis and therapy. Am Fam Physician 2005;72:2237-2242, 2247-2248.

51. Pfeffer G, Bacchetti P, Deland J: Comparison of custom and prefabricated orthoses in the initial treatment of proximal plantar fasciitis. Foot Ankle Int 1999;20:214-221.

52. Crawford F, Thomson C: Interventions for treating plantar heel pain. Cochrane Database Syst Rev 2003;(3). Available at http://www.mrw.interscience.wiley.com/cochrane/clsysrev/articles/CD000416/frame.html.

SECTION 5

Special Tests and Procedures

CHAPTER 39

Exercise Prescription

CPT David D. Farnsworth, MD,
and Michael Cannon, MD, MS

All parts of the body if used in moderation and exercised in labors to which each is accustomed, become thereby healthy and well developed, and age slowly; but if unused and left idle, they become libel to disease, defective in growth, and age quickly.

—*Hippocrates*

KEY POINTS

- Regular exercise in all patients should use at least 1000 kcal of energy weekly; this has been shown to decrease all-cause mortality by 20% to 30%.

- In addition to meeting goals for prevention, an exercise prescription should be tailored to meet an individual's specific needs for cardiorespiratory fitness, chronic disease treatment, weight control, recreation, and/or competition.

- An exercise prescription should be customized to minimize side effects for each patient, with the most significant side effect being cardiovascular events and the most common detrimental outcome being musculoskeletal injuries. Side-effect risks specific to any individual's own health profile should be addressed.

- Components of the exercise prescription, including the exercise mode, intensity, duration, frequency, and progression of activity, must be reviewed periodically to ensure that the plan continues to maximize benefits and compliance and to minimize side effects as an individual's health profile, abilities, and life circumstances change over time.

INTRODUCTION

The effectiveness of exercise as a disease-modifying and preventive health measure is a topic of renewed interest in medicine. It has been estimated that as many as 1 in 10 Americans die prematurely of diseases that are directly related to physical inactivity,[1] including coronary artery disease, which is the leading killer in the United States.[2] The 1991 National Health Interview Survey—Health Promotion/Disease Prevention reported that 22% of adults engage in light to moderate physical activity for at least 30 minutes per day; 54% are somewhat active but do not meet the current recommendations; and 24% are completely sedentary (reporting no physical activity over the past month).[3] In 1996, the seminal study of the exercise patterns of Americans performed by the Centers for Disease Control and Prevention (CDC) reported that more than 60% of Americans were not regularly active and

that 25% more were not active at all.[4] As the trend toward inactivity increases in America and the incidence of chronic health conditions continues to rise among both children and adults, the importance of prescribing attainable and effective exercise programs to patients has never been greater.

Recent evidence supports the use of a variety of different exercise strategies at lower levels of effort as effective prevention and treatment modalities. In conjunction with standard protocols for achieving physical fitness, these recent findings elucidate a broad array of programs from which individual exercise prescriptions can be customized to better fit a patient's lifestyle and needs. Evidence-based, effective exercise prescriptions can be formulated to address the recreational, preventive, and disease-modifying needs of individual patients in ways that maximize the likelihood of success.

Exercise goals

Exercise prescriptions can serve two main functions in a clinical setting, each of which may have a different dose—response relationship: (1) the treatment and prevention of diseases; and (2) cardiorespiratory fitness attainment, improvement, and maintenance. Cardiorespiratory fitness is defined as a component of physiologic fitness that relates to the ability of the circulatory and respiratory systems to supply oxygen during sustained physical activity.[4] Whereas all patients should have a program for disease prevention, the exercise prescription may be customized to meet many other patient goals (i.e., competition, recreation, disease treatment, or weight loss). Most research has focused on the threshold for obtaining health benefits, and it has been shown that significant health benefits may be obtained from moderate-intensity activity **(Table 39.1).** An interesting finding of this research was that health benefits may be obtained without significantly improving fitness or losing weight. Conversely, at higher intensities and durations, cardiorespiratory fitness may be improved without significantly improving health benefits **(Figure 39.1).**

Current guidelines for disease prevention and treatment

In 1996, the Surgeon General reported the following: "Significant health benefits can be obtained by including a moderate amount of physical activity (e.g., 30 minutes of brisk walking or raking leaves, 15 minutes of running, or 45 minutes of playing volleyball) on most, if not all, days of the week." As a corollary, the reports noted that greater health benefits would likely be obtained by increasing either the duration or intensity of the exercise.[4]

Table 39.1 The Benefits of Exercise

Health Problem	Sources of Evidence (Category)
All-cause mortality	C
Cardiovascular disease	
prevention/treatment	C
Hypertension (HTN)	
prevention/treatment	A
Hyperlipidemia	
prevention/treatment	B
Type II diabetes mellitus	
prevention/treatment	C
Obesity	
prevention	C
treatment	A
Colon cancer	
prevention	C
COPD (chronic obstructive pulmonary disease)	
treatment	D
Low back pain	
prevention	B
treatment	C
Osteoporosis	
prevention/treatment	A
Rheumatic disease	
treatment	D

Evidence categories:

A—Evidence from end points of a well-designed, randomized clinical trial (RCT) that provide a consistent pattern of findings. Requires a substantial number of studies involving a large number of participants.

B—Evidence from endpoints of intervention that include only a limited number of RCTs, post hoc or subgroup analysis of RCTs, or meta-analysis of RCTs. Pertains when few randomized trials exist: they are small; and the trial results are somewhat inconsistent.

C—Evidence is from outcomes of uncontrolled or nonrandomized trials or from observational studies.

Adapted form Chakravarthy MV, Booth FW: Hot Topics: Exercise. Philadelphia, Hanley & Belfus, Inc., 2003, pp 71-72.

In 2001, the American College of Sports Medicine (ACSM) along with the American Heart Association and the CDC revised guidelines that were similar to those published by the Surgeon General, reporting that activity of moderate intensity in several 10-minute to 15-minute sessions over the course of a day would provide the same health benefits as a single 30-minute session.[5,6] The ACSM further specified their recommendations for weight control, concluding that overweight individuals should increase the duration of activity to 45 minutes of exercise per day to facilitate weight loss and prevent weight regain. The Institute of Medicine has subsequently recommended an even longer duration (60 minutes) of moderate-intensity exercise to prevent weight gain.[7]

EVIDENCE

Over the past decade, several significant studies have been performed to assess the health benefits of low-level exercise, which has resulted in various recommendations. These studies have shown that it is possible to prevent heart disease, stroke, and certain types of cancer (colon and breast) and to reduce type II diabetes incidence by 30% with 3 or more hours of moderate-intensity physical activity per week. Exercise has been shown to reduce the risk of all-cause mortality by 20% to 30% and of cardiovascular disease by 20%.[4,8]

The Women's Health Initiative Observational Study[9] was a large, randomized, controlled clinical trial that monitored more than 70,000 postmenopausal women from 1994 to 1998. The women were stratified into five groups on the basis of their self-reported exercise level, which was quantitated both by intensity and time spent exercising. These groups were evaluated for the incidence of coronary events, including death from coronary causes, nonfatal myocardial infarction, coronary revascularization, angina, congestive heart failure, stroke, and carotid revascularization.

The results of this study revealed a stepwise increase in health benefits with increasing levels of exercise. The age-adjusted analysis, controlled for other risk factors, showed that women who walked at least 2.5 hours per week had a relative risk reduction of nearly 30% as compared with those who did not walk at all. Furthermore, women who engaged in both walking and vigorous exercise had a greater benefit than those who engaged in either alone. It was determined that, for walking to be beneficial, it had to occur at a pace of 2 to 3 mph. Casual walking slower than 2 mph was not shown to be beneficial as compared with rarely or never walking.

The Women's Health Study[10] monitored the exercise habits of about 40,000 female health professionals who were 45 years of age

Figure 39.1 Health benefits of exercise intensity. CV, cardiovascular.

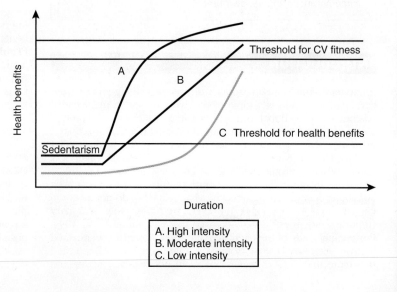

A. High intensity
B. Moderate intensity
C. Low intensity

and older from 1992 to 1999. The purpose of this study was to determine the amount of exercise needed to produce a cardioprotective benefit, with primary end points of myocardial infarction, coronary bypass surgery, or coronary angioplasty.

It was found that as little as 1 hour of walking per week was shown to produce a significant reduction in relative risk of 51%. Unlike the Women's Health Initiative study, walking at paces slower than 2 mph was also shown to produce benefit as compared with not walking regularly (relative risk reduction, 44%). Time spent walking predicted the degree of risk reduction, but walking pace did not.

The Physicians' Health Study[11] was a large, prospective clinical trial of 21,271 physicians with a primary end point of new-onset diabetes. The study concluded that, when obese individuals become physically active, the risk of chronic health conditions began to return to that of the unfit, normal-weight individual. As compared with physicians with a body mass index (BMI) of less than 23 kg/m^2, physicians with a BMI that was higher than 26.4 kg/m^2 had a sevenfold increased risk of developing type II diabetes if they exercised vigorously (defined as any activity that resulted in working up a sweat) less than once per week. This increased risk was reduced to fourfold among physicians of equal BMI (> 26.4 kg/m^2) who exercised vigorously more than once per week. Thus, these findings suggest that physical activity independent of obesity lowers the risk of type II diabetes.

The Harvard Alumni Health Study[12] monitored the cardiovascular risk factors (including exercise habits) of 12,000 middle-aged men from 1977 to 1993. No significant reduction in the risk of coronary artery disease was associated with increasing levels of energy expenditure in light and moderate intensity activities. A significant risk reduction of 13% was associated with walking more than 3 miles per week, but increasing the amount of walking to 12 miles per week produced no additional benefit.

Additional studies have confirmed these results and shown benefits of moderate-intensity exercise. The Nurses' Health Study[13] found that women who walked briskly (moderate intensity) for 3 hours per week or at high intensity for 1.5 hours per week, had a relative risk reduction of 30% to 40% for myocardial infarction as compared with sedentary women. The Railroad study[14] reported a 30% to 40% greater risk of dying of coronary artery disease or of any cause among participants who were sedentary as compared with those who expended more than 1000 kcal per week participating in leisure-time physical activity. However, LaCroix and colleagues[15] found that walking more than 4 hours per week was associated with fewer hospitalizations than walking less than 1 hour per week.

Results have been variable in the investigations of the amounts of exercise needed to attain exercise-related weight loss and to prevent weight regain. The National Weight Control Registry[16] reviewed the record of 629 women and 155 men who lost an average of 30 kg and maintained a minimum weight loss of 13.6 kg for 5 years. These individuals had an energy expenditure of approximately 2800 kcal per week or about 1.5 hours of brisk walking per day. However, other studies have found that shorter amounts of physical activity can also have a beneficial effect on weight control. For example, a 1-year clinical trial of 173 postmenopausal women with an average BMI of 30.5 kg/m^2 found that women in the intervention group, who exercised an average of 25 minutes per day, experienced an average BMI reduction of 0.3 kg/m^2, whereas the BMI of the women in the control group increased by 0.3 kg/m^2.[17]

ENERGY EXPENDITURE GOALS

In addition to supporting the use of routine exercise to meet preventive and treatment goals to improve health, the previously described studies have also provided data to support the specific energy expenditure goals required to attain these benefits. The net caloric expenditure of an activity is determined by the interaction of intensity, duration, and frequency. The caloric thresholds for increasing cardiorespiratory fitness, losing weight, and reducing the risk of chronic disease are all different. Home exercise prescriptions should be designed with these energy expenditure goals in mind.

The ACSM recommends a target range of 150 to 400 kcal of exercise energy expenditure each day, which, at the lower end, yields roughly 1000 kcal per week of energy expenditure (assuming 6 to 7 days of exercise per week). This is associated with a 20% to 30% decrease in the risk of all-cause mortality.[6]

For attaining overall health benefits, the low end of energy expenditure (150 kcal/day) or 30 minutes of moderate-intensity exercise (a 2 to 3 mph walk) on all or most days of the week should be the minimum level of activity. This exercise need not be continuous to obtain these health benefits.[18] A variety of activities can be used to attain these goals (see **Table 39.2** for the energy expenditures of various physical activities). For weight control in overweight or obese patients, a weekly energy expenditure of 2100 to 2800 kcal[19,20] or 45 to 90 minutes of daily exercise may be required.[21] Cardiorespiratory fitness is maintained by continuous exercise three times weekly for 20 minutes minimum at an intensity of at least 60% of peak predicted exercise capacity; it is not defined by energy expenditure. However, those exercising for fitness exceed the minimum 1000 kcal per week goal for overall health benefits. Additional health benefits accrue from this increased exercise load.[6]

FORMULATING THE EXERCISE PRESCRIPTION

The fundamental components of an exercise prescription are the mode, intensity, duration, frequency, and progression of physical activity. After the specific exercise goals are defined for an individual, the strategy for best meeting those goals can be developed. A well-defined plan must also include an understanding of the potential barriers to implementing the plan for any individual, including preventing potential side effects and applying behavioral modification strategies to minimize these barriers.

Mode/type of exercise

A pre-exercise assessment is essential to determining the activities that maximize exercise benefits and minimize the risks of injury. The most important factors that influence the choice of activity are the patient's interests, his or her current activity level and capabilities, injury history, and history of medical conditions. Walking tends to be a good choice for most people, and it is the most-studied mode of exercise; walking at speeds exceeding 2 mph has been shown to produce the greatest health benefits. Activities that involve the large muscle groups in a rhythmic, continuous nature have been shown to produce the greatest increase in cardiorespiratory fitness.

Barriers to engaging in an exercise prescription may be avoided by customizing activity to a patient's interests and capabilities. This would include an initial assessment of what activities a patient is already doing, what activities he or she enjoys, and what activities can be done without further training. It may also be helpful to encourage alternating modes of activity to reduce boredom and decrease the chance of injury.

To minimize the risk of injury, a thorough health history that includes a family and personal history indicative of cardiovascular risk **(Box 39.1)** and past musculoskeletal injuries should be performed on all patients. Activities specific for each patient's medical conditions can then be chosen to minimize risk and maximize health benefits. For example, obese patients and those

Table 39.2 Energy Expenditures for Various Activities

Activity	METs*	Kilocalories**
Aerobic dancing	6-9	440-660
Bowling	2-4	150-300
Calisthenics	3-8	220-600
Canoeing (leisure)	3-6	220-440
Cycling (<10 mph)	3-6	220-440
Cycling (>10 mph)	6-8	440-600
Dancing	3-7	220-510
Desk Work	1.5-2.5	110-180
Fishing (sitting)	1.5-3	110-220
Fishing (standing/casting)	3-6	220-440
Football (touch)	6-10	440-740
Golf (walking)	2-3	150-220
Handball	8-12	600-880
Hiking (cross-country)	3-7	220-510
Lawn mowing	3-8	220-600
Running at 5 mph	8.7	640
Running at 6 mph	10.2	750
Running at 10 mph	16.3	1200
Sexual intercourse	2-5	150-370
Shoveling	4-7	300-510
Shuffleboard	2-3	150-220
Skating (ice/roller)	5-8	370-600
Skiing (cross-country)	6-12	440-880
Skiing (downhill)	5-8	370-600
Soccer	5-12	370-880
Softball	3-6	220-440
Stair climbing	4-8	300-600
Swimming (moderate)	4-6	300-440
Swimming (fast treading)	6-8	440-600
Tennis	4-9	300-660
Volleyball	3-6	220-440
Walking at 2 mph	2	150
Walking at 4 mph	4.5	330
Walking at 4 mph (uphill)	6	440

*1 MET = resting metabolic rate, 3.5 mL of C_1 per kg per minute.
**The kilocalories expended during a particular activity are based on a person weighing 70 kg (154 lb).
One kilocalorie = approximately 200mL of C_2 consumed.
mph, miles per hour.
Gauer RL, O'Connor FG: How to write an exercise prescription. Available at http://www.hooah4health.com/toolbox/exRx/default.htm.
Jones TF, Eaton CB: Am Fam Physician 1995;52:543-550.
ACC/AHA Guidelines for Exercise Testing: A report of the American College of Cardiology/American Heart Association Task Force on Practice Guidelines. Gibbons RJ, Balady GJ, Beasley JW, et al: J Am Coll Cardiol 1997;30:260-315.
Pollock ML, Wilmore JH (eds): Exercise in Health and Disease: Evaluation and Prescription for Prevention and Rehabilitation, 2nd ed. Philadelphia, Saunders, 1990, pp 239-369.
Squires RW, Gau GT, Miller TD, Allison TG, Lavie CJ: Mayo Clin Proc 1990;65:731-755.

who have degenerative joint disease will not be capable of following a regimen that prescribes activities that result in repetitive high impact on the knees. There are certain subsets of patients in whom the risk of activity exceeds the benefits **(Box 39.2).**

For athletes, the principle of training specificity should be considered when formulating an exercise prescription. Exercises involving one set of muscles may improve overall fitness without significantly improving performance in sporting activities that require the use of other muscle groups. For example, although swimming is low impact and an excellent method of maintaining cardiorespiratory fitness, it will not significantly improve

Box 39.1: American Heart Association Consensus Panel Recommendations for Preparticipation Athletic Screening

Family History
1. Premature sudden cardiac death
2. Heart disease in surviving relatives less than 50 years old

Personal History
3. Tobacco use
4. Dyslipidemias
5. Age and gender
6. Diabetes mellitus
7. Obesity
8. Heart murmur
9. Systemic hypertension
10. Fatigue
11. Syncope or near syncope
12. Excessive or unexplained exertional dyspnea
13. Exertional chest pain

Physical Examination
14. Heart murmur (supine/standing)
15. Femoral arterial pulses (to exclude coarctation of aorta)
16. Stigmata of Marfan's syndrome
17. Brachial blood pressure measurement (sitting)

Adapted from Maron BJ, Thompson PD, Puffer JC, et al: Circulation 1996;94:850-856.

Box 39.2: Absolute Contraindications to Exercise

- Unstable angina pectoris
- Recent electrocardiogram changes
- Uncontrolled cardiac arrhythmias
- Malignant ventricular tachycardia
- Decompensated congestive heart failure
- Critical aortic stenosis (symptomatic)
- Known cerebral aneurysms
- Dissecting aortic aneurysm
- Recent myocardial infarction
- Third-degree heart block
- Myocarditis or pericarditis
- Thrombophlebitis
- Acute pulmonary embolism
- Untreated high-risk proliferative retinopathy
- Recent significant retinal hemorrhage
- Uncontrolled hypertension
- Uncontrolled metabolic disease, including diabetes
- Current febrile illness
- Acute renal failure

From Maron BJ, Zipes DP, et al: J Am Coll Cardiol 2005;45:1312-1375.

road-racing ability. Traditional aerobic training programs may fail to meet the goals of athletes who are interested in improving strength and endurance specific to their sport.

Exercise intensity

Intensity is the most complex aspect of an exercise prescription. Like the mode of activity, intensity must take into account a patient's goals and health status. Although increased cardiorespiratory fitness and health benefits do increase with increased exercise intensity, so too does the risk for musculoskeletal and cardiac side effects. For each individual, a benefit–risk balance must be understood to maximize the patient's improvement in health. The standard recommendation for exercise intensity in a healthy patient who wishes to achieve the health benefits of exercise is to exercise at 50% of his or her peak predicted exercise capacity.[3,4,6] Those patients wishing to achieve a goal of cardiorespiratory fitness should exercise at 60% to 90% of their maximum predicted exercise capacity. However, because exercise at these higher intensities increases the risk for injury and cardiovascular side effects, most patients should be started at a lower intensity. For example, for deconditioned, sedentary patients without contraindicating health conditions, exercise should begin at a low intensity (i.e., 40% to 50% of predicted peak exercise capacity).

Most patients do not require formal exercise testing to define their peak exercise capacity. Monitoring heart rate changes with exercise and/or using a standardized scale of perceived exertion are two commonly employed methods.

Two heart-rate methods for determining exercise intensity are commonly used as a result of their ease of use. To use the standard method **(Table 39.3),** a patient simply calculates his or her maximal heart rate, which is then multiplied by the prescribed intensity level. For example, the target heart rate for a deconditioned 50-year-old overweight male who has been prescribed an intensity of 50% would be 85 bpm based on the following see calculations:

$$\text{Maximal heart rate} = 220 - 50 = 170$$
$$\text{Target heart rate} = 170 \times 0.50 = 85 \text{ bpm}$$

The Karvonen (heart rate reserve) method uses an individual's resting heart rate to more closely approximate the desired intensity level. Using this method to calculate the rate for an athletic 30-year-old male with a resting heart rate of 60 bpm and a prescribed intensity level of 80%, the target heart rate would be 164 bpm (see the calculation below). Note that this is a higher target heart rate than

Table 39.3 The Heart Rate Methods for Determining Peak Exercise Intensity

Standard Method

THR = MHR × desired intensity level

MHR = 220 − age

THR = target heart rate; MHR = maximal heart rate

Benefits: Ease of use. (Patients can easily monitor their own intensity while exercising.)

Limitations: Often significantly underestimates the MHR in patients who are on calcium channel blockers and beta blockers and in the elderly.

Karvonen Method

First calculate the heart rate reserve (HRR) = MHR − RHR.

THR = (MHR − RHR) × % intensity + RHR

RHR = resting heart rate

Benefits: More closely matched to the VO_2 max (i.e., 60%-80% THR = 60%-80% VO_2 max), especially in the more fit individual.

Limitations: Difficult for patients to use.

Box 39.3: The Borg Scale

6: No exertion at all

7: Extremely light

9: Very light

11: Light

13: Moderate

15: Hard

17: Very hard

19: Extremely hard

20: Maximum all-out effort with absolutely nothing being held in reserve

From Borg G (ed): An Introduction to Borg's RPE-Scale. Ithaca, NY, Mouvement Publications, 1985.

would be calculated using the standard method (maximal heart rate × 0.8 = 152). Target heart rate = (190 - 60) × 0.80 + 60 = 164.

Patients can be instructed to measure their carotid pulse if they are unable to palpate a radial pulse during various stages of exercise. Commercial monitors may also be recommended for those who find it difficult to monitor their own pulse.

Another approach to measuring exercise intensity is the rating of perceived exertion scale, which measures the subjective interpretation of the exercise experience. This may be a more preferable method of measuring exercise intensity for patients who are taking β-blockers and calcium-channel blockers, and it provides the advantage of uninterrupted exercise. The original scale, called the *Borg scale*, involves 15 grades from 6 to 20, with each level associated with a verbal description of perceived intensity **(Box 39.3).** The original scale was studied in a young population and correlated with the actual heart rate at a given level of work. Because heart rate maximums decline with age, the actual heart rate and the rating of perceived exertion do not correlate well in the older population. Within each age group, however, this scale has been shown to exhibit a linear relationship between work intensity and heart rate.[22]

Duration

The duration of activity prescribed will depend on the energy expenditure goals, the mode of exercise, the intensity goals, the sport-specific training protocols, and the time constraints of an individual's schedule. Exercise duration and intensity combine to define energy expenditure for each session of exercise. Exercise at high intensity for a shorter duration can accomplish similar energy expenditures to exercise of shorter intensity and longer duration. To achieve the benefits of disease prevention, 30 minutes of moderate-intensity exercise (i.e., 50% predicted peak exercise), which need not be continuous, is generally the goal. For those who want to improve cardiorespiratory fitness, a minimum of 20 minutes of continuous exercise at an intensity of at least 60% of predicted peak exercise is required.[23]

Several studies have shown that multiple short intervals of exercise produce health benefits that are equal to those of a single 30-minute session.[23] Likewise, cardiorespiratory fitness likewise has been shown to improve somewhat with short-duration, high-intensity exercise.[18,24-26]

Frequency

Recent recommendations from the Surgeon General and the ACSM/CDC are for 30 minutes of moderate-intensity physical activity on most if not all days of the week for health-related benefits.[27] Those individuals who exercise at the higher intensities (i.e., 60% to 90% predicted exercise capacity) will be able to improve or maintain their health in three sessions weekly, whereas those involved in lower-intensity programs may need to exercise 5 or more days a week to meet caloric expenditure goals. Deconditioned individuals will find improvements in cardio-respiratory fitness by exercising only one to two times per week, whereas conditioned individuals will find little cardiorespiratory improvement at a frequency below twice weekly.[27]

Improvement in cardiovascular fitness tends to plateau at frequencies between three and five times per week.[27] Exercising 6 days a week should be reserved for competitive athletes, and exercise on all days of the week is not recommended as a result of the abrupt increase in musculoskeletal injuries that occurs with daily exercising.[6]

Progression of physical activity

After an exercise program has been initiated, the rate and means of progression to the goal exercise level will become the focus of subsequent visits. The recommended rate of progression will depend on the patient's age, health status, and tolerance of current activity. Patients who are exercising for the health benefits associated with an exercise regimen can often achieve these benefits without progression of their exercise regimen. Conversely, activity progression for athletes and patients desiring weight loss might be the most important aspect of their exercise prescriptions. The ACSM recommends three stages of progression: initial, improvement, and maintenance.[6]

Initial stage

For those individuals who are not able to begin at the ACSM/CDC recommendations of 30 minutes per day on most days of the week, both duration and frequency may need to be adjusted to an appropriate starting point. For a sedentary patient, the recommendation is to start with 15 minutes of moderate-intensity exercise (40% to 50%) on 3 to 4 days per week. During the initial stage, the focus is on limiting muscle soreness and injury while building up muscle and bone tolerance. A 10-minute warm up with or without stretching should precede exercise, and stretching after exercise should be emphasized to prevent fatigue and injury. The initial stage usually lasts between 4 and 6 weeks.

Improvement stage

This stage focuses on increasing levels of exercise until the recommended 30 minutes on most or all days of the week is achieved. After this goal is met, focus should be turned to increasing exercise intensity to the upper range for health-related benefits (50% to 70%). Duration should then be gradually increased at a rate of no faster than 70% per week. Intensity should be increased incrementally with interval training (i.e., increasing the intensity during one workout per week until all workouts are at the same intensity). This stage typically lasts from 4 to 8 months, but it is dictated by the rate of adaptation to the increased workload.

Maintenance stage

This stage begins after the preestablished fitness goals have been achieved and focuses on maintaining duration, frequency, and intensity at the level required to meet the initial goals.

Exercise goals change over time as do the ability to perform certain activities; thus, the exercise prescription must reflect the changing needs of each patient to maintain the maximal health and recreational benefits over time.

THE SIDE EFFECTS OF EXERCISE

Although for most individuals the benefits of physical activity significantly outweigh the risks, there are potential detrimental effects

Table 39.4 Prevalence of Physical Activity-Related Injury

Activity	Injury Prevalence
Walking	1%-12%
Running/jogging	24%-85%
Aerobics	1.5%-48.7%
Bicycling	1%-34%
Swimming	No data
Weight lifting	3.3%
Racquet sports	No data

Hootman, JM: The Epidemeology of Physical Activity-related Musculoskeletal Injuries: Part I. Epidemiology Supercourse. University of Pittsburgh, Penn, 2002.

of an exercise regimen. The most significant are cardiac events related to exercise, and the most common are exercise-induced musculoskeletal injuries, both of which represent significant barriers to physical activity.

Musculoskeletal injuries

The most common adverse effects of activity are musculoskeletal injuries and the resulting potential for the development of traumatic osteoarthritis. Certain groups of people, such as the elderly and women, may not engage in physical activity because they fear pain and injury.[28] Musculoskeletal injury has also been identified as one of the major risk factors leading to relapse from an exercise regimen.

Little research has been done to estimate the prevalence of activity-related musculoskeletal injuries in the general population. However, a 1998 study conducted by the National Center for Injury Prevention and the CDC surveyed a broad national sample of US adults and provided estimates of the injury prevalence associated with a few commonly prescribed activities[29] **(Table 39.4).** Those who are most at risk for developing musculoskeletal injuries are individuals who engage in high-intensity exercise. High-load mechanical forces resulting from overtraining or repetitive overuse can lead to bone microfractures, muscle and tendon fiber tears, and a localized connective tissue swelling/spasm cycle induced by ischemia. Exercising more frequently than 6 days per week increases the risk of injury, but so does infrequent exercise.[6] Additionally, longer durations of exercise increase injury risk, and certain activities carry their own risks (e.g., bicycling, boxing, and skiing).

The prevention of musculoskeletal injures commonly consists of a stretching program that is focused on improving flexibility. Although stretching programs have been shown to improve activities of daily living and increase flexibility, stretching before exercise has not been proven to prevent injury, and it may actually predispose an individual to injury by increasing muscle laxity.[30] Stretching after a 5-minute to 10-minute warmup and stretching after exercise have both been shown to reduce the incidence of injury. Stretching should be a slow, sustained movement to the first-perceived level of tightness, and it should last for 15 to 30 seconds.

Cardiovascular events

Cardiovascular side effects are much less common than musculoskeletal injuries during activity, but they are also much more serious and concerning. Common cardiovascular side effects include myocardial infarction, aortic dissection, silent ischemia in diabetics, and sudden death. It has been estimated that between 4% and 10%

of all myocardial infarctions are associated with physical activity.[31,32] The most common causes for sudden death, however, vary by age group. Among older athletes, the most common cause of sudden death coronary artery disease, which is an uncommon cause among younger athletes.[33,34]

A complete evaluation of cardiac risks should be included before every exercise prescription. Individuals with significant risk discovered from family history, personal history, or physical examination require further cardiac testing before starting an exercise program (see Box 39.1).

Disease-specific effects

Individuals with certain health problems may have other side-effect risks with exercise. For example, diabetics with peripheral neuropathy can be at risk for foot wounds and injuries incurred during running or biking, including falls related to their loss of sensation. Patients with retinopathy are at increased risk for vitreous hemorrhage and retinal detachment[35] and should therefore avoid high-impact or contact sports.

THE CHALLENGE OF BEHAVIOR MODIFICATION

Perhaps the most challenging aspect of medicine is achieving behavior changes in patients. Whether it involves discussing safe sexual practices with a teenager, convincing a 30 pack-year smoker to quit, or confronting an overweight, sedentary individual about the need to exercise, behavior modification can be a daunting task for physicians. Training and stature in the community place physicians in a unique position to provide comprehensive activity counseling. The goal of an individualized exercise prescription is to improve health while meeting the specific additional exercise needs of a particular person. It is important to assess not only how the patient health history affects the exercise prescription but also how a patient's interest level and his or her opportunities for exercise can be enhanced to limit barriers to achieving healthy levels of activity.

Several studies have assessed the effectiveness of health care providers for counseling patients to determine if these efforts result in behavior modification. These studies have shown that physician counseling in a primary care setting has been effective for short-term changes in physical activity level, but adherence to change is more difficult.[36] Two such studies are the Physician-based Assessment and Counseling for Exercise (PACE) study,[37] which was developed by the CDC, and the Industrywide Network for Social, Urban, and Rural Efforts INSURE study.[38] The PACE program used an "exercise assessment algorithm" to determine a patient's activity status, which is used to define the patient as a "precontemplator," a "contemplator," or an "active" person. The *precontemplator* (roughly 10% of patients) does not exercise nor do they intend to start in the near future. The *contemplator* (50% of patients) either has considered starting an exercise program or is doing so infrequently. The *active* individual (40% of patients) is near or already has achieved physical activity standards. Other assessments to determine cardiovascular risk status and level of motivation or goals may then be used. This information is useful for the determination of counseling strategies, the starting point, and the end point of the exercise prescription. Evidence suggests that the PACE program is practical and effective for increasing physical activity among patients who are counseled in the primary care setting. The INSURE project addressed the need to shift physician behavior toward an increased role in exercise counseling. This intervention showed that medical education seminars in combination with reimbursement for prevention counseling heightened physician involvement with counseling patients and resulted in an increased percentage of patients who subsequently started exercising.

Special populations
The athletic patient

Competitive athletes are a particularly unique subset of patients defined as individuals who "participate in an organized team or individual sport that requires competition against others as a central component, places a high premium on excellence and achievement, and requires some form of systematic (and usually intense) training."[39] Traditional sports training programs for athletes have focused on improving fitness through long-duration, submaximal training sessions, regardless of the individual sport-specific musculoskeletal and metabolic demands. However, most team sports demand short bursts of high-intensity activity interspersed with periods of inactivity. Many of the effects of training on fitness (including peak exercise capacity improvement, conditioning bradycardia, and blood lactate levels) are muscle specific as a result of intracellular enzymatic adaptations.[6,40] These principles can be used by health professionals to formulate a sport-specific high-intensity interval training prescription. High-intensity interval training involves short 2-minute to 5-minute bursts of sport-specific activity (e.g., skating, biking, swimming, sprinting) at near-maximal intensity (i.e., a Borg rating of 18 or 19, 90% to 100% of peak exercise capacity, or a target heart rate of 90% to 100% intensity by the Karvonen calculation) followed by an equal duration of rest.[41] High-intensity interval training is an effective means of providing additional improvement in cardiovascular fitness and performance for elite athletes.[41]

Two categories of formal exercise testing are commonly used to measure and track the cardiorespiratory fitness of athletes: maximal and submaximal exercise testing. These tests are generally quantitated as a peak exercise capacity, which measures the maximum volume of oxygen that the body can take in, deliver, and use in 1 minute. Maximal exercise testing is considered the gold standard for measuring peak exercise capacity, and it is defined by the plateau in oxygen consumption with further increase in workload.[42] Maximal testing requires an athlete to reach his or her maximal exercise capacity without being limited by fatigue or musculoskeletal problems, and it additionally requires trained staff and expensive equipment, including electrocardiogram monitoring and/or open-circuit spirometry.[43] As a result of these limitations, submaximal exercise testing is more widely used in a general practice setting. Submaximal testing determines the heart-rate response to steady-state exercise at a submaximal workload to predict a peak exercise capacity. It is limited by several assumptions, including the athlete's ability to maintain steady-state exercise, and by medications that alter the heart rate.[6]

Athletes are prone to overtraining with regard to both intensity level and frequency of training, and this can lead to overuse injury. Training more than 6 days per week has been shown to significantly increase injury.[44] The increase in physiologic capacity plateaus after training exceeds 3 days a week. Athletes who present with signs or symptoms of overtraining **(Box 39.4)** should be evaluated for signs of exercise dependence. The obligatory exerciser is a person who has a compulsion or addiction to exercise and who will continue to do so despite pain and injury caused by overtraining.[45] These are highly motivated people who often exercise several times a day and/or for extremely long durations. They may also display addictive and compulsive behaviors in other areas. The physician may help prevent overtraining injuries by formulating an exercise prescription that focuses on achieving appropriate amounts of recovery, mandatory days of rest, eating a healthy diet, and educating the patient about the body's needs for optimal performance **(Table 39.5)**.

The diabetic patient

Type II diabetes makes up approximately 90% to 95%[46] of all cases of diabetes, and it has recently been classified as an epidemic by the CDC.[47] Exercise has been shown to be an essential part of

Box 39.4: Signs and Symptoms of Overtraining

- Persistent fatigue
- Greater-than-normal muscle soreness
- Weight loss
- Decreased performance
- Frequent illness
- Poor wound and injury healing
- Sleep disturbance
- Decreased appetite
- Impaired concentration
- Moodiness: anxiety, apathy, or hostility
- Shin splints
- History of stress fractures
- Amenorrhea

From Harmon KG, Hawley CJ, Rubin A, Schoene RB: Phys Sportsmed 2003;31:25-31.

achieving good glycemic control. Exercise improves insulin sensitivity, lowers blood pressure, improves lipid profiles, decreases body fat, and decreases insulin requirements. To achieve these health benefits, the ACSM and the American Diabetes Association recommend a minimum expenditure of 1000 kcal/week during physical activity for patients with type II diabetes.[48] The management of type I diabetes during exercise is particularly challenging, requiring frequent monitoring of blood glucose and insulin adjustments; therefore, it is recommended that a physician with experience with managing type I diabetes be consulted before a patient with this condition starts an exercise program.

Before a patient with diabetes participates in an exercise program, a careful evaluation of the cardiovascular, renal, and visual systems is recommended as a result of the potential complications associated with exercise. Most patients with diabetes die from complications of atherosclerosis; therefore, a cardiovascular risk assessment is recommended for all diabetic patients before they begin to exercise.[49] Because diabetics often have silent ischemia, angina may not be a good predictor of cardiovascular complications, and a baseline electrocardiogram is recommended for all diabetic patients before they begin exercise. Any abnormalities should be assessed with stress testing and/or evaluated by a cardiologist. Both the American Diabetes Association and the American Heart Association recommend routine stress testing every 5 years after the age of 35 years for all type II diabetics. Diabetics with hypertension need good control of both conditions before they begin to exercise. A fundoscopic examination looking for microaneurysms, proliferative retinopathy, and cotton-wool spots is also recommended because a rapid lowering of blood sugar or a rapid increase in blood pressure can precipitate worsening retinopathy.[50]

Table 39.5   Exercise Prescription for Athletes

Maximizing Benefits	Minimizing Side Effects
Prescribe activities that use muscle groups specific to the sport	Mandate rest days to avoid fatigue-associated injuries
Use high-intensity interval training (HIT) as a sport-specific means of improving cardiorespiratory fitness	Vary workouts by intensity and mode
Educate on the benefits of rest to achieve maximal performance	Watch for sings of overtraining
	Avoid training in weather extremes

Table 39.6   Exercise Prescription for Diabetes

Maximizing Benefits	Minimizing Side Effects
Start at lower intensity (40% HRR) and progress to the recommended level (50%-70% HRR). Weightlift with light to moderate weights and high repetitions. Resistance exercise improves insulin sensitivity to about the same extent as aerobic exercise.	Avoid exercising when fasting blood glucose is > 250 with ketosis. Avoid activity with blood glucose > 300. Get a preparticipation ECG, eye exam, monofilament test for peripheral neuropathy, and creatinine level. Avoid weight-bearing activities in patients with insensitive feet (monofilament log is positive). Avoid high-intensity exercise and weight training if proliferative retinopathy is present. Eat some extra carbs prior to exercise if blood glucose < 100. Keep hydrated—early and often (2 full glasses 2 hours prior to exercise). Avoid exercise at the weather extremes. Always wear good shoes, and check your feet for blisters after exercise. Wear a diabetic bracelet or tag when exercising, or always exercise with a friend who is aware of your condition.

ECG, electrocardiogram; HRR, heart rate reserve.

The exercise prescription for diabetics should follow the general outline of mode, intensity, duration, and progression. Diabetics should start at a lower intensity (around 40% of the heart rate reserve) and progress to the recommended 50% to 70% of the heart rate reserve.[51] Resistance training should also be prescribed for diabetics because it has been shown to improve insulin sensitivity to roughly the same extent as aerobic exercise.[52] Weight loss is not necessary to benefit from the effects of physical activity on glucose tolerance and insulin clearance rates.[20] Exercise should be avoided on days when the fasting blood glucose is greater than 250 mg/dL or when ketosis is present **(Table 39.6)**.

The obese patient

The exercise prescription for the obese should emphasize total energy expenditure and the prevention of weight gain. Although a return to ideal body weight would be optimal, regardless of weight loss, meeting the recommendations for exercise will improve the health-related benefits. Modest reductions in weight loss have been associated with significant improvements in hypertension and lipid profiles in the obese.[53] Exercise improves body composition by replacing fat with muscle, especially through resistance training. To maintain weight loss, a significant amount of kilocalories must be expended per week (2500 to 2800 kcal), which generally translates into 45 to 90 minutes of moderate-intensity physical activity per session.

Table 39.7   Exercise Prescription for Obesity

Maximizing Benefits	Minimizing Side Effects
Start at a intensity and duration comfortable for the patient. Manipulate intensity and duration to achieve a high total weekly energy expenditure > 2000 kcal. Exercise combined with diet control is more effective at maintaining weight loss than diet alone.	Test for diabetes and screen for cardiovascular side effects. Alternate between weight-bearing and non—weight-bearing activities. Avoid outdoor exercise during hot weather. Avoid exercise that place strain on the back (e.g., push-ups, squats, sit-ups).

Table 39.8 Exercise Prescription for Hypertension

Maximizing Benefits	Minimizing Side Effects
A limited increase in aerobic activity has significant benefits in preventing and treating hypertension. Daily exercise can aid in optimizing control of hypertension for patients already on antihypertensives. Resistance training is a recommended secondary exercise mode with lower weights, higher repetitions, and techniques that limit Valsalva.	Avoid exercise if the resting blood pressure is > 200/110. Screen for cardiovascular disease. Beware of dehydration if on diuretics. Beware of orthostasis if on beta blockers.

Many of the side effects of exercise for the overweight or obese patient result from the increased health risks associated with obesity. Obese patients are more likely to suffer from arthritis, cardiovascular disease, and diabetes, and they therefore may be subject to the risks of exercise with these conditions.[54] In addition, obese patients have an increased risk of musculoskeletal injury, low back pain, and hyperthermia during exercise.[6,55] Initially, the prescribed mode, intensity, and duration may need to begin below the recommendations for health benefits and weight loss to avoid side effects. They can then progress over the course of several weeks to achieve energy expenditure goals **(Table 39.7)**.

The hypertensive patient

The Framingham Heart Study has estimated that 75% of hypertension in men and 65% of hypertension in women is directly attributable to excess body weight.[56] For patients in the prehypertensive range (systolic blood pressure, 120 to 139 mm Hg; diastolic blood pressure, 80 to 89 mm Hg), lifestyle management including an exercise prescription is the recommended initial treatment. Exercise prescriptions should follow the same general outline as the standard population, with added emphasis on a frequency of most or all days of the week to gain the benefit of acute blood pressure lowering. Exercising at intensities in the moderate range (40% to 70% of the heart rate reserve) appears to reduce blood pressure as much as exercise at higher intensities.[57] Exercise should also be added to patients with a systolic blood pressure in the higher ranges (>160 mm Hg) only after medication management has been initiated. Exercise should be avoided if the resting blood pressure exceeds 220/100 mm Hg.

Although resistance training should not be used as a primary exercise mode in hypertensive patients, contrary to popular belief, weight training is recommended as an adjunct exercise for these individuals. Resistance should be low, involve a great number of repetitions, and use techniques that minimize the Valsalva maneuver to maximize benefits and minimize blood pressure elevations during exercise[58] **(Table 39.8)**.

CONCLUSION

Evidence-based physical activity counseling must become an integral component of routine patient care in the primary care setting to limit health risks of an increasingly sedentary population and to fully use exercise as an effective treatment for a number of chronic medical problems. Patients should be informed of the significant health benefits derived from moderate-intensity exercise and

should be involved in formulating an individualized exercise program. Translating these guidelines into practice may be the most effective approach to improving our nation's health.

REFERENCES

1. Hahn RA, Teutsch SM, Rothenberg RB, et al: Excess deaths from nine chronic diseases in the United States, 1986. JAMA 1990;264:2654-2659.
2. American Heart Association: Heart Disease and Stroke Statistics—2005 Update. Dallas, American Heart Association, 2005.
3. Pate RR, Pratt M, Blair SN, et al: Physical activity and public health: a recommendation from the Centers for Disease Control and Prevention and the American College of Sports Medicine. JAMA 1995;273:402-407.
4. US Department of Health and Human Services: Physical Activity and Health: A Report of the Surgeon General. Atlanta: US Department of Health and Human Services, Centers for Disease Control and Prevention, National Center for Chronic Disease Prevention and Health Promotion, 1996.
5. Jakicic JM, Clark K, Coleman E, et al: American College of Sports Medicine position stand. Appropriate intervention strategies for weight loss and prevention of weight regain for adults. Med Sci Sports Exerc 2001;33:2145-2156.
6. Whaley MH, Brubaker PH, Otto RM, et al, for the American College of Sports Medicine: ACSM's Guidelines for Exercise Testing and Prescription, 7th ed. Philadelphia, Lippincott Williams & Wilkins, 2006, p 7.
7. Institute of Medicine: Dietary reference intakes for energy, carbohydrate, fiber, fat, fatty acids, cholesterol, protein, and amino acids. Washington, DC: National Academies Press, 2002.
8. Volk B, Holman JR: Exercise: how much is enough for cardiovascular health? Consultant 2006;46(6):589-593.
9. Manson JE, Greenland P, LaCroix AZ, et al: Walking compared with vigorous exercise for the prevention of cardiovascular events in women. N Engl J Med 2002;347:716-725.
10. Lee IM, Rexrode KM, Cook NR, et al: Physical activity and coronary heart disease in women: is "no pain, no gain" passé? JAMA 2001;285:1447-1454.
11. Manson JE, Nathan DM, Krolewski AS, et al: A prospective study of exercise and incidence of diabetes among US male physicians. JAMA 1992;268:63-67.
12. Sesso HD, Paffenberg RS Jr, Lee IM: Physical activity and coronary heart disease in men: the Harvard Alumni Health Study. Circulation 2000;102:975-980.
13. Manson JE, Hu FB, Rich-Edwards JW, et al: A prospective study of walking as compared with vigorous exercise in the prevention of coronary heart disease in women. N Engl J Med 1999;341:650-658.
14. Slattery ML, Jacobs DR Jr, Nichamn MZ: Leisure time physical activity and coronary heart disease death. The US Railroad Study. Circulation 1989;79:304-311.
15. LaCroix AZ, Leville SG, Hecht JA, et al: Does walking decrease the risk of cardiovascular disease hospitalizations and death in older adults? J Am Geriatr Soc 1996;44:113-120.
16. Klem ML, Wing RR, McGuire MT, et al: A descriptive study of individuals successful at long-term maintenance of substantial weight loss. Am J Clin Nutr 1997;66:239-246.
17. Irwin ML, Yasui Y, Ulrich CM, et al: Effect of exercise on total and intra-abdominal body fat in postmenopausal women: a randomized trial. JAMA 2003;289:323-330.
18. Debusk RF, Stenestrand U, Sheehan M, et al: Training effects of long versus short bouts of exercise in healthy subjects. Am J Cardiol 1990;65:1010-1013.
19. Fogelholm M, Kukkonen-Harjula K, Nenonen A, et al: Effects of walking training on weight maintenance after a very-low-energy diet in premenopausal obese women. Arch Intern Med 2000;160:2177-2184.
20. Chakravarthy MV, Booth FW: Hot Topics: Exercise. Philadelphia, Hanley & Belfus, 2003.
21. Saris WH, Blair SN, VanBook MA, et al: How much physical activity is enough to prevent unhealthy weight gain? Outcomes of the IASO 1st Stock Conference and consensus statement. Obes Rev 2003;4:101-114.
22. Borg G. An Introduction to Borg's RPE-Scale. Ithaca, NY, Mouvement Publications, 1985.
23. Pollock ML, Gaesser GA, Butcher JD: The recommended quality and quantity of exercise for developing and maintaining cardiorespiratory and muscular fitness, and flexibility in healthy adults. Med Sci Sports Exerc 1998;30:975-991.
24. Murphy MH, Hardman AE: Training effect of short and long bouts of brisk walking in sedentary women. Med Sci Sports Exerc 1998;30:152-157.
25. Jakicic JM, Wung RR, Butler BA, et al: Prescribing exercise in multiple short bouts versus one continuous bout: effects on adherence; CR fitness and weight loss in overweight women. Int J Obes Relat Metab Disord 1995;19:893-901.
26. Tabata I, Nishimura K, Kouzaki M, et al: Effects of moderate-intensity endurance and high-intensity intermittent training on anaerobic capacity and VO_2 max. Med Sci Sports Exerc 1996;28:1327-1330.
27. Gettman LR, Pollock ML, Durstine JL, et al: Physiological responses of men to 1, 3, and 5 day per week training programs. Res Q 1976;47:638-646.
28. Hootman JM: The epidemiology of physical activity-related musculoskeletal injuries. Available at www.pitt.edu/~super1/lecture/cdc0341/001.htm. Accessed July 19, 2007.
29. Powell KE, Heath GW, Kresnow MJ, et al: Injury rates from walking, gardening, weightlifting, outdoor bicycling, and aerobics. Med Sci Sport Exerc 1998;30(8):1246-1249.

30. Pope RP, Herbert RD, Kirwan JD, Graham BJ: A randomized trial of preexercise stretching for prevention of lower-limb injury. Med Sci Sports Exerc 2000;32(2):271-277.
31. Giri S, Thompson PD, Kiernan FJ, et al: Clinical and angiographic characteristics of exertion-related acute myocardial infarction. JAMA 1999;282(18):1731-1736.
32. Mittleman MA, Maclure M, Tofler GH, et al: Triggering of acute myocardial infarction by heavy exertion: protection against triggering by regular exercise. N Engl J Med 1993;329(23)1677-1683.
33. Maron BJ: Sudden death in young athletes. N Engl J Med 2003;349:1064-1075.
34. Burke AP, Farb A, Virmar R, et al: Sports-related and non-sports-related sudden cardiac death in young adults. Am Heart J 1991;121:568-575.
35. Devlin JT, Ruderman N: Diabetes and exercise: the risk-benefit profile revisited. In Ruderman N, Devlin JT, Schneider SH, Krisra A (eds): Handbook of Exercise in Diabetes. Alexandria, VA, American Diabetes Association, 2002.
36. Eakin EG, Glasgow RE, Riley KM: Review of primary care-based physical activity intervention studies: effectiveness and implications for practice and future research. J Fam Pract 2000;49(2):158-168.
37. Centers for Disease Control and Prevention: Project PACE: Physician's Manual: Physician-Based Assessment and Counseling for Exercise. Atlanta, Centers for Disease Control and Prevention, 1992.
38. Logsdon DN, Lazaro CM, Meier RV: The feasibility of behavioral risk reduction in primary medical care. Am J Prev Med 1989;5:249-256.
39. Maron BJ, Zipes DP, et al: 36th Bethesda Conference eligibility recommendations for competitive athletes with cardiovascular abnormalities. J Am Coll Cardiol 2005;45:1312-1375.
40. Henriksson J, Reitman JS: Time course of changes in human skeletal muscle succinate dehydrogenase and cytochrome oxidase activities and maximal oxygen uptake with physical activity and inactivity. Acta Physiol Scand 1977;99:91-97.
41. Laursen PB, Jenkins DG: The scientific basis for high-intensity interval training: optimising training programmes and maximising performance in highly trained endurance athletes. Sports Med 2002;32:53-73.
42. McArdle WD, Katch FI, Katch VL. Exercise Physiology: Energy, Nutrition, and Human Performance, 2nd ed. Philadelphia, Lea & Febiger, 1990.
43. Noonan V, Dean E: Submaximal exercise testing: clinical application and interpretation. Phys Ther 2000;80:782-807.
44. American College of Sports Medicine Position Stand. The recommended quantity and quality of exercise for developing and maintaining cardiorespiratory and muscular fitness, and flexibility in healthy adults. Med Sci Sports Exerc 1998;30:975-991.
45. Yates A. Compulsive Exercise and Eating Disorders: Toward an Integrated Theory of Activity. New York, Brunner/Mazel, 1991.
46. Centers for Disease Control and Prevention: National Diabetes Fact Sheet: General Information and National Estimates on Diabetes in the United States, 2005. Atlanta, GA, US Department of Health and Human Services, Centers for Disease Control and Prevention, 2005.
47. Mokdad AH, Bowman BA, Ford ES, et al: The continuing epidemics of obesity and diabetes in the United States. JAMA 2001;286:1195-1200.
48. American College of Sports Medicine Position Stand. Exercise and type 2 diabetes. Med Sci Sports Exerc 2000;32(7):1345-1360.
49. Beckman JA, Creager MA, Libby P: Diabetes and atherosclerosis: epidemiology, pathophysiology, and management. JAMA 2002;287:2570-2581.
50. Aiello LM, Cavakkerano J, Aiello LP, et al: Retinopathy. In Ruderman NB, Devlin JT (eds): The Health Professional's Guide to Diabetes and Exercise. Alexandria, American Diabetes Association, 1995, pp 143-152.
51. American Diabetes Association Position Statement. Standards of medical care in diabetes–2006. Diabetes Care 2006;29:S4-S42.
52. Ivy JL: Role of exercise training in the prevention and treatment of insulin resistance and non-insulin-dependent diabetes mellitus. Sports Med 1997;24:321-336.
53. American College of Sports Medicine Position Stand: Appropriate intervention strategies for weight loss and prevention of weight regain for adults. Med Sci Sports Exerc 2001;33:2145-2152.
54. Field AE, Coakley EH, Must A, et al: Impact of overweight on the risk of developing common chronic diseases during a 10-year period. Arch Intern Med 2001;161: 1581-1586.
55. Haymes EM, McCormick RJ, Buskirk ER: Heat tolerance of exercising lean and obese prepubertal boys. J Appl Physiol 1975;39:457-461.
56. Garrison RJ, Kanel WB, Stokes J 3rd, et al: Incidence and precursors of HTN in young adults: the Framingham Offspring Study. Prev Med 1987;16:235-251.
57. Fagard R: Exercise characteristics and the blood pressure response to dynamic physical training. Med Sci Sports Exerc 2001;33:S484-S492.
58. American College of Sports Medicine Position Stand: Exercise and hypertension. Med Sci Sports Exerc 2004;36:533-553.

CHAPTER 40

Cardiovascular Testing

David A. Djuric, MD, and Francis G. O'Connor, MD, MPH

KEY POINTS

- Treadmill stress testing is a safe procedure when done properly, with the risk of death during or immediately after a test estimated at less than 0.01%.[1]
- Clinical guidelines suggest that physicians perform 50 exercise stress tests to qualify for privileges and that they perform at least 25 tests per year to maintain clinical competency.[3]
- The Bruce protocol is the most commonly used protocol for clinical exercise testing.[3]
- When performed on the appropriate patient and coupled with clinical information, the exercise stress test has an estimated 50% sensitivity and 90% specificity for the detection of obstructive coronary artery disease.[4]
- There is general consensus and strong evidence that exercise testing is justified in adults with an intermediate pretest probability of disease.

INTRODUCTION

Clinical exercise testing is defined as a cardiovascular stress test that uses either treadmill or bicycle exercise in conjunction with electrocardiographic and blood-pressure monitoring. The American College of Cardiology and the American Heart Association (ACC/AHA) Task Force on Practice Guidelines (Committee on Exercise Testing) have published guidelines (most recently updated in 2002) about the performance and interpretation of clinical exercise stress testing. As with any procedure, several factors must be considered when determining the appropriateness of an exercise test and its usefulness for predicting the outcome of both symptomatic and asymptomatic patients: (1) the expertise of the professional and technical staff performing and interpreting the study; (2) the sensitivity, specificity, and accuracy of the chosen technique; (3) the cost/benefit analysis when comparing the accuracy of this technique versus a more expensive imaging test; (4) how the results of this test will affect clinical decision making; and (5) the potential benefit of patient reassurance.[1]

Exercise stress testing is widely used in primary care settings to assess physical fitness, determine functional capacity, diagnose cardiac disease, reassess known cardiac disease, develop an exercise prescription, and assist with cardiac rehabilitation. When clinical exercise testing is used in an appropriate patient population, the procedure is exceptionally safe; however, myocardial infarction and death can occur in as many as 1 in 2500 tests.[2] Therefore, physicians must use sound clinical judgment when referring patients for exercise testing or conducting stress testing themselves. Clinical guidelines suggest that physicians perform 50 exercise stress tests to qualify for privileges and that they perform at least 25 tests per year to maintain clinical competency[3] **(Box 40.1).**

INDICATIONS AND CONTRAINDICATIONS

Exercise testing may be used for diagnostic, prognostic, or therapeutic indications. The majority of exercise testing is used for diagnostic purposes to evaluate adults with known or suspected ischemic heart disease. The ACC/AHA Task Force on Practice Guidelines (Committee on Exercise Testing) has identified a classification system for common indications for exercise stress testing:

> Class I: general consensus/evidence that testing is justified
> Class II: divergence of opinion on utility (IIa, in favor; IIb, less evidence)
> Class III: agreement that testing is not warranted[1]

Box 40.2 outlines the current recommendations from the ACC/AHA Task Force pertaining to the diagnosis of obstructive coronary artery disease. In this capacity, the exercise test is most useful for patients with an intermediate pretest probability of obstructive coronary artery disease based on the patient's age, gender, and symptoms **(Table 40.1).** As indicated in Table 40.1, the test is most appropriate for patients who are experiencing symptoms, from the younger patient who has classic angina symptoms to middle-aged and elderly patients with atypical angina symptoms to elderly patients with seemingly noncardiac chest pain. However, testing may be helpful for evaluating asymptomatic patients who have multiple risk factors that indicate a moderate risk of an adverse cardiac event within 5 years. It may be used diagnostically for patients who are involved in high-risk occupations (e.g., pilots, police officers). Additionally, testing may be indicated for patients with sedentary lifestyles who wish to start a vigorous exercise program. It is generally not appropriate to use exercise testing as a diagnostic tool for patients with a high pretest probability of disease; however, exercise testing may be used for prognostic purposes in such cases. Although exercise testing is typically the initial diagnostic test of choice regardless of gender, it is worth

Box 40.1: Required Equipment for Stress Testing

- Exercise device: treadmill or bicycle ergometer
- Electrocardiogram (ECG) monitor
- ECG recorder
- ECG leads
- ECG pads
- ECG paper
- Razor
- Blood-pressure cuff
- Stethoscope
- Defibrillator
- Resuscitative medications

Box 40.2: Exercise Testing to Diagnose Obstructive Coronary Artery Disease

Class I
Adult patients (including those with complete right bundle-branch block or less than 1 mm of resting ST depression) with an intermediate pretest probability of coronary artery disease on the basis of gender, age, and symptoms (specific exceptions are noted under Classes II and III)

Class IIa
Patients with vasospastic angina

Class IIb
1. Patients with a high pretest probability of coronary artery disease by age, symptoms, and gender
2. Patients with a low pretest probability of coronary artery disease by age, symptoms, and gender
3. Patients with less than 1 mm of baseline ST depression and who are taking digoxin
4. Patients with electrocardiographic criteria for left ventricular hypertrophy and less than 1 mm of baseline ST depression.

Class III
1. Patients with the following baseline electrocardiogram abnormalities:
   - Pre-excitation (Wolff–Parkinson–White) syndrome
   - Electronically paced ventricular rhythm
   - More than 1 mm of resting ST depression
   - Complete left bundle-branch block
2. Patients with a documented myocardial infarction or prior coronary angiography demonstrating significant disease have an established diagnosis of coronary artery disease; however, ischemia and the subsequent risk of cardiac event can be determined by testing

From Gibbons RJ, Balady GJ, Bricker JT, et al: ACC/AHA 2002 guideline update for exercise testing: a report of the American College of Cardiology/American Heart Association Task Force on Practice Guidelines (Committee on Exercise Testing). 2002. American College of Cardiology (Web site). Available at www.acc.org/clinical/guidelines/exercise/dirindex.htm.

noting that, as a diagnostic tool, it has been shown to be less accurate among women as a result of a higher percentage of false-positive results (10% difference in diagnostic accuracy) (LOE: meta-analysis).[1]

The second most common use for exercise testing is for risk stratification and the prognosis of patients with known coronary artery disease **(Box 40.3).** In these patients, exercise testing is considered but one component of the evaluation. The results of the test must be used in conjunction with data collected from the clinical examination, laboratory tests, and imaging studies. The patient's risk is determined by his or her risk factors, symptoms, functional capability, and evidence and severity of ischemic changes on the exercise test. The size of the coronary artery lesion is typically proportional to the degree of ST segment depression, the number of involved ECG leads, and the duration of depression in recovery. However, unlike the resting ECG, tracings taken during stress testing cannot localize the at-risk areas on the basis of the involved leads (LOE: B).[4] The most commonly used prognostic tool is the Duke Treadmill Score (DTS), which is discussed later in this chapter.

Exercise testing is additionally used for prognostic assessment in post–myocardial infarction patients **(Box 40.4).** Patients typically undergo a submaximal test 4 to 6 days after the myocardial infarction for prognostic assessment, activity prescription, and the evaluation of medical therapy. If not conducted at 4 to 6 days, a symptom-limited test may be performed at about 2 to 3 weeks. These tests additionally provide guidance for early cardiac

rehabilitation and assess the patient's ability to perform daily activities. Finally, the exercise test is repeated at 3 to 6 weeks for a repeat prognostic assessment if the initial test was submaximal.

Exercise testing can also be useful for assessing functional capacity. For the sports medicine physician, this can be an

Table 40.1 Pretest Probability of Coronary Artery Disease by Age, Gender, and Symptoms

Age (y)	Gender	Typical/Definite Angina Pectoris	Atypical/Probable Angina Pectoris	Nonanginal Chest Pain	Asymptomatic
30-39	Men	Intermediate	Intermediate	Low	Very low
	Women	Intermediate	Very low	Very low	Very low
40-49	Men	High	Intermediate	Intermediate	Low
	Women	Intermediate	Low	Very low	Very low
50-59	Men	High	Intermediate	Intermediate	Low
	Women	Intermediate	Intermediate	Low	Very low
60-69	Men	High	Intermediate	Intermediate	Low
	Women	High	Intermediate	Intermediate	Low

From Gibbons RJ, Balady GJ, Bricker JT, et al: ACC/AHA 2002 guideline update for exercise testing: a report of the American College of Cardiology/American Heart Association Task Force on Practice Guidelines (Committee on Exercise Testing). 2002. American College of Cardiology (Web site). Available at www.acc.org/clinical/guidelines/exercise/dirindex.htm. Based on Diamond GA, Forrester JS: N Engl J Med 1979;300:1350-1358.

Box 40.3: Risk Assessment and Prognosis in Patients with Symptoms or a Prior History of Coronary Artery Disease

Class I

1. Patients undergoing initial evaluation with suspected or known coronary artery disease, including those with complete right bundle-branch block or less than 1 mm of resting ST depression (specific exceptions are noted under Class IIb)

2. Patients with suspected or known coronary artery disease that has been previously evaluated and who are now presenting with a significant change in clinical status

3. Low-risk unstable angina patients 8 to 12 hours after presentation who have been free of active ischemic or heart failure symptoms

4. Intermediate-risk unstable angina patients 2 to 3 days after presentation who have been free of active ischemic or heart failure symptoms

Class IIa

Intermediate-risk unstable angina patients who have initial cardiac markers that are normal, a repeat electrocardiogram without significant change, cardiac markers 6 to 12 hours after the onset of symptoms that are normal, and no other evidence of ischemia during observation

Class IIb

1. Patients with the following resting ECG abnormalities:

   - Pre-excitation (Wolff–Parkinson–White) syndrome
   - Electronically paced ventricular rhythm
   - 1 mm or more of resting ST depression
   - Complete left bundle-branch block or any interventricular conduction defect with a QRS duration of more than 120 msec

2. Patients with a stable clinical course who undergo periodic monitoring to guide treatment

Class III

1. Patients with a severe comorbidity that is likely to limit life expectancy and/or their candidacy for revascularization

2. High-risk unstable angina patients

From Gibbons RJ, Balady GJ, Bricker JT, et al: ACC/AHA 2002 guideline update for exercise testing: a report of the American College of Cardiology/American Heart Association Task Force on Practice Guidelines (Committee on Exercise Testing). 2002. American College of Cardiology (Web site). Available at www.acc.org/clinical/guidelines/exercise/dirindex.htm.

Box 40.4: After Myocardial Infarction

Class I

1. Before discharge for prognostic assessment, activity prescription, evaluation of medical therapy (submaximal at about 4 to 76 days; exceptions are noted under Classes IIb and III)

2. Early after discharge for prognostic assessment, activity prescription, evaluation of medical therapy, and cardiac rehabilitation if the predischarge exercise test was not done (symptom limited, about 14 to 21 days; exceptions are noted under Classes IIb and III)

3. Late after discharge for prognostic assessment, activity prescription, evaluation of medical therapy, and cardiac rehabilitation if the early exercise test was submaximal (symptom limited, about 3 to 6 weeks; exceptions are noted under Classes IIb and III)

Class IIa

After discharge for activity counseling and/or exercise training as part of cardiac rehabilitation for patients who have undergone coronary revascularization

Class IIb

- Patients with the following ECG abnormalities:
- Complete left bundle-branch block
- Pre-excitation syndrome
- Left ventricular hypertrophy
- Digoxin therapy
- More than 1 mm of resting ST-segment depression
- Electronically paced ventricular rhythm
- Periodic monitoring for patients who continue to participate in exercise training or cardiac rehabilitation

Class III

1. Severe comorbidity that is likely to limit life expectancy and/or candidacy for revascularization

2. At any time to evaluate patients with acute myocardial infarction who have uncompensated congestive heart failure, cardiac arrhythmia, or noncardiac conditions that severely limit their ability to exercise

3. Before discharge to evaluate patients who have already been selected for or who have undergone cardiac catheterization (Although a stress test may be useful before or after catheterization to evaluate or identify ischemia in the distribution of a coronary lesion of borderline severity, stress imaging tests are recommended.)

From Gibbons RJ, Balady GJ, Bricker JT, et al: ACC/AHA 2002 guideline update for exercise testing: a report of the American College of Cardiology/American Heart Association Task Force on Practice Guidelines (Committee on Exercise Testing). 2002. American College of Cardiology (Web site). Available at www.acc.org/clinical/guidelines/exercise/dirindex.htm.

important tool to aid in the development of an exercise prescription or for activity counseling. These activities may include return-to-work evaluations, disability assessments, and prognosis assessments. Studies have shown that, even among patients without known coronary artery disease, low levels of aerobic fitness are an independent risk factor for all-cause and cardiovascular mortality (LOE: A).[5,6] One such study showed that the highest all-cause and cardiovascular mortality was seen among men with an exercise capacity of less than 4.4 METs, whereas those who averaged greater than 9.2 METs had no deaths during the study period (LOE: A).[7] A second study of 3679 men with coronary artery disease (CAD) referred for exercise testing showed that those with an exercise capacity of less than 4.9 METs had a relative risk of death of 4.1 as compared with those with a capacity of 10.7 METs during an average follow-up of 6.2 years (LOE: A).[8] The National Exercise and Heart Disease Project that followed patients after myocardial infarction showed that, for every 1 MET increase in exercise capability, there was a 10% decrease in all-cause mortality over a 19-year period, regardless of the study group.[9] Further specific recommendations from the ACC/AHA Task Force are referenced in the guidelines update for exercise testing.[1]

The ACC/AHA guidelines outline the absolute and relative contraindications to exercise testing (Box 40.5). These guidelines are designed to ensure the safety of the patient, and they are the responsibility of the physician performing the pretest clearance.

Box 40.5: Contraindications to Exercise Testing

Absolute
- Acute myocardial infarction (within 2 days)
- High-risk unstable angina
- Uncontrolled cardiac arrhythmias causing symptoms or hemodynamic compromise
- Severe symptomatic aortic stenosis
- Uncontrolled symptomatic heart failure
- Acute pulmonary embolus or pulmonary infarction
- Acute myocarditis or pericarditis
- Acute aortic dissection

Relative
- Left main coronary stenosis
- Moderate stenotic valvular heart disease
- Electrolyte abnormalities
- Severe arterial hypertension (systolic blood pressure >200 mm Hg or diastolic blood pressure >110 mm Hg)
- Tachyarrhythmias or bradyarrhythmias
- Hypertrophic cardiomyopathy and other forms of outflow tract obstruction
- Mental or physical impairment leading to inability to exercise adequately
- High-degree atrioventricular block

From Gibbons RJ, Balady GJ, Bricker JT, et al: ACC/AHA 2002 guideline update for exercise testing: a report of the American College of Cardiology/American Heart Association Task Force on Practice Guidelines (Committee on Exercise Testing). 2002. American College of Cardiology (Web site). Available at www.acc.org/clinical/guidelines/exercise/dirindex.htm.

EVALUATION

Pretest procedure

An overview of exercise treadmill testing is presented in **Box 40.6.** The reader is encouraged to reference this overview while reading the following sections detailing test performance.

The physician has a number of responsibilities during exercise testing. Before the procedure, the physician is responsible for the pretest evaluation, clearance, and selection of the proper protocol. During the test, the physician must ensure proper patient preparation, perform the test, and terminate it at the appropriate time. After the test, the physician must help the patient to recover and then interpret the test results. Patient evaluation and clearance starts with a thorough history and physical that focus especially on any cardiovascular symptoms or past medical problems. This history is especially important for determining whether the patient has any contraindications for undergoing the exercise test. Chest pain symptoms must be fully elucidated and then characterized as angina, atypical angina, or atypical chest pain. The chest pain history should clarify whether the patient is experiencing unstable angina. The physician determines whether there is a history of exercise-induced syncope or presyncope or if the patient has any symptoms that are consistent with viral myocarditis, pericarditis, or unstable congestive heart failure. Any risk factors for coronary artery disease **(Table 40.2)** are also noted. The physician should review the results of any previous cardiac testing and discuss any problems with previous tests.

Additionally, the physician should obtain a thorough medication history and discuss any orthopedic problems that may affect ambulation or make some testing protocols difficult. It is essential to have an understanding of the patient's exercise history and capabilities to properly select the testing protocol. Finally, the physician should ask about any significant family history of cardiac, pulmonary, or metabolic disease and about any family history of sudden death.

The physician should conduct a thorough physical examination, paying special attention to any concerning findings in the patient's history and cardiopulmonary examination. In particular, the physician should document bilateral blood pressure measurements, the pulse pressure, the carotid upstroke evaluation, carotid bruits, and simultaneous radial–femoral pulses. Cardiopulmonary auscultation should include attention to the second heart sound and a determination of the presence of any murmurs, gallops, rubs, or clicks. Murmurs that are suggestive of hypertrophic cardiomyopathy or aortic stenosis are of particular concern. The examination should exclude signs of decompensated congestive heart failure.

Before administering the test, the physician must obtain informed consent from the patient. Consent forms vary among institutions; however, all must give the patient enough information to ensure that he or she understands the purpose, procedure, risks, benefits, and alternatives to the testing. The consent form should also outline the confidentiality of the patient information as described in the Health Insurance Portability and Accountability Act of 1996.

Before the test, the patient is given preliminary instructions about the procedure. The patient should be instructed to eat little or no food for at least 2 to 3 hours before the test and to ensure adequate fluid intake over the day leading up to the test. To be well rested for the test, the patient should be advised to avoid strenuous exercise on the day of the test. The patient should wear loose-fitting, nonrestrictive clothing and running shoes to allow for ease of movement. If the test is performed on an outpatient basis, the patient should be asked to consider bringing someone to drive him or her from the appointment in the event that the patient is too tired to drive after the test. Specific instructions should be given regarding antihypertensive or antianginal medications.

If the test is being performed for diagnostic purposes, the patient may need to taper from those medications to ensure that they do not alter the sensitivity of ischemic ECG changes. If the test is being performed for functional purposes, there is likely no need to discontinue these medications because the exercise response should mimic the responses during regular exercise. On the basis of the information obtained during the history and physical and the purpose of the test itself, an appropriate exercise protocol will be selected.

Conducting the test

On arrival, the physician or technician conducts an equipment safety check to ensure that the system is in good working order. If the patient's history was obtained before the appointment for the exercise test, the physician should again explore with the patient any changes in chest pain symptoms to ensure that any atypical chest pain has not progressed to unstable angina between the initial evaluation and the test itself. Any findings on the pretest assessment should be confirmed and reassessed. Verify that the informed consent form has been signed, and give the patient an additional opportunity to ask any questions. The patient is then given a demonstration of the equipment and shown appropriate treadmill walking. The physician discusses the indications for test termination as well **(Box 40.7).**

The patient's skin is prepped for ECG lead placement, which includes shaving appropriate locations and removing any lotions, oils, or dead skin cells. ECG leads are placed as shown in **Figure 40.1,** and the electrodes are placed in the standard positions for obtaining a routine 12-lead ECG, except the limb leads are

Box 40.6: Exercise Treadmill Testing

Procedure Pretest Checklist
- Perform equipment and safety check.
- Obtain informed consent.
- Complete pretest history and physical examination.
- Enter patient information into the exercise test system.
- Prepare the skin and place the electrodes.
- Connect the exercise testing monitor to the electrodes.
- Secure the blood-pressure cuff on the appropriate arm.
- Obtain a resting blood-pressure reading and an electrocardiogram (ECG) with the patient in a supine position.
- Review the resting 12-lead ECG for any recent changes.
- Obtain a blood-pressure reading and an ECG with the patient standing.
- Provide instructions and demonstrate the appropriate use of the treadmill:
    - Instruct patient to use the handrails only for balance and to not grip them tightly.
    - Encourage the patient to maintain an upright position and to take long strides.
    - Remind the patient that his or her blood pressure will be checked during each stage.
    - Remind the patient to use the Borg scale.
- Complete any other tests (e.g., fingerstick glucose, pulse oximetry).
- Answer the patient's final questions before beginning the testing.

Conducting the Procedure
- Assist the patient onto the testing equipment (i.e., treadmill or bicycle).
- Provide a warmup period to ensure the patient's comfort with the apparatus.
- When the patient is comfortable, initiate the testing protocol.
- Ensure continuous monitoring of the heart rate, blood pressure, and ECG as well as of symptoms.
- Record the ECG during the last 15 seconds of each stage or each 2-minute period if using a ramp protocol.
- Record the heart rate during the last 5 seconds of each stage or each 2-minute period if using a ramp protocol.
- Record the blood pressure during the last 45 seconds of each stage or each 2-minute period if using a ramp protocol.

- Record any symptoms as they occur.
- Terminate the exercise portion of the test as appropriate.
- Record the patient's ECG immediately after exercise.
- Place the patient in a supine position while continuing monitoring.
- Auscultate the patient for cardiovascular changes associated with ischemia.
- Record an ECG at 1 minute into and every 2 minutes during recovery.
- Record the heart rate every minute during recovery.
- Record the blood pressure immediately after exercise and then every 2 minutes during recovery.
- Terminate the test after any ECG changes have returned to baseline and when the heart rate and blood pressure are stable.

Physician Responsibilities/Required Knowledge
- Appropriate indications for exercise testing
- Alternative physiologic cardiovascular tests
- Appropriate contraindications, risks, and risk assessment for testing
- Recognize and treat complications of exercise testing
- Competence in basic and advanced cardiac life support
- Various exercise protocols and the indications for each
- Basic exercise physiology
- Recognize and treat serious cardiac arrhythmias
- Cardiovascular medications and their effects on the hemodynamic response to exercise
- Principles and details of exercise testing
- End points of exercise testing and indications for terminating the exercise test
- Specificity, sensitivity, and diagnostic accuracy of exercise testing
- How to apply Bayes' theorem to interpret test results
- Normal ECG changes in response to exercise
- Conditions and circumstances that can lead to false-positive, indeterminate, or false-negative test results
- Prognostic value of exercise testing
- Alternative or supplementary diagnostic procedures to exercise testing and when they should be used
- The concept of metabolic equivalent and the estimation of exercise intensity

placed in modified locations to minimize the effects of movement. The arm leads are placed on the respective lateral front shoulders on the anterior deltoids, and the leg leads are placed on the respective upper abdominal quadrants. Alternatively, the leg leads can be placed with the right-leg electrode over the lower lumbar spine and the left-leg electrode placed directly below the umbilicus. An appropriately sized blood pressure cuff is placed firmly on the patient's arm for obtaining serial blood pressures.

Baseline measurements are now collected. The patient is instructed to lie recumbent on his or her back while a supine ECG, blood pressure, and heart rate are obtained. Next, the patient stands while an ECG, blood pressure, and heart rate are taken in this position.

The patient is helped on to the treadmill and given a low-level warm up to ensure comfort on the treadmill. After the patient is

comfortable, he or she is told that the protocol will now be initiated. During exercise, the patient's blood pressure, heart rate, ECGs, and signs and symptoms are continuously monitored. The ECG is followed continuously on the monitor and recorded during the last 15 seconds of each stage or the last 15 seconds of each 2-minute time period if a ramp protocol is used. The heart rate is monitored continuously and recorded during the last 5 seconds of every minute. Blood pressure is measured and recorded during the last 45 seconds of each stage or of each 2-minute time period if using a ramp protocol. Signs and symptoms are monitored continuously and recorded when observed. In addition to this monitoring data, any adverse symptoms or abnormal ECG changes are noted. During exercise, the patient is warned of upcoming stage changes.

Table 40.2 Coronary Artery Disease Risk Factor Thresholds

Risk Factor	Defining Criteria
Positive	
Family history	Myocardial infarction, cardiovascular revascularization, or sudden death before 55 years of age in father or other male first-degree relative or before 65 years of age in mother or other female first-degree relative
Cigarette smoking	Current smoker or smoker who quit within the previous 6 months
Hypertension	Blood pressure more than 140/90 mm Hg or taking an antihypertensive medication
Hypercholesterolemia	Total cholesterol more than 200 mg/dL, high-density lipoprotein cholesterol less than 35 mg/dL, low-density lipoprotein cholesterol more than 130 mg/dL, or on lipid-lowering medication
Impaired fasting glucose	Fasting blood glucose more than 110 mg/dL on at least two occasions
Obesity	Body mass index greater than 30 kg/m^2 or waist girth of more than 100 cm
Sedentary lifestyle	No regular exercise or no exercise accumulating 30 minutes or more of moderate physical activity on most days of the week
Negative	
High serum high-density lipoprotein cholesterol	High-density lipoprotein cholesterol greater than 60 mg/dL

From American College of Sports Medicine: Guidelines for Exercise Testing and Prescription, 6th ed. Philadelphia, Lea and Febiger, 2000.

The ACC/AHA guidelines provide absolute and relative indications for terminating the exercise testing (see Box 40.7). Additionally, the test may be stopped after the patient reaches a percentage of the predicted maximal heart rate (usually 85%). However, there exists a wide spectrum with regard to maximal heart rate, and, therefore, the "target" heart rate may be submaximal for some patients but unobtainable for others. Thus, the committee highly recommends using symptom-limited stress testing as well as the end points outlined in **Box 40.8.** The absolute indications are unambiguous, whereas the relative indications do allow the physician to use clinical judgment when deciding whether to terminate the exercise portion of the test.

After the completion of the exercise portion of the test, the patient is immediately placed in the supine position. This acutely increases the workload of the heart by increasing the preload, and, therefore, it may precipitate ischemic abnormalities that are not seen while the patient is upright. During this recovery phase, the ECG is continuously monitored and recorded immediately after exercise, during the last 15 seconds of the first minute of recovery, and then every 2 minutes. The heart rate is continuously monitored and recorded during the last 5 seconds of every minute. The blood pressure is measured and recorded immediately after exercise and then every 2 minutes. Again, signs and symptoms are continuously monitored and recorded as observed. Additionally, the physician auscultates the patient immediately after exercise for any abnormal heart findings, such as a new heart murmur or a third heart sound. The physician also auscultates the lungs for

Box 40.7: Indications for Terminating Exercise Testing Absolute

Absolute
- Drop in systolic blood pressure of >10 mm Hg from baseline blood pressure despite an increase in workload when accompanied by other evidence of ischemia
- Moderate to severe angina
- Increasing nervous system symptoms (e.g., ataxia, dizziness, or near syncope)
- Signs of poor perfusion (cyanosis or pallor)
- Technical difficulties in monitoring the electrocardiogram or the systolic blood pressure
- Subject's desire to stop
- Sustained ventricular tachycardia
- ST elevation of ≥1.0 mm in leads without diagnostic Q waves (other than in V1 or aVR)

Relative
- Drop in systolic blood pressure of >10 mm Hg from baseline blood pressure despite an increase in workload in the absence of other evidence of ischemia
- ST or QRS changes such as excessive ST depression (>2 mm of horizontal or downsloping ST-segment depression) or marked axis shift
- Arrhythmias other than sustained ventricular tachycardia, including multifocal premature ventricular contractions, triplets of premature ventricular contractions, supraventricular tachycardia, heart block, or bradyarrhythmias
- Fatigue, shortness of breath, wheezing, leg cramps, or claudication
- Development of bundle-branch block or interventricular conduction delay that cannot be distinguished from ventricular tachycardia
- Increasing chest pain
- Hypertensive response (>250 mm Hg and/or diastolic blood pressure >115 mm Hg)

From Gibbons RJ, Balady GJ, Bricker JT, et al: ACC/AHA 2002 guideline update for exercise testing: a report of the American College of Cardiology/American Heart Association Task Force on Practice Guidelines (Committee on Exercise Testing). 2002. American College of Cardiology (Web site). Available at www.acc.org /clinical/guidelines/exercise/dirindex.htm.

signs of bronchoconstriction as a possible cause of chest pain. The physician should also auscultate for new-onset rales and monitor for symptoms that are suggestive of acute-onset congestive heart failure. The recovery period with monitoring continues until the patient is stable and any ST-segment changes have returned to baseline, which usually takes 8 to 10 minutes. This completes the test, and the monitoring equipment may be removed while the test is interpreted **(Box 40.9).**

The treadmill and bicycle ergometer protocols are compared in **Figure 40.2.**

INTERPRETATIONS

Clinical and hemodynamic responses

Interpretation of the exercise test requires the analysis and interpretation of both the electrocardiographic measurements and the nonelectrocardiographic observations related to myocardial ischemia. All of these findings contribute to the prognosis or extent of

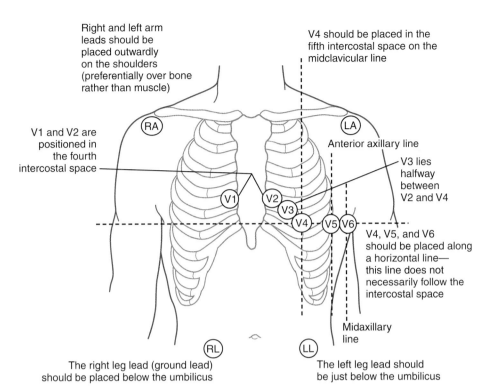

Right and left arm leads should be placed outwardly on the shoulders (preferentially over bone rather than muscle)

V4 should be placed in the fifth intercostal space on the midclavicular line

V1 and V2 are positioned in the fourth intercostal space

Anterior axillary line

V3 lies halfway between V2 and V4

V4, V5, and V6 should be placed along a horizontal line—this line does not necessarily follow the intercostal space

Midaxillary line

The right leg lead (ground lead) should be placed below the umbilicus

The left leg lead should be just below the umbilicus

Figure 40.1 Electrocardiogram lead placement. (From American Heart Association Scientific Statement: Circulation 2001;104:1694-1740.)

disease. The non-ECG findings that should be evaluated include blood pressure and heart rate response, the presence or absence of symptoms, the presence or absence of dysrhythmias, aerobic capacity, and perceived exertion. By assimilating all of this information with the pretest probability, the clinician can determine the probability that the patient has coronary artery disease and the severity of the disease and thus predict the prognosis and likelihood of future adverse cardiac events. With this information, the physician can provide recommendations regarding future management, such as deciding between revascularization and medical management.

The first information provided by the patient is the presence of symptoms. Chest pain, claudication, shortness of breath, and wheezing are each important findings. Exercise-induced anginal symptoms are a component of the DTS, and they may or may not correlate with ischemic ECG changes. Typical angina with ischemic ECG changes is an indication for termination of the test.[1] Other symptoms that are indicative of underlying cardiovascular disease may exist without angina or ECG changes and, thus, may presage underlying coronary artery disease. In the same manner, a patient's appearance may be helpful in his or her assessment. Light perspiration, peripheral cyanosis, and a decrease in skin temperature may indicate poor tissue perfusion as a result of inadequate cardiac output with resulting vasoconstriction. Fatigue is a normal and expected response to exercise; however, fatigue at lower levels of exertion relates to poor exercise capacity. Fatigue can be measured using the Borg or category–ratio scale shown in **Table 40.3.** A Borg scale rating of more than 18 suggests that the patient has achieved maximal exercise, and values of more than 15 to 16 suggest that the anaerobic threshold has been exceeded.[10]

Box 40.8: The Written Report

- Patient's demographics (age, gender, comorbidities)
- Patient's medications (to include whether they were taken prior to testing)
- Indications for testing
- Baseline heart rate, blood pressure, and any electrocardiogram abnormalities
- Protocol used
- Exercise time
- Reason for terminating test
- Heart rate response
- Blood pressure response
- Symptoms reported during test
- Dysrhythmias or ectopy
- Functional aerobic capacity (METs)
- ECG changes with exercise or recovery (type, location, and in which stage)
- Goal achieved: maximal versus submaximal
- Presence or absence of myocardial ischemia (positive or negative test)
- Duke Treadmill Score (if indicated)

Box 40.9: Techniques and Equipment for Exercise Testing

- Bruce
- Cornell
- Balke-Ware
- ACIP
- mACIP
- Naughton
- Weber
- Bicycle ergometry

Figure 40.2 Exercise stress testing protocols.

Functional class	Clinical status	O₂ Cost ml/kg/min	Mets	Bicycle ergometer (70 kg, kpm/min)	Bruce 3 min stages mph / % gr	Balke-Ware % grade at 3.3 mph (1 min stages)	USAFSAM mph / % gr	*Slow USAFSAM mph / % gr	McHenry mph / % gr	Stanford % grade at 3 mph	Stanford % grade at 2 mph	ACIP mph / % gr	CHF mph / % gr	Mets
Normal and I	Healthy, dependent on age, activity	56.0	16		5.5 / 20	26, 25								16
		52.5	15		5.0 / 18	24, 23								15
		49.0	14	1500		22, 21								14
		45.5	13		4.2 / 16	20, 19						3.4 / 24.0		13
		42.0	12	1350		18, 17				22.5				12
		38.5	11	1200		16, 15	3.3 / 25		3.3 / 21	20.0		3.1 / 24.0		11
	Sedentary healthy	35.0	10	1050	3.4 / 14	14, 13			3.3 / 18	17.5		3.0 / 21.0	3.4 / 14.0	10
		31.5	9	900		12, 11	3.3 / 20		3.3 / 15	15.0		3.0 / 17.5	3.0 / 15.0	9
		28.0	8	750		10, 9			3.3 / 12	12.5	17.5	3.0 / 14.0	3.0 / 12.5	8
II		24.5	7		2.5 / 12	8, 7	3.3 / 15	2 / 25	3.3 / 9	10.0	14.0	3.0 / 10.5	3.0 / 10.0	7
		21.0	6	600		6, 5		2 / 20	3.3 / 6	7.5	10.5	3.0 / 7.0	3.0 / 7.5	6
III	Limited	17.5	5	450	1.7 / 10	4, 3	3.3 / 10	2 / 15		5.0	7.0	3.0 / 3.0	2.0 / 10.5	5
		14.0	4	300	1.7 / 5	2, 1	3.3 / 5	2 / 10	2.0 / 3	2.5	3.5	2.5 / 2.0	2.0 / 7.0	4
IV	Symptomatic	10.5	3		1.7 / 0		3.3 / 0	2 / 5		0		2.0 / 0.0	2.0 / 3.5	3
		7.0	2	150			2.0 / 0	2 / 0					1.5 / 0.0	2
		3.5	1										1.0 / 0.0	1

1 Watt = 6.1 Kpm/min

Table 40.3   Borg Scale for Rating Perceived Exertion

Rating of Perceived Exhaustion	New Rating Scale
6: Very, very light	0: Nothing at all
7	0.5: Very, very weak
8	1: Very weak
9: Very light	2: Weak
10	3: Moderate
11: Fairly light	4: Somewhat strong
12	5: Strong
13: Somewhat hard	6
14	7: Very strong
15: Hard	8
16	9
17: Very hard	10: Very, very strong
18	—Maximal
19: Very, very hard	

From American Heart Association Scientific Statement: Circulation 2001;104:1694-1740.

The physical examination with cardiopulmonary auscultation immediately after exercise can elucidate an exercise-induced left ventricular dysfunction through new cardiac gallops or precordial bulge. Any new murmur may also represent valvular disease or papillary muscle dysfunction, whereas new-onset rales are indicative of acute congestive heart failure.

Exercise or aerobic capacity is also an important prognostic indicator. The most accurate measurement of aerobic capacity is with a direct measurement of maximal oxygen consumption. Gas analysis increases the expense when added to the stress system, and it may not be widely available for routine testing. When unavailable, the best estimate of exercise capacity is the measurement of the work effort, which is expressed in METs. Figure 40.2 shows the conversion of exercise time per protocol to METs. Studies have shown that a low exercise tolerance portends an increased risk of all-cause and cardiovascular mortality, whereas those patients with a good exercise tolerance have a lower risk of adverse cardiovascular events (LOE: A).[5-9]

Maximal heart rate can be predicted using a number of different equations that are based on age, with the most common being 220 minus the patient's age (e.g., for a 35-year-old patient, 220 − 35 = 185 bpm). Although these equations have been validated with large study groups, there is still significant individual variability. There is a high likelihood for error when extrapolating the age-adjusted submaximal predicted maximal heart rate. Therefore, achieving the predicted maximal heart rate should not be an absolute end point or suggestive of a maximal effort. Additionally, heart rate response to exercise may be influenced by a number of factors; a rapid rise in the heart rate could be the result of deconditioning, anemia, metabolic disorders, or dehydration. A relatively slow heart rate could be attributed to training, enhanced stroke volume, or medications (e.g., β-blockers).[11] Although the maximal heart rate is a highly variable factor in exercise testing, there are two significant abnormalities that should be evaluated. Chronotropic incompetence (i.e., the inability to raise heart rate above 120 bpm with exercise) is associated with the presence of heart disease and increased mortality (LOE: A).[12,13]

A delayed decrease in the heart rate during recovery (<12 bpm at 1 minute into recovery) after a maximal exercise test is a predictor of increased mortality (LOE: B).[14]

Blood-pressure response to exercise should consist of a progressive increase in systolic blood pressure and a stable or slightly decreased diastolic blood pressure, thereby widening the pulse pressure. The increase in systolic pressures is typically 10 ± 2 mm Hg per MET.[11] In younger age groups, men typically have a higher systolic blood pressure; however, by 70 years of age, that difference has disappeared, and the blood-pressure response should be similar in both genders.[11] A relative indication to terminate testing is a hypertensive response, which is defined as a systolic blood pressure of more than 250 mm Hg or a diastolic blood pressure of more than 115 mm Hg.[1] An inadequate rise in systolic blood pressure with increasing exercise or a drop in the systolic blood pressure of more than 10 mm Hg is also considered an abnormal test, and, when not accompanied by other signs of ischemia, it is a relative indication to terminate testing. These conditions can result from aortic outflow obstruction, severe left ventricular dysfunction, myocardial ischemia, and certain medications. When found with other measures of ischemia, exercise-induced hypotension is an indicator of a poorer prognosis, with a positive predictive value of 50% for left main or three-vessel disease, and it represents an absolute indication for test termination (LOE: B).[10,15] During the recovery phase, the normal blood-pressure response is a progressive decline in systolic blood pressure; however, if the patient is recovering in an upright position, systolic pressures may fall abruptly as a result of venous pooling in the lower extremities. At 3 minutes into the recovery period, a systolic blood pressure/peak systolic blood pressure ratio of more than 0.90 is abnormal, with a diagnostic accuracy for coronary artery disease of 75% (LOE: review).[16]

One indicator of myocardial oxygen demand is the rate-pressure product or double product (maximal systolic blood pressure × heart rate). With this equation, a normal peak exercise value should be greater than 25,000. Typical stable angina should manifest with signs and symptoms at a reproducible double product that is additionally known as the *anginal threshold*. Lower anginal thresholds correlate with more severe ischemic disease. This is helpful when evaluating exercise capacity for an exercise prescription to ensure that exercise levels remain below this threshold.

Electrocardiographic response

Although many ECG changes are representative of ischemia, there are also a number of normal exercise-induced ECG responses that may be seen during exercise testing, most prominently during maximal exercise.

The P-wave magnitude increases significantly in the inferior leads, and there may be some minor P-wave morphology changes with the superposition of the P and T waves in successive beats. There should be no significant changes in the duration of the P wave.[10]

The PR segment shortens and slopes downward in the inferior leads. These changes have been attributed to atrial repolarization, and they may cause a false-positive ST segment depression in the inferior leads.[10]

The Q wave should demonstrate a slightly increased negative deflection in the septal leads. The R wave should decrease in amplitude, most noticeably in the lateral leads, and this should last into the first minute of recovery. Also in the lateral leads, the S wave deflection becomes more negative and greater in depth. As the R wave decreases in amplitude, the S wave increases in depth. Overall, the QRS complex may shorten minimally.[10]

The J point (J junction), which is the point that distinguishes the QRS complex from the ST segment, becomes depressed, with a return to normal during recovery. The depressed J point will initially depress the ST segment; however, the ST segment should rapidly upslope back to baseline in less than 80 msec. Patients with early repolarization characterized by baseline J point elevation may develop an isoelectric J point with exercise, which is also a normal finding.[10]

The T wave gradually decreases in amplitude during early exercise. At maximum exercise, the T wave begins to increase in amplitude, and, at 1 minute into recovery, the T-wave amplitude should be back to pre-exercise levels. The T-wave changes can be seen in all leads. The QT interval will also decrease with increasing heart rates.[10]

There should be no significant changes to the U wave; however, at heart rates of more than 130 bpm, the U wave may be difficult to discern as a result of its approximation of the T and P waves.[10]

The most common manifestation of exercise-induced myocardial ischemia is ST-segment depression. The standard criteria diagnosing myocardial ischemia is 1 mV or more of horizontal or downsloping ST segment depression as compared with the PQ junction at 80 msec after the J point (60 msec in heart rates of more than 130 bpm) that is present for three consecutive beats.[10] This criteria balances the specificity and sensitivity to provide an appropriate positive predictive value in an intermediate-risk patient. An upsloping depression of more than 1.5 mm at 80 msec is also considered diagnostic for myocardial ischemia.[17] Slowly upsloping ST-segment depression of less than 1.5 mm but more than 0.7 mm, a downsloping or horizontal depression of 0.5 mm to 1.0 mm, or an elevation of 0.5 mm to 1.0 mm is suggestive of myocardial ischemia and should be further evaluated with other ECG and clinical variables.[18] The ST-segment depression does not localize the ischemia to a specific area of myocardium. The more leads involved in the depression, the earlier the time of appearance, the duration of the ECG changes, and the greater the amplitude of the depression at low workloads all confer a greater extent of the ischemia; however, the ischemia cannot be localized from these ECG changes (LOE: B).[6] Although exercise-induced ischemic ECG changes often persist into recovery, changes can arise after the completion of exercise. These depressions seen only during the recovery phase have the same predictive power as changes seen only during exercise at 85% of the maximum predicted heart rate.[17,18] Although

ST-segment changes can occur in any leads, the best diagnostic group of leads for determining myocardial ischemia are leads I, aVR, V4, V5, and V6, with V5 being the single best lead to monitor. The inferior leads II, III, and AVR are sensitive for diagnosing ischemia; however, isolated depression in these leads is more often a false positive as a result of atrial repolarization (LOE: B).[6] The interpretation of changes in the ST segment can be affected by abnormalities in the resting ECG, such as bundle-branch blocks and left ventricular hypertrophy. Patients with a left bundle-branch block or left ventricular hypertrophy with significant baseline repolarization changes should be referred for an exercise test that is complemented by echocardiography or nuclear imaging to enhance the diagnostic accuracy.[10] An example of ST-segment depressions is shown in **Figure 40.3.**

An exercise-induced ST segment elevation of greater than 0.1 mV that remains persistently elevated at 80 msec (or 60 msec) after the J point in three consecutive beats may occur in an infarcted area of myocardium where Q waves are present or in a noninfarct territory without Q waves. ST elevation without Q waves is an uncommon finding, and it represents either a severe proximal transmural ischemic process or a severe coronary artery spasm (Prinzmetal angina). Unlike ST-segment depressions, elevations in the ST segment do localize the infarcting area of myocardium. Prior myocardial infarction is the most frequent cause of exercise-induced ST-segment elevation in leads with Q waves. These elevations may represent ischemic areas adjacent to severe hypokinetic or akinetic areas from the previous myocardial infarction or the development of a ventricular aneurysm. Concomitant ST-segment depression and elevation during a single test may represent multivessel disease or reciprocal changes and thus require follow-up with imaging techniques to distinguish between the two.[10,17]

In addition to the ST-segment changes, there are infrequent abnormal ECG findings that can be used as markers of ischemia during testing[19]:

- A prolonged P-wave duration of more than 20 msec from baseline
- The decreased amplitude or disappearance of the septal Q wave during maximal exercise
- The increased amplitude of the R wave at maximal exercise (best seen in V4 or V5)

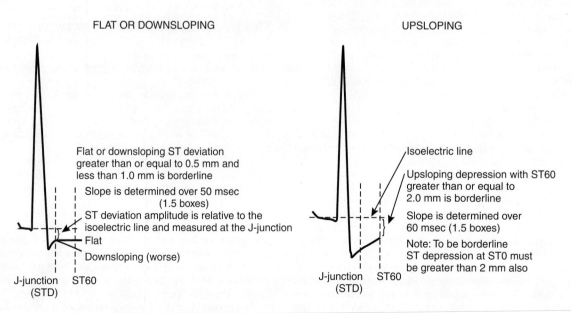

FLAT OR DOWNSLOPING

Flat or downsloping ST deviation greater than or equal to 0.5 mm and less than 1.0 mm is borderline

Slope is determined over 50 msec (1.5 boxes)

ST deviation amplitude is relative to the isoelectric line and measured at the J-junction

Flat

Downsloping (worse)

J-junction (STD)   ST60

UPSLOPING

Isoelectric line

Upsloping depression with ST60 greater than or equal to 2.0 mm is borderline

Slope is determined over 60 msec (1.5 boxes)

Note: To be borderline ST depression at ST0 must be greater than 2 mm also

J-junction (STD)   ST60

Figure 40.3 ST segment evaluation. (From American Heart Association Scientific Statement: Circulation 2001;104:1694-1740.)

- The increased duration of the QRS complex or an exercise-induced bundle-branch block in an older patient (may be seen in younger patients without CAD)

Benign supraventricular arrhythmias commonly occur during exercise testing. Various cardiovascular medications, alcohol, caffeine, and nicotine can all promote arrhythmias. Additionally, in patients with CAD, the inability to supply sufficient oxygen with increased sympathetic tone and myocardial oxygen demand during exercise can precipitate arrhythmias.[10] Ectopic atrial beats or short runs of supraventricular tachycardia have no diagnostic or prognostic significance for obstructive CAD. Likewise, isolated unifocal premature ventricular contractions commonly occur during exercise, and they are not always indicative of CAD. A cohort study of 29,244 patients with a mean age of 56 ± 11 years who were referred for symptom-limited exercise testing without a history of heart failure, valvular disease, or arrhythmias monitored the patients for frequent ventricular ectopy during and after exercise as defined by seven or more premature ventricular contractions per minute, ventricular bigeminy or trigeminy, ventricular couplets or triplets, ventricular tachycardia, ventricular flutter, torsades de pointes, or ventricular fibrillation. Those patients with frequent ventricular ectopy during recovery had a statistically significant increase in risk of death (hazard ratio, 1.5) that was not seen in those with ectopy only during exercise.[20] It is thought that the period immediately after exercise is especially dangerous for arrhythmogenicity as a result of the elevated levels of catecholamine and generalized vasodilation. The peripheral vasodilation and decreased preload leads to decreased cardiac perfusion while the heart rate remains elevated, thereby exacerbating ischemia.

The most popular and widely validated tool to calculate the patient's prognosis following exercise stress testing is the DTS (LOE: B).[21,22] This score allows providers to identify patients who are at high risk for future cardiovascular events and who thus require more significant intervention as compared with those who can be treated with medical management. The DTS correlates three indices obtained with a Bruce protocol with prognosis: exercise time, maximal ST segment depression, and angina index (0, no angina; 1, typical angina; 2, test terminated as a result of angina). The DTS is then determined with the following equation:

$$\text{Score} = \text{Minutes} - \text{exercised} - (5 \times \text{Maximal ST depression}) - (4 \times \text{Angina index})$$

Mark and colleagues developed the above prognostic treadmill exercise score in 2942 consecutive patients referred to Duke for cardiac catheterization over a 10-year period. They then validated that score prospectively in 613 outpatients who were referred for exercise testing. The nomogram shown in **Figure 40.4** shows the prognostic relations validated by the DTS. Patients with a score of +5 or greater are placed in the low-risk group, with an annual cardiac mortality of 0.25% to 0.5%; Patients with score of −10 to +4 are placed in the moderate group, with an annual cardiac mortality of 1.25% to 2%, whereas patients with a score of −11 or less

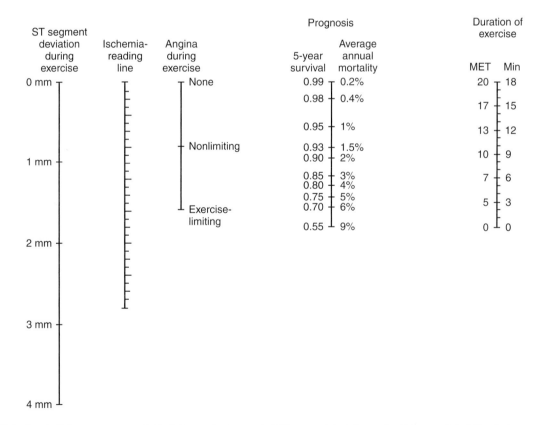

Figure 40.4 Duke Treadmill Score nomogram. 1, Mark the maximal amount of ST-segment deviation on the ST-segment deviation during exercise line. 2, Mark the observed degree of angina on the angina line. 3, Connect the points on the ST-segment deviation line and the angina line. 4, Mark the duration of exercise from the Bruce protocol on the duration line. 5, Connect the duration of exercise point with the point at which the ST segment deviation/angina line crosses the ischemia reading line. 6, Where that line crosses the prognosis line is the patient's 5-year survival and average annual mortality. (From Gibbons RJ, Balady GJ, Bricker JT, et al: ACC/AHA 2002 guideline update for exercise testing: a report of the American College of Cardiology/American Heart Association Task Force on Practice Guidelines [Committee on Exercise Testing]. 2002. American College of Cardiology [Web site]. Available at www.acc.org/clinical/guidelines/exercise/dirindex.htm.)

are placed in the high-risk group, with an average annual mortality of 5.0% to 7.0% (LOE: B).[22]

At the completion of interpretation, the provider should provide a written evaluation of the interpretation that addresses all of the pertinent positive and negative findings of the test. Items to discuss in the written report are outlined in Box 40.8.

PITFALLS, COMPLICATIONS, CONTROVERSIES, RISKS, AND BENEFITS

Confounding variables in interpretation

When comparing studies that excluded patients with left ventricular hypertrophy with repolarization abnormalities with the studies that included patients with this ECG finding, no significant effect on the sensitivity of the exercise test was found (72% versus 67%); however, the left ventricular hypertrophy slightly decreased the average specificity (77% versus 69%). Because there is no change in the sensitivity, if there is less than 1 mm of baseline ST depression, the ACC/AHA still recommends that a standard exercise test be the initial test, with more advanced testing only indicated for those with abnormal results.[1]

Baseline ST segment abnormalities can be the result of a number of causes that are unrelated to CAD, including repolarization abnormalities, cardiac hypertrophy, Wolff–Parkinson–White syndrome, Lown–Ganong–Levine syndrome, mitral valve prolapse, pericarditis, digitalis effect, and female gender. Any baseline abnormality in the ST segment makes the interpretation of the exercise test more difficult, and it may produce a false-positive result. Resting ST segment depression without an identifiable cause is a marker for adverse cardiac events in males. A study of 223 male patients showed males with baseline ST-segment depression had almost twice the prevalence of severe coronary artery disease as compared with males without (30% versus 16%). In these patients, additional exercise-induced ST-segment depression of 2 mm or downsloping of 1 mm in ST-segment depression during recovery were reliable markers of severe coronary disease (likelihood ratio, 3.4; sensitivity, 67%; specificity, 80%) (LOE: B).[1] As discussed previously, another possible cause of a false-positive result is coronary artery spasm in a patient without underlying coronary artery disease. In this case, the patient would typically experience significant anginal symptoms with associated ST-segment elevation; however, cardiac catheterization would demonstrate no stenosis.

Left bundle-branch block can produce exercise-induced ST-segment depression of up to 1 cm that is not associated with ischemia, and no amount of ST-segment depression confers diagnostic significance. ST-segment elevation, however, is abnormal with a left bundle-branch block, and it is associated with infarct.[1]

Exercise-induced ST-segment depression usually occurs in right bundle-branch block across the anterior chest leads (V1 through V3), and it is not associated with ischemia; however, the lateral and inferior leads should be similar to a normal resting ECG. Therefore, exercise-induced ST-segment depression in any of these leads is abnormal. Unlike left bundle-branch block, right bundle-branch block does not affect the sensitivity, specificity, or predictive value of the test (LOE: B).[1]

Digoxin produces a nonischemic ST-segment depression response to exercise in 25% to 40% of healthy adult patients, with the rate increasing with age. The patient must abstain from taking digoxin for 2 weeks before testing to eliminate this abnormal response.[1]

For routine exercise testing, discontinuation of β-blocker or calcium-channel blocker therapy is typically unnecessary. Although patients taking these medications exhibited a significant decrease in maximal heart rate, there was no difference in test performance among patients who were referred for the evaluation for CAD.[1] For routine testing, the risk of discontinuing the β-blockers/calcium-channel blockers among patients with hypertension or with possible symptoms of ischemia likely outweighs the benefits; however, if continued, the medication may reduce the diagnostic and prognostic value of the test as a result of the blunted heart rate response. The decision to hold medication must be made carefully on an individual basis to avoid a possible rebound effect.

Other antihypertensive and vasodilating medications can affect the test by altering the hemodynamic response of blood pressure. The acute administration of nitrates can decrease the anginal symptoms and expected ST-segment depression associated with ischemia. Although diuretics have little effect on heart rate and cardiac performance, their use may lead to electrolyte abnormalities such as hypokalemia and thus interfere with interpreting the ST segment and T waves; they may also cause increased ectopy and exacerbate muscle fatigue.[10]

Other errors that may result in a false-negative result include the patient's inability to achieve an adequate workload (which is why achieving a maximum predicted heart rate is not an ideal indication for test termination), not monitoring a sufficient number of leads, minimal single-vessel disease, adequate collateral circulation, or technical/observer error. Most systems will provide the observer with a signal-averaged ECG tracing in addition to the raw data to help minimize beat-to-beat variability and movement artifact. If there is significant variability, the signal averaging may underestimate or overestimate the ST-segment changes. Therefore, to prevent error, the provider should also monitor the raw data in addition to the averaged output.

CONCLUSION

Cardiac exercise stress testing is a safe procedure when performed properly. Primary care sports medicine clinicians, with appropriate training, can conduct exercise stress testing in the outpatient or inpatient setting and derive a great deal of clinical information. The data obtained from clinical exercise stress testing can assist in managing patients confronted with disease, investigaing those with exercise-related symptoms, and promoting healthy lifestyles by assisting with writing exercise prescriptions.

REFERENCES

1. Gibbons RJ, Balady GJ, Bricker JT, et al: ACC/AHA 2002 guideline update for exercise testing: a report of the American College of Cardiology/American Heart Association Task Force on Practice Guidelines (Committee on Exercise Testing). 2002. American College of Cardiology (Web site). Available at www.acc.org/clinical/guidelines/exercise/dirindex.htm.
2. Stuart RJ Jr, Ellestad MH: National survey of exercise testing facilities. Chest 1980;77:94-97.
3. Schant RC, Gottlieb CF, Leonard JJ, et al: Clinical competence in exercise testing: a statement for physicians from the ACP/ACC/AHA task force on clinical privileges in cardiology. Circulation 1990;40:1884-1888.
4. Tavel ME, Shaar C: Relation between the electrocardiographic stress test and degree and location of myocardial ischemia. Am J Cardiol 1999;84:119-124.
5. Blair SN, Kohl HW 3rd, Paffenbarger RS Jr, et al: Physical fitness and all-cause mortality. A prospective study of healthy men and women. JAMA 1989;262:2395-2401.
6. Blair SN, Kohl HW 3rd, Barlow CE, et al: Changes in physical fitness and all-cause mortality. A prospective study of healthy and unhealthy men. JAMA 1995;273:1093-1098.
7. Vanhees L, Fagard R, Thijs L, et al: Prognostic significance of peak exercise capacity in patients with coronary artery disease. J Am Coll Cardiol 1994;23:358-363.
8. Myers J, Prakash M, Foelicher V, et al: Exercise capacity and mortality among men referred for exercise testing. N Engl J Med 2002;346:793-801.

9. Dorn J, Naughton J, Imamura D, et al: Results of a multicenter randomized clinical trial of exercise and long-term survival in myocardial infarction patients: the national exercise and heart disease project (NEHDP). Circulation 1999;100:1764-1769.

10. Fletcher GF, Balady GJ, Amsterdam EA: Exercise standards for testing and training: a statement for healthcare professionals from the American Heart Association. Circulation 2001;104:1694-1740.

11. Whaley MH, Brubaker PH, Otto RM (eds): ACSM's Guidelines for Exercise Testing and Prescription/American College of Sports Medicine, 7th ed. Philadelphia, Lippincott Williams & Wilkins, 2000.

12. Ellestad MH: Chronotropic incompetence. The implications of heart rate response to exercise (compensatory parasympathetic hyperactivity?). Circulation 1996;93:1485-1487.

13. Lauer MS, Francis GS, Okin PM, et al: Impaired chronotropic response to exercise stress testing as a predictor of mortality. JAMA 1999;281:524-529.

14. Nishime EO, Cole CR, Blackstone EH, et al: Heart rate recovery and treadmill exercise score as predictors of mortality in patients referred for exercise ECG. JAMA 2000;284:1392-1398.

15. Dubach P, Froelicker VF, Klein J, et al: Exercise-induced hypotension in a male population: criteria, causes, and prognosis. Circulation 1988;78:1380-1387.

16. Taylor AJ, Beller GA: Postexercise systolic blood pressure response: clinical application to the assessment of ischemic heart disease. Am Fam Physician 1998;58:1126-1130.

17. Ellestad MH: Stress Testing: Principles and Practice, 5th ed. New York, Oxford University Press, 2003.

18. Rywik TM, Zink RC, Gittings NS, et al: Independent prognostic significance of ischemic ST-segment response limited to recovery from treadmill exercise in asymptomatic subjects. Circulation 1998;97:2117-2122.

19. Evans CH, Harris G, Menold V: A basic approach to the interpretation of the exercise test. Primary Care 2001;28:73-97.

20. Froikis JP, Pothier CE, Blackstone EH: Frequent ventricular ectopy after exercise as a predictor of death. N Engl J Med 2003;348:781-790.

21. Mark DB, Hlatky MA, Harrell FE Jr, et al: Exercise treadmill score for predicting prognosis in coronary artery disease. Ann Intern Med 1987;106:793-800.

22. Mark DB, Shaw L, Harrell FE Jr, et al: Prognostic value of a treadmill exercise score in outpatients with suspected coronary artery disease. N Engl J Med 1991;325:849-853.

Testing for Maximal Aerobic Power

Patricia A. Deuster, PhD, MPH, and Yuval Heled, PhD

KEY POINTS

- Maximal oxygen uptake (VO_{2max}) serves as an index of cardiorespiratory function, general health, and aerobic fitness.
- The methodology for measuring or estimating VO_{2max} should be appropriate for the population of interest, the rationale of the testing, and the individual and/or group's occupation and physical condition.
- A valid measure of VO_{2max} requires the activation of large muscle groups, such as those used during running, cycling, or climbing.
- Maximal aerobic capacity can be estimated from both submaximal exercise and nonexercise prediction tests, but it should be measured when accurate results are needed, such as for research.
- A plateau in oxygen intake despite an increase in workload is considered the primary criterion for VO_{2max}.

INTRODUCTION

Maximal aerobic power or maximal oxygen uptake (VO_{2max}) is a measure of the maximum amount of oxygen that an individual can use per unit of time during strenuous physical exertion at sea level. It is an important measure for several reasons: (1) it serves as an index of cardiovascular and pulmonary function; (2) it characterizes the functional capacity of the cardiopulmonary system to transport oxygen to the working muscles; and (3) it is one of the limiting factors in endurance performance. Maximal aerobic power is typically expressed in absolute power as L/min^{-1} or normalized for body weight as $mL/kg^{-1}/min^{-1}$. An individual's VO_{2max} can be measured or estimated by a variety of techniques, including treadmill running, cycle ergometry, arm cranking, stair stepping, rowing, and walking. However, the gold standard is progressive treadmill testing by running to exhaustion. The most common way to

measure VO_{2max} is by open-circuit spirometry whereby the individual breathes in ambient air and then the exhaled air is measured and analyzed. The amount of oxygen consumed (VO_2) can be computed on the basis of the composition of the inspired air by quantifying the volume (V) and oxygen (O_2) content of the expired air.

The objectives of this chapter are as follows: (1) to provide an overview of maximal and submaximal exercise testing; (2) to present selected criteria for documenting that a true maximal value is achieved; and (3) to describe different ways of measuring and estimating VO_{2max}.

MAXIMAL OXYGEN UPTAKE AND EXERCISE TESTING

Maximal oxygen uptake

By definition, *maximal oxygen uptake* is the highest VO_2 achieved when a person is working at maximal capacity.[1,2] Classically, VO_2 reaches a plateau and does not increase further, even with an increase in external workload. Absolute values, which are typically expressed in liters per minute (L/min^{-1}), may range from as low as $1.0\ L/min^{-1}$ (or lower in patients with cardiovascular disease) up to $6\ L/min^{-1}$ (or even higher in large, well-trained individuals). Because two individuals of quite different sizes may have the same absolute VO_{2max} value, VO_{2max} is often normalized for body weight and expressed as $mL/kg^{-1}/min^{-1}$; this allows for between-person comparisons. Values for VO_{2max} may range from a low of 10 to a high of 80 or more $mL/kg^{-1}/min^{-1}$.

Principles of exercise testing

Although VO_{2max} testing is appropriate for all healthy people and it provides important information about aerobic fitness and cardiopulmonary health, it should be emphasized that absolute and relative contraindications to performing exercise tests have been established by the 2002 American College of Cardiology/American Heart Association Task Force on Practice Guidelines. These contraindications are provided in **Table 41.1.** When an exercise test is conducted, certain requirements must be met to obtain a valid measure of VO_{2max}, Including the following: (1) the exercise must involve large muscle groups; (2) the rate of work must be measurable and reproducible; (3) the conditions must be standardized; and

The opinions and assertions expressed herein are those of the authors and should not be construed as reflecting those of the Uniformed Services University of the Health Sciences.

Table 41.1 Contraindications to Exercise Testing from the 2002 American College of Cardiology/American Heart Association Task Force on Practice Guidelines*

Absolute	Relative[†]
Acute myocardial infarction (within 2 days)	Left main coronary stenosis
High-risk unstable angina	Moderate stenotic valvular heart disease
Uncontrolled cardiac arrhythmias causing symptoms or hemodynamic compromise	Electrolyte abnormalities
Symptomatic severe aortic stenosis	Severe arterial hypertension[‡]
Uncontrolled symptomatic heart failure	Tachyarrhythmias or bradyarrhythmias
Acute pulmonary embolus or pulmonary infarction	Hypertrophic cardiomyopathy and other forms of outflow tract obstruction
Acute myocarditis or pericarditis	Mental or physical impairment leading to inability to exercise adequately
Acute aortic dissection	
High-degree atrioventricular block	

*www.acc.org/qualityandscience/clinical/guidelines/exercise/dirindex.htm.
†Relative contraindications can be superseded if the benefits of exercise outweigh the risks.
‡In the absence of definitive evidence, the committee suggests cutoff points for systolic blood pressure of >200 mm Hg and/or diastolic blood pressure of >110 mm Hg.

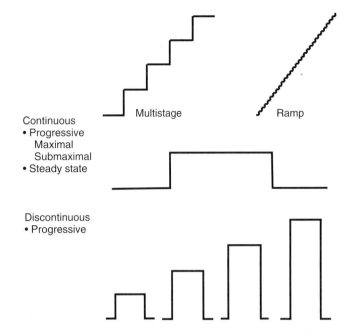

Figure 41.1 Various types of exercise testing methodologies: continuous (progressive multistage), ramp, steady state, and discontinuous.

(4) the mode of exercise should be tolerated by most people.[2-4] In addition, the test should be independent of the motivation or specific skill sets of the individual.[1,4] Furthermore, all maximal exercise tests should begin with a warm up so that the individual has adapted to a submaximal level before moving up to maximal exercise.[3]

A variety of test methodologies, with these principles considered, have emerged over the years to either measure or estimate maximal aerobic power. These methodologies include continuous progressive tests with 2-minute to 3-minute stages, continuous progressive tests with less than 2-minute stages (ramp tests), continuous steady-state tests, and discontinuous progressive tests.[2] **Figure 41.1** provides a graphic view of these various test methodologies. Whereas steady-state protocols are always submaximal, progressive tests can be either submaximal or maximal. When submaximal tests are conducted, only an estimate of VO_{2max} can be obtained.

Types of tests

Significant efforts have been devoted to examining various exercise paradigms so that the most suitable test for achieving VO_{2max} can be used.[2,5-11] **Table 41.2,** which provides a comparison of different modalities, shows that treadmill running with a grade is the preferred approach to achieving VO_{2max}.[9-11] It is important to note that the magnitude of the differences across test modalities depends in part on the sport preference of the subject being tested. For example, a VO_{2max} obtained during arm cranking approached 80% of the value obtained during arm and leg work combined, but only in a trained canoeist.[5,6] Similarly, the upper range for upright cycling applies primarily to those who are trained cyclists.[2,12]

Treadmill tests for maximal aerobic power

Exercise on a treadmill is a very common approach for measuring VO_{2max}. As such, a variety of treadmill test protocols have been described.[2-4,13-17] Some tests use a constant speed and impose incremental grade changes; these include the Balke,[13] Taylor,[4] and Stanford[1] tests. Kyle and colleagues[18] described a continuous version of the Taylor test that uses 2.5%-increment increases in grade with a constant speed. The choice of speed (6 to 8 mph) is determined from the heart rate after a 10-minute warm up. This is an excellent test that can be used with the criteria that are described later for documenting whether VO_{2max} is achieved.

Other test protocols change both grade and speed or just speed. The most commonly used test is the one described by Bruce and colleagues.[3] Although the time to complete the Bruce protocol is minimal, it imposes marked increases in both speed and grade, which many people find difficult. By contrast, the original Balke protocol,[1] which uses 2%-increment increases in grade coupled with 3-minute stages, takes a long time to achieve VO_{2max}. Modified versions of both protocols can be used, depending on the population of interest. Clearly smaller-grade increments and a slow speed are preferred for older and/or deconditioned persons, whereas large work increments and high speeds may be suitable for young and highly active populations. Figure 41.2 provides a range of the relative VO_2 values expected for various speeds and grades. This information can provide the tester with an estimate of

Table 41.2 Maximal Values Achieved during Various Types of Maximal Exercise Tests

Types of Exercise	Percentage of Maximal Oxygen Uptake
Uphill running	100%
Horizontal running	95%-98%
Upright cycling	90%-96%
Supine cycling	82%-85%
Arm cranking	62%-80%
Cross-country skiing	100%-104%
Step test	97%
Swimming	85%

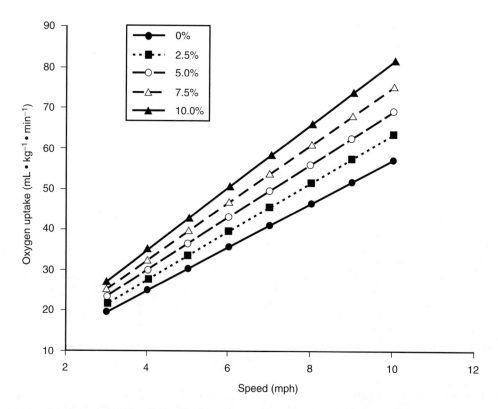

Figure 41.2 Oxygen uptake values expected for various speeds and grades as determined by the American College of Sports Medicine's formulas for metabolic calculations.

what to expect at a given speed and grade despite significant individual variation as a result of biomechanics, body composition, and other such characteristics.

Cycle ergometer tests for maximal aerobic power

Although similar principles can be applied to cycle ergometer tests, the cycle ergometer differs from the treadmill in that work rates are weight independent, and the two primary variables are cycling rate and resistance. These factors determine the power or work per unit of time, which is expressed in watts (W). If VO_2 is measured during a steady state at various cycling rates, a linear relation between a change in VO_2 and the work rate is typically noted: the range of 9 to 12 mL of $O_2/min^{-1}/W^{-1}$ depends on the rate of work incrementation[19]; **Figure 41.3** depicts the relationship between W and VO_2 for cycling ergometry. This relationship can be used to estimate VO_{2max} when actual measurements are not possible, although some variability between persons will always be noted. For traditional cycle ergometer tests, a cycling rate of 50 revolutions/rotations per minute (rpm) is often used, but some subjects find this rate too slow at low resistance settings. In all cases, the person should have a warm up with either no load or a minimal load (25 W) before any progressive increase in resistance. Each progressive stage should be between 1 and 3 minutes in length, and the step increments should range between 25 and 60 W, depending on the characteristics of the population. Williams and colleagues[20] recently found that adolescent boys could achieve VO_{2peak} during only 90 seconds of a maximal intensity cycle sprint. Accordingly, a supramaximal test may present an alternative to the traditional incremental cycle exercise test to exhaustion when assessing maximal aerobic power. For a detailed description of other cycle and treadmill exercise test protocols, the reader should refer to the American College of Sports Medicine's *Guidelines for Exercise Testing and Prescription.*[1]

Criteria for documenting the attainment of maximal aerobic power

When a maximal aerobic power test is conducted, it is important to document whether a true VO_{2max} has been achieved. Such a determination begins with an understanding of the physiologic responses to severe exercise and assessing selected parameters that have been designated as criteria for a VO_{2max} test. The criteria allow the tester to decide whether the obtained value should be considered the VO_{2max} or a peak VO_2 (VO_{2peak}). As noted previously, a plateau in VO_2 or only a small increase in VO_2 with an increase in external workload is considered the primary criterion. Secondary criterion include measures of blood (or plasma) lactate, respiratory exchange ratio (RER), heart rate, and perceived exertion.[1,21,22]

CRITERIA FOR MAXIMAL AEROBIC POWER

A plateau in oxygen uptake

A plateau in oxygen intake despite an increase in workload is considered the primary criterion for VO_{2max}. If a plateau in VO_2 is observed, VO_{2max} has been achieved. However, this criterion is not always achieved.[18,20,23-28] Various factors influence the quantification of VO_{2max}, including between-subject variability and absolute increases in grade and speed. Meyers and colleagues[29] suggested that a plateau phenomenon is not always seen with various protocols because of the sampling interval selected (e.g., breath by breath; 5-, 10-, or 15-second averages) and the magnitude of the work increments for each exercise stage. Many efforts have been undertaken to define precise criterion for attaining a plateau. In one of the early studies performed by Taylor and colleagues[4] 115 subjects ran at a speed of 7 mph on a given grade (0% to 12.5%) for 3 minutes; the grade was increased by

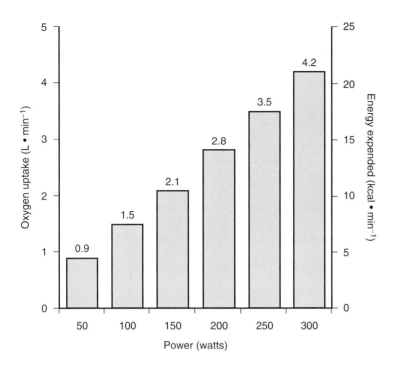

Figure 41.3 Predicted amount of oxygen consumed requirements for various power outputs (watts) on a cycle ergometer. Note that these requirements are independent of body weight.

2.5% until the subject could go no longer; the grade increases were typically carried out on different days or after a period of rest. With this protocol, it was shown that a 2.5%-grade increase typically resulted in a rise of approximately 300 mL/min^{-1} in VO$_2$. However, at a certain point, higher levels of exercise, which were different for each person, did not elicit the 300 mL/min^{-1} increase. On the basis of this information, it was determined that an increase of less than 150 mL/min^{-1} or 2.1 mL/kg^{-1}/min^{-1} in VO$_2$ at the next higher work rate marked a plateau. The authors of the study concluded that a grade increase was preferable to speed increases for achieving a plateau. In addition, they demonstrated that 93.9% of persons tested achieved the designated plateau.[4]

It is important to note that other investigators have not always found that such a high percentage of persons achieve a plateau. The percentage of adults achieving a plateau ranges from 25% of men and women[26,30] to 72.5% of men.[18] The numbers are similar for children, with 25%[27] to 33%[28] of prepubertal children achieving a plateau during treadmill exercise and cycle ergometry, respectively. For most studies, VO$_{2peak}$ values do not differ from VO$_{2max}$ values. Thus, although a plateau is not seen for many people as a result of various factors, VO$_{2peak}$ may be considered a valid index of VO$_{2max}$. Although no consensus has been reached over the years, this criterion is still considered by many to be the gold standard or the primary criterion. Because a plateau is not consistently observed, the secondary criteria described here have evolved.

Blood lactate levels

In the absence of a true plateau in VO$_2$, a rise in blood lactate has been used to demonstrate a maximal effort.[1,12] As the workload continues to rise and the person nears a maximal effort, blood lactate levels increase as a result of accelerated glycolysis, an increase in the recruitment of fast-twitch muscle fibers, a reduction in liver blood flow, and/or an elevation in plasma epinephrine concentration.[1,2,12] These observations were first made by Astrand,[12] who noted that, in the absence of a visible plateau, lactate values along with a subject-reported stress level could be used to document the attainment of a true VO$_{2max}$.[2,12]

Although identifying a standard cutoff for blood lactate levels has been difficult, the values derived from Astrand's earliest studies suggesting a cutoff of 7.9 to 8.4 mmol/L[2,12] are still accepted today. Subsequent investigators have noted that 8 mM is a reasonable criterion value.[21,22,31,32] Cumming and Borysyk[31] and Stachenfeld[32] found that 78% of their test subjects achieved lactate levels of more than 8 mmol/L. Moreover, 8 mmol/L was the best criterion in terms of specificity and positive predictive value as compared with other secondary criteria.[32] Current standards vary, but a value of 8 mmol/L or greater appears to be consistent with research studies and is well accepted by researchers in general.

Respiratory exchange ratio

The respiratory quotient and the RER are both calculated as the ratio of the volume of carbon dioxide (CO$_2$) produced to the volume of oxygen (O$_2$) used, or VCO$_2$/VO$_2$. The respiratory quotient, which typically ranges between 0.7 and 1.0, is an indicator of metabolic fuel or substrate use in tissues; it must be calculated under resting or steady-state exercise conditions. A ratio of 0.7 is indicative of mixed fat use, whereas a ratio of 1.0 indicates the exclusive use of carbohydrates.[33] Thus, during low-intensity, steady-state exercise, the respiratory quotient and the RER are typically between 0.80 and 0.88, when fatty acids are the primary fuel.

As the intensity of the exercise increases and carbohydrates become the dominant or primary fuel, the respiratory quotient and the RER increase to between 0.9 and 1.0. Because the respiratory quotient reflects tissue substrate use, it cannot exceed 1.0. By contrast, the RER, which reflects the respiratory exchange of CO$_2$ and O$_2$, commonly exceeds 1.0 during strenuous exercise. During non–steady-state, strenuous exercise, the volume of CO$_2$ production rises as a result of hyperventilation and the increased buffering of blood lactic acid derived from skeletal muscles; thus, the RER no longer reflects substrate usage but rather high ventilation rates and blood lactate levels.[2,22,33]

Because RER reproducibly increases during exercise, it is considered a parameter that can document maximal effort. Issekutz,[33] who was the first to propose the use of RER as a criterion for VO$_{2max}$, noted that it must exceed 1.15. A higher value may suggest a more accurate assessment of VO$_{2max}$. The 1.15 value appears to be reasonable, although not all persons are able to achieve it. Studies have noted values of 1.00, 1.05, 1.10, and 1.13 as criterion for maximal performance,[21,22] but, at present, no clear consensus has been reached.

Age-predicted maximal heart rate

The widely recognized linear relationship between heart rate and VO_2 has encouraged the use of estimated maximal heart rate as a criterion for achieving VO_{2max}. Attaining a target percentage of the age-predicted maximal heart rate is one of the most widely recognized criterion.[21,22] Unfortunately, the traditional equation used to estimate maximal heart rate (220 − Age) was derived from approximately 10 different studies, and most tested subjects were less than 65 years of age.[34] Additionally, the equation was never validated for adults who were more than 60 years of age, and it may underestimate maximal heart rate among older adults by more than 20 beats per minute (bpm). For this reason, the American College of Sports Medicine and others have recommended that heart rate should not be used alone but rather in conjunction with other secondary criteria.[1,21,22] In 2001, Tanaka and colleagues[34] published a new equation for estimating age-predicted maximal heart rate (208 − 0.7 × Age), but whether it will prove to be less variable at all ages remains to be determined.

Borg scale or rating of perceived exertion

The Borg scale is the most widely used method for quantifying perceived exertion. It was designed to increase in a linear fashion as exercise intensity increased and to parallel the apparent linearity of VO_2 and heart rate with workload.[35,36] The original Borg scale ranges from 6 to 20, with each number anchored by a simple and understandable verbal expression. The specific numbers of the scale were intended to be a general representation of actual heart rate such that, when a person was exercising at 130 bpm, a perceived exertion of 13 should be reported. Similarly, if the perceived exertion were 19, a heart rate of around 190 would be expected. The scale was not intended to be exact but rather to be an aid in the interpretation of perceived exertion.

Studies have demonstrated a good correlation between the rating of perceived exhaustion and VO_2.[37,38] Eston and colleagues[37] obtained rating of perceived exhaustion values during a graded exercise test and reported a good correlation between heart rates and VO_2 when the reported rating of perceived exhaustion was between 13 and 17. An rating of perceived exhaustion value of 17 or greater should be accepted as meeting the criterion for achieving VO_{2max}.

Since the initial scale was developed, a variant scale using 0 to 10 as the numeric ratio has been proposed. This scale, which has not been widely accepted, is suitable for examining subjective symptoms, such as breathing difficulties.[35] However, the original 15-point rating of perceived exhaustion scale remains the standard for use as a criterion for VO_{2max}. **Table 41.3** provides the ratings for the original and new Borg scales.

Recommended criteria for testing

The criteria for VO_{2max} were initially established for a discontinuous treadmill test with 2.5% increases in grade. To date, the criteria for a plateau have not been redefined for other specific tests, but the 150 mL/min^{-1} increase continues to be used. Because the attainment of a true plateau is not an absolute prerequisite, some combination of secondary criterion may be preferable. The criteria presented in **Table 41.4** are offered as a guide, and it is suggested that at least two (and preferably three) of the four secondary criteria be met. If a true plateau is noted, then this alone would be

Table 41.3 The Original and New Borg Scales for the Rating of Perceived Exertion

	Original Scale		*Ratio Scale*
6	No exertion at all	0	Nothing at all
7	Extremely light	0.5	Very, very weak
8		1	Very weak
9	Very light	2	Weak
10		3	Moderate
11	Light	4	Somewhat strong
12		5	Strong
13	Somewhat hard	6	
14		7	Very strong
15	Hard (heavy)	8	
16		9	
17	Very hard	10	Very, very strong
18		*	Maximal
19	Extremely hard		
20	Maximal exertion		

sufficient for documenting VO_{2max}. If the criteria are not met, then the test results would be considered to reflect VO_{2peak}.

PREDICTING MAXIMAL AEROBIC POWER

Laboratory measurements are the only way to accurately quantify VO_{2max}. Nevertheless, this procedure does pose some limitations, such as the space and equipment available, the expertise of the technician, and the health condition of the subject. These factors have led to the development of multiple "prediction" tests that can be conducted in clinical, commercial, and/or outdoor arenas. Current prediction tests can be divided into three types, depending on the situation: (1) maximal effort prediction tests; (2) submaximal effort prediction tests; (3) nonexercise prediction tests. Understanding the advantages, disadvantages, and limitations of each test can be important for determining the most appropriate test to use for a given environment, a specific population, and a particular need.

Maximal prediction tests

Maximal prediction tests, although designed to reduce the problems associated with "true" VO_{2max} tests, do require the subject to perform a given protocol to maximal effort. Some aspect of performance is then used to predict VO_{2max} on the basis of the values collected from a sample study. Although cycling and arm ergometry can also be used, the most common maximal prediction

Table 41.4 Criteria for Documenting a Maximal Effort Test*

Increase in amount of oxygen consumed is less than 150 mL/min^{-1} or 2.1 mL/kg^{-1}/min^{-1} with a 2.5% grade increase

Blood lactate ≥8 mM

Respiratory exchange ration ≥1.15

Increase in heart rate to within ± 10 bpm for estimated maximal for age

Borg scale rating (Perceived Exertion)

*If the first criterion is not met, then at least three of the remaining four should be met.

tests involve running because the tests can be performed in a variety of ways: (1) run a required distance as quickly as possible; (2) run as far as possible within a set time; (3) perform a shuttle/track run; or (4) run on a treadmill and use the time run during a standard maximal treadmill test.

One of the best-known examples of a prediction test is the Cooper 12-minute field performance test.[39] Subjects are required to run on a level surface (usually a measured track) for 12 minutes, and the distance (D = meters covered) is recorded. Cooper found that VO_{2max} could be predicted on the basis of a regression equation with a considerable reliability (r = 0.897), and, as a result, this test has been used by many health professionals. Correlation coefficients (r) between this test and actual VO_{2max} measures are typically around 0.87 to 0.89.[39,40] The following regression equation can be used to estimated VO_{2max} from the distance covered in 12 minutes[1]:

$$VO_{2max}(\text{in } mL/kg^{-1}/min^{-1}) = D \times 0.02233 - 11.3$$

Another commonly used walking/running test is the 1.5-mile run: subjects must complete 1.5 miles in as short a time as possible. The time (T) required to complete the distance is used to predict the VO_{2max} of the individual.[1,40,41] Correlations between this test and actual VO_{2max} measures range from 0.73 to 0.92.[1,40,42] The equation for the 1.5-mile run (T = time) is as follows:

$$VO_{2max}(\text{in } mL/kg^{-1}/min^{-1}) = (483/T) + 3.5$$

Variations on the 1.5-mile run that include variables other than time have also been developed.[1,42,43] For example, the Rockport 1-mile walk test uses body weight, age, gender, and heart rate.[1,42,43] Fortunately, these tests yield essentially comparable values, and it is incumbent upon the tester as to which test will be easier and most feasible to conduct.

Another test that has been used with children and that is useful for runners in training include the shuttle/track run test. This test involves having the individual start running at a certain speed and cover a fixed distance (20 to 400 meters) multiple times for a specified time.[44-47] After each distance, the speed is increased or the time allotted to complete each shuttle is reduced. This reduction in time (or increase in speed) is continued until the subject can no longer keep pace. The speed achieved can then be used to predict the individual's VO_{2max} from regression formulas. Correlations between values obtained from these tests and actual measurements range from 0.83 to 0.98.[44-47] The formula for estimating VO_{2max} from the 20-meter shuttle[46] (S = speed in km/h) is as follows:

$$VO_{2max}(\text{in } mL/kg^{-1}/min^{-1}) = 5.857 \times S - 19.458$$

Another way to estimate VO_{2max} is by measuring the time that a person stays on a treadmill during a standardized maximal exercise test. For each of the major maximal effort treadmill protocols, regression equations to predict VO_{2max} from time have been developed. For example, for the Bruce protocol, regression equations with correlations between 0.86 and 0.92 have been developed for active men, sedentary men, men with coronary heart disease, and healthy adults.[3,15-17] One of the more general equations for predicting VO_{2max} from the time it takes to complete the Bruce protocol was reported by Pollack and all[16] (T = time in minutes) is as follows:

$$VO_{2max}(\text{in } mL/kg^{-1}/min^{-1}) = 4.326 \times T - 4.66$$

Regression equations, like that for the Bruce protocol, have also been developed with a reasonable degree of accuracy for the Balke and Ellestad protocols.[3,15-17] Such equations can be developed within any test facility from a particular standardized protocol. However, it must be remembered that prediction equations are typically specific for a population and should thus be used with caution when working with another group of individuals. Gender, age, race/ethnicity, and perceived functional ability may be important in such prediction equations.

One cycle ergometry test for predicting VO_{2max} uses maximal work rate (W), body weight (kg), and age (yr).[48] This progressive test uses a constant pedal rate (60 rpm) with incremental increases in work rate (15 W/min^{-1}) until the subject can no longer sustain 60 rpm. The equations used to predict VO_{2max} for men and women are as follows:

Men: VO_{2max} in $mL/min^{-1} = 10.51 \times W + 6.35 \times kg$
$- 10.49 \times yr + 519.3$
Women: VO_{2max} in $mL/min^{-1} = 9.39 \times W + 7.7 \times kg$
$- 5.88 \times yr + 136.7$

The above-mentioned tests are all examples of prediction tests that involve maximal effort. Each has a specific use, depending on the goals and the population of interest, but each also has the inherent problems and/or errors that come with any prediction equation.

Submaximal prediction tests

Individuals who are less fit, who are just starting an exercise program, or who are recovering from medical conditions often cannot tolerate a maximal effort. In response to the need to test such populations, submaximal prediction tests have evolved. These tests, which can be either constant load, steady-state, or progressive tests, have at least four advantages over maximal exertion tests, including the following: (1) they are physically less demanding; (2) they take less time to perform; (3) they are safer to conduct; and (4) they can often be performed with large groups. However, to accomplish this, some accuracy is sacrificed.

Most submaximal tests use heart rate for the estimation of VO_{2max}. Åstrand and Ryhming[49] were among the first to report a linear relationship between heart rate and VO_2, and, on the basis of this relationship, they recommended the use of heart rate to predict VO_{2max}. Thus, heart rate provides the theoretic basis behind most submaximal tests: when a subject works at submaximal levels, heart rate is used to predict a maximal performance either by extrapolation to maximal heart rate or from heart rate at a known power output.

The relationship between heart rate and workload is particularly important for progressive, submaximal cycle ergometry protocols. One typical progressive protocol uses four incremental, 2-minute stages, with the initial workload based on the body weight of the subject and his or her self-reported activity level.[50] For example, a 95-kg, physically active subject would complete the four-stage protocol by pedaling at 50 rpm for work rates of 50, 100, 150, and 200 W. The subject's heart rates at each work rate are plotted, and the line of best fit is determined: the point on the line that coincides with the estimated maximal heart rate would provide an estimate of VO_{2max} **(Figure 41.4).** Other progressive tests, such as those with stair steppers, treadmills, and seated rowing machines in which power outputs are known, have been used in a similar manner.[51,52]

Steady-state submaximal effort tests are also commonly used for the prediction of VO_{2max}. Treadmills, track walking/running, stair steppers, cycle ergometers, bench steps, rowing machines, and squat repetitions have all been used.[1,41-43,49,51,53-57] Although there are obvious differences among these tests, there are also similarities: each requires a steady-state work rate and a measure of the subject's heart rate upon the completion of the test. From there, heart rate may either be used alone to predict VO_{2max} from a

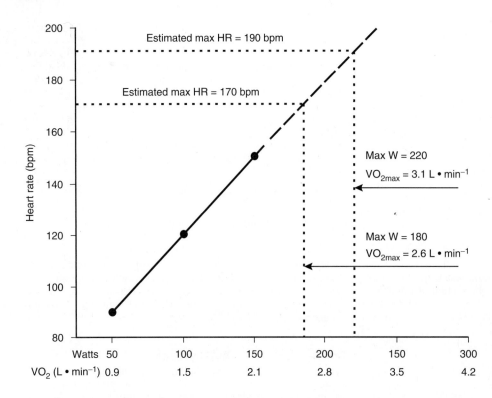

Figure 41.4 Extrapolation of maximal oxygen uptake from estimated maximal heart rate and work rate on a cycle ergometer test.

nomogram [49,57] or in conjunction with other variables, such as age, weight, gender, and other variables from a regression equation.[41-43,51,53-56] One of the first nomograms for predicting VO_{2max} from heart rate at submaximal workloads was derived by Åstrand and Ryhming from cycle, stair-stepping, and treadmill-running data.[49] Although their nomogram is still used, it has been modified for use with other populations.[57,58]

In addition to nomograms, regression equations have been developed to predict VO_{2max} on the basis of individuals walking/jogging on a treadmill at submaximal levels,[54] stepping up and down stairs for a set time,[41,53,56] jogging 1 mile on a track,[42] or by using heart rate and activity counts from triaxial accelerometry.[59] Swain and colleagues[60] proposed a new method for estimating VO_{2max} on the basis of VO_2 reserve and heart rate at the end of a 6-minute submaximal cycle ergometry protocol that elicited 65% to 75% of heart rate reserve; the correlation between measured and predicted VO_{2max} was 0.89. Petrella and colleagues[56] described a safe and simple self-paced step test that could be conducted in a doctor's office to predict aerobic fitness in adults who are more than 65 years of age; the correlation with VO_{2max} was reported to be 0.93 for females and 0.91 for males.

Lastly, although submaximal exercise prediction tests do serve an important role in estimating VO_{2max}, all of them are somewhat variable with regard to their accuracy because their predictive value relies on an accurate estimate of maximal heart rate. Unfortunately, there is inherent error in estimating maximal heart rate. As noted previously, maximal heart rate can be estimated as 220 − Age (as a low estimate) or 210 − 0.5 × Age (as a higher estimate). However, despite these equations, the true maximal heart rate can still be higher or lower by as much as 20 to 30 bpm (one standard deviation: 10 to 12), depending on the subject's age and training.[1,50] Moreover, these equations assume that the decline in maximal heart rate for a given age is uniform. Clearly, an erroneous estimate of maximal heart rate can markedly affect the estimate. For example, in Figure 41.4, if the estimated maximal heart rate were 190 bpm, then the estimated VO_{2max}

would be 3.1 L/min^{-1}, whereas, if the true maximal heart rate were only 170 bpm, then the VO_{2max} would be 2.6 L/min^{-1}. If a person weighed 70 kg and the values were normalized for body weight, then the relative VO_{2max} values would be 44.2 and 37.1 mL/kg^{-1}/min^{-1}, respectively, for the 190 and 170 maximal heart rates.

Nonexercise prediction tests

The value of cardiorespiratory fitness as an indicator of all-cause mortality has been reported,[61] and, as such, the need to estimate VO_{2max} noninvasively has increased. Prediction equations that use nonexercise parameters such as age, body composition, gender, level of physical activity, and the subject's perceived functional ability to walk, jog, or run given distances have emerged.[62,63] The reliability of these newer nonexercise prediction tests shows promise. For example, George and colleagues[63] found that a questionnaire-based regression equation predicted VO_{2max} with a correlation of 0.85 in a sample of physically active college students. Similarly, Heil and colleagues[62] developed an equation for men and women between the ages of 20 and 79 years and noted a correlation of 0.88 for the generalized equation (men and women together). The equation included percent body fat, age, gender, and an activity code derived from personal statements about activity level. Although this equation appears to be useful because of its wide age range, very few of the subjects were highly fit, and it may be best for a fairly sedentary population.

Malek and colleagues developed equations to predict VO_{2max} from age, height, weight, and exercise frequency, intensity, and duration in aerobically trained women[64] and men,[65] but these are population specific. Overall, nonexercise prediction tests have one distinct advantage: they can be administered without the requirements of equipment, supervision, or any inconvenience to the subject. However, as with all regression equations, generalization to a population other than the one from which it was derived remains questionable.

Table 41.5 Normative Values (Percentile) for Maximal Aerobic Power for Men and Women by Age*

Age in Years	Poor (≤10)	Fair (10-30)	Average (30-70)	Good (70-90)	Excellent (≥90)
Men					
20-29	<35	35-41	42-49	50-55	>55
30-39	<33	33-39	40-47	48-52	>52
40-49	<31	31-36	37-45	46-51	>51
50-59	<30	30-35	36-41	42-49	>49
≥60	<27	27-31	32-37	38-44	>44
Women					
20-29	<28	28-33	34-41	42-49	>49
30-39	<27	27-31	32-39	40-46	>46
40-49	<25	25-30	31-36	37-43	>43
50-59	<22	22-27	28-33	34-38	>38
≥60	<20	20-23	24-31	32-35	>35

*American College of Sports Medicine Aerobic Power Standards for men and women.

NORMATIVE AND POPULATION VALUES FOR MAXIMAL AEROBIC POWER

The American College of Sports Medicine has published normative values for VO_{2max} by age and gender so that individual values can be classified to into one of five groups: (1) poor (well below average); (2) fair (below average); (3) average; (4) good (above average); and (5) excellent (well above average)[1] **(Table 41.5).** The importance of VO_{2max} cannot be overemphasized with respect to health: low aerobic power or low cardiovascular fitness is associated with higher morbidity and mortality for all causes.[61] Data from 1999 to 2000 and 2001 to 2002 National Health and Nutrition Examination Surveys showed that approximately 11.3% of non-Hispanic whites and 22.9% of non-Hispanic blacks between 20 and 49 years of age had estimated VO_{2max} values that were in the American College of Sports Medicine's poor category (below 30 mL/kg^{-1}/min^{-1}).[66] Non-Hispanic black women had the lowest VO_{2max} values such that 30.9% were in the poor category.[66] Of note is the finding that 33.6% of adolescents have poor aerobic fitness.[67] Thus, despite the importance of maximal aerobic power, the distribution of estimated VO_{2max} values from the National Health and Nutrition Examination Surveys indicates low fitness among most of the US population.

CONCLUSION

In summary, maximal aerobic power or VO_{2max} is an extremely valuable measure of cardiovascular and pulmonary function, work capacity, and endurance performance. It can be directly measured using a standardized maximal treadmill or cycle ergometer protocol, or it can be predicted using a maximal or submaximal protocol or regression equation. A variety of protocols for predicting VO_{2max} are readily available, and many are extremely easy to administer. All tests have certain advantages and limitations that should be considered by the test administrator. Care must be taken to only use a prediction equation on a population that is comparable in terms of age, gender, ethnicity, and fitness level because each prediction equation was based on results derived from a particular population and thus it may not apply to a population with different characteristics.

REFERENCES

1. Whaley MH, Brubarker PH, Otto RM (eds): ACSM's Guidelines for Exercise Testing and Prescription, 7th ed. Baltimore, Lippincott Williams & Wilkins, 2006.
2. Astrand PO, Rodahl K. Textbook of Work Physiology: Physiological Bases of Exercise, 4th ed. Windsor, Canada, Human Kinetics, 2003.
3. Bruce RA, Kusumi F, Hosmer D: Maximal oxygen intake and nomographic assessment of functional aerobic impairment in cardiovascular disease. Am Heart J 1973;85(4):546-562.
4. Taylor HL, Buskirk E, Henschel A: Maximal oxygen intake as an objective measure of cardio-respiratory performance. J Appl Physiol 1955;8(1):73-80.
5. Astrand PO, Saltin B: Maximal oxygen uptake and heart rate in various types of muscular activity. J Appl Physiol 1961;16:977-981.
6. Bergh U, Kanstrup IL, Ekblom B: Maximal oxygen uptake during exercise with various combinations of arm and leg work. J Appl Physiol 1976;41(2):191-196.
7. Brahler CJ, Blank SE: VersaClimbing elicits higher VO2max than does treadmill running or rowing ergometry. Med Sci Sports Exerc 1995;27(2):249-254.
8. Gleser MA, Horstman DH, Mello RP: The effect on Vo2 max of adding arm work to maximal leg work. Med Sci Sports 1974;6(2):104-107.
9. Kasch FW, Phillips WH, Ross WD, et al: A comparison of maximal oxygen uptake by treadmill and step-test procedures. J Appl Physiol 1966;21(4):1387-1388.
10. Nagle FJ, Richie JP, Giese MD: VO2max responses in separate and combined arm and leg air-braked ergometer exercise. Med Sci Sports Exerc 1984;16(6):563-566.
11. Secher NH, Ruberg-Larsen N, Binkhorst RA, et al: Maximal oxygen uptake during arm cranking and combined arm plus leg exercise. J Appl Physiol 1974;36(5):515-518.
12. Astrand PO: Quantification of exercise capability and evaluation of physical capacity in man. Prog Cardiovasc Dis 1976;19(1):51-67.
13. Balke B, Ware RW: An experimental study of physical fitness of Air Force personnel. U S Armed Forces Med J 1959;10(6):875-888.
14. Ellestad MH, Allen W, Wan MC, et al: Maximal treadmill stress testing for cardiovascular evaluation. Circulation 1969;39(4):517-522.
15. Froelicher VF Jr, Brammell H, Davis G, et al: A comparison of three maximal treadmill exercise protocols. J Appl Physiol 1974;36(6):720-725.
16. Pollock ML, Bohannon RL, Cooper KH, et al: A comparative analysis of four protocols for maximal treadmill stress testing. Am Heart J 1976;92(1):39-46.
17. Pollock ML, Foster C, Schmidt D, et al: Comparative analysis of physiologic responses to three different maximal graded exercise test protocols in healthy women. Am Heart J 1982;103(3):363-373.
18. Kyle SB, Smoak BL, Douglass LW, et al: Variability of responses across training levels to maximal treadmill exercise. J Appl Physiol 1989;67(1):160-165.
19. Hansen JE, Casaburi R, Cooper DM, et al: Oxygen uptake as related to work rate increment during cycle ergometer exercise. Eur J Appl Physiol Occup Physiol 1988;57(2):140-145.
20. Williams CA, Ratel S, Armstrong N: Achievement of peak VO2 during a 90-s maximal intensity cycle sprint in adolescents. Can J Appl Physiol 2005;30(2):157-171.
21. Duncan GE, Howley ET, Johnson BN: Applicability of VO2max criteria: discontinuous versus continuous protocols. Med Sci Sports Exerc 1997;29(2):273-278.
22. Howley ET, Bassett DR Jr, Welch HG: Criteria for maximal oxygen uptake: review and commentary. Med Sci Sports Exerc 1995;27(9):1292-1301.
23. Noakes TD: Maximal oxygen uptake: "classical" versus "contemporary" viewpoints: a rebuttal. Med Sci Sports Exerc 1998;30(9):1381-1398.
24. Noakes TD: Implications of exercise testing for prediction of athletic performance: a contemporary perspective. Med Sci Sports Exerc 1988;20(4):319-330.
25. St Clair Gibson A, Lambert MI, Hawley JA, et al: Measurement of maximal oxygen uptake from two different laboratory protocols in runners and squash players. Med Sci Sports Exerc 1999;31(8):1226-1229.
26. Day JR, Rossiter HB, Coats EM, et al: The maximally attainable VO2 during exercise in humans: the peak vs. maximum issue. J Appl Physiol 2003;95(5):1901-1907.
27. Gürsel Y, Sonel B, Gok H, et al: The peak oxygen uptake of healthy Turkish children with reference to age and sex: a pilot study. Turk J Pediatr 2004;46(1):38-43.
28. Rivera-Brown AM, Alvarez M, Rodriguez-Santana JR, et al: Anaerobic power and achievement of VO2 plateau in pre-pubertal boys. Int J Sports Med 2001;22(2):111-115.
29. Myers J, Walsh D, Sullivan M, et al: Effect of sampling on variability and plateau in oxygen uptake. J Appl Physiol 1990;68(1):404-410.
30. Fielding RA, Frontera WR, Hughes VA, et al: The reproducibility of the Bruce protocol exercise test for the determination of aerobic capacity in older women. Med Sci Sports Exerc 1997;29(8):1109-1113.
31. Cumming GR, Borysyk LM: Criteria for maximum oxygen uptake in men over 40 in a population survey. Med Sci Sports 1972;4(1):18-22.
32. Stachenfeld NS, Eskenazi M, Gleim GW, et al: Predictive accuracy of criteria used to assess maximal oxygen consumption. Am Heart J 1992;123(4 Pt 1):922-925.
33. Issekutz BJ, Birkhead NC, Rodahl K: Use of respiratory quotients in assessment of aerobic work capacity. J Appl Physiol 1962;17(1):47-50.
34. Tanaka H, Seals DR, Monahan KD, et al: Regular aerobic exercise and the age-related increase in carotid artery intima-media thickness in healthy men. J Appl Physiol 2002;92(4):1458-1464.

35. Borg GA: Psychophysical bases of perceived exertion. Med Sci Sports Exerc 1982;14(5):377-381.

36. Borg GA, Noble B: Perceived exertion. In Wilmore J (ed): Exercise and Sport Science Reviews. New York, Academic Press, 1974, pp 131-153.

37. Eston RG, Davies BL, Williams JG: Use of perceived effort ratings to control exercise intensity in young healthy adults. Eur J Appl Physiol Occup Physiol 1987;56(2):222-224.

38. Glass SC, Knowlton RG, Becque MD: Accuracy of RPE from graded exercise to establish exercise training intensity. Med Sci Sports Exerc 1992;24(11):1303-1307.

39. Cooper KH: A means of assessing maximal oxygen intake. Correlation between field and treadmill testing. JAMA 1968;203(3):201-204.

40. McNaughton L, Hall P, Cooley D: Validation of several methods of estimating maximal oxygen uptake in young men. Percept Mot Skills 1998;87(2):575-584.

41. Zwiren LD, Freedson PS, Ward A, et al: Estimation of VO2max: a comparative analysis of five exercise tests. Res Q Exerc Sport 1991;62(1):73-78.

42. George JD, Vehrs PR, Allsen PE, et al: VO2max estimation from a submaximal 1-mile track jog for fit college-age individuals. Med Sci Sports Exerc 1993;25(3):401-406.

43. Kline GM, Porcari JP, Hintermeister R, et al: Estimation of VO2max from a one-mile track walk, gender, age, and body weight. Med Sci Sports Exerc 1987;19(3):253-259.

44. Berthoin S, Pelayo P, Lensel-Corbeil G, et al: Comparison of maximal aerobic speed as assessed with laboratory and field measurements in moderately trained subjects. Int J Sports Med 1996;17(7):525-529.

45. Leger L, Boucher R: An indirect continuous running multistage field test: the Universite de Montreal track test. Can J Appl Sport Sci 1980;5(2):77-84.

46. Leger LA, Lambert J: A maximal multistage 20-m shuttle run test to predict VO2 max. Eur J Appl Physiol Occup Physiol 1982;49(1):1-12.

47. Naughton LM, Cooley D, Kearney V, et al: A comparison of two different shuttle run tests for the estimation of VO2max. J Sports Med Phys Fitness 1996;36(2):85-89.

48. Storer TW, Davis JA, Caiozzo VJ: Accurate prediction of VO2max in cycle ergometry. Med Sci Sports Exerc 1990;22(5):704-712.

49. Astrand PO, Ryhming I: A nomogram for calculation of aerobic capacity (physical fitness) from pulse rate during sub-maximal work. J Appl Physiol 1954;7(2):218-221.

50. Lockwood PA, Yoder JE, Deuster PA: Comparison and cross-validation of cycle ergometry estimates of VO2max. Med Sci Sports Exerc 1997;29(11):1513-1520.

51. Holland G, Hoffman J, Vincent W: Treadmill vs. steptreadmill ergometry. Phys Sportsmed 1990;18:79-85.

52. Beneke R: Anaerobic threshold, individual anaerobic threshold, and maximal lactate steady state in rowing. Med Sci Sports Exerc 1995;27(6):863-867.

53. Roy JL, Smith JF, Bishop PA, et al: Prediction of maximal VO2 from a submaximal StairMaster test in young women. J Strength Cond Res 2004;18(1):92-96.

54. Ebbeling CB, Ward A, Puleo EM, et al: Development of a single-stage submaximal treadmill walking test. Med Sci Sports Exerc 1991;23(8):966-973.

55. Inoue Y, Nakao M: Prediction of maximal oxygen uptake by squat test in men and women. Kobe J Med Sci 1996;42(2):119-129.

56. Petrella RJ, Koval JJ, Cunningham DA, et al: A self-paced step test to predict aerobic fitness in older adults in the primary care clinic. J Am Geriatr Soc 2001;49(5):632-638.

57. Teraslinna P, Ismail AH, MacLeod DF: Nomogram by Astrand and Ryhming as a predictor of maximum oxygen intake. J Appl Physiol 1966;21(2):513-515.

58. Macsween A: The reliability and validity of the Astrand nomogram and linear extrapolation for deriving VO2max from submaximal exercise data. J Sports Med Phys Fitness 2001;41(3):312-317.

59. Plasqui G, Westerterp KR: Accelerometry and heart rate as a measure of physical fitness: proof of concept. Med Sci Sports Exerc 2005;37(5):872-876.

60. Swain DP, Parrott JA, Bennett AR, et al: Validation of a new method for estimating VO2max based on VO2 reserve. Med Sci Sports Exerc 2004;36(8):1421-1426.

61. Blair SN, Kohl HW 3rd, Paffenbarger RS Jr, et al: Physical fitness and all-cause mortality. A prospective study of healthy men and women 1989;262(17):2395-2401.

62. Heil DP, Freedson PS, Ahlquist LE, et al: Nonexercise regression models to estimate peak oxygen consumption. Med Sci Sports Exerc 1995;27(4):599-606.

63. George JD, Stone WJ, Burkett LN: Non-exercise VO2max estimation for physically active college students. Med Sci Sports Exerc 1997;29(3):415-423.

64. Malek MH, Housh TJ, Berger DE, et al: A new nonexercise-based VO2(max) equation for aerobically trained females. Med Sci Sports Exerc 2004;36(10):1804-1810.

65. Malek MH, Housh TJ, Berger DE, et al: A new non-exercise-based Vo(2)max prediction equation for aerobically trained men. J Strength Cond Res 2005;19(3):559-565.

66. Duncan GE, Li SM, Zhou XH: Cardiovascular fitness among U.S. adults: NHANES 1999-2000 and 2001-2002. Med Sci Sports Exerc 2005;37(8):1324-1328.

67. Carnethon MR, Gulati M, Greenland P: Prevalence and cardiovascular disease correlates of low cardiorespiratory fitness in adolescents and adults. JAMA 2005;294(23):2981-2988.

CHAPTER 42

Exercise-Induced Asthma Testing

Rochelle M. Nolte, MD, and Christopher J. Lettieri, MD

KEY POINTS

- Self-reported symptoms are not reliable for identifying exercise-induced asthma.
- The International Olympic Committee Medical Commission and the United States Anti-Doping Agency require that all athletes who will use a β-agonist before competition must have objective evidence of exercise-induced asthma.
- Although a pharmacologic challenge such as methacholine can diagnose exercise-induced asthma in some instances, a negative test cannot definitively rule out asthma, and a physiologic bronchoprovocative test should be performed if an athlete is having symptoms.
- False negatives may occur if exercise-induced asthma screening is done by a physiologic challenge with inadequate exercise or environmental stress. This may lead to the need for repeat testing or for referral for methacholine challenge testing in an athlete with symptoms but with a negative test result.
- False positives can occur with all bronchoprovocative testing, and any diagnosis that is in doubt should be confirmed by another means.

INTRODUCTION

Exercise-induced asthma (EIA) is characterized by symptoms of coughing, wheezing, shortness of breath, and/or chest tightness either during or after exercise[1] **(Table 42.1).** EIA is also associated with airway obstruction as evidenced by a drop in forced expiratory volume in 1 second (FEV_1). There are two commonly used terms: *EIA* and *exercise-induced bronchospasm*.[1] In patients with underlying asthma, it is thought that the mechanism of action is an inflammatory process, and occasionally the term *EIA* is used to refer to an exacerbation in a patient with persistent asthma. The term *exercise-induced bronchospasm* is sometimes used to refer to bronchial obstruction as a result of exercise in a person who does not have persistent asthma, and the mechanism may be

The views expressed in this chapter are those of the authors and are not to be interpreted as the views of the US Army, the US Coast Guard, or the US Public Health Service.

something other than an inflammatory process.[1] For the purposes of this chapter, EIA will refer to both categories **(Box 42.1).**

The overall incidence of EIA is estimated to be 12% to 15% (LOE: B).[2] It is estimated that 90% of patients with asthma have EIA and that 35% to 40% of patients with allergic rhinitis have EIA. The remainder of the general population is estimated to have an incidence of EIA that ranges from 3% to 16%.[2,3] The estimated prevalence of EIA in some selected populations is listed in **Table 42.2.**

Patients with previously diagnosed persistent asthma appear to have chronic inflammatory changes that may require daily treatment with inhaled corticosteroids. Exercise may initiate a cascade of inflammatory events that leads to bronchoconstriction in patients with underlying asthma. Patients with underlying asthma can also have an exacerbation precipitated by chemical irritants (e.g., chlorine in pools, the high levels of nitrogen dioxide in ice arenas[4,5]). Patients with persistent asthma also seem to have more severe exacerbations than individuals who only have exercise-induced symptoms. The rare fatal asthma exacerbations associated with exercise often involve excessive mucus production and mucus plugging in patients with underlying persistent asthma.[6] Patients with previously diagnosed persistent asthma may also be more prone to emotional stimuli, and they may have an exacerbation that is precipitated by competition anxiety.[6]

Patients who do not have persistent asthma but who only have exercise-induced symptoms appear to be more at risk of developing EIA with exposure to cold or dry air. The precise mechanism of EIA is not exactly known, but it is postulated that the high minute ventilation associated with aerobic activity may dry and cool the airways of the athletes or possibly lead to the release of mediators that cause bronchoconstriction. Another theory is that the rewarming of the airways after exercise leads to the dilatation of the small vessels that wrap around the bronchial tree and that the influx of warm blood leads to fluid exudation from the blood vessels into the submucosa of the airway wall, which leads to mediator release with subsequent bronchoconstriction. There is also some evidence that inflammation may be involved, but it does not appear to be as extensive in patients with EIA as it is in patients with chronic asthma.[3]

Exercise typically results in airway dilation, even among asthmatics. As such, dyspnea that occurs shortly after the onset of exercise is unlikely to result from bronchoconstriction. In individuals with an early onset of dyspnea, causes other than asthma, such as deconditioning and cardiac disease, should be considered. In susceptible individuals, exercise may result in transient

Table 42.1 Symptoms of Exercise-Induced Asthma

Cough during or after exercise

Wheezing during or after exercise

Shortness of breath during or after exercise

Chest tightness during or after exercise

Congestion or excessive mucus production during or after exercise

Excessive fatigue with training

Feeling "out of shape" for the current level of training

Chest pain or headache (atypical symptoms)

Abdominal pain, cramps, or nausea (atypical symptoms)

Table 42.2 Prevalence of Exercise-Induced Asthma in Selected Populations[10]

Patients with chronic asthma	90%
Patients with allergic rhinitis	35% to 40%
Patients without asthma or allergic rhinitis	3% to 16%
1984 US Olympic Team	11%
1996 US Summer Olympic Team	20%
1998 US Winter Olympic Team	23%
Basketball players	12%
Finnish runners	9%
Figure skaters	30% to 35%
Cross-country skiers	55%

bronchospasm and precipitate asthma symptoms. Bronchospasms typically peak 5 to 10 minutes after stopping exercise. The diagnosis should be considered for a patient with an exercise limitation who reports cough, shortness of breath, wheezing, and chest discomfort during or shortly after exercise.

In May 2001, the International Olympic Committee Medical Commission (IOC-MC) held a workshop to examine asthma and the use of β-agonists. The workshop concluded the following:

- At recent Olympic Games, there had been a large increase in the number of athletes who notified officials of their need to inhale a β-agonist.
- Some athletes may have been misdiagnosed and may not have had EIA.
- There is no scientific evidence to confirm that inhaled β-agonists enhance performance in the doses that are required to inhibit EIA.

Box 42.1: Checklist Box

- Take a thorough history.
- Perform a thorough physical examination.
- Follow up any abnormalities that are found on cardiac or pulmonary examination.
- Follow up any treatment of any evidence of allergies or respiratory infections.
- Perform spirometry.
- If spirometry at rest is abnormal, evaluate and treat the condition as persistent asthma.
- If spirometry at rest is normal, perform challenge testing.
- Instruct the patient about medications to be withheld and to avoid exercise or caffeine on the day of testing.
- Ensure that a portable spirometer is ready to be taken to the field, that it has an appropriate power source, and that it is set up to record and store prechallenge and (numerous) postchallenge trials
- Ensure that mouthpieces are available to take to the field or that an appropriate cleaning technique can be performed.
- Ensure that a nose clip is ready to be taken to the field.
- Ensure that an inhaled bronchodilator is available for treating clinically significant dyspnea.
- Ensure that everything that is needed for data collection is in place and working correctly. Even if it is, have a backup plan (e.g., hand copying all of the results on the display screen while you are in the field in case there is a glitch in the system when you get back to the office to download the results).

- A skewed distribution of notifications of β-agonist use by sport was observed, with a higher prevalence in endurance sports.
- The geographic distribution of notifications of inhaled β-agonists was markedly skewed, but it correlated well with the reported prevalence of asthma symptoms in the corresponding countries.
- There is some evidence that the daily use of an inhaled β-agonist may result in tolerance to the medication.
- Inhaled corticosteroids may be underused among the athletes who are notifying officials of the use of β-agonists.
- Eucapnic voluntary hyperventilation (EVH) was considered to be the optimal laboratory-based challenge to confirm that an athlete has EIA.
- When they are administered systemically, β-agonists do have anabolic effects.[7]

For the 2002 Olympic Games in Salt Lake City, Utah, and for all Olympic Games since, the IOC-MC has required objective evidence of EIA for all athletes planning to use an inhaled β-agonist before competition.[8] A note from a treating physician stating that the athlete has EIA is no longer acceptable because a report of symptoms has not been found to be a reliable way to make the diagnosis of EIA.[1,9] The IOC-MC requires testing with either a bronchodilator test that demonstrates the reversibility of bronchoconstriction with the administration of an inhaled bronchodilator measured with spirometry or with a bronchial provocation test for athletes who only have symptoms with exercise.

The acceptable bronchial provocation tests must all demonstrate a fall in FEV_1. Peak expiratory flow measurements (such as those commonly obtained in primary care clinics with a peak flow meter) are unacceptable. The acceptable bronchial provocation tests include EVH, the inhalation of a hypertonic aerosol such as saline or mannitol, methacholine challenge, and an exercise challenge test, either in the laboratory or in the field.[10,11]

The thresholds that define a positive bronchial provocation test are arbitrarily determined. **Table 42.3** lists different values that are used by various organizations to diagnose EIA. Typically, a challenge is done by measuring a baseline FEV_1 and then measuring the decrease in FEV_1 after the challenge. Setting the threshold for diagnosis at a lower decrement increases the sensitivity of the test but decreases the specificity. Setting the threshold for diagnosis at a higher decrement increases specificity but decreases sensitivity.

Eliasson and colleagues[12] evaluated the sensitivity and specificity of four techniques: indoor exercise challenge on a cycle ergometer, methacholine challenge, EVH with dry gas, and EVH with cold gas. The study looked at 20 patients without known chronic asthma who presented with symptoms of EIA. They were compared with 20 controls in the randomized crossover study. The threshold for each of the tests that yielded 100% specificity was a drop in FEV_1 of 9% for indoor exercise challenge (which led to a

Table 42.3 Pulmonary Function Testing Criteria for the Diagnosis of Asthma[7,12-17]

	Bronchodilator Response	Exercise Testing	Methacholine Challenge	Eucapnic Voluntary Hyperventilation
American Thoracic Society	12% and 200 cc improvement in FEV_1 or FVC	10% decrease in FEV_1 after exercise	20% decrease in FEV_1 at 8 mg/mL	12% decrease in FEV_1 after 6 minutes of hyperpnea in dry air
International Olympic Committee Medical Commission	12% improvement in FEV_1	10% decrease in FEV_1 after exercise	20% decrease in FEV_1 at 4 mg/mL	10% decrease in FEV_1 after 6 minutes of hyperpnea in dry air
US Army	15% improvement in FEV_1	15% decrease in FEV_1 after exercise	20% decrease in FEV_1 at 4 mg/mL	15% decrease in FEV_1 after 6 minutes of hyperpnea in dry air
US Air Force	15% improvement in FEV_1	None stated	None stated	None stated
US Navy/Marines	None stated	None stated	None stated	None stated
US Coast Guard	None stated	None stated	None stated	None stated

FEV_1, forced expiratory volume in 1 second; FVC, forced vital capacity.

sensitivity of only 10%); 15% for methacholine challenge (which was 55% sensitive); 11% for dry gas EVH (with 50% sensitivity); and 12% for cold gas EVH (with 35% sensitivity). They determined that the indoor exercise challenge was not sensitive enough to be used to rule out EIA. For the other tests, thresholds that were thought to give the best ratio of specificity and sensitivity were 12% for methacholine challenge (95% specific and 65% sensitive); 5% for dry gas EVH (80% specific and 75% sensitive); and 5% for cold gas EVH (90% specific and 80% sensitive).[12]

Bronchodilator testing

Bronchodilator testing is done by having the patient perform baseline spirometry (when off of caffeine and all medications that may affect the test and at least 4 hours after any physical exercise), administering an inhaled bronchodilator (e.g., a β_2-agonist), and then repeating the spirometry. The reversibility of airflow obstruction is established by an increase in FEV_1 or forced vital capacity (for specific levels, see the Interpretations section later in this chapter).

Although a bronchodilator challenge can be used as evidence of EIA, it can give a false-negative result in some athletes. Athletes who only have symptoms after exercise may not show any increase in FEV_1 after administration of a β_2-agonist at rest. If an athlete who has shown no increase in FEV_1 with a bronchodilator challenge is complaining of symptoms of EIA, an exercise challenge is recommended.

Methacholine challenge testing

A fall in FEV_1 of 20% or more from baseline is considered to be a positive methacholine challenge.[7] As with the bronchodilator testing, a negative result with a methacholine challenge does not necessarily exclude EIA, and an alternate provocative test should be used if an athlete has symptoms. Although the methacholine challenge test is a commonly used bronchoprovocative test for the diagnosis of asthma, it is thought that some athletes with EIA may have a trigger that is precipitated by intense physical activity but not by a pharmacologic challenge.

Although methacholine challenge testing is currently the most common airway challenge performed in the United States, it is not widely available in most primary care offices, and it may require referral to a pulmonologist or to a large clinic that has the facilities to perform full pulmonary function testing.

Eucapnic voluntary hyperventilation testing

EVH is considered positive when a fall in FEV_1 of 10% or more is recorded after a 6-minute period of hyperpnea in dry air.[7]

EVH testing requires the subject to hyperventilate dry air containing 5% carbon dioxide at room temperature for 6 minutes at a target ventilation of 30 times the subject's FEV_1.[11] EVH can induce EIA symptoms in athletes by having them breathing at a ventilation rate that is equivalent to or higher than most forms of exercise.[11] As with exercise, a variety of mediators are likely to be involved in the response. EVH is suggested as an alternative to exercise challenge testing. It is not as commonly performed as a methacholine challenge, and it may require referral to a large pulmonary clinic or a tertiary care medical center for testing, but the IOC-MC considers it to be the optimal laboratory-based challenge to confirm that an athlete has EIA.[7]

Exercise challenge testing (laboratory based)

The response to an exercise challenge is considered abnormal or suggestive of EIA when there is a fall in FEV_1 of 10% or more as compared with baseline during the first 30 minutes after exercise. A fall in FEV_1 of 15% is considered highly suggestive and specific for EIA. Exercise challenge testing done in a laboratory usually consists of spirometry or pulmonary function testing before and after (usually immediately after and then 5, 10, 15, 20, and 30 minutes after exercise) a standard exercise protocol on either a treadmill or a cycle ergometer. Having patients do their exercise challenge test in a laboratory setting ensures that the temperature, humidity, and level of exertion can all be monitored and controlled, but there are some drawbacks. False-negative results are possible in a laboratory setting for patients who may have symptoms only at high levels of exertion during competition or intense training that cannot be simulated in the laboratory or for patients who have an environmental precipitant that is present while they are competing or training but not in the laboratory.

Exercise challenge testing (sport specific/field based)

A sport-specific exercise challenge is another option, and it can be a more sensitive tool to diagnose EIA in some athletes, especially if an environmental trigger from the training environment is contributing to their symptoms. An exercise challenge test in the field uses the same criteria for fall in FEV_1 to make the diagnosis of EIA as a laboratory-based challenge test. A field-based exercise challenge is done by having the athlete perform his or her sport at the level of intensity and in the conditions in which he or she has experienced symptoms. The test is done by taking a portable spirometer to the athlete's area of training or competition and having the athlete perform spirometry before competing or training and then repeating the spirometry after competition (or simulated competition). The athlete should be exercising at a level of intensity that is high enough to precipitate symptoms. Having the athlete in his or her usual training environment—whether it is an indoor pool, an ice arena, or an outdoor ski area—seems to increase the sensitivity, but conditions such as temperature or humidity outside and chlorine or nitrogen dioxide levels inside cannot always be predicted or controlled. As such, the test may need to be repeated.

EVALUATION

Diagnosing EIA starts with a thorough history from the athlete regarding his or her symptoms. History taking should focus on when the athlete has symptoms and what the relationship of those symptoms is to exercise. Any symptoms that are not related to exercise should be noted (e.g., nocturnal symptoms), as should any seasonal variation. The age at which the athlete first noted symptoms is important, as is any history of any allergic symptoms, aspirin allergy, nasal polyposis, or eczema. Any specific triggers (e.g., temperature, dry air, specific indoor pools or arenas) should also be noted. A family history of asthma, atopic dermatitis, or other related problems should be asked about. When distinguishing EIA from other causes of shortness of breath while exercising, the history can be quite helpful. A lack of physical fitness may lead to shortness of breath that progresses through the exercise session but that improves with the cessation of activity. However, the symptoms of EIA generally persist after the cessation of exercise. Evaluating for risk factors of vocal cord dysfunction is important, especially in patients who appear to have EIA that is refractory to treatment.

A thorough physical examination should be performed. Although the examination will usually be normal, evaluating for signs of allergies and nasal polyps as well as for cardiac or pulmonary abnormalities is important. Auscultation of the heart for murmurs, gallops, or thrills; of the glottis for an inspiratory wheeze; and of the lungs for abnormal sounds or prolonged expiration should be performed.

After a thorough history and physical examination, spirometry should be performed. If spirometry at rest shows baseline obstruction, a trial of reversibility with an inhaled bronchodilator is indicated. If the pattern is reversible (and the patient is not having an acute exacerbation or trigger), then the patient has persistent asthma, and he or she should have all of his or her symptoms addressed and be evaluated for daily treatment with inhaled corticosteroids. If spirometry at rest is normal, the athlete may still have EIA, and some challenge testing should be performed **(Boxes 42.2 and 42.3).**

For a list of tests that are commonly used to diagnose EIA in the United States, see **Table 42.4.** There are many portable and handheld spirometers available today. Any spirometer used should meet the standards of the American Thoracic Society. The ideal spirometer for field testing will be durable, easily transported, electrically safe, able to work at different temperatures and humidity levels, hygienic, accurate, able to hold a record of tracings until they can be downloaded and printed, and easy to use.

If possible, having the athlete complete a trial of spirometry in the office before proceeding with field testing is helpful because this gives the athlete a chance to be coached and to learn how to do the spirometry correctly, and it increases the chances of having an accurate test when in the field.

The patient should be instructed to withhold some medications before the exercise challenge test. Leukotriene antagonists should be withheld for 4 days. Long-acting bronchodilators,

---

Box 42.2: Indications for Testing for Exercise-Induced Asthma

- Any typical symptoms of exercise-induced asthma
- Atypical symptoms that may be related to exercise-induced asthma, such as fatigue, muscle cramps, abdominal pain, sore throat, or feeling "out of shape" for the current level of training and conditioning
- To confirm a suspected diagnosis of exercise-induced asthma
- To provide objective evidence of exercise-induced asthma before the use of a bronchodilator during competition in any event in accordance with International Olympic Committee or United States Olympic Committee guidelines
- To evaluate athletes who exercise in high-risk environments (e.g., cold dry air, ice arenas, indoor pools)
- To monitor the effectiveness of treatment

---

antihistamines, and nedocromil should be withheld for 2 days. Short-acting bronchodilators should be withheld for 8 hours. No inhaled corticosteroids or cromolyn should be used on the day of testing (some recommend withholding inhaled corticosteroids for 1 week before testing). On the day of the test, the patient should avoid caffeine, and he or she should not exercise before reporting for the testing session.

The athlete should perform spirometry (with the results of the best of three trials used) before the exercise session. If the testing is being done at an actual competition, the pretest spirometry should be done before any warm up exercises are done. The athlete should proceed with his or her normal warm up routine and competition.

It has been shown that an exercise session does not need to be longer than about 6 to 8 minutes to produce symptoms as long as

---

Box 42.3: Contraindications for Testing for Exercise-Induced Asthma

- Acute illness that may affect test results
- Exercise during the previous 4 hours
- Hemoptysis
- Nausea and vomiting
- Acute vertigo
- Recent pneumothorax
- Recent thoracic surgery
- Known aortic aneurysm
- Recent abdominal surgery
- Recent eye surgery
- Recent myocardial infarction or unstable angina
- Stroke within the previous 3 months
- Pregnancy
- Uncontrolled hypertension (systolic blood pressure >200 mm Hg or diastolic blood pressure >100 mm Hg)
- The patient has not correctly followed instructions for withholding medications
- The patient is unwilling to cooperate with testing (the test is effort dependent)

Table 42.4 Tests Currently Used for the Diagnosis of Exercise-Induced Asthma in the United States

Bronchodilator challenge testing

Methacholine challenge testing

Eucapnic voluntary hyperventilation

Laboratory-based exercise challenge testing

Sport-specific field-based exercise challenge testing

the exercise is done at high intensity. The exercise session should mimic the athlete's competition environment (or the training environment, if that is where the symptoms are occurring) as closely as possible. If it is logistically possible, the exercise challenge can be done at an actual competition. In some cases, this could be an exercise session of more than an hour for some endurance events, or it may be less than a minute long for some winter sports (e.g., downhill skiing, speed skating).

After the exercise session, repeat spirometry should be done at intervals 5, 10, 15, 20, and 30 minutes after exercise, with three trials performed at each interval. There are many different proposed intervals for the after-exercise testing, from every 3 minutes starting at 2 minutes after exercise to every 10 minutes for 30 minutes. Most recommended regimens involve intervals of 5 to 10 minutes for the 30 minutes after exercise. The postexercise spirometry may be discontinued if the FEV_1 has hit a nadir and returned to baseline on subsequent testing. For example, if the trial at 10 minutes was 20% below baseline but the trials at 15 and 20 minutes had improved and returned to the pre-exercise baseline, then the 30-minute postexercise test can be skipped. Care should be taken to avoid having the intervals be so frequent or numerous that the athlete tires and is not capable of giving an adequate effort to produce accurate results.

An inhaled bronchodilator should be available to be administered at any time to reverse clinically significant dyspnea or to treat a patient who has not recovered to within 10% of baseline by the end of the testing session.

TECHNIQUES AND EQUIPMENT

- Evaluate the patient for contraindications, and review his or her medications.
- Counsel the patient about the examination and what it is being used for, and ensure that the patient understands and consents to the testing.
- Instruct the patient to withhold all appropriate medications and to avoid exercise and caffeine before testing.
- Ensure that the patient has been adequately coached regarding how to do the spirometry and that he or she demonstrates proper technique.
- Calibrate the machine according to the instructions for the particular instrument.
- Enter all of the patient's demographic data (e.g., sex, height, age) according to the instructions that accompany the spirometer.
- Ask the patient if he or she would like to urinate before the test.
- Provide a nose clip for the patient, and ensure that it is in place.
- Have the patient take three normal tidal volume breaths.
- Have the patient take a maximal inhalation.
- Have the patient place the mouthpiece into his or her mouth.
- Have the patient perform a forced maximal expiration by instructing the patient to blow as hard and as fast as he or she can. Coach and encourage the patient by emphatically saying

"Breathe, breathe, breathe," "Faster, faster, faster," "Go, go, go," or something similar until the forced vital curve flattens out (the test should last for at least 6 seconds)

- At the end of the maximal exhalation, have the patient do a maximal inhalation.
- Repeat this process for three trials to check the reproducibility of the results.
- Repeat this entire sequence at each of the postexercise testing intervals, and ensure that the results are recorded.
- Ensure that an inhaled bronchodilator is available to treat any clinically significant dyspnea that is precipitated by the exercise session.

INTERPRETATIONS

Table 42.3 lists the diagnostic criteria of the IOC-MC, the American Thoracic Society, and the different branches of the US military for the various tests used to diagnose EIA.

Bronchodilator testing

The American Thoracic Society and the IOC-MC have slightly different diagnostic criteria for diagnosing asthma when using a bronchodilator test. According to the American Thoracic Society, a patient should have symptoms that are suggestive of asthma, and he or she should have a spirometry measurement that shows obstruction at baseline that is reversible with an inhaled bronchodilator. The IOC-MC does not specify what symptoms a patient must demonstrate or that the baseline spirometry must be below normal. In other words, if an athlete has a baseline spirometry of 100% of predicted at baseline and improves to 112% of predicted after treatment with an inhaled bronchodilator, then he or she meets the IOC-MC's established criteria for being able to use an inhaled bronchodilator before competition. A bronchial reversibility test is considered positive if there is an increase of 12% or more of the baseline FEV_1 or forced vital capacity and if the increase exceeds 200 mL after that administration of an inhaled β_2-agonist.[7]

Eucapnic voluntary hyperventilation testing

The IOC-MC considers EVH to be the optimal laboratory-based challenge for confirming that an athlete has EIA. The EVH test is considered positive when a fall in FEV_1 of 10% or more from baseline is recorded after a 6-minute period of hyperventilation in dry air.[7]

Exercise challenge testing

The response to the exercise challenge is considered positive when there is a fall in FEV_1 of 10% or more as compared with baseline during the first 30 minutes after exercise for either a laboratory-based or a field-based test according to the IOC-MC.[7] According to the American Thoracic Society, a fall in FEV_1 of 15% is more specific for EIA, but a 10% fall is a reasonable threshold for diagnosis because healthy subjects generally demonstrate an increase in FEV_1 after exercise.[13]

Methacholine challenge testing

Before a methacholine challenge test, all of the medications mentioned previously should be held. Corticosteroids in particular should be held for 1 week before testing. A methacholine challenge test is considered positive by the IOC-MC if there is a fall in FEV_1 of 20% or more from baseline at a dose that is less than

Table 42.5   Risks and Benefits of Testing for Exercise-Induced Asthma

Risks	Benefits
Danger to patient if testing is done with one of the contraindications present	Provides proper diagnosis of exercise-induced asthma for athletes, thus permitting proper management
Risk of precipitating a clinically significant asthma attack	Can help exclude exercise-induced asthma, thus preventing inappropriate prescribing of medications
Risk of not being able to get results if all needed equipment is not present and functioning properly	Provides needed documentation for athletes participating in events sanctioned by the International Olympic Committee and United States Olympic Committee who will use an inhaled bronchodilator before competition
Risk of distracting athlete if testing is done during actual competition	
Risk of false-positive or false-negative results if procedure is not properly followed	Provides a baseline against which future testing can be done when an athlete is being treated
Time-consuming test to do in the field	Provides results that can be used to educate the athlete about his or her condition

or equal to 2 μmol, 400 mcg (PD_{20}); after the inhalation of a solution with a concentration that is less than or equal to 4 mg/mL (PC_{20}); or after the inhalation of a maximum of 40 breath units when the subject is not taking inhaled corticosteroids.[7]

Occasionally, a patient who is taking inhaled or oral corticosteroids may be a candidate for a methacholine challenge test. For patients who have been taking inhaled steroids for at least 3 months, the PD_{20} should be less than or equal to 6.6 μmol, 1320 mcg, or the PC_{20} should be less than or equal to 13.2 mg/mL or to the inhalation of a maximum of 130 breath units to be accepted as proof of airway hyperresponsiveness, according to the IOC-MC.[7]

PITFALLS, COMPLICATIONS, CONTROVERSIES, RISKS, AND BENEFITS

For the risks and benefits of testing for EIA, see **Table 42.5.**

- Provocative testing may precipitate a clinically significant asthma attack. The testing physician should ensure that measures are available to treat a possible attack by having an inhaled bronchodilator available and by having the ability to provide emergency care or to call for emergency transport, if needed.
- Presumptive treatment with an inhaled bronchodilator before exercise on the basis of history is still advocated by some. This may be acceptable if the following conditions are present:

  - The athlete has had a physical examination that excludes any cardiac or other serious causes of his or her symptoms.
  - The athlete has never had an attack that required emergency medical treatment.
  - The athlete is going to return for reevaluation to see if the symptoms do indeed improve with the use of the bronchodilator.

- The athlete has no intention of participating in any sporting event sanctioned by the IOC or the United States Olympic Committee.
- The athlete has no intention of doing something in the future (e.g., applying to a military academy, entering an occupation with strict physical entrance requirements) that would be precluded by a diagnosis of asthma or the prescription of an inhaled bronchodilator. If the athlete does have contradictory intentions, spirometry should be performed to ensure that the diagnosis of asthma is correct because it may have a significant adverse effect on a young person's future.

- Evaluating for EIA by measuring peak expiratory flow rates using a peak flow meter:

  - This is easier for many providers because peak flow meters are more affordable than spirometers.
  - A peak flow meter is easier to use in the field because the athlete can be given his or her own peak flow meter and taught how to measure for a decrease in peak flow after exercise.
  - These meters can only be used by reliable and motivated patients because testing is extremely effort dependent. The peak expiratory flow rate is considered unreliable and insensitive for the diagnosis of asthma, and it is not recommended as a diagnostic test
  - This test cannot be used to confirm the diagnosis of any athlete competing in events that are sanctioned by the IOC or the United States Olympic Committee or that are monitored by the World Anti-Doping Agency or the United States Anti-Doping Agency.
  - This test should not be used for any individual who may in the future want to do something that would be precluded by being diagnosed with asthma or being prescribed an inhaled bronchodilator, such as applying to a military academy or entering an occupation with strict physical entrance requirements. If the patient wishes to do one of these things, then spirometry should be performed to confirm that the diagnosis is correct, because the results could have significant adverse effects on a young person's future.

- Vocal cord dysfunction frequently mimics the symptoms of EIA. Patients with vocal cord dysfunction are often misdiagnosed as having EIA, which leads not only to the inappropriate use of medications (with unnecessary exposure to side effects) but also to a risk of progressing to the use of other medications with more significant side effects as the patient proves to be unresponsive to traditional treatments.
- There is some controversy about the IOC-MC's policy of requiring objective evidence of EIA because there is no scientific evidence to confirm that inhaled β$_2$-agonists enhance performance in the doses that are required for treatment.[5,6]

CONCLUSION

EIA can cause functional limitations for athletes. While a presumptive diagnosis can be made and short-acting bronchodilators used empirically prior to exercise, this diagnosis should be confidently established when possible. There are conditions that can mimic EIA, and patients not experiencing an expected response to therapy should be evaluated further. While there are pharmacologic and physiologic bronchoprovocative tests that are sensitive and specific for airway hyperreactivity, both false negatives and false positives can occur and the results should always be correlated with the clinical picture.

REFERENCES

1. Storms WW: Review of exercise-induced asthma. Med Sci Sports Exerc 2003;35:1464-1470.
2. Rupp NP: Diagnosis and management of exercise-induced asthma. Phys Sportsmed 1996;24:1-9.
3. Storms WW: Asthma associated with exercise. Immunol Allergy Clin North Am 2005;25:31-43.
4. Pope JS, Koenig SM: Pulmonary disorders in the training room. Clin Sports Med 2005;24:541-564.
5. Witten A, Solomon C, Abbritti E, et al: Effects of nitrogen dioxide on allergic airway responses in subjects with asthma. J Occup Environ Med 2005;47:1250-1259.
6. Fields KB, Reimer CD: Chapter 22: Pulmonary problems in athletes. In Fields KB, Fricker PA (eds): Medical Problems in Athletes. Malden, Massachusetts, Blackwell Science, 1997, pp 136-150.
7. International Olympic Committee Medical and Scientific Department: Beta2 adrenoceptor agonists and the Olympic Games in Turin, 2005. E-mail address: beta2@olympic.org.
8. Weiler JM: Why must Olympic athletes prove that they have asthma to be permitted to take inhaled beta$_2$-agonists? J Allergy Clin Immunol 2003;111:36-37.
9. Holzer K, Bruckner P: Screening of athletes for exercise-induced bronchoconstriction. Clin J Sport Med 2004;14:134-138.
10. Rundell KW, Wilber RL, Szmedra L, et al: Exercise-induced asthma screening of elite athletes: field versus laboratory exercise challenge. Med Sci Sports Med 2000;32:309-320.
11. Anderson SD, Argyros GJ, Magnussen H, Holzer K: Provocation by eucapnic voluntary hyperpnoea to identify exercise-induced bronchoconstriction. Br J Sports Med 2001;35:344-347.
12. Eliasson AH, Phillips YY, Rajagopal KR, Howard RS: Sensitivity and specificity of bronchial provocation testing: an evaluation of four techniques in exercise-induced bronchospasm. Chest 1992;102:347-355.
13. American Thoracic Society: Lung function testing: selection of reference values and interpretative strategies. Am Rev Respir Dis 1991;144:1202-1218.
14. Headquarters, Department of the Army: Army Regulation 40-501: Standards of Medical Fitness. May 29, 2007.
15. Secretary of the Air Force: Air Force Instruction 48-123: Medical Examinations and Standards. 2001.
16. Medical Department, US Navy: NAVMED p. 117: Manual of the Medical Department, US Navy. August 12, 2005.
17. Directorate of Health and Safety, US Coast Guard: Commandant Instruction Manual 6000. IC Change 2. July 13, 2007.

OTHER READINGS

Barreiro TJ, Perillo I: An approach to interpreting spirometry. Am Fam Physician 2004;69:1107-1114.

Crapo RO, Casaburi R, Coates AL, et al: Guidelines for methacholine and exercise challenge testing—1999. Am J Respir Crit Care Med 2000;161:309-329.

Zakynthinos SG, Koulouris NG, Roussos C: Chapter 5: Respiratory system mechanics and energetics. In Mason RJ, Murray JF (Hon), Broaddus VC, Nadel JA (Hon) (eds): Murray and Nadel's Textbook of Respiratory Medicine, 4th ed. Philadelphia, WB Saunders, 2005, pp 87-130.

Gait Analysis

Timothy L. Switaj, MD, and Francis G. O'Connor, MD, MPH

KEY POINTS

- Videotaped observational gait analysis (VOGA) is a safe procedure with a long history of involvement in the analysis of children with gait disorders and adults with complex neuromuscular disorders.
- VOGA has emerged as a useful technique for the analysis of athletes, and it can be complemented by computer software packages that permit advanced biomechanical assessments.
- VOGA can aid the clinician with identifying subtle biomechanical patterns that may not be present on static examination and that can lead to running injuries.
- VOGA can be useful not only when designing a therapeutic plan for rehabilitation or orthotic fabrication but also when assessing a therapeutic intervention.
- Multiple studies show that observations are moderately reliable, even for those examiners with significant experience. Computer software has helped to decrease the variability in the interpretation of data.

INTRODUCTION

The practice of gait analysis has been around for at least a century, but only recently, with the advancement of technology, has gait analysis been practical for the office setting and the nonelite athlete. Before the advent of technology, gait analysis was performed without the assistance of computers or videography, and interpretation relied solely on the clinical experience of the observer. Multiple studies in the nonmedical literature show repeatedly that observations are moderately reliable and that heightened clinical experience increases the reliability of the examiner's observations.[1-4]

Just as technology has helped to advance the practice of medicine in many other disciplines, it has substantially aided the practice of gait analysis. Gait analysis is now more reliable as computers help to make measurements and videography allows for the frame-by-frame observation of movements. It is also a more practical and affordable application in the clinical practice setting for nonelite athletes. In addition to the advantages provided by videotaping the session, computer technology aids in the interpretation of data through the complex measurements of angles, forces, and electromyography. Videotaped observational gait analysis (VOGA) allows for the measurement and interpretation of kinematics, movement patterns, and kinetics as well as of the forces involved in producing those movements, such as joint forces and ground reaction forces.

Overall, the predominance of the literature regarding VOGA is in the setting of physical therapy and rehabilitation for patients after a stroke and for children with neuromuscular disorders such as cerebral palsy. These studies have looked at patients with gross gait abnormalities in laboratories with very sophisticated equipment rather than at patients with only slight deviations from biomechanical norms in outpatient sports medicine clinics. However, VOGA is finding an increasing role in the practical evaluation of runners and other athletes who present for running-related injuries or pain. As such, more evidence-based research is needed to examine the uses of this tool in the outpatient sports medicine setting. This chapter will serve to provide an overview of VOGA that includes the equipment needed, the planning of a VOGA session, and the analysis of the data obtained **(Box 43.1).**

INDICATIONS AND CONTRAINDICATIONS

VOGA has an ever-widening breadth of uses in modern medicine. For many years, VOGA has been used in rehabilitation clinics to aid in the development and monitoring of rehabilitation programs for people after strokes, for children with congenital muscular abnormalities, and for hosts of other patients. More recently, it has become commonly used in attempts to identify subtle patterns of kinematic or kinetic abnormalities during dynamic periods that are not visible on static examinations to diagnose, prevent, or treat running injuries. It is also commonly used for the assessment of orthotic prescriptions as well as for assessing improvement in a therapy program. The military is using VOGA more and more for the assessment and monitoring of patients after they have sustained traumatic limb amputations and now have prostheses. VOGA can also be used with the assistance of pressure monitors for the evaluation of compartment syndrome, with examiners looking for foot drop during the taping session. Contraindications are few, but they mirror those of a patient who is being considered for graded exercise testing or another treadmill evaluation. **Box 43.2** gives a summary of common indications and contraindications for VOGA testing.

Box 43.1: Videotaped Observational Gait Analysis Checklist

- Identify a patient that may benefit from a videotaped observational gait analysis session.
- Evaluate the patient first with a history, a physical examination, and radiographs as needed, and ensure that no contraindications exist for the patient to perform on a treadmill.
- Discuss the procedure with the patient, and schedule the session.
- Ensure that all equipment is available and working properly and that the room has adequate lighting.
- Obtain consent from the patient for the session.
- Reinterview and examine the patient before starting the session, and ask the patient about any changes since the office visit that could affect the session.
- Place retroflective tape on bony landmarks.
- Perform a static evaluation of the patient with and without shoes.
- Perform a dynamic evaluation of the patient on a treadmill with and without shoes as per taping session protocol.
- Review the tape, and record results on an available data collection form.
- Interpret the data either manually or with the aid of computer software.
- Identify any deficiencies that are found in the data interpretation.
- Devise a therapeutic plan to resolve deficiencies and implement a plan.
- Arrange for follow up and possible repeat videotaped observational gait analysis session to monitor the progress of therapy.

EVALUATION

To discuss abnormalities in gait that are identified using videotaped analysis, it is essential to understand the normal biomechanics of gait during both walking and running because there are significant differences between the two.

Box 43.2: Indications and Contraindications for Videotaped Observational Gait Analysis Testing

Indications
- Detection of subtle dynamic abnormalities in kinematics or kinetics that are not found on static evaluation
- Evaluation for compartment syndrome
- Development and monitoring of physical therapy programs
- Assessment of orthotics and shoe wear
- Evaluation of limb prostheses after amputation

Contraindications
- Known significant coronary artery disease
- Recent myocardial infarction
- Known obstructive disease that is being medically managed
- Orthopedic or other conditions with which the patient would not be able to perform on a treadmill
- Respiratory conditions such as asthma or chronic obstructive pulmonary disease that may be exacerbated by exercising on a treadmill

A gait cycle occurs from the initial contact of one foot with the surface until the recontact of that foot with the surface, and it is divided into two distinct phases: the stance phase and the swing phase. During walking, the major action occurs in the stance limb. Alternatively, during running, the majority of the force is supplied by the swing arm and leg. The stance phase starts when the foot contacts the surface. The swing phase starts at the toe off of the foot that just finished the stance phase.

The stance phase makes up 60% of the walking gait cycle and is divided into four subphases: loading response, midstance, terminal stance, and preswing. Each subphase accounts for approximately 15% of the total gait cycle and 25% of the stance phase during walking. Loading response begins with the initial contact of the foot with the surface, and it is a period during which both feet are on the ground, thus providing a double support to the frame. Midstance occurs when the initial-contact foot makes full contact with the surface, at which time single support occurs as the other limb enters the swing phase. Single support occurs for as long as the other limb is in the swing phase. Terminal stance is when the initial contact foot is preparing to lift off of the surface. Preswing, which is the final subphase of the stance phase, is a second period during which double support occurs.

The swing phase makes up the remaining 40% of the walking gait cycle; it begins with toe off and ends with initial contact. It is subdivided into the initial swing, midswing, and terminal swing. During walking, initial swing and terminal swing each occupy about 20% of the gait cycle, and the swing phase occurs in the limb opposite the one that is in the stance phase.

Although it contains both a stance and a swing phase, the running gait cycle is very different, most notably in that the stance phase only occupies 40% of the gait cycle, whereas the swing phase occupies the remaining 60%. The stance phase during running has only two subphases: absorption and propulsion. Midstance is now the point at which absorption becomes propulsion. During running, the swing phase gets divided into two subphases: initial swing and terminal swing, with midswing being the point of transition between the two. Initial swing is the first 75% of the swing phase, with terminal swing making up the remaining 25%. Instead of double support periods (of which there are two during the walking gait cycle), running contains two periods of double float during which neither limb is in contact with the surface. These periods of double float are found at the beginning and end of the swing phase of the running gait cycle.

In addition to understanding the stance and swing phases of the gait cycle, one must also understand several other terms: *stride length, step length*, and *cadence. Stride length* is defined as occurring from the initial contact of one foot with the surface to the initial contact of the other foot with the surface. This is limited, and it has a maximal length as a result of a person's leg length, height, and overall abilities. *Step length* is one complete gait cycle, and *cadence* is the number of steps that occur during a given period. Generally, cadence varies from person to person and between men and women, with women having a natural cadence of six to nine steps per minute more than men. As one runs faster, initially step length increases, and this is followed closely by an increase in cadence. As mentioned, stride length has a finite maximal length up to which point an increase in stride length correlates with increased speed; however, after attaining that maximal stride length, increases in speed only occur with increases in cadence.

Kinematics

Kinematics is defined as the independent motion of joints or body segments. They occur without an outside force acting on the joint or body segment. As with the gait cycle, there are significant

Table 43.1 Normal Range-of-Motion Values for Lower-Extremity Joints during Running

Phase	Joint	Range of Motion
Foot strike to midstance	Hip	45 to 20 degrees of flexion at midstance
	Knee	20 to 40 degrees of flexion by midstance
	Ankle	5 degrees of plantarflexion to 10 degrees dorsiflexion
Midstance to take off	Hip	20 degrees of flexion to 5 degrees of extension
	Knee	40 to 15 degrees of flexion
	Ankle	10 to 20 degrees of dorsiflexion
Follow through	Hip	5 to 20 degrees of hyperextension
	Knee	15 to 5 degrees of flexion
	Ankle	20 to 30 degrees of plantarflexion
Forward swing	Hip	20 to 65 degrees of flexion
	Knee	5 to 130 degrees of flexion
	Ankle	30 to 0 degrees of plantarflexion
Foot descent	Hip	65 to 40 degrees of flexion
	Knee	130 to 20 degrees of flexion
	Ankle	0 to 5 degrees of dorsiflexion to 5 degrees of plantarflexion

Reproduced from McPoil TG, Cornwall MW: Applied sports biomechanics in rehabilitation: running. In Zachazewski JE, Magee DJ, Quillen WS (eds): Athletic Injuries and Rehabilitation. Philadelphia, WB Saunders, 1996, p 356.

differences in the kinematics of walking and running, and these generally manifest as increased joint range of motion (ROM) during running. The differences in joint kinematics are primarily in the sagittal plane during running, with little to no difference in joint motion within the coronal or transverse planes.[5] As an athlete runs and increases speed, the hips and knees increase flexion, and this is accompanied by an increase in ankle dorsiflexion, which results in a lower center of gravity.[6] Normal ROM values can be found in **Table 43.1**.

The hip has an overall increase in ROM as one goes from walking to running, and this is manifested by an increase in flexion and a decrease in extension. During walking, the hip generally flexes about 37 degrees and extends to 6 degrees, thus giving a total ROM of 43 degrees.[7] During running, the hip increases flexion to about 46 degrees, and it rarely extends beyond neutral. Maximal extension occurs at the point of take off, with maximal flexion during the terminal swing. At the same time, the pelvis begins with 8 degrees of external rotation at initial contact and converts to 8 degrees of internal rotation at take off.[5] The motion of the hip in the coronal plane does not significantly change as velocity increases.

The knee is similar to the hip in that the primary changes occur with sagittal ROM manifested with an increase in flexion and a decrease in extension. The knee flexes during absorption while running. The average knee ROM during walking is 60 degrees, and it increases to 63 degrees with running. Walking flexion is 64 degrees, with −8 degrees of extension; during running, flexion increases to 79 degrees, and extension increases to −16 degrees.[6] Neutral position does not occur in the knee during walking or running. At initial contact, the knee is flexed approximately 10 degrees during walking and 35 degrees with running.[6] At the midstance of running, the knee reverses motion to enter the propulsive phase.

The ankle primarily goes through plantarflexion and dorsiflexion during the gait cycle. During a normal walking gait cycle, the ankle plantarflexes to 18 degrees and dorsiflexes to about 12 degrees.[7] However, during running, the overall ROM of the ankle increases to about 50 degrees, with increased hip and knee flexion limiting the amount of plantarflexion and producing rapid dorsiflexion during the propulsion phase. The joints of the foot have motion that is not as simple as that of the ankle joint. Most of the foot joints have either biplanar or triplanar motion. Pronation and supination are triplanar motions. Pronation encompasses dorsiflexion, abduction, and eversion, whereas supination involves plantarflexion, adduction, and inversion. Multiple joints in the foot have triplanar motions that include the following: subtalar, oblique midtarsal, longitudinal midtarsal, and fifth ray. The first ray is triplanar, but, instead of displaying traditional pronation and supination, it shows dorsiflexion with adduction and inversion as well as plantarflexion with abduction and eversion. The metatarsophalangeal joints are biplanar with dorsiflexion and plantarflexion accompanied by abduction and adduction to about 10 degrees. Interphalangeal joints move in a similar fashion to the metatarsophalangeal joints; however, their abduction and adduction are even more limited. A summary of the normal kinematics of joints and body segments during the walking gait cycle can be found in **Figure 43.1**.

Kinetics

Kinetics (as opposed to kinematics) looks at the forces that cause movement. There are internal forces, such as muscular activity, and external forces, such as ground reactions. Muscle forces uniformly increase during running, with an increase in muscle activity and muscle activity duration that occurs in all muscles. Ground reactive forces are more complex and can best be measured using a force plate and by looking at shoe wear patterns during the static examination.

There are three components to ground reactive forces: fore–aft, medial–lateral, and vertical. Vertical is the most significant component for the gait cycle and its resultant forces on the body. The vertical forces produced during walking are routinely 1.3 to 1.5 times the body weight, occurring in peaks during the loading response and preswing.[7] With running, these forces increase to three to four times the body weight, and they are distributed through the stance phase, with a small impact force during the first 20% of stance and the rest of the force distributed throughout the remainder of the stance phase.[7] Fore–aft forces can best be described as breaking and propulsion. Breaking occurs during the first half of the stance phase, whereas propulsion occurs during the last half. The maximum fore–aft forces only reach about 30% of body weight. Medial–lateral forces are very small and seemingly insignificant, with maximums of only about 10% of body weight.

The videotaped observational gait analysis session

A VOGA session needs to be a systematic process that is performed in the same way with every taping session. It starts with the preparation of the equipment to ensure that all equipment is in good working order with normal functionality. After ensuring that the equipment is ready, the examiner must begin to prepare the patient for the VOGA session. The patient needs to be in the appropriate attire for exercise and to have with them their usual running shoes. The patient should be prepared with the placement of retroflective tape strips on the bony landmarks of the body as illustrated in **Figure 43.2**.

The observation of the patient's posture and gait when he or she enters the room can provide useful information. After this, a static assessment should be performed. Regardless of the order in which the static assessment is performed, there are certain aspects that always need to be completed. These include the

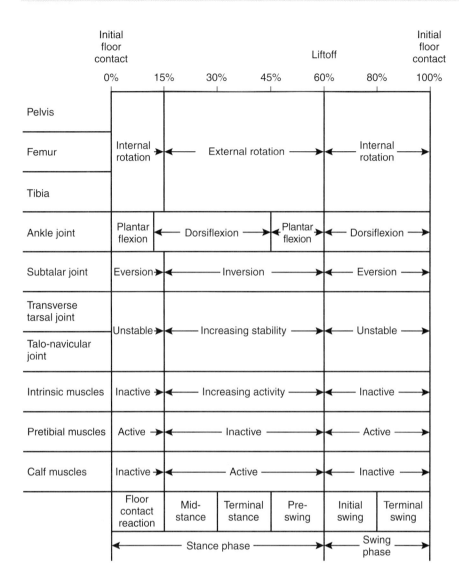

	0%	15%	30%	45%	60%	80%	100%
	Initial floor contact				Liftoff		Initial floor contact
Pelvis							
Femur	Internal rotation	←— External rotation —→			Internal rotation		
Tibia							
Ankle joint	Plantar flexion	←— Dorsiflexion —→		Plantar flexion	←— Dorsiflexion —→		
Subtalar joint	Eversion	←——— Inversion ———→			←— Eversion —→		
Transverse tarsal joint / Talo-navicular joint	Unstable	←— Increasing stability —→			←— Unstable —→		
Intrinsic muscles	Inactive	←— Increasing activity —→			←— Inactive —→		
Pretibial muscles	Active	←——— Inactive ———→			←— Active —→		
Calf muscles	Inactive	←——— Active ———→			←— Inactive —→		
	Floor contact reaction	Mid-stance	Terminal stance	Pre-swing	Initial swing	Terminal swing	
	←————————— Stance phase —————————→				←—— Swing phase ——→		

Figure 43.1 The kinematics of the normal gait cycle. (Redrawn from Mann RA, Hagy J: Am J Sports Med 1980;8[5]:345-350.)

inspection of the patient's shoes for their wear pattern, an examination of the patient's feet and their arches, and the examination of stance both with and without the wearing of shoes. One should evaluate the spine for curvature, the pelvis and shoulders for rotation or tilt, and the legs to determine if there is an underlying leg-length discrepancy. A systematic approach should be taken when inspecting the remainder of the patient's body before the exercise portion of the examination is begun.

After the static assessment is complete, the patient can step onto the treadmill to begin the gait assessment. Several protocols have been devised to yield specific lengths of videotaping each section of the body from different views; **Table 43.2** describes one such protocol.[8] The protocol should ensure that the entire body is imaged in both static and motion positions from the sagittal, coronal, and transverse positions. Sagittal views will provide data about pelvic tilt, hip and knee flexion/extension, and ankle dorsiflexion/plantarflexion, whereas the coronal views describe pelvic obliquity, hip abduction/adduction, knee varus/valgus, and foot inversion/eversion. The transverse plane can be used to determine the abnormal rotation of the pelvis, femur, tibia, and feet.[9] Initially, the treadmill should be set with a 0 degree inclination and at a pace that is determined by the patient to be his or her comfortable pace. This needs to be a logical, systematic, and predetermined protocol that is

well known to all staff involved in the session. The grade and pace may need to be adjusted with regard to the patient's complaint. For example, if the patient notes pain only with running uphill, then one would want to tape the patient's movements while he or she is running on a graded incline. The session should be performed first with the patient barefoot, and then the entire session should be repeated with the patient wearing his or her usual running shoes.

TECHNIQUES AND EQUIPMENT

A good, reliable VOGA session starts with adequate preparation, which is always begun with ensuring that one has the appropriate equipment for the study to be performed. To start, one needs an appropriate clinical setting in which to perform VOGA. The room needs to be large enough to incorporate the treadmill, the computer equipment, a bed or examination table, the patient, the observer, and his or her necessary staff. Although rare (especially given the low exercise stress of VOGA), there is the theoretic risk of a cardiac event or fainting, and, thus, one should have a bed or examination table available and know where the nearest cardiac emergency cart is located.

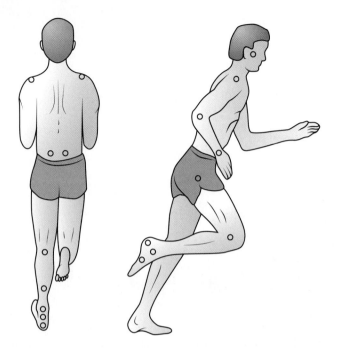

Figure 43.2 The placement of retroflective tape on bony landmarks. (From O'Connor FG, Hoke B, Torrance A: Video gait analysis. In O'Connor FB, Wilder RP [eds]: Textbook of Running Medicine. New York, McGraw-Hill, 2001, p 59.)

There is no specific treadmill type or model that is better than others for the performance of VOGA; however, some characteristics need to be considered during the purchase of the treadmill. It needs to be of good quality, with the ability to provide speeds of 10 to 12 miles per hour and grades of 10% to 20%. The treadmill needs to be placed in the room so that the observer is able to have a good view of the patient from all necessary angles.

In the past, the examiner needed a camera that had frame-by-frame recording and zoom features as well as a recorder to make a tape of the session and then play it back. In today's modern world, a digital video camera encompasses all of these features in one small package. A tripod is helpful to provide a stable platform for the camera to record the patient's movements. Ideally, the tripod should be sturdy and able to be set for a camera height of 18 inches above the ground.

To perform the VOGA session, the patient must be in appropriate attire and wearing his or her usual running shoes. Retroflective tape needs to be available to mark the bony landmarks on the patient's body. A computer is also necessary with a monitor or TV screen that is an adequate size for seeing the retroflective tape to make measurements on the basis of these markings. There are software packages available to assist with data collection and the interpretation of the session; however, they can be expensive to purchase, and training may be required to master their use. A printer is necessary so that results can be printed for ease of interpretation and for placement in the patient's medical record. If computer software is not available to assist with interpretation, a data collection or scoring sheet is needed.

Data collection

Data collection can be made easier with either the use of computer software or the use of a kinematic gait analysis form. Many different forms are available for use, depending on the patient being studied; the available forms may need to be tailored to the appropriate clinical setting. Retroflective tape markers placed strategically on bony landmarks of the patient's body will allow for ease of angular measurements while watching the videotaped session **(Table 43.3)**. It is important that one uses retroflective markers because the use of reflective markers can make it more difficult to visualize the landmarks on video replay, and this increases the likelihood of the misinterpretation of the data. The use of markers with adhesive backgrounds poses the additional difficulty of skin irritation as a result of the adhesive backings.

Table 43.2 Taping Session Protocol

Static Posture: Head to Feet

Anterior, 10 seconds

Lateral, 10 seconds

Posterior, 10 seconds

Posterior View

Head to feet, 30 seconds

Hips to feet, 30 seconds

Lower leg and rear foot

  Shoes on, 30 seconds

  Shoes off (walking), 30 seconds

  Shoes off (running), 30 seconds

Lateral View

Head to feet, 30 seconds

Hips to feet, 30 seconds

Anterior View (Optional)

Head to feet, 30 seconds

Hips to feet, 30 seconds

Lower leg and feet, 30 seconds

Reproduced from Hoke BR, Lefever-Button SL: When the Feet Hit the Ground, Everything Changes. Level Two: Take the Next Step. Toledo, OH, American Physical Rehabilitation Network, 1994, p 75.

Table 43.3 Retroflective Taping Landmarks

Position	Body Part	Landmark
Lateral	Head	Zygomatic arch
	Shoulder	Acromion
	Elbow	Lateral epicondyle
	Wrist	Ulnar styloid
	Hip	Greater trochanter
	Knee	Central femoral condyle
	Ankle	Fibular malleolus
	Foot	Lateral border parallel to floor
Posterior	Lower back	Posterior sacroiliac spine
	Knee	Popliteal fossa
	Lower leg	Bisection of the distal third of the tibia/fibula
	Foot	Calcaneal bisection
Anterior	Hip	Anterior sacroiliac spine
	Patella	Midpoint
	Lower leg	Tibial tuberosity
	Foot	Midline of second metatarsal

Modified from Hoke BR, Lefever-Button SL: When the Feet Hit the Ground, Everything Changes. Level Two: Take the Next Step. Toledo, OH, American Physical Rehabilitation Network, 1994, p 76.

The use of the retroflective markers allows for the easy measurements of angles between bony landmarks, but it does not allow for the evaluation of the movement of the bony structures.

INTERPRETATION

Just as with the VOGA taping session, the interpretation of the data to arrive at the results of the study requires a systematic process to ensure that no abnormality is missed. To be able to identify abnormal patterns identified during the VOGA session, it is essential to understand normal motion parameters. Subtle abnormalities in displacement, rotation, and ROM can suggest causes of running problems.

The patient's head should sit straight on his or her shoulders, with no rotation or anterior or posterior displacement seen during the gait cycle. Vertical displacement should not exceed 4 cm. The earlobe should remain in line with the tip of the shoulder at all times. Torticollis, muscular weakness, and prior trauma can be suggested by the abnormal carrying of the head during the gait cycle. Leg-length discrepancies are suggested by the excessive vertical displacement of the head as a result of an early heel lift during the gait cycle. The shoulders should move in a symmetric pattern; any abnormality in this area could indicate a contralateral lower-extremity injury. Normal elbow carry for the recreational runner is 80 to 110 degrees of flexion, with excess flexion leading to wasted energy. Arm movements that cross the midline are suggestive of pelvic rotation, and they can impair forward progression while the athlete is running.

The trunk must be examined not only for rotation but also for forward, backward, and lateral lean. The trunk should be neutral in a vertical position with no forward or backward lean. Forward leaning while running may indicate weak back musculature or tight hip flexors, whereas a lateral lean of more than 4 cm can indicate a leg-length discrepancy or hip abductor weakness. Excessive external rotation of the hip can be an indicator of tight hip flexors, whereas excessive internal rotation may be evident in a patient with piriformis syndrome.

Normal ranges of motion for the lower-extremity joints are found in Table 43.1. The hip must be observed not only for flexion and extension but also for rotation. Hip rotation cannot be directly measured using a standard VOGA session because an overhead view would be required. However, it can be inferred from multiple other views during the session. Rotation should not exceed 8 degrees, and pelvic drop should not exceed 4 degrees. The examiner must be on the lookout for evidence of tight hip flexors, which are demonstrated by excessive external rotation at the hip as well as weak hip abductors, which could lead to iliotibial band syndrome.

When looking at the knee, the most important value is the cushioning flexion range, which is a calculation performed by subtracting the position of the knee at foot strike from its position at maximum stance flexion; quadriceps weakness is suggested when this value is less than 20 to 25 degrees. Hamstring weakness can be suggested by swing phase knee flexion of less than 115 to 120 degrees. The identification of ankle plantarflexion and dorsiflexion can provide a lot of information about the gait. Marked plantarflexion at heel strike can indicate anterior tibialis weakness or, more concerning, a drop foot resulting from an exertional compartment syndrome. Gastrocsoleus inflexibility or anterior tibial impingement, which are the more likely conditions of the ankle, are suggested by limited dorsiflexion. When limited dorsiflexion is combined with early heel off, one can suspect plantar fasciitis, metatarsalgia, or hallux limitus as possible complications.

Finally, during the interpretation of VOGA data, one must not neglect the foot. Two joints exist in the foot that need consideration: the subtalar joint and the midtarsal joint. Normal foot motion through the gait cycle starts with slight subtalar supination at heel strike followed by rotation into pronation up to a maximum of 6 to 8 degrees toward the end of contact. Resupination occurs during the midstance, peaking just before toe off during propulsion. The subtalar joint pronates early during the swing phase and then hovers near neutral for the remainder of the phase.

When discussing the midtarsal joint, one must talk about its position with regard to two axes: the longitudinal and the oblique. At contact, supination occurs around the longitudinal axis, with pronation around the oblique axis. During midstance, the longitudinal axis becomes progressively more pronated, whereas the oblique axis remains unchanged. Full pronation around both axes occurs at heel off, and this is followed by progressive supination around the oblique axis during propulsion, which is maximal at toe off. Early during the swing phase, the joint pronates around the oblique axis. Later during this phase, it supinates around the longitudinal axis.

Subtalar motion can be measured by placing tape at the proximal calcaneus and another several centimeters distal to yield the calcaneal angle. Normal ranges are as follows: 6 degrees of inversion at foot strike; 6 to 8 degrees of eversion at maximal pronation; neutral at heel lift; and 6 to 8 degrees of inversion at toe off. Excessive pronation is defined as persistent eversion during heel off.

Another parameter that can be helpful when looking at the foot is the assessment of the angle of gait. This can be assessed best using a posterior view of the feet. Excessively wide gaits (> 1.5 inches) can suggest iliotibial band syndrome. Excessive external rotation of the foot (> 7 degrees) can indicate torsional abnormalities, a weak posterior tibialis, or limited dorsiflexion, possibly from an equinus deformity. Heel whips can also be identified by observing for exaggerated rotatory twisting of the heel after heel rise. Circumduction, or the accompanying lifting of the affected extremity with rotation, can indicate weakness of the anterior tibialis, joint restriction, or weak hip flexors.

If the patient does not respond to therapies that address the abnormalities found during a VOGA session, one must consider other methods of evaluation and treatment. One possibility is that of force-plate analysis of the foot and consideration for orthotics. Many different commercially available systems exist, and one must be informed about the system that is available for use.

CONCLUSION

VOGA is becoming more frequently available to the sports medicine provider at the individual clinic level. This technique is not just being used on elite athletes or complicated rehabilitation patients with known gait abnormalities. If a physician is to perform VOGA, he or she must have a defined protocol for the taping session with the proper equipment and preparation. The abnormalities found during the interpretation of data from a VOGA session can provide a target for the treatment of patients with running difficulties. Subtle differences in rotation, displacement, and angles can lead to a diagnosis that may have eluded the provider without the aid of VOGA. Data interpretation needs to be systematic in its performance by trained observers, with the normal ranges for the values being measured always kept in mind. Although the reliability of VOGA is considered moderate at best, increasing technology is allowing for greater ease of data gathering and interpretation; this makes it less expensive to perform and thus an option for the recreational runner with unidentifiable abnormalities.

REFERENCES

1. Brunnekreef JJ, van Uden CJ, van Moorsel S, Kooloos JG: Reliability of videotaped observational gait analysis in patients with orthopedic impairments. BMC Musculoskelet Disord 2005;6:17.
2. Eastlack ME, Arvidson J, Snyder-Mackler L, et al: Interrater reliability of videotaped observational gait-analysis assessments. Phys Ther 1991;71(6):465-472.
3. Krebs DE, Edelstein JR, Fishman S: Reliability of observational kinematic gait analysis. Phys Ther 1985;65(7):1027-1033.
4. Wren TA, Rethlefsen SA, Healy BS, et al: Reliability and validity of visual assessments of gait using a modified physician rating scale for crouch and foot contact. J Pediatr Orthop 2005;25(5):646-650.
5. Ounpuu S: The biomechanics of running: a kinematic and kinetic analysis. Instr Course Lect 1990;39:305-318.
6. Mann RA, Hagy J: Biomechanics of walking, running and sprinting. Am J Sports Med 1980;8(5):345-350.
7. Ounpuu S: The biomechanics of walking and running. Clin Sports Med 1994;13(4):843-863.
8. Hoke BR, Lefever-Button SL: When the Feet Hit the Ground, Everything Changes. Level Two: Take the Next Step. Toledo, OH, American Physical Rehabilitation Network, 1994.
9. Harris GF, Wertsch JJ: Procedures for gait analysis. Arch Phys Med Rehabil 1994;75(2):216-225.

OTHER READINGS

Birrer RB, Buzermanis S, Dellacorte MP, et al: Biomechanics of running. In O'Connor FG, Wilder RP (eds): Textbook of Running Medicine. New York, McGraw-Hill, 2001, p 11.
Cavanagh PR, Lafortune MA. Ground reaction forces in distance running 1980; 13(5):397-406.
Kopf A: Clinical gait analysis—methods, limitations and possible applications. Acta Med Austriaca 1998;25(1):27-32.
Novacheck TF: Walking, running, and sprinting: a three-dimensional analysis of kinematics and kinetics. Instr Course Lect 1995;44:497-506.
Thordarson DB: Running biomechanics. Clin Sports Med 1997;16(2):239-247.

CHAPTER 44

Concussion Testing and Management

Scott A. Playford, MD

KEY POINTS

- Sport-related concussions are common and underreported.
- Concussions produce a complex cascade of neurotransmitter release and ion flux in the brain. This cascade results in cognitive as well as physical symptoms that may last for minutes to months.
- Continued reevaluation is essential. No athlete should return to play or practice while still symptomatic.
- Care and treatment must be individualized for each concussed athlete. There is no universal algorithm.
- Many sideline assessment tools and neurocognitive tests for sport-related concussion are available, but no test or screening tool replaces good clinical judgment by the physician.

INTRODUCTION

Concussion is one of the most difficult problems faced by health care professionals on the sideline. It is a high-risk injury that is complicated by emotional responses and legal ramifications, but it is commonly treated using guidelines built on opinion, experience, and very little direct science. Additional challenges come from the difficulty of diagnosing a concussion, assessing symptom resolution, and relying on the individual athlete for symptom reporting. Concussion is something that the sideline physician will see and must learn to recognize and manage properly. The primary goals of correct concussion assessment and management are to identify immediate neurologic emergencies that require further intervention, prevent catastrophic outcomes, and avoid or limit cumulative injury.

DEFINITION

A good measure of the level of controversy for an injury or condition is the difficulty involved with defining it. In 1966, the Committee of Head Injury Nomenclature of the Congress of Neurological Surgeons developed a consensus definition of concussion as "a clinical syndrome characterized by immediate and transient post traumatic impairment of neural function

The views expressed in this chapter are those of the author and do not necessarily reflect the official policy or position of the Department of the Navy, the Department of Defense, or the US Government.

due to brainstem involvement."[1] Over the years, the definition and features continued to be debated and modified. The First International Symposium on Concussion in Sports convened in Vienna, Austria, in November 2001 and proposed a much more thorough definition.[2] The group defined a sports concussion as

a complex pathophysiological process affecting the brain, induced by traumatic biomechanical forces. Several common features that incorporate clinical, pathologic and biomechanical injury constructs that may be utilized in defining the nature of a concussive head injury include:

1. Concussion may be caused either by a direct blow to the head, face, neck, or elsewhere on the body with an "impulsive" force transmitted to the head.
2. Concussion typically results in the rapid onset of short-lived impairment of neurologic function that resolves spontaneously.
3. Concussion may result in neuropathological changes but the acute clinical symptoms largely reflect a functional disturbance rather than structural injury.
4. Concussion results in a graded set of clinical syndromes that may or may not involve loss of consciousness. Resolution of the clinical and cognitive symptoms typically follows a sequential course.
5. Concussion is typically associated with grossly normal structural neuroimaging studies.

In November 2004, the Second International Conference on Concussion in Sport met in Prague, Czech Republic, and, after review, recommended no changes to the previous definition from the Vienna conference but did add a note that "in some cases post-concussive symptoms may be prolonged or persistent."[3]

To add to the confusion, the term *mild traumatic brain injury* is being used more in recent literature. This term is derived from the assessment of a head injury based on the Glasgow Coma Scale. The Glasgow Coma Scale assesses the individual in the areas of post-injury eye response, verbal response, and motor response and assigns a score from 3 to 15, with 3 being the worst and 15 being the best. A score of 13 to 15 is considered "mild brain injury."[4]

INCIDENCE

Determining the true incidence of concussion has been a challenge for a number of reasons. The two most common sources of data are from surveys and emergency department visits. Surveys tend to underestimate the number of concussions as a result of recall bias and a lack of education about concussion signs and symptoms. Emergency department data have varied widely partly because of the lack of consensus about the definitions of concussion and mild traumatic brain injury. In addition, statistics from emergency departments will not effectively represent the true occurrence of athletic head injury, because the vast majority of sports concussions do not get seen in the emergency department. Various sports governing bodies have begun to monitor the rate of concussions and to establish reporting systems such as the National Collegiate Athletic Association Injury Surveillance System, which provides a more accurate source of sports-related data but still tends to underestimate the incidence when self-reporting is relied on.

Surveys of high school sports shows that the majority of injuries occur among football players. One group collected data from 10 different high school sports over the 1995 to 1997 season and documented 23,566 reportable injuries in 75,298 player seasons (i.e., one person on one team in one season).[5] Of the sports monitored, football had the highest rate, with 34.6% of players being injured or a case rate of 8.1 per 1000 athlete exposures (i.e., one athlete participating in one game or practice). Although numbers of concussions were not specifically listed, 13.3% of the football injuries were classified as head, neck, or spine trauma, and 10.3% were labeled as "neurotrauma."[5]

A secondary analysis of data regarding emergency department visits in the National Hospital Ambulatory Medical Care Survey for the period of 1998 to 2000 showed that, out of 70,900 emergency department visits, 878 (1.23%) were for mild traumatic brain injury.[6] On the basis of this information, the authors estimated the national number of emergency department visits for mild traumatic brain injury to be approximately 1,350,000 or 503.1 per 100,000.

On the basis of survey and surveillance data, the number of traumatic brain injuries in the United States from sports-related activities has been estimated at 300,000 annually.[7] One study of high school athletes estimated the annual rate of concussion to be 17.15 per 100,000 or 0.17 per 1000 athlete exposures.[8] Many believe this to be a significant underestimation, so another group studied 1532 high school football players and administered a confidential survey. At the end of the season, 15.3% of the players reported sustaining a concussion during that season, but only 47.3% of those injured said that they reported it.[9]

Data from the National Collegiate Athletic Association Injury Surveillance System show a much higher estimate at the collegiate level. National Collegiate Athletic Association data from 2004 to 2005 show the rate of concussion to be 1.24 per 1000 athlete exposures for soccer.[10] Data from the system for football show the rate to be 0.44 per 1000 for practices[11] and 3.91 per 1000 athlete exposures for games.[12] A group compared the Injury Surveillance System data with an Internet-based collection technique and still suggests an underestimation. For 2001 to 2002, the Injury Surveillance System showed the concussion rate for games to be 2.64 per 1000 and the total for both games and practices to be 0.49 per 1000, but the Internet-based data showed a game rate of 5.56 per 1000 and a total of 0.74 per 1000.[13]

The Athletic Injury Monitoring System collected data about injuries in American football in high school and college during the 1997 and 1998 seasons. They found a total of 595 reported concussions (273 high school and 322 college), which accounted for 10% of the total injuries reported.[14] They extrapolated that, with an estimated 1.08 million participants in organized football in the United States, there would be approximately 43,000 football-related concussions annually in the nation. From their survey, the rates of concussion (practice and games) were 0.56 per 1000 athlete exposures for high school and 0.58 per 1000 athlete exposures for college.[14]

PATHOPHYSIOLOGY

Despite the long time that the clinical syndrome of concussion has been recognized and the amount of research that has been performed, the pathophysiologic basis of concussion is still largely a mystery. The majority of concussions are minor and result in full recovery in a short period of time, so most concussed athletes do not present to medical centers for imaging or other testing. As a result, most human studies on traumatic brain injury have involved more severe head injury rather than minor trauma from athletic participation. Although this may give some insight into the post-injury cascade that takes place, it is unclear how it translates to sports concussions. More prospective studies have been done in recent years, but usually with only small numbers and often with conflicting results.

Creating models for experimental concussion presents more of a problem. Ethical considerations prohibit human testing, so animal models have been the primary source of knowledge about the early and late effects of concussion. Although this provides important information and new directions for research, there are a number of limitations. Aside from the differences in the structure and anatomy that changes the way animals handle head trauma as compared with humans, the ability to interpret amnesia and other cognitive changes in animals is poor at best. With that being said, animal studies have provided researchers with a much better understanding of the cellular and biochemical changes that take place after traumatic brain injury. In recent years, with the development of cerebral microdialysis, researchers have been able to make the jump from animal models to direct observation in the human brain.[15]

Traumatic brain injury is caused by either static or dynamic loads (the head is either fixed or free to move). Forces applied to the brain can be categorized as compressive, tensile, or shearing. Compressive forces are usually the best tolerated, whereas shearing forces are the least tolerated.[16] Concussion usually results from an acceleration–deceleration force that is applied to the moving brain. This creates a shearing force or a distortion of the vascular and neural elements of the brain. In animal models, rotational forces (particularly in the coronal plane) are more often implicated.[17] Increased intracranial pressure has not been correlated with concussion.[17]

On the cellular level, there has been a better elucidation of posttraumatic events. After the traumatic event, there is a large release of excitatory amino acids acting as neurotransmitters. Of these excitatory amino acids, glutamate has been the most studied, and it is thought to be the major player.[18,19] When glutamate reacts with specific receptors on neural tissue, sodium–potassium pumps are activated, thereby causing an influx of sodium, chloride, and calcium, which leads to cellular swelling and damage.[18,20] Along with the glutamate release, there is a large extracellular increase in potassium that likely adds to electrophysiologic alterations.[18,21,22]

With the neurotransmitter and ion flux, cellular metabolism also appears to be affected. Animal models have shown a brief period of increased metabolism and hyperglycolysis followed by a longer-lasting metabolic depression with hypoglycolysis.[18,19,23-25] Because the increase in metabolism is accompanied by a decrease in cerebral blood flow, there is an accumulation of lactic acid. Human studies, although having small numbers, suggest that traumatic brain injury in humans also produces focal alterations in the blood–brain barrier,[26] and they confirm an initial increase in glucose metabolism that is followed by a more prolonged depression.[19,27,28] These changes in ion concentrations and cellular metabolism represent cellular changes that, although still ongoing, put the brain at a relatively increased risk for further injury with repeated trauma. As a result, further research is being done to more clearly define the sequence and timeline of the injury

Table 44.1 Common Signs and Symptoms of Concussion

Signs	Symptoms
• Loss of consciousness or impaired conscious state	• Headache or pressure in the head
• Vacant stare or glassy eyes	• Nausea
• Appears dazed or confused	• Dizziness or balance problems
• Slow to answer questions or follow instructions	• Visual problems (e.g., seeing stars or flashing lights, double or fuzzy vision)
• Easily distracted, poor concentration, unable to focus	• Sensitivity to light or noise
• Disorientation to game, score, or opposing team	• Feeling "dinged," "foggy," "dazed," or lightheaded
• Inappropriate playing behavior (e.g., running in the wrong direction)	• Feeling slowed down or fatigued
• Slurred or incoherent speech	• Hearing problems (e.g., ringing in the ears)
• Lack of coordination or clumsiness	• Depressed mood or anxiety
• Significantly decreased playing ability	• Irritability or low frustration tolerance
• Inappropriate emotional reactions (e.g., laughing or crying)	• Sleep disturbances
• Memory deficits (e.g., forgets plays, unable to recall three out of three words or objects)	• Feeling more emotional
• Vomiting	• Lack of attention or concentration difficulty
• Changes in personality or typical behavior	• Memory problems
• Convulsive movements or motor phenomena (e.g., tonic posturing)	

cascade and to attempt to correlate the pathophysiologic changes with the clinical symptoms. This will allow clinicians to more effectively develop guidelines for a safe return to play.

Another area of great interest and increasing research is the identification of useful serum biochemical markers (biomarkers) that are specific to brain injury. Biomarkers have been used for many years for other conditions, such as the measurement of creatine kinase and troponin for cardiac muscle injury. A number of biomarkers for neural injury have been investigated, but the one that has shown the most promise so far is S100B. It is the major low-affinity calcium-binding protein in astrocytes, and it is released with astrocyte injury and death.[29] S100B release is immediate and short lived, so delayed testing in patients with minor head trauma may not be useful. Small studies have shown an increase in serum S100B levels in individuals suffering a mild traumatic brain injury as compared with healthy controls[30] and a correlation of serum S100B levels with the degree of injury and the time to recovery.[29,31-33] Unfortunately, as many small studies have also shown a poor correlation between measured serum S100B and symptom severity or persistence.[34,35] To add to the confusion, a group measured serum S100B levels in 61 teenage amateur soccer players after 55 minutes of controlled heading and found a small increase as compared with other exercising players without heading,[36] thereby raising the question of normal cutoffs for exertion versus injury.

FEATURES

The identification of a concussed player is often difficult. Although a loss of consciousness is usually readily apparent, as previously stated, this is often not present. In other cases of concussion, the diagnosis is made on the basis of the report of symptoms by the player or the observation of abnormalities or deficits by teammates, coaches, or medical staff. Some features of concussion are easy to observe, such as stumbling, slurred speech, or vomiting. Other features, such as an impairment in memory or concentration, may not be as obvious unless specifically tested for. Amnesia is usually described as anterograde or retrograde. Anterograde amnesia, which is often called *short-term memory loss*, involves intact memory up to the event but difficulty with maintaining new memories after the concussive event. Retrograde amnesia involves the inability to remember events

that occurred before the concussive injury. **Table 44.1** lists the common signs and symptoms of a concussed athlete.[3,37,38]

GRADING

Grading or categorizing concussions on the basis of severity is another source of controversy. Many grading scales have been proposed over the years, with variable acceptance. Unfortunately, the grading scales are primarily based on expert opinion and little evidence. The three most commonly accepted and quoted grading scales are those of Cantu (developed in 1986, revised in 2001),[39] those of the Colorado Medical Society,[40] and the American Academy of Neurologists guidelines.[38] **Table 44.2** summarizes the scales and compares their similarities and differences.

One primary difference that can be seen when comparing these scales is the relative importance of the loss of consciousness. For many years, physicians have believed and perpetuated the idea that a loss of consciousness indicated a more severe injury to the brain and thus a worse outcome. There have also been studies that support this assumption, although they often have very small numbers of participants.[41] More recently, additional studies have been done that suggest that it is posttraumatic amnesia rather than loss of consciousness that is a marker for more significant injury or prolonged recovery.[42-44] This is reflected in Cantu's revisions in 2001, in which he differentiated between brief and prolonged loss of consciousness. In 2004, during the International Conference on Concussion in Sport in Prague, this issue was discussed, and the consensus opinion was that loss of consciousness as a symptom would not necessarily classify an injury as being more severe.[3] This decision was in agreement with the conclusion from Vienna in 2001, which stated that injury grading scales should be abandoned and instead combined measures of recovery developed to determine injury severity or prognosis and to guide return to play decisions on an individual basis.[2,3] The members proposed a new classification scheme for management purposes that distinguished concussion as either simple or complex.[3]

Simple concussion

The athlete suffers an injury that resolves without complication over a period of 7 to 10 days. Other than limiting play or training

Table 44.2   Common Concussion Grading Systems

Concussion Grade	Cantu (2001 Revision)	Colorado Medical Society (1991)	American Academy of Neurologists (1997)
Grade 1 (mild)	No LOC PTA or postconcussion signs and symptoms that clear in less than 30 minutes	Transient mental confusion No PTA No LOC	No LOC Transient confusion Symptoms or abnormalities clear in <15 minutes
Grade 2 (moderate)	LOC lasting <1 minute and PTA or Postconcussion signs and symptoms lasting longer than 24 hours	No LOC Confusion with PTA	No LOC Symptoms or abnormalities last >15 minutes
Grade 3 (severe)	LOC lasting >1 minute or PTA lasting >24 hours or Postconcussion signs and symptoms lasting >7 days	Any LOC, however brief	Any LOC, either brief (seconds) or prolonged (minutes)

LOC, loss of consciousness; PTA, posttraumatic amnesia.

while symptomatic, the athlete requires no other intervention and has no long-term sequelae.

Complex concussion

The athlete suffers persistent symptoms, including a return of symptoms with exertion. A concussion is also considered to be complex if the athlete exhibits specific sequelae, such as a prolonged loss of consciousness (> 1 minute), concussive convulsions, or prolonged cognitive impairment after the injury. Athletes with multiple concussions or those who have repeat concussions with progressively less force may also be included in this group. These athletes may have additional management considerations, and they may require a more thorough workup.

MANAGEMENT

Preparation

As with any potentially serious injury, concussion occurrence should be considered and planned for before the sporting event. Emergency action plans and procedures should be in place and reviewed with the medical and training staff ahead of time. Special equipment such as a backboard and straps for spinal immobilization should be inspected, and practice drills should be done so that everyone is familiar with the equipment. Emergency transport procedures should also be considered and disseminated.

Standardized testing

When the Quality Standards Subcommittee of the American Academy of Neurology met in 1996 and published its practice parameters for the management of concussions in 1997, the panel of experts presented a recommendation for future research to develop "a valid, standardized, systematic sideline evaluation designed for the immediate assessment of concussion in athletes."[38] In response to the challenge, later in 1996, the Standard Assessment of Concussion was developed and tested. The goal was to design an evaluation tool to be used on the sideline by athletic trainers and similar personnel for the immediate assessment of athletes who were suspected of having a concussion.[45] The test was designed to be sensitive and specific enough for sports concussion but also easy to learn and quick to administer. Another potential obstacle came from the practice effect exhibited when a test was repeated on the same athlete. The *practice* or *learning effect* occurs when an athlete's test performance improves with repeated exposures to the same test. The developers of the Standard Assessment of Concussion created three forms

of the examination to allow for repeated assessment of the same player while limiting the practice effect.[45]

A number of other checklists and evaluation tools have been developed, with variable acceptance and use. In 2004, the Prague conference set out to improve on the available tests by combining eight different existing tools (including the Standard Assessment of Concussion) into one new standardized tool called the Sport Concussion Assessment Tool[3] **(Figure 44.1 and Box 44.1).**

An additional complication with the development and use of sideline assessment tools has been the establishment of standard scores and norms. Because these tests are used across the spectrum of ages and economic and educational levels, it is impossible to present a set of normative data for use as standard comparison. As a result, high-risk athletes should be tested with whatever standardized tool is chosen before the start of the season. An individual baseline can then be established for each athlete and used for comparison when the athlete is retested after an injury. Choosing a tool with alternate forms will reduce the likelihood of practice effect.

On-field evaluation

Immediate evaluation is similar to any other emergency and should first involve the assessment of the airway, breathing, and circulation. The level of consciousness of the injured athlete should next be assessed. If the athlete is unconscious or unable to respond appropriately or cooperate with the examination, cervical spine precautions should be taken. If he or she is complaining about any neck pain or shows any focal neurologic deficits in the extremities, the neck should be immobilized and the protocol for cervical spine injury followed. In this event, the helmet should not be removed, and the athlete should be strapped onto a backboard with the pads and helmet in place. The goal of the on-field evaluation is to quickly differentiate between neurologic emergencies that require transport for further workup or stabilization and less-severe injuries that can be evaluated on the sideline.

Sideline evaluation

On the sideline, the physician should get a more detailed history and perform a more complete examination. The physician should try to delineate the mechanism of injury and identify symptoms such as a history of loss of consciousness or the presence of posttraumatic amnesia (PTA). The examination should look for focal neurologic deficits as well as any alteration in cognitive functions, such as memory, attention span, concentration, or speed of information processing. The athlete should not be left alone, and he or she should be reassessed at regular intervals because many concussed athletes will have a delayed onset of signs and symptoms.

This tool represents a standardized method of evaluating people after concussion in sport. This tool has been produced as part of the Summary and Agreement Statement of the Second International Symposium on Concussion in Sport, Prague 2004.

Sport concussion is defined as a complex pathopsychological process affecting the brain, induced by traumatic biomechanical forces. Several common features that incorporate clinical, pathological, and biomechanical injury constructs that may be utilized in defining the nature of a concussive head injury include:
1. Concussion may be caused either by a direct blow to the head, face, neck, or elsewhere on the body with an "impulsive" force transmitted to the head.
2. Concussion typically results in the rapid onset of short-lived impairment of neurological function that resolves spontaneously.
3. Concussion may result in neuropathological changes, but the acute clinical symptoms largely reflect a functional disturbance rather than structural injury.
4. Concussion results in a graded set of clinical syndromes that may or may not involve loss of consciousness. Resolution of the clinical and cognitive sypmtoms typically follows a sequential course.
5. Concussion is typically associated with grossly normal structural neuroimaging studies.

Postconcussion Symptoms
Ask athletes to score themselves based on how they feel now. It is recognized that a low score may be normal for some athletes, but clinical judgment should be exercised to determine if a change in symptoms has occurred following the suspected concussion event.

It should be recognized that the reporting of symptoms may not be entirely reliable. This may be due to the effects of a concussion or because the athlete's passionate desire to return to competition outweighs the natural inclination to give an honest response.

If possible, ask someone who knows the athlete well about changes in affect, personality, behavior, etc.

Remember, concussion should be suspected in the presence of ANY ONE or more of the following:
• Symptoms (such as headache), or
• Signs (such as loss of consciousness), or
• Memory problems.
Any athlete with a suspected concussion should be monitored for deterioration (ie, should not be left alone) and should not drive a motor vehicle.

For more information see the "Summary and Agreement Statement of the Second International Symposium on Concussion in Sport" in:
Clinical Journal of Sport Medicine 2005;15(2):48–55
British Journal of Sports Medicine 2005;39(4):196–204
Neurosurgery 2005, in press
The Physician and Sportsmedicine 2005;33(4):29–44
This tool may be copied for distribution to teams, groups, and organizations.

The SCAT Card
(Sport Concussion Assessment Tool)
Athlete Information

What is a concussion? A concussion is a disturbance in the function of the brain caused by a direct or indirect force to the head. It results in a variety of symptoms (like those listed below) and may, or may not, involve memory problems or loss of consciousness.

How do you feel? You should score yourself on the following symptoms, based on how you feel now.

Postconcussion Symptom Scale

	None		Moderate			Severe	
Headache	0	1	2	3	4	5	6
"Pressure in head"	0	1	2	3	4	5	6
Neck pain	0	1	2	3	4	5	6
Balance problems or dizzy	0	1	2	3	4	5	6
Nausea or vomiting	0	1	2	3	4	5	6
Vision problems	0	1	2	3	4	5	6
Hearing problems/ringing	0	1	2	3	4	5	6
"Don't feel right"	0	1	2	3	4	5	6
Feeling "dinged" or "dazed"	0	1	2	3	4	5	6
Confusion	0	1	2	3	4	5	6
Feeling slowed down	0	1	2	3	4	5	6
Feeling like "in a fog"	0	1	2	3	4	5	6
Drowsiness	0	1	2	3	4	5	6
Fatigue or low energy	0	1	2	3	4	5	6
More emotional than usual	0	1	2	3	4	5	6
Irritability	0	1	2	3	4	5	6
Difficulty concentrating	0	1	2	3	4	5	6
Difficulty remembering	0	1	2	3	4	5	6

(Follow-up symptoms only)

Sadness	0	1	2	3	4	5	6
Nervous or anxious	0	1	2	3	4	5	6
Trouble falling asleep	0	1	2	3	4	5	6
Sleeping more than usual	0	1	2	3	4	5	6
Sensitivity to light	0	1	2	3	4	5	6
Sensitivity to noise	0	1	2	3	4	5	6
Other:	0	1	2	3	4	5	6

What should I do?
Any athlete suspected of having a concussion should be removed from play, and then seek medical evaluation.

Signs to watch for:
Problems could arise over the first 24–48 hours. You should not be left alone and must go to a hospital at once if you:
• Have a headache that gets worse
• Are very drowsy or can't be awakened (woken up)
• Can't recognize people or places
• Have repeated vomiting
• Behave unusually or seem confused; are very irritable
• Have seizures (arms and legs jerk uncontrollably)
• Are unsteady on your feet; have slurred speech.
Remember, it is better to be safe. Consult your doctor after a suspected concussion.

What can I expect?
Concussion typically results in the rapid onset of short-lived impairment that resolves spontaneously over time. You can expect that you will be told to rest until you are fully recovered (that means resting your body and your mind). Then, your doctor will likely advise that you go through a gradual increase in exercise over several days (or longer) before returning to sport.

Figure 44.1 The Sport Concussion Assessment Tool.

The SCAT Card
(Sport Concussion Assessment Tool)
Medical Evaluation

Name: _____   Date: _____

Sport/Team: _____   Mouth guard? Y   N

1) SIGNS
Was there loss of consciousness or unresponsiveness?	Y	N
Was there seizure or convulsive activity?	Y	N
Was there a balance problem/unsteadiness?	Y	N

2) MEMORY
Modified Maddocks questions (check correct)

At what venue are we? __; Which half is it? __; Who scored last? __
What team did we play last? __; Did we win last game? __

3) SYMPTOM SCORE
Total number of positive symptoms (from reverse side of the card) = ___

4) COGNITIVE ASSESSMENT
5 word recall

		Immediate	Delayed
	(Examples)		(after concentration tasks)
Word 1_____	cat	__	__
Word 2_____	pen	__	__
Word 3_____	shoe	__	__
Word 4_____	book	__	__
Word 5_____	car	__	__

Months in reverse order:
Jun-May-Apr-Mar-Feb-Jan-Dec-Nov-Oct-Sep-Aug-Jul (circle incorrect)
or
Digits backward (check correct)

5-2-8	3-9-1	____
6-2-9-4	4-3-7-1	____
8-3-2-7-9	1-4-9-3-6	____
7-3-9-1-4-2	5-1-8-4-6-8	____

Ask delayed 5-word recall now

5) NEUROLOGICAL SCREENING
	Pass	Fail
Speech	____	____
Eye motion and pupils	____	____
Pronator drift	____	____
Gait assessment	____	____

*Any neurological screening abnormality necessitates
formal neurological or hospital assessment*

6) RETURN TO PLAY
Athletes should not be returned to play the same day of injury.
When returning athletes to play, they should follow a stepwise
symptom-limited program, with stages of progression. For example:
1. Rest until asymptomatic (physical and mental rest)
2. Light aerobic exercise (eg, stationary cycling)
3. Sport-specific exercise
4. Non-contact training drills (start light resistance training)
5. Full contact training after medical clearance
6. Return to competition (game play)

There should be approximately 24 hours (or longer) for each stage, and
the athlete should return to stage 1 if symptoms recur. Resistance
training should only be added in the later stages. Medical clearance
should be given before return to play.

Instructions:
This side of the card is for the use of medical doctors, physical
therapists, or athletic trainers. In order to maximize the
information gathered from the card, it is strongly suggested
that all athletes participating in contact sports complete a
baseline evaluation prior to the beginning of their competitive
season. This card is a suggested guide only for sport
concussion and is not meant to assess more severe forms of
brain injury. **Please give a COPY of this card to athletes for
their information and to guide follow-up assessment.**

Signs:
Assess for each of these items and circle
Y (yes) or N (no)

Memory: If needed, questions can be modified to make them
specific to the sport (eg, "period" versus "half").

Cognitive Assessment:
Select any 5 words (an example is given). Avoid choosing
related words such as "dark" and "moon," which can be
recalled by means of word association. Read each word at a
rate of one word per second. The athlete should not be
informed of the delayed testing of memory (to be done after
the reverse months and/or digits). Choose a different set of
words each time you perform a follow-up exam with the same
candidate.

Ask the athlete to recite the months of the year in reverse
order, starting with a random month. Do no start with
December or January. Circle any months not recited in the
correct sequence.

For digits backward, if correct, go to the next string length.
If incorrect, read trial 2. Stop after incorrect on both trials.

Neurological Screening:
Trained medical personnel must administer this examination.
These individuals might include medical doctors, physical
therapists, or athletic trainers. Speech should be assessed for
fluency and lack of slurring. Eye motion should reveal no
diplopia in any of the 4 planes of movement (vertical,
horizontal, and both diagonal planes). The pronator drift is
performed by asking patients to hold both arms in front of
them, palms up, with eyes closed. A positive test is pronating
the forearm, dropping the arm, or drifting away from midline.
For gait assessment, ask the patient to walk away from you,
turn, and walk back.

Return to Play:
A structured, graded exertion protocol should be developed
and individualized on the basis of sport, age, and the
concussion history of the athlete. Exercise or training should
be commenced only after the athlete is clearly asymptomatic
with physical and cognitive rest. Final decision for clearance to
return to competition should ideally be made by a medical
doctor.

For more information see the "Summary and Agreement
Statement of the Second International Symposium on
Concussion in Sport" in:
Clinical Journal of Sport Medicine 2005;15(2):48–55
British Journal of Sports Medicine 2005;39(4):196–204
Neurosurgery 2005, in press
The Physician and Sportsmedicine 2005; 33(4):29–44

Figure 44.1   Continued

Box 44.1: Concussion Testing Checklist

- Check the preseason cognitive testing scores.
- Use sideline testing to look for a change from baseline.
- Repeat testing after recovery.
- Consider more in-depth neuropsychologic testing.
- Use testing with multiple versions to avoid practice effect.
- Correlate testing with an examination; never allow a symptomatic athlete to return to play.
- Remember to check the airway, breathing, and circulation and to consider cervical spine precautions.

The American Academy of Neurology summary statement recommends repeat examinations every 5 minutes.[38] As with the initial on-field examination, the primary goal is to identify neurologic emergencies that require additional medical evaluation or intervention. If the athlete is showing persistent symptoms, worsening symptoms, focal neurologic deficits, or an alteration in level of consciousness, he or she should be transported for further evaluation. Intracranial hemorrhage is the leading cause of death from athletic head injury, and athletes with an epidural hematoma often will have a lucid period before the hematoma reaches a fatal size over 30 to 60 minutes.[16]

After the event

Appropriate counseling after the competition is essential. The athlete should be educated about his or her condition and its implications. Intracranial hemorrhage from an epidural hematoma, a subdural hematoma, a subarachnoid hemorrhage, or an intracerebral hematoma may have a delayed onset, and coaches, roommates, or parents need to be instructed about signs and symptoms to watch for. Warning signs and an emergency plan should be reviewed with the athlete and anyone who will be caring for or staying with the injured athlete (e.g., parents). Follow-up plans should also be discussed and arranged. The athlete should be instructed about complete rest, which may include mental rest as well (e.g., no homework, classes, or tests).

Imaging

Because concussions are generally not associated with any structural abnormalities, neuroimaging is usually not required. A number of imaging modalities are available, including computed tomography scanning, magnetic resonance imaging, functional magnetic resonance imaging, positron emission tomography, single-photon emission computed tomography, electroencephalography, and evoked potentials. They are indicated on the basis of symptoms or examination findings.[3,46]

NEUROPSYCHOLOGIC TESTING

Because the return-to-play decision continues to be an area of disagreement and controversy, efforts have been made to establish more objective, scientifically based decisions regarding when it is safe to allow a player to resume practice and play. As previously discussed, it is universally accepted that no injured athlete should return to play while still symptomatic, but, because most postconcussive symptoms are subjective and rely on the athlete's report, reliability is questionable. Neuropsychologic testing has been examined as the potential objective solution to the provider's

dilemma. This type of testing has been used for many years by neuropsychologists to detect and quantify residual effects after traumatic brain injury. There are more than 20 different batteries of tests that measure various aspects of cognitive function, including concentration, motor dexterity, information processing, visual memory, verbal memory, executive function, and brain stem function.[47] Traditionally, neuropsychologists test psychologic functioning and some sensory and motor functioning as well. Because the testing is time consuming and expensive and because it requires interpretation by a neuropsychologist, it has had limited usefulness in the sports setting. Recently the neurocognitive portions of the testing have been modified and grouped to be more useful for the patient with a sports concussion, and its use has grown to include the National Football League, the National Hockey League, and increasing numbers of colleges, universities, and high schools.[47] Tests have shown various abnormalities in the concussed athlete, including those involving maintaining and distributing attention, alterations in balance and stability, information processing, reaction times, verbal learning, and memory (LOE: D).[47-51] These findings may be present despite the absence of subjective complaints by the athlete. Gait stability studies have shown that concussed athletes may learn to compensate for altered stability and show no deficits on gait testing. If the individual is challenged with a second task, such as one involving memory or concentration while undergoing gait testing, the instability will be unmasked (LOE: D).[48,52] As with sideline concussion assessment tools, to optimize the use of neuropsychologic testing, the athlete must be tested before the start of the season to establish an individual baseline for future comparison.

Computers have opened new doors for neuropsychologic testing. Recently, more companies have developed commercial computer-based and Internet-based testing tools. For a fee, schools or teams can purchase program software or access to Internet-based programs. Each athlete completes a brief computerized test before the start of the season to establish a neurocognitive baseline, and this information is then stored in a computer database. If a head injury occurs, the injured player repeats the test, and the physician receives an automated report back from the program or the company comparing the preinjury and postinjury performances. The goal is to simply determine if there has been a change from baseline functioning rather than to produce data that require complex interpretation, so reports are often a simple "yes" or "no." Companies currently marketing programs include CogState (CogState Ltd, Victoria, Australia), Headminder (Headminder Inc, New York City), and ImPACT (University of Pittsburgh Medical Center Sports Medicine Concussion Program). The programs are all designed to be administered with little training because the athletes are self-guided through the computerized test. The systems also include randomization to help reduce the practice effect from repeated use on the same athlete.[52] The tests have not been compared head to head, so when choosing one of the products, the physician and athletic staff should consider the reliability of the testing, the validation that the tests detect subtle changes from sports-related concussions, and the clinical utility in the setting in which the test will be used. Although the companies developing the software have put out some data regarding reliability and validity, studies are ongoing.[53] Computerized neuropsychologic testing shows promise, but it is too early to call its use the standard of care; nothing replaces good clinical judgment by a physician.

In its position statement regarding the management of sports-related concussions, the National Athletic Trainers' Association proposes that neuropsychologic testing offers a good adjunct to the clinical assessment of a concussed athlete but that it should not be used as the only means to determine the return to play. The Association discusses the potential benefits of the commercial computerized programs, but it makes no formal recommendation regarding their use. It is recommended that some sort of baseline neurocognitive testing should be done before the start of the season.[54] The Prague consensus also discusses the potential benefits of neuropsychologic testing, but it cautions that, in the symptomatic concussed athlete, testing "adds nothing to the return-to-play decisions and it may contaminate the testing process by allowing for practice effects to confound the results."[3]

COMPLICATIONS

Second-impact syndrome

Second-impact syndrome (SIS) occurs when an athlete who sustains a head injury (e.g., a concussion or a cerebral contusion) sustains a second head injury before the symptoms of the first one have fully cleared. The second injury is often minor or incidental, and the result is the rapid development of increased intracranial pressure from vascular engorgement and edema; this syndrome carries a mortality rate of approximately 50%.[16] In the United States, most reports of SIS have been in football players, but it has also been noted in hockey players and boxers.[55] It is most commonly described as occurring among adolescents males (between 14 and 16 years of age), and it is almost unheard of among adults.[55,56] SIS was first described in 1973,[57] and the term *second-impact syndrome* was first used to describe the condition in 1984.[58] The syndrome is believed to be related to the loss of the autoregulation of cerebral blood flow that results in vascular engorgement and a rapid increase in intracranial pressure, which is similar to the malignant brain edema found in children after a traumatic head injury.[16,55,59] More recent evidence suggests that cytotoxic or cellular edema, which is related to the postconcussive altered membrane permeability and ion transport, is also a significant contributor to the condition.[60-62]

As a result of the high morbidity and mortality rates, SIS has received a lot of attention over the years, and it has provided the major impetus for the development of accurate athlete-assessment tools and return-to-play guidelines. Many experts question the existence of SIS as a separate and discrete syndrome as opposed to a variant of the malignant brain edema of children. Some researchers have reviewed published cases of SIS using strict diagnostic criteria and failed to find convincing evidence of either an initial head injury or a repeat blow.[56,63] Clearly this has many implications, and research is ongoing.

Repeat concussions

It has been commonly presumed and taught over the years that athletes who suffer a concussion are at an increased risk of repeat concussion in the future, but evidence has been lacking. More recent studies have attempted to determine if this is in fact true and if so, to quantify the risk. One study looking at data from high school and college football players over two consecutive seasons recorded 572 concussions. They found that, among high school players who had a history of concussion, 18% sustained another concussion as compared with only 3% of players with no history. In the college athletes, 16% of players with a history of concussion suffered a repeat concussion as compared with only 3% of those with no such history. The calculated relative risk showed that concussion was 5.8 times more likely among individuals with a history of concussion (LOE: D).[64] Another study of college football players examining 184 concussed athletes found that those athletes with a history of three or more concussions during the previous 7 years were three times more likely to sustain another concussion (LOE: D).[65] One big question that still remains unanswered is whether the increased risk of repeat concussion is actually the result of pathoanatomic changes that lead to an increase in susceptibility. Alternatively, the higher risk may be related to

behavioral components such as more aggressive play, poor athletic technique, or less supervision.

Cumulative effects

Another source of conflicting opinion is the long-term effects of concussion and the cumulative effects of repeated concussions. As with other aspects of concussion, results of studies have not been consistent. One study compared children with brain injuries with children with orthopedic injuries over an average of 4 years and found an increased incidence of cognitive and behavioral problems in those children who had severe traumatic brain injury as compared with the strictly orthopedic group. The authors failed to show a statistical difference between the moderate traumatic brain injury group and the group without brain injury, which raises questions about whether this would be a concern in athletic head injuries.[66]

With regard to repetitive concussions, some studies failed to show a significant cumulative effect (LOE: D).[67-69] The majority of research, however, suggests that concussed athletes who have a history of concussion are more symptomatic and require more time to recover (LOE: D).[65,70-76] One study of high school athletes identified four markers of concussion severity as positive loss of consciousness, retrograde amnesia, anterograde amnesia, and confusion. They found that athletes with a history of three or more concussions were more than nine times more likely to exhibit three or four of the abnormal markers when they sustained a subsequent concussion (LOE: D).[76]

Chronic traumatic brain injury has long been described in boxing as *dementia pugilistica, traumatic encephalopathy*, or *"punch drunk" syndrome*. Severity has been linked to the length of the boxer's career, and it ranges from affective changes and psychiatric disturbances to a permanent decrease in cognitive function and Parkinson-like symptoms.[74,77] Chronic traumatic brain injury is being described more in other sports as well, including soccer and football.[74] A survey of 2552 retired professional football players found that those with a history of three or more concussions had a fivefold greater prevalence of being diagnosed with mild cognitive impairment as compared with those with no history of concussion (LOE: D).[75]

An area of growing interest with regard to long-term outcomes is that of apolipoprotein E, a gene with three primary alleles. The ε-4 allele has been linked to poor neurocognitive outcomes after various types of brain injury. Studies of professional boxers with chronic traumatic brain injury have shown that those with the most severe impairments are more likely to have the apolipoprotein E ε-4 allele.[78] Other studies have linked the apolipoprotein E ε-4 genotype to poorer recovery after traumatic brain injury.[79] A study of mild traumatic brain injury suggested that the presence of the apolipoprotein E ε-4 allele might be associated with worse initial presentation but failed to show any relation to recovery rate or prolonged symptoms.[80] There was also no association with the presence of the apolipoprotein E ε-4 genotype and diffuse brain edema in children.[81] The link with athletic concussions is still being studied. The implication of being able to predict which athletes are at risk for long-term cognitive impairment is enticing but not yet a reality.

Postconcussive syndrome

Postconcussive syndrome criteria are described in the *Diagnostic and Statistical Manual of Mental Disorders, 4th edition*, of the American Psychiatry Association. The syndrome is characterized by persistent headache, an inability to concentrate, irritability, fatigue, vertigo, emotional lability, and disturbances in gait, sleep, and vision.[82,83] It usually follows a more severe concussion (a loss of consciousness of less than 5 minutes or prolonged posttraumatic amnesia), but the time to onset and the course is not well defined or universally agreed upon.[82]

TREATMENT

The treatment of concussion is another area with little supporting research. The standard approach has been complete rest until all symptoms resolve. If impairments in cognition, memory, or concentration are present, the concussed athlete may also require mental rest as well. For high school and college students, this may require consultation with coaches, teachers, and/or guidance counselors. One study compared 6 days of bed rest with routine exertional avoidance and found some improvement in subjective dizziness immediately after the concussion but otherwise no effect on the recovery curve or the development of prolonged symptoms (LOE: B).[84]

Pharmacologic intervention has not proven to be useful for the treatment of concussion. Several options have been studied, including corticosteroids, antioxidants, glutamate receptor antagonists, and calcium-channel antagonists, but unfortunately no agent has been found to alter the course of mild traumatic brain injury.[85] Antidepressants may be useful for treating prolonged postconcussive symptoms such as depression or affective changes.

Return to play

As with the grading of concussions, this is an area of disagreement and variation. One unifying theme that should always apply is that no concussed athlete should ever resume play while still symptomatic. As previously discussed, the presence of symptoms reflects

ongoing alterations of the neural cells and tissue and represents a period of vulnerability for further injury. All decisions related to return to play should involve a physician and should be individualized for the athlete in question.

For mild concussions, many experts agree that it is safe to return to play on the same day as the injury. The athlete's history of concussions should be taken into consideration. Cantu, the American Academy of Neurologists, and the Colorado Medical Society all agree that an athlete who suffers a mild concussion and who is asymptomatic may resume play, but they caution that the athlete should be monitored for 15 to 20 minutes first because symptoms may have a delayed onset.[38-40] If the injured athlete is asymptomatic after an adequate period of observation, he or she should have an exertional challenge (e.g., push-ups or running on the sideline) before being allowed to return to play. If symptoms return with exertion, the player should remain out. **Table 44.3** shows additional recommendations that are based on the three previously discussed grading scales.[38-40]

Initially, 1 week was chosen as an arbitrary timeline on the basis of experience and practice. Researchers have since attempted to more accurately determine the recovery curve. Studies of college and professional athletes have shown that the majority of concussed athletes have a resolution of symptoms and return to baseline in 3 to 7 days (LOE: D).[69,70,86] Concussed high school athletes have shown a trend toward longer recovery times (LOE: D).[44,86] Studies involving neuropsychologic testing have raised more questions, with some showing resolution in 5 to 10 days but others showing persistent alterations in several measurements up to 14 days out among both high school and college athletes, despite the resolution of subjective complaints by the players (LOE: D).[47,68,87]

Table 44.3   Return-to-Play Guidelines by Concussion Grading System

Concussion Grade	Number of Concussion Suffered	Cantu	Colorado Medical Society	American Academy of Neurologists
Grade 1 (mild)	First	Return to play after 1 symptom-free week End season if computed tomography scanning or magnetic resonance imaging abnormal	Remove from contest May return to same contest or practice if symptom free for at least 20 minutes	Remove from contest May return to play if symptom free within 15 minutes
Grade 1 (mild)	Second	Return to play in 2 weeks after 1 symptom-free week	May not return to contest or practice May return after 1 symptom-free week	May not return to contest or practice May return to play after 1 symptom-free week
Grade 1 (mild)	Third	End season May return to play next season if no symptoms	End season May return to play in 3 months if without symptoms	
Grade 2 (moderate)	First	Return to play after 1 symptom-free week	May not return to contest or practice May return to play after 1 symptom-free week	May not return to contest or practice May return to play after 1 full symptom-free week Computed tomography scanning or magnetic resonance imaging recommended if symptoms or signs persist
Grade 2 (moderate)	Second	May not return for a minimum of 1 month May return to play then if symptom free for 1 week Consider ending season	Consider ending season May return in 1 month if symptom free	May not return to contest or practice May return to play after at least 2 symptom-free weeks End season if any computed tomography scanning or magnetic resonance imaging abnormalities

Continued

Table 44.3   Return-to-Play Guidelines by Concussion Grading System—cont'd

Concussion Grade	Number of Concussion Suffered	Cantu	Colorado Medical Society	American Academy of Neurologists
Grade 2 (moderate)	Third	End season May return to play next season if without symptoms	End season May return to play next season if without symptoms	
Grade 3 (severe)	First	May not return to play for a minimum of 1 month May return to play then after 1 symptom-free week	May not return to contest or practice Transport to hospital for evaluation May return to play in 1 month after 2 symptom-free weeks	May not return to contest or practice Transport to hospital if unconscious or in the presence of neurologic abnormality Computed tomography scanning or magnetic resonance imaging recommended if posttraumatic symptoms or signs persist If loss of consciousness is brief (seconds), may return to play in 1 week if no symptoms or signs If loss of consciousness is prolonged (minutes), return to play after 2 symptom-free weeks
Grade 3 (severe)	Second	End season May return to play next season if no symptoms	End season May return to play next season if no symptoms	May not return to contest or practice May return to play after a minimum of 1 symptom-free month End season if any computed tomography scanning or magnetic resonance imaging abnormalities
Grade 3 (severe)	Third		End season Strongly discourage any return to contact or collision sports	

Recent expert consensus statements recommend a more individualized approach and suggest a stepwise progression with the return to play as shown in **Table 44.4**.[3,88] With this approach, the athlete should proceed to the next level as long as he or she is asymptomatic. However, if any symptoms return, the athlete will drop back to the previous asymptomatic level and try to advance again in 24 hours. For mild concussions, this process will normally take 1 week to complete (1 to 2 days at each level), but it should be tailored for the individual athlete.

Table 44.4   Prague Conference Recommendations for Return to Play after Concussion

Level	Action
1	No activity, complete rest Once asymptomatic, proceed to step 2
2	Light aerobic exercise such as walking or stationary cycling No resistance training
3	Sport-specific exercise Progressive addition of resistance training at steps 3 or 4
4	Noncontact training drills
5	Full-contact training after medical clearance
6	Game play

CONTROVERSIES

- Most recommendations regarding concussion management have been based on expert opinion and little clinical research.
- Presentation and symptom resolution after a concussion are highly variable and difficult to predict. Postconcussive amnesia may be more indicative of significant injury than loss of consciousness.
- Subtle neurochemical changes in the brain after a concussion may put the injured athlete at an increased risk for more severe injury, including death from SIS.
- Historically, neuropsychologic testing has been used to assess for changes and deficits after more severe central nervous system insults, such as stroke or Alzheimer's dementia. Studies are ongoing to determine whether these tests are sensitive enough to detect the often subtle changes associated with sports-related concussion.
- Computerized neuropsychologic testing is quick and easy, but the increased accessibility may lead to its use in lieu of proper assessment and disposition by a physician.

REFERENCES

1. Committee on Head Injury Nomenclature of the Congress of Neurological Surgeons: Glossary of head injury including some definitions of injury to the cervical spine. Clin Neurosurg 1966;12:386-394.
2. Aubry M, Cantu R, Dvorak J, et al: Summary and agreement statement of the 1st International Symposium on Concussion in Sport, Vienna 2001. Clin J Sport Med 2002;12(1):6-11.

3. McCrory P, Johnston K, Meeuwisse W, et al: Summary and agreement statement of the 2nd International Conference on Concussion in Sport, Prague 2004. Br J Sports Med 2005;39(4):196-204.

4. Teasdale G, Jennett B: Assessment of coma and impaired consciousness. A practical scale. Lancet 1974;2(7872):81-84.

5. Powell JW, Barber-Foss KD: Injury patterns in selected high school sports: a review of the 1995-1997 seasons. J Athl Train 1999;34(3):277-284.

6. Bazarian JJ, McClung J, Shah MN, et al: Mild traumatic brain injury in the United States, 1998-2000. Brain Inj 2005;19(2):85-91.

7. Thurman DJ, Branche CM, Sniezek JE: The epidemiology of sports-related traumatic brain injuries in the United States: recent developments. J Head Trauma Rehabil 1998;13(2):1-8.

8. Schulz MR, Marshall SW, Mueller FO, et al: Incidence and risk factors for concussion in high school athletes, North Carolina, 1996-1999. Am J Epidemiol 2004; 160(10):937-944.

9. McCrea M, Hammeke T, Olsen G, et al: Unreported concussion in high school football players: implications for prevention. Clin J Sport Med 2004;14(1):13-17.

10. National Collegiate Athletic Association Injury Surveillance System (Web site): Injury summary—body part by injury type: National, Men's Soccer, games 2004-2005. Available at www1.ncaa.org/membership/ed_outreach/health-safety/iss/Natl_Reports_2004_05/MSOC_CompBody.pdf. Accessed December 16, 2006

11. National Collegiate Athletic Association Injury Surveillance System (Web site): Injury summary—body part by injury type: National, Football, games 2004-2005. Available at www1.ncaa.org/membership/ed_outreach/health-safety/iss/Natl_Reports_2004_05/FB_COMPBODY_2005.pdf. Accessed December 16, 2006.

12. National Collegiate Athletic Association Injury Surveillance System (Web site): Injury summary—body part by injury type: National, Football, practices 2004-2005. Available at http://www1.ncaa.org/membership/ed_outreach/health-safety/iss/Natl_Reports_2004_05/FB_PRACBODY_2005.pdf. Accessed December 16, 2006.

13. Booher MA, Wisniewski J, Smith BW: Comparison of reporting systems to determine concussion incidence in NCAA Division I collegiate football. Clin J Sport Med 2003;13(2):93-95.

14. Zemper ED: A two-year prospective study of cerebral concussion in American football. Res Sports Med 2003;11:157-172.

15. Hillered L, Vespa PM, Hovda DA: Translational neurochemical research in acute human brain injury: the current status and potential future for cerebral microdialysis. J Neurotrauma 2005;22(1):3-41.

16. Cantu RC: Athletic head injuries. Clin Sports Med 1997;16(3):531-542.

17. McCrory P, Johnston KM, Mohtadi NG, et al: Evidence-based review of sport-related concussion: basic science. Clin J Sport Med 2001;11(3):160-165.

18. McIntosh TK: Neurochemical sequelae of traumatic brain injury: therapeutic implications. Cerebrovasc Brain Metab Rev 1994;6(2):109-162.

19. Povlishock JT, Katz DI: Update of neuropathology and neurological recovery after traumatic brain injury. J Head Trauma Rehabil 2005;20(1):76-94.

20. Yoshino A, Hovda DA, Katayama Y, et al: Hippocampal CA3 lesion prevents postconcussive metabolic dysfunction in CA1. J Cereb Blood Flow Metab 1992;12(6):996-1006.

21. Katayama Y, Kawamata T, Tamura T, et al: Calcium-dependent glutamate release concomitant with massive potassium flux during cerebral ischemia in vivo. Brain Res 1991;558(1):136-140.

22. Katayama Y, Becker DP, Tamura T, et al: Massive increases in extracellular potassium and the indiscriminate release of glutamate following concussive brain injury. J Neurosurg 1990;73(6):889-900.

23. Kubota M, Nakamura T, Sunami K, et al: Changes in local cerebral glucose utilization, DC potential and extracellular potassium in various degree of experimental cerebral contusion. No To Shinkei 1989;41(8):799-805.

24. Yoshino A, Hovda DA, Kawamata T, et al: Dynamic changes in local cerebral glucose utilization following cerebral conclusion in rats: evidence of a hyper- and subsequent hypometabolic state. Brain Res 1991;561(1):106-119.

25. Richards HK, Simac S, Piechnik S: Uncoupling of cerebral blood flow and metabolism after cerebral contusion in the rat. J Cereb Blood Flow Metab 2001;21(7):779-781.

26. Korn A, Golan H, Melamed I, et al: Focal cortical dysfunction and blood-brain barrier disruption in patients with Postconcussion syndrome. J Clin Neurophysiol 2005;22(1):1-9.

27. Bergsneider M, Hovda DA, Shalmon E, et al: Cerebral hyperglycolysis following severe traumatic brain injury in humans: a positron emission tomography study. J Neurosurg 1997;86(2):241-251.

28. Hovda DA, Lee SM, Smith ML, et al: The neurochemical and metabolic cascade following brain injury: moving from animal models to man. J Neurotrauma 1995;12(5):903-906.

29. Berger RP: The use of serum biomarkers to predict outcome after traumatic brain injury in adults and children. J Head Trauma Rehabil 2006;21(4):315-333.

30. de Kruijk JR, Leffers P, Menheere PP, et al: S-100B and neuron-specific enolase in serum of mild traumatic brain injury patients. A comparison with health controls. Acta Neurol Scand 2001;103(3):175-179.

31. Herrmann M, Curio N, Jost S: Release of biochemical markers of damage to neuronal and glial brain tissue is associated with short and long term neuropsychological outcome after traumatic brain injury. J Neurol Neurosurg Psychiatry 2001; 70(1):95-100.

32. Stranjalis G, Korfias S, Papapetrou C: Elevated serum S-100B protein as a predictor of failure to short-term return to work or activities after mild head injury. J Neurotrauma 2004;21(8):1070-1075.

33. Savola O, Hillbom M: Early predictors of post-concussion symptoms in patients with mild head injury. Eur J Neurol 2003;10(2):175-181.

34. Bazarian JJ, Zemlan FP, Mookerjee S, et al: Serum S-100B and cleaved-tau are poor predictors of long-term outcome after mild traumatic brain injury. Brain Inj 2006;20(7):759-765.

35. Stapert S, de Kruijk J, Houx P, et al: S-100B concentration is not related to neurocognitive performance in the first month after mild traumatic brain injury. Eur Neurol 2005;53(1):22-26.

36. Mussack T, Dvorak J, Graf-Baumann T, et al: Serum S-100B protein levels in young amateur soccer players after controlled heading and normal exercise. Eur J Med Res 2003;8(10):457-464.

37. Collins MW, Lovell MR, Mckeag DB: Current issues in managing sports-related concussion. JAMA 1999;282(24):2283-2285.

38. Practice parameter: the management of concussion in sports (summary statement). Report of the Quality Standards Subcommittee. Neurology 1997;48(3):581-585.

39. Cantu RC: Posttraumatic retrograde and anterograde amnesia: pathophysiology and implications in grading and safe return to play. J Athl Train 2001;36(3):244-248.

40. Report of the Sports Medicine Committee: Guidelines for the Management of Concussion in Sports. Denver, Colorado, Colorado Medical Society, 1990 (revised May 1991).

41. McCrea M, Kelly JP, Randolph C, et al: Immediate neurocognitive effects of concussion. Neurosurgery 2002;50(5):1032-1040.

42. Lovell MR, Iverson GL, Collins MW, et al: Does loss of consciousness predict neuropsychological decrements after concussion?. Clin J Sport Med 1999;9(4):193-198.

43. Collins MW, Iverson GL, Lovell MR, et al: On-field predictors of neuropsychological and symptom deficit following sports-related concussion. Clin J Sport Med 2003; 13(4):222-229.

44. Lovell MR, Collins MW, Iverson GL, et al: Recovery from mild concussion in high school athletes. J Neurosurg 2003;98(2):296-301.

45. McCrea M, Kelly JP, Kluge J, et al: Standardized assessment of concussion in football players. Neurology 1997;48(3):586-588.

46. Johnston KM, McCrory P, Mohtadi NG, et al: Evidence-based review of sport-related concussion: clinical science. Clin J Sport Med 2001;11(3):150-159.

47. Grindel SH, Lovell MR, Collins MW: The assessment of sport-related concussion: the evidence behind neuropsychological testing and management. Clin J Sport Med 2001;11(3):134-143.

48. van Donkelaar P, Osternig L, Chou LS: Attentional and biomechanical deficits interact after mild traumatic brain injury. Exerc Sport Sci Rev 2006;34(2):77-82.

49. Collins MW, Fields M, Lovell MR, et al: Relationship between postconcussion headache and neuropsychological test performance in high school athletes. Am J Sports Med 2003;31(2):168-173.

50. Gosselin N, Theriault M, Leclerc S, et al: Neurophysiological anomalies in symptomatic and asymptomatic concussed athletes. Neurosurgery 2006;58(6):1151-1161.

51. Collie A, Makdissi M, Maruff P, et al: Cognition in the days following concussion: comparison of symptomatic versus asymptomatic athletes. J Neurol Neurosurg Psychiatry 2006;77(2):241-245.

52. Parker TM, Osternig LR, Van Donkelaar P, et al: Gait stability following concussion. Med Sci Sports Exerc 2006;38(6):1032-1040.

53. Randolph C, McCrea M, Barr WB: Is neuropsychological testing useful in the management of sport-related concussion? J Athl Train 2005;40(3):139-152.

54. Guskiewicz KM, Bruce SL, Cantu RC, et al: National Athletic Trainers' Association position statement: management of sport-related concussion. J Athl Train 2004;39(3):280-297.

55. Cantu RC: Recurrent athletic head injury: risks and when to retire. Clin Sports Med 2003;22(3):593-;603, x.

56. McCrory P: Does second impact syndrome exist? Clin J Sport Med 2001;11(3):144-149.

57. Scheider RC. Head and neck injuries in football: mechanisms, treatment, and prevention. Baltimore, Williams & Wilkins, 1973, pp 35-43.

58. Saunders RL, Harbaugh RE: The second impact in catastrophic contact-sports head trauma. JAMA 1984;252(4):538-539.

59. Bruce DA, Alavi A, Bilaniuk L, et al: Diffuse cerebral swelling following head injuries in children: the syndrome of "malignant brain edema." J Neurosurg 1981;54(2):170-178.

60. Marmarou A, Fatouros PP, Barzo P, etal: Contribution of edema and cerebral blood volume to traumatic brain swelling in head-injured patients. J Neurosurg 2000;93(2):183-193. Erratum in J Neurosurg 2001;94(2):349.

61. Barzo P, Marmarou A, Fatouros P, et al: Cerebral edema and changes of cerebral blood volume in patients with head injuries. Orv Hetil 2002;143(27):1625-1634.

62. Unterberg AW, Stover J, Kress B, et al: Edema and brain trauma. Neuroscience 2004;129(4):1021-1029.

63. McCrory PR, Berkovic SF: Second impact syndrome. Neurology 1998;50(3):677-683.

64. Zemper ED: Two-year prospective study of relative risk of a second cerebral concussion. Am J Phys Med Rehabil 2003;82(9):653-659.

65. Guskiewicz KM, McCrea M, Marshall SW, et al: Cumulative effects associated with recurrent concussion in collegiate football players: the NCAA Concussion Study. JAMA 2003;290(19):2549-2555.

66. Yeates KO, Armstrong K, Janusz J, et al: Long-term attention problems in children with traumatic brain injury. J Am Acad Child Adolesc Psychiatry 2005;44(6):574-584.

67. Iverson GL, Brooks BL, Lovell MR, et al: No cumulative effects for one or two previous concussions. Br J Sports Med 2006;40(1):72-75.

68. Macciocchi SN, Barth JT, Littlefield L, et al: Multiple concussions and neuropsychological functioning in collegiate football players. J Athl Train 2001;36(3):303-306.

69. Pellman EJ, Lovell MR, Viano DC, et al: Concussion in professional football: neuropsychological testing—part 6. Neurosurgery 2004;55(6):1290-1303.

70. McCrea M, Guskiewicz KM, Marshall SW, et al: Acute effects and recovery time following concussion in collegiate football players: the NCAA Concussion Study. JAMA 2003;290(19):2556-2563.

71. Wall SE, Williams WH, Cartwright-Hatton S, et al: Neuropsychological dysfunction following repeat concussions in jockeys. J Neurol Neurosurg Psychiatry 2006; 77(4):518-520.

72. Moser RS, Schatz P, Jorda BD: Prolonged effects of concussion in high school athletes. Neurosurgery 2005;57(2):300-306.

73. Iverson GL, Gaetz M, Lovell MR, et al: Cumulative effects of concussion in amateur athletes. Brain Inj 2004;18(5):433-443.

74. Rabadi MH, Jordan BD: The cumulative effect of repetitive concussion in sports. Clin J Sport Med 2001;11(3):194-198.

75. Guskiewicz KM, Marshall SW, Bailes J, et al: Association between recurrent concussion and late-life cognitive impairment in retired professional football players. Neurosurgery 2005;57(4):719-726.

76. Collins MW, Lovell MR, Iverson GL, et al: Cumulative effects of concussion in high school athletes. Neurosurgery 2002;51(5):1175-1179.

77. Guterman A, Smith RW: Neurological sequelae of boxing. Sports Med 1987; 4(3):194-210.

78. Jordan BD, Relkin NR, Ravdin LD, et al: Apolipoprotein E epsilon4 associated with chronic traumatic brain injury in boxing. JAMA 1997;278(2):136-140.

79. Friedman G, Froom P, Sazbon L, et al: Apolipoprotein E-epsilon4 genotype predicts a poor outcome in survivors of traumatic brain injury. Neurology 1999;52(2):244-248.

80. Liberman JN, Stewart WF, Wesnes K, et al: Apolipoprotein E epsilon 4 and short-term recovery from predominantly mild brain injury. Neurology 2002; 58(7):1038-1044.

81. Quinn TJ, Smith C, Murray L, et al: There is no evidence of an association in children and teenagers between the apolipoprotein E epsilon4 allele and post-traumatic brain swelling. Neuropathol Appl Neurobiol 2004;30(6):569-575.

82. Putukian M, Echemendia RJ: Psychological aspects of serious head injury in the competitive athlete. Clin Sports Med 2003;22(3):617-630, xi.

83. Brown SJ, Fann JR, Grant I: Postconcussional disorder: time to acknowledge a common source of neurobehavioral morbidity. J Neuropsychiatry Clin Neurosci 1994;6(1):15-22.

84. de Kruijk JR, Leffers P, Meerhoff S, et al: Effectiveness of bed rest after mild traumatic brain injury: a randomised trial of no versus six days of bed rest. J Neurol Neurosurg Psychiatry 2002;73(2):167-172.

85. McCrory P: New treatments for concussion: the next millennium beckons. Clin J Sport Med 2001;11(3):190-193.

86. Field M, Collins MW, Lovell MR, et al: Does age play a role in recovery from sports-related concussion? A comparison of high school and collegiate athletes. J Pediatr 2003;142(5):546-553.

87. McClincy MP, Lovell MR, Pardini J, et al: Recovery from sports concussion in high school and collegiate athletes. Brain Inj 2006;20(1):33-39.

88. Canadian Academy of Sport Medicine Concussion Committee: Guidelines for assessment and management of sport-related concussion. Clin J Sport Med 2000;10(3):209-211.

CHAPTER 45

Running Shoes: Assessment and Selection

Charles W. Webb, DO, FAAFP,
and Marc A. Childress, MD

KEY POINTS

- Try on more than one shoe.
- Briefly jog in each shoe (with the agreement of the salesperson, of course).
- Purchase running shoes that are a half-size larger than your street shoes; make sure that there is at least a thumb's width of space between your longest toe and the end of the shoe.
- Never purchase a shoe if it does not feel perfect the moment that you put it on: there is no "break-in" period for running shoes.

INTRODUCTION

Equipment and apparel have become inseparable aspects of modern athletics. In some cases, these items may be critical to the sport, but, in far more situations, these products are designed to augment and protect athletes during the course of their endeavors. This is certainly the case with running shoes. Although the human body is perfectly capable of running and jogging without shoes, nearly all runners today elect to use shoes for a variety of reasons, including protection from the running surface, the prevention of injury, or the improvement of performance. As opposed to the barefooted competitors of ancient times, runners today face a dizzying array of options for sport-specific footwear. Additionally, it is difficult to find objective and useful information to guide runners in their decision-making process. For any physician who cares for both active and prospective runners, it can be very helpful to have a good basic knowledge of available products and to know how to counsel patients with regard to the selection of appropriate footwear. This chapter is designed to provide a background on the design and function of running shoes and a framework for creating a helpful running shoe prescription.

BUSINESS AND INDUSTRY CONCERNS

Like so many aspects of medicine, footwear is big business. Shoe manufacturers spend billions of dollars annually to market their products, which are highly linked to sponsored events and athletes. Additionally, each company is extremely aggressive in attempting to convince runners that their proprietary components provide superior performance. A close inspection of marketing techniques and published information will reveal a paucity of objective information for the making of these distinctions. From a business perspective, this makes perfect sense. Consider the analogy of competing medications within the same class. Rarely will patients and physicians be provided with the results of head-to-head trials because these trials are either never attempted or simply never published as a result of a lack of overwhelming evidence. Additionally, in an unregulated industry (in contrast with the US Food and Drug Administration approval processes), there is often no interest in pursuing these types of investigations because there is no enforced accountability or need to prove efficacy.

With footwear, this is made all the more interesting by the dynamics of fashion and sports culture. It is often impossible to gauge function from a simple visual inspection. Shoes that are innovative and well designed may be bland and appear rather simple, whereas poorly made shoes can easily be flashy and attractive. This can make the process of assessing shoes more difficult for patients and physicians alike.

Runners are often extremely loyal to a certain brand. This can be the case for providers as well, especially if they have a background in running. Care must be taken to maintain some objectivity when making recommendations to patients regarding footwear choices. The running culture is full of anecdotal advice that covers training regimens, nutrition, apparel, and footwear. In an attempt to be a consistent and unbiased source of advice to patients, physicians need to be cognizant of the lack of clinical information and outcome data for many of the factors that will be discussed here.

Despite these concerns, there are some tenets that have gained universal acceptance in the market (if not in the clinical world). Although research continues in the field of biomechanics and in the relationship of materials and technology to footwear, the industry currently works within the framework that is described below.

RUNNING SHOE ANATOMY

Running shoe components can be discussed in three basic segments. From top to bottom, these are as follows **(Figure 45.1):**

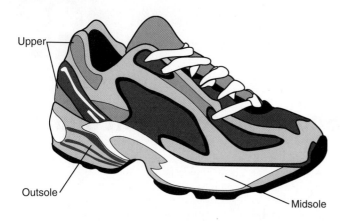

Figure 45.1 Basic figure of a running shoe.

Outsole: A rubber or composite layer that comes in contact with the running surface.
Midsole: A foam layer that provides cushioning and support. It can also contain extra support or cushioning devices.
Upper: The part of the shoe that secures the foot to the shoe and that provides additional support. This is the layer that contains the laces and the tongue of the shoe.

Outsoles are typically constructed of one of two rubber compounds: blown rubber and carbon rubber. Blown rubber is lighter and it offers a subtle benefit in cushioning, but it is less durable. Carbon rubber is slightly heavier and denser and thus more durable. Heavier runners (> 180 pounds) or runners who are maintaining higher mileage (> 30 miles) may benefit from a carbon rubber outsole, whereas most others will not compromise the integrity of the shoe with the more typical blown-rubber outsole. Many manufacturers are experimenting with other composite materials for outsoles, such as clear polymers, integrated midsole ethylene vinyl acetate polymers, and molded plastic frames. Most of these options will still include a rubber compound at the contact surface. Flexibility can be enhanced or diminished by outsole design. Flex grooves, separate outsole plates, and other methods to maintain the natural flex point at the ball of the foot will often be incorporated. Many of these measures will have little effect,[1] but, in some situations (e.g., excessive heel flare, which is common in trail shoes), they may increase the velocity of pronation and exacerbate instability injuries.[2]

Midsole design varies widely among manufacturers, and this is often where the marketed cushioning options will be found. Although there is a profound lack of data to this effect, there appears to be no clear difference in injury prevention among the proprietary methods of cushioning. These include air pads, encapsulated gels, lower-density ethylene vinyl acetate pads, arched plastic plates, silicone honeycomb pads, suspension fibers, and others. Some of these substances will offer a subjective difference in the sense of cushioning, but there is little evidence to support a clinical difference. Although impact dispersion may not be clearly affected by these inserts, there is a demonstrable difference in the durability of the midsole when various devices are used. Foam rubber products such as ethylene vinyl acetate are quickly susceptible to compression and loss of memory.[3] The addition of air, gel, or plastic devices can prolong the cushioning life span of the midsole by virtue of higher material memory. The variety of these devices is remarkable, and often manufacturers will incorporate numerous named compounds or devices into the same shoe **(Table 45.1)**.

Most manufacturers will also use the midsole to incorporate various stability devices, most of which are designed to help bolster support on the medial aspect of the shoe. There are a few

Table 45.1 A Sample of Various Midsole Technologies on the Market Today

Device	Manufacturer	Description
Air	Nike	Inert gas encapsulated in a polyurethane shell
DMX	Reebok	Communicating air chambers
Adiprene	Adidas	Proprietary ethylene vinyl acetate
Hydroflow	Brooks	Encapsulated gel fluid
GRID	Saucony	Cartridge of synthetic strings under tension
ARC	Avia	Plastic arch
Wave	Mizuno	Plastic series of arches
N-ergy	New Balance	Varied pressure chambers

examples on the market of shoes that truly attempt to compensate for underpronators. Because underpronating feet tend to be high arched and rigid, they benefit less from addition lateral stability and more from appropriate cushioning. For medial stability devices (which are often referred to as *medial posts*), most shoes will use a higher-density form of the midsole material. This is often denoted by a darker color (usually varying shades of gray). This is not a universal rule, but it is often helpful for locating shoes with extra medial support. Some shoes that are designed for those with more excessive stability needs will incorporate a semirigid thermoplastic polyurethane device into the medial portion of the midsole, thus further minimizing the amount of allowable pronation.

Various manufacturers have also used a midsole cutout under the junction of the midfoot and the hindfoot junction. This serves to reduce weight as well as (in theory) to allow the foot to flex and roll in a more natural pattern. There is little objective evidence to suggest that this is helpful in the area of injury prevention. Some will place thermoplastic polyurethane devices here to control the amount of this motion between the hindfoot and the forefoot. Flexibility at the forefoot has long been touted as critical to a natural and efficient gait, although it is questionable whether the flexion of the forefoot is affected to any significant degree by the midsole as opposed to the natural degree of flexibility of the foot itself.[4]

Upper design is often driven by the stylistic emphasis of the shoe, but there are some important functional factors as well. Around the heel, the shoe will have a "heel counter" that serves to cradle the heel and to hold the heel firmly to the rest of the shoe (most times there is a very slight angle into the foot to prevent slippage). The heel counter stiffness varies with the overall stability of the shoe, and it can range from nearly fixed in some motion-control shoes to crushable in some racing flats. Ensure that the heel counter does not create friction at either of the malleoli or at the Achilles tendon because these are common areas of complaint in poor-fitting running shoes. The counter should not come in contact with the malleoli in running shoes (as opposed to other athletic footwear, which may envelope the ankle in an attempt to provide additional support). The vamp, which is the middle portion of the upper that the laces are tied into, should be comfortable and flexible. The tongue should line up over the highest point of the foot, and it should feel very well cushioned. If the foot feels constricted around this area during standing, then the shoe is either too narrow or the laces are too tight. The toe box is the area between the vamp and the front portion of the shoe. This should allow enough room laterally for the foot to feel flat and relaxed, and it should be long enough for an additional thumb's width of space from the tip of the longest toe to the end of the shoe when standing straight (see the sizing tips discussed later in this chapter).

Another component to consider is the insole (or sock liner), which is most often a removable piece. This piece is designed to provide a smooth and soft contour for the sole of the foot. Most insoles will include a porous foam material with a fabric overlay. This portion of the shoe can have a significant impact in the non-–weight-bearing or standing comfort of a shoe. However, the cushion provided by this layer has little impact relative to the forces that are encountered during running. This is one of the best reasons to "test jog" in a shoe before purchase because the degree of comfort when running can be significantly different than the comfort noted when sitting or standing.

LASTING

Each manufacturer uses a proprietary model of a human foot to build the shoe around. This template, or "last," varies per brand and even from model to model within certain companies. Factors such as heel and forefoot width, arch placement, and shoe curvature will be affected by the last that is used in the construction of each particular shoe. This accounts for the large variety of fits encountered by different models and brands. Additionally, each shoe will follow a predetermined shape along the contact area of the shoe; this is designed to complement the normal amount of curve seen in the footprint of the human foot. When advertised, shoes will often be grouped into one of three categories: curved, semi-curved, and straight. Typically, curved lasts are more flexible and better matched to high-arched (pes cavus) feet. Semi-curved shoes are the most common, following the natural curvature of the most common foot type. Straight lasted shoes are designed as exactly that, with a reduction in the amount of curvature and often better accommodating those with significant pes planus; these runners may have greater needs for support and motion control. Certain brands have used unique lasting to cater to certain specific foot types, offering shoes that are designed to fit female runners, narrow feet, flatter or wider feet, and so on **(Figure 45.2).**

The term *last* also applies to the manner in which the upper is secured to the midsole. Shoes will generally be constructed in one of three fashions: board lasted, slip lasted, and combination lasted. Board lasted shoes have an insole board that runs the length of the shoe, with attachments to the upper at the sides. Slip lasting involves a circumferential wrap of the upper in a moccasin (or "slipper") style that adheres more directly to the midsole.

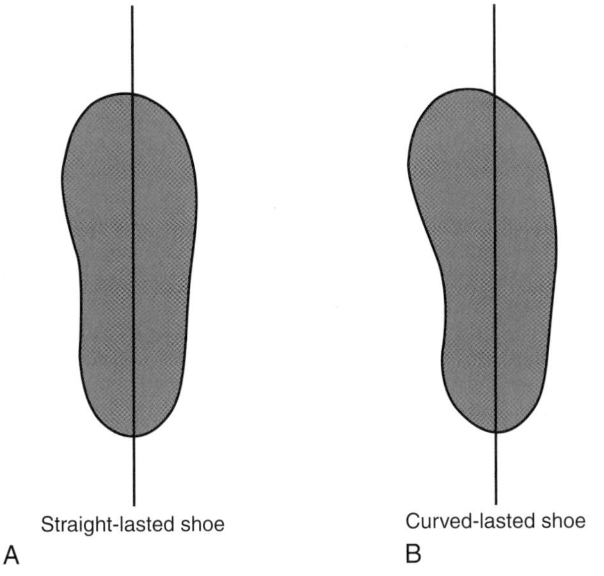

Combination lasted shoes are typically slip lasted in the forefoot, with an insole board in the hindfoot and midfoot. Board lasting is more commonly used in shoes that are designed for motion control because the process offers greater stability and less flexibility. Likewise, slip lasting is used in highly flexible shoes that cater to higher-arched runners. Combination lasted shoes are designed to match runners who desire the fit benefits of slip lasting but who may require the added stability of the board lasting. The differences in the type of lasting are usually easily visible on removal of the insole **(Figure 45.3).**

Because information about each model's construction is often not readily available to the public or clinicians, it is critically important that the patient try on multiple brands and models within those brands. Even within the appropriate genre of running shoe (e.g., cushion, stability, motion control), a shoe constructed for a differently shaped foot can create problems ranging from minor discomfort to increased slippage and friction to more significant injury.

The combination of design and materials in each of the portions of the shoe described previously make for a unique fit and feel for each available shoe on the market. The degree of difference depends in great part on the foot and the gait type of the runner. These are the factors that can be helpful when recommending certain features in the hopes that injuries can be reduced.

USE OF THE RUNNING SHOE PRESCRIPTION

Although there is a decent amount of information regarding the kinematic effects of some of the design features discussed previously,[5] there remains a gap between this body of information and its application to shoes that are available on the market.

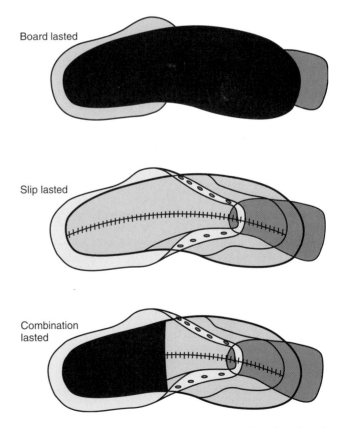

Board lasted

Slip lasted

Combination lasted

Figure 45.2 Examples of shoes that are straight lasted (*A*) and curve lasted (*B*).

Straight-lasted shoe

Curved-lasted shoe

A

B

Figure 45.3 Schematic views of shoes that are board lasted, slip lasted, and combination lasted.

In addition, there is often significant disagreement in these studies on the basis of the method of testing. For the most part, the biomechanical studies do not publish data regarding commercially available shoes or shoe components, and it can be difficult to translate the results of these studies into appropriate recommendations for branded shoes on the market.

As a result, physicians have fewer resources available to make evidence-based suggestions regarding footwear. Thus, it has been found that the best practical suggestions are made on the basis of design divisions in the industry. When making a recommendation or even a prescription, it is suggested that certain patient characteristics be evaluated to best match with the various types of running shoes on the market. The following segment of this chapter describes a stepwise patient assessment for a running shoe prescription. This form guides recommendations on the basis of easily identified genres and factors that are available from major shoe companies. An example form is included. The goals of this form and this discussion are to equip patients with both the information and the vocabulary that will help guide them to the most appropriate shoe. A helpful prescription should include recommendations that could be easily understood by both the patient and the supplier. Runners are increasingly seeking information from the Internet, and many retailers have incorporated helpful questionnaires that guide runners to matching shoes.[6] Although there is certainly no recognized format for such a prescription, the listed items can be helpful for both runners and salespeople **(Table 45.2).**

Background information

The initial questions listed relate to the durability needed from the shoe. Heavier runners (> 180 lbs) may benefit from more durable midsole (polyurethane) and outsole (carbon rubber) materials. The same may also be said for higher mileage runners (> 20 to 30 miles/week). However, keep in mind that the use of these denser materials in lighter runners may decrease the amount of cushioning, even if only in a subjective way. It is important to ask about orthotic use, even if the patient is using over-the-counter products. This may help highlight certain features that would be beneficial in the shoes. Runners who use prescription orthotic products need to have them available when they are trying on new shoes because many shoes are not well designed to accommodate the additional width and height of many orthotics. It is also not uncommon to see runners who use over-the-counter orthotic devices that may or may not be helpful. There is a considerable amount of discussion regarding the efficacy of these inserts.[7]

Foot analysis

The next section involves having the patient stand with his or her back to you and his or her heels at eye level (it is recommended that the examiner be lowered rather than having the patient elevated). The typical heel will usually be in slight pronation (hindfoot valgus) and then swing into a more varus position upon rising onto the toes. Heels that remain in valgus upon rising will most likely need medial support, but they may also need evaluation for the root of their hindfoot rigidity (e.g., previous injury, coalition). Heels that start and remain in varus are usually high-arched rigid feet, and good shoes for these feet will need to maximize cushioning.

The images seen on the prescription form represent a relief of the standing foot. They can be obtained in a variety of ways, including simple visualization (and possibly tracing the contact area) or having the patient wet his or her feet in a basin and then stand on an absorbent surface (e.g., a brown paper bag, a dark towel, a Chux pad) to see the area of weight-bearing contact. The basic spectrum involves pes planus (flatfeet) through pes

Table 45.2 Running Shoe Prescription

Patient Name: _____

Height: _____

Weight: _____

Average weekly miles: _____

Average pace (if known): _____

Orthotics: Y/N

Standing Foot Analysis

Resting ankle

_____ Neutral

_____ Pronated

_____ Supinated

With heel raise

_____ Neutral

_____ Pronated

_____ Supinated

Circle One*

A   B   C

Foot-Strike Analysis

(Preferably jogging/running gait rather than walking gait)

(If performed, please note the method of analysis [i.e., treadmill, flat ground, examination of previous footwear].)

Method: _____

_____ Heel strike

_____ Midfoot strike

_____ Forefoot strike

Recommendations (Check one from each category)

_____ Normal/stability (This is for most neutral runners with normal arches, and it incorporates a moderate amount of support in combination with good cushioning.)

_____ Motion control (This is for lower-arched runners who may roll toward the inside of their feet while running; it also incorporates good cushioning.)

_____ Cushion (This is for higher-arched runners with more rigid feet who may stay on the outside of their feet while running.)

_____ Normal durability (This is for low to mid mileage runners who are light to normal build for their weight.)

_____ Extra durability (This is for heavier runners or those who run more miles.)

_____ Heel striker

_____ Midfoot striker

_____ Forefoot striker

*Examples of arches of human foot. *A,* Normal. The forefoot and heel are connected by a curved band that is about 2 inches wide. *B,* Flat. A large impression or a very little arch. *C,* High. The forefoot and heel are connected by a very narrow strip.

cavus (high-arched feet). It is important to remember that, contrary to the belief of many patients, high-arched feet do not provide more cushioning to the body. In fact, these feet are often rigid and inflexible. Thus, patients with high arches typically will be less likely to overpronate, and they may in some cases underpronate (supinate). As mentioned previously, few shoes target underpronation specifically, but the emphasis should be on maximizing cushioning. Most shoes that target these runners will be labeled as *cushion shoes.* By contrast, the flatfooted arch often allows for sufficient cushioning, so shoes can help control the amount of pronation that these feet tend to exhibit; these shoes are usually described as *motion-control shoes.* For those with feet that would appear to fall in the middle of the spectrum, the bulk of the market is targeted at providing a comfortable mix of stability and cushioning; these will often be described as *stability shoes.*

Gait assessment

Gait assessment is the next segment of the prescription. Although much is made of pronation and supination (underpronation) in runners, it is important to remember that these are normal motions of the natural gait. The difference between an athlete with a neutral gait and one that might benefit from correction is sometimes subtle, and it depends in great part on whether the natural gait is causing pain or injury. Upon foot strike, the heel is typically the first to make contact at the lateral aspect. This is important to evaluate for runners who may make contact at the midfoot or the forefoot because this can affect the need for support and cushioning.

In ideal circumstances, this part of the evaluation would be performed on a dedicated treadmill with computer and video equipment to assess the moment-by-moment strike and roll of the foot. However, for the vast majority of clinic situations, this is nowhere near reality. If time and facilities allow, having the patient run on a regular treadmill can allow for similar visualization. However, without the aid of slow-motion cameras, it is difficult to visualize each of the components of the stride. For more details about gait analysis, see Chapter 43. Another way of assessing the gait is through an examination of the patient's last pair of running shoes. It is far preferable to have a pair of shoes that have been primarily for running because the gait is often quite different from that seen when walking and running. However, this is often not possible, especially if patients are seeking an initial recommendation.

The normal gait cycle includes foot strike at the lateral aspect of the heel. Upon impact, the heel will undergo pronation as the body moves forward over the foot. As the leg arcs forward, the weight of the body is transferred through the midfoot, by which time the foot has undergone a mild amount of supination, thus distributing the weight more evenly over the ball of the foot. Through flexion at the metatarsophalangeal joints, the foot rolls up onto the toes, and it is again pushed into the air. This cycle is repeated with every stride.

This is where the examination of the previous footwear can be very helpful. By evaluating the wear patterns, one can estimate the average distribution of force in the shoe over time. For example, most shoes will wear first over the lateral heel. As discussed previously, this is consistent with the neutral gait. However, if there is a significant amount of tread wear and midsole breakdown on the medial side of the heel, this may suggest overpronation. As the physician looks further forward on the shoe, he or she should see that, by the ball of the foot, the wear pattern is fairly even. Again, excessive wear to the inside is consistent with overpronation. Likewise, a wear pattern that started normally in the lateral heel and that continued laterally into the ball of the foot suggests underpronation. Look at the toe to see that wear is fairly even, often

focused at the longest toe. Having the old shoes can also allow for a brief examination for some of the other items emphasized in this chapter. Separation of the midsole from the upper in the ball of the foot suggests that the shoe may have been too narrow. Stressed or broken seams at the toes can be an indicator that the patient needs a larger size.

With all of this information, it is helpful to make simple recommendations that are understandable to both the patient and the salesperson. Time rarely allows for a full explanation of each part of the evaluation, so it can be helpful to include on the prescription a brief explanation of why the recommendations are being made.

GENERAL TIPS

Sizing

Be sure to recommend that your patients try shoes that are one half to one full size larger than their street shoes. Also recommend that the shoes be tried on either at the end of the day or soon after running or exercise. Feet swell during exercise, and the repeated impact of the running stride can slightly stretch the feet lengthwise. Shoes that are too small can lead to toenail damage, and they can severely impair the foot's ability to attenuate shock throughout the natural arc of the foot. Shoes that are too narrow can lead to blisters and to forefoot and toe pain, and they can limit the natural flex points at the metatarsophalangeal joints. Allow at least a thumb's width of space between the end of the longest toe (not always the great toe) and the front end of the shoe. In addition, if the ball of the foot feels constricted, look at wider shoes or other brands.

Lacing

Recommend that patients try various heights of lacing. Rarely do all of the uppermost eyelets need to be used. These recommendations apply to those individuals with heel slippage that results from very narrow hindfeet. If shoes are laced excessively high or tightly, pain along the anterior ankle joint may result, sometimes with distal nerve irritation (i.e., "lace bite"). There are a variety of lacing styles available for different foot types; these will not be covered here, but they can be found on the Internet. Keep in mind that these are not universal solutions. There is little objective evidence that these are helpful, but there is no harm in experimenting as long as the foot is secure.

In-store tips

It is imperative that patients try on more than one shoe before making a purchase. Recommend that patients try different brands and different models. There is no shoe that will cater appropriately to every runner, especially in the area of fit. If the shoe does not feel great immediately and feel better than all of the other options, then it is not the right shoe. Please emphasize this point of the immediate sensation. Unlike other footwear, there is no break-in period for running shoes. If there are any points of stiffness, pressure, or friction, then these will likely only worsen. Encourage patients to be as extensive when testing the shoe as the salesperson will allow. Some stores will allow and even encourage short jogs in or around the store before purchasing.

Regarding price, there are a few tips worth remembering. The most expensive shoe is not necessarily the best shoe. Although the prices of shoes have increased as a whole, a 1988 study suggested that there was no appreciable difference in injury avoidance between shoes that cost less than $25 and those that cost more than $40.[8] The numbers used are likely to be less relevant today, but the premise remains.

Many patients will be tempted to shop for running footwear through the Internet or catalogs. Many of these Web sites and sales resources are great sources of information for guiding runners to the appropriate shoes; however, it must be emphasized that the only time when it is appropriate to purchase a pair of shoes without trying them on is if the shoe is identical in model and size to a pair in which the athlete has already successfully run. Shoes from the same brand and even the same model in a different generation can have a significantly different fit, road feel, and level of flexibility.

Shoe life span

Most shoes are designed to offer adequate protection through 300 to 500 miles.[9] This depends again on the makeup of the shoe and the weight of the runner. In lower-mileage runners, these distances may not be reached within 6 months. The effective life of some of the cushioning materials can also deteriorate over time, regardless of use. For this reason, recommend a mileage cutoff or roughly 6 months of time, whichever comes first. Other signs that shoes may need to be replaced are the ability to sense small rocks and seams in the road through the sole of the shoe as well as a stinging or slapping sensation when the forefoot of the shoe hits the ground. Shoe life can also be affected by weather conditions. Moisture and cold temperatures have both been implicated in a reduced life span.[10]

SPECIAL CONSIDERATIONS

Older runners

Although the natural heel pad is excellent for providing a significant amount of shock attenuation, it is known to atrophy and lose elasticity with age.[11] Additionally, the normal human gait cycle is well suited to absorb additional shock through the degree of flexion in the feet and legs. Older (approximately 60 years old) and younger (approximately 20 to 30 years old) subjects are biomechanically different in the way that they run.[12] For example, older runners use shorter steps at a higher frequency and display smaller knee ranges of motion, higher vertical impact speeds, higher peak impact forces, and higher initial loading rates than younger runners. These findings demonstrate that the older runner may be less able to compensate for the repeated stresses of distance running, and this may even explain the higher incidence of overuse injuries in this population.[13] Accordingly, cushioning becomes a more important consideration when prescribing running shoes for older runners.

Female runners

Many shoe companies have become sensitive to the athletic needs of women and are promoting footwear that has a narrower fit for women. The female foot has a narrower Achilles tendon, a narrower heel in relation to the forefoot, and a foot that is narrower in general than the male counterpart. Women have been historically noted to have larger Q angles than men,[14] although this may be over estimated.[15] Women have the following differences from men while running: the impact in their vertical ground force reaction; peak tibial acceleration; maximal pronation; peak pronation velocity; and peak pressures and peak pressure rates.[16] In the recent past, women's shoes were based on a scaled-down version of lasts derived from the male foot anatomy. However, more manufacturers are now producing shoes solely for women that are designed with the previously mentioned factors having been addressed.

REFERENCES

1. Stacoff A, Reinschmidt C, Nigg BM, et al: Effects of shoe sole construction on skeletal motion during running. Med Sci Sports Exerc 2001;33(2):311-319.
2. Nigg BM, Morlock M: The influence of lateral heel flare of running shoes on pronation and impact forces. Med Sci Sports Exerc 1987;19(3):294-302.
3. Verdejo R, Mills NJ: Heel-shoe interactions and the durability of EVA foam running-shoe midsoles. J Biomech 2004;37(9):1379-1386.
4. Oleson M, Adler D, Goldsmith P: A comparison of forefoot stiffness in running and running shoe bending stiffness. J Biomech 2005;38(9):1886-1894.
5. Frederick EC: Kinematically mediated effects of sport shoe design: a review. J Sports Sci 1986;4(3):169-184.
6. www.roadrunnersports.com
7. Nigg BM, Stergiou P, Cole G: Effect of shoe inserts on kinematics, center of pressure, and leg joint moments during running. Med Sci Sports Exerc 2003;35(2):314-319.
8. Gardner LI Jr, Dziados JE, Jones BH, et al: Prevention of lower extremity stress fractures: a controlled trial of a shock absorbent insole. Am J Public Health 1988 Dec;78(12):1563-1567.
9. Cook SD, Kester MA, Brunet ME, Haddad RJ Jr: Biomechanics of running shoe performance. Clin Sports Med 1985;4(4):619-626.
10. Dib MY, Smith J, Bernhardt KA, et al: Effect of environmental temperature on shock absorption properties of running shoes. Clin J Sport Med 2005;15(3):172-176.
11. Hsu TC, Wang CL, Tsai WC, et al: Comparison of the mechanical properties of the heel pad between young and elderly adults. Arch Phys Med Rehabil 1998;79(9):1101-1104.
12. Bus SA: Ground reaction forces and kinematics in distance running in older-aged men. Med Sci Sport Exerc 2003;35:1167-1175.
13. Egermann M, Brocai D, Lill CA, Schmitt H: Analysis of injuries in long-distance triathletes. Int J Sports Med 2003;24(4):271-276.
14. Tillman MD, Bauer JA, Cauraugh JH, Trimble MH: Differences in lower extremity alignment between males and females. Potential predisposing factors for knee injury. J Sports Med Phys Fitness 2005;45(3):355-359.
15. Grelsamer RP, Dubey A, Weinstein CH: Men and women have similar Q angles: a clinical and trigonometric evaluation. J Bone Joint Surg Br 2005;87(11):1498-1501.
16. Henning EM: Gender differences for running in athletic footwear. In Hennig E, Stacoff A (eds): Proceedings of the 5th Symposium on Footwear Biomechanics. Zurich, Switzerland, 2001, p 44.

CHAPTER 46

Compartment Syndrome Testing

Brandon D. Larkin, MD, and Janiece N. Stewart, MD

KEY POINTS

- Compartment syndrome is a common cause of exertional leg pain in athletes, and clinical diagnosis alone is unreliable.
- Successful compartment pressure testing requires a thorough knowledge of anatomy.
- The Pedowitz criteria are the generally accepted guidelines for the diagnosis of chronic exertional compartment syndrome. However, debate exists regarding the accuracy of the currently used diagnostic criteria.
- Numerous alternative noninvasive investigative methods (e.g., magnetic resonance imaging, bone scanning, near-infrared spectroscopy, and technetium-99m methoxyisobutyl isonitrile perfusion imaging) have been studied and shown to have variable diagnostic values.

INTRODUCTION

Chronic leg pain in athletes is a common complaint that is often difficult to diagnose because several distinct pathologic processes may present with similar characteristics. Although the range of potential diagnoses is wide, medial tibial stress syndrome, stress fracture, chronic exertional compartment syndrome (CECS), nerve entrapment, and popliteal artery entrapment syndrome are the most common causes of exercise-related leg pain in athletes[1] **(Table 46.1).** Several studies have investigated the prevalence of individual diagnoses to explain exercise-related lower leg pain, and the findings are somewhat contradictory on the basis of the patient populations studied. A retrospective review of 150 athletes with chronic leg pain found that CECS was the most prevalent condition, with an incidence of 33%; this was followed by stress fractures in 25% and medial tibial stress syndrome in 13% (LOE: D).[2] Another study of 98 patients with recurrent anterior leg pain caused by either sports or trauma noted a 42% incidence of medial tibial stress syndrome, a 27% incidence of CECS, and a 13% incidence of peroneal nerve entrapment (LOE: D).[3] Regardless of distribution, a thorough knowledge of the anatomy and biomechanics of the lower extremities is necessary to successfully determine the most likely cause in a specific case and to develop an efficient, appropriate diagnostic plan and treat-ment regimen.

CECS is a common cause of exercise-induced lower leg pain in athletes. With this condition, pain is the result of elevated intramuscular pressure within an anatomic compartment. Four individual compartments exist in the lower leg: the anterior compartment, the lateral compartment, the superficial posterior compartment, and the deep posterior compartment. Housed within each of these compartments are muscles, nerves, and blood vessels, which are enclosed by fibrous fascia. During activity, muscle size may increase by 20%, thereby causing a compression of the components of the compartment if the surrounding fascia is of limited compliance.[4] This in turn leads to symptoms of pain and numbness in the area of the affected musculature or distally as a result of nerve compression.

Pathophysiology

The pathophysiology of CECS is not well understood. In normal athletes, intracompartmental pressure may rise threefold- to fourfold during exercise, but it rapidly returns to normal within a few minutes.[5] In athletes with CECS, however, there is a higher increase in pressure for a longer duration. Four factors have been identified that may, in combination, contribute to this difference: (1) an inelastic nature of the fascial sheath; (2) an increased skeletal muscle volume as a result of blood flow and edema; (3) muscle hypertrophy during exercise; and (4) gait-related dynamic contraction factors.[6]

The combination of these factors causes a transient rise in compartment pressure that eventually compromising the microcirculatory status. As blood flow decreases below the level that is needed to meet metabolic demands, tissue ischemia results, and the athlete experiences symptoms of pain, numbness, and weakness.[7]

EVALUATION

History

The hallmark of CECS is its reproducibility. The classic presentation involves recurrent leg cramping, burning, or aching pain and tightness during exercise over a specific component of the leg at a predictable point of activity, increasing in severity if that activity persists and resolving within minutes of the cessation of exercise. A longer period of rest is required for the complete resolution of a pain episode. CECS is most commonly associated with overuse injury in well-conditioned athletes, particularly runners.[8] Prolonged periods of rest do not result in a lack of pain when

Table 46.1   Differential Diagnosis for Chronic Exertional Compartment Syndrome

Diagnosis	Presentation	Diagnostic Studies
Stress fracture	Localized tenderness over the tibia; pain with bending stress	Plain x-ray, magnetic resonance imaging, bone scanning
Medial tibial stress syndrome	Pain on resisted plantarflexion and inversion along the posteromedial aspect of the tibia	Bone scanning, magnetic resonance imaging
Peripheral nerve entrapment	Tingling or numbness in a specific nerve distribution	Electromyelogram, nerve conduction study
Popliteal artery entrapment syndrome	Pain and coolness after excessive dorsiflexion and plantarflexion	Arteriogram
Radiculopathy	Sensory deficits; weakness	Electromyelogram, central nervous system evaluation

activity later ensues,[9] so athletes may actually completely stop their participation in the provocative sports. Pain is usually constant and unrelated to ground contact. Approximately 75% to 95% of patients present with bilateral symptoms (LOE: B).[10] Nonsteroidal anti-inflammatory medications are thought to be largely ineffective.[8]

Pain associated with the anterior and lateral compartments is typically described as occurring over the anterolateral aspect of the shin, with occasional radiation to the anterior ankle and the dorsum of the foot. Pain in the mid and upper calf is usually referred to the superficial posterior compartment, where deep posterior compartment pain lies over the medial shin or the distal calf, often spreading to the medial arch of the foot.[9]

Numbness, tingling, and weakness may also occur, and these may be the only presenting complaints, which indicate the involvement of the affected compartment's resident nerve. The athlete often notes a feeling of altered foot strike while running as a result of the transient weakness of the affected nerve's musculature.[11]

Physical examination

Another hallmark of CECS is a lack of physical signs at rest.[9] There may be a palpable firmness and/or fascial muscle herniation in the affected compartment, but little else is usually evident. Therefore, all patients with historic features that are indicative of CECS should undergo an exercise challenge test followed by a postexercise examination.[7] Ideally, the actual provoking activity (i.e., running, roller-blading, elliptical machine) should be performed during this testing. After the reproduction of the discomfort, the athlete should be assessed for tenderness, tightness, or swelling over the affected compartment. A full vascular and neurologic examination should be performed that includes sensation to light touch and strength testing.

Abnormal neurologic findings may clue the examiner in as to the identity of the affected nerve and, therefore, the compartment involved.[9] Anterior compartment involvement after exercise may display weakness of dorsiflexion or toe extension, paresthesias over the dorsum of the foot, numbness in the first web space, or even transient or persistent foot drop.[12] Sensory changes over the anterolateral aspect of the leg and weakness of ankle inversion may indicate lateral compartment involvement. Superficial posterior compartment symptomatology includes dorsolateral foot sensory deficits and weakness of plantar flexion, and deep posterior compartment involvement may lead to plantar foot paresthesias and weakness of toe flexion and ankle inversion.[7]

The patient should have normal dorsalis pedis and posterior tibialis pulses after exercise challenge testing. If these are decreased from baseline, a vascular cause such as popliteal artery entrapment should be considered.[7]

Despite a history that is suggestive of CECS, no physical examination finding can firmly establish the diagnosis. Numerous other causes can result in similar symptoms. A false-positive rate of 74% on the basis of clinical examination has been reported (LOE: D).[3] Therefore, diagnosis that is based only on clinical presentation

increases the risk of misdiagnosis, delayed diagnosis, and inappropriate therapy.[13] Most studies emphasize the need for intramuscular pressure measurement during the diagnostic process. Targeted testing can be performed on the basis of the history if the clinical presentation indicates the involvement of a specific compartment. A vague location of symptoms may necessitate the testing of all four compartments of the leg **(Table 46.2).**

TECHNIQUES AND EQUIPMENT

Testing strategies

Compartment pressure testing is an invasive procedure. Successful and uncomplicated performance of this test requires a thorough knowledge of the anatomy of the compartments to be entered to avoid contact with vital neurovascular structures. Two types of intracompartmental pressure measurement strategies have been used. Dynamic testing makes use of a slit catheter inserted into the compartment before exercise and attached to the athlete's leg. Using this technique, the examiner is able to continuously monitor pressure changes during exercise and to correlate symptoms with objective data.[6] However, dynamic testing is not without problems. Catheter placement in the compartment is difficult to maintain during exercise. Also, the attachment of the apparatus to the patient may restrict the natural gait. In addition, dynamic testing does not allow the athlete to run on his or her usual training

Table 46.2   Indication and Contraindications for Compartment Pressure Testing

Indications	Contraindications
Clinical evidence of chronic exertional compartment syndrome:	History of a bleeding disorder or anticoagulation
• Recurrent exercise-induced leg discomfort that increases with continued exercise and resolves with rest	Rash or infection of the overlying skin
• Tight, cramping, or squeezing ache over a specific compartment area	
• Numbness, tingling, or weakness of the leg or foot	
Exercise challenge testing provoking signs of chronic exertional compartment syndrome:	
• Firmness or tenderness to palpation of an anatomic compartment of the leg	
• Weakness in an anatomic nerve distribution	
• Loss of sensation to light touch in an anatomic nerve distribution	

surface because it may only be performed on a treadmill, and it does not allow for the simultaneous testing of multiple compartments. Many have found the results of the dynamic measurement technique to be inconsistent and difficult to interpret because values vary substantially from patient to patient (LOE: B).[14]

Static compartment pressure testing is currently the most common technique employed for the determination of pathology. Static pressure measurements are obtained via a needlestick both before and after exercise. This technique allows the athlete to move freely during activity and affords some degree of freedom to accurately reconstruct actual training conditions and location. In addition, several compartments on both legs can be measured, which is often necessary if the clinical presentation is vague. However, this method does require two to three needlesticks per compartment tested.

Equipment

Numerous apparatuses have been used to measure compartment pressures in both static and dynamic testing. Techniques employed include a needle manometer, a slit catheter, a wick catheter, continuous infusion, and a solid-state transducer intracompartmental catheter.[6,15] A commonly used device is the Stryker Intracompartmental Pressure Monitor (Stryker Corporation, Kalamazoo, Mich) **(Figure 46.1).** It is a battery-operated, handheld, digital fluid pressure monitor that has been found to be more accurate and easier to use than the needle manometer.[16] It is compatible with both static and dynamic testing. Its convenience and, more importantly, its reproducibility between examiners make it an appropriate tool for the busy clinical office setting.[7,17]

Anatomy

As mentioned previously, a thorough understanding of the anatomy of the compartment to be studied is imperative for safe and effective compartment pressure testing. The leg contains four anatomically distinct compartments, each bound by bone and fascia

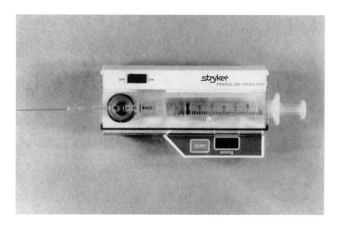

Figure 46.1 Stryker handheld compartment pressure monitor. (From Canale ST [ed]: Campbell's Operative Orthopaedics, 10th ed. St. Louis, Mosby, 2003.)

and each containing a major nerve **(Figure 46.2).** The anterior compartment contains muscles that are used to extend the toes and to dorsiflex the ankle. It contains the extensor hallucis longus, the extensor digitorum longus, the peroneus tertius, and the anterior tibialis muscles as well as the deep peroneal nerve. The blood supply is from the anterior tibial artery. The lateral compartment houses the muscles that are responsible for the eversion of the foot: the peroneus longus and brevis. It also contains the superficial peroneal nerve as well as branches of the peroneal artery. The plantarflexors of the foot—the gastrocnemius, the soleus, and the plantaris—are contained in the superficial posterior compartment along with the sural nerve. The deep posterior compartment contains the muscles of toe flexion, ankle plantarflexion, and ankle inversion, which are the flexor hallucis longus, the flexor digitorum longus, and the posterior tibialis muscles. The posterior tibial nerve and the posterior tibial artery are also located within the deep posterior compartment.

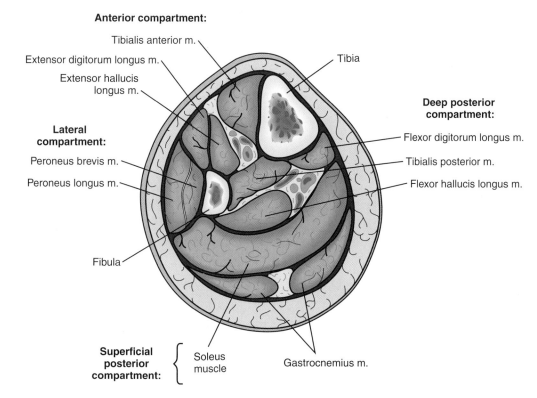

Figure 46.2 Axial anatomy of the lower extremity. m., muscle. (Redrawn from Scuderi, McCann [eds]: Sports Medicine: A Comprehensive Approach. Philadelphia, Mosby, 2005.)

Anterior compartment:
Tibialis anterior m.
Extensor digitorum longus m.
Extensor hallucis longus m.
Tibia

Lateral compartment:
Peroneus brevis m.
Peroneus longus m.

Deep posterior compartment:
Flexor digitorum longus m.
Tibialis posterior m.
Flexor hallucis longus m.

Fibula

Superficial posterior compartment: Soleus muscle
Gastrocnemius m.

Although all compartments can be affected and often are affected in combination, most studies have found the distribution of pathology to be relatively consistent. Anterior compartment syndrome is the most common (45%), followed by the deep posterior compartment (40%), the lateral compartment (10%), and the superficial posterior compartment (5%).[18]

Some describe a separate and distinct fifth compartment that is encompassed by the fascia surrounding the posterior tibialis muscle and that may be important in CECS.[11] However, recent studies have called into question the consistency of this anatomic finding, describing it alternatively as a subcompartment that is only occasionally demonstrable in cadaveric investigation. Regardless of its classification, the area may display a separate increase in intramuscular pressure, and it should likely be an important target of surgical treatment (LOE: E).[19]

The procedure (Box 46.1)

1. Obtain written informed consent from the patient after explaining the risks and benefits of the procedure.
2. The Stryker pressure monitor is a reusable device that requires a disposable set of accessories that are packaged together. This set should include a sterile 18-gauge needle, a diaphragm chamber, and a syringe filled with 3 mL of normal saline. Additional equipment includes sterile gloves, alcohol swabs, gauze, Betadine solution, a 25-gauge needle and syringe for the instillation of local anesthesia, and 1% xylocaine without epinephrine. Bupivacaine 0.5% solution should also be used for local anesthesia if the patient's symptoms require an extended period of time to occur to avoid repeated injections of the shorter-acting anesthetic.[7]
3. Have the patient lie relaxed in the supine position with the knees extended and the ankle in a vertical position.
4. Identify the desired compartments, and sterilize the overlying skin with alcohol and Betadine.
5. Anesthetize the column of tissue between the skin and fascia with 1 to 3 mL of 1% lidocaine without epinephrine, taking care to avoid penetration through the fascia and into the compartment.
6. Prepare the Stryker monitor for insertion by connecting the provided disposable syringe, the sterile needle, and the diaphragm transducer (see Figure 46.1). Press the syringe to fill the diaphragm and needle until a drop of saline is expressed from the needle tip and no air bubbles are visible in the diaphragm. Power on the monitor, and depress the "zero" button to clear the unit.
7. Orient the device at a 90-degree angle to the skin to be entered. Immediately before inserting the needle into the extremity, zero the device again, ensuring that the angle of entry is maintained as the "zero" button is depressed.
8. Insert the needle at 90 degrees into the anesthetized skin, through the subcutaneous tissue and fascia, and into the compartment. There is a palpable "pop" as the fascia is breached. Approaches for individual compartments are described later in this chapter.
9. After the needle has entered the compartment, instill a small amount of saline to ensure a solid column of fluid. Allow a few moments for the monitor to equilibrate. Record the measurement, and remove the needle.
10. To approach the anterior compartment, palpate the tibialis anterior just lateral to the anterior tibial border, and insert the needle at the level of the mid third of the tibia **(Figure 46.3)**. Just above the interosseous membrane sits the neurovascular bundle, which contains the deep peroneal nerve, the anterior tibial artery, and the veins and which should be avoided.
11. To approach the lateral compartment, palpate the muscle bellies of the peroneus longus and brevis at the same mid-tibial level as the anterior approach **(Figure 46.4)**. Needle insertion should be at the midpoint between the head of the fibula and the lateral malleolus. The intramuscular septum between the anterior and lateral compartments is usually apparent with deep palpation from the anterior tibia laterally. The angle of entry into the lateral compartment is typically parallel with the examination table.

Box 46.1: Checklist of Procedure

- Obtain written informed consent after discussing risks and benefits with the patient.
- Gather and assemble equipment.
- Position the patient supine with the knees extended and the ankles in a vertical position.
- Sterilize the overlying skin.
- Anesthetize the skin and the subcutaneous tissue.
- Prepare the Stryker monitor by instilling saline to fill the diaphragm and needle.
- Power on the monitor, and zero the unit.
- Orient the device at a 90-degree angle to the skin, and zero the device again.
- Insert the needle through the skin, the subcutaneous tissue, and the fascia and into the compartment.
- Instill a small amount of saline, and wait for the monitor to equilibrate.
- Record the measurement, and remove the needle.
- Repeat the procedure in all compartments that are suspicious for involvement.
- Cover the needle sites with bandages.
- Have the patient exercise until symptoms occur and until the point at which he or she would normally discontinue exercise as a result of pain.
- Repeat the procedure in all involved compartments at 1 minute and 5 minutes after exercise.
- Dispose of the needles in a biohazard container.
- Advise the patient about postprocedure care.

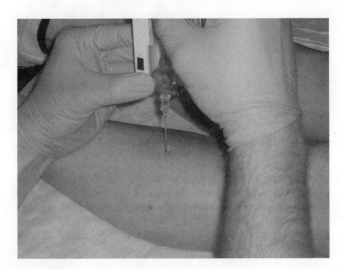

Figure 46.3 Anterior approach.

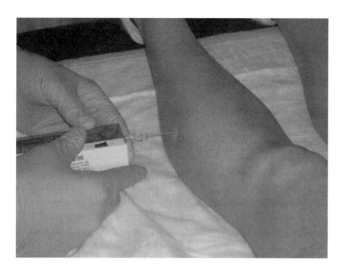

Figure 46.4 Lateral approach.

12. To approach the superficial posterior compartment, palpate the muscle bellies of the gastrocnemius and the soleus. Approach this compartment from the medial side just posterior to the medial border of the tibia, avoiding the small saphenous vein and the medial and lateral sural cutaneous nerves **(Figure 46.5)**. It is helpful to flip the monitor so that the display faces the examiner during this approach.

13. To approach the deep posterior compartment, continue advancing the needle after completing testing of the superficial compartment, closely approximating the posterior aspect of the tibia. A second "pop" is felt when the deep compartment is entered. A vascular bundle containing the peroneal artery and veins lies medial to the posterior border of the fibula. A neurovascular bundle with the tibial nerve, the posterior tibial artery, and veins lies in the posterior aspect of the compartment behind the tibialis posterior muscle.

14. Cover the needle sites with bandages.

15. Have the patient perform the provocative activity until typical symptoms are fully reproduced,[20] usually to the point at which the athlete would normally discontinue exercise as a result of pain. It is important to use provocative activities that are as similar to the pain-provoking exercise as possible (LOE: E).[21]

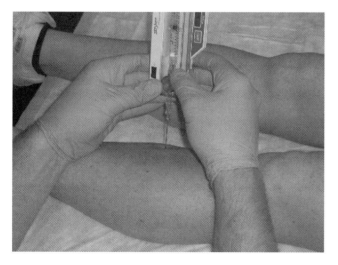

Figure 46.5 Superficial and deep posterior approach.

16. Compartment pressures should be measured again at 1 minute after exercise or as soon as possible after the onset of symptoms. The procedure should be repeated 5 minutes into the rest period (LOE: B).[14] Entry into each compartment should use the same needle holes that were used during pre-exercise testing.

17. Dispose of the needles in a biohazard container.

18. Advise the patient about postprocedure care. Bleeding, signs of infection, or neurologic complaints should signal a need to return for evaluation and treatment.

INTERPRETATION

Findings that are consistent with the diagnosis of CECS are an elevated resting compartment pressure obtained before exercise, a marked elevation of postexertion pressure, and/or a delayed return to normal pressure several minutes into the rest period.

The most commonly accepted criteria for the accurate diagnosis of CECS were described by Pedowitz and colleagues.[13] One or more of the following criteria must be met in addition to an appropriate history and physical examination (LOE-B):

- Pre-exercise compartment pressure of 15 mm Hg or more
- 1-minute postexercise compartment pressure of 30 mm Hg or more
- 5-minute postexercise compartment pressure of 20 mm Hg or more

There is a fair amount of controversy regarding the most accurate threshold for the diagnosis of CECS. Although the Pedowitz criteria are generally considered to be the standard scale, several studies have used differing or additional criteria. Reports of normal values for resting intracompartmental pressure even vary as a result of such variables as operator experience, the catheter type, the volume of the instilled fluid, the position of the leg and foot of the subject, the type of exercise performed, and the timing of the measurement.

Although Pedowitz and colleagues consider a pressure of less than 15 mm Hg to be normal in a resting compartment, other authors have found that a measurement of less than 10 mm Hg may be a more accurate normal value at rest.[20] The same study proposed that levels of greater than 20 mm Hg at 1 minute and greater than 20 mm Hg at 5 minutes and an intracompartmental pressure normalization time of greater than 15 minutes are adequate criteria, with the latter being the most reliable for diagnosing CECS in adolescent athletes (LOE: B). Several authors agree that delayed pressure normalization time may be the most appropriate indicator of pathology.[14] If symptoms are fully reproduced during provocative exercise testing, the subjective relief of pain by the athlete—and, thus, the return of the compartment pressure to normal (LOE: D)[22]—has been found to occur after a period of 20 minutes of rest.[20] Therefore, the measurement of compartment pressure at 15 minutes after exercise would seem to be appropriate if findings at 5 minutes after exercise are equivocal.[1]

Although the Pedowitz criteria are, for the most part, commonly agreed on, they are based on a comparison with 210 normal anterior muscle compartments that were tested during the study's data collection. With CECS of the posterior compartment, there is considerably more disagreement about the proper cutoff values.[9] However, most clinicians use the same criteria for the anterior compartment and other compartments.[23]

Because of the variability in the interpretation of the results of compartment pressure testing, positive pressure tests alone are insufficient to make the diagnosis and should never replace a thorough history and physical examination.

Other diagnostic modalities

Because results of compartment pressure testing are interpreted differently and objective criteria are the focus of continuing debate, the search for other diagnostic methods is vigorous, especially for a noninvasive modality. Other tools that have been employed include the triple-phase bone scan, magnetic resonance imaging (MRI), near-infrared spectroscopy, and technetium-99m methoxyisobutyl isonitrile perfusion imaging.

Bone scanning may show decreased radionuclide uptake in or near the affected area, thereby supporting the diagnosis of decreased blood flow and thus elevated intracompartmental pressure. The characteristic pattern also displays increased tracer concentration superior and inferior to the abnormality.[15] MRI may be useful for the diagnosis of CECS as a result of its sensitivity to changes in water distribution in skeletal muscle. If tissue edema is involved in pressure elevation in individual compartments, post-exercise MRI may be able to detect the increased water content (LOE: C).[24] Although MRI is sensitive, its specificity remains questionable because it may display findings that are similar to those of metabolic rhabdomyolysis, muscle lesions, or even changes in normal muscle caused by exercise.[24] Studies question the diagnostic value of MRI with regard to its ability to consistently confirm CECS (LOE: D).[25] Nevertheless, if the limitations of these modalities are taken into account, bone scanning and MRI offer diagnostic alternatives for the athlete who is hesitant to consent to the more invasive compartment pressure testing procedure.

Near-infrared spectroscopy is an indirect, noninvasive method of investigating CECS in which the degree of the deoxygenation of muscle tissue as a result of exercise can be measured. It is based on the discovery of ischemia caused by increased intracompartmental pressure that causes an increased extraction of oxygen from arterial blood by muscle, thereby resulting in decreased venous oxyhemoglobin content. The tissue oxygen saturation is thought to reflect the oxygen saturation of venous blood because most of the blood content of tissue is in the venous compartment. Recent studies have shown that patients with the clinical complaints and elevated compartment pressures that are typical of CECS show a larger decrease in tissue oxygen saturation on near-infrared spectroscopy and a longer period of recovery to normal levels than do healthy controls (LOE: C).[26] In addition, spectroscopy approaches the sensitivity of intracompartmental pressure testing for diagnosis (LOE: D).[25] However, because it depends on light absorption through tissue to measure muscle oxygenation, near-infrared spectroscopy is limited in its usefulness for very dark-skinned athletes.[26]

Technetium-99m methoxyisobutyl isonitrile perfusion testing evaluates the uptake of a radiolabeled intravenous solution by peripheral muscles. Uptake is determined by blood flow and inhibited by hypoxia, thus making it useful for detecting muscle ischemia. Case reports exist that illustrate a visually apparent decrease in its concentration in muscles that are contained in compartments with elevated pressures after exercise as compared with imaging at rest (LOE: E).[27] Technetium-99m methoxyisobutyl isonitrile imaging requires the visual interpretation of concentration within the compartment, and its results were not found to be identical to invasive compartment pressure testing. Further study is needed to determine its place in the diagnosis of CECS.

UPPER EXTREMITY COMPARTMENT SYNDROME

Although CECS in the lower extremity is well described in the literature, there is a relative dearth of discussion regarding its involvement in the upper extremity. A likely reason for this is the rarity of the condition among athletes. When it does occur, its typical presentation is tightness and pain in the forearm (not related to trauma) that occurs during a steady increase in activity. As is seen in lower extremity compartment syndrome, pain relents within minutes of the cessation of the exercise. Dyesthesias and weakness may also occur in the distal extremity. Affected athletes include those with repetitive arm motion, including tennis players,[28] weight-lifters,[29] and motorcyclists.[30]

Because of its rarity, the diagnosis of CECS in the upper extremities is often delayed. Physical examination findings may include the swelling and palpable tenderness of the affected musculature after exercise. These findings may be elicited during the examination after repetitive resisted range-of-motion exercises of the elbow, wrist, and/or fingers.[28]

Numerous techniques for compartment pressure testing of the upper extremity have been described. The insertion of a catheter into the individual compartments of the forearm has been used for the measurement of compartment pressures before, during, and 15 to 30 minutes after repetitive exercise to the point at which symptoms recur (LOE: E).[30] Others instruct the patient to perform maximal isometric contractions of the affected muscle group for 5 seconds; recording compartmental pressures during this effort and again shortly after exercise ceases to determine whether an immediate return to baseline has occurred (LOE: E).[28]

Although there is no consensus regarding the best method for the measurement of upper extremity compartment pressure, there is also none concerning which values are to be considered diagnostic.[31] It has been suggested that a resting pressure of greater than 15 mm Hg or a 5-minute postexercise pressure of greater than 25 mm Hg is pathologic (LOE: E).[29] Others suggest that the period of greater than 15 minutes for the recovery of pressure to the baseline level after exercise is more indicative (LOE: E).[32] They point out that resting baseline pressures are often quite variable and intensely technique dependent and that they therefore should not be used as diagnostic criteria.

As with lower-extremity CECS, clinical factors are most important for diagnosis. However, objective studies do provide supportive data and thus should be used when appropriate (**Boxes 46.2, 46.3, 46.4, and 46.5**).

Box 46.2: Pitfalls

Errors in Measurement[7]

- Calibration of the monitor at an inconsistent angle on repeat testing
- Inconsistency of knee and ankle joint positioning on repeat testing
- Application of external pressure on the compartment while stabilizing the extremity

Errors in Diagnosis

- Unnecessary surgical procedure that may lead to further complications
- Recurrence of pain after a "curative" surgical procedure

Box 46.3: Complications

- Postprocedure bruising, swelling, and pain
- Neurologic sequelae from nerve injury
- Bleeding from damage to local vasculature

Box 46.4: Controversies

- Timing of postexercise testing
- Accurate diagnostic criteria
- Dynamic versus static testing

Box 46.5: Risks and Benefits

Risks

- Infection
- Scarring at the site of the injection
- Damage to the surrounding neurovascular structures
- Reaction to the local anesthesia

Benefits

- Accurate diagnosis
- Avoidance of an unnecessary surgical procedure

REFERENCES

1. Edwards PH, Wright ML, Hartman JF: A practical approach for the differential diagnosis of chronic leg pain in the athlete. Am J Sports Med 2005;33(8):1241-1249.
2. Clanton TO, Solcher BW: Chronic leg pain in the athlete. Clin Sports Med 1994;13(4):743-759.
3. Styf J: Diagnosis of exercise-induced pain in the anterior aspect of the lower leg. Am J Sports Med 1988;16(2):165-169.
4. Touliopolous S, Hershman EB: Lower leg pain. Diagnosis and treatment of compartment syndromes and other pain syndromes of the leg. Sports Med 1999;27(3):193-204.
5. Walker WC: Lower leg pain. In Lillegard WA, Butcher JD, Rucker KS (eds): Handbook of Sports Medicine: A Symptom-Oriented Approach, 2nd ed. Boston, Butterworth-Heinemann, 1999, p 251.
6. McDermott AG, Marble AE, Yabsley RH, et al: Monitoring dynamic anterior compartment pressures during exercise. A new technique using the STIC catheter. Am J Sports Med 1982;10(2):83-89.
7. Glorioso JE, Wilckens JH: Exertional leg pain. In O'Connor FG, Wilder RP (eds): Textbook of Running Medicine. New York, McGraw-Hill, 2001, p 95.
8. Turnipseed W, Detmer DE, Girdley F: Chronic compartment syndrome. An unusual cause for claudication. Ann Surg 1989;210(4):557-562.
9. Blackman PG: A review of chronic exertional compartment syndrome in the lower leg. Med Sci Sports Exerc 2000;32(3 Suppl):S4-S10.
10. Kiuru MJ, Mantysaari MJ, Pihlajamaki HK, et al: Evaluation of stress-related anterior lower leg pain with magnetic resonance imaging and intracompartmental pressure measurement. Mil Med 2003;168(1):48-52.
11. Dammann GG, Albertson KS: Surgical considerations in the leg. In O'Connor FG, Sallis RE, Wilder RP, et al (eds): Sports Medicine: Just the Facts. New York, McGraw-Hill, 2005, p 373.
12. Detmer DE, Sharpe K, Sufit RL, et al: Chronic compartment syndrome: diagnosis, management, and outcomes. Am J Sports Med 1985;13(3):162-170.
13. Pedowitz RA, Hargens AR, Mubarak SJ, et al: Modified criteria for the objective diagnosis of chronic compartment syndrome of the leg. Am J Sports Med 1990;18(1):35-40.
14. Rorabeck CH, Bourne RB, Fowler PJ, et al: The role of tissue pressure measurement in diagnosing chronic anterior compartment syndrome. Am J Sports Med 1988;16(2):143-146.
15. Wilder RP, Sethi S: Overuse injuries: tendinopathies, stress fractures, compartment syndrome, and shin splints. Clin Sports Med 2004;23(1):55-81.
16. Awbrey BJ, Sienkiewicz PS, Mankin HJ: Chronic exercise-induced compartment pressure elevation measured with a miniaturized fluid pressure monitor. A laboratory and clinical study. Am J Sports Med 1988;16(6):610-615.
17. Hutchinson M, Ireland M: Chronic exertional compartment syndrome—gauging pressure. Phys Sportsmed 1999;27;101.
18. Edwards P, Myerson M: Exertional compartment syndrome of the leg: steps for expedient return to activity. Phys Sportsmed 1996;24;31-37.
19. Hislop M, Tierney P, Murray P, et al: Chronic exertional compartment syndrome: the controversial "fifth" compartment of the leg. Am J Sports Med 2003;31(5):770-776.
20. Garcia-Mata S, Hidalgo-Ovejero A, Martinez-Grande M: Chronic exertional compartment syndrome of the legs in adolescents. J Pediatr Orthop 2001;21(3):328-334.
21. Padhiar N, King JB: Exercise induced leg pain-chronic compartment syndrome. Is the increase in intra-compartment pressure exercise specific? Br J Sports Med 1996;30(4):360-362.
22. Styf J, Korner L, Suurkula M: Intramuscular pressure and muscle blood flow during exercise in chronic compartment syndrome. J Bone Joint Surg Br 1987;69(2):301-305.
23. Tzortziou V, Maffulli N, Padhiar N: Diagnosis and management of chronic exertional compartment syndrome (CECS) in the United Kingdom. Clin J Sport Med 2006;16(3):209-213.
24. Eskelin MK, Lotjonen JM, Mantysaari MJ: Chronic exertional compartment syndrome: MR imaging at 0.1 T compared with tissue pressure measurement. Radiology 1998;206(2):333-337.
25. van den Brand JG, Nelson T, Verleisdonk EJ, et al: The diagnostic value of intracompartmental pressure measurement, magnetic resonance imaging, and near-infrared spectroscopy in chronic exertional compartment syndrome: a prospective study in 50 patients. Am J Sports Med 2005;33(5):699-704.
26. Mohler LR, Styf JR, Pedowitz RA, et al: Intramuscular deoxygenation during exercise in patients who have chronic anterior compartment syndrome of the leg. J Bone Joint Surg Am 1997;79(6):844-849.
27. Owens S, Edwards P, Miles K, et al: Chronic compartment syndrome affecting the lower limb: MIBI perfusion imaging as an alternative to pressure monitoring: two case reports. Br J Sports Med 1999;33(1):49-51.
28. Berlemann U, al-Momani Z, Hertel R: Exercise-induced compartment syndrome in the flexor-pronator muscle group. A case report and pressure measurements in volunteers. Am J Sports Med 1998;26(3):439-441.
29. Hider SL, Hilton RC, Hutchinson C: Chronic exertional compartment syndrome as a cause of bilateral forearm pain. Arthritis Rheum. 2002;46(8):2245-2246.
30. Goubier JN, Saillant G: Chronic compartment syndrome of the forearm in competitive motor cyclists: a report of two cases. Br J Sports Med 2003;37(5):452-453; discussion 453-454.
31. Kumar PR, Jenkins JP, Hodgson SP: Bilateral chronic exertional compartment syndrome of the dorsal part of the forearm: the role of magnetic resonance imaging in diagnosis: a case report. J Bone Joint Surg Am 2003;85-A(8):1557-1559.
32. Garcia Mata S, Hidalgo Ovejero A, Martinez Grande M: Bilateral, chronic exertional compartment syndrome of the forearm in two brothers. Clin J Sport Med 1999;9(2):91-99.

Electrodiagnostic Testing

Jimmy D. Bowen, MD, FAAPMR, CSCS

KEY POINTS

- A careful history and physical examination of the patient is not replaced but rather is complemented by electrodiagnostic testing.
- The electrodiagnostic evaluation is a continuation and an extension of the clinical investigation.
- Electrodiagnostic evaluation allows for the clinical use of nerves and the probing of muscles to localize lesions that are demonstrated by the weaknesses, sensory losses, and reflex changes of the physical examination.
- Electrodiagnostic evaluation helps to determine the type and chronology of an abnormality.
- Like the clinical examination, the electrodiagnostic evaluation is dependent on the evaluator.

INTRODUCTION

"Since the measuring device has been constructed by the observer... we have to remember that what we observe is not nature itself, but nature exposed to our method of questioning."

—*Werner Karl Heisenberg[1]*

A 16-year-old high school football strong safety reports to your office with his second stinger in the last month **(Figure 47.1).** Four weeks before the visit, he was making a chop tackle, hitting the running back with his right shoulder, when he noted that his neck bent laterally to the left. He had an immediate lancinating pain down his right arm, and he was unable to raise his arm. He became weak in that arm, and the athletic trainer held him out for 2 weeks, until his strength returned to normal. During his second game after returning, he dove in in front of a running back to make a tackle. His head hit the running back's thigh, and his head and neck went into lateral flexion and extension to the right. He again experienced immediate lancinating pain and an inability to raise his arm. He reports to your office with improving aching right proximal arm pain. On clinical examination, he is weak in the external rotators of the shoulder, the deltoid, the biceps, the supinator, and the radial wrist extensors. He has no sensory deficit.

The above description is of a stinger or burner, which is a very common injury in football. In fact, it may have affected as many as 65% of college football players at one time or another.[2] Much controversy exists regarding this pinch–stretch injury of the cervical C5-C6 nerve roots or of the more distal upper trunk brachial plexopathy. Is this player's injury proximal at the nerve root level or more distal at the upper trunk? What is the prognosis for the return of strength and return to play? An electrodiagnostic examination (EDX) may be the definitive test for answering these questions for this athlete and his parents.[3]

THE ELECTRODIAGNOSTIC EXAMINATION

EDX is not the "black box" from which the physiatrist or neurologist[4] produces magical explanations for some mysterious neurologic or muscle ailment, although at times it may seem that way. EDX can be a great tool for evaluating athletes with neuromuscular problems. This chapter will provide the sports medicine specialist with a basis for requesting and understanding the EDX. To appropriately refer a patient for EDX, it is important to understand the when, why, and how to facilitate the most productive consultation for the patient. To understand the basic concepts associated with the EDX, it is important to understand the basics of nerve, muscle, and neuromuscular junction physiology as well as the anatomy and examination of the neurologic and musculoskeletal systems. From this information, an understanding of the application of the EDX and its components is achievable.

In almost every article, chapter, or textbook about electrodiagnosis, two statements are consistently observed:

- A careful history and physical examination of the patient is not replaced but rather is complemented by EDX.
- The EDX is a continuation and an extension of the clinical investigation.

The EDX allows for the clinical use of nerves and muscles to localize lesions that have been demonstrated by the weaknesses, sensory losses, and reflex changes found during a physical examination. It also can help with the determination of the type and chronology of an abnormality.

Like the clinical examination, the EDX is dependent on the evaluator.[3,4] If the evaluator is skilled and confident with localizing neuromuscular lesions on the clinical examination, is there any additional useful information gained by requesting EDX? If the

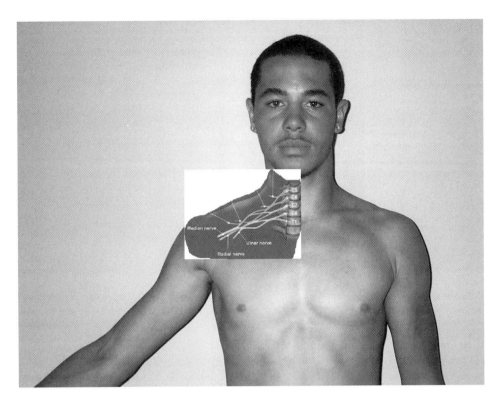

Figure 47.1 Right brachioplexus superimposed on athlete with a history of a stinger.

evaluator is less skilled or confident with the examination, he or she may not be able to frame requests and questions in anatomic terms and therefore may not get the information desired. In these cases, it may be advisable for the patient to be referred to a physiatrist, a neurologist, or a nonphysician practitioner for a clinical evaluation before any request for EDX[4,5] **(Box 47.1).**

Indications for electrodiagnostic testing

Press and Young[6] gave some useful generalizations for the indications for EDX: (1) to establish or confirm a clinical diagnosis; (2) to localize nerve lesions; (3) to determine the extent and chronicity of nerve injury; (4) to use the information obtained for anatomic study correlation; and (5) to provide information that will be useful when making decisions about return to play and prognosis, remembering that the best indication of return to play is the athlete's functional ability in reproducible sport-specific activities.[7]

Box 47.1: The Electrodiagnostic Evaluation

The electrodiagnostic evaluation should include the following:

- A history
- A physical examination
- Directed nerve conduction studies
- Complementary needle electrode examination
- A table of results
- A written summary of the results with evaluator interpretation
- A discussion of potential causes of the impairment
- A written direction for further evaluation
- The prognosis regarding any impairment recognized

Limitations of electrodiagnostic testing

EDX does not replace a competent history and physical examination.[3,8-10] If the mechanism of injury, the time course of the injury, the history of the athlete, and the physical examination are sensitive and specific when correlated to the present injury, then the diagnosis may be unequivocal and the EDX may be of little or no additional value. If the diagnosis is equivocal, however, EDX can substantially alter, confirm, and clarify it.[11]

Because of the changes that occur after an injury to the nervous system, the timing of the EDX is essential for providing the best information about the injury. Because of the changes that occur pathophysiologically after a nerve injury, it may become necessary to use serial studies to fully evaluate the degree and prognosis of the injury. In addition, there are some relative contraindications to EDX, including open wounds in the area being tested and a pending muscle biopsy. The use of pacemakers or defibrillators and patients with coagulopathy, lymphedema, or anasarca would pose relative contraindications to the use of EDX,[12] although these patients would rarely present in as members of the athletic patient population.

WHAT TO KNOW ABOUT NEUROANATOMY AND PHYSIOLOGY

In simplistic terms, the typical EDX investigates problems that are associated with the physiology and function of the peripheral nervous system.[13] The nerves of the peripheral nervous system are essentially insulated bundles of wires that are bound together and insulated inside a cable that can transmit electricity in any direction that the cable runs. The sensory system of the peripheral nervous system receives an electrical impulse and transmits this electrical "message" to the central nervous system for modulation and interpretation. The motor system takes an impulse—action potential—from the central nervous system, directing it to the neuromuscular junction, where the message is transformed to an electrochemical transmission across the junction. Upon receipt at the muscle, the message is transmitted

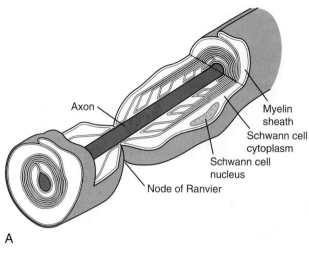

A

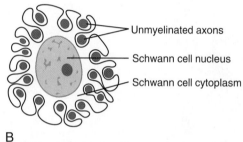

B

Figure 47.2 Myelination. *A*, A myelinated axon demonstrating the circumferential wrapping of the myelin sheath insulating the nerve along its length (except for the node of Ranvier). There is one Schwann cell per internode. *B*, One Schwann cell may provide a modicum of myelination for multiple axons in unmyelinated nerves. (From Dumitru D, Amato A, Zwarts M: Electrodiagnostic Medicine, 2nd ed. Philadelphia, Hanley & Belfus, 2002, p 15.)

through ionic changes, thus causing depolarization, propagation of the action potential, and eventual muscle action.

Within each nerve, there may be sensory fibers (afferent), motor fibers (efferent), or both. Fibers (axons) differ with regard to their activity, size, and amount of insulation (myelin) **(Figure 47.2)**. The axons are analogous to the wires in our previous description. Nutrition for the axon and the removal of wastes are provided by movement within the axon cellular material (axoplasm), which is

known as *axoplasmic flow*. The nutrition center for a sensory nerve is the dorsal root ganglion, which is located at or distal to the neuroforamina of the spine. The nutrition center for the motor unit and motor nerve is in the ventral spinal cord at the alpha motor neuron. The larger the axon, the faster electrical transmission occurs. The myelin of the axon is maintained by Schwann cells. Myelin provides for the salutatory propagation of the electrical impulse at the nodes of Ranvier, significantly increasing the velocity of transmission of the electrical impulse. The EDX primarily tests the large myelinated axons that make up the nerves of the peripheral nervous system.

Types of nerve injury

According to Seddon, nerve injuries can be divided into three classes: neuropraxia, axonotmesis, and neurotmesis[13,14] **(Table 47.1)**. Neuropraxia represents a failure of nerve conduction (usually reversible) that is caused by metabolic or microstructural abnormalities without disruption of the axon. It in essence represents an injury to the myelin. If it is severe, salutatory conduction is disrupted, and a conduction block occurs. If it is less than severe, a focal slowing of conduction may occur, as seen in focal nerve entrapments such as carpal tunnel syndrome. Axonotmesis represents an injury to the myelin and the axon with the preservation of the nerve supportive connective tissue (endoneurium), which results in axonal degeneration (Wallerian) distal to the injury. A common example is a stinger, which that may represent a fifth-level or sixth-level cervical radicular injury or a proximal upper trunk brachial plexus injury. Neurotmesis is the partial or complete transection of the nerve that causes discontinuity of the myelin and the axons proximally and distally and that leads to distal Wallerian degeneration of the nerve.

COMPONENTS OF THE ELECTRODIAGNOSTIC EXAMINATION

The EDX should consist of a history, a physical examination, directed nerve conduction studies, complementary needle electrode examination, a table of results, a written summary of the results with evaluator interpretation, a discussion of the potential causes of the impairment, a written direction for further evaluation, and, finally, the prognosis regarding any impairment recognized. The integration of these components provides a meaningful diagnostic conclusion. This is what the physician is requesting and what the athlete or patient is purchasing.

A solid understanding of the process helps the physician to better enlighten and educate the athlete regarding what to

Table 47.1 Nerve Pathophysiology and Classification

Type	Pathology	Electrodiagnostic Examination Changes	Recovery
Neuropraxia	Local myelin injury; primarily large fibers; axonal continuity; no Wallerian degeneration	Conduction velocity slowing across segment; distal latency prolonged across segment; loss of amplitude across segment; preservation of amplitude distal; needle examination normal	Weeks to months
Axonotmesis	Disruption of axonal continuity with Wallerian degeneration; endoneurium may be intact	Loss of amplitude proximal and distal; needle examination with spontaneous activity; needle examination with abnormal motor units	Months to years; axonal regeneration required for recovery; prognosis dependent on intact endoneurium
Neurotmesis	Disruption of entire nerve	No response proximal or distal; needle examination with spontaneous activity; needle exam without recruitable motor units	Surgical modification of nerve ends required; prognosis guarded and dependent on the nature of the injury and local factors

expect during the evaluation. The evaluation is at worst painful and at best mildly uncomfortable, depending on the cooperation of the patient and the skill of the electrodiagnostician.[15] The testing is also relatively expensive in terms of time and money. Therefore, getting the most out of the examination is important.

The EDX is divided into two complementary portions: the nerve conduction studies and the electromyography. The nerve conduction studies involve exciting the nerves electrically with externally applied safe pulses over various points along a nerve and measuring the obtained responses. This type of testing evaluates the large myelinated axons found within a nerve. The electromyography evaluation represents an electrophysiologic assessment of the motor unit.[16] Electromyography involves recording the electrical activity of a muscle at rest and during activity by inserting needle electrodes into multiple areas of a muscle and recording the electrical activity of a small number of fibers of a single motor unit with each pass or needle advancement.

A motor unit represents the anatomic unit of the anterior horn cell (alpha motor neuron), its axon, the neuromuscular junction, and all of the muscle fibers innervated by the axon **(Figure 47.3)**. The motor unit is influenced by inputs from the brain and the spinal cord (upper motor neuron) as well as afferent inputs from the periphery, such as position sensors in joints, Golgi tendon organs, and muscle spindles. The result is the ability of the muscles to have the various contraction patterns that are necessary for functional activity that is under the control of the central nervous system.[16]

PRINCIPLES OF NERVE CONDUCTION STUDIES

Nerve conduction studies evaluate the fastest 20% of the fibers, and the aim is to investigate and document focal abnormalities in the length of a mixed, motor, or sensory nerve. During this evaluation, the following questions are given attention:

- Is the fastest conduction velocity normal?
- Is the summated action potential response measured under the recording electrodes of normal size and shape?
- Does the response seen alter in size, shape, or duration when evaluating the response using different stimulation points?

Normal values for the nerve conduction studies are age matched and temperature controlled from published studies or specific laboratory determinations.[12] Clinically it is useful to study the motor and sensory functions of the peripheral nerves separately. However, most peripheral nerves are mixed nerves. Fortunately, at their distal ends, all mixed nerves form discrete motor and sensory branches, which can be studied separately.[12-14,17]

Specific techniques

Motor conduction studies evaluate the motor nerve or the motor portion of a compound nerve by electrically stimulating a proximal portion of the nerve and recording a summated voltage response from the stimulated muscle fiber action potentials through the use of recording electrodes placed over the belly (motor end point) of a specific muscle that is innervated by the nerve. The voltage response recorded is known as a *compound muscle action potential (CMAP)*. This CMAP is the digital summation of near synchronous muscle action potentials recorded from a common area of muscle. This summated action potential is achieved by sequentially elevating the voltage or current used to stimulate a nerve to a supramaximal level such that all possible stimulation is achieved as demonstrated by no change in the CMAP (i.e., it does not get any larger). The criteria measured from a CMAP are the latency, the amplitude, and the duration **(Figure 47.4)**. The latency represents the onset of the summated response after the stimulus. The amplitude is measured by the change from the baseline to the peak of the action potential. The duration represents the time from the action potential's deflection from the baseline until its return to the baseline.

The stimulus is usually done at a distal and proximal point along a nerve. The more proximal stimulus produces a similar-looking action potential (amplitude and shape) if the nerve is normal, except the latency should be greater from the proximal point. By measuring the distance between the two stimulation points, the conduction velocity of the fastest axons can be determined. The technique is usually orthodromic, which means that the stimulus and the recording are in the normal direction of propagation of a motor response.

Sensory conduction studies demonstrate a sensory nerve action potential from supramaximally stimulating sensory fibers and

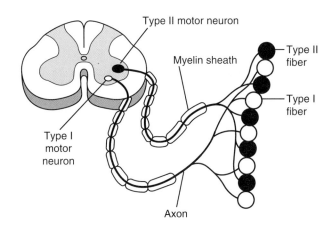

Figure 47.3 Two motor units (type I and type II fibers). Note that the fibers from one motor unit are interspersed with those from another motor unit. (From Dumitru D, Amato A, Zwarts M: Electrodiagnostic Medicine, 2nd ed. Philadelphia, Hanley & Belfus, 2002, p 267.)

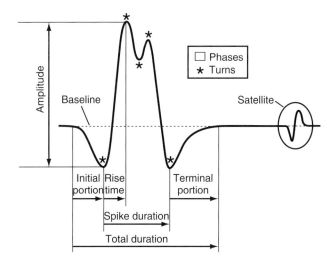

Figure 47.4 Motor unit action potential morphology. A schematic representation of a single motor unit action potential with the various subcomponents delineated. (From Dumitru D, Amato A, Zwarts M: Electrodiagnostic Medicine, 2nd ed. Philadelphia, Hanley & Belfus, 2002, p 43.)

recording the results more distally along a nerve's path. This may be done orthodromically or antidromically. The term *antidromically* refers to the stimulus being proximal and the recording distal for a sensory nerve, which is the opposite of the normal sensory propagation. It has to be remembered that, when a nerve is stimulated through the stimulating electrodes, the propagation of electricity is in both directions along the nerve path.[13] Again, the amplitude, latency, duration, and conduction velocity can be observed, recorded, calculated, and compared with known normals.

The responses of F waves are used to evaluate the most proximal portions of a motor nerve axon, which cannot be accessed in a normal motor nerve conduction studies. When the motor nerve action is stimulated, the propagation is in both directions, thus giving rise to the CMAP distally and causing the alpha motor neuron and the axon hillock to be depolarized proximally. The proximal stimulus propagation gives rise to different axon populations backfiring and sending a variable late response that is recorded at the same distal electrodes that measured the CMAP. This late response is most reliable if 10 to 20 firings are recorded and the minimal reproducible latency is measured.[12,13] Because of the great length of transmission, a small focal change may not be appreciated. However, in patients with conditions such as Guillain–Barré syndrome (acute inflammatory demyelinating polyradicular neuropathy), in whom the proximal portions of the nerve are affected by demyelination, the F-wave response may be the testing of choice.

Nerve conduction study results

Nerve conduction studies provide pathophysiologic information that evaluates the length of a nerve. The pathology of a peripheral nerve affects the axons or myelin either exclusively, predominately, or in combination. During the evaluation of the nerve action potentials of the motor or sensory nerves if there is axon loss, a reduction in the CMAP or sensory nerve action potential amplitude may be seen when stimulating across and distal to the injury site. For the CMAP, this represents fewer functioning motor axons connected to muscle fibers. The latency and conduction velocity remain relatively normal unless the largest axons are affected. The timing of testing becomes important after an axonal injury, because the distal portions of the axon will be normal for days until Wallerian degeneration occurs.

Demyelination causing a slowing or blocking of conduction will prolong the latency of the action potential and slow the conduction velocity when stimulation occurs across the demyelination site. The amplitude may also be affected when stimulation occurs across the site, but it may be normal distal to the demyelination site.[9] Stimulation proximal or distal to an area of neurotmesis demonstrates no action potential after Wallerian degeneration occurs.

Electromyography (needle examination)

The needle examination makes use of a needle electrode that is inserted into a muscle to evaluate the lower motor neuron pathway.[13,18] However, it does not evaluate the sensory pathway. Conventional needles record from a radius of about 1 mm; within this radius may be 100 muscle fibers. A motor unit may have hundreds of motor fibers associated with it throughout a muscle. Within the 1 mm, the needle may "see" four to six fibers of a single motor unit. An electromyographer becomes skilled at interpreting the appearance of the muscle activity as well as the sound of the activity. The muscle is evaluated both at rest, when it is normally silent, and during voluntary muscle activity. If there is spontaneous activity in a resting muscle, it may represent a lesion or a disease process that affects the axons of the motor unit or the muscle itself.

The types of spontaneous activity are fibrillation potentials, positive sharp waves, fasciculations, complex repetitive discharges, and myotonic and myokymic discharges. With the activation of the muscle, motor units can be analyzed to evaluate and distinguish between neuropathic and myopathic processes. The motor units are evaluated for size (amplitude and duration), complexity (phases), and recruitment. The patient is asked to minimally activate a muscle, which should result in a few recorded motor units. The early recruited waveforms are usually small and have a frequency of 6 to 10 Hz, which is represented by consistent spikes or discharges. As the activity increases, other motor units are recruited.

Spontaneous activity normally begins to occur in muscle that has been denervated. Within 2 to 3 weeks after the activity of the axon is reduced or eliminated, the muscle fibers associated with the motor unit become supersensitive, producing acetylcholine receptors over the whole muscle fiber and not just the neuromuscular junction. The effect is to render the muscle fiber supersensitive to acetylcholine, which results in spontaneous discharges. It is detected with the electromyography electrode as a muscle fiber fibrillation or positive sharp wave. These are graded by the number of different fibrillations (the density of the fibers affected) and by the persistence throughout the muscle from a scale of 0 to 4+.[19] Complex repetitive discharges represent the ephaptic transmission (time-linked cross talk) of a stereotyped group of single-fiber potentials that begin and end abruptly and that have a constant frequency between 1 and 100 Hz. They occur predominately in neuropathic disease. Fasciculations arise from the discharge of a single motor unit occurring at irregular intervals.[20] They may be visible (if superficial) at the skin. The fasciculations may resemble a voluntary muscle potential, except they are not under voluntary control. Fasciculations may be benign or associated with motor neuron disease, radiculopathy, and neuropathy. Myotonic discharges are seen with myotonic dystrophies and channelopathies. They vary in frequency and size, but they characteristically sound like a dive bomber or a two-cycle motorcycle. Myokymia is a regular or irregular discharge of groups of motor units that produce a "flickering" in muscle and that may be seen in the face of individuals with demyelinating disease such as multiple sclerosis or tumors of the brain stem.

The pattern and recruitment of voluntary muscle action potentials helps distinguish myopathy from neuropathy and acute neuropathy from chronic neuropathy. Reduced recruitment is usually distinguished by the presence of large motor units firing at high rates before the next motor unit is recruited. This represents the presence of motor units that have reinnervated through the branching of nerves, which usually represents neurogenic injury. Early recruitment represents small fibers that are typically noted at a low frequency before the next fiber is recruited, and, with minimal voluntary activity, many fibers are recruited. In effect, small ineffective fibers require more fibers firing earlier to generate force. This usually represents a primary muscle disease.

By isolating a single motor unit on a display, amplitude, duration, and number of phases can be measured. With primary muscle disease, the motor unit potentials will be small and of short duration. With an axonotmetic injury to the nerve, there is Wallerian degeneration. Intact axons will sprout collaterals, thus reinnervating areas of muscle that had been denervated. Early during reinnervation, the motor unit potentials may show increased complexity and increased duration as a result of the difference in axonal maturity. As the collateral sprouts mature and become more organized, the complexity (or phases) is reduced and the motor unit potentials will become large in amplitude and duration, thus demonstrating the increased amount of muscle fibers that are activated through the collateral sprouting of one axon. By combining the presence of spontaneous activity and the appearance of motor unit potentials, acute, subacute, and chronic denervation and reinnervation may be distinguished.

CONCLUSION

The use of an EDX as an adjunct for the care of an athlete may produce a reliable tool for evaluating pathology within the neuromuscular system. To get the most out of an EDX study, it is important to realize the examiner-dependent nature of the clinical examination, to provide referral-directed questions, and to develop effective communication with the patient about the prognosis. Understanding the examination of the neuromuscular system, the pathophysiology of the nerve injury or the neuromuscular disease, and the components of a requested EDX will make a physician a more complete sports medicine specialist.

REFERENCES

1. Heisenberg WK: Physics and Philosophy. Copenhagen, George Allen and Unwin, 1958.
2. Torg JS: Cervical spine injuries in the adult. In DeLee JC, Drez D Jr, Miller MD (eds): DeLee & Drez's Orthopaedic Sports Medicine: Principles and Practice, 2nd ed. Philadelphia, WB Saunders, 2003, pp 797-799.
3. Fuller G: How to get the most out of nerve conduction studies and electromyography. J Neurol Neurosurg Psychiatry 2005;76(suppl II):ii41-ii46.
4. Dillingham TR, Pezzin LE, Rice JB: Electrodiagnostic services in the United States. Muscle Nerve 2004;29(1):198-204.
5. Spielholz NI: Electrodiagnostic services in the United States. Muscle Nerve 2004;30(4):510-511.
6. Press JM, Young JL: Electrodiagnostic evaluation of spine problems. In Gonzalez EG, Materson RS (eds): The Nonsurgical Management of Acute Low Back Pain. New York, Demos Vermande, 1997, pp 191.
7. Feinberg JH: Burners and stingers. Phys Med Rehabil Clin North Am 2000;11(4):771-783.
8. Hogan CJ, Degnan GC: An orthopedic surgeon's guide to interpreting electromyography. Am J Orthop Oct 2001;30(10):745-750.
9. Dillingham TR: Electrodiagnostic approach to patients with suspected radiculopathy. Phys Med Rehabil Clin N Am 2002;13(3):567-588.
10. Dillingham TR: Electrodiagnostic approach to patients with weakness. Phys Med Rehabil Clin N Am 2003;14(2):163-184.
11. Haig AJ, Tzeng H-M, Lebreck DM: The value of electrodiagnostic consultation for the patient with upper extremity nerve complaints: a prospective comparison with the history and physical examination. Arch Phys Med Rehabil 1999;80:1273-1281.
12. Mallik A, Weir AI: Nerve conduction studies: essentials and pitfalls in practice. J Neurol Neurosurg Psychiatry 2005;76(suppl II):ii23-ii31.
13. Dumitru D, Amato AA, Zwarts MJ: Electrodiagnostic Medicine, 2nd ed. Philadelphia, Hanley and Belfus, 2002.
14. Akunthota V, Tobey J: Electrodiagnostic testing. In O'Connor F, Sallis R, Wilder R, St. Pierre P, (eds): Sports Medicine: Just the Facts. McGraw-Hill, 2004, pp 111-117.
15. Strommen JA, Daube JR: Determinants of pain in needle electromyography. Clin Neurophysiol 2001;112(8):1414-1418.
16. Barkhaus PE, Nandedkar SD: EMG evaluation of the motor unit: the electrophysiologic biopsy. http://emedicine.com/neuro/topic610.htm. Accessed January 2005.
17. Robinson LR, Stolp-Smith KA: Paresthesias and focal weakness: the diagnosis of nerve entrapment. In AAEM Annual Assembly. Vancouver, BC, Johnson Printing, 1999.
18. Mills KR: The basics of electromyography. J Neurol Neurosurg Psychiatry 2005;76(suppl II):ii32-ii35.
19. Kraft GH: Fibrillation potential amplitude and muscle atrophy following peripheral nerve injury. Muscle Nerve 1990;13:814-821.
20. Layzer RB: The origin of muscle fasciculations and cramps. Muscle Nerve 1994;17(4):1243-1249.

Therapeutic and Diagnostic Injections and Aspirations

Thomas M. Howard, MD, and LCDR Leslie H. Rassner, MD

KEY POINTS

- Injections and aspirations can be valuable diagnostic and therapeutic tools in the management of musculoskeletal complaints.
- There is mixed evidence to support and refute the value and accuracy of various musculoskeletal injections.
- Before being given any injection, the patient must give informed consent regarding the potential benefits, risks, and alternatives to the procedure.
- The provider should have adequate familiarity with the anatomic landmarks and procedure technique before attempting a musculoskeletal injection.
- Pertinent radiographs should be ordered and reviewed before performing a musculoskeletal injection.

INTRODUCTION

Musculoskeletal injections can be very satisfying procedures for both providers and patients. Injections may be diagnostic, therapeutic, or both.

The management of musculoskeletal injury should always begin with a pathoanatomic diagnosis. The next steps in treating injury include controlling inflammation, promoting healing, increasing fitness, controlling abuse, and returning to activity.[1] Since the 1950s, intra-articular, peritendinous, and bursal steroid injections have been used for a variety of musculoskeletal disorders, targeting their anti-inflammatory effects to specific areas.[2] The decreased pain associated with a successful injection can allow the completion of rehabilitative therapy, which promotes healing, increases fitness, and ultimately results in the successful return to activity.

The views expressed in this chapter are those of the authors and do not necessarily reflect the official policy or position of the Department of the Navy, the Department of Defense, or the US Government.

Despite the ubiquitous use of steroid injections, the perception of therapeutic efficacy and safety varies widely and among patients and practitioners.[3] The original publications of the rheumatologic pioneers of steroid injections relied on retrospective, uncontrolled, nonblinded case series of their clinical experience.[4] As experience and research designs progressed, questions of side effects, cartilage damage, and risks versus benefits arose. Studies have contradicted original reports of the efficacy of many common musculoskeletal injections.[3,5,6] Additionally, the literature continues to vary with regard to medications used, injection techniques, whether steroid placement is confirmed objectively, outcome measures, and the length of follow up, thus making meta-analysis difficult.[5,7,8]

During the past decade, the accuracy of the techniques themselves has been called into question by radiographic surveillance for correct injection placement, with experienced providers rating between 37% and 70% accuracy for intra-articular injections.[9,10] Simultaneously, studies are correlating pain relief with the accuracy of the injection placement.[9] This brings into question the significance of previous, well-designed, prospective, controlled, and blinded studies that lacked radiographic confirmation of medication placement.[6]

In summation, concerns about injection accuracy and efficacy highlight the importance of proper training in injection techniques and the thorough counseling of each patient with regard to the risks, benefits, and alternatives of these procedures.

INDICATIONS

Musculoskeletal aspirations and injections can be both diagnostic and therapeutic. Aspirations allow for the diagnostic evaluation of synovial fluid using gross appearance and laboratory analysis **(Table 48.1)**. Joint aspirations of tense effusions are also therapeutic, relieving pain and returning a functional range of motion.

Steroid injections of the joints and soft tissue can reduce the pain of various rheumatologic diseases and musculoskeletal injuries and allow for the completion of physical therapy.[6] The short-term benefit of intra-articular corticosteroids for the treatment of knee osteoarthritis is well established (LOE: B).[7] For the treatment of rheumatoid arthritis, intra-articular triamcinolone has been shown to relieve pain in the injected joint for at least 6 months in 50% of patients (LOE: B).[11,12] In a study of patients

Table 48.1 Synovial Fluid Analysis

Classification (with Examples)	Appearance	White Blood Cells per μL	Polymorphonuclear Leukocytes (%)	Crystals
Normal	Clear to straw-colored	<150	<25	No
Noninflammatory osteoarthritis, patellofemoral syndrome, traumatic arthritis, early rheumatoid arthritis, hyperparathyroidism	Yellow, transparent	<3000	<30	No
Inflammatory rheumatoid arthritis, lupus erythematosus, Reiter's syndrome, rheumatic fever	Yellow, cloudy, or bloody	3000-75,000	>50	No
Infectious bacterial, mycobacterial, fungal	Yellow, purulent	50,000-200,000	>90	No
Crystal-induced gout, pseudogout	Cloudy, turbid	50,000-200,000	<90	Yes
Hemorrhagic traumatic arthritis, ligamentous disruption (e.g., anterior cruciate ligament tear, fracture), anticoagulation, thrombocytopenia	Reddish-brown	50-10,000	<50	No

Data from O'Connell T: Interpreting Tests From Joint Aspirates. Philadelphia, Elsevier Science, 2002.

with microscopy-confirmed gout, intra-articular triamcinolone acetonide resulted in the resolution of pain by 24 hours in 50% of patients and improvement in pain at 48 hours in 100% of patients (LOE: D).[13]

The additional discussion of the evidence of efficacy for other conditions will be discussed with the corresponding procedure techniques.

MEDICATIONS

Corticosteroid mode of action and effects

Corticosteroids inhibit the synthesis of cytokine genes and proinflammatory mediators such as nitric oxide and prostaglandins. Corticosteroids effectively inhibit the activation, migration, and recruitment of immune cells and fibroblasts.[6] The therapeutic value of these effects remains controversial **(Table 48.2).**

Steroids are meant to form crystals in tissues and to be slowly absorbed with time, thereby causing their prolonged anti-inflammatory effect.[14] Locally injected corticosteroids are partially absorbed systemically. The systemic effects of the steroid depend on the solubility, dose, and duration of treatment **(Table 48.3).**

In 1951, the use of injected steroids for the palliative treatment of inflamed joints, bursa, and tendon sheaths began.[4] Corticosteroids are thought to stabilize the intimal cells of the synovium, protect vessels, improve circulation by decreasing edema formation, and stabilize chondroblasts.[15] Additionally, intra-articular corticosteroids inhibit leukocyte secretion from the synovium, thereby increasing the concentration of hyaluronic acid in the joint and increasing the viscosity of the synovial fluid.[3]

The anti-inflammatory effects of steroids are commonly thought to break the cycle of inflammation and damage postulated to occur continuously in patients with chronic overuse tendinitis.[2,16] However, histopathologic animal studies have shown tendon degeneration and an absence of inflammatory cells as soon as 2 to 3 weeks after tendon insult.[17] The terms *tendinosis* and

Table 48.2 Corticosteroids Used for Joint and Soft-Tissue Injection

Corticosteroid	Proprietary Name	Effect Onset	Dose Equivalent for Large Joint (Knee or Shoulder)
Short Acting			
Betamethasone acetate	Soluspan	Rapid	12 mg
Intermediate Acting			
Triamcinolone acetonide	Kenalog	Variable	40 mg
Dexamethasone sodium phosphate	Decadron	Rapid	4 mg
Long Acting			
Dexamethasone acetate	Decadron LA	Variable	8 mg
Triamcinolone hexacetonide	Aristospan	Variable	20 mg
Methylprednisolone acetate	Depo-Medrol	Very slow	80 mg

Data from Snibbe JC, Gambardella RA: Clin Sports Med 2005;24(1):83-91; Eberhard BA, Sison MC, Gottlieb BS, Ilowite NT: J Rheumatol 2004;31(12):2507-2512; O'Connor FG, Sallis RE, Wilder RP, St. Pierre P: Sports Medicine: Just the Facts. New York, McGraw-Hill, 2005; Derendorf H, Mollmann H, Gruner A, et al: Clin Pharmacol Ther 1986;39(3):313-317; Paluska SA: Indications, Contraindications, and Overview for Aspirating or Injecting a Joint or Related Structure. Philadelphia, Elsevier Science, 2002; Balogh Z, Ruzsonyi E: Scand J Rheumatol Suppl 1987;67:80-82; Pyne D, Ioannou Y, Mootoo R, Bhanji A: Clin Rheumatol 2004;23(2):116-120.

Table 48.3   Corticosteroid Adverse Outcomes

Complication	Rates
Local	
Postinjection flare of pain	2%-10%
Skin depigmentation	Rare
Fat atrophy	Rare, <0.006%
Joint or soft-tissue infection	Rare, <0.001-0.072%*
Nerve damage	Few case reports
Weight-bearing tendon rupture or atrophy	Unknown
Cartilage deterioration	Unknown
Necrotizing fasciitis	Few case reports
Pneumothorax (shoulder region injections)	Rare
Systemic	
Facial flushing	15%
Syncope or temporary dizziness	Rare, <0.003%
Transient paresis or dysphoria	Rare
Allergic reactions (anaphylaxis and urticaria)	Rare, <1.0%
Fall in erythrocyte sedimentation rate or C-reactive protein	Unknown
Hyperglycemia in diabetics	Unknown
Cushingoid state†	Rare
Adrenal crisis	Case report
Uterine bleeding	Unknown
Sickle-cell crisis	Few case reports
Psychiatric events (e.g., hallucinations, dysphonia)	Few case reports

*Rates vary in literature between 1 in every 20,000 and 1 in every 50,000.[22]
†Cushingoid state involves iatrogenic hypothalamic—pituitary—adrenal axis suppression with moon face, buffalo hump, weight gain, and disturbance of the menstrual cycle.[39]
Data from Saunders S: Injection Techniques in Orthopaedic and Sports Medicine, 2nd ed. Philadelphia, WB Saunders, 2002; O'Connor FG, Sallis RE, Wilder RP, St. Pierre P: Sports Medicine: Just the Facts. New York, McGraw-Hill, 2005; Rogojan C, Hetland ML: Clin Rheumatol 2004;23(4):373-375; Pattrick M, Doherty M: Br Med J (Clin Res Ed) 1987;295(6610):1380; Karsh J, Yang WH: Ann Allergy Asthma Immunol 2003;90(2):254-258; Kumar N, Newman RJ: Br J Gen Pract 1999;49(443):465-466.

tendinopathy more accurately describe the collagen disruption and myofibroblastic differentiation of the tenocytes found on biopsy in classic "tendinitis" conditions such as Achilles tendinitis and lateral epicondylitis (LOE: D).[6,17,18]

With this shift in the understanding of the pathology of tendon disorders, the mechanisms of action of corticosteroids in musculoskeletal overuse injuries must be reconsidered. Corticosteroids cause the decreased production of collagen and extracellular matrix proteins by fibroblasts. Therefore, their effect might be mediated through the inhibition of the production of collagen, other extracellular matrix molecules, and granulation tissue at sites of tendon pain and injury. The pain of tendinopathy has been suggested to result from the stimulation of nociceptors by chemicals released from damaged and degrading tissue. Corticosteroids might alter the release of these noxious chemicals or the behavior of the pain receptors.[6]

Corticosteroid risks and complications (see Table 48.3)
Local

- Postinjection flare of pain ("steroid flare")
  - Postinjection inflammatory symptoms may occur, which are thought to result from the intracellular ingestion of steroid crystals.[19]
  - Onset may occur as soon as 2 hours after injection, and pain resolves by 72 hours postinjection; it may be treated with ice and acetaminophen or oral nonsteroidal anti-inflammatory drugs.
  - Patients with pain beyond 36 hours should be evaluated to rule out iatrogenic infection.[20]
- Dermatologic changes: depigmentation and fat atrophy
  - Depigmentation is rare and most cases recover pigmentation in 2 to 12 months; it can occur up to 4 months after injection.
  - Depigmentation is more common among dark-skinned individuals, with repeated injections, and when using long-acting, relatively insoluble preparations.[21]
  - Some authors recommend using shorter-acting corticosteroids when treating dark-skinned individuals to reduce the risk of this complication.[16]
- Joint or soft-tissue infection
  - Infection rates vary by study from 1 in every 10,000 to 1 in every 50,000 with the use of thorough alcohol swabbing in one study and unspecified precautions in another (LOE: D).[21,22]
  - Elderly patients with debilitating disuse or patients receiving immunosuppressive therapy are more prone to this complication (LOE: D).[14]
- Nerve damage
  - Damage to nerves can be in two types: direct mechanical injury to the nerve and its fascicles or chemical neuritis induced by the steroid agent. Nerves located superficially under the skin are more vulnerable to injury (LOE: D).[23]
  - Partial laceration of the nerve by the needle can result in the formation of a neuroma.
  - The steroid can deposit around the nerve, leaving a chalky, whitish material that is found on subsequent operative exploration.
- Weight-bearing tendon rupture
  - Injections of the Achilles tendon and plantar fascia have been associated with increased rates of tendon rupture.[6,24] It is difficult to assess whether this association is the result of damage from the injection itself or from the extent of the underlying tendon disease that necessitated injection.[25,26] Healthy rabbits receiving retrocalcaneal intrabursal and peritendinous Achilles corticosteroid injection showed significantly weaker Achilles tendons with lower forces needed to rupture them than were seen in uninjected controls.[27] This study raises the concern that peritendinous corticosteroid injection might not be without risk.
- Cartilage deterioration
  - The intra-articular administration of corticosteroids relieves the pain and swelling associated with various arthropathies.[2]
  - In one randomized controlled trial comparing intra-articular triamcinolone with saline injected every 3 months for 2 years, radiologic examination did not show any difference in joint deterioration (LOE: B).[28] In a study of 21 children and adolescents, treatment with intra-articular corticosteroid suppressed synovial inflammation and caused a reversal of pannus formation as demonstrated by magnetic resonance imaging with contrast. Thirteen months after intra-articular steroid injection, no adverse effects on growth or statural height were observed (LOE: B).[8]

This study group suggested that steroids might suppress the synovial membrane genes that play a role in articular cartilage destruction in rheumatologic disease states.[8]

- Animal studies of intra-articular steroid injection of normal joints have shown a reduction in the proteoglycan content of the articular cartilage matrix, alterations in cartilage metabolic processes, and, at high doses, organelle distortion and disruption.[15,29] An equine study with artificially induced full-thickness cartilage defects showed lower quality replacement tissue in methylprednisolone-acetate–treated joints as compared with those treated with placebo.[15]
- Necrotizing fasciitis
  - There are three case reports of this condition after steroid injection.[30]
  - In general, necrotizing fasciitis is associated with diabetes mellitus, obesity, advancing age, and atherosclerosis. Necrotizing fasciitis can be associated with an initiating injury such as a burn, laceration, or abrasion. In some cases, no evidence of an initiating injury has been found.[30]
- Needle trauma
  - With improper technique, it is possible to cause a pneumothorax and direct traumatic damage to articular cartilage.[20]

Systemic
- Facial flushing
  - There is a generally accepted rate of 2% to 10% (LOE: D).[20]
  - In a study specifically addressing facial flushing after intra-articular injection, the rate of flushing was 40%, with 15% reporting it to be unpleasant. Facial flushing was more common among women but independent of age, underlying disease process, and prior vasomotor instability (LOE: D).[31]
- Allergic reactions
  - Immediate and delayed sensitivity allergic reactions have been documented as a reaction to anesthetic and corticosteroid preparations.[32,33] A patient without a previous reaction to local anesthetics or injected corticosteroids may still develop anaphylaxis after a musculoskeletal injection. Patients with a history of asthma and/or aspirin intolerance may be at an increased risk for an allergic reaction.[34]
  - In one study, clinical allergic manifestations observed after the injection of hydrocortisone included urticaria (0.12%), bronchospasms and angioedema (0.015%), and local urticaria (0.16%) (LOE: D).[35]
  - The onset of symptoms can vary from a few hours to 2 to 3 days after acute exposure.[32]
  - In a review of anaphylaxis case reports, all cases resolved with acute treatment, which included intravenous steroids and epinephrine (LOE: E).[36]
- Hyperglycemia in diabetics
  - This is a temporary side effect of the suppression of the hypothalamic–pituitary axis.[16] Hyperglycemia parallels the initial suppression of endogenous hydrocortisone the first week after injection, resolving by 2 weeks postinjection with the return of normal endogenous hydrocortisone levels (LOE: C).[37]
- Cushing's syndrome
  - The systemic absorption of corticosteroids can result in hypercortisolism as well as suppression of the hypothalamic pituitary axis.[38] Iatrogenic Cushing's syndrome can manifest with moon face, buffalo hump, gain of weight, and disturbance of the menstrual cycle.[39]
  - Iatrogenic Cushing's syndrome has been demonstrated for up to 5 months after triamcinolone injection. The duration of adrenal suppression has been demonstrated to last up to 8 months (LOE: E).[38] In case reports, all signs and symptoms have resolved spontaneously with time (LOE: E).[39]
- Glaucoma
  - This is a reported potential complication, but it is rare in practice.
- Neuropsychiatric events
  - Neuropsychiatric side effects are similar to those of oral steroids. These side effects usually occur among older patients with underlying medical conditions, but they are not limited to patients with psychiatric histories (LOE: E).[22,40,41]

ANESTHETIC SELECTION
- Local anesthetics: lidocaine 1% or 2%; bupivacaine 0.25%, 0.50%, or 0.75%.
- Anesthetic with epinephrine is not used in any aspirations or injections. Radiologists may use epinephrine in their arthrogram protocols.[42]
- Lidocaine has duration of action of roughly 1 hour as compared with the 8-hour duration of action of bupivacaine. A study of steroid injections for overuse injuries demonstrated a statistically significant pain reduction from bupivacaine for up to 6 hours postinjection (LOE: A).[43]
- Single-use vials are preferable to multidose vials as a result of concerns about potential allergic reactions to parabens preservatives. Parabens can precipitate at the injection site and potentially lead to a postinjection flare.[16,44]

VISCOSUPPLEMENTATION
Hyaluronic acid is a polysaccharide chain made of disaccharide units and glucuronic acid secreted by the synovium into the joint space. In patients with knee osteoarthritis, the concentration and molecular weight of hyaluronic acid are reduced, thereby resulting in lower joint lubrication and possibly increased shear forces. Hyaluronic acid also has anti-inflammatory effects.[3]

Hyaluronic acid injected intra-articularly has a half-life of 24 hours.[45] The intra-articular injection is thought to possibly affect the synthesis of hyaluronic acid by synovial fibroblasts.[45] Hyaluronic acid injections have not been shown to be more effective than steroids for reducing knee osteoarthritis pain at 3 or 6 months (LOE: B and A, respectively).[45,46] Because the aspiration of knee effusions alone has been shown to reduce knee osteoarthritis pain, it is difficult to interpret the results of trials against placebo because the aspiration alone may be part of the beneficial effect.[47] One study also showed a 15% complication rate with hyaluronic acid injections, which serves as a reminder that viscosupplementation is not a procedure without risk.[48] Viscosupplementation is an option for patients in whom conservative treatment has failed.

CONTRAINDICATIONS TO INJECTIONS
Absolute contraindications[16,20]
- Cellulitis or broken skin over the injection site
- Septic effusion of a bursa or periarticular structure (except in diagnostic aspirations)
- Acute systemic infection (do not inject patients with a febrile illness)

- History of a reaction to any components of the injection solution
- Prosthetic joint
- Intra-articular fracture site (hematoma blocks are safely and routinely used for anesthesia when reducing nonarticular fractures)
- Unstable joint
- Reluctant patient
- Children (select patients with rheumatologic conditions may be injected by experienced specialists[11])

Relative contraindications[16,20]

- Patient who is anticoagulated or who has a coagulopathy (if you must inject, correct coagulopathy first)
- Poorly controlled diabetes
- Immunosuppressed
- Psychogenic pain
- Severe anxiety
- Lack of response to prior injections

INJECTION PRECAUTIONS

Informed consent
- Always explain the benefits, risks, and alternatives to the procedure. Document the patient's informed consent.

Aseptic technique
- Use clean, dry hands.
- Use prepacked, sterile, disposable needles and syringes.
- Use single-dose vials of medication when possible.
- Do not touch the patient's skin after marking and cleansing the injection site. A retracted pen tip or needle cap may be used to mark the skin before cleansing. Pen ink should not be used for injection site marking because it will be wiped away by cleansing.
- Isopropyl alcohol may be used for cleansing for extra-articular injections. As a rule, intra-articular injections and aspirations requiring culture require Betadine skin preparation.[49]
- When performing intra-articular injection, aspirate to check that the fluid does not look infected.
- It is generally accepted that masks and gowns are not used.[16,49]

General precautions
- Question the patient about drug allergies before the injection.
- Before performing an injection for a musculoskeletal complaint, order and review pertinent radiographs.
- Do not exceed maximum doses of anesthetics: lidocaine 200 mg (20 mL of 1.0% or 10 mL of 2.0%) and bupivacaine 150 mg (60 mL of 0.25% or 30 mL of 0.5%).
- Limit injections into a weight-bearing joint to no more than three injections per year (LOE: E).[20]
- Do not inject steroid in more than two large joints at one time or use more than the equivalent dose of 16 mg of dexamethasone or 80 mg of triamcinolone in multiple soft-tissue or smaller joint injections. Limit injection to one joint in those patients who are at risk for adrenal suppression or systemic reactions to corticosteroids (i.e., those taking oral steroids, those who are immunosuppressed, diabetics, and the elderly; this is the author's opinion and based on case reports) (LOE: E).

- Do not inject against resistance. Resistance may represent the placement of the needle tip in a ligament or tendon.
- Advise patients that ice, acetaminophen, and nonsteroidal anti-inflammatory drugs (NSAIDS) may be used postinjection to prevent or treat any symptoms of steroid flare.

Allergy/anaphylaxis precautions (LOE: E)[16]
- All patients should be observed for 30 minutes after injection.
- Anaphylaxis may begin with any of the following symptoms:
  - Flushing, itchy skin, or urticaria
  - Nervousness/confusion
  - Nausea and/or vomiting
  - Abdominal pain
  - Hypotension
  - Tachycardia
  - Respiratory difficulties or distress from angioedema or bronchospasm
  - Convulsions
  - A feeling of impending catastrophe
- Outpatient clinic recommended emergency supplies[16]
  - Cardiopulmonary resuscitation mask and disposable airways
  - EpiPen
  - Diphenhydramine (oral and injectable)
  - Consider intravenous supplies and fluids, intravenous steroids, and oxygen if the practice setting can support it

SHOULDER INJECTION AND ASPIRATION TECHNIQUES

Acromioclavicular joint
Indication
This treatment is indicated for the relief of pain related to acromioclavicular (AC) degenerative disease and subacute AC separation.

Evidence
In one uncontrolled, retrospective study, 81% of patients that underwent steroid joint injection for AC arthropathy failed to obtain long-term relief from the injection. Sixty-seven percent of patients progressed on to distal clavicle excisions for persistent pain (LOE: D).[50]

Anatomy
The AC joint is typically angled at an approximately 45-degree angle directed midline caudally. The capsule lies just below the subcutaneous tissue.

The AC joint is best found by first palpating the supraspinatus fossa (pictured in the subacromial injection as the concavity in which the thumb rests during that injection). From the fossa, move anterior to find the flare of the distal clavicle. Pushing down on the distal clavicle while the finger is over the AC joint verifies its location. Shoulder abduction can be helpful during palpation.

Procedure (Figure 48.1)
- The patient is seated.
- After sterile Betadine preparation, the needle is inserted at the superior–lateral AC joint and directed inferior–medially.
- The injection may be difficult with significant degenerative joint disease. It is often helpful to view the patient's radiograph before the injection.

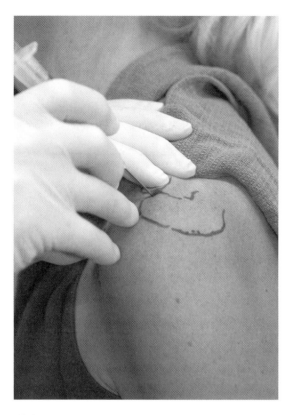

Figure 48.1 Acromioclavicular joint.

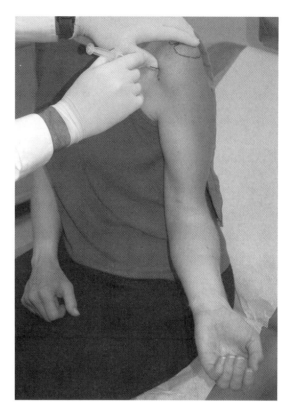

Figure 48.2 Proximal biceps tendon.

- To ensure appropriate placement in AC joint, aspirate after injection. This will return some medication to the syringe and confirm proper placement.

Precautions
- This can be a difficult injection in a severely arthritic joint.

Aftercare
- Protection and rest for 7 days
- This injection may be repeated in 6 weeks if less than 50% relief has been obtained.
- Needle size: 25 gauge, ½ to 1 inch
- Medication: ½ mL dexamethasone acetate (8 mg/mL) or ½ mL triamcinolone (40 mg/mL) in 2 to 3 mL of lidocaine (1%)

Proximal biceps tendon
Indication
This is used for the relief of pain related to biceps tendinitis.

Anatomy
The greater tuberosity of the humerus lies in a direct line with the lateral epicondyle of the elbow. The bicipital groove is just medial to the greater tuberosity. The bicipital groove can be located by moving 1 to 1¼ inches caudal from the anterolateral edge of the acromion.

Procedure (Figure 48.2)
- The patient is seated.
- After an alcohol preparation, the needle is inserted parallel to the biceps tendon in the bicipital groove. The depth should be ¾ to 1 inch, and the injection is should flow freely, without resistance. If bony resistance of the humerus is felt, pull back slightly.

Precautions
- Avoid direct injection into the tendon.

Aftercare
- Limited use of the extremity for 7 days, avoiding all lifting
- Needle size: 25 gauge, 1½ inch
- Medication: ½ mL of triamcinolone (40 mg/mL) and 1 to 2 mL of anesthetic

Intra-articular shoulder
Indication
Use this treatment for the relief of pain associated with osteoarthritis, undersurface supraspinatus tendinitis/partial thickness tear, or adhesive capsulitis.

Evidence
Two studies with radiographic confirmation of injection demonstrated accuracy rates of 36.8% and 42% for the anterior injection approach (LOE: B and D, respectively).[9,51] One study noted no resistance to flow with all injections, highlighting that the free flow of medication with injection does not automatically confirm correct placement (LOE: D).[51]

Cochrane meta-analysis found that intra-articular steroid injection for adhesive capsulitis may be beneficial (LOE: B).[52] A randomized controlled trial also found benefit from intra-articular shoulder joint distension with steroid placement (LOE: B).[53]

Anatomy
The coracoid process lays inferomedial to the AC joint. The capsule of the glenohumeral joint lies just deep to the coracoid process from an anterior approach. The glenohumeral joint is appreciated by internally and externally rotating the shoulder.

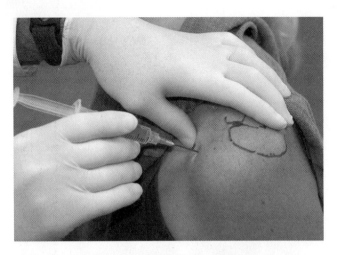

Figure 48.3 Intra-articular shoulder, anterior approach.

Procedure: Anterior approach (Figure 48.3)

- The patient is in a seated position.
- After Betadine preparation, the needle is introduced 1 cm lateral and 1 cm inferior to the coracoid process. Gentle passive internal rotation of the shoulder after the placement of the needle will confirm location by causing paradoxic motion of the needle.

Procedure: Posterior approach (Figure 48.4)

- The patient is in a seated position.
- After Betadine preparation, the needle is introduced 2 to 3 cm inferior to the posterolateral corner of the acromion and directed anteriorly in the direction of the coracoid process. The injection should be performed slowly but with consistent pressure.

Precautions

- Anatomic landmarks must be ensured to avoid the placement of the needle too far medially (risk of pneumothorax) or inferiorly (risk of vascular or neurologic injury).
- An aspiration should be done to ensure that the needle has not been placed in a blood vessel.
- Decrease the volume of injected anesthetic in cases of adhesive capsulitis to meet resistance.

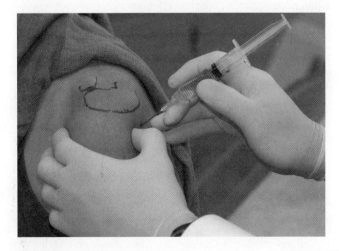

Figure 48.4 Intra-articular shoulder, posterior approach.

Aftercare

- The patient should avoid heavy use and rehabilitation exercises for 7 days after injection. Codman's pendulum exercises may be started without delay.
- The area may be iced for 15 minutes every 4 to 6 hours to control pain.
- Needle size: 25 gauge, 1½ inch.
- Medication: 1 mL dexamethasone acetate (8 mg/mL) or 1 mL triamcinolone (40 mg/mL) in 7 to 8 mL of lidocaine (1%).

Subacromial space
Indication

This treatment is used for the reduction of pain resulting from the inflammation of the supraspinatus tendon or the subacromial bursa or from lateral impingement.

Evidence

One meta-analysis reported that subacromial injection for rotator cuff disease may be beneficial, although the effect may be small and not well maintained (LOE: B).[52] Another meta-analysis concluded that subacromial injections of corticosteroids are effective for the improvement for rotator cuff tendinitis for up to a 9-month period (LOE: B).[54] Subacromial injection accuracy rates range from 29% to 87% success with blind (not guided by radiology) injection (LOE: B, D, B, and B, respectively).[9,51,55,56] A physical examination demonstrating the postinjection relief of symptoms on repeat Neer and Hawkins impingement testing does not confirm subacromial bursal placement because pain relief can occur with the injection of either the subacromial bursa or the deltoid muscle (LOE: B).[55] Radiologically confirmed subacromial injection placement does show a statistically significant "great benefit" as compared with injections that are determined to be inaccurately placed (LOE: B).[9] At 6 weeks of follow-up, sonographic-guided subacromial injections similarly confirmed significantly less pain and increased shoulder function as compared with blind injection (LOE: B).[57]

Another study of blind subacromial steroid injection for impingement syndrome compared no injection, one injection, and two injections given 10 days apart. This study did not confirm injection placement, and it involved all patients completing physical therapy. At 1 month of follow-up, only the two-injection group had a significant reduction in pain. By 3 months of follow-up, there was no significant difference in pain among the three groups (LOE: B).[58]

Anatomy

The subacromial space is formed by the acromial arch (the acromion and the coracoacromial ligament) superolaterally, the supraspinatus muscle inferiorly, the clavicle anteriorly, and the spine of the scapula posteriorly. The subacromial space is a potential space that is occupied by subacromial bursa. The posterolateral corner of the acromion is a landmark for this injection.

Procedure (Figure 48.5)

- The patient is seated with his or her back straight and the shoulders back and relaxed. An assistant may apply downward traction on the arm during the injection to increase the subacromial space.
- The posterolateral corner of the acromion is palpated. Approximately 1 inch (i.e., a thumb's width) inferiorly, a mark should be made with a ballpoint pen retracted tip.
- After alcohol skin preparation, the needle is introduced into the mark, bevel up in a slightly cephalad angulation, and pointed toward the AC joint. If bony resistance is felt, the needle is most likely hitting the acromion, and it should be redirected inferiorly. Insertion depth is approximately 1 to 1½ inch.

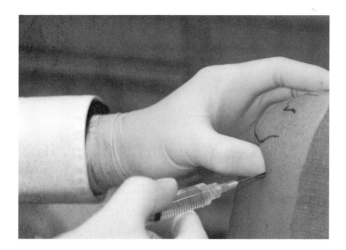

Figure 48.5 Subacromial space.

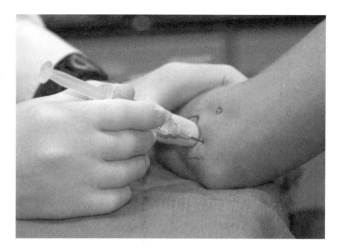

Figure 48.6 Intra-articular elbow joint.

Precautions

- Do not inject if the medicine does not flow freely. Consider withdrawing and reestablishing landmarks.

Aftercare

- The patient should avoid heavy use and rehabilitation exercises for 7 days after injection. Codman's pendulum exercises may be started without delay.
- The patient must be counseled that subacromial injections are performed in conjunction with the continuation or initiation of a rehabilitation exercise program. Patients who do not complete rehabilitation will likely have relapse of pain within 1 to 3 months of the corticosteroid injection.
- Needle size: 21 or 22 gauge, 1½ inch (One author uses 25 gauge, 1½ inch.)
- Medication: 1 mL dexamethasone acetate (8 mg/ml) or 1 mL triamcinolone (40 mg/mL) in 3 mL of lidocaine (1%) and 3 mL of bupivacaine 0.25%

ELBOW INJECTION AND ASPIRATION TECHNIQUES

Intra-articular elbow joint (see Chapter 20, Elbow Injuries)
Indication
This procedure is performed to confirm the diagnosis of fracture with an aspiration of the hemarthrosis, to relieve the tension and pain of traumatic hemarthrosis, and to restore the range of motion (mostly flexion).

Anatomy
The capsule of the elbow joint contains the three joints: the radiohumeral joint, the radioulnar joint, and the humeroulnar joint. Joint swelling typically produces a visible lateral bulge.

Procedure (Figure 48.6)
- The patient is seated with the forearm supported and pronated.
- The radial head, lateral epicondyle, and olecranon are identified. The entry point is marked at the center of the triangle formed by these three structures.
- After Betadine skin preparation, the needle is inserted parallel to the skin through the radial collateral ligament and to a depth

of approximately ¾ to 1 inch into the synovial cavity, aspirating while advancing.
- If bone is encountered prematurely, local anesthetic may be injected. The needle is withdrawn ¼ inch and redirected.
- If aspiration at a depth of 1 inch does not return fluid, the needle bevel is rotated 180 degrees and the aspiration reattempted.
- For a fracture, a 1-mL to 2-mL volume of anesthetic may be injected at the termination of aspiration, with the needle hub stabilized with a hemostat while changing syringes.

Aftercare
- 2 to 3 days of relative rest with protection of the extremity
- After 2 to 3 days, the patient should start increasing the range of motion within the limits of pain using gentle stretching.
- Physical therapy with passive mobilization techniques may be used.
- Needle size: 21 to 22 gauge, 1½ inch.
- Medication: 1 to 2 mL of lidocaine 1% or 2%.

Lateral epicondylitis/lateral tennis elbow
Indication
This treatment is indicated if lateral epicondylitis has not resolved with conservative therapy. The pain and tenderness of lateral epicondylitis is located in the extensor carpi radialis brevis tendon at its origin on the lateral epicondyle.

Evidence
Corticosteroid injection has been shown to have short-term effectiveness for approximately 2 to 6 weeks (LOE: B).[6] At 1 year of follow-up, the outcomes of the injection group are similar to those of the control group (LOE: B).[59]

Anatomy
The radial head is appreciated by pronation and supination of the elbow, and the lateral humeral epicondyle is proximal to the radial head. The common extensor tendon, which is composed of the extensor carpi radialis brevis, the extensor digitorum, the extensor digiti minimi, and the extensor carpi ulnaris, originates at the lateral epicondyle. The extensor carpi radialis brevis origin is one fingerbreadth inferior and medial to the lateral epicondyle of the humerus.

Procedure (Figure 48.7)
- The patient may be supine or seated with the forearm supinated.
- The area of maximal tenderness should be marked.

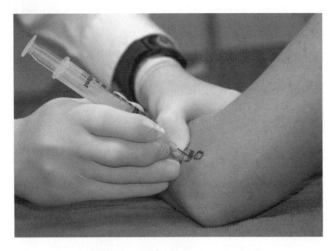

Figure 48.7 Lateral epicondylitis.

- After alcohol skin preparation, solution is injected in a wide, wagon-wheel pattern around the point of maximum tenderness, which is also the insertion point of the extensor tendons.
- If resistance is felt, the needle should be slightly withdrawn.

Precautions
- Avoid injection into subcutaneous fat because this may cause fat atrophy.
- Superficial injection may cause skin discoloration.

Aftercare
- Protected use of arm for 7 days
- Iontophoresis and deep friction may be begun immediately.
- An initial physical therapy program should consist of stretching and icing that progresses over 2 to 3 weeks from gripping exercises to isometric exercises of the wrist extensors.
- Needle size: 25 gauge, ⅝ inch.
- Medication: ½ to 1 mL dexamethasone acetate (8 mg/mL) or ½ to 1 mL triamcinolone (40 mg/mL) in 2 mL of lidocaine (1%)

Medical epicondylitis/golfer's elbow
Indication
This procedure is done for medial epicondylitis that has not resolved with conservative therapy, including counterforce bracing, equipment modification, and physical therapy. It may also be used to treat pain and inflammation occurring in the common flexor and pronator tendons at their insertion on the medial epicondyle.

Evidence
In a randomized, prospective, double-blinded study, steroid injection of medial epicondylitis statistically reduced pain at 6 weeks of follow-up. At 3 months and 1 year of follow-up, the study had insufficient power to determine a significant difference between groups (LOE: A).[60]

Anatomy
The medial epicondyle is best palpated with the elbow flexed to 90 degrees.

Procedure (Figure 48.8)
- The patient is seated with the humerus externally rotated and the forearm supinated and resting comfortably on a tray or table. The elbow is flexed approximately 60 degrees.

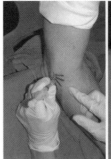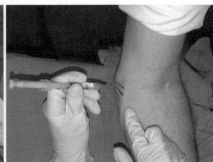

Figure 48.8 Medial epicondylitis.

- The point of maximal tenderness, which is roughly a ½-inch distal to the medial epicondyle, is marked.
- After alcohol preparation, the needle is inserted at the mark and the solution is injected in a wide, wagon-wheel pattern around the point of maximum tenderness.
- If resistance is felt, the needle should be slightly withdrawn.

Precautions
- Avoid injection into the ulnar nerve.
- Avoid injection into subcutaneous fat (this may cause fat atrophy).
- Superficial injection may cause skin discoloration.

Aftercare
- Protected use of arm for 7 days
- Iontophoresis and deep friction may be begun immediately.
- An initial physical therapy program should consist of stretching and icing that progresses over 2 to 3 weeks from gripping exercises to isometric exercises of the wrist flexors.
- The injection can be repeated in 6 weeks if less than 50% pain relief is obtained or rehabilitation exercises are poorly tolerated.
- Needle size: 25 gauge, ⅝ inch.
- Medication: ½ mL dexamethasone acetate (8 mg/mL) or ½ mL triamcinolone (40 mg/mL) in 1 to 2 mL of lidocaine (1%).

Olecranon bursitis
Indication
This is used in cases of inflammation of the bursal sac overlying the olecranon.

Evidence
In a study of 47 patients with traumatic olecranon bursitis, patients who were aspirated without corticosteroid injection experienced delayed recovery but no complications from aspiration. Patients who were injected with triamcinolone after aspiration had a rapid recovery but suffered from complications including infection, skin atrophy, and chronic local pain (LOE: B).[61]

Anatomy
The olecranon bursa is approximately the size of a golf ball, and it is located between the olecranon process of the ulna and the overlying skin.

Procedure (Figure 48.9)
- The patient is seated with the elbow supported and flexed 90 degrees.
- Identify and mark the distal base of the bursa.
- Apply Betadine preparation and drape to area. Using a 25-gauge to 27-gauge needle, inject 0.5 mL of anesthetic over the bursa. Enter

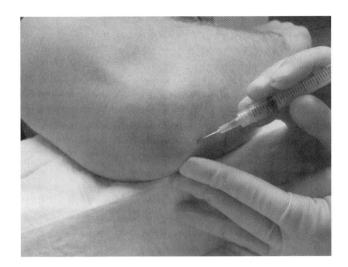

Figure 48.9 Olecranon bursa.

the bursal sac with an 18-gauge needle parallel to the skin with the bevel outward, aspirating while advancing. When the bursal fluid is reached, rotate the bevel 180 degrees. Aspirate the contents of bursal sac, applying manual pressure as needed to completely decompress the contents.

- If infection is suspected, send the fluid for laboratory evaluation.
- If infection is not suspected, the spiration syringe may be detached, stabilizing the needle within the sac with a hemostat. Corticosteroid is then injected into the bursal sac.
- After the procedure, the site is dressed with sterile dressing, and a compression bandage is applied for 24 hours.

Precautions

- Betadine preparation and sterile technique are crucial to prevent the creation of a septic bursitis from an aseptic one.
- If suspicious fluid is aspirated, do not inject steroid until after a laboratory fluid analysis is complete to rule out infection.

Aftercare

- Compression bandage for 24 hours to prevent fluid reaccumulation.
- Protect elbow for 3 days with bulky dressing.
- Limit use of extremity for 7 days.
- Needle size: for anesthetic, 25 to 27 gauge, ⅝ inch; for aspiration, 18 gauge, 1½ inch
- Medication: lidocaine 1% or 2%, ½ ml for local anesthesia; optional: ½ to 1 mL triamcinolone (40 mg/mL) in 1 to 2 mL of lidocaine (1%) for intrabursal injection

HAND AND WRIST INJECTION AND ASPIRATION TECHNIQUES

Carpal tunnel syndrome
Indication

Injections in this area are for the reduction of flexor tendon inflammation to result in the reduction of pain and median nerve compression of carpal tunnel syndrome. Symptom relief from injection can be used to confirm the diagnosis. Night splinting may be used as an alternative treatment or in conjunction with a corticosteroid injection.[62]

Evidence

In one study, about 50% of the injected median nerves became more painful within 6 months, and 90% became more painful within 18 months. At 2 years of follow up, only 8% of the injected median nerves remained symptomatically improved (LOE: B).[63]

In a prospective, randomized, open, controlled clinical trial, an average of two local steroid injections was as effective as surgical decompression for the symptomatic relief of carpal tunnel syndrome at 1 year (LOE: B).[64]

In a prospective, randomized, controlled clinical trial, night splints worn almost every night provided symptomatic relief and improved sensory and motor conduction velocities at 1 year of follow up. By comparison, local corticosteroid injections had no long-term benefit for the relief of complaints or for electrophysiologic findings (LOE: B).[62]

Anatomy

The carpal tunnel is formed by the proximal carpal row and the flexor retinaculum. The carpal tunnel contains the flexor digitorum profundus, the flexor digitorum superficialis, the flexor pollicis longus, the flexor carpi radialis, and the median nerve. The flexor retinaculum is as wide at the thumb, and its proximal edge lies at the distal wrist crease.

The median nerve lies immediately under the palmaris longus tendon at the midpoint of the wrist medial (ulnar) to the flexor carpi radialis tendon. Not every patient will have a palmaris longus. If it is not present, ask the patient to press the tip of the thumb to the tip of the little finger. The crease formed at the midpoint of the palm points to the median nerve location within the carpal tunnel.

Procedure (Figure 48.10)

- The patient may be positioned seated or supine. The wrist is positioned palm up in a neutral position. The dorsum of the hand can be rested on a folded towel.
- After alcohol skin preparation, the needle is inserted just proximal to the distal flexor crease and medial (ulnar) to the palmaris longus (or above the landmark for the median nerve within the carpal tunnel). The needle is placed at a 45-degree angle and directed distally toward the index finger. The authors inject proximal to distal; however, some providers use the same landmarks but inject distal to prox-imal. The needle is placed through the flexor retinaculum, and a pop may be felt. The depth of penetration should be approximately 1 inch. Medication should flow freely with minimal pressure.
- If pain or paresthesias are reported in the palm or fingertips during needle placement, the needle should be withdrawn and reangled before reinsertion.

Aftercare

- Rest for a few days and then resumption of normal activities
- A night splint may be used to prevent the patient from sleeping in wrist flexion.
- Wrist motion may be limited for 3 to 4 weeks with a Velcro wrist immobilizer with a metal stay.
- Corticosteroid injection can be repeated if symptoms have not improved by 50%.
- Needle size: 25 or 27 gauge, ⅝ inch
- Medication: 1 mL triamcinolone (40 mg/mL) in 1 mL of lidocaine (1%) and 1 mL of bupivacaine

First carpometacarpal joint arthritis
Indication

This treatment is indicated in the presence of arthritis of the base of the thumb with associated pain, swelling, and bony deformity.

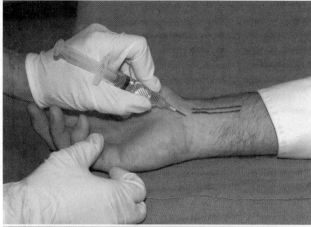

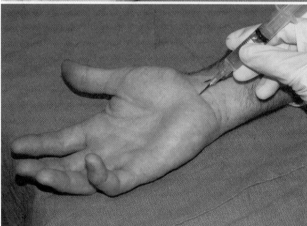

Figure 48.10 Carpal tunnel.

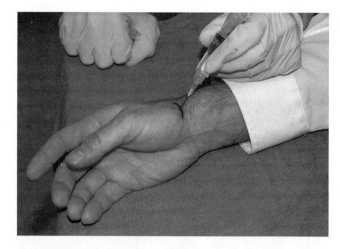

Figure 48.11 First carpometacarpal joint.

Evidence

In a randomized, double-blinded, controlled trial, no benefit of ultrasound-guided corticosteroid carpometacarpal joint injection was found over placebo in moderate to severe carpometacarpal osteoarthritis (LOE: A).[65]

Anatomy

The first carpometacarpal joint is the articulation between the first metacarpal and the trapezium. The joint line is found by passively flexing and extending the thumb while palpating for the joint space on the dorsum of the wrist at the apex of the snuffbox. The radial artery lies at the base of the snuffbox.

Procedure (Figure 48.11)

- The hand is rested in a neutral position on its side with the thumb up. Traction is pulled distally on the thumb by the examiner or an assistant to increase the joint space.
- After Betadine skin preparation, the needle is inserted at the marked joint line in the apex of the snuffbox, inserting perpendicularly to a depth of ½ to ⅝ inch into the joint space.
- If bone is encountered at a superficial depth, the needle is withdrawn and redirected. The steroid is deposited in a bolus.
- If the radial artery is encountered, withdraw and apply direct pressure for 5 minutes. Reenter ¼ inch to either side.
- Entering the joint capsule can be difficult, especially when severe arthritis is present. Local anesthetic can be used to infiltrate the area before joint injection.

Aftercare

- Activity should be avoided for 3 days.
- Thumb motion can be restricted for 3 to 4 weeks with taping, a dorsal hood splint, or a thumb spica splint.
- Injection may be repeated in 6 weeks if symptoms have not improved by 50%.
- Needle size: 25 gauge, ⅝ inch
- Medication: ½ mL triamcinolone (40 mg/mL) in ½ to 1 mL of lidocaine (1%)

de Quervain's tenosynovitis
Indication

Treatment in this area is used to reduce pain in the extensor pollicis brevis and the abductor pollicis longus tendons at the level of the radial styloid process to allow adequate rehabilitation and tissue healing. Patients who fail to improve with dorsal hood splint or thumb spica immobilization or with symptoms lasting more than 6 weeks may be candidates for injection.

Evidence

In a study of pregnant and breastfeeding women, splinting alone did not provide a satisfactory relief of the pain associated with activities of daily living. In these women, corticosteroid provided complete relief of pain (LOE: C).[66]

A meta-analysis comparing de Quervain's treatments calculated cure rates of 83% with injection alone, 61% with injection and splint, 14% with splint alone, and 0% with rest or nonsteroidal anti-inflammatory drugs (LOE: D).[67] Another study also found the added value of splinting with injection to be debatable (LOE: D).[68]

Anatomy

Extensor pollicis brevis and abductor pollicis tendons are contained in the first dorsal wrist compartment. Tendons form the dorsal and volar boundaries of the anatomic snuffbox. The two tendons of the first dorsal compartment can be best identified when the thumb is held in extension.

Procedure (Figure 48.12)

- The patient may be seated or supine, with the wrist in a vertical position with the radial side up. This may be accomplished by resting the wrist over a folded towel.

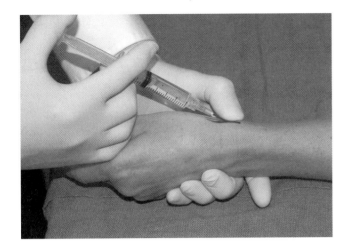

Figure 48.12   de Quervain's tenosynovitis.

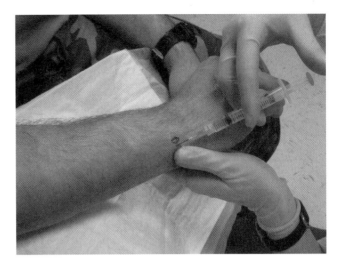

Figure 48.13   Extensor carpi ulnaris.

- The tendons should be identified and marked at the level of the radial styloid process, which is usually the point of maximal tenderness.
- After alcohol skin preparation, the needle is inserted at the mark with the bevel up and directed proximally at a 30-degree angle nearly parallel to the tendons. If a gap between the tendons is appreciable, the needle should be inserted into this gap.
- The needle should be inserted ¼ inch and then the plunger should be aspirated and gently pushed. If resistance in encountered, the needle should be pulled back and the process repeated.
- A thumb on the radial styloid may feel the injection fluid "bubbling" along the sheath.

Precautions
- Avoid injection into subcutaneous fat (this may cause fat atrophy).
- Superficial injection may cause skin discoloration. Thin women are at the greatest risk for fat atrophy and skin discoloration.[16]

Aftercare
- Some authors recommend protection from use and direct pressure for 3 days after injection followed by restricted use with splint or immobilizer for 3 to 4 weeks.[69] These authors do not feel that protection and restriction are mandatory.
- The injection can be repeated after 6 weeks if symptoms have not improved by 50%, but the risk of skin and subcutaneous fat atrophy may be greater or permanent.[69]
- Needle size: 25 to 27 gauge, ½ to 1 inch
- Medication: ¼ to ½ mL dexamethasone acetate (8 mg/mL) or ¼ to ½ mL triamcinolone (40 mg/mL) in ¾ to 1 mL of lidocaine (1%)

Extensor carpi ulnaris
Indication
This treatment is used for ulnar wrist pain related to the inflammation of the extensor carpi ulnaris tendon.

Anatomy
The extensor carpi ulnaris is palmar to the ulnar styloid in the sixth dorsal compartment. The extensor carpi ulnaris tendon palpable at the distal ulna with swelling in the sheath is often appreciated several centimeters proximal from this point.

Procedure (Figure 48.13)
- The patient is seated with the palm down and the hand and wrist supported.
- After alcohol skin preparation of the medial wrist at the distal ulna, the needle is inserted at the distal ulna and directed proximally. Solution should be palpable as it fills the extensor carpi ulnaris sheath.

Precautions
- Avoid injection into subcutaneous fat (this may cause fat atrophy).
- Superficial injection may cause skin discoloration.

Aftercare
- Relative rest of the upper extremity for 7 days
- Needle size: 25 gauge, 1½ inch
- Medication: ¼ to ½ mL dexamethasone acetate (8 mg/mL) or ¼ to ½ mL triamcinolone (40 mg/mL) in 2 to 3 mL of lidocaine (1%)

Ganglion cyst
Indication
This treatment is given in the presence of a symptomatic ganglion cyst. The cyst is an abnormal accumulation of synovial or tenosynovial fluid that has leaked from its normal confines and caused a subcutaneous inflammatory reaction and subsequent cyst wall formation. This type of cyst is also known as a "Bible bump."

Evidence
Aspiration combined with steroid injection and temporary immobilization has a success rate of approximately 40%. The success rate of surgical excision is approximately 80% (LOE: B).[70] In tropical Africa, a prospective study without controls used intralesional hyaluronidase injection in combination with aspiration, and this resulted in a 5% recurrence rate at 6 months of follow up (LOE: D).[71]

Anatomy
Most dorsal ganglions are located directly over the scaphoid. Cysts are more prominent when the wrist is flexed.

Procedure

- The hand and wrist are prone with the wrist flexed 30 to 45 degrees over a rolled towel.
- Local anesthetic may be placed in the subcutaneous tissue adjacent to the cyst (approximately ½ mL with a 25-gauge to 27-gauge needle). Alternatively, ethyl chloride spray just before needle insertion may be used for skin anesthesia.
- After alcohol skin preparation, the 18-gauge aspiration needle is inserted bevel up at the proximal base of the cyst, away from visible veins and tendons. The needle is advanced into the cyst center parallel to the skin. The depth is rarely more than ⅜ inch from the surface.
- The needle is rotated 180 degrees. The viscous contents are aspirated with a 10-mL syringe and manual tissue pressure to the sides of the cyst.
- After aspiration, the needle hub is held in place with a hemostat while the aspiration syringe is exchanged for a steroid-filled syringe using sterile technique. Steroid should flow easily into the aspirated cyst.
- Some physicians follow fluid aspiration by dry needling rather than steroid injection. Dry needling is thought to encourage scar formation and discourage the reaccumulation of cyst fluid.

Precautions

- Dictated by the location of the ganglion and the surrounding structures
- Surgical consultation is recommended for nerve paresthesias or a significant loss of range of motion.
- In one author's experience, this injection involves a greater risk for fat atrophy and skin pigment changes (LOE: E).

Aftercare

- Wrist motion should be restricted for 3 to 4 weeks, avoiding lifting, gripping, grasping, and vibration; a Velcro wrist brace may be worn for protection from these activities.
- Injection can be repeated at 6 weeks if fluid reaccumulates. However, it would also be appropriate to refer the patient for surgery after a failed aspiration/injection as a result of the higher success rate of surgical excision.[70]
- Needle size: for cyst aspiration and steroid placement, 18 gauge, 1½ inch; for local anesthetic, 25 to 27 gauge, ⅝ inch
- Medication: ¼ mL of triamcinolone (40 mg/mL) in ½ mL of lidocaine (1%)

Intersection syndrome
Indication

This treatment is performed in the presence of painful crepitus of the intersection of the muscle bellies of the extensor pollicis brevis and the adductor pollicis longus overlying the tendons of the extensor carpi radialis brevis and the extensor carpi radialis longus, 4-cm proximal to the distal radius.

Anatomy

The anatomy of this area was described in the previous section about ganglion cysts.

Procedure (Figure 48.14)

- The patient is seated with the palm pronated and resting on a flat surface. Identify the intersection with slow wrist radial deviation and thumb extension. Enter the skin from the radial border at a shallow angle, directing under the bellies of the extensor pollicis brevis and the adductor pollicis longus.

Precautions

- Avoid venous injection.
- Superficial injection may cause skin discoloration.

Aftercare

- Needle size: 25 to 27 gauge, ½ to 1 inch
- Medication: 10 to 20 mg triamcinolone acetonide with ½ to 1 mL lidocaine

Triangular fibrocartilage complex
Indication

Chronic ulnar-sided wrist pain as a result of a tear or degeneration of the triangular fibrocartilage complex is the reason for this treatment.

Anatomy

Triangular fibrocartilage complex fills the space between the distal ulna (ulnar styloid) and the proximal medial carpus.

Procedure (Figure 48.15)

- The patient sits with the palm down and the hand supported.
- After alcohol skin preparation, solution is injected via a medial approach. The needle is inserted just distal to the ulnar styloid.

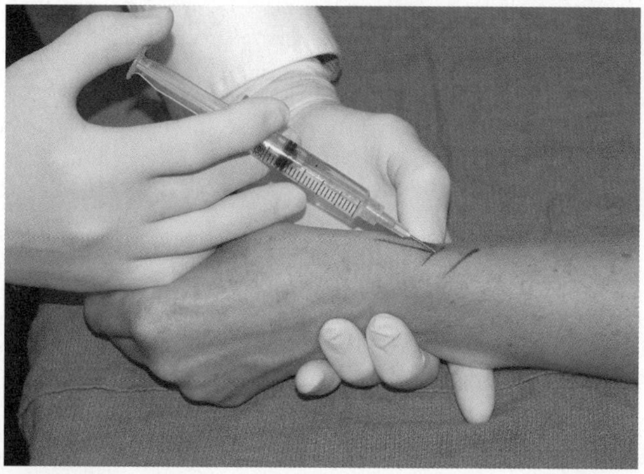

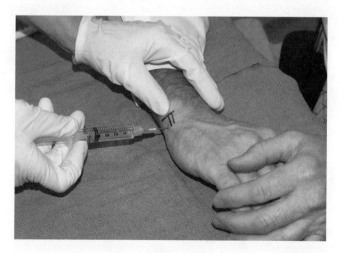

Figure 48.14 Intersection syndrome.

Figure 48.15 Triangular fibrocartilage complex.

Aftercare

- Limited use of extremity for 1 week; avoidance of flexion and ulnar deviation
- Needle: 25 gauge, 1½ inch
- Medication: ½ to 1 mL dexamethasone acetate (8 mg/mL) or ½ to 1 mL triamcinolone (40 mg/mL) in 2 to 3 mL of lidocaine (1%)

Trigger finger/stenosing tenosynovitis
Indication

This treatment is given in the presence of painful catching or locking of finger with active flexion and a palpable nodule at the first annular pulley of the flexor mechanism.

Evidence

A literature review shows a success rate of 67% to 98% with up to three injections. In one retrospective review of diabetics, the success rate was lower (50%) with up to three injections (LOE: D).[72]

Anatomy

A tender flexor tendon nodule of the flexor digitorum superficialis, typically just proximal to metacarpophalangeal joint, is found. This nodule will translate with active flexion/extension of the affected digit beneath the first annular pulley, just proximal to the metacarpophalangeal joint.

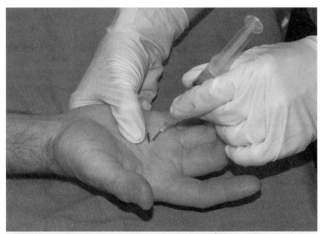

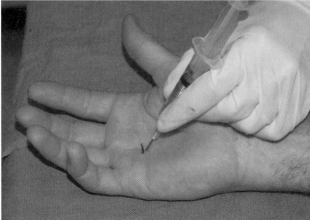

Figure 48.16   Trigger finger.

Procedure (Figure 48.16)

- The patient may be seated or supine.
- The site of the injection is marked proximal to the distal palmar crease and just proximal to the metacarpophalangeal joint.
- After alcohol skin preparation, the needle is inserted bevel up at a 45-degree angle into the nodule, parallel to the tendon, and directed proximally toward the arm. When an increased, rubbery resistance is felt at approximately a ¼ inch depth, the plunger should be gently pushed. The solution is injected just atop the tendon and underneath the tenosynovial sheath. Occasionally a slight pop is felt when entering the sheath.
- If there is resistance to injection, the needle may be in the tendon. The needle should be slightly withdrawn, aspirated, and reinjected when the plunger moves freely.
- Some authors recommend insertion proximal to distal palmar crease and injecting directed toward the fingertips.[16,69]

Precautions

- Ensure that pain is not the result of infectious flexor tenosynovitis.
- Infectious flexor tenosynovitis is evidenced by intense pain with any attempt to flex or extend, by the finger held in flexion for comfort, by uniform swelling involving the entire finger (in contrast with localized swelling in local inflammation), and by percussion tenderness along the course of the tendon sheath.
- There is a risk of tendon rupture.
- Avoid injection into subcutaneous fat (this may cause fat atrophy).
- These authors recommend a maximum of two injections after which the patient should be considered for evaluation for surgical release.[69]

Aftercare

- No restriction required.
- Some physicians recommend restriction and buddy taping for 2 days.
- Injection can be repeated after 5 to 6 weeks if symptoms have not improved dramatically.
- Needle size: 25 to 27 gauge, ½ to 1 inch
- Medication: ¼ mL dexamethasone acetate (8 mg/mL) or ¼ mL triamcinolone (40 mg/mL) in ¾ mL of lidocaine (1%)

HIP AND PELVIS INJECTION AND ASPIRATION TECHNIQUES

Coccyx
Indication

Pain and inflammation of the coccyx and the coccygeal ligaments at the articulation with the sacrum result in this use of this treatment.

Evidence

In a prospective randomized study of coccydynia treatments, local steroid injection had a success rate of 60% as compared with an 85% success rate with manipulation and corticosteroid injection. Patients with persistent pain went on for coccygectomy, with a success rate of 90% (LOE: B).[73]

Anatomy

At the termination of the sacrum inferiorly lies the coccyx. Full palpation of the coccyx and examination of the sacrococcygeal joint require a bimanual transrectal examination.

Procedure

- The patient lies in a lateral decubitus position with the hips and knees fully flexed. Alternatively, the patient may lie prone over a small pillow.
- Using a bimanual rectal examination technique, the sacrococcygeal joint is identified and marked externally.
- An assistant may be required to place upward traction on the buttock to expose the gluteal crease.
- After alcohol skin preparation, the needle is inserted ½ to 1 inch inferior to joint in the midline at a 70-degree angle cephalad. The needle is advanced until the bony end point is reached (approximately ½ to 1 inch), and it is then withdrawn slightly. Steroid is peppered into the tender ligaments.

Precautions

- Patients who are more than 50 years of age with pain in the sacrococcygeal area must undergo a rectal and pelvic examination to rule out anorectal or pelvic pathology.

Aftercare

- Relative rest for 3 days.
- Avoid sitting on hard surfaces. (Patients may use a ring cushion for sitting.)
- Needle size: 25 gauge, 1½ inch.
- Medication: ½ to 1 mL dexamethasone acetate (8 mg/mL) or ½ to 1 mL triamcinolone (40 mg/mL) in 1 to 2 mL of lidocaine (1%).

Ischial bursitis
Indication

This treatment is used for pain and inflammation of the ischial bursa.

Anatomy

The ischium is the attachment point of the bicep femoris, and it can involve both semitendinosis and semimembranosus. The sciatic nerve lies lateral to the ischium about a third of the way between the ischium and the greater trochanter.

Procedure

- The patient lies in the lateral decubital position with the affected side up and the hip flexed to 90 degrees. The provider stands behind the patient.
- Identify the ischium and the point of maximal tenderness. Inject down to but not into the junction of the bone and the tendon.

Precautions

- Avoid injection into the tendon or the sciatic nerve, which lies deep and posterior to the trochanter.

Aftercare

- Relative rest from heavy hamstring strengthening, hill running, or speed work/sprinting for 1 week
- Needle size: 25 gauge, 1½ inch
- Medication: ½ to 1 mL triamcinolone (40 mg/mL) in 3 mL of lidocaine (1%)

Piriformis
Indication

This treatment is used for the chronic pain of piriformis syndrome. Consider the diagnostic injection of lidocaine only before steroid injection.

Anatomy

The piriformis originates from the lateral border of the sacrum and inserts into the posterior aspect of the greater trochanter of the femur.

The sciatic nerve is very close to the central aspect of the muscle, with the nerve passing over the muscle in most cases and through or below in a small percentage of patients.

Procedure

- The position is similar to that used for ischial injection, with the patient in the lateral decubital position with affected side up and the hip flexed to 90 degrees.
- Identify the point of maximal tenderness and insert the needle for injection. If the point of maximal tenderness is directly in the middle, consider performing this treatment with ultrasound or fluoroscopic guidance.

Precautions

- Avoid injection into the sciatic nerve.

Aftercare

- Relative rest from heavy hamstring strengthening, hill running, or speed work/sprinting for 1 week
- Needle size: 25 gauge, 1½ inch
- Medication: diagnostic, 2 mL lidocaine with 2 mL bupivacaine; therapeutic, ½ mL triamcinolone (40 mg/mL) in 1 to 2 mL of lidocaine 1%

Sacroiliac joint
Indication

Pain and inflammation of sacroiliac strain and sacroiliitis persisting beyond 6 weeks are indications for this treatment.

Evidence

Periarticular injection of methylprednisolone for the treatment of pain in the region of the sacroiliac joint in nonspondylarthropathic patients significantly reduced pain at 1 month of follow-up as compared with saline-injected controls (LOE: B).[74] Generally this injection is thought to be more successful with fluoroscopic, computed tomography, or magnetic resonance imaging guidance (LOE: D).[74,75]

Anatomy

The sacroiliac joint is formed by the articulation of the sacrum with the ileum. The dimples at the top of the buttocks overlie the posterior superior iliac spines. The sacroiliac joints are caudal and medial to the posterior superior iliac spines. The joint is angled obliquely posteroanteriorly.

Procedure

- The patient is positioned fully prone.
- The sacroiliac joint is marked 1 inch caudal to the posterior superior iliac spines and 1 inch lateral from midline.
- After Betadine skin preparation, the needle is placed at the mark and angled obliquely lateral at a 45-degree angle. The needle is passed between the ilium and sacrum until ligamentous resistance is felt, which occurs at a depth of 1½ to 2½ inches.
- If bone is encountered before 1½ inches, the needle is withdrawn 1 inch and redirected approximately 5 degrees until maximum depth is achieved without encountering bone.
- Medication may be deposited in a bolus or by peppering the capsule.

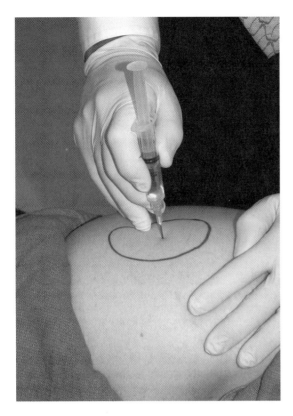

Figure 48.17 Greater trochanteric bursa.

Precautions
- True sacroiliitis may be associated with a spondyloarthropathy. A rheumatologic workup may be indicated for some patients.

Aftercare
- The patient should avoid direct pressure, bending, lifting, and all unnecessary walking and standing for 3 days.
- Core and lower back exercises are begun after acute pain has resolved.
- Injection may be repeated in 6 weeks if pain persists.
- Needle size: 21 or 22 gauge, 1½ to 3½ inches
- Medication: 1 mL triamcinolone (40 mg/mL) in 2 mL of lidocaine

Trochanteric bursitis
Indication
This treatment is used for pain relief of trochanteric bursitis to allow for participation in physical therapy, exercise, and continued activities of daily living.[3]

Anatomy
Up to three separate bursae are located along the superior margin of the greater trochanter between the iliotibial band and the greater trochanter.

Evidence
In an observational study, corticosteroid injection was an effective therapy for trochanteric bursitis, with 61.3% of patients reporting improvement in pain at 26 weeks of follow up (LOE: D).[76]

Procedure (Figure 48.17)
- The patient lies in a lateral decubitus position with the injection site superior. The patient is draped to expose the lateral hip.

- Palpate the soft tissue at the superior margin of the trochanter to identify it, and make a mark at the point of maximal tenderness with the retracted tip of a ballpoint pen.
- After alcohol skin preparation, insert the needle at the mark and perpendicular to the skin. When bone is reached, withdraw slightly and aspirate. Inject the solution in a wagon-wheel pattern, peppering the bursa.
- If paresthesias are reported, the needle should be withdrawn and reinserted laterally.
- The anesthetic will transiently irritate the bursa, and this will reproduce the patient's symptoms.

Precautions
- Avoid injection of the sciatic nerve, which lies deep and posterior to the trochanter.

Aftercare
- The patient must complete a physical therapy program to prevent relapse.
- Needle size: 25 gauge, 1½ inch length at minimum, preferably 2 inches or longer
- Medication: 1 to 2 mL dexamethasone acetate (8 mg/mL) or 1 to 2 mL triamcinolone (40 mg/mL) in 4 mL of lidocaine (1%)

KNEE INJECTION AND ASPIRATION TECHNIQUES

Iliotibial band friction syndrome
Indication
This treatment is done for the relief of pain related to the acute or chronic irritation of the iliotibial band as it crosses the lateral femoral condyle.

Anatomy
The iliotibial band arises from the tensor fascia latae muscle in the lateral buttocks and runs along the lateral leg to its insertion at Gerdy's tubercle on the anterolateral tibia. Irritation typically occurs at the point of contact with the lateral femoral condyle.

Procedure (Figure 48.18)
- The patient may be seated or in the lateral decubitus position.
- The point of maximal tenderness is identified and marked.

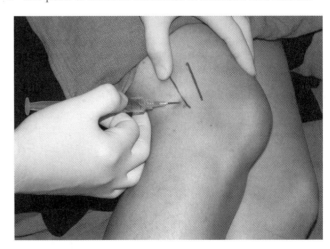

Figure 48.18 Iliotibial band.

- After alcohol skin preparation, the needle is inserted into the mark and angled posterior and slightly medial. The injection depth is just above the periosteum. If bone is contacted, withdraw the needle slightly, aspirate, and then inject.
- Medication is peppered in the area. The intent is to inject between the epicondyle and the iliotibial band.
- It is important to not inject the iliotibial band itself. If resistance is felt, redirect the needle.

Precautions
- Be aware that the common peroneal nerve is posterior and medial to the tendon of the biceps femoris.
- Avoid injection into subcutaneous fat (this may cause fat atrophy).
- Superficial injection may cause skin discoloration.

Aftercare
- Rest from aggravating activity for 1 week
- Needle size: 25 gauge, ⅝ inch
- Medication: ½ to 1 mL dexamethasone acetate (8 mg/mL) or ½ to 1 mL triamcinolone (40 mg/mL) in 3 mL of lidocaine (1%)

Intra-articular knee
Indication
This treatment is indicated for the relief of pain caused by degenerative joint disease or tense hemarthrosis. Joint aspiration may be diagnostic with fluid analysis. After trauma, aspiration can assist with the narrowing of the differential diagnosis of processes that result in synovitis as compared with hemarthrosis (see Table 48.1).

Evidence
In patients with chronic arthritis, corticosteroid injection can reduce pain and synovitis, with results lasting up to 1 year (LOE: D).[8] Corticosteroid treatment as compared with saline injection every 3 months showed no significant increase in joint-space narrowing and a trend toward a reduction in pain for up to 2 years (LOE: A).[77]

In meta-analysis, intra-articular steroid injections were shown to be useful for reducing pain from osteoarthritis of the knee for up to 4 weeks. These authors concluded that the beneficial effect is unlikely to continue beyond that time (LOE: B).[28]

A prospective randomized study comparing a complete synovial fluid aspiration and intra-articular corticosteroid injection with injection alone indicated that arthrocentesis reduces the risk for arthritis relapse in rheumatoid arthritis patients. At the end of the study, there were 23% relapses in the arthrocentesis group and 47% in the no arthrocentesis group (P = .001) (LOE: B).[78]

Anatomy
The joint is formed by the articulation of the tibia, the femur, and the patella. There is a continuous space from the suprapatellar pouch to the patellar tendon insertion.

Procedure
- Multiple approaches are possible. The knee should be thoroughly prepped with Betadine, and sterile techniques should be employed. Lidocaine (1 mL) may be superficially peppered at the site of injection/aspiration for anesthesia.
- Use an anterior, seated approach **(Figure 48.19):**
  - The patient is seated with the knee flexed to 90 degrees.
  - The needle is inserted on either the lateral or medial border of the patellar tendon at a 45-degree angle to the sagittal plane. The needle is directed toward the center of the knee

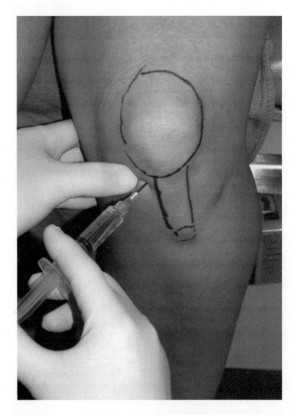

Figure 48.19 Intra-articular knee, anterior seated.

medially, posteriorly, and slightly cephalad at a depth of approximately 1¼ to 1½ inch.
- The injection should flow freely. Any resistance prompts needle repositioning.
- Use a lateral suprapatellar approach **(Figure 48.20):**
  - With the patient supine, the superior lateral margin of the patella is palpated.
  - The needle is inserted one fingerbreadth superior and one fingerbreadth below the superolateral corner of the patella.
  - The medication is instilled at this point.
    This approach is also used for aspiration, which is accomplished with a 60-mL syringe.
- If an infectious cause is not suspected, after aspiration the syringe may then be replaced with a syringe containing the steroid solution and injected through the same needle.

Precautions
- Avoid injection into the anterior cruciate ligament because this is quite painful.
- Limit steroid injections to three to four injections in a 12-month period. Repetitive injection can lead to a softening of the cartilage and further damage.
- Avoid injection into subcutaneous fat (this may cause fat atrophy).
- Superficial injection may cause skin discoloration.

Aftercare
- After corticosteroid injection, relative rest for 7 days
- After aspiration for tense effusion, apply compression dressing.
- Crutches with advancement from no weight bearing to toe-touch ambulation may be dictated by patient pain.
- Needle size: for injection, 21 to 22 gauge, 1½ inch; for aspiration, 18 to 22 gauge, 1½ inch; for local anesthetic before injection, 25 gauge, ⅝ inch

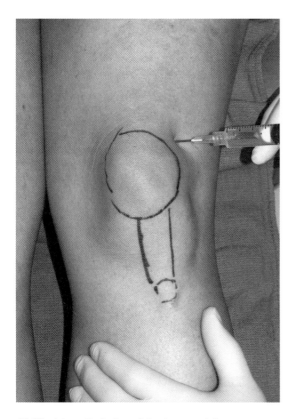

Figure 48.20 Intra-articular knee, lateral suprapatellar.

• Medication: 1 mL dexamethasone acetate (8 mg/mL) or 1 mL triamcinolone (40 mg/mL) in 3 to 5 mL of lidocaine (1%)

Pes anserine bursitis
Indication
Pain and inflammation of pes anserine bursitis is a reason for this treatment.

Anatomy
The pes anserine bursa lies just posterior to and beneath the combined tendon insertion of the "sergeant" or "SGT" group of hamstring muscles: the sartorius, the gracilis, and the semi-tendinosis. The tendons of this group insert on the medial aspect of the tibia below the joint line.

Procedure (Figure 48.21)
• The pes anserine combined tendon can be identified by making the patient strongly flex the knee against resistance. Tendons can be followed distally to their insertion. The pes anserine bursa is found as an area of tenderness just proximal to the insertion point. The point of maximal tenderness is marked.
• The patient may be seated or supine for injection.
• After alcohol skin preparation, the needle is inserted just lateral to the mark and angled posterior and medial. Insert the needle to the bone, and then withdraw slightly. The goal is to inject between the tibia and the pes anserine tendons. The depth of injection is approximately ¼ inch.
• If resistance to injection is felt, withdraw and redirect the needle.

Precautions
• Be aware that most pes anserine bursitis is associated with medial degenerative joint disease or meniscal pathology and

that it has been seen with proximal tibial stress fractures. Consider evaluation for these conditions in addition to pes anserine injection.
• Avoid injection into subcutaneous fat (this may cause fat atrophy).
• Superficial injection may cause skin discoloration.

Aftercare
• Avoid overuse activities for a minimum of 1 week.
• After 1 week, begin a graduated stretching and strengthening program.
• Needle size: 25 gauge, ⅝ inch
• Medication: ½ mL of triamcinolone with 1 mL of lidocaine and 1 mL of bupivacaine

FOOT AND ANKLE INJECTION AND ASPIRATION TECHNIQUES

Great toe metatarsophalangeal joint
Indication
Pain and limited motion of the first metatarsophalangeal joint are indications for this treatment.

Evidence
In patients with metatarsophalangeal joint synovitis, intra-articular steroid injection improved or completely resolved pain in 93% of subjects.[79]

Anatomy
The joint can be best located by palpating the metatarsal head while passively flexing and extending the toe.

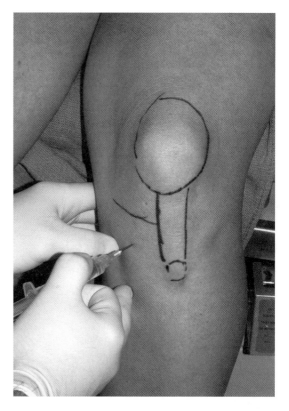

Figure 48.21 Pes anserine bursa.

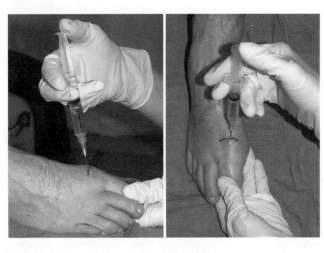

Figure 48.22   First metatarsophalangeal joint.

Procedure (Figure 48.22)
- The patient is supine with the foot supported.
- The joint line is marked. An assistant should provide traction to the toe, plantarflexing it about 30 degrees with some distraction to open up the joint space dorsally.
- After Betadine skin preparation, insert the needle perpendicularly into the joint space. Deposit the solution as a bolus.

Precautions
- Avoid hitting bone or injecting into the extensor hallucis longus tendon.

Aftercare
- Avoid excessive weight bearing for 1 week.
- May tape first and second toes together with a pad between them.
- Needle size: 25 gauge, ⅝ inch
- Medication: ½ mL triamcinolone (40 mg/mL) or dexamethasone (8 mg/mL) in 1 mL of a lidocaine/bupivacaine mix.

Intra-articular ankle
Indication
This treatment is given for pain from soft-tissue impingement, synovitis, or chronic capsulitis.

Anatomy
The medial to anterior tibialis tendon is found in the hollow between the medial malleolus and the articulation between the tibia and the talus.

Procedure (Figure 48.23)
- The patient is seated or lying supine with a towel beneath the knee. Place the foot in slight 20-degree plantarflexion to increase the medial joint space. An assistant can distract the ankle joint.
- After Betadine skin preparation, the needle is inserted just medial to the tibialis anterior tendon into the anteromedial recess, parallel to the plafond and at a 45-degree angle to the sagittal plane. The depth of insertion is approximately 1 to 1½ inches.

Precautions
- Avoid injection into the dorsalis pedis artery.

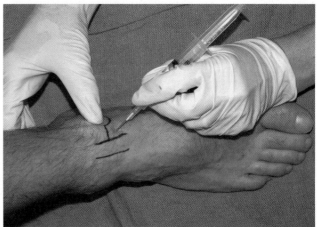

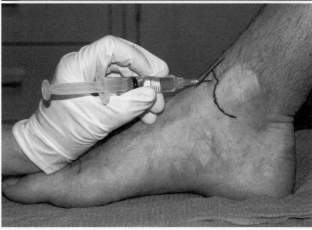

Figure 48.23   Intra-articular ankle.

Aftercare
- Avoid excessive weight bearing activities for 1 week.
- Needle size: 25 gauge, 1 to 1½ inch
- Medication: ½ mL triamcinolone (40 mg/mL) or ½ mL dexamethasone (8 mg/mL) with 3 to 5 mL of lidocaine (1%)

Morton's neuroma
Indication
Treatment is given for the pain of perineuronal fibrosis of an interdigital nerve, usually between the second and third metatarsal heads, which is known as *Morton's neuroma*.

Anatomy
Neuroma is typically between and slightly plantar to the metatarsal heads.

Procedure (Figure 48.24)
- The patient is supine with a pillow under the knee to allow the foot to be slightly plantarflexed.
- The point of maximal tenderness is marked, and it is usually ½ inch proximal to the web space.
- After alcohol skin preparation, the needle is inserted dorsally at the mark and entered between the metatarsal heads. The needle is advanced perpendicularly through the transverse tarsal ligament. The depth of the insertion is approximately ½ inch.
- After the giving way or popping of passing through the ligament is felt, the steroid is injected.

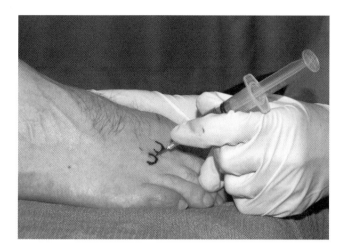

Figure 48.24   Morton's neuroma.

Precautions

- Patients are at risk for interdigital nerve injury.

Aftercare

- Rest for 3 days, avoiding weight-bearing activities
- Needle size: 25 gauge, 1 inch
- Medication: ½ mL of triamcinolone (40 mg/mL) or ½ mL of dexamethasone (8 mg/mL) in 2 mL of lidocaine

Plantar fascia
Indication

This treatment is given for the relief of pain caused by the inflammation of the plantar fascia origin that is recalcitrant to conservative management.

Anatomy

Plantar fascia originates at the anterior plantar calcaneous and fans out at its distal insertion on the mid metatarsals. This structure forms, in part, the medial longitudinal arch.

Procedure (Figure 48.25)

- These authors have found the medial approach to be significantly less painful than the plantar approach (LOE: E).
- The patient is supine.

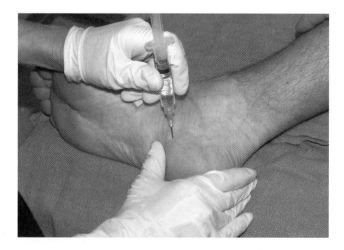

Figure 48.25   Plantar fascia.

- Prepare the skin with alcohol. The patient actively dorsiflexes the foot and great toe, which will accentuate the medial margin of the plantar fascia.
- Palpate the medial calcaneal tuberosity, and insert the needle superior to the plantar fascia. Spread the medication in a fanlike pattern at the origin of the fascia.
- If pain is felt radiating across2 the heel or arch or if significant resistance is felt, withdraw the needle and reinsert it at slightly altered angle, or recheck for landmarks.

Precautions

- There is an association with rupture of the plantar fascia and previous steroid injection, with one study documenting a rupture rate of 10% with injection (LOE: D).[24,80] Rupture can lead to chronic pain as a result of the loss of integrity of the foot arch (LOE: D).[81]
- Avoid injection into the heel fat pad because this may cause fat atrophy.
- Superficial injection may cause skin discoloration.
- Avoid the median plantar nerve.

Aftercare

- Heel support is recommended for at least 1 week after injection.
- No running for 1 week, and avoid excessive weight bearing.
- Needle size: 25 to 27 gauge, 1 to 1½ inch
- Medication: ½ mL dexamethasone acetate (8 mg/mL) or ½ mL triamcinolone (40 mg/mL) in 3 mL of lidocaine (1%)

Tarsal tunnel
Indication

This treatment is given for medial foot pain and paresthesia with a positive Tinel's sign over the tarsal tunnel. Consider diagnostic anesthetic injection before steroid injection.

Anatomy

The tarsal tunnel is posterior and inferior to the medial malleolus and beneath the deltoid ligament. Within the tunnel pass "Tom, Dick, and a very nervous Harry": the tibialis posterior, the flexor digitorum longus, the posterior tibial artery, the tibial nerve, and the flexor hallucis longus. The tibial nerve should be approximately 4 cm from the medial malleolus.

Procedure (Figure 48.26)

- Palpate the area of pain that reproduces distal neurologic symptoms, and inject there.

Precautions

- Avoid the injection of nerves, tendons, and the posterior tibial vein.
- Avoid injection into subcutaneous fat (this may cause fat atrophy).

Aftercare

- The patient is placed in a walking boot for 7 days.
- Needle size: 25 gauge, ⅝ inch
- Medication: ½ ml of dexamethasone (8 mg/mL) or triamcinolone (40 mg/mL) in 1 to 2 mL of lidocaine

SOFT-TISSUE INJECTION AND ASPIRATION TECHNIQUES

Myofascial trigger points
Indication

This treatment is used for the diagnosis and treatment of myofascial trigger points.

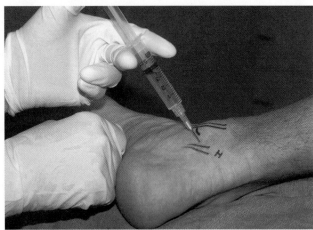

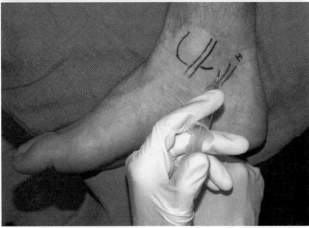

Figure 48.26 Tarsal tunnel.

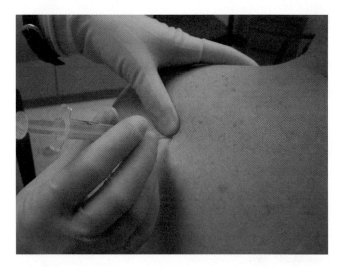

Figure 48.27 Trigger point.

- After alcohol skin preparation, the needle is inserted at the mark, perpendicular to the skin. The needle is passed 1 to 1½ inches through the fascia until giving way or the pop of entering muscle is felt or until the patient perceives the needle as being in the "right spot."
- The solution is deposited using a fanning approach. The patient should perceive an increase in pain as the fluid is injected. The physician may palpate a local muscle twitch or triggering when the trigger point is hit.

Precautions
- Knowledge of the anatomy of the injection site is crucial to avoid vascular and nervous structures.

Aftercare
- May initiate acupressure, ice, and therapeutic exercises without delay
- May repeat injection in 1 to 2 weeks
- Needle size: 25 to 27 gauge, 1 to 1½ inch
- Medication: 1½ mL of lidocaine/bupivacaine mix at each trigger point **(Table 48.4)**

Anatomy
Trigger points are palpable fusiform nodules that run parallel to the fibers of a muscle.

Procedure (Figure 48.27)
- Tender nodules are found and marked. Up to 10 to 15 trigger points can be treated during one visit. Do not exceed the maximum doses of anesthetics or lidocaine (200 mg: 20 mL of 1.0% or 10 mL of 2.0%).

Table 48.4 Recommended Corticosteroid and Anesthetic Dosages for Injection

| Site | Needle Gauge and Length (Inches) | Steroid Volume (mL) (Choose One) | | Anesthetic Total Volume (mL)* |
		Triamcinolone Acetate (40 mg/mL)	Dexamethasone Acetate (8 mg/mL)	
Shoulder				
Acromioclavicular joint	25, ½ to 1	½	½	2 to 3
Biceps tendon	25, 1½	½		1 to 2
Intra-articular shoulder	25, 1½	1	1	7 to 8
Subacromial space	22-25, 1½	1	1	6
Elbow				
Intra-articular elbow	21 to 22, 1½			1 to 2
Lateral epicondylitis	25, ⅝	½ to 1	½ to 1	2
Medial epicondylitis	25, ⅝	½	½	1 to 2
Olecranon bursa	18,† ⅝ to 1½	½ to 1		1 to 2
Wrist/Hand				
Carpal tunnel	25 or 27, 1	1		2
Carpometacarpal joint	25, ⅝	½		½ to 1
de Quervain's tenosynovitis	25 to 27, ½ or ⅝	¼ to ½	¼ to ½	¾ to 1
Extensor carpi ulnaris	25, ⅝	¼ to ½	¼ to ½	2 to 3
Ganglion cyst	18,† ⅝ to 1½	¼		½
Triangular fibrocartilage complex	25 to 27, ½ to 1	½ to 1	½ to 1	2 to 3
Trigger finger	25 to 27, ½ to 1	¼	¼	¾
Hip/Pelvis				
Coccyx	25, 1½	½ to 1	½ to 1	1 to 2
Ischial bursa	25, 1½	½ to 1		3
Sacroiliac joint	21 or 23, 1½ to 3½	1		2
Trochanteric bursa	25, 1½ to >2	1 to 2	1 to 2	4
Knee				
Iliotibial Band	25, ⅝	½ to 1	½ to 1	3
Intra-articular knee	See text	1	1	3 to 5
Pes anserine bursa	25 to 27, 1 to 1½	½		2
Foot/Ankle				
First metatarsophalangeal joint	25, ⅝	½	½	1
Intra-articular ankle	25, 1 to 1½	½		3 to 5
Morton's neuroma	25, 1	½	½	2
Plantar fascia	25 to 27, 1 to 1½	½	½	3
Tarsal tunnel	25, ⅝	½	½	1 to 2
Soft Tissue				
Trigger points	25 to 27, 1 to 1½			1½

*Lidocaine 1% or 2% and/or bupivacaine 0.25% or 0.5%.
†A smaller needle is used for local anesthetic.
Adapted from O'Connor FG, Sallis RE, Wilder RP, St. Pierre P: Sports Medicine: Just the Facts. New York, McGraw-Hill, 2005.

REFERENCES

1. O'Connor FG, Howard TM, Fieseler CM, Nirschl RP: Managing overuse injuries: a systematic approach. Phys Sportsmed 1997;25(5).

2. Hollander JL: Intrasynovial corticosteroid therapy in arthritis. Md State Med J 1970;19(3):62-66.

3. Snibbe JC, Gambardella RA: Use of injections for osteoarthritis in joints and sports activity. Clin Sports Med 2005;24(1):83-91.

4. Hollander JL: Intra-articular hydrocortisone in arthritis and allied conditions; a summary of two years' clinical experience. J Bone Joint Surg Am 1953;35-A(4):983-990.

5. Labelle H, Guibert R, Joncas J, et al: Lack of scientific evidence for the treatment of lateral epicondylitis of the elbow. An attempted meta-analysis. J Bone Joint Surg Br 1992;74(5):646-651.

6. Paavola M, Kannus P, Jarvinen TA, et al: Treatment of tendon disorders. Is there a role for corticosteroid injection? Foot Ankle Clin 2002;7(3):501-513.

7. Bellamy N, Campbell J, Robinson V, et al: Intraarticular corticosteroid for treatment of osteoarthritis of the knee. Cochrane Database Syst Rev 2005;(2):CD005328.

8. Huppertz HI, Tschammler A, Horwitz AE, Schwab KO: Intraarticular corticosteroids for chronic arthritis in children: efficacy and effects on cartilage and growth. J Pediatr 1995;127(2):317-321.

9. Eustace JA, Brophy DP, Gibney RP, et al: Comparison of the accuracy of steroid placement with clinical outcome in patients with shoulder symptoms. Ann Rheum Dis 1997;56(1):59-63.

10. Jones A, Regan M, Ledingham J, et al: Importance of placement of intra-articular steroid injections. BMJ 1993;307(6915):1329-1330.

11. Eberhard BA, Sison MC, Gottlieb BS, Ilowite NT: Comparison of the intraarticular effectiveness of triamcinolone hexacetonide and triamcinolone acetonide in treatment of juvenile rheumatoid arthritis. J Rheumatol 2004;31(12):2507-2512.

12. Honkanen VE, Rautonen JK, Pelkonen PM: Intra-articular glucocorticoids in early juvenile chronic arthritis. Acta Paediatr 1993;82(12):1072-1074.

13. Fernandez C, Noguera R, Gonzalez JA, Pascual E: Treatment of acute attacks of gout with a small dose of intraarticular triamcinolone acetonide. J Rheumatol 1999;26(10):2285-2286.

14. Grillet B, Dequeker J: Intra-articular steroid injection. A risk-benefit assessment. Drug Saf 1990;5(3):205-211.

15. Shoemaker RS, Bertone AL, Martin GS, et al: Effects of intra-articular administration of methylprednisolone acetate on normal articular cartilage and on healing of experimentally induced osteochondral defects in horses. Am J Vet Res 1992;53(8):1446-1453.

16. Saunders S. Injection Techniques in Orthopaedic and Sports Medicine, 2nd ed. Philadelphia, WB Saunders, 2002.

17. Khan KM, Cook JL, Kannus P, et al: Time to abandon the "tendonitis" myth. BMJ 2002;324(7338):626-627.

18. Khan KM, Cook JL, Bonar F, et al: Histopathology of common tendinopathies. Update and implications for clinical management. Sports Med 1999;27(6):393-408.

19. Berger RG, Yount WJ: Immediate "steroid flare" from intraarticular triamcinolone hexacetonide injection: case report and review of the literature. Arthritis Rheum 1990;33(8):1284-1286.

20. O'Connor FG, Sallis RE, Wilder RP, St. Pierre P: Sports Medicine: Just the Facts. New York, McGraw-Hill, 2005.

21. Rogojan C, Hetland ML: Depigmentation—a rare side effect to intra-articular glucocorticoid treatment. Clin Rheumatol 2004;23(4):373-375.

22. Charalambous CP, Tryfonidis M, Sadiq S, et al: Septic arthritis following intra-articular steroid injection of the knee—a survey of current practice regarding antiseptic technique used during intra-articular steroid injection of the knee. Clin Rheumatol 2003;22(6):386-390.

23. Stahl S, Kaufman T: Ulnar nerve injury at the elbow after steroid injection for medial epicondylitis. J Hand Surg [Br] 1997;22(1):69-70.

24. Sellman JR: Plantar fascia rupture associated with corticosteroid injection. Foot Ankle Int 1994;15(7):376-381.

25. Mahler F, Fritschy D: Partial and complete ruptures of the Achilles tendon and local corticosteroid injections. Br J Sports Med 1992;26(1):7-14.

26. Read MT: Safe relief of rest pain that eases with activity in achillodynia by intrabursal or peritendinous steroid injection: the rupture rate was not increased by these steroid injections. Br J Sports Med 1999;33(2):134-135.

27. Hugate R, Pennypacker J, Saunders M, Juliano P: The effects of intratendinous and retrocalcaneal intrabursal injections of corticosteroid on the biomechanical properties of rabbit Achilles tendons. J Bone Joint Surg Am 2004;86-A(4):794-801.

28. Godwin M, Dawes M: Intra-articular steroid injections for painful knees. Systematic review with meta-analysis. Can Fam Physician 2004;50:241-248.

29. Papachristou G, Anagnostou S, Katsorhis T: The effect of intraarticular hydrocortisone injection on the articular cartilage of rabbits. Acta Orthop Scand Suppl 1997;275:132-134.

30. Birkinshaw R, O'Donnell J, Sammy I: Necrotising fasciitis as a complication of steroid injection. J Accid Emerg Med 1997;14(1):52-54.

31. Pattrick M, Doherty M: Facial flushing after intra-articular injection of steroid. Br Med J (Clin Res Ed) 1987;295(6610):1380.

32. Pollock B, Wilkinson SM, MacDonald Hull SP: Chronic urticaria associated with intra-articular methylprednisolone. Br J Dermatol 2001;144(6):1228-1230.

33. Ijsselmuiden OE, Knegt-Junk KJ, van Wijk RG, van Joost T: Cutaneous adverse reactions after intra-articular injection of triamcinolone acetonide. Acta Derm Venereol 1995;75(1):57-58.

34. Karsh J, Yang WH: An anaphylactic reaction to intra-articular triamcinolone: a case report and review of the literature. Ann Allergy Asthma Immunol 2003;90(2):254-258.

35. Kendall P: Untoward effects following local hydrocortisone injection. Ann Phys Med 1958;4:170-175.

36. Mace S, Vadas P, Pruzanski W: Anaphylactic shock induced by intraarticular injection of methylprednisolone acetate. J Rheumatol 1997;24(6):1191-1194.

37. Derendorf H, Mollmann H, Gruner A, et al: Pharmacokinetics and pharmacodynamics of glucocorticoid suspensions after intra-articular administration. Clin Pharmacol Ther 1986;39(3):313-317.

38. Kumar S, Singh RJ, Reed AM, Lteif AN: Cushing's syndrome after intra-articular and intradermal administration of triamcinolone acetonide in three pediatric patients. Pediatrics 2004;113(6):1820-1824.

39. Jansen TL, Van Roon EN: Four cases of a secondary Cushingoid state following local triamcinolone acetonide (Kenacort) injection. Neth J Med 2002;60(3):151-153.

40. Daragon A, Vittecoq O, Le Loet X: Visual hallucinations induced by intraarticular injection of steroids. J Rheumatol 1997;24(2):411.

41. Robinson DE, Harrison-Hansley E, Spencer RF: Steroid psychosis after an intra-articular injection. Ann Rheum Dis 2000;59(11):927.

42. Wellings RM, Davies AM, Pynsent PB, Cassar-Pullicino VN: A comparison of a conventional non-ionic contrast medium (iohexol) alone and with adrenaline and an iso-osmolar non-ionic contrast medium (iotrolan) in computed tomographic arthrography of the shoulder. Br J Radiol 1994;67(802):941-944.

43. Kannus P, Jarvinen M, Niittymaki S: Long- or short-acting anesthetic with corticosteroid in local injections of overuse injuries? A prospective, randomized, double-blind study. Int J Sports Med 1990;11(5):397-400.

44. O'Connell T: Interpreting Tests From Joint Aspirates. Philadelphia, Elsevier Science, 2002.

45. Tasciotaoglu F, Oner C: Efficacy of intra-articular sodium hyaluronate in the treatment of knee osteoarthritis. Clin Rheumatol 2003;22(2):112-117.

46. Leopold SS, Redd BB, Warme WJ, et al: Corticosteroid compared with hyaluronic acid injections for the treatment of osteoarthritis of the knee. A prospective, randomized trial. J Bone Joint Surg Am 2003;85-A(7):1197-1203.

47. Charalambous CP: Corticosteroid compared with hyaluronic acid injections for the treatment of osteoarthritis of the knee. J Bone Joint Surg Am 2004;86-A(4):874, author reply 874.

48. Evanich JD, Evanich CJ, Wright MB, Rydlewicz JA: Efficacy of intraarticular hyaluronic acid injections in knee osteoarthritis. Clin Orthop Relat Res 2001;(390):173-181.

49. Paluska SA: Indications, Contraindications, and Overview for Aspirating or Injecting a Joint or Related Structure. Philadelphia, Elsevier Science, 2002.

50. Jacob AK, Sallay PI: Therapeutic efficacy of corticosteroid injections in the acromioclavicular joint. Biomed Sci Instrum 1997;34:380-385.

51. Sethi PM, Kingston S, Elattrache N: Accuracy of anterior intra-articular injection of the glenohumeral joint. Arthroscopy 2005:21(1):77-80.

52. Buchbinder R, Green S, Youd JM: Corticosteroid injections for shoulder pain. Cochrane Database Syst Rev 2003;(1):CD004016.

53. Khan AA, Mowla A, Shakoor MA, Rahman MR: Arthrographic distension of the shoulder joint in the management of frozen shoulder. Mymensingh Med J 2005;14(1):67-70.

54. Arroll B, Goodyear-Smith F: Corticosteroid injections for painful shoulder: a meta-analysis. Br J Gen Pract 2005;55(512):224-228.

55. Yamakado K: The targeting accuracy of subacromial injection to the shoulder: an arthrographic evaluation. Arthroscopy 2002;18(8):887-891.

56. Esenyel CZ, Esenyel M, Yesiltepe R, et al: The correlation between the accuracy of steroid injections and subsequent shoulder pain and function in subacromial impingement syndrome. Acta Orthop Traumatol Turc 2003;37(1):41-45.

57. Naredo E, Cabero F, Beneyto P, et al: A randomized comparative study of short term response to blind injection versus sonographic-guided injection of local corticosteroids in patients with painful shoulder. J Rheumatol 2004;31(2):308-314.

58. Akgun K, Birtane M, Akarirmak U: Is local subacromial corticosteroid injection beneficial in subacromial impingement syndrome? Clin Rheumatol 2004;23(6): 496-500.

59. Hay EM, Paterson SM, Lewis M, et al: Pragmatic randomised controlled trial of local corticosteroid injection and naproxen for treatment of lateral epicondylitis of elbow in primary care. BMJ 1999;319(7215):964-968.

60. Stahl S, Kaufman T: The efficacy of an injection of steroids for medial epicondylitis. A prospective study of sixty elbows. J Bone Joint Surg Am 1997; 79(11):1648-1652.

61. Weinstein PS, Canoso JJ, Wohlgethan JR: Long-term follow-up of corticosteroid injection for traumatic olecranon bursitis. Ann Rheum Dis 1984;43(1):44-46.

62. Sevim S, Dogu O, Camdeviren H, et al: Long-term effectiveness of steroid injections and splinting in mild and moderate carpal tunnel syndrome. Neurol Sci 2004;25(2):48-52.

63. Girlanda P, Dattola R, Venuto C, et al: Local steroid treatment in idiopathic carpal tunnel syndrome: short-term and long-term efficacy. J Neurol 1993;240(3): 187-190.

64. Ly-Pen D, Andreu JL, de Blas G, et al: Surgical decompression versus local steroid injection in carpal tunnel syndrome: a one-year, prospective, randomized, open, controlled clinical trial. Arthritis Rheum 2005;52(2):612-619.

65. Meenagh GK, Patton J, Kynes C, Wright GD: A randomised controlled trial of intra-articular corticosteroid injection of the carpometacarpal joint of the thumb in osteoarthritis. Ann Rheum Dis 2004;63(10):1260-1263.

66. Avci S, Yilmaz C, Sayli U: Comparison of nonsurgical treatment measures for de Quervain's disease of pregnancy and lactation. J Hand Surg [Am] 2002; 27(2):322-324.

67. Richie CA 3rd, Briner WW Jr: Corticosteroid injection for treatment of de Quervain's tenosynovitis: a pooled quantitative literature evaluation. J Am Board Fam Pract 2003;16(2):102-106.

68. Lane LB, Boretz RS, Stuchin SA: Treatment of de Quervain's disease: role of conservative management. J Hand Surg [Br] 2001;26(3):258-260.

69. Anderson BC. Guide to Arthrocentesis and Soft Tissue Injection, 1st ed. Philadelphia, Elsevier, 2005.

70. Limpaphayom N, Wilairatana V: Randomized controlled trial between surgery and aspiration combined with methylprednisolone acetate injection plus wrist immobilization in the treatment of dorsal carpal ganglion. J Med Assoc Thai 2004;87(12): 1513-1517.

71. Otu AA: Wrist and hand ganglion treatment with hyaluronidase injection and fine needle aspiration: a tropical African perspective. J R Coll Surg Edinb 1992; 37(6):405-407.

72. Griggs SM, Weiss AP, Lane LB, et al: Treatment of trigger finger in patients with diabetes mellitus. J Hand Surg [Am] 1995;20(5):787-789.

73. Wray CC, Easom S, Hoskinson J: Coccydynia. Aetiology and treatment. J Bone Joint Surg Br 1991;73(2):335-338.

74. Luukkainen RK, Wennerstrand PV, Kautiainen HH, et al: Efficacy of periarticular corticosteroid treatment of the sacroiliac joint in non-spondylarthropathic patients with chronic low back pain in the region of the sacroiliac joint. Clin Exp Rheumatol 2002;20(1):52-54.

75. Karabacakoglu A, Karakose S, Ozerbil OM, Odev K: Fluoroscopy-guided intraarticular corticosteroid injection into the sacroiliac joints in patients with ankylosing spondylitis. Acta Radiol 2002;43(4):425-427.

76. Shbeeb MI, O'Duffy JD, Michet CJ Jr, et al: Evaluation of glucocorticosteroid injection for the treatment of trochanteric bursitis. J Rheumatol 1996;23(12):2104-2106.

77. Raynauld JP, Buckland-Wright C, Ward R, et al: Safety and efficacy of long-term intraarticular steroid injections in osteoarthritis of the knee: a randomized, double-blind, placebo-controlled trial. Arthritis Rheum 2003;48(2):370-377.

78. Weitoft T, Uddenfeldt P: Importance of synovial fluid aspiration when injecting intra-articular corticosteroids. Ann Rheum Dis 2000;59(3):233-235.

79. Trepman E, Yeo SJ: Nonoperative treatment of metatarsophalangeal joint synovitis. Foot Ankle Int 1995;16(12):771-777.

80. Acevedo JI, Beskin JL: Complications of plantar fascia rupture associated with corticosteroid injection. Foot Ankle Int 1998;19(2):91-97.

81. Saxena A, Fullem B: Plantar fascia ruptures in athletes. Am J Sports Med 2004;32(3):662-665.

82. Balogh Z, Ruzsonyi E: Triamcinolone hexacetonide versus betamethasone. A double-blind comparative study of the long-term effects of intra-articular steroids in patients with juvenile chronic arthritis. Scand J Rheumatol Suppl 1987;67:80-82.

83. Pyne D, Ioannou Y, Mootoo R, Bhanji A: Intra-articular steroids in knee osteoarthritis: a comparative study of triamcinolone hexacetonide and methylprednisolone acetate. Clin Rheumatol 2004;23(2):116-120.

84. Kumar N, Newman RJ: Complications of intra- and peri-articular steroid injections. Br J Gen Pract 1999;49(443):465-466.

Ergogenic Aids

Jeffrey L. Levy, DO; Jorge Cabrera, MD, PhD; Sean Thomas, MD;
and Fred H. Brennan, Jr, DO, FAOASM, FAAFP

KEY POINTS

- Athletes of all levels and ages use ergogenic aids.
- The majority of ergogenic aids have been poorly researched or have not been shown to produce the advertised results. However, a few do have some ergogenic potential in certain individuals.
- The Dietary and Supplement Health Education Act puts the onus on the Food and Drug Administration to prove that supplements are harmful. The manufacturers can produce and advertise the product as long as they do not state that it is for medicinal use.
- Anabolic steroids and ephedrine are two ergogenic aids that have been studied extensively and that have definite adverse effects.
- The use of ergogenic aids is associated with high-risk behavior and should be screened for during the preparticipation examination.

INTRODUCTION

Athletes have long attempted to find the one thing that will give them "the edge" in competition. Whether it is the type of equipment they use, the training aids employed, or the use of performance-enhancing substances, getting that edge over their opponents is the ultimate goal. Ergogenic substances are commonly used by athletes who seek to gain such a competitive edge. Anything that enhances energy production, use, or recovery can be considered ergogenic. Ergogenic aids can be classified into five categories: (1) mechanical aids (e.g., longer spikes on cleats); (2) psychologic aids (e.g., hypnosis); (3) physiologic aids (e.g., blood doping); (4) pharmacologic aids (e.g., androgenic anabolic steroids); and (5) nutritional supplements (e.g., creatine). From a medical standpoint, the use of physiologic, pharmacologic, and nutritional aids can be dangerous. Quality, unbiased research is difficult to find in the lay literature, and athletes are often taking these nutritional supplements at significantly higher doses than recommended.

The role of the medical professional must be to counsel the athlete about the following: (1) the safe use (or nonuse) of these

substances; (2) the lack of regulation of supplement contents; and (3) the potential short-term and long-term side effects. In addition, athletes who use ergogenic aids are more likely to engage in other high-risk behaviors, such as heavy drinking, drunk driving, and unprotected intercourse.[1] As such, inquiring about supplement usage is an integral part of the preparticipation examination, and it will lead the clinician during further counseling.

History

Trying to find a substance to improve performance is not a new concept, nor it is necessarily illegal. For example, the ancient Greeks ate mushrooms to enhance performance; animal hearts were eaten during the medieval times to increase courage; Hitler had testosterone injected into his troops to increase their aggressiveness; and Dr. Charles Edward Brown-Séquard claimed to reverse his own aging process by the self-injection of testicular extracts. The modern day Olympics were a liftoff point for the common use of androgenic anabolic steroids (AASs). Dr. John Ziegler was a US physician for the Olympic team who tried to invent a safer AAS than what the Soviet Union Olympic athletes were using during the 1950s. He developed dianabol, a modified form of testosterone that subsequently was found to have significant adverse side effects.[2] Since then, there has been continued development and production of many potentially dangerous substances. In many of our favorite sports, there are athletes who consume, inject, apply, and inhale all types and forms of supplements.

Regulation

The Dietary Health and Education Act of 1994 permits the marketing and sales of supplements without regulation as long as there is no medicinal purpose advertised. For example, if caffeine is labeled as a drug for the treatment of migraine headaches, the pharmaceutical company is required to do extensive studies of its efficacy and safety before the US Food and Drug Administration (FDA) will allow its use. However, if a supplement manufacturer claims that caffeine is helpful for "burning fat" but does not promote any medicinal purpose, then there is no FDA oversight or regulation required. The onus is on the FDA, which cannot possibly review the thousands of products available, to prove that the supplement is safe or dangerous in the form in which it is being sold. The lack of FDA oversight and regulation

Box 49.1: Documented Testing Programs

- United States Olympic Committee: www.usoc.org
- United States Anti-Doping Agency (official administrator of drug testing for the United States Olympic committee): www.usantidoping.org
- World Anti-Doping Agency (official administrator of drug testing for the International Olympic Committee: www.wada-ama.org/en/prohibitedlist.ch2 (this site contains the current list of prohibited substances)
- NCAA Web site home page: www2.ncaa.org/index.php
- NCAA Web site for drug testing information: www2.ncaa.org/legislation_and_governance/eligibility_and_conduct/drug_testing.html
- National Center For Drug Free Sport (the official administrator of drug testing for the NCAA): www.drugfreesport.com/home.asp

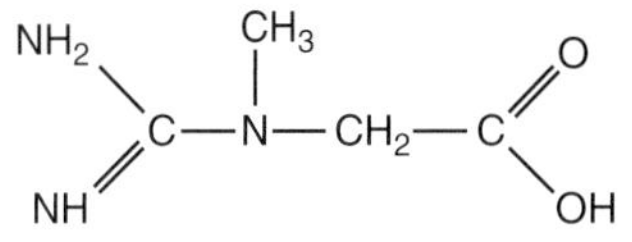

Figure 49.1 Creatine structure. (From Hettiarachchy J: The efficacy and safety of creatine monohydrate [Web site]. Available at altmed.creighton.edu/creatine/background.htm. Accessed July 27, 2007.)

permits potentially harmful supplements (albeit not intentionally) to be sold to susceptible individuals who are seeking a performance advantage.

The athlete's view

Today's athlete is in a precarious position because there is some scientific and medical data that certain ergogenic aids can modestly improve performance and are likely safe to take. The major professional sporting leagues—the National Collegiate Athletic Association (NCAA), the US Olympic Committee, and the International Olympic Committee (IOC)—all have well-documented testing programs, and their lists of banned substances can be found on their Web sites **(Box 49.1).** One major problem with supplements is that what is listed on the package does not always correlate with what is actually contained within. The IOC performed a study of 634 nonhormonal nutritional supplements that were manufactured in different countries around the world, and 94 (15%) of these were found to contain nonlabeled testosterone or nandrolone, which would have resulted in a positive drug test for the athlete.[3] Notably, 45 of these positive results came from manufacturers in the United States. The IOC's position is that athletes should refrain from all supplement use to avoid ingesting any unknown contaminant. However, this is unlikely to be the athlete's position. For example, two different polls[4,5] from the 1980s and the 1990s posed this question of Olympic athletes: "If you could take a pill that would guarantee victory but would subsequently kill you, would you take it?" In both polls, more than 50% of the athletes questioned said that they would take such a pill! In addition, if they could take it without subsequently dying, more than 95% of the athletes said that they would take it. The results of these polls are evidence that athletes are not only willing to cheat but they are willing to take something that is potentially fatal in order to win.

CREATINE

Background

Creatine **(Figure 49.1)** has been one of the most popular nutritional supplements since its commercial availability began during the early 1990s with a reported use among young athletes that ranges up to 78%.[6] Even before this popularization, the Soviet Union and other Eastern Bloc countries during the 1970s began using it as an ergogenic aid.[7] It was not until the 1992 Olympic Games in Barcelona that it came into public view. Several athletes were reported to be using creatine as an ergogenic aid, including 100-meter gold-medal winner Linford Christie and 400-meter hurdles gold-medal winner Salley Gunnell. The following summarizes the biochemical pathway, its purported use, and a review of some of the most recent literature about both the ergogenic effects and side effects of creatine.

Creatine is an amino acid that is produced endogenously in the kidney, liver, and pancreas from methionine, L-arginine, and glycine. Approximately 95% of the substance is located in the skeletal muscle, and the remaining 5% is found in the kidney, the liver, and the brain. The endogenous biosynthesis of creatine in the liver and kidneys produces about 1 to 2 g daily, and an additional 1 to 2 g is absorbed via the small intestine from the consumption of meats and/or fish.[8,9] Creatine serves as an energy sink for the production of phosphocreatine, which reversibly catalyzes the transfer of the high-energy phosphate group in adenosine diphosphate to form adenosine triphosphate. Because of the limited amount of cytosolic adenosine triphosphate molecules in skeletal muscle, this phosphocreatine reserve is essential during periods of rapid and intense skeletal muscle contractions. From a single coupled reaction, the breakdown of phosphocreatine generates adenosine triphosphate quickly and reversibly. Without this pool of phosphocreatine, much less adenosine triphosphate would be generated during this period, cytosolic adenosine triphosphate would be used up within 2 to 3 seconds, and skeletal-muscle fatigue would ensue.[10,11] It follows that a bigger store of phosphocreatine in muscle should reduce fatigue. There are currently two forms of creatine that are marketed widely; creatine ethyl ester and creatine monohydrate-based supplements. The exogenous consumption of either of these forms causes two physiologic effects: (1) the suppression of the endogenous production of creatine; and (2) the significant augmentation of the total creatine "pool" (LOE: C, C, A, and C for 14 through 17, respectively).[8,12-17] The endogenous inhibition of creatine production may continue for weeks after supplementation because total creatine levels can remain elevated for up to 1 month (LOE: C and C, respectively).[18,19] The question of whether an increased amount of total creatine from creatine supplementation translates into improved athletic performance has been debated since its commercial introduction during the 1990s.

Reported uses

Creatine in weight lifting is thought to enable athletes to train at a higher rate of intensity for a longer period of time, which translates into an increase in the number of repetitions and an increase in the amount of weight lifted. In theory, if more repetitions are achieved during a workout, a higher degree of protein synthesis will be stimulated. Bodybuilders regularly take creatine supplements to increase their muscle mass and to have the power and strength for vigorous weight lifting. Competitors such as cyclists and runners rely on creatine during training, and competition use it for its ability to improve athletic endurance. Creatine supplementation is also used by runners for longer-distance events, such as the 1000 meter. However, long-distance runners may be less inclined to supplement with creatine because of its muscle-bulking effect.

Performance studies

Although variable loading and maintenance protocols exist for creatine, there is a consensus that total creatine stores in muscle are augmented by supplementation (LOE: C, C, A, and C for 14 through 17, respectively).[8,12-17] Interestingly, the variable increases in creatine stores, which may range from 0% percent (known as "nonresponders") to 40%, depend on factors such as the level of presupplementation creatine stores, the proportion of muscle fiber types (type II versus type I), muscle size, insulin sensitivity, exercise intensity, and so on (LOE: C).[14] With this in mind, an increase in total creatine should lead to elevated energy stores, increased muscle size, and, ultimately, enhanced performance. Numerous studies address whether creatine is an effective ergogenic aid. It is important to note the diversity of loading regimens, the number of days loaded, and parameters assayed across all of these studies. One reported outcome of creatine supplementation in male athletes between 18 and 35 years of age is an increase in fat-free mass of 1 to 2 kg (LOE: C, C, B, C, A, C, and C for 19 through 25, respectively).[14,19-25] This initial gain in mass occurred within several days of supplementation, and it is thought to be the result of water retention. Cell hydration induces protein synthesis and/or acts to reduce protein degradation. Creatine's osmotic hydration of myocytes and its effects on protein synthesis or degradation continues to be examined in vitro and in vivo.[26-30] Does this increase in fat-free mass translate to improved performance? A review of current literature over the past 5 years shows the variety of studies done on various parameters, and, therefore, for simplification, the information was organized on the basis of the event and the level of evidence. **Table 49.1** organizes the studies that are listed in references 31 through 67.

Although creatine supplementation has yielded inconsistent results when applied to competitive swimming, the strongest studies to support its effectiveness comes from two recent randomized, double-blind, crossover studies in which the creatine supplementation group decreased their finish times in swimming sprints (LOE: A and A, respectively).[34,35] The consensus of evidence from Table 49.1 regarding creatine supplementation for sprints and cycling showed no significant difference in any of the parameters studied, which included maximal voluntary isometric torque and muscle activation, fatigue, running velocity, and/or recovery from dynamic exercise. The most recent studies of aerobic/endurance-type sports demonstrate that creatine supplementation does not increase muscle oxidative capacity and consequently does not alter performance during endurance types of exercise. However, creatine does appear to increase weight lifting ability (LOE: A, A, and A, respectively).[63,65,67] The results indicated that creatine supplementation increased muscle strength in strong association with the estimated creatine uptake and body mass (i.e., the greater the uptake, the greater the performance gains). In addition, most studies did report an increase in fat-free mass in the range of 1 to 2 kg during the loading dose of creatine. There is debate regarding whether this is from fluid shifts or an actual increase in muscle.

It is important to note that most of the studies reviewed from 2000 through 2006 had small sample sizes; variability with regard to the level of fitness, age, and/or gender; and the confounding variable of heterogeneity from responders versus nonresponders to creatine. All of these factors may contribute to differences in the results that have been published to date.

Safety

The safety profile for creatine is based on several small studies and a handful of longitudinal studies that have looked at the side effects. The most common systems evaluated include the cardiac system; the renal system; the gastrointestinal system, including liver abnormalities, nausea, and vomiting; and the musculoskeletal system. Because of its osmotic potential, there was some concern that fluid retention as a result of creatine use could elevate a person's blood pressure. The following two studies have evaluated the short-term effect of creatine on blood pressures, with both showing no significant changes. In a double-blind study, there was no effect of short-term creatine supplementation on systolic, diastolic, or mean blood pressure among young male and female subjects (LOE: A).[68] Similarly, a longer-term study demonstrated no alterations in blood pressure with creatine supplementation (LOE: B).[69] Renal function also does not appear to be affected in athletes with no prior renal abnormalities. This evidence comes from two studies, which showed that short-term as well as

Table 49.1 Data from 2000 through 2006

Swimming		Sprints/Cycling		Endurance/Aerobic		Power/Weight Lifting	
Author	**Level of Evidence**	**Author**	**Level of Evidence**	**Author**	**Level of Evidence**	**Author**	**Level of Evidence**
Theodorou[31]	C	Hoffman[37]	B	Santos[53]	C	Chilibeck[59]	B
Mendes[32]	C	Ahmun[38]	A	Biwer[54]	C	Candow[60]	C
Anomasiri[33]	B	Gill[39]	A	Van Loon[55]	B	Volek[61]	C
Mero[34]	A	Ostojic[40]	B	Cox[56]	A	Kilduff[62]	C
Selsby[35]	A	Kinugasa[41]	A	Syrotuik[57]	B	Ayoama[63]	A
Dawson[36]	B	Eckerson[42]	C	Bennett[58]	C	Kutz[64]	A
		Kocak[43]	B			Chwalbinska-Moneta[65]	C
		Delecluse[44]	A			Warber[66]	C
		Lehmkuhl[45]	B			Kilduff[67]	A
		Ziegenfuss[46]	B				
		Cottrell[47]	B				
		Preen[48]	A				
		Finn[49]	A				
		Skare[50]	C				
		Deutekom[51]	A				
		Schedel[52]	C				

long-term creatine supplementation did not alter the glomerular filtration rate (LOE: C and C, respectively).[70,71] Given the large population of athletes who consume creatine, there are scarce reports of renal damage (LOE: E).[72] Similarly, there is a lack of evidence to suggest that short-term creatine supplementation has a negative effect on thermoregulatory responses during exercise. It is important to point out that creatine supplementation with fluid restriction or rapid weight loss may contribute to decreased plasma volume and altered fluid balance that would make the athlete more prone to heat exhaustion (LOE: A and C, respectively).[73,74] Anecdotal reports of liver dysfunction, muscle cramping, nausea, and vomiting have not been proven in clinical trails.[73,74]

Testing and policies
Currently creatine supplementation is not banned by any sports organization, including the NCAA, the IOC, and the World Anti-Doping Agency. The question remains whether any nutritional practice that enhances performance violates the spirit of competitive sports. It is important to consider that creatine supplementation is a practice similar to carbohydrate loading, which is well accepted. There is also a concern that creatine supplementation could cause a gateway effect, whereby athletes who have learned to take creatine are more prone and willing to use dangerous or banned substances.

STEROIDS
Background
AASs are synthetic derivatives of the male hormone testosterone **(Figure 49.2).** Since first being isolated in 1935, AASs have been chemically altered either by the alkylation of the 17-α position or the carboxylation of the 17-β hydroxyl group to maximize the anabolic effects of the drug, to minimize the androgenic effects, and to elude detection by current methods.[75] As a result of these modifications, the pharmacodynamic and pharmacokinetic properties have altered their half-life and degradation, thereby resulting in an analogue that has a higher serum concentration for longer periods of time than its parent compound testosterone. The use of testosterone and its analogue as an ergogenic aid dates back to the early 1960s, when it was traditionally reserved for elite power athletes such as football players, weight lifters, track and field athletes, and bodybuilders.[76] AASs have made their way to the high school level as evidenced by surveys reporting that 4% to 6% of seniors (including females) admit to using steroids at some point during their lives (LOE: cross-sectional surveys).[77-80] Contrary to the strong propaganda in athletic circles that testosterone was a potent ergogenic aid, several studies in eugonadal males reported questionable effects of testosterone and its derivatives on muscle size and performance (LOE: A and A, respectively).[81,82] This was further reinforced in 1977, when the American College of Sports Medicine position on steroid use stated that there was no conclusive scientific evidence that steroid

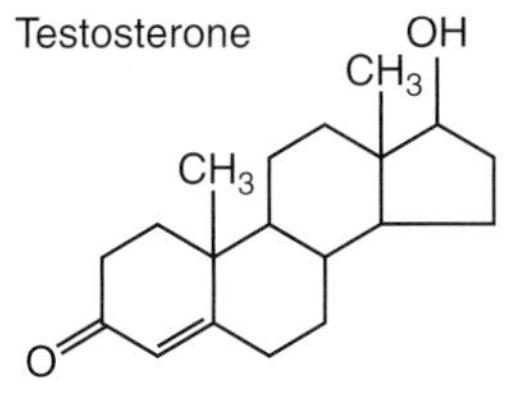

Figure 49.2 Testosterone molecule. (From White Tiger Productions: The cholesterol primer. Available at www.raw-milk-facts.com/cholesterol_primer_T3.html. Accessed July 27, 2007.)

enhanced or hindered athletic performance. As a result of the questionable previous study designs and prevailing new evidence about the administration of supraphysiologic doses of testosterone on eugonadal males, it is now generally accepted that androgenic steroids do increase muscle mass and strength (LOE: B, C, B, B, B, and C, respectively).[83-88]

This discussion about steroids will focus primarily on testosterone and its effects; however, any pertinent information about other derivatives will be presented as needed. Testosterone is synthesized primarily in the testes, with a minor contribution by the adrenal glands. Similar to other compounds within the testosterone pathway (e.g., cortisol and aldosterone), testosterone binds to an intracellular receptor that associates directly with DNA and activates transcription and translation. Although anabolic steroids are receptor specific, there is some cross-reactivity with mineralocorticoid and glucocorticoid receptors. It is this cross-specificity of receptors that may explain the anticatabolic effects of AASs as well as their water-retaining side effects. Once in the cell, testosterone is converted via an enzymatic cascade to androstenediol, to estrogen via aromatase, or to dihydrotestosterone (an even more potent androgen) via 5-α reductase.

Reported uses
Steroids are known to improve performance in sports, which is the main reason why many competitive athletes use them. However, among competitive bodybuilders and even the general population, steroids have been used for aesthetic reasons, such as to increase their muscle size and to reduce body fat. The perception that male football players, weight lifters, and sprinters are the sole consumers of anabolic steroids is misleading and dangerous. Both white-collar and blue-collar workers, females and, most alarmingly, adolescents are using steroids to look, perform, and feel better, regardless of the dangers.[77,78]

Performance studies
Studies have examined the effects of testosterone on hypogonadal, eugonadal, and older males. Studies done on hypogonadal males used replacement/physiologic doses of testosterone and reported a significant increase in fat-free mass and muscle strength (LOE: C, B, B, B, and C, respectively).[84-88] Supraphysiologic doses of androgenic steroids have been investigated by several groups with regard to their effects eugonadal males and older males (LOE: B, A, and B, respectively).[89-91] As with hypogonadal males, the extent of both fat-free mass and strength increase was greater at higher doses of testosterone in eugonadal males when diet and exercise were controlled (LOE: B, A, and B, respectively).[89-91] Replacement-dose therapy in older males also increased lean body mass, increased some measured parameter of muscle strength, or both (LOE: C, C, B, C, and A, respectively).[92-97] The above studies showed a strong correlation between an increase in both muscle size and tension, which suggests that more is involved than just increased fluid retention. Instead, it appears that exogenous testosterone administration produced more contractile components in the muscle fiber. It is inferred that this increase in contractile units will help athletes in sports that require power, such as weight lifting and track and field. It is noteworthy that, in one study, testosterone administration did not improve performance in endurance events (LOE: B).[98] The caveat that must be understood for the studies referenced above is that they do not simulate the doses taken by athletes. The dosage of AASs may range from several hundred milligrams to several grams per day. Athletes commonly "stack" more than one type of steroid and combine steroids with a presumed nonsteroidal ergogenic aid; they then markedly increase their training duration and intensity to maximize the desired anabolic effect.

Safety

The side-effect profile of anabolic steroids is extensive. Some of these side effects will largely depend on the chemical modifications made to the parent structure. As can be seen in several underground steroid handbooks, steroids have differing half-lives and functions, such as "bulking" versus "cutting." In addition, the side effect profile can vary from mildly to severely hepatotoxic.[99] It is worth noting that oral steroids are mostly alkylated on the 17-carbon position, which gives them the second-pass effect through the liver and makes them highly hepatotoxic. Because the liver is the primary site of detoxification of these alkylated steroids, prolonged and heavy use may lead to hepatocellular hyperplasia, transaminitis, increased alkaline phosphatase and lactate dehydrogenase, and hepatocellular/intrahepatic cholestasis, all of which can lead to hepatic failure.[100-103]

The effects of AASs are not exclusive to the liver. The heart is also affected, with reports of acquired hypertrophic cardiomyopathy, increased risk of arrhythmias, sudden death, myocardial infarction, and stroke. (LOE: E and E for 107 and 108, respectively).[104-108] Lipid profiles are also altered, with decreased high-density lipoprotein cholesterol levels and elevated low-density lipoprotein cholesterol levels.[109,110] When these arthrogenic properties are combined with testosterone-induced increases in erythropoiesis and alterations of endothelial and platelet function, the stage is set for thrombus formation and, thus, for myocardial infarction and stroke.[111,112]

More common side effects include acne from the activation of sebaceous glands, gynecomastia as a result of testosterone aromatization, and testicular atrophy from the feedback suppression of the hypothalamus–pituitary–testes axis.[113,114] In addition, there have been reports of disabling tendon ruptures of the triceps, biceps, and bilateral quadriceps in users of AASs (LOE: E and E, respectively).[115,116] This may be the result of a paradoxic effect of high-dose AASs producing dysplastic collagen fibrils that may weaken tendons (LOE: E and E, respectively).[115,116]

The psychiatric effects of steroids are controversial. Anecdotal reports of "roid rage" have brought awareness to the association between anabolic steroid use and bouts of anger. Previous studies used low androgen doses, lacked placebo control or blinding, and included competitive athletes, including some with preexisting psychopathology. In a randomized, double-blind study of 43 individuals who were exposed to high doses of testosterone, there was no statistical difference between the placebo and treatment groups (LOE: A).[117]

In females, the administration of high-dose testosterone results in a number of reversible changes, including menstrual irregularities and breast atrophy, as well as permanent virilizing effects, such as male-pattern baldness, deepening of the voice, hirsutism, and clitoromegaly.[113]

Testing and policies

The established protocol for steroid testing involves the purification of the substance from the urine or serum and then subjecting it to gas or liquid chromatography and mass spectrometry. The NCAA currently uses a ratio of testosterone to epitestosterone of 6:1; however, this ratio varies with certain organizations, such as the National Football League, for which a 4:1 ratio is a presumptive positive test and 10:1 ratio is a conclusively positive test (National Football League Policy on Anabolic Steroids and Related Substances, 2005).[195] Numerous techniques have been used to attempt to prevent the detection of a prohibited drug or to compromise the integrity of the drug test. Some cited methods include providing false urine samples (urine substitution), contaminating the urine sample with chemicals, using diuretics to dilute urine samples, taking masking agents (e.g., probenecid), and using epitestosterone either systemically or in the urine to artificially alter the testosterone-to-epitestosterone ratio.

As a result of concerns about the growing illicit market, an increase in the prevalence of abuse, and the growing evidence of the harmful long-term effects of steroid use, Congress placed anabolic steroids into Schedule III of the Controlled Substances Act in 1991.

The IOC, the NCAA, and many professional sports leagues, including Major League Baseball, the National Basketball Association, the National Football League, and the National Hockey League, have banned the use of steroids by athletes because of the potentially dangerous side effects and because they give the user an unfair advantage. The consequences for each sport vary. For example, major league baseball will suspend a player who tests positive for steroids for 10 days for a first offense, 30 days for a second offense, 60 days for a third offense, and a full year for a fourth offense. In the National Football League, players are suspended for four games for a first offense, six games for a second offense, and a minimum of one year for a third offense.

ADRENAL ANDROGENS

Background

Dehydroepiandrosterone (DHEA) and androstenedione are adrenal androgens secreted by the adrenal cortex and precursors to the production of testosterone in the testes. DHEA was introduced as an over-the-counter supplement during the 1980s, and it was marketed as an antiaging prohormone with various beneficial effects. It was removed in 1985 by the FDA because of a lack of clinical efficacy or safety, but it returned into the commercial market with the passage of the federal Dietary Supplement Health and Education act in 1994. Serum levels of DHEA in a 70-year-old person are only 20% of those seen in a young adult. The theory was that the supplementation of this prohormone may slow aging, prevent heart disease, and decrease obesity.[118] Recently, DHEA has fallen out of favor as an ergogenic aid, and it instead has been advertised as a "fountain of youth." This is demonstrated in the lay literature, in which there is little mention of DHEA as an ergogenic substance.[99]

Androstenedione, which is a downstream derivative of DHEA, has received much more recognition and popularity as an ergogenic aid. This was probably helped by the admission of professional baseball player Mark McGwire's testimony of his use of androstenedione during his record-breaking season. Much like testosterone, androstenedione was used by Eastern Bloc countries during the 1970s as an anabolic precursor hormone because of its presumed ability to elevate serum testosterone levels.

The basis for using DHEA and androstenedione as an ergogenic aid was derived from a study in which nonathletic women were given either 100 mg of DHEA or 100 mg of androstenedione.[119] The results indicated that both prohormones elevated testosterone levels. Women who took DHEA had testosterone levels that rose from under 199 ng/dL to 280 ng/dL within 60 minutes. Testosterone levels in the androstenedione group rose to as high as 660 ng/dL during the same time period, which was approximately three times the normal level. The androstenedione-induced testosterone increase lasted several hours and remained at peak levels for just a few minutes. The results of this 44-year-old study, along with the recent headlines of top name athletes using these substances, remains the major marketing impetus for these supplements.

Reported uses

DHEA is used by athletes in an attempt to elevate serum testosterone and ultimately to increase muscle mass and strength. Despite the lack of sufficient scientific evidence, DHEA has also been advertised as a cure-all. Purported benefits include weight loss and the primary prevention of cancer, atherosclerosis, Alzheimer disease, Parkinson disease, and diabetes. Advocates of DHEA recommend it to slow the effects of aging. Androstenedione promoters claim that it enhances athletic performance and strength by increasing testosterone production and subsequent muscle mass.

Performance studies

A consistent finding of several studies of DHEA and androstenedione is that both short-term and long-term supplementation do not alter body composition or improve athletic performance. DHEA has been shown to increase androstenedione levels but not testosterone levels, and it does not positively alter the adaptations associated with resistance training in young men (LOE: C, A, and A, respectively).[120-122] Interestingly, androstenedione appears to have a dimorphic affect, with increases in serum testosterone concentration in women; however, in eugonadal men, there are not significant increases (LOE: B and A, respectively).[123,124] It is also noteworthy that the transient elevations in testosterone that did occur were accompanied by greater increases in circulating estrogen(s) (LOE: C and B for 125 and 127, respectively).[125-127] Studies with 8 to 12 weeks of supplementation with androstenedione or androstenediol showed no effect on body composition or physical performance (LOE: B and A, respectively).[128,129] As compared with a control group, androstenedione did not improve muscle protein synthesis among young eugonadal men as measured by muscle biopsy and phenylalanine enrichment (LOE: C).[130] In the light of this research and several years of marketing as a prohormone, it appears that both the scientific and athletic communities are in general agreement that DHEA and androstenedione are weak ergogenic aids at best.[99]

Safety

The interpretation of data regarding the safety of both prohormones becomes more difficult when it is unclear what dosages are being consumed by recreational and professional athletes. In addition, there are only a few studies that have pursued long-term side effects, perhaps because of these substances' lack of efficacy as ergogenic aids. From the studies that have been published, the consensus among the literature is that there are significant increases in blood estrone and estradiol levels with oral androstenedione supplementation (LOE: B and C, respectively).[127,130] This increase in serum estrogens is presumed to cause feminizing effects in males that may be irreversible. By contrast, in women, androstenedione supplementation has been shown to instead produce an elevation of testosterone levels, thereby elevating the risk of virilization (LOE: A, A, and C, respectively).[122,124,125] Other studies have focused on the effects of blood lipid levels. Similar to testosterone supplementation, DHEA and androstenedione caused significant reductions in high-density lipoprotein levels, which is an independent risk factor for cardiac disease (LOE: A, A, and C, respectively).[124,129,130]

The potential health concerns from using prohormones such as DHEA and androstenedione have not been thoroughly evaluated by the scientific community. As such, the long-term effects are generally unknown. Ultimately, it appears that the risks outweigh the advertised benefits, especially for elite athletes because these prohormones can cause a positive test for AASs on random drug testing.

Testing and policies

Both DHEA and androstenedione are banned by the IOC. Furthermore, androstenedione is banned by the NCAA and the National Football League. One reason why athletes chose

androstenedione as a performance-enhancing agent was because traces of the substance diminished within hours or days, thereby making detection nearly impossible. Androstenedione may disrupt the balance between testosterone and epitestosterone from a ratio of 2:1 or 3:1 to about 14:1. Per IOC regulations, testosterone levels above a 6:1 ratio are considered positive and result in penalties and suspension for the athletes.

HUMAN GROWTH HORMONE AND INSULIN-LIKE GROWTH FACTOR 1

Background

Human growth hormone (HGH) is a polypeptide that consists of 191 amino acids. Researchers and doctors have been studying the effects of HGH in children for years. HGH was originally used to treat children who were abnormally small and not developing as they should because of HGH deficiency, Turner's syndrome, or other metabolic issues such as chronic renal failure (LOE: A and B for 131 and 134, respectively).[131-135] Similar to DHEA, there is a decline in the production of endogenous HGH as one ages, and it is estimated that the total amount of HGH secreted by a 60-year-old man is half that of a 20-year-old man. The assumption was that replacement with exogenous HGH to serum levels comparable to that of a much younger person would rejuvenate elderly subjects.

HGH is secreted in a pulsatile manner from the anterior pituitary with its maximal secretion during a 24-hour cycle at nighttime and, during the lifetime, at puberty. In addition to these diurnal variations in serum levels, arginine as well as exercise have been shown to stimulate HGH secretion.[135,136] Scientific research and genetic engineering have provided recombinant HGH (rHGH), which is available in a variety of forms such as a spray, pill, or injection, as opposed to cadaveric HGH, which is still available for purchase in Eastern European countries on the black market. Injections are extremely expensive, averaging $3000 and upward per month, depending on the dosage administered, with some athletes taking up to 20 times the prescribed dosage.[137] As with any pharmaceutical agent that has anabolic potential, the scope of use for HGH is no longer limited for idiopathic short stature in children. The use of HGH as an ergogenic aid has been on the rise over the last decade, with approximately 5% of American high school students using it as an anabolic agent.[138,139] Olympic-caliber athletes have been found with ampules of rHGH. In addition to its reported anabolic effects by athletes, it is also an optimal performance-enhancing agent to use because of its difficulty to assess in serum or urine.

Unlike other ergogenics, HGH and insulin-like growth factor 1 (IGF-1) are peptides, and, therefore, they are subject to processes such as degradation and precipitation if not diluted properly. Both rHGH and recombinant IGF-1 are discussed in this section because, similar to DHEA and androstenedione, they are mediators of the same pathways. IGF-1 is a downstream hormone that is produced in the liver and activated by HGH. In contrast with the lipophilic steroid molecules, HGH and IGF-1 circulate in serum and activate membrane-bound receptors to trigger a signaling cascade. This leads to some of the known actions of HGH in the body, including increasing amino acid uptake in skeletal muscle and activating lipolysis, gluconeogenesis, and glucogenolysis.[140]

Reported uses

HGH and IGF-1 have been marketed for multiple uses, including fat loss, antiaging effects, muscle growth, and improved sexual potency. In athletics, rHGH and IGF-1 are injected intramuscularly and thought to cause localized muscle growth. These polypeptides have short half-lives of approximately 10 minutes because of the endogenous proteases in blood.[99] Professional bodybuilders often stack HGH and IGF-1 with insulin to minimize the insulin resistance caused by these agents.

Performance studies

The interest in HGH as an anabolic agent was propagated by two studies that reported increased muscle mass and a decreased fat-to-muscle ratio in elderly men after the administration of replacement-dose HGH (LOE: C and B, respectively).[141,142] After a 10-week administration of HGH (0.02 mg/kg/day), strength did not increase in any of the muscle groups as compared with controls, despite an increase in lean mass and a decrease in fat mass among patients who were more than 60 years of age (LOE: A).[143] In addition, there were no morphologic changes in muscle fibers in the HGH-treated subjects (LOE: A and A, respectively).[143,144] A similar lack of effect was also seen after 16 weeks of treatment (LOE: B).[145] Several studies have investigated whether an anabolic effect of HGH can be demonstrated in athletes. Among young men, resistance exercise with or without HGH resulted in similar increments in muscle size, strength, and muscle protein synthesis (LOE: C).[146] This study was corroborated by two other studies in which short-term HGH treatment did not increase the rate of muscle protein synthesis, reduce the rate of whole-body protein breakdown, or have any effect on maximal concentric contraction (LOE: A for 148).[147,148] The increase in fat-free mass with HGH treatment was probably the result of an increase in lean tissue other than skeletal muscle, fluid retention, the accumulation of connective tissue, or any combination of the three.

Aside from its reported anabolic effects, HGH has alleged properties of being an excellent lipolytic agent. Although body fat is not an issue for most athletes, bodybuilders in particular strive to achieve a "ripped" look for competition by taking several performance-enhancing agents including HGH. A study with rHGH in endurance-trained athletes increased lipolysis and fatty acid availability at rest, during, and after exercise (LOE: A and C, respectively).[149,150] Despite the lack of compelling data as an ergogenic aid, HGH has a reputation among athletes for enhancing performance and decreasing fat. As a result, the IOC has made a concerted effort to detect illegal doping with HGH, thus legitimizing some of the unsubstantiated claims of its ergogenic potential by athletes.

IGF-1 is a downstream mediator of HGH. There are no studies in the literature regarding its use among athletes or its effects on muscle growth parameters, strength, or body composition. Underground literature reports that, when HGH and IGF-1 are stacked together with insulin or AASs, the result is a potent combination.[99] However, similar to HGH, the use of this peptide is cost prohibitive, partially as a result of the limited supplies available and a prevalence of counterfeit IGF-1.

Safety

The side effects of the chronic use of exogenous supraphysiologic doses of rHGH on individuals with normal serum HGH levels have not been studied. A model in which the deleterious effects of excessive HGH secretion can be studied exists: patients with acromegaly. In these individuals, HGH secretion is often 100 times that of normal, resulting in cardiac abnormalities such as concentric wall hypertrophy and diastolic dysfunction. In addition, the supraphysiologic doses of HGH induce lipolysis and cause elevations of serum free fatty acids that are high enough to induce arrhythmias.[156,157] Other disorders that occur more frequently with acromegaly include hypertension, diabetes, abnormal lipid metabolism, respiratory disease, osteoarthritis, breast cancer, and colorectal cancer. These factors result in the greater morbidity and mortality rates found in this population (LOE: D for 152).[151-155]

The more common side effects noted with replacement-dose rHGH are fluid retention and mild increases in blood pressure (LOE: A).[158] The effects of replacement-dose rHGH on low-density lipoprotein cholesterol and total cholesterol are variable, although no alterations in high-density lipoprotein cholesterol or triglyceride levels have been shown.[159] Musculoskeletal problems such as myopathies, carpal tunnel syndrome, and acromegaly have been reported with the use of exogenous HGH (LOE: A for 148).[147,148] In addition, a retrospective cohort study of patients treated with human pituitary growth hormone showed significantly higher risks of mortality from colorectal cancer, Hodgkin's disease, and cancer in general.[160]

The black market has become a source of cheap HGH via the selling of cadaveric extracted HGH, most notably in Europe. With the extraction of cadaveric HGH, prion diseases (e.g., the invariably fatal Creutzfeld–Jakob disease) have become more prevalent. Its production has thus been banned in most countries (LOE: A).[148]

In summary, the evidence for an HGH-induced increase in human skeletal muscle protein and maximum voluntary muscle force is minimal. It appears that HGH treatment as an ergogenic aid would be a detriment rather than an aid to athletic performance as a result of water retention, carpal tunnel compression, insulin resistance, myopathies, and cardiomyopathies. In addition, whether prolonged HGH treatment alone or in combination with other agents used by athletes (e.g., anabolic steroids, β-agonists) is associated with other adverse effects has yet to be evaluated. The use of HGH as an antiaging agent for elderly individuals is also suspect because it is limited by the induction of insulin resistance and carpal tunnel compression.

Although IGF-1, as a downstream mediator of HGH, is presumed to be more potent as an ergogenic aid than HGH, the major impediment to its widespread use is its cost and availability. As advances in recombinant DNA technology progress, recombinant proteins such as HGH and IGF-1 will become the next line of ergogenics to replace AASs in the current doping arsenal.

Testing and policies

The use of rHGH is considered doping, and it is banned by the IOC, the National Football League, the National Hockey League, and Major League Baseball. The likelihood of detecting rHGH is very limited as a result of its short half life of several minutes, and it is therefore believed to be undetectable by most laboratories. At the present time, the amino acid sequences of pituitary-derived HGH and rHGH are so similar that it is difficult to discriminate between endogenous and exogenous HGH. Thus, no official test is implemented in the doping control procedures, and the only situation when athletes were found guilty of doping with rHGH arose from the actions of customs officers or policemen who arrested athletes who were carrying ampules with them.

STIMULANTS

Ephedra
Background
Ephedra is a sympathomimetic amine that has been used for thousands of years for upper respiratory ailments, asthma, and weight loss. It is structurally similar to amphetamines, and it has commonly been used alone or in combination with caffeine to improve athletic performance. Its mechanisms of action include the direct stimulation of the β-adrenergic receptors and the indirect stimulation of receptors for dopamine and norepinephrine release. This results in an increase in blood pressure, heart rate, and subsequent cardiac output to the muscles, heart, and brain, which theoretically could be an ergogenic effect. In addition, as a result of the catecholamine release, there may be a delayed perception of fatigue.

Reported uses

Ephedrine, which is the major alkaloid of the ephedra plant, has long been used in Chinese medicine and subsequently here in the United States for respiratory symptoms. It has also been used as a weight-loss supplement and an aid to delay fatigue, to increase energy, and to increase fat-free mass by athletes of all levels.[161] It was the major ingredient in a vast array of supplements that accounted for more than $1.3 billion in sales in 2001.[162]

Performance studies

A landmark meta-analysis of the data concerning ephedra and ephedrine has been performed and was published both as a government document and in the *Journal of the American Medical Association*. This study played a major role in the banning of ephedra and it derivatives from over-the-counter products.

The RAND Corporation was commissioned by the federal government to investigate ephedra and ephedrine. Their meta-analysis, called the RAND report (LOE: meta-analysis),[163,164] reviewed 52 controlled trials of the use of these substances, specifically evaluating their efficacy and safety when used for weight loss and for enhanced athletic performance. Many of the studies found were not included in the analysis as a result of poor methodology and high attrition rates. Nevertheless, a very modest increase in weight loss of 2 pounds (as compared with placebo) was found as well as a small improvement in the short-term athletic performance when taking an ephedrine/caffeine combination after a one-time dose.[163] No studies for weight-loss were conducted for more than 6 months, so no conclusions regarding long-term use could be made.[163] In addition, the *Journal of the American Medical Association* report found that taking ephedrine and caffeine together resulted in increased muscle endurance, but only during the first three repetitions of a leg-extension exercise.[164]

The vast majority of literature shows no significant effect of ephedra or ephedrine on athletic performance or on any other parameters, such as strength, oxygen uptake, or time to exhaustion (LOE: review).[165] The conclusions of both analyses were that there was a small increase in weight loss and no significant data available to determine efficacy to improve athletic performance.

Safety

In the *Journal of the American Medical Association* review data of 50 trials, there was a 2.2-fold to 3.6-fold increase in the odds of developing adverse psychiatric, autonomic, cardiovascular, or gastrointestinal symptoms with ephedra or ephedrine.[164] Between 1997 and 1999, the FDA received 140 adverse-event reports associated with the use of ephedra and its derivatives.[166] A review was done at that time to determine the true relationship of the events and ephedra. The results showed that 31% of cases were definitely or probably related to the use of supplements containing ephedra-type alkaloids, and another 31% were possibly related (LOE: D).[167] Cardiovascular effects (i.e., hypertension, tachycardia) were the most common at 47%, and central nervous system effects (i.e., stroke, seizure) occurred in 18%. Possibly most concerning was the finding that 26% of the definite, probable, or possible groups had permanent injury or death.[167]

In addition, impaired thermoregulation as a result of vasoconstriction and subsequent heat injuries is possible. The deaths of Steve Bechler of the Baltimore Orioles, Kory Stringer of the Minnesota Vikings, and Rashidi Wheeler of Northwestern University's football team were all associated with ephedra and exercising in extreme heat.[168]

Testing and policies

Ephedra and its associated compounds have been banned by the majority of amateur and professional sporting leagues. As of April 2004, it has been illegal to manufacture or sell ephedra and its derivatives over the counter in the United States; however, these substances are still widely available via the Internet. Although these substances were banned by the NCAA during the mid 1990s, testing in collegiate athletes began a few years ago after results of a 2001 NCAA study revealed that 3.9% of their athletes reported the use of ephedra over the previous 12 months.[162]

Caffeine
Background

Caffeine is a methylxanthine alkaloid that has well-documented ergogenic effects; it is subsequently the ergogenic aid that is most widely used by athletes. It is postulated that it works by three different mechanisms: (1) it increases free fatty acid production, which spares muscle glycogen and increases available energy; (2) it enhances muscle function and endurance by increasing calcium release from the sarcoplasmic reticulum; and (3) it antagonizes adenosine receptors with subsequent lipolysis and increased catecholamine release for increased energy sources and decreases in perceived fatigue.[169] Caffeine and other less-well-known stimulants have essentially replaced ephedra in many ergogenic supplements.

Reported uses

Athletes use caffeine to increase time to exhaustion in prolonged submaximal exercise. In addition, because it has replaced ephedrine, it has the same advertised uses of increased fat-free mass and increased weight loss. At lower doses, it may enhance hand control and concentration.

Performance studies

Because caffeine has been used for such a long period of time and is legal, it is one of the best-studied supplements. The vast majority of studies support its ergogenic effects on prolonged exercise and endurance (LOE: review).[170] The studies have a great deal of heterogeneity in that they test athletes of diverse levels, in varying endurance sports, with different doses of caffeine. It seems as if the ergogenic effect is best at lower doses, as seen in a study by Graham and Spriet in which endurance was enhanced at 85% of maximal oxygen consumption for trained runners at 3 to 6 mg/kg of caffeine but not at higher levels (LOE: C).[171] Additional studies have noted ergogenic effects at higher doses, but the maximal effect was noted at the 3 to 6 mg/kg level.[170]

For short bursts of exercise, the data is a bit more inconsistent but still supportive. Bruce and colleagues found that 6 to 9 mg/kg of caffeine improved the times of competitive rowers during a 2000-meter time trial (LOE: C).[172] A similar study of a female crew team found the same improved times at levels of 6 to 9 mg/kg (LOE: C).[173] A confounding variable in these studies may be the level of athlete. For example, Collomp and colleagues documented that sprint swimming times improved after caffeine ingestion only in well-trained swimmers and not in recreational athletes (LOE: C).[174] In addition, athletes who are caffeine naïve may have enhanced responses as compared with chronic caffeine users.

Safety

Caffeine appears to be safe, particularly at the levels that are noted to be ergogenic (i.e., low levels of approximately 3 to 6 mg/kg) (LOE: review).[170] However, at higher doses, gastrointestinal disturbance, cardiac palpitations, dizziness, headache, fatigue, tremor, jitteriness, anxiety, and loss of concentration are just a few of the common side effects (LOE: review).[169]

For athletes, the diuretic property of caffeine is a marked concern because decreased volume status puts the athlete at risk of clinical dehydration, possible electrolyte imbalance, and abnormal temperature regulation. However, studies show that exercise seems to mitigate the diuretic effect (LOE: review).[170]

No significant dehydration, perspiration, or temperature abnormalities have been seen during exercise nor is there a change in expected urine output or electrolyte balance. There is no evidence of any volume status abnormality associated with caffeine and exercise.

Testing and policies
Because caffeine use is ubiquitous in the world, the IOC removed it from their banned drug list in 2004. However, the NCAA still restricts its use and has a level of 15 µg/mL in urine as the cutoff for positive tests.[169] Testing for a commonly used and socially accepted drug is difficult at best. Beyond the prevalence of use, the testing of urine samples may not be indicative of true serum levels because each individual has different filtration and absorption rates. In addition, the level for a positive test is set so high that it is unlikely to prevent its usage. If someone were to test positive, the adverse side effects would likely negate the positive ergogenic effects. As an example, to obtain the levels needed for a positive test, approximately 8 cups of coffee, each containing 100 mg of caffeine, would have to be ingested within 1 hour of testing. At this level, the possibility of palpitation, gastrointestinal upset, and headache increase significantly. In most people, 300 to 500 mg of caffeine is required to achieve ergogenic serum levels; this is far below the established banned limit.

β-HYDROXY-β-METHYLBUTYRATE

β-Hydroxy-β-methylbutyrate (HMB) is a derivative of the branched-chain amino acid leucine, and it is found naturally in catfish, citrus fruits, and breast milk. It is considered to be anabolic as well as anticatabolic. Past research has been met with significant scrutiny because many of the positive studies were performed by the patent holder and have not been reproduced.[175] Quality studies are still scant regarding its efficacy.

Nonetheless, HMB is thought to be anabolic because it is converted to 3-hydroxy-3-methyl-glutaryl-CoA, with subsequent use in the cellular production of cholesterol (LOE: review).[176] As the muscle hypertrophies with training, there is a lack of cholesterol for the cell membrane and, therefore, a lack of muscle growth. After supplementation with HMB, more cholesterol is produced, and muscle hypertrophy can ensue. HMB is theorized to be anticatabolic and to quicken recovery after a workout by preventing muscle proteolysis during exercise.[176] Studies of cellular markers (e.g., lactate dehydrogenase, creatine phosphokinase) for muscle damage have supported this decrease in muscle breakdown theory (LOE: A).[177]

Reported uses
HMB is used by athletes to decrease their recovery time and to increase their muscle mass. In addition, HMB has been used by older exercisers to prevent age-associated muscle mass loss.

Performance studies
A meta-analysis reviewed nine randomized, placebo-controlled studies. HMB was given orally (3 g/d) for at least 3 weeks (LOE: meta-analysis).[178] The major limitations of this meta-analysis were that the patent holder performed the study and that the studies included were of lower quality. Nonetheless, significant increases in lean body mass and muscle strength were noted.

In another randomized, placebo-controlled study, 75 men and women were evaluated after 4 weeks of 3 g/d of HMB and resistance training three times a week. The treated group had a significant increase in strength and fat-free mass, regardless of sex or previous training status (LOE: B).[179]

Other studies have not found the same results. A well-done, randomized, double-blind, placebo-controlled study by Slater and colleagues of 27 well-trained men found no significant change in body composition or strength after 6 weeks of HMB as compared with the placebo group (LOE: A).[180] Both groups increased these parameters, but this was attributed to the strict athletic diet and proper training.

At best, the data has been mixed and requires more study. HMB could theoretically be ergogenic, but it is relatively new, and it is a good example of a supplement that has been poorly studied. Nonetheless, when reviewing the available literature, two points are important to note: (1) the concomitant use of creatine and HMB has been reported to increase lean body mass and strength, but the literature is sparse, and this combination requires further study; and (2) the gains noted by supplementation have typically been seen among untrained individuals who are undergoing resistance training.[176]

Safety
Although there is not a great deal of literature available at this time, no adverse effects have been found. A review of lipid studies, hepatic enzymes, renal function, and hematologic indices has not been shown to have them adversely affected after 6 to 8 weeks of HMB.[176]

Testing and policies
There is presently no testing for HMB by any organization and thus no related policies.

ERYTHROPOEITIN AND OTHER RELATED SUBSTANCES

Background
Erythropoietin (EPO) is a hormone that is produced naturally in the body to stimulate red blood cell production in the bone marrow. Multiple recombinant forms of human EPO (rHuEPO) have been developed as antianemic agents for chronic renal failure. They have also been used to treat anemia in other disease states, such as acquired immunodeficiency syndrome, cancer, chemotherapy, and prematurity. Different forms include rHuEPO-α, rHuEPO-β, and rHuEPO-ω. Darbepoetin-α, which is also known as *novel erythropoiesis protein*, is a synthetic compound that was developed through research into the structural features of EPO.[181] The uses of these agents by Olympians and competitive cyclists have prompted attention being paid to their use as an ergogenic aid. Gene-activated EPO has recently been approved for the same indications, and other agents that are under investigation include oral forms of EPO, gene therapy, EPO mimetics, inhibitors of hematopoietic cell phosphatase, allosteric effectors of hemoglobin, hemoglobin oxygen carriers, and perfluorochemicals.[181]

Reported uses
Through increases in hemoglobin and hematocrit, there is an increase in oxygen-carrying capacity and a subsequent improvement in the performance of endurance sports.

Performance studies
Several studies have shown an increase in the maximal oxygen consumption of anemic hemodialysis patients as well as that of healthy subjects (LOE: review).[182] In healthy subjects, it also

improved run time to exhaustion.[182] Earlier studies of blood doping have shown that there is a direct correlation between hemoglobin concentration and maximal oxygen consumption.[181] Increased maximal oxygen consumption is directly correlated with improved aerobic performance.

Safety

There have been several documented adverse effects related to the use of rHuEPO, including the following: red cell aplasia as a result of the formation of antierythropoietin antibodies (LOE: D),[183] thrombotic vascular events, and hypertension (LOE: review).[184] Animal studies have shown the development of anemia after the cessation of intensive treatment with EPO.[185] The deaths of 18 Dutch and Belgian cyclists from 1987 to 1990 may have resulted from the use of EPO (LOE: D).[186]

Testing and policies

All EPOs, darbepoetin-α, and perfluorochemicals are banned by the IOC and the NCAA. Several methods of detection are available for rHuEPO and darbepoetin-α. Perfluorochemicals are only tested for in special circumstances.

DIURETICS

Background

Diuretics are an integral part of treating hypertension in both sedentary and athletic individuals. Their primary mode of action affects the movement of fluids and electrolytes within the kidney. Each diuretic works in a specified location within the nephron. The result is a loss of total body fluid and acute weight loss. Acetazolamide is also well known for its use in preventing and treating altitude sickness. It works on various aspects of the respiratory cycle, with its primary effects being on ventilation and maximal oxygen consumption.

Reported uses

Most diuretic use is in conjunction with sports that require strict weight control. Through the diuresis of free water, there is an acute reduction in weight. There is also a theoretic advantage in sports such as sprinting, in which a lower body weight could improve performance. Acetazolamide's effects on the respiratory system could improve athletic performance at higher altitudes. Finally, some athletes take diuretics to dilute the concentrations of other banned substances within their urine; this technique is called *masking*. There are several other substances that affect the urinary tract that can be used for masking, but their use is beyond the scope of this chapter.

Performance studies

Diuretic-induced dehydration is of significant concern. Studies have shown a detrimental effect of diuretic-induced dehydration on the performance of distance runners (>1500 meters) (LOE: C).[187] Performance degradation can occur at even modest levels of dehydration (<2% of body weight) (LOE: review).[188] A study evaluating the effects of acute weight loss through diuretic-induced dehydration did not demonstrate a detrimental or beneficial effect on the performance of a small sample of sprinters (LOE: C).[189]

Safety

Diuretic use is considered a significant risk factor for the development of heat injuries. Heat injury remains the third leading cause of death among high school athletes, but it is felt that heat-related pathology and morbidity are underreported among athletes.[190] Kidney failure has been reported among athletes who are using diuretics for the treatment of hypertension. Hypokalemia is another problem that can result from the use of diuretics. The use of diuretics for weight loss and weight control among athletes has been documented on several occasions, and it has included competitors at Olympic, collegiate, and high school levels. However, surveys of high school and collegiate wrestlers that were completed in 1999 were compared with historic controls from the 1980s, and it was found that there is an overall lower incidence of dangerous weight-management techniques (LOE: cross-sectional surveys).[191,192] Studies have shown acetazolamide to be safe and effective for the prevention of acute mountain sickness in both Himalayan trekkers and travelers at moderate altitudes who are not undergoing vigorous exercise (LOE: A and A, respectively).[193,194]

Testing and policies

The IOC and the NCAA have banned diuretics and other masking agents. They are easily detected in urine samples with the use of multiple techniques.

CONCLUSION

Medical personnel providing support to today's athlete are challenged by the large number of different substances reported to enhance performance, the changing marketing tactics, the lengths patients will go to be successful, and the rapidly decreasing age of athletes. With screening and education, athletes can be protected from possibly harming themselves or being barred from competition. Working toward this goal should be initiated during the pre-participation examination and then regularly discussed during office or training room visits. Providing performance study data and safety information may significantly decrease the likelihood of adverse outcomes.

REFERENCES

1. Stephens MB, Olsen C: Ergogenic supplements and health risk behaviors. J Fam Pract 2001;50:696-699.
2. McDevitt ER: Sports pharmacology. In DeLee JC, Drez D Jr, Miller MD (eds): DeLee and Drez's Orthopaedic Sports Medicine: Principles and Practice, 2nd ed. Philadelphia, WB Saunders, 2003, pp 471-492.
3. Geyer H, Parr MK, Mareck U, et al: Analysis of non-hormonal nutritional supplements for anabolic-androgenic steroids--results of an international study. Int J Sports Med 2004;25(2):124-129.
4. Mirkin G: Eating for competing. Semin Adolesc Med 1987;3:177-183.
5. Bamberger M, Yaeger D: Over the edge. Sports Illustrated. 1997;April 14:61-70.
6. Pearce PZ: Sports supplements: a modern case of caveat emptor. Curr Sports Med Rep 2005;4(3):171-178.
7. Kalinski MI: State-sponsored research on creatine supplements and blood doping in elite Soviet sport. Perspect Biol Med 2003;46(3):445-451.
8. Walker JB: Creatine: biosynthesis, regulation and function. Adv Enzymol Relat Areas Mol Biol 1979;50:177-242.
9. Wyss M, Kaddurah-Daouk R: Creatine and creatinine metabolism. Physiol Rev 2000;80(3):1107-1213.
10. Connett RJ: Analysis of metabolic control: new insights using scaled creatine kinase model. Am J Physiol 1988;254(6 Pt 2):R949-R959.
11. Meyer RA, Sweeney HL, Kushmerick MJ: A simple analysis of the "phosphocreatine shuttle. Am J Physiol 1984;246(5 Pt 1):C365-C377.
12. Hoberman HD, Sims EAH, Peter JH: Creatine and creatine metabolism in the normal male adult studied with the aid of isotopic nitrogen. J Biol Chem 1948;172:45-58.
13. Harris RC, Soderlund MK, Hultman E: The effect of oral creatine supplementation on running performance and during maximal short term exercise in man. J Physiol 1993;467:74.

14. Greenhaff PL, Bodin K, Soderlund K, Hultman E: Effect of oral creatine supplementation on skeletal muscle phosphocreatine resynthesis. Am J Physiol 1994;266(5 Pt 1):E725-E730.

15. Balsom PD, Soderlund K, Sjodin B, Ekblom B: Skeletal muscle metabolism during short duration high-intensity exercise: influence of creatine supplementation. Acta Physiol Scand 1995;154(3):303-310.

16. Gordon A, Hultman E, Kaijser L, et al: Creatine supplementation in chronic heart failure increases skeletal muscle creatine phosphate and muscle performance. Cardiovasc Res 1995;30:413-418.

17. Hultman E, Soderlund K, Timmons JA, et al: Muscle creatine loading in men. J Appl Physiol 1996;81(1):232-237.

18. Febbraio MA, Flanagan TR, Snow RJ, et al: Effect of creatine supplementation on intramuscular TCr, metabolism and performance during intermittent, supramaximal exercise in humans. Acta Physiol Scand 1995;155(4):387-395.

19. Balsom PD, Harridge SD, Soderlund K, et al: Creatine supplementation per se does not enhance endurance exercise performance. Acta Physiol Scand 1993;149(4):521-523.

20. Earnest CP, Snell PG, Rodriguez R, et al: The effect of creatine monohydrate ingestion on anaerobic power indices, muscular strength and body composition. Acta Physiol Scand 1995;153(2):207-209.

21. Green AL, Simpson EJ, Littlewood JJ, et al: Carbohydrate ingestion augments creatine retention during creatine feeding in man. Acta Physiol Scand 1996;158:195-202.

22. Vandenberghe K, Goris M, Van Hecke P, et al: Long-term creatine intake is beneficial to muscle performance during resistance training. J Appl Physiol 1997;83(6):2055-2063.

23. Kreider RB, Ferreira M, Wilson M, et al: Effects of creatine supplementation on body composition, strength, and sprint performance. Med Sci Sports Exerc 1998;30(1):73-82.

24. Maganaris CN, Maughan RJ: Creatine supplementation enhances maximum voluntary isometric force and endurance capacity in resistance trained men. Acta Physiol Scand 1998;163(3):279-287.

25. Snow RJ, McKenna MJ, Selig SE, et al: Effect of creatine supplementation on sprint exercise performance and muscle metabolism. J Appl Physiol 1998;84(5):1667-1673.

26. Ingwall JS, Morales MF, Stockdale FE: Creatine and the control of myosin synthesis in differentiating skeletal muscle. Proc Natl Acad Sci U S A 1972;69(8):2250-2253.

27. Ingwall JS, Morales MF, Stockdale FE, Wildenthal K: Creatine: a possible stimulus skeletal cardiac muscle hypertrophy. Recent Adv Stud Cardiac Struct Metab 1975;8:467-481.

28. Ingwall JS: Creatine and the control of muscle-specific protein synthesis in cardiac and skeletal muscle. Circ Res 1976;38(5 suppl 1):I115-I123.

29. Parise G, Mihic S, MacLellelan D, et al: Creatine monohydrate supplementation does not increase whole body or mixed muscle fractional protein synthetic rates in males and females. Med Sci Sport Exerc 2000;32:S289.

30. Haussinger D, Lang F, Gerok W: Regulation of cell function by the cellular hydration state. Am J Physiol 1994;267(3 Pt 1):E343-E355.

31. Theodorou AS, Havenetidis K, Zanker CL, et al: Effects of acute creatine loading with or without carbohydrate on repeated bouts of maximal swimming in high-performance swimmers. J Strength Cond Res 2005;19(2):265-269.

32. Mendes RR, Pires I, Oliveira A, Tirapegui J: Effects of creatine supplementation on the performance and body composition of competitive swimmers. J Nutr Biochem 2004;15(8):473-478.

33. Anomasiri W, Sanguanrungsirikul S, Saichandee P: Low dose creatine supplementation enhances sprint phase of 400 meters swimming performance. J Med Assoc Thai 2004;87(suppl 2):S228-S232.

34. Mero AA, Keskinen KL, Malvela MT, Sallinen JM: Combined creatine and sodium bicarbonate supplementation enhances interval swimming. J Strength Cond Res 2004;18(2):306-310.

35. Selsby JT, Beckett KD, Kern M, Devor ST: Swim performance following creatine supplementation in Division III athletes. J Strength Cond Res 2003;17(3):421-424.

36. Dawson B, Vladich T, Blanksby BA: Effects of 4 weeks of creatine supplementation in junior swimmers on freestyle sprint and swim bench performance. J Strength Cond Res 2002;16(4):485-490.

37. Hoffman JR, Stout JR, Falvo MJ, et al: Effect of low-dose, short-duration creatine supplementation on anaerobic exercise performance. J Strength Cond Res 2005;19(2):260-264.

38. Ahmun RP, Tong RJ, Grimshaw PN: The effects of acute creatine supplementation on multiple sprint cycling and running performance in rugby players. J Strength Cond Res 2005;19(1):92-97.

39. Gill ND, Hall RD, Blazevich AJ: Creatine serum is not as effective as creatine powder for improving cycle sprint performance in competitive male team-sport athletes. J Strength Cond Res 2004;18(2):272-275.

40. Ostojic SM: Creatine supplementation in young soccer players. Int J Sport Nutr Exerc Metab 2004;14(1):95-103.

41. Kinugasa R, Akima H, Ota A, et al: Short-term creatine supplementation does not improve muscle activation or sprint performance in humans. Eur J Appl Physiol 2004;91(2-3):230-237.

42. Eckerson JM, Stout JR, Moore GA, et al: Effect of two and five days of creatine loading on anaerobic working capacity in women. J Strength Cond Res 2004;18(1):168-173.

43. Kocak S, Karli U: Effects of high dose oral creatine supplementation on anaerobic capacity of elite wrestlers. J Sports Med Phys Fitness 2003;43(4):488-492.

44. Delecluse C, Diels R, Goris M: Effect of creatine supplementation on intermittent sprint running performance in highly trained athletes. J Strength Cond Res 2003;17(3):446-454.

45. Lehmkuhl M, Malone M, Justice B, et al: The effects of 8 weeks of creatine monohydrate and glutamine supplementation on body composition and performance measures. J Strength Cond Res 2003;17(3):425-438.

46. Ziegenfuss TN, Rogers M, Lowery L, et al: Effect of creatine loading on anaerobic performance and skeletal muscle volume in NCAA Division I athletes. Nutrition 2002;18(5):397-402.

47. Cottrell GT, Coast JR, Herb RA: Effect of recovery interval on multiple-bout sprint cycling performance after acute creatine supplementation. J Strength Cond Res 2002;16(1):109-116.

48. Preen D, Dawson B, Goodman C, et al: Pre-exercise oral creatine ingestion does not improve prolonged intermittent sprint exercise in humans. J Sports Med Phys Fitness 2002;42(3):320-329.

49. Finn JP, Ebert TR, Withers RT, et al: Effect of creatine supplementation on metabolism and performance in humans during intermittent sprint cycling. Eur J Appl Physiol 2001;84(3):238-243.

50. Skare OC, Skadberg, Wisnes AR: Creatine supplementation improves sprint performance in male sprinters. Scand J Med Sci Sports 2001;11(2):96-102.

51. Deutekom M, Beltman JG, de Ruiter CJ, et al: No acute effects of short-term creatine supplementation on muscle properties and sprint performance. Eur J Appl Physiol 2000;82(3):223-229.

52. Schedel JM, Terrier P, Schutz Y: The biomechanic origin of sprint performance enhancement after one-week creatine supplementation. Jpn J Physiol 2000;50(2):273-276.

53. Santos RV, Bassit RA, Caperuto EC, Costa Rosa LF: The effect of creatine supplementation upon inflammatory and muscle soreness markers after a 30km race. Life Sci 2004;75(16):1917-1924.

54. Biwer CJ, Jensen RL, Schmidt WD, Watts PB: The effect of creatine on treadmill running with high-intensity intervals. J Strength Cond Res 2003;17(3):439-445.

55. van Loon LJ, Oosterlaar AM, Hartgens F, et al: Effects of creatine loading and prolonged creatine supplementation on body composition, fuel selection, sprint and endurance performance in humans. Clin Sci (Lond) 2003;104(2):153-162.

56. Cox G, Mujika I, Tumilty D, Burke L: Acute creatine supplementation and performance during a field test simulating match play in elite female soccer players. Int J Sport Nutr Exerc Metab 2002;12(1):33-46.

57. Syrotuik DG, Game AB, Gillies EM, Bell GJ: Effects of creatine monohydrate supplementation during combined strength and high intensity rowing training on performance. Can J Appl Physiol 2001;26(6):527-542.

58. Bennett T, Bathalon G, Armstrong D 3rd, et al: Effect of creatine on performance of militarily relevant tasks and soldier health. Mil Med 2001;166(11):996-1002.

59. Chilibeck PD, Stride D, Farthing JP, Burke DG: Effect of creatine ingestion after exercise on muscle thickness in males and females. Med Sci Sports Exerc 2004;36(10):1781-1788.

60. Candow DG, Chilibeck PD, Chad KE, et al: Effect of ceasing creatine supplementation while maintaining resistance training in older men. J Aging Phys Act 2004;12(3):219-231.

61. Volek JS, Ratamess NA, Rubin MR, et al: The effects of creatine supplementation on muscular performance and body composition responses to short-term resistance training overreaching. Eur J Appl Physiol 2004;91(5-6):628-637.

62. Kilduff LP, Pitsiladis YP, Tasker L, et al: Effects of creatine on body composition and strength gains after 4 weeks of resistance training in previously nonresistance-trained humans. Int J Sport Nutr Exerc Metab 2003;13(4):504-520.

63. Ayoama R, Hiruma E, Sasaki H: Effects of creatine loading on muscular strength and endurance of female softball players. J Sports Med Phys Fitness 2003;43(4):481-487.

64. Kutz MR, Gunter MJ: Creatine monohydrate supplementation on body weight and percent body fat. J Strength Cond Res 2003;17(4):817-821.

65. Chwalbinska-Moneta J: Effect of creatine supplementation on aerobic performance and anaerobic capacity in elite rowers in the course of endurance training. Int J Sport Nutr Exerc Metab 2003;13(2):173-183.

66. Warber JP, Tharion WJ, Patton JF, et al: The effect of creatine monohydrate supplementation on obstacle course and multiple bench press performance. J Strength Cond Res 2002;16(4):500-508.

67. Kilduff LP, Vidakovic P, Cooney G, et al: Effects of creatine on isometric bench-press performance in resistance-trained humans. Med Sci Sports Exerc 2002;34(7):1176-1183.

68. Mihic S, MacDonald JR, McKenzie S, Tarnopolsky MA: Acute creatine loading increases fat-free mass, but does not affect blood pressure, plasma creatinine, or CK activity in men and women. Med Sci Sports Exerc 2000;32(2):291-296.

69. Peteers BM, Lantz CD, Mayhew JL: Effect of oral creatine monohydrate and creatine phosphate supplementation on maximal strength indices, body composition, and blood pressure. J Strength Cond Res 1999;13:3-9.

70. Poortmans JR, Auquier H, Renaut V, et al: Effect of short-term creatine supplementation on renal responses in men. Eur J Appl Physiol Occup Physiol 1997;76(6):566-567.

71. Poortmans JR, Francaux M: Long-term oral creatine supplementation does not impair renal function in healthy athletes. Med Sci Sports Exerc 1999;31(8):1108-1110.

72. Koshy KM, Griswold E, Schneeberger EE: Interstitial nephritis in a patient taking creatine. N Engl J Med 1999;340(10):814-815.

73. Mendel RW, Blegen M, Cheatham C, et al: Effects of creatine on thermoregulatory responses while exercising in the heat. Nutrition 2005;21(3):301-307.

74. Oopik V, Paasuke M, Timpmann S, et al: Effect of creatine supplementation during rapid body mass reduction on metabolism and isokinetic muscle performance capacity. Eur J Appl Physiol Occup Physiol 1998;78(1):83-92.

75. Shahidi NT: A review of the chemistry, biological action, and clinical applications of anabolic-androgenic steroids. Clin Ther 2001;23(9):1355-1390.

76. Yesalis CE, Bahrke MS: Anabolic-androgenic steroids and related substances. Curr Sports Med Rep 2002;1(4):246-252.

77. Yesalis CE, Barsukiewicz CK, Kopstein AN, Bahrke MS: Trends in anabolic-androgenic steroid use among adolescents. Arch Pediatr Adolesc Med 1997;151(12):1197-1206.

78. Buckley WE, Yesalis CE 3rd, Friedl KE, et al: Estimated prevalence of anabolic steroid use among male high school seniors. JAMA 1988;260(23):3441-3445.

79. Wilson JD: Androgen abuse by athletes. Endocr Rev 1988;9(2):181-199.

80. Bardin CW: The anabolic action of testosterone. N Engl J Med 1996;335(1):52-53.

81. Tricker R, Casaburi R, Storer TW, et al: The effects of supraphysiological doses of testosterone on angry behavior in healthy eugonadal men—a clinical research center study. J Clin Endocrinol Metab 1996;81(10):3754-3758.

82. Yesalis CE, Bahrke MS: Anabolic-androgenic steroids and related substances. Curr Sports Med Rep 2002;1(4):246-252.

83. Bhasin S, Storer TW, Berman N, et al: The effects of supraphysiologic doses of testosterone on muscle size and strength in normal men. N Engl J Med 1996;335(1):1-7.

84. Brodsky IG, Balagopal P, Nair KS: Effects of testosterone replacement on muscle mass and muscle protein synthesis in hypogonadal men—a clinical research center study. J Clin Endocrinol Metab 1996;81(10):3469-3475.

85. Katznelson L, Finkelstein JS, Schoenfeld DA, et al: Increase in bone density and lean body mass during testosterone administration in men with acquired hypogonadism. J Clin Endocrinol Metab 1996;81(12):4358-4365.

86. Wang C, Eyre DR, Clark R, et al: Sublingual testosterone replacement improves muscle mass and strength, decreases bone resorption, and increases bone formation markers in hypogonadal men—a clinical research center study. J Clin Endocrinol Metab 1996;81(10):3654-3662.

87. Wang C, Swerdloff RS, Iranmanesh A, et al: Testosterone Gel Study Group: Transdermal testosterone gel improves sexual function, mood, muscle strength, and body composition parameters in hypogonadal men. J Clin Endocrinol Metab 2000;85(8):2839-2853.

88. Snyder PJ, Peachey H, Berlin JA, et al: Effects of testosterone replacement in hypogonadal men. J Clin Endocrinol Metab 2000;85(8):2670-2677.

89. Bhasin S, Storer TW, Berman N, et al: Testosterone replacement increases fat-free mass and muscle size in hypogonadal men. J Clin Endocrinol Metab 1997;82(2):407-413.

90. Griggs RC, Pandya S, Florence JM, et al: Randomized controlled trial of testosterone in myotonic dystrophy. Neurology 1989;39(2 Pt 1):219-222.

91. Young NR, Baker HW, Liu G, Seeman E: Body composition and muscle strength in healthy men receiving testosterone enanthate for contraception. J Clin Endocrinol Metab 1993;77(4):1028-1032.

92. Tenover JS: Effects of testosterone supplementation in the aging male. J Clin Endocrinol Metab 1992;75(4):1092-1098.

93. Morley JE, Perry HM 3rd, Kaiser FE, et al: Effects of testosterone replacement therapy in old hypogonadal males: a preliminary study. J Am Geriatr Soc 1993;41(2):149-152.

94. Sih R, Morley JE, Kaiser FE, et al: Testosterone replacement in older hypogonadal men: a 12-month randomized controlled trial. J Clin Endocrinol Metab 1997;82(6):1661-1667.

95. Urban RJ, Bodenburg YH, Gilkison C, et al: Testosterone administration to elderly men increases skeletal muscle strength and protein synthesis. Am J Physiol 1995;269(5 Pt 1):E820-E826.

96. Snyder PJ, Peachey H, Hannoush P, et al: Effect of testosterone treatment on body composition and muscle strength in men over 65 years of age. J Clin Endocrinol Metab 1999;84(8):2647-2653.

97. Tenover JL: Experience with testosterone replacement in the elderly. Mayo Clin Proc 2000;75(suppl):S77-S81; discussion S82.

98. Casaburi R, Storer T, Bhasin S: Androgen effects on body composition and muscle performance. In Bhasi S, Gabelnick H, Spieler JM, et al (eds): Pharmacology, Biology, and Clinical Applications of Androgens: Current Status and Future Prospects. New York, Wiley-Liss, 1996, pp 283-288.

99. Rea A: Chemical Muscle Enhancement: Bodybuilder's Desk Reference: Bad Boys Fitness. 2002.

100. Bagatell CJ, Bremner WJ: Androgens in men—uses and abuses. N Engl J Med 1996;334(11):707-714.

101. Gurakar A, Caraceni P, Fagiuoli S, Van Thiel DH: Androgenic/anabolic steroid-induced intrahepatic cholestasis: a review with four additional case reports. J Okla State Med Assoc 1994;87(9):399-404.

102. Soe KL, Soe M, Gluud C: Liver pathology associated with the use of anabolic-androgenic steroids. Liver 1992;12(2):73-79.

103. Foster ZJ, Housner JA: Anabolic-androgenic steroids and testosterone precursors: ergogenic aids and sport. Curr Sports Med Rep 2004;3(4):234-241.

104. Hartgens F, Kuipers H: Effects of androgenic-anabolic steroids in athletes. Sports Med 2004;34(8):513-554.

105. Hartgens F, Rietjens G, Keizer HA, et al: Effects of androgenic-anabolic steroids on apolipoproteins and lipoprotein (a). Br J Sports Med 2004;38(3):253-259.

106. Urhausen A, Albers T, Kindermann W: Are the cardiac effects of anabolic steroid abuse in strength athletes reversible? Heart 2004;90(5):496-501.

107. McNutt RA, Ferenchick GS, Kirlin PC, Hamlin NJ: Acute myocardial infarction in a 22-year-old world class weight lifter using anabolic steroids. Am J Cardiol 1988;62(1):164.

108. Frankle MA, Eichberg R, Zachariah SB: Anabolic androgenic steroids and a stroke in an athlete: case report. Arch Phys Med Rehabil 1988;69(8):632-633.

109. Haupt HA, Rovere GD: Anabolic steroids: a review of the literature. Am J Sports Med 1984;12(6):469-484.

110. Parssinen M, Seppala T: Steroid use and long-term health risks in former athletes. Sports Med 2002;32(2):83-94.

111. Ferenchick G, Schwartz D, Ball M, Schwartz K: Androgenic-anabolic steroid abuse and platelet aggregation: a pilot study in weight lifters. Am J Med Sci 1992;303(2):78-82.

112. Urhausen A, Torsten A, Wilfried K: Reversibility of the effects on blood cells, lipids, liver function and hormones in former anabolic-androgenic steroid abusers. J Steroid Biochem Mol Biol 2003;84(2-3):369-375.

113. Kutscher EC, Lund BC, Perry PJ: Anabolic steroids: a review for the clinician. Sports Med 2002;32(5):285-296.

114. Maravelias C, Dona A, Stefanidou M, Spiliopoulou C: Adverse effects of anabolic steroids in athletes. A constant threat. Toxicol Lett 2005;158(3):167-175.

115. Cope MR, Ali A, Bayliss NC: Biceps rupture in body builders: three case reports of rupture of the long head of the biceps at the tendon-labrum junction. J Shoulder Elbow Surg 2004;13(5):580-582.

116. Freeman BJ, Rooker GD: Spontaneous rupture of the anterior cruciate ligament after anabolic steroids. Br J Sports Med 1995;29(4):274-275.

117. Tricker R, Casaburi R, Storer TW, et al: The effects of supraphysiological doses of testosterone on angry behavior in healthy eugonadal men—a clinical research center study. J Clin Endocrinol Metab 1996;81(10):3754-3758.

118. Schulman C, Lunenfeld B: The ageing male. World J Urol 2002;20(1):4-10.

119. Mahesh VB, Greenblatt RB: Isolation of dehydroepiandrosterone and 17alpha-hydroxy-delta5-pregenolone from the polycystic ovaries of the Stein-Leventhal syndrome. J Clin Endocrinol Metab 1962;22:441-448.

120. Brown GA, Vukovich MD, Sharp RL, et al: Effect of oral DHEA on serum testosterone and adaptations to resistance training in young men. J Appl Physiol 1999;87(6):2274-2283.

121. Brown GA, Vukovich MD, Martini ER, et al: Endocrine responses to chronic androstenedione intake in 30- to 56-year-old men. J Clin Endocrinol Metab 2000;85(11):4074-4080.

122. Wallace MB, Lim J, Cutler A, Bucci L: Effects of dehydroepiandrosterone vs androstenedione supplementation in men. Med Sci Sports Exerc 1999;31(12):1788-1792.

123. Flynn MA, Weaver-Osterholtz D, Sharpe-Timms KL, et al: Dehydroepiandrosterone replacement in aging humans. J Clin Endocrinol Metab 1999;84(5):1527-1533.

124. Morales AJ, Haubrich RH, Hwang JY, et al: The effect of six months treatment with a 100 mg daily dose of dehydroepiandrosterone (DHEA) on circulating sex steroids, body composition and muscle strength in age-advanced men and women. Clin Endocrinol (Oxf) 1998;49(4):421-432.

125. Rasmussen BB, Volpi E, Gore DC, Wolfe RR: Androstenedione does not stimulate muscle protein anabolism in young healthy men. J Clin Endocrinol Metab 2000;85(1):55-59.

126. Ziegenfuss TN, Berardi JM, Lowery LM: Effects of prohormone supplementation in humans: a review. Can J Appl Physiol 2002;27(6):628-646.

127. Leder BZ, Longcope C, Catlin DH, et al: Oral androstenedione administration and serum testosterone concentrations in young men. JAMA 2000;283(6):779-782.

128. King DS, Sharp RL, Vukovich MD, et al: Effect of oral androstenedione on serum testosterone and adaptations to resistance training in young men: a randomized controlled trial. JAMA 1999;281(21):2020-2028.

129. Broeder CE, Quindry J, Brittingham K, et al: The Andro Project: physiological and hormonal influences of androstenedione supplementation in men 35 to 65 years old participating in a high-intensity resistance training program. Arch Intern Med 2000;160(20):3093-3104.

130. Brown GA, Dewey JC, Brunkhorst JA, et al: Changes in serum testosterone and estradiol concentrations following acute androstenedione ingestion in young women. Horm Metab Res 2004;36(1):62-66.

131. Fine RN, Sullivan EK, Tejani A: The impact of recombinant human growth hormone treatment on final adult height. Pediatr Nephrol 2000;14(7):679-681.

132. Lanes R: Growth velocity, final height and bone mineral metabolism of short children treated long term with growth hormone. Curr Pharm Biotechnol 2000;1(1):33-46.
133. Germak JA: Growth hormone therapy in children with short stature: is bigger better or achievable? Indian J Pediatr 1996;63(5):591-597.
134. Saenger P, Attie KM, DiMartino-Nardi J, et al: Metabolic consequences of 5-year growth hormone (GH) therapy in children treated with GH for idiopathic short stature. Genentech Collaborative Study Group. J Clin Endocrinol Metab 1998;83(9):3115-3120.
135. Vimalachandra D, Craig JC, Cowell CT, Knight JF: Growth hormone treatment in children with chronic renal failure: a meta-analysis of randomized controlled trials. J Pediatr 2001;139(4):560-567.
136. Hunter WM, Fonseka CC, Passmore R: Growth hormone: important role in muscular exercise in adults. Science 1965;150(699):1051-1053.
137. Consitt LA, Copeland JL, Tremblay MS: Endogenous anabolic hormone responses to endurance versus resistance exercise and training in women. Sports Med 2002;32(1):1-22.
138. Koch JJ: Performance-enhancing: substances and their use among adolescent athletes. Pediatr Rev 2002;23(9):310-317.
139. Rickert VI, Pawlak-Morello C, Sheppard V, Jay MS: Human growth hormone: a new substance of abuse among adolescents? Clin Pediatr (Phila) 1992;31(12):723-726.
140. Juhn M: Popular sports supplements and ergogenic aids. Sports Med 2003;33(12):921-939.
141. Marcus R, Butterfield G, Holloway L, et al: Effects of short term administration of recombinant human growth hormone to elderly people. J Clin Endocrinol Metab 1990;70(2):519-527.
142. Rudman D, Feller AG, Nagraj HN, et al: Effects of human growth hormone in men over 60 years old. N Engl J Med 1990;323:1-6.
143. Taaffe DR, Pruitt L, Reim J, et al: Effect of recombinant human growth hormone on the muscle strength response to resistance exercise in elderly men. J Clin Endocrinol Metab 1994;79(5):1361-1366.
144. Taaffe DR, Jin IH, Vu TH, et al: Lack of effect of recombinant human growth hormone (GH) on muscle morphology and GH-insulin-like growth factor expression in resistance-trained elderly men. J Clin Endocrinol Metab 1996;81(1):421-425.
145. Yarasheski KE, Zachwieja JJ, Campbell JA, Bier DM: Effect of growth hormone and resistance exercise on muscle growth and strength in older men. Am J Physiol 1995;268:E268-E276.
146. Yarasheski KE, Campbell JA, Smith K, et al: Effect of growth hormone and resistance exercise on muscle growth in young men. Am J Physiol 1992;262(3 Pt 1):E261-E267.
147. Yarasheski KE, Zachwieja JJ, Angelopoulos TJ, Bier DM: Short-term growth hormone treatment does not increase muscle protein synthesis in experienced weight lifters. J Appl Physiol 1993;74(6):3073-3076.
148. Deyssig R, Frisch H, Blum WF, Waldhor T: Effect of growth hormone treatment on hormonal parameters, body composition and strength in athlete. Acta Endocrinol (Copenh) 1993;128(4):313-318.
149. Healy ML, Gibney J, Pentecost C, et al: Effects of high-dose growth hormone on glucose and glycerol metabolism at rest and during exercise in endurance-trained athletes. J Clin Endocrinol Metab 2006;91(1):320-327.
150. Wee J, Charlton C, Simpson H, et al: GH secretion in acute exercise may result in post-exercise lipolysis. Growth Horm IGF Res 2005;15(6):397-404.
151. Hayward RP, Emanuel RW, Nabarro JD: Acromegalic heart disease: influence of treatment of the acromegaly on the heart. Q J Med 1987;62(237):41-58.
152. Bengtsson BA, Eden S, Ernest I, et al: Epidemiology and long-term survival in acromegaly. A study of 166 cases diagnosed between 1955 and 1984. Acta Med Scand 1988;223(4):327-335.
153. Sacca L, Cittadini A, Fazio S: Growth hormone and the heart. Endocr Rev 1994;15(5):555-573.
154. Jenkins PJ, Fairclough PD, Richards T, et al: Acromegaly, colonic polyps and carcinoma. Clin Endocrinol (Oxf) 1997;47(1):17-22.
155. Orme SM, McNally RJ, Cartwright RA, Belchetz PE: Mortality and cancer incidence in acromegaly: a retrospective cohort study. United Kingdom Acromegaly Study Group. J Clin Endocrinol Metab 1998;83(8):2730-2734.
156. Kurien VA, Yates PA, Oliver MF: The role of free fatty acids in the production of ventricular arrhythmias after acute coronary artery occlusion. Eur J Clin Invest 1971;1(4):225-241.
157. Opie LH: Fatty acids and sudden death. Am Heart J 1973;85(4):575.
158. Salomon F, Cuneo RC, Hesp R, Sonksen PH: The effects of treatment with recombinant human growth hormone on body composition and metabolism in adults with growth hormone deficiency. N Engl J Med 1989;321(26):1797-1803.
159. Maison P, Griffin S, Nicoue-Beglah M, et alMetaanalysis of Blinded Randomized Placebo-Controlled Trials: Impact of growth hormone (GH) treatment on cardiovascular risk factors in GH-deficient adults: a Metaanalysis of Blinded, Randomized, Placebo-Controlled Trials. J Clin Endocrinol Metab 2004;89(5):2192-2199.
160. Swerdlow AJ, Higgins CD, Adlard P, Preece MA: Risk of cancer in patients treated with human pituitary growth hormone in the UK, 1959-85: a cohort study. Lancet 2002;360(9329):273-277.
161. Geiger JD: Adverse events associated with supplements containing ephedra alkaloids. Clin J Sports Med 2002;12:263.
162. Keisler BD, Hosey RG: Ergogenic aids: an update on ephedra. Curr Sports Med Rep 2005;4:231-235.
163. FDA Evidence Reports Number 76: Ephedra and ephedrine for weight loss and athletic performance enhancement: clinical efficacy and side effects (Web site). Available at www.fda.gov/bbs/topics/NEWS/ephedra/summary.html. Accessed July 27, 2007.
164. Shekelle PG, Hardy ML, Morton SC, et al: Efficacy and safety of ephedra and ephedrine for weight loss and athletic performance: a meta-analysis. JAMA 2003;289(12):1537-1545.
165. Congeni J, Miller S: Supplements and drugs used to enhance athletic performance. Pediatr Clin North Am 2002;49:435-461.
166. Miller SC: Safety concerns regarding ephedrine-type alkaloid-containing dietary supplements. Mil Med 2004;169:87-93.
167. Haller CA, Benowitz NL: Adverse cardiovascular and central nervous system events associated with dietary supplements containing ephedra alkaloids. N Engl J Med 2000;343:1833-1888.
168. Krome CN, Tucker AM: Cardiac arrhythmia in a professional football player. Phys Sportsmed 2003;30(12):21-25.
169. Paluska SA: Caffeine and exercise. Curr Sports Med Rep 2003;2:213-219.
170. Graham TE: Caffeine and exercise: metabolism, endurance and performance. Sports Med 2001;31:785-807.
171. Graham TE, Spriet LL: Metabolic, catecholamine and exercise performance responses to various doses of caffeine. J Appl Physiol 1995;78:867-874.
172. Bruce CR, Anderson ME, Fraser SF, et al: Enhancement of 2000m rowing performance after caffeine ingestion. Med Sci Sports Exerc 2000;32:1958-1963.
173. Anderson ME, Bruce CR, Fraser SF, et al: Improved 2000-m rowing performance in competitive oarswomen after caffeine ingestion. Int J Sport Nutr Exerc Metab 2000;10(4):464-475.
174. Collomp K, Ahmaidi S, Chatard JC, et al: Benefits of caffeine ingestion on sprint performance in trained and untrained swimmers. Eur J Appl Physiol 1992;64:377-380.
175. Juhn MS: Popular sports supplements and ergogenic aids. Sports Med 2003;33:921-939.
176. Palisin T, Stacy JJ: Beta-hydroxy-beta-methylbutyrate and its use in athletics. Curr Sports Med Rep 2005;4:220-223.
177. Jowko E, Ostaszewski P, Jank M, et al: Creatine and beta-hydroxy-beta-methylbutyrate (HMB) additively increase lean body mass and muscle strength during a weight training program. Nutrition 2001;17:558-566.
178. Nissen SL, Sharp RL: Effect of dietary supplements on lean mass and strength gains with resistance exercise: a meta-analysis. J Appl Physiol 2003;94:651-659.
179. Panton LB, Rathmacher JA, Baier S, Nissen SL: Nutritional supplementation of the leucine metabolite beta-hydroxy-beta-methylbutyrate (HMB) during resistance training. Nutrition 2000;16:734-739.
180. Slater G, Jenkins D, Logan P, et al: Beta-hydroxy-beta-methylbutyrate does not affect changes in strength or body composition during resistance training in trained men. Int J Sport Nutr Exerc Metab 2001;11:384-396.
181. Gaurdard A, Varlet-Marie E, Bressolle F, et al: Drugs for increasing oxygen transport and their potential use in doping. Sports Med 2003;33(3):187-212.
182. Sawka MN, Joyner MJ, Miles DS, et al: American College of Sports Medicine position stand. The use of blood doping as an ergogenic aid. Med Sci Sports Exerc 1996;28:i-viii.
183. Casadevall N, Nataf J, Viron B, et al: Pure red-cell aplasia and antierythropoietin antibodies in patients treated with recombinant erythropoietin. N Engl J Med 2002;346(7):469-475.
184. Raine AE: Hypertension, blood viscosity and cardiovascular morbidity in renal failure: implications of erythropoietin therapy. Lancet 1988;I(8577):97-100.
185. Piron M, Loo M, Gothot A, et al: Cessation of intensive treatment with recombinant human erythropoietin is followed by secondary anemia. Blood 2001;97(2):442-448.
186. Leigh-Smith S: Blood boosting. Br J Sports Med 2004;38:99-101.
187. Armstrong LE, Costill DL, Fink WJ: Influence of diuretic-induced dehydration on competitive running performance. Med Sci Sports Exerc 1985;17(4):456-461.
188. Casa DJ, Armstrong LE, Hillman SK, et al: National Athletic Trainers' position statement: fluid replacement for athletes. J Athl Train 2000;35(2):212-224.
189. Watson G, Judelson DA, Armstrong LE, et al: Influence of diuretic-induces dehydration on competitive sprint and power performance. Med Sci Sports Exerc 2005;37(7):1168-1174.
190. Coris EE, Ramirez AM, Van Durme DJ: Heat illness in athletes: the dangerous combination of heat, humidity and exercise. Sports Med 2004;34(1):9-16.
191. Oppliger RA, Steen SA, Scott JR: Weight loss practices of college wrestlers. Int J Sport Nutr Exerc Metab 2003;12(1):29-46.
192. Kiningham RB, Goreflo DW: Weight loss methods of high school wrestlers. Med Sci Sports Exerc 2001;33(5):810-813.
193. Gertsch JH, Basnyat B, Johnson WE, et al: Randomised, double blind, placebo controlled comparison of ginkgo biloba and acetazolamide for the prevention of acute mountain sickness among Himalayan trekkers: the prevention of high altitude illness trial (PHAIT). BMJ 2004;328(7443):797.
194. Carlsten C, Swenson ER, Rouss S: A dose response study of acetazolamide for acute mountain sickness prophylaxis in vacationing tourist at 12,000 feet (3600 m). High Alt Med Biol 2004;5(1):33-39.
195. National and Related Football League Policy on Anabolic Steroids and Related Substances, Procedures Regarding Testosterone. 2007, p11.

CHAPTER 50

Evidence-Based Regenerative Injection Therapy (Prolotherapy) in Sports Medicine

K. Dean Reeves, MD; Bradley D. Fullerton, MD, FAAPMR; and Gaston Topol, MD

KEY POINTS

· The treatment of sports injuries to the point of restoration of full sports performance is an obvious goal in sports medicine. However, healing is the preferred goal because returning connective tissue to normal strength allows for a durable return to full sports performance.

· Regenerative injection therapy (prolotherapy) is the injection of growth factors or growth factor production stimulants to promote the regeneration of normal cells and tissue. Inflammation is not required, and scarring is not the result.

· Open-label clinical trials have been uniformly positive in outcome, but double-blind clinical trials have been hampered by a needling control that does not appear to be a placebo. Recent studies are making use of a noninjection control.

· Making use of consecutive patient data from athletes with career-threatening injuries (i.e., chronic groin strain in soccer or rugby players) that are not responsive to other treatments is a recommended study approach to assess regenerative injection therapy's ability to reverse otherwise permanent conditions. This is an avenue for the critical assessment of regenerative injection therapy's potential.

· Serial high-resolution ultrasound images are limited somewhat by uniformity of technique, but they offer a way to follow healing from regenerative injections.

INTRODUCTION

The treatment of sports injuries to the point of restoration of full sports performance is an obvious goal in sports medicine. Healing, however, is the preferred goal because returning connective tissue to normal strength allows for a durable return to full sports performance.

Given the advancements in the knowledge of the degenerative nature of chronic sprain or strain and the ability of high-definition ultrasound to demonstrate the objective healing of soft tissue, the use of prolotherapy, which is also called *regenerative injection therapy* (RIT), is expected to greatly accelerate in the next decade. This chapter will cover the pathology of injury; the current treatment methods and their limitations; and the rationale, basic science, and clinical studies of prolotherapy/RIT. In the latter section, it will also introduce two areas of particularly pertinent research approaches in sports medicine: the treatment of connective-tissue–based, career-threatening injuries and the use of high-resolution ultrasound to document healing.

PATHOLOGY OF INJURY

During sports participations, tendons are subjected to unpredictable mechanical loads as they transmit forces to bone. Ligaments are likewise unpredictably stressed as they attempt to hold bony structures together at a fixed length. These mechanical loads, when excessive, lead to unhealthy changes in tendon or ligament structures. Numerous terms have been used to describe these unhealthy changes. *Tendinitis* implies inflammation, and *tendinosis* implies degeneration. Because inflammation and degeneration can only be confirmed via biopsy, the generic term *tendinopathy* is proposed as perhaps the best descriptive term.[1]

Mechanical testing of tendon specimens has provided a stress-strain curve, and this curve demonstrates that collagen fibers uncrimp by 2% stretch of a tendon and microscopically rupture beginning at 4% to 8% stretch. Beyond 8% stretch, macroscopic tears are noted, and, beyond 12%, complete rupture is likely.[1] Repetitive submaximal loading can cause microscopic injuries that, through the failure of individual collagen fibers, reduce the effective cross-sectional area of the tendon or ligament and thus make it more susceptible to failure.[2]

CURRENT TREATMENT METHODS AND THEIR LIMITATIONS

Although the structure, composition, and mechanical properties of the tendon can change favorably in response to altered mechanical loading conditions, that response is not consistently favorable, even in animal models. For example, although the strength of the insertion site may increase after long-term training,[3] the maximum stress of failure of the tendon may still decrease.[4]

Although appropriate training or exercise produces positive effects on tendons, long-term repetitive loading often produces inflammatory mediators such as prostaglandin E2 and degradative enzymes such as matrix metalloproteinase 1 and 3, even when loads are within the strength limits of the tendon.[5] Other factors such as vascular supply, age, and genetics can also contribute to tendinopathy, which helps explain how it can occur in sedentary people.[6]

It has been observed that rest is limited in its efficacy for bringing about healing in tendons in part because tendon metabolic activity is only 13% of muscle; this leads to an extended healing period that is not practical for the athlete.[7] Eccentric exercise appears to offer benefit in tendinopathy, and it has been used since the 1980s.[8] Mechanical loading with certain magnitudes and frequencies may enhance tendon repair and remodeling via fibroblast stimulation.[9]

The major goal of clinicians when treating acute musculoskeletal injuries is to return athletes to their preinjury level of function, ideally in the shortest time possible and without compromising tissue-level healing.[10] Inflammation can lead to the degradation of intact collagen and to viable cell death, thus potentially increasing the functional deficit and recovery period. Nonsteroidal anti-inflammatory drugs (NSAIDs) are the most frequently used pharmacologic substances for the treatment of tendinopathy.[11] It was logical years ago to assume, without rigorous clinical study or sufficient basic science backing, that inflammation might be harmful during healing, and thus treatment with anti-inflammatory medications or the injection of such should be helpful. However, it has been shown in animal studies that merely limiting neutrophil and leukocyte numbers after injury does not necessarily improve tendon function or strength.[12] A key issue is that many cellular and subcellular events that occur during the inflammatory response lead to the production and release of a plethora of growth factors that trigger the healing phase.[13] During the late 1990s, basic science evidence began accumulating about the negative effects of NSAIDs on fibroblast growth.[14] In 2001, Elder and colleagues published a sentinel article showing that a COX-2 inhibitor impaired the repair of the medial collateral ligament in rats after induced injury.[15] NSAIDs likely vary in their degree of inhibition of fibroblast growth, as Riley and colleagues showed with human patella and flexor tendon cells.[16] There is currently no randomized, controlled trial evidence of the tissue-level effects of cyclooxygenase inhibitors on acute musculoskeletal injuries.[10] Further questions regarding the use of these agents have been raised given the links between NSAIDs and adverse cardiovascular events.[10] It is fair to state that care needs to be taken before presumptively interfering with the natural processes of the healing cascade. It is now accepted that, when fracture healing or spine fusion is desired, NSAIDs should be avoided.[17] Current recommendations are to begin limiting the use of certain NSAIDs in soft-tissue injuries,[18] and, as nonselective NSAIDs are further investigated, these recommendations may expand. Cohen and colleagues' recent publication showing that both traditional and COX-specific NSAIDs significantly inhibited tendon-to-bone healing in a study of rotator cuff repair in rats is particularly sobering.[19] Given the questionable effects of oral anti-inflammatory drugs on soft tissue, it is understandable that the anti-inflammatory effects on critical growth factors are particularly profound if an anti-inflammatory solution is injected. Thus, the intratendinous injection of corticosteroids leads to negative rather than positive mechanical effects, such as reduced tensile strength and a loss of viscoelasticity in tendons.[20,21]

CURRENT DEFINITION AND POPULAR NON—CONNECTIVE TISSUE USES OF PROLOTHERAPY/RIT

Since 1995, the definition of prolotherapy has changed.[22] The prior definition of prolotherapy concentrated on the injection of inflammatory solutions to induce growth. However, as our understanding of the direct use of growth factors and multiple ways to stimulate them has expanded, the definition of prolotherapy is best described simply as RIT, or, more specifically, as "the injection of growth factors or growth factor production stimulants to promote regeneration of normal cells and tissue."[23] The most widespread form of RIT is the injection of erythrocyte growth factor (erythropoietin) to cause red cell proliferation in patients with chronic anemia and, more recently, in preparation for an acute loss of blood such as occurs during surgical procedures.[24]

At this point, the question has become more complicated: Although virtually all physicians are ordering the injection of growth factors for non—soft-tissue applications, what is the evidence for injection of growth factor or growth factor production stimulators in sports medicine conditions such as degeneration in tendons, ligaments, or cartilage?

Growth stimulation through single growth-factor injection

Wang and colleagues describe the "application of growth factors that stimulate cell proliferation and extracellular matrix synthesis in tendinopathy,"[25] and they cited Molley and colleagues regarding this description.[26]

To confirm its practical usefulness, growth-factor injection should cause a microscopic or macroscopic change in structure, a measurable mechanical improvement in the local structure, and an improved functionality of the animal or human. All three of these have not been studied systematically for any single growth factor. However, primary publication findings do show the following:

Microscopic or macroscopic change in structure from single growth-factor injection

1. Improved collagen structure from the injection of insulin-like growth factor (IGF-1) in injured or degenerated animal tendons[27]
2. Increase in the amount of tendon callus in transected rat Achilles tendon via the injection of bone morphogenetic proteins 13 and 14[28]
3. Increase in cell proliferation and gene expression of procollagen types I and III when bone morphogenetic protein 12 is added to human patellar tendon fibroblast cultures[29]

Measurable mechanical improvement in the local structure due to a single growth-factor injection

1. Improved tensile strength in transected tendons via the injection of cartilage-derived morphogenetic protein 2[30]
2. Increase in failure load of transected and repaired Achilles tendon by a single injection of transforming growth factor β[31]

Improved pain or function of the animal or human via single growth-factor injection

1. Improved walking pattern after the injection of IGF-1 in simulated Achilles-equivalent injury in rat tendon[32]

Summary of single growth-factor injection

Single growth factor use has been studied at the animal level, but no single growth factor has been studied enough to demonstrate all key elements of macroscopic or macroscopic change in structure, improved mechanics, or improved pain or function in either animals or humans.

Providing multiple simultaneous growth factors by injection: Emphasis on thrombin-stimulated platelet aggregates

The most important complexity thus far discovered about growth factors is that they work in coordination and cooperation with each other. For example, IGF-1 primarily stimulates fibroblast migration and proliferation and increased collagen production; transforming growth factor β regulates cell migration and the binding tendencies of collagen; vascular endothelial growth factor is heavily related to angiogenesis; platelet-derived growth factor stimulates IGF-1 production and has a role in tissue remodeling; and basic fibroblast growth factor stimulates angiogenesis and regulates cell migration and proliferation. In addition, increasing the breaking energy of a healing tendon is a verifiable effect of several growth factors (IGF-1, transforming growth factor β and platelet-derived growth factor).[26] Tsubone and colleagues demonstrated that all major growth factors are expressed within 10 days after tendon injury but by different cell types and in different locations (i.e., some in tendon cells [platelet-derived growth factor, vascular endothelial growth factor] and some in inflammatory cells only [epidermal growth factor, IGF, basic fibroblast growth factor]).[33] Intervention with a growth-factor injection will ideally be done with an awareness of this healing timeline when each factor is expressed.

Injecting multiple growth factors simultaneously may be done with combinations of artificially produced (recombinant) growth factors. For example, Thomopoulos and colleagues demonstrated that platelet-derived growth factor BB and basic fibroblast growth factor in combination led to more proliferation effect than either factor demonstrated individually.[34] Another method of injecting multiple growth factors simultaneously is by injecting thrombin-activated platelet concentrates (platelet-rich plasma), which contain the chief growth factors for connective tissue. Platelet-rich plasma, when activated by thrombin, can also serve to stimulate further growth-factor production by cells that are exposed to the solution.[35] The results from the injection of thrombin-activated platelet concentrates are as follows.

Microscopic or macroscopic changes in structure from the injection of multiple growth factors through thrombin-activated platelet aggregates

1. Human tendon fibroblasts exposed to activated platelet concentration react by proliferation.[35]

Measurable mechanical improvement in the local structure from the injection of multiple growth factors via thrombin-activated platelet aggregates

1. After transection repair and the injection of platelet concentrate in postsurgical hematoma, the Achilles tendon equivalent in rats improved 30% more in strength and stiffness than did the control group.[36]
2. The normal patellar tendon of the rabbit, when injected directly with autologous blood, improved significantly in strength as compared with noninjected control tendon; it also maintained normal morphology.[37]

Improved pain or function of the animal or human from the injection of multiple growth factors via thrombin-activated platelet aggregates

1. In patients with refractory tennis elbow symptoms, autologous blood injections eliminated pain even during strenuous activity in 22 out of 28 subjects (LOE: D).[38]

Summary of multiple growth-factor injection using thrombin-activated platelet aggregates

The provision of multiple growth factors more closely simulates natural healing and is attainable via thrombin-activated platelet concentrate. Microscopic evidence of proliferation, measurable mechanical improvement in animals, and improved function in a human application (tennis elbow) have been described in recent studies but require repetition to confirm the results.

Providing multiple simultaneous growth factors by stimulating their production: Emphasis on noninflammatory dextrose

Diabetic research into the effects of elevated glucose levels on human fibroblasts and other cells has provided much of the in vitro basic science for such an alternative.

A normal human cell contains only 0.1% dextrose. Normal human cells, when exposed to an extracellular d-glucose (dextrose) concentration of as little as 0.5%, begin to produce platelet-derived growth factor,[39] transforming grown factor β,[40,41] epidermal growth factor,[42] basic fibroblast growth factor,[43] IGF,[44] and connective tissue growth factor.[41] Note that these growth factors are pertinent to the growth of tendon, ligament, and cartilage but not to bone.[45] Dextrose from 0.5% to 10% continues to be noninflammatory in nature. This is evidenced by the peripheral vein tolerance of hypertonic dextrose up to 10%. Ten percent dextrose has been studied sparingly because the standard concentration in clinical use for many years has been 12.5%, and it has generally been accepted (but not proven) that 12.5% dextrose is the minimum concentration that will stimulate the inflammatory cascade for a more vigorous growth effect. However, it is important to demonstrate that something as simple and ubiquitous in the body as dextrose, when concentrated, can create a stimulation of growth by noninflammatory means. In short, we truly have a prototype for noninflammatory, inexpensive growth stimulation. What we know about noninflammatory, dextrose growth is summarized by the following:

Microscopic or macroscopic changes in structure due to noninflammatory dextrose exposure

1. Cell proliferation and collagen synthesis increase has been demonstrated in human renal cortical fibroblasts (0.6% dextrose).[46]

Measurable mechanical improvement in the local structure by the injection of noninflammatory dextrose

1. In a pilot study, consecutive patients with anterior cruciate ligament laxity as measured by mechanical arthrometer (KT-1000) were injected with 9 mL of simple 10% dextrose at 0, 2, and 4 months. Subsequently, they were injected as needed if they were symptomatic at 6, 8, and 10 months (LOE: C).[47] Sixteen patients were included in this trial, and 14 of 16 had moderate to severe osteoarthritis as demonstrated by osteophyte formation and minimal (<3 mm) residual cartilage. Despite this, at 1 year, the difference in KT-1000-measured anterior displacement

from side to side improved 54%, and 9 out of 16 patients no longer tested as having laxity using standard KT-1000 criteria.

Improved pain or function of the animal or human from the injection of noninflammatory dextrose

1. In the previously described study involving patients with anterior cruciate ligament laxity and concomitant knee osteoarthritis, patients were followed for 3 years using intention-to-treat criteria without data dropout. Walking pain improvement at 1 year was 40%, subjective swelling improved 52%, and range of motion improved by 14.1 degrees.

2. A double-blind, placebo-controlled study was conducted on patients with knee osteoarthritis (LOE: A).[48] One hundred eleven knees were injected with 9 mL of 10% dextrose at 0, 2, and 4 months. Knee pain had been present for an average of more than 8 years, an average of less than 3 mm of cartilage remained, and 35 out of 111 knees were bone on bone in at least one compartment. Walking pain reduced 35%, subjective swelling reduced by 45%, knee buckling episodes reduced by 67%, and range-of-motion improvement was 13.2 degrees with three injections of dextrose solution. Control solution injection led to improvements as well, but multivariate analysis demonstrated that the dextrose solution was superior ($P = 0.028$).

3. A double-blind, placebo-controlled study of patients with finger osteoarthritis was also conducted (LOE: A).[49] Subjects were patients with finger osteoarthritis as determined by standard radiographic criteria and who had had pain for more than 5 years. In this study, symptomatic finger joints were injected with 0.25 to 0.5 mL of 10% dextrose on both sides of each joint at 0, 2, and 4 months; and this resulted in a 42% improvement in grip pain and 8 degrees of improvement in the flexion range of motion. The study demonstrated the superior results of dextrose as compared with placebo with regard to pain ($P = 0.027$) and flexibility of joints ($P = 0.003$) at 6 months.

Summary of basic science and clinical research on the injection of noninflammatory dextrose

Dextrose elevation to as little at 0.6% in vitro stimulates human cells to produce key growth factors, and it has been demonstrated to cause cell proliferation in renal fibroblasts. In addition, it has been shown in pilot studies to tighten loose anterior cruciate ligaments and to be safe and probably effective therapeutically by two double-blind studies in patients with osteoarthritis. More basic science data and the repetition of double-blind studies are recommended. If simple dextrose stimulates the production of all key growth factors for ligament, tendon, and cartilage, it would be an inexpensive method of noninflammatory growth stimulation that may prove to be cost-effective for the long term.

Providing multiple simultaneous growth factors by stimulating their production: Emphasis on the use of brief inflammatory cascade activation

Although the stimulation of growth without inflammation has some advantages, the most cost-effective approach to RIT may involve the use of the natural inflammatory route of growth factor stimulation. This inflammatory cascade is also briefly stimulated after a significant injury, but smaller (overuse) sports injuries create damage and do not stimulate the healing

cascade at all.[25] Thus, growth-factor production is either time limited or does not occur at all in many sports-related injuries. When the inflammatory cascade is stimulated by injury, cell death and tissue stretch need to be corrected. However, growth-factor stimulation by brief inflammation does not require significant damage to the tissue in question, and, thus, positive changes in structure and function can occur without having to correct the negative effects of injury. The primary solutions in clinical use for inflammatory cascade initiation have been dextrose 12.5% to 25% (which becomes inflammatory at those levels), phenol from 0.5% to 1.25%, and sodium morrhuate 0.1% to 1%. Research in the area of inflammation induction for repair has been hampered by limited research funding as a result of the inexpensive solutions being used; differences in technique among investigators sometimes leading to incorrect injection methods, which can be counterproductive (LOE: A)[50]; and the lack of a placebo control because the trauma of needling and microbleeding have led to significant benefit in a number of cases (LOE: B).[51]

Microscopic or macroscopic changes in structure after injection to briefly activate an inflammatory cascade

1. After the injection of Sylnasol into the rabbit Achilles equivalent, 40% macroscopic thickening as compared with the opposite leg control at 9 months postinjection was seen.[52]

2. Macroscopic increase in the size of the attachment of rabbit Achilles tendon equivalent to bone was found 9 months after the injection of Sylnasol as compared with the opposite control leg.[52]

3. An increase in ligament fibril diameter of rabbit medial collateral ligament was demonstrated after injection with sodium morrhuate as compared with saline-injected control.[53]

4. An increase in the number of cells in rabbit patellar and Achilles tendons occurs when they are injected with sodium morrhuate as compared with saline-injected control.[54]

Measurable mechanical improvement in local structure after injection to briefly activate an inflammatory cascade

1. Increases in thickness of 28%, in mass of 47%, and in ligament-to-bone-junction strength of 27% were seen in rabbit medial collateral ligament that was injected with sodium morrhuate as compared with saline-injected control.[53]

2. Increases in the diameter of rabbit patellar and Achilles tendons were seen when they were injected with sodium morrhuate as compared with saline-injected control.[54]

3. An increase in the strength of the rabbit patellar ligament of 36% was seen when it was injected once with sodium morrhuate 5% as compared with saline control.[55]

4. Injection of knees with phenol 1.25%, dextrose (glucose) 12.5%, and glycerin 12.5% (P2G)[56] resulted in a highly significant decrease in laxity, as measured by AP drawer testing with the Genucom knee apparatus.

Improved pain or function of the animal or human after injection to briefly activate an inflammatory cascade

Many studies have been conducted, but only those with 25 or more patients, the name of the solution used, the percentage of improvement, and the percentage of patients with pain resolved or pain measured with a visual analog scale are summarized here.

1. Older case series in chronic back pain patients (not clearly stated as consecutive patients):
   a. A subjective average pain improvement of more than 50% with Sylnasol injection was seen among 100 adults with low back pain and sacroiliac laxity (LOE: D).[57]
   b. Complete pain relief was seen in 48% of 42 adults with low back pain who were injected with Sylnasol (LOE: D).[58]
   c. The resolution of pain was seen in 82% of 267 adult patients with low back pain who were injected with Sylnasol/pontocaine or zinc/phenol (LOE: D).[59]
   d. Among 136 adults with low back pain who were injected with P2G, 45% experienced pain relief of more than 75% (LOE: D).[60]
   e. Of 43 adults with low back pain who were injected with sodium morrhuate, more than 75% pain relief was experience by 72% of patients (LOE: D).[61]
2. Older case series in chronic neck or head pain patients (not clearly stated as consecutive patients):
   a. Eighty-two patients with chronic neck sprain with pain were injected with P2G, and good to excellent pain reduction was seen in 82% of them (LOE: D).[62]
   b. Three hundred twenty-two patients with posttraumatic headache with pain that had lasted an average of 4 years were injected with Sylnasol, phenol/dextrose/glycerine, or zinc sulfate. Good to excellent pain elimination was seen among 59% of these patients (LOE: D).[63]
3. Recent double-blind studies with clear methods in low back pain patients:
   a. Eighty-one patients with chronic back pain were treated with P2G in lidocaine or with saline. Pain improvement of 60% as compared with 23% in control was seen at 6 months ($P < 0.001$) (LOE: A).[64]
   b. Chronic back pain in 81 patients was treated with P2G in lidocaine or saline with lidocaine. Pain improvement of 53% as compared with 38.5% in controls was seen at 6 months ($P = 0.056$) (LOE: A).[65]
   c. Chronic back pain in 74 patients was treated with P2G in lidocaine or 0.5% lidocaine in saline. Incorrect injection sites using inflammatory solution led to worse results in the active group (5% improvement in pain) and less than a placebo result in the control group (15% improvement in pain) (LOE: A).[50]
   d. One hundred ten patients with chronic back pain were injected with dextrose 20% in 0.2% lidocaine or 0.2% lidocaine. Incomplete injection method with deep sacroiliac ligament not treated for four sessions and inferior sacroiliac and sacrospinous/sacrotuberous ligaments not treated. A more than 50% reduction in pain was noted among 46% of glucose patients as compared with 36% of control patients. This difference was not significant, but results were durable at 2 years in both groups, thus indicating strongly that needling has a therapeutic effect even without proliferant included in the solution (LOE: A).[66]

Summary of basic science and clinical research on the injection of inflammatory proliferants

RIT using an inflammatory solution has received considerable clinical research attention for many years. Animal studies regarding microscopic and macroscopic changes are missing for dextrose and P2G, but they have been performed with sodium morrhuate. Mechanical changes in thickness, mass, and the strength of the ligament have been studied only with sodium morrhuate,[53] but tightening of knee laxity by an arthrometric measure has been demonstrated in a pilot study using P2G.[56] Case reports over many years demonstrate the safety of inflammatory solution

injection for both low back and neck pain, and they suggest efficacy.[67] However, double-blind studies with P2G or dextrose for back pain have been hampered by design flaws, including treatments simultaneous to injection,[64,65] incomplete injection technique,[66] improper patient selection leading to incorrect area injection,[50] a control that is not a placebo,[50,64-66] and the inclusion of patients who are receiving compensation for disability.[50] Nevertheless, treatment in each study resulted in considerable and sustainable improvement in pain and function. Similar to acupuncture and manipulation, true placebo controls for studies in RIT are difficult to design and expensive for investigators without usual funding sources for research.

Using regenerative injection therapy for the treatment of connective-tissue–based, career-threatening injuries in sports medicine (example of inflammatory dextrose use)

Conditions that are critically blocking full performance in the athlete and that are not amenable to surgery or that would require long periods of sports cessation are suitable for consecutive patient study using noninflammatory or inflammatory proliferant solutions. An example is a study by Topol and colleagues of 24 consecutive elite athletes (22 rugby and 2 soccer) with career-threatening or, potentially, career-ending chronic groin pain preventing full sports participation that was nonresponsive to therapy with graded sports reintroduction.[23] Patients received monthly injection of 12.5% dextrose and 0.5% lidocaine in adductor and abdominal insertions and the symphysis pubis, depending on palpation tenderness. Injections were given until complete resolution or lack of improvement for two consecutive treatments occurred. A mean of 2.8 treatments were given. A reduction in the visual analog pain scale score for pain with sports was from a mean of 6.3 to 1.0 ($P < 0.0001$), and the reduction in the Nirschl pain phase scale score was from 5.25 to 0.79 ($P < 0.0001$). Twenty out of 24 patients had no pain in the groin at an average follow-up time of 17 months, and 22 out of 24 patients were no longer restricted with regard to sports participation, with a success rate of return to elite sports of 92% (LOE: D).

Further such studies are forthcoming and will likely involve the use of brief inflammatory cascade stimulation; this appears to be not only economical and safe, but it also has been the best studied in both animals and humans.

Use of high-resolution ultrasound to document changes after proliferant injection
Case 1: Complete Achilles tendon rupture

A sectional study was recently published by Lazzara using radiographic imaging (magnetic resonance imaging and high-resolution ultrasound) to document healing (LOE: E).[68] The subject was a 26-year-old former European national soccer player who, during a soccer tournament, ruptured her Achilles tendon with a 1.1-cm gap; this was treated with casting in plantarflexion and no weight bearing for 60 days. The player refused surgery against medical advice, and she opted for proliferant injection. Strict avoidance of weight bearing was continued, and RIT was performed approximately every 10 days for 8 treatments over 3 months using 15% dextrose and 3.75% sodium morrhuate. Palpable filling in of the gap was noted by the second treatment visit, and, by 6 weeks (after three treatments), high-resolution ultrasound demonstrated newly formed tendon bridging the gap. Magnetic resonance imaging obtained at the tenth week after treatment onset showed an intact Achilles tendon. The athlete was jogging and aggressively stretching her Achilles tendon by 4 months. Clearly this was an instance in which surgery was the preferred alternative for treatment, and yet it serves to illustrate the potential for radiographic confirmation of soft-tissue healing by brief inflammatory cascade stimulation. Radiographic findings are found in the original source manuscript, but the following cases have ultrasound images available.

Case 2: A 61-year-old male golfer with extensor tendinosis

This patient had 3 years of left lateral elbow pain and 2 years of extension deficit in his elbow range, and he had received 3 steroid injections. His chief complaint was difficulty playing golf. On examination, he had a firm end feel to extension at -10 degrees, and there was pain over the common extensor insertion and the radial head. Magnetic resonance imaging was diagnostic for common extensor tendinosis. **Figure 50.1** shows a high-resolution ultrasound of the elbow in pronation at three different points in time. The images on the left and right are identical, but the images on the right are labeled anatomically: A is the radial head; the line labeled B is the bony narrowing between the lateral epicondyle and the capitulum of the humerus (the rounded portion of the end of the humerus that articulates with the radial head); C represents movement up the bone toward the lateral epicondyle; and E, which is only seen clearly in the bottom right view, is along the side of the capitulum of the humerus, which is better seen after proliferant injection. This patient received 9 injection sessions beginning on November 29, 2004. Several treatments were with dextrose 15%, and two included 0.5% sodium morrhuate. Common extensor entheses, annular ligament, radial collateral ligament, and capsular entheses were injected. The clinical result by August 15, 2005, was an extension range gain to -2 to -3 degrees, no pain on palpation, and no functional limitations. The serial ultrasounds demonstrate hypoechoic (dark) areas of tissue separation or insufficiency and edema (D is the common extensor tendon). By the time of the ultrasound on August 15, the entire region above the bones was more densely populated with organized connective tissue fibers. It is interesting to note that the capitulum (although it is not seen well on the first two ultrasounds) appears to move closer to the radial head, and dynamic ultrasound showed that radial head subluxation ceased as treatment progressed. This appears to correlate with the range-of-motion loss at treatment onset that also resolved with treatment. Note also that, although bony growth factors are not stimulated by injection, the typical effects after treatment with proliferant include a periosteal reaction that allows for the better visualization of contours of bone and an increased echogenicity of the soft tissue as edema resolves and tissue becomes more tightly packed.

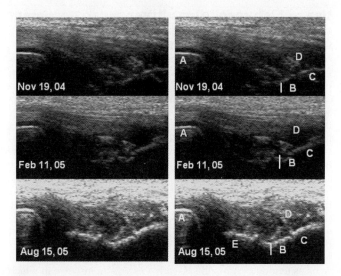

Figure 50.1 Extensor tendinosis changes with regenerative injection therapy.

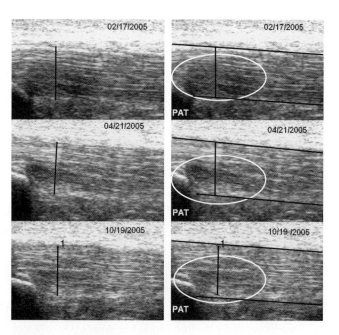

Figure 50.2 Patellar tendinosis changes with regenerative injection therapy.

Case 3: A cyclist with patellar tendinosis

A 40-year-old male competitive cyclist was first seen in November 2004 because he could not run or handle rough terrain or sustained hills as a result of knee pain. He had history of remote distal realignments (patellofemoral tracking type surgery). Pain was at the inferior patella and over the tibial tuberosity. He was treated on February 17, 2005, and April 21, 2005, with an injection of 15% dextrose over the patellar tendon origin on the inferior patella pole and its insertion over the tibial tuberosity. Complete symptom resolution occurred with the last follow-up evaluation on January 23, 2006, at which point the patient was training for the racing season. **Figure 50.2** shows a high-resolution ultrasound at the time of the first two sessions and at 6-month follow-up on October 19, 2005. On the right side of the figure are the same images but with red outlining the patellar tendon to depict its thickness. In addition, the yellow circle surrounds an area of hypoechogenicity. From February 17, 2005, through October 19, 2005, an increase in the echogenicity of the tendon is demonstrated.

Case 4: An 85-year-old male patient with bicipital tendinosis

Although this patient was not an athlete in the competitive sense, he was quite active for 85 years of age. This patient had chronic, worsening anterior shoulder pain. The initial examination on May 16, 2005, showed that the bicipital tendon and the surrounding region were painful to palpation. The patient received three treatments consisting of the injection of 15% dextrose around the bicipital region on May 27, June 17, and July 8, 2005, without regard for whether the injections were precisely extratendinous or intratendinous because the injections are always given on bone in successive rows. **Figure 50.3** shows a longitudinal ultrasound through the bicipital tendon at the time of the first evaluation and at follow-up on August 18, 2005. On the right side are the labeled images. Deltoid muscle thickness is represented by A in the figure, and the degree of decrease in the swelling in the deltoid is easily seen by the decrease in thickness by August 18. The long head of the bicipital tendon is outlined in yellow on the right, and,

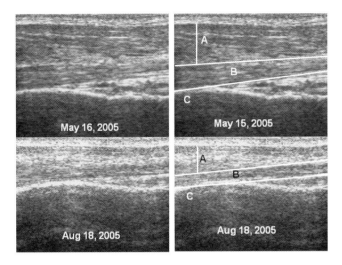

Figure 50.3 Biceps tendinosis changes with regenerative injection therapy (longitudinal view).

between May and August, the tendon changes shape to become more linear as edema decreases in the proximal portion. Again, an echogenicity increase throughout the region is seen. The point marked *C* is the proximal humerus at the distal onset of the bicipital groove. **Figure 50.4** is a transverse ultrasound image at the distal bicipital groove showing the subscapularis entheses as *A*, the lesser tubercle at *B*, the greater tubercle labeled *E*, and the deltoid thickness labeled *F*. The area labeled *C* is a hypoechoic area just outside the biceps tendon, and it is seen to decrease in echogenicity between May 16 and August 18, 2005. The point marked *D* is the biceps tendon itself in transverse view. The decrease in edema both in the overlying tissue and in the tendon itself is clearly seen along with an increase in the density of the bicipital tendon.

Cases 2 through 4 were performed in the same clinic by the same clinician. At each follow-up, the ultrasound examination, the patient position, the probe pressure, and the machine settings (including transmit and gain) were reproduced exactly as they had been during the prior study. In other words, the amount of sound transmitted by the probe was the same at each study; thus, the increase in tissue signal is felt to be related solely to an increase in tissue density.

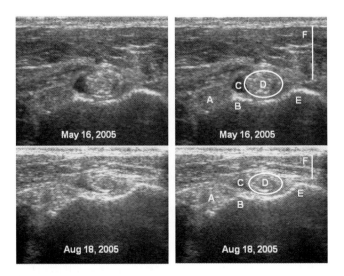

Figure 50.4 Biceps tendinosis changes with regenerative injection therapy (transverse view).

SUMMARY OF BASIC SCIENCE AND CLINICAL WORK IN PROLOTHERAPY/REGENERATIVE INJECTION THERAPY

Single growth-factor use is not likely to be fruitful as a result of the importance of cooperation among various growth factors. Multiple growth-factor provision by platelet concentrate is promising but limited in the area treatable by the volume of purified platelet concentrate. Noninflammatory dextrose appears to provide clinical benefit in both joint and ligament applications, and it is quite inexpensive. Inflammatory proliferant injection should be more potent than noninflammatory dextrose injection due to the multiplication effects of stimulating the inflammatory cascade. However, the occasional truly inflammatory process may be flared by such inflammatory proliferant solutions. Many studies have been performed to address growth stimulation and have covered all of the described approaches, and many more are desired. The biggest forces driving prolotherapy/RIT toward common usage are its low cost, its ability to actually tighten loose connective tissue, its promising effects on joints, its potential for widespread use in athletics to truly repair overuse injuries and partial tears, and its ability to objectively demonstrate radiographic healing with the increasing use of musculoskeletal ultrasound. It is likely that this will be the century for RIT in sports medicine. Although methods for prolotherapy performance are not the intent of this chapter, **Boxes 50.1 and 50.2** present indications, contraindications, pitfalls, and complications for the interested reader. A recommended text is by Hackett and colleagues,[69] and recent chapters addressing technique are found in *Pain Procedures in Clinical Practice*[70] and Waldman's *Pain Management*.[71]

Box 50.1: Indications and Contraindications for Regenerative Injection Therapy

Indications
1. Pain from chronic sprain or strain impairing athletic performance
2. Connective tissue laxity impairing athletic performance (i.e., shoulder capsular laxity, wrist laxity, anterior cruciate ligament laxity, repetitive ankle inversion tendency)
3. Pain from career sport or activity impairing rest and quality of life

Contraindications
1. Potential local infection
2. Allergies (i.e., to local anesthetics if they are used or to shellfish if sodium morrhuate is used); phenol is used digestively and can have no allergy; corn allergy does not appear to be an issue or very rarely (dextrose is made from corn)
3. Local inflammatory process: noninflammatory proliferants would be suggested, potentially after deinflammation with steroid
4. Injection of a prosthetic joint (on principle as a result of increased morbidity in the event of a rare infection); injection around a prosthetic joint as a result of external joint pain sources may be necessary
5. Patient on anticoagulation with an elevated international normalized ratio (it is preferable to have coumadin held before injection similar to other injection procedures); intraspinal hematomas have never been reported but hemarthrosis and hematomas have been either in those with an elevated international normalized ratio or in those taking Lovenox

---

Box 50.2: Pitfalls and Complications of Regenerative Injection Therapy

Needling Risks (Depending on the Portion of the Body Being Treated)

1. Septic joint: This appears to be similar to steroid injection risk at a rate of 1 in 10,000 to 1 in 40,000 for intra-articular injections.

2. Spinal headache: This is estimated to occur in 1 in 300 low back procedures with lumbosacral junction treatment.

3. Peripheral nerve contact: As a result of the ubiquitous presence of small nerve branches and the occasional contact of larger nerve branches, nerve irritation will occur rarely with treatment. Burning pain reactions are typical, lasting from days to several months.

4. Pneumothorax: This is estimated to occur in about 1 in 20,000 needle insertions in the thoracic region.

Solution Risks

1. Stiffness and soreness after treatment: Typically this will last from 1 to 3 days but will occasionally last longer. It is important to have patient contact the physician if flare lasts for more than 10 days because this can be counterproductive in patients with chronic pain.

2. Allergy: Any physician performing injection should prepare for such a reaction and check, in particular, for shellfish allergy before administering sodium morrhuate.

3. Chemical arachnoiditis: This appears to occur with midline injection only of stronger proliferants such as phenol and when boluses in the midline exceed 0.5% or the concentration of phenol exceeds 1.25%. However, this is rare and almost always temporary. Nevertheless, paraspinal injections anywhere near the neural foramina should be with a lesser solution or with small doses and a careful emphasis on concentration limits.

CONCLUSION

Suboptimal healing may lead to elimination of symptoms and return to full sport. However, suboptimal tissue leaves the athlete with a decrease in tensile strength of the damaged tissue or relative laxity with stretch of fixed length nerve endings. These effects increase susceptibility of the athlete to repetitive injury or rupture, can reflexly inhibit full performance, and create a regional stiffness, even without associated pain. All these are threats to a full and enjoyable carrer for the elite athlete and can increase the potential for chronic pain after retirement. Much remains to be discovered about stimulating regeneration and blocking degeneration after acute or chronic sports injuries. However, current agents appear capable of restoring connective tissue organization, as seen by ultrasonographic confirmation. The choice of agents will depend on such factors as speed of healing needed, cost efficacy, and the stage of the season.

Education on the basic science of connective tissue injuries and training on how to choose and apply the most cost-effective method of regenerative injection therapy will best be achieved in the context of routine physical medicine and rehabilitation training. Ultrasonographic documentation of lesion reversal may ultimately be used to monitor healing efficacy in this age of evidence-based medicine.

REFERENCES

1. Wang JH: Mechanobiology of tendon. J Biomech 2006;39:1563-1582.
2. Kirkendall DT, Garrett WE: Function and biomechanics of tendons. Scand J Med Sci Sports 1997;7:62-66.
3. Woo SL, Gomez MA, Amiel D, et al: The effects of exercise on the biomechanical and biochemical properties of swine digital flexor tendons. J Biomech Eng 1981;103:51-56.
4. Soslowsky LJ, Thomopoulos S, Tun S, et al: Overuse activity injures the supraspinatus tendon in an animal model: a histologic and biomechanical study. J Shoulder Elbow Surg 2000;9:79-84.
5. Kjaer M: Role of extracellular matrix in adaptation of tendon and skeletal muscle to mechanical loading. Physiol Rev 2004;84:649-698.
6. Young JS, Kumta SM, Maffulli N: Achilles tendon rupture and tendinopathy: management of complications. Foot Ankle Clin 2005;10:371-382.
7. Zernicke RF, Garhammer J, Jobe FW: Human patellar-tendon rupture. J Bone Joint Surg Am 1977;59:179-183.
8. Stanish WD, Rubinovich RM, Curwin S: Eccentric exercise in chronic tendinitis. Clin Orthop Relat Res 1986;208:65-68.
9. Kannus P, Jozsa L, Natri A, Jarvinen M: Effects of training, immobilization and remobilization on tendons. Scand J Med Sci Sports 1997;7:67-71.
10. Warden SJ: Cyclo-oxygenase-2 inhibitors: beneficial or detrimental for athletes with acute musculoskeletal injuries? Sports Med 2005;35(4):271-283.
11. Saltzman CL, Tearse DS: Achilles tendon injuries. J Am Acad Ortho Surg 1998;6:316-325.
12. Marsolais D, Cote CH, Frenette J: Nonsteroidal anti-inflammatory drug reduces neutrophil and macrophage accumulation but does not improve tendon regeneration. Lab Invest 2003;83(7):991-999.
13. Marsolais D, Frenette J: Inflammation and tendon healing. Med Sci 2005;21(2):181-186.
14. Sun R, Gimbel HV, Liu S, et al: Effect of diclofenac sodium and dexamethasone on cultured human Tenon's capsule fibroblasts. Ophthalmic Surg Lasers 1999;30(5):382-388.
15. Elder CL, Dahners LE, Weinhold PS: A cyclooxygenase-inhibitor impairs ligament healing in the rat. Am J Sports Med 2001;29(6):801-810.
16. Riley GP, Cox M, Harrall RL, et al: Inhibition of tendon cell proliferation and matrix glycosaminoglycan synthesis by non-steroidal anti-inflammatory drugs in vitro. J Hand Surg 2001;26(3):224-228.
17. Dahners LE, Mullis BH: Effects of nonsteroidal anti-inflammatory drugs on bone formation and soft-tissue healing. J Am Acad Orthop Surg 2004;12(3):139-143.
18. Paoloni JA, Orchard JW: The use of therapeutic medications for soft-tissue injuries in sports medicine. Med J Aust 2005;183(7):384-388.
19. Cohen DB, Kawamura S, Ehteshami J, et al: Indomethacin and celecoxib impair rotator cuff tendon-to-bone healing. Am J Sports Med 2006;34(3):362-369.
20. Kennedy J, Willis RB: The effects of local steroid injections on tendons: a biomechanical and microscopic correlative study. Am J Sports Med 1976;4:11-21.
21. Nirschl RP: Elbow tendinosis/tennis elbow. Clin Sports Med 1992;11(4):851-870.
22. Reeves KD: Technique of prolotherapy. In Lennard TA (ed): Physiatric Procedures in Clinical Practice. Philadelphia, Hanley and Belfus, 1995, pp 57-70.
23. Topol GA, Reeves KD, Hassanein K: Efficacy of dextrose prolotherapy in elite male kicking-sport athletes with chronic groin pain. Arch Phys Med Rehabil 2005;86(4):697-702.
24. Price S, Pepper JR, Jaggar SI: Recombinant human erythropoietin use in a critically ill Jehovah's witness after cardiac surgery. Anesth Analg 2005;101(2):325-327.
25. Wang JH, Losifidis MI, Fu FH: Biomechanical basis for tendinopathy. Clin Orthop Relat Res 2006;443:320-322.
26. Molloy T, Wang Y, Murrell G: The roles of growth factors in tendon and ligament healing. Sports Med 2003;33:381-394.
27. Dahlgren LA, van der Meulen MC, Bertram JE, et al: Insulin-like growth factor-1 improves cellular and molecular aspects of healing in a collagenase-induced model of flexor tendinitis. J Orthop Res 2003;20:910-919.
28. Aspenberg P, Forslund C: Bone morphogenetic proteins and tendon repair. Scand J Med Sci Sports 2000;10:372-375.
29. Fu SC, Wong YP, Chan BP, et al: The roles of bone morphogenetic protein (BMP) 12 in stimulating the proliferation and matrix production of human patellar tendon fibroblasts. Life Sci 2003;72:2965-2974.
30. Forslund C, Aspenberg P: Improved healing of transected rabbit Achilles tendon after a single injection of cartilage-derived morphogenetic protein-2. Am J Sports Med 2003;31:555-559.
31. Kashiwagi K, Mochizuki Y, Yasunaga Y, et al: Effects of transforming growth factor-beta 1 on the early stages of healing of the Achilles tendon in a rat model. Scand J Plast Reconstr Surg Hand Surg 2004;38(4):193-197.
32. Kurtz CA, Loebig TG, Anderson DD, et al: Insulin-like growth factor I accelerates functional recovery from Achilles tendon injury in a rat model. Am J Sports Med 1999;27:363-369.
33. Tsubone T, Moran SL, Amadio PC, et al: Expression of growth factors in canine flexor tendon after laceration in vivo. Ann Plast Surg 2004;53(4):393-397.
34. Thomopoulos S, Harwood FL, Silva MJ, et al: Effect of several growth factors on canine flexor tendon fibroblast proliferation and collagen synthesis in vitro. J Hand Surg 2005;30(3):441-447.
35. Anitua E, Andia I, Sanchez M, et al: Autologous preparations rich in growth factors promote proliferation and induce VEGF and HGF production by human tendon cells in culture. J Orthop Res 2005;23(2):281-286.

36. Aspenberg P, Virchenko O: Platelet concentrate injection improves Achilles tendon repair in rats. Acta Orthop Scand 2004;75(1):93-99.
37. Taylor MA, Norman TL, Clovis NB, et al: The response of rabbit patellar tendons after autologous blood injection. Med Sci Sports Exerc 2002;34(1):70-73.
38. Edwards SG, Calandruccio JH: Autologous blood injections for refractory lateral epicondylitis. J Hand Surg 2003;28A(2):272-278.
39. Di Paolo S, Gesualdo L, Ranieri E, et al: High glucose concentration induces the overexpression of transforming growth factor-beta through the activation of a platelet-derived growth factor loop in human mesangial cells. Am J Pathol 1996;149(6):2095-2106.
40. Oh JH, Ha H, Yu MR, et al: Sequential effects of high glucose on mesangial cell transforming growth factor-beta 1 and fibronectin synthesis. Kidney Int 1998;54(6):1872-1878.
41. Murphy M, Godson C, Cannon S, et al: Suppression subtractive hybridization identifies high glucose levels as a stimulus for expression of connective tissue growth factor and other genes in human mesangial cells. J Biol Chem 1999;274(9):5830-5834.
42. Fukuda K, Kawata S, Inui Y, et al: High concentration of glucose increases mitogenic responsiveness to heparin-binding epidermal growth factor-like growth factor in rat vascular smooth muscle cells. Arterioscler Thromb Vasc Biol 1997;17(10):1962-1968.
43. Ohgi S, Johnson PW: Glucose modulates growth of gingival fibroblasts and periodontal ligament cells: correlation with expression of basic fibroblast growth factor. J Periodontal Res 1996;31(8):579-588.
44. Pugliese G, Pricci F, Locuratolo N, et al: Increased activity of the insulin-like growth factor system in mesangial cells cultured in high glucose conditions. Relation to glucose-enhanced extracellular matrix production. Diabetologia 1996;39(7):775-784.
45. Woo SL, Hildebrand K, Watanabe N, et al: Tissue engineering of ligament and tendon healing. Clin Orthop Relat Res 1999;367S:312-314.
46. Jones SC, Saunders HJ, Qi W, et al: Intermittent high glucose enhances cell growth and collagen synthesis in cultured human tubulointerstitial cells. Diabetologia 1999;42(9):1113-1119.
47. Reeves KD, Hassanein K: Long term effects of dextrose prolotherapy for anterior cruciate ligament laxity: a prospective and consecutive patient study. Altern Ther Health Med 2003;9(3):58-62.
48. Reeves KD, Hassanein K: Randomized prospective double-blind placebo-controlled study of dextrose prolotherapy for knee osteoarthritis with or without ACL laxity. Altern Ther Health Med 2000;6(2):68-80.
49. Reeves KD, Hassanein K: Randomized prospective placebo controlled double blind study of dextrose prolotherapy for osteoarthritic thumbs and finger (DIP, PIP and trapeziometacarpal) joints: evidence of clinical efficacy. J Altern Complement Med 2000;6(4):311-320.
50. Dechow E, Davies RK, Carr AJ, et al: A randomized, double-blind, placebo-controlled trial of sclerosing injections in patients with chronic low back pain. Rheumatology 1999;38(12):1255-1259.
51. Altay T, Gunal I, Ozturk H: Local injection treatment for lateral epicondylitis. Clin Orthop 2002;398:127-130.
52. Hackett GS. Ligament and Tendon Relaxation Treated by Prolotherapy, 3rd ed. Springfield, IL, Charles C. Thomas, 1956.
53. Liu YK, Tipton CM, Matthes RD, et al: An in-situ study of the influence of a sclerosing solution in rabbit medial collateral ligaments and its junction strength. Connect Tissue Res 1983;11:95-102.
54. Maynard JA: Morphological and biochemical effects of sodium morrhuate on tendons. J Orthop Res 1985;3(2):236-248.
55. Aneja A, Karas SG, Weinhold PS, et al: Suture plication, thermal shrinkage, and sclerosing agents: Effects on rat patellar tendon length and biomechanical strength. Am J Sports Med 2005;33(11):1729-1734.
56. Ongley MJ, Dorman TA, Eek BC, et al: Ligament instability of knees: a new approach to treatment. Man Med 1988;3:152-154.
57. Bahme BB: Observations on the treatment of hypermobile joints by injection. J Am Osteopath Assoc 1945;45:101-109.
58. Blaschke JA: Conservative management of intervertebral disc injuries. J Okla State Med Assoc 1961;54:494-501.
59. Myers A: Prolotherapy treatment of low back pain and sciatica. Bull Hosp Joint Dis 1961;22:48-55.
60. Peterson TH: Injection treatment for back pain. Am J Orthop Surg 1963;246:320-321.
61. Schwartz RG, Segedy N: Prolotherapy: a literature review and retrospective study. J Neurol Orthop Med Surg 1991;12:220-223.
62. Hackett GS, Huang TC: Prolotherapy for headache. Headache 1962;2:20-28.
63. Kayfetz DO, Blumenthal LS, Hacket GS, et al: Whiplash injury and other ligamentous headache: its management with prolotherapy. Headache 1963;3:21-28.
64. Ongley MJ, Klein RG, Dorman TA, et al: A new approach to the treatment of chronic low back pain. Lancet 1987;2:143-146.
65. Klein RG, Bjorn CE, DeLong B, et al: A randomized double-blind trial of dextrose-glycerine-phenol injections for chronic low back pain. J Spinal Disord 1993;6:23-33.
66. Yelland MJ, Glasziou PP, Bogduk N, et al: Prolotherapy injections, saline injections, and exercises for chronic low-back pain: a randomized trial. Spine 2004;29(1):9-16.
67. Rabago D, Best TM, Beamsley M, Patterson J: A systematic review of prolotherapy for chronic musculoskeletal pain. Clin J Sport Med 2005;15(5):376-380.
68. Lazzara MA: The non-surgical repair of a complete Achilles tendon rupture by prolotherapy: biological reconstruction. A case report. J Orthop Med 2005;27(3):128-132.
69. Hackett GS, Hemwall GA, Montgomery GA. In Hemwall Gustav A (ed): Ligament and Tendon Relaxation Treated by Prolotherapy, 5th ed. IL, Oak Park, 1992.
70. Reeves KD: Prolotherapy: basic science, clinical studies, and technique. In Lennard TA (ed): Pain Procedures in Clinical Practice, 2nd ed. Philadelphia, Hanley and Belfus, 2000, pp 172-190.
71. Reeves KD: Prolotherapy: injection of growth factors or growth factor production stimulants to grow normal cells or tissue. In Waldman SD (ed): Pain Management. Philadelphia, Elsevier, 2006, pp 1106-1127.

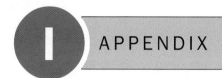

APPENDIX

Team Physician Consensus Statement

SUMMARY

The objective of the Team Physician Consensus Statement is to provide physicians, school administrators, team owners, the general public, and individuals who are responsible for making decisions regarding the medical care of athletes and teams with guidelines for choosing a qualified team physician and an outline of the duties expected of a team physician. Ultimately, by educating decision makers about the need for a qualified team physician, the goal is to ensure that athletes and teams are provided the very best medical care.

The Consensus Statement was developed by the collaboration of six major professional associations concerned about clinical sports medicine issues: American Academy of Family Physicians, American Academy of Orthopaedic Surgeons, American College of Sports Medicine, American Medical Society for Sports Medicine, American Orthopaedic Society for Sports Medicine, and the American Osteopathic Academy of Sports Medicine. These organizations have committed to forming an ongoing project-based alliance to "bring together sports medicine organizations to best serve active people and athletes."

EXPERT PANEL

Stanley A. Herring, MD, Chair, Seattle, Washington
John A. Bergfeld, MD, Cleveland, Ohio
Joel Boyd, MD, Edina, Minnesota
William G. Clancy, Jr, MD, Birmingham, Alabama
H. Royer Collins, MD, Phoenix, Arizona
Brian C. Halpern, MD, Marlboro, New Jersey
Rebecca Jaffe, MD, Chadds Ford, Pennsylvania
W. Ben Kibler, MD, Lexington, Kentucky
E. Lee Rice, DO, San Diego, California
David C. Thorson, MD, White Bear Lake, Minnesota

TEAM PHYSICIAN DEFINITION

The team physician must have an unrestricted medical license and be an MD or DO who is responsible for treating and coordinating

Reprinted with permission of the project-based alliance for the advancement of clinical sports medicine, which is comprised of the American Academy of Family Physicians, the American Academy of Orthopaedic Surgeons, the American College of Sports Medicine, the American Medical Society for Sports Medicine, the American Orthopaedic Society for Sports Medicine, and the American Osteopathic Academy of Sports Medicine, © 2000. Supported by an unrestricted educational grant from Knoll Pharmaceuticals.

the medical care of athletic team members. The principal responsibility of the team physician is to provide for the well being of individual athletes—enabling each to realize his/her full potential. The team physician should possess special proficiency in the care of musculoskeletal injuries and medical conditions encountered in sports. The team physician also must actively integrate medical expertise with other health care providers, including medical specialists, athletic trainers, and allied health professionals. The team physician must ultimately assume responsibility within the team structure for making medical decisions that affect the athlete's safe participation.

QUALIFICATIONS OF A TEAM PHYSICIAN

The primary concern of the team physician is to provide the best medical care for athletes at all levels of participation. To this end, the following qualifications are necessary for all team physicians:

- Have an MD or DO in good standing, with an unrestricted license to practice medicine
- Possess a fundamental knowledge of emergency care regarding sporting events
- Be trained in cardiopulmonary resuscitation
- Have a working knowledge of trauma, musculoskeletal injuries, and medical conditions affecting the athlete

In addition, it is desirable for team physicians to have clinical training, experience, and administrative skills in some or all of the following:

- Specialty Board certification
- Continuing medical education in sports medicine
- Formal training in sports medicine (fellowship training, board-recognized subspecialty in sports medicine [formerly known as a certificate of added qualification in sports medicine])
- Additional training in sports medicine
- Fifty percent or more of practice involving sports medicine
- Membership and participation in a sports medicine society
- Involvement in teaching, research, and publications relating to sports medicine
- Training in advanced cardiac life support
- Knowledge of medical/legal, disability, and workers' compensation issues
- Media skills training

DUTIES OF A TEAM PHYSICIAN

The team physician must be willing to commit the necessary time and effort to provide care to the athlete and team. In addition, the team physician must develop and maintain a current, appropriate knowledge base of the sport(s) for which he/she is accepting responsibility. The duties for which the team physician has ultimate responsibility include the following:

- Medical management of the athlete
- Coordinate preparticipation screening, examination, and evaluation
- Manage injuries on the field
- Provide medical management of injury and illness
- Coordinate rehabilitation and return to participation
- Provide for proper preparation for safe return to participation after an illness or injury
- Integrate medical expertise with other health care providers, including medical specialists, athletic trainers, and allied health professionals
- Provide for appropriate education and counseling regarding nutrition, strength and conditioning, ergogenic aids, substance abuse, and other medical problems that could affect the athlete
- Provide for proper documentation and medical record keeping
- Administrative and logistical duties
- Establish and define the relationships of all involved parties
- Educate athletes, parents, administrators, coaches, and other necessary parties of concerns regarding the athletes
- Develop a chain of command
- Plan and train for emergencies during competition and practice
- Address equipment and supply issues
- Provide for proper event coverage
- Assess environmental concerns and playing conditions

EDUCATION OF A TEAM PHYSICIAN

Ongoing education pertinent to the team physician is essential. Currently, there are several state, regional, and national stand-alone courses for team physician education. There are also many other resources available. Information regarding team-physician––specific educational opportunities can be obtained from the organizations under Conclusion.

Team physician education is also available from other sources such as: sport-specific (e.g., National Football League Team Physician's Society) or level-specific (e.g., United States Olympic Committee) meetings; National Governing Bodies' (NGB) meetings; state and/or county medical society meetings; professional journals; and other relevant electronic media (Web sites, CD-ROMs).

CONCLUSION

American Academy of Family Physicians (AAFP)
11400 Tomahawk Creek Pkwy
Leawood, KS 66211-2672
1-800-274-2237

American Academy of Orthopaedic Surgeons (AAOS)
6300 N River Rd
Rosemont, IL 60018
1-800-346-AAOS

American College of Sports Medicine (ACSM)
401 W Michigan St
Indianapolis, IN 46202-3233
317-637-9200

American Medical Society for Sports Medicine (AMSSM)
11639 Earnshaw
Overland Park, KS 66210
913-327-1415

American Orthopaedic Society for Sports Medicine (AOSSM)
6300 N River Rd, Suite 200
Rosemont, IL 60018
847-292-4900

American Osteopathic Academy of Sports Medicine (AOASM)
7611 Elmwood Ave, Suite 201
Middleton, WI 53562
608-831-4400

This Consensus Statement establishes a definition of the team physician and outlines a team physician's qualifications, duties, and responsibilities. It also contains strategies for the continuing education of team physicians. Ultimately, this statement provides guidelines that best serve the health care needs of athletes and teams.

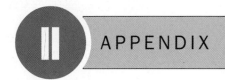

Sports and Physical Activity in Youth

Bernard Purcell, MS, and Mark B. Stephens, MD, MS

KEY POINTS

- The number of overweight children and adolescents in the United States has quadrupled over the last 30 years.
- Both inactivity and overeating play a role in rising obesity levels. The impact of inactivity seems to be the most critical.
- An individual's habitual level of physical activity is directly related to all-cause mortality. Physical activity reduces the risk for cardiovascular disease, diabetes, hypertension, osteoporosis, and obesity and has beneficial effects on mental and emotional health as well.
- If the present trend of inactivity and overweight continues, the current generation of children will be the first in modern American history to have a life-expectancy shorter than its parents.
- Physicians can combat overweight by helping to address barriers to activity and consistently counseling their patients regarding the benefits of an active lifestyle.
- Specifically, physicians should: (1) accurately assess activity levels among youth; (2) identify and help patients to overcome barriers to physical activity; and (3) create patient-specific solutions to promote physical activity.

INTRODUCTION

The United States is in the midst of an epidemic of overweight. A central contributing factor to this epidemic is a decline in average physical activity levels among children. Despite the proven benefits of physical activity, American youth are less physically active than ever before. Predictably, as physical activity decreases, overweight increases. The American College of Sports Medicine,[1] the Centers for Disease Control and Prevention,[2] *Healthy People 2010*,[3] and the Surgeon General's Call to Action[4] have all issued recommendations aimed at reversing the trend of inactivity-related overweight. Despite expert recommendations, activity levels continue to decline and children continue to gain excess weight.

The benefits of exercise are seen at the earliest ages of childhood development. Improved cardiovascular health,[5] reduced risk of hypertension[5] and diabetes,[6] and improved self-esteem[7] are but a few of the positive elements of routine physical activity. Although levels of activity naturally decline as a person ages,

behaviors established during childhood persist into adulthood.[8] Therefore, regular bouts of physical activity during childhood translate to an active adult lifestyle. Because of this, physicians must know the benefits of physical activity, recognize barriers to an active lifestyle, and implement patient-centered solutions to promote physical activity among America's youth.

WHAT IS THE STATUS QUO?

Over the past three decades, the prevalence of overweight children and adolescents between the ages of 6 and 19 has quadrupled.[9] Levels of physical activity among American youth have concurrently dropped as exercise is replaced by sedentary behaviors. American teens now average only 12 minutes of vigorous activity per day. Television, video and computer games, and mechanized personal transport (i.e., elevators and cars) have eliminated or reduced the energy expenditure associated with routine daily activities.

WHY IS EXERCISE IMPORTANT?

The health benefits of activity are numerous. An individual's habitual level of physical activity is the most significant determinant of all-cause mortality.[10] Physical activity specifically reduces the risk for cardiovascular disease,[11] diabetes,[6] hypertension,[11] osteoporosis,[6] and obesity.[12]

Physical activity positively impacts mental health as well. Regular physical activity reduces levels of stress and anxiety, improves self-esteem, and improves body image.[7] Adolescents who are not physically active are more likely to engage in high-risk behaviors such as cigarette use, drug use, and engage in early sexual activity.[3]

WHY DON'T YOUTH EXERCISE?

Many factors contribute to the lack of sufficient physical activity among American youth.

School factors

The past two decades have seen a precipitous decline in physical activity during high school. This includes leisure time activity as well as school-based activity.[13] Although roughly 70% of

12-year-old to 13-year-old children meet recommended activity levels, only 40% of youth between the ages of 18 to 21 years reach this level of activity.[14] Currently, less than half of all students are enrolled in dedicated physical education classes.[14] Of those who are enrolled, only one third attend class daily. The students who do attend physical education often do not engage in sufficiently vigorous activity during class. Many students stand around awaiting instructions or engage only in short bursts of intermittent activity.[21] Physical education attendance correlates positively with an active adult lifestyle.[14] Thus, it is important that clinicians advocate for physical education programming within their local community schools.

Personal factors

Personal characteristics, such as gender and educational level also correlate with individual activity levels. Distinct differences in levels of physical activity exist between males and females. Males are more likely than females to routinely engage in physical activity.[6] For example, during physical education class males spend more time engaged in physical activity than do females. Additionally, more males participate in after-school sports programs. This trend of gender differences in physical activity in males begins in childhood and continues throughout adolescence.[3]

Another personal factor impacting routine levels of physical activity is "athletic perception." This phenomenon occurs as a shift from generalized physical activity ("play") to specific sporting events ("organized sports") during childhood and adolescence. Paradoxically, although participation of organized sports is growing, overall rates of physical activity and fitness are decreasing. Whether it is a child's self-perception of athleticism, the perception of a coach, or the perception of a parent, the translation of physical activity to sports eliminates certain children or adolescents from participation. Some children do not have the athletic ability or competitive drive to participate in high-level sports. In this case, self-elimination is likely. As opportunities for formal sports participation increase, chances for informal physical activities or recreational sports often become less available to youths, thus further eliminating opportunities for activity.

Educational level also predicts an individual's habitual level of physical activity. Lower educational levels and poor school performance correlate with decreased physical activity among both boys and girls.[15,16] Interestingly, higher grades in physical education correlate positively with future activity levels.[15] Maternal education level also positively influences the activity levels of children.[16]

Cultural factors

Family is the primary cultural determinant of a child's habitual level of physical activity. Family size, parental activity levels, and housing location influence childhood activity levels.[27] In general, children in large families are more likely to be physically active than children living in small families. Urban youth are more likely to be active than those from rural settings.[16] Paradoxically, children living on farms engage in the lowest amount of leisure-time physical activity.[28] Children also follow the examples of their parents. Children with inactive and overweight parents are more likely to be overweight and inactive themselves.

Physical activity levels differ among ethnic and racial groups as well. In the United States, Hispanic and African American youth have lower rates of physical activity and higher rates of obesity than non-Hispanic whites[3,18] **(Figure App-II.1).**

Social factors also influence the activity of children and adolescents. Socioeconomic status is one of the strongest predictors of activity levels. Children of lower socioeconomic status are the least likely to engage in routine physical activity.[16]

Environmental factors

Environment factors also influence levels of activity in children and adolescents. The availability and proximity of safe opportunities for activity may influence a child's desire to engage in leisure or spontaneous activity. Parks or recreation centers provide an environment that fosters physical activity. Children who use a recreation center are more likely to achieve regular bouts of moderate to vigorous activity than those who do not.

Finally, television, video games, and home computers are major determinants of physical activity levels among children. Time spent watching television, surfing the Internet, or playing video games inversely correlates with activity levels.[4,19] A majority of American households have at least one television. Seventy percent of high-school students watch 1 hour of television a day; 43% watch 2 or more hours a day.[20] It follows, therefore, that physical activity levels are inversely correlated with television viewing. Children should be encouraged to limit video gaming, computer time (outside of homework activities), and television viewing to less than a total of 1 hour per day.

WHAT CAN BE DONE?

General guidelines

In response to decreasing levels of childhood physical activity, several professional organizations have released position statements to promote exercise. The American College of Sports Medicine recommends 15 to 60 minutes of moderate to vigorous physical activity on most (preferably all) days of the week.[1] The Centers for Disease Control and Prevention recommend 30 minutes or more of physical activity within the normal daily routine for improving wellness.[2] *Healthy People 2010* recognized the lack of activity among children and set specific goals to increase activity level[3] **(Table App-II.1).** The Surgeon General's Call to Action to Combat Disease and Obesity emphasizes that physical activity improves overall health and wellness by affecting obesity, cholesterol levels, heart disease, and anxiety.[4] Although each of these guidelines offers a particular view of physical activity, all are consistent in recommending that children obtain 30 minutes of moderate to vigorous physical activity on most (preferably all) days of the week.

The physician's role

Physicians play a central role in promoting activity. Physicians can make a huge impact by candidly discussing the problem of physical inactivity and overweight with young patients and their parents. Unfortunately, routine discussion of the importance of physical activity occurs in only 15%-20% of visits with overweight children. To help promote activity physicians should do the following: (1) accurately assess activity levels; (2) identify and help to overcome barriers to physical activity; and (3) create patient-specific solutions to promote physical activity.

Assessing a patient's activity level

For physicians to offer valid counseling to improve physical activity, they must first be able to evaluate a child's current level of physical activity. This can be done through direct patient observation, mechanical device recordings (pedometers or heart rate monitors), or patient/parent self-reporting. Each of these methods has advantages and disadvantages in terms of feasibility, labor requirements, and reporting error. For practical purposes, parent or youth self-reporting is the easiest to use.

Identifying and overcoming barriers

It is important to identify individual patient barriers to physical activity. Scholastic, personal, cultural, and environmental factors

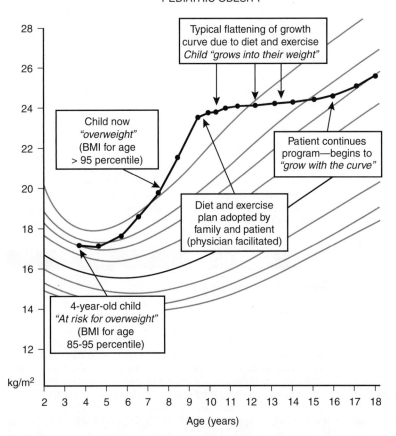

WHY DIET AND EXERCISE WORK FOR
PEDIATRIC OBESITY

Typical flattening of growth
curve due to diet and exercise
Child "grows into their weight"

Child now
"overweight"
(BMI for age
> 95 percentile)

Patient continues
program—begins to
"grow with the curve"

Diet and exercise
plan adopted by
family and patient
(physician facilitated)

4-year-old child
"At risk for overweight"
(BMI for age
85-95 percentile)

kg/m²

Age (years)

Figure App-II.1 Diet and exercise are effective treatments for pediatric obesity. A typical case of pediatric obesity responding to a lifestyle modification program. The growth chart used is the Centers for Disease Control and Prevention body mass index for age for boys who are 2 to 20 years of age. (From Levin S: Arch Pediatr Adolesc Med 2003;157:816-820.)

all affect an individual's exercise participation. Identifying and addressing these barriers is a key step in improving a child or adolescent's activity habits.

Creating patient-specific solutions

Well-child visits, preparticipation physical examinations, and general wellness examinations provide perfect opportunities for preventive counseling. Approximately 80% of children and adolescents visit a physician each year, and most believe their physician to be a credible source of health information.[21] Preventive office-based counseling has a positive effect on physical activity patterns.[22] Unfortunately, most opportunities for counseling are consistently missed by physicians. In more than 60% of visits from 1997 to 2000, preventive counseling was not documented.[23]

It is important, therefore, to create a specific, age-appropriate activity program for each patient. Throughout youth, children and adolescents differ with regard to both physical and mental maturity. Activity should be prescribed in a developmentally appropriate

manner for each patient. Unorganized play such as running, tumbling, and catching on safe, flat surfaces is appropriate for early childhood. Early adolescents understand rules and have improved coordination. For this age group, sports like football, basketball, and ice hockey are appropriate. Older adolescents should participate in activities of personal preference, whether team sports or an individual activities. Physicians should support their patients' involvement in activities in which continued participation is most likely.

PACE+: One example

One practical program that physicians can use is the Patient-Centered Assessment and Counseling for Exercise + Nutrition (PACE +) program. PACE + was developed to provide physicians with an accurate, rapid method for assessing activity. PACE + also serves as a guide for counseling related to physical activity and nutrition. This program combines computer-based assessment, clinical counseling, and phone and mail contact to promote patient

---

Table App-II.1   Physical Activity Goals for Children—*Healthy People 2010*

Population Goals	School System Goals	Inactivity Goals
Increase the number of adolescents achieving 30 min/day of moderate physical activity	Increase the number of public and private schools requiring physical education classes	Reduce the number of adolescents viewing ≥2 hours/day of television or screen-based media
Increase the number of adolescents achieving 30 min/day of vigorous physical activity	Increase the number of adolescents active in physical education classes	Increase the number of trips made by bicycle or walking

From the US Department of Health and Human Services: Healthy People 2010: Understanding and Improving Health. Washington, DC, US Department of Health and Human Services, US Government Printing Office, 2000.

wellness. PACE + is tailored to each youth and is an effective tool for improving physical activity and nutritional practices.[21] PACE + is a feasible and effective tool for improving adolescent activity (www.paceproject.org/home.html).

SPECIAL CONSIDERATIONS

Risks of exercise: Sudden cardiac death

Exercise is not without risk. Exercise-associated sudden cardiac death is the primary catastrophic risk associated with physical activity in young athletes. Fortunately, the incidence of this is quite low (1 in 200,000 to 1 in 300,000). However, if young people choose not to exercise regularly, many more will suffer premature death from complications of diabetes and other obesity-related illness. In fact, if the current trajectory of inactivity and obesity continues, the current generation of children will be the first in modern American history to have a life-expectancy that is shorter than that of their parents.[24]

The preparticipation physical examination is an excellent opportunity for screening young athletes for risks for sudden cardiac death (see Chapter 2, Preparticipation Examination). Patients with a history of exertional syncope are at greater risk for a sudden cardiac event, and should be screened with either an electrocardiogram or an echocardiogram. Additionally, patients with a family history of sudden cardiac death before the age of 50 years should undergo further testing. Cardiac murmurs that change with characteristic physical maneuvers should also be evaluated.[25] Primary care providers should have a very low threshold for specialty referral in patients with a concerning history or unusual examination findings.

Risks of exercise: Musculoskeletal injury

Another risk associated with physical activity is musculoskeletal injury. The risks of injury are low, however, compared with the benefits of exercise. Nevertheless, childhood injuries can be associated with significant morbidity and occasionally long-term disability as adults. During the preparticipation examination, physicians should focus on injury prevention. Specifically, patients and their parents should be counseled about the proper use of protective equipment and appropriate training regimens. Injury prevention is a relatively new science that attempts to design exercise equipment, institute rule changes, and create training programs to provide maximal protection against injury.

Atkins or South Beach: Is dieting appropriate for kids?

Dieting is an effective means of losing weight in adults and if safely implemented, is also effective for children and adolescents. As trends in overweight continue, however, entrepreneurs have flooded the market with weight-loss diets, raising the concern for what constitutes an appropriate weight-loss diet for children. A developing child requires a full complement of nutrients, so dieting in children and adolescents must be carefully monitored. Fruit, vegetable, and calcium consumption must be maintained. Caloric intake must also be maintained to meet resting metabolic needs. If carefully implemented, "diets" allow children to "grow into their weight"[26] (see Figure App-II.1[26]).

If taken to extremes or not closely monitored, however, diets represent a danger to children. The high-school athlete who is attempting to make weight or the adolescent female who wants to achieve a particular physiognomy are at particular risk.[27] If a child or adolescent participates in unhealthy weight-loss behaviors such as ingesting diet pills, vomiting, or fasting, he or she can severely affect his or her physical maturation, bone health, and tissue homeostasis.[28] Although dieting can be an effective tool for weight loss among children, appropriate medical oversight is always recommended.

Weight training in children and adolescents

Weight training in adults stimulates muscle hypertrophy. The effects of resistance training during childhood and adolescence, however, have been debated for years. Injury to the growing skeleton, tissue fatigue, and lack of effectiveness have been cited as factors recommending against weight training in youths.[29] However, recent data suggest that, although the risk of injury is a very serious concern, weight training produces significant strength and health-related benefits among children and adolescents.[30] Increases in strength are the result of improved motor unit activation, muscle coordination, fiber recruitment, and neuronal firing.[30] In addition to increasing strength, weight training can also improve bone density and cardiorespiratory fitness, reduce blood lipid levels, and increase motor skills.

Young athletes should always use exercises with safe amounts of weight and proper technique in a supervised environment. Overtraining should be avoided.

Female athlete triad

Modern society overemphasizes extremely lean physiques for young women.[31] Accordingly, female athletes are at particular risk for the development of disordered eating habits as they attempt to meet particular physical standards or excel in sport. Female athletes participating in sports such as gymnastics, figure skating, diving, ballet, and running are at the highest risk for developing the female athlete triad.[31]

The female athlete triad results from the combined effects of disordered eating and excessive physical activity. It consists of disordered eating, amenorrhea (or oligomenorrhea), and osteoporosis. Inadequate nutrition contributes to delayed or absent menstrual periods and improper bone development,[32] and excessive physical activity contributes to menstrual irregularities.

Physicians should use opportunities such as the preparticipation physical to screen for this condition. Amenorrhea is a red flag for the female athlete triad. Physical signs of disordered eating include lanugo, periodontal disease, and tooth-enamel loss. Surveys such as the Eating Disorder Inventory, the Eating Disorder Attitude Test, and the Eating Disorder Examination can help confirm disordered eating practices.[32]

Ergogenic sports supplements

History is replete with stories of athletes trying to gain an advantage over their competitors. Supplements ranging from mushrooms to cocoa beans to the designer steroid tetrahydrogestrinone have been used to gain this competitive edge.[33] An ergogenic aid is defined as any substance that has the ability to "create work." Three of the most popular ergogenic aids will be discussed here: anabolic steroids, human growth hormone, and creatine. The first two are illegal without a physician's prescription for a specific medical condition.

Ergogenic sports supplement use has been documented in professional sports such as baseball, football, weight lifting, and track. However, with 30 million children and adolescents in the United States participating in organized sports, ergogenic aid use in this younger and more vulnerable cohort has risen significantly.[33] Physicians should discuss issues of safety and efficacy with adolescents in a confidential manner. Unfortunately, many patients will choose to use supplements despite counseling. Therefore, understanding what is legal, safe, and available adds credibility to the discussion. Many adolescents do not know the proper dosage or the possible ramifications of the use of ergogenic aids.

Anabolic-androgenic steroids

Anabolic-androgenic steroids (AASs) are synthetic testosterone derivatives. Taken either orally or via intramuscular injection, AASs increase lean muscle mass and explosive strength. While AASs are illegal in all sports, between 4% and 11% of male and approximately 2.5% of female high-school–aged adolescents currently use AASs.[34] Overall, one in four anabolic steroid users begins to use during adolescence.[33] Side effects of AASs include physical (e.g., testicular atrophy, hepatic damage, cardiac events, masculinization in females), psychological (e.g., extreme levels of aggression and mood altering), and societal (e.g., punishment under federal law) consequences.[33] The drive for perfection, recognition, and highly competitive college scholarships are all motivators for young athletes to use performance-enhancing supplements. Vanity is another common reason adolescents use ergogenic sports supplements: one third of high-school–age students cited appearance as the primary motivation for using AASs.[35]

The preparticipation physical is a good opportunity for both screening and education. AAS side effects can be used to identify potential users. Significant muscle mass gains, mood swings, testicular atrophy, acne, and increased aggression all suggest potential AAS use. Clear, confidential, nonjudgmental information about the effects and consequences of AAS use should be provided.

Human growth hormone

Human growth hormone (HGH) is a relatively new performance-enhancing supplements. HGH decreases subcutaneous fat, creating a more toned appearance. Its muscular effects, however, are minimal. Although effective medically for the promotion of growth among patients who are deficient in HGH, when it is used as a supplement, HGH actually weakens skeletal muscle.[35] Health implications of adolescents taking HGH include premature physeal closure and hypertension. Additionally, HGH use is illegal and banned in all sports.

Creatine

Creatine is one of the most widely used performance-enhancing supplements. More than 2500 tons were manufactured and consumed in 1999 alone.[34] Creatine, unlike AASs or HGH, is legal and can be purchased over the counter as a nutritional supplement. Endogenous creatine stores reside primarily in skeletal muscle and are essential for muscle contraction. Exogenous creatine is thought to improve anaerobic exertion by allowing for faster muscle recuperation and improved power output. In adults, improvements in muscle mass and strength, as well as delays in fatigue, have been observed with creatine use.[35]

However, the long-term effects of creatine use are largely unknown. There are scientific data available about the effects of creatine in youth. Despite this, many adolescents use creatine. Safe levels of creatinine intake are not well studied for the adolescent athlete. **(Table App-II.2).**

Table App-II.2   Guidelines for Creatine Use

Loading Phase	Maintenance Phase	Hydration Precautions
5 g creatine monohydrate taken 4 times a day for 4-6 days	2 g creatine monohydrate taken once daily for 3 months	Drink 6-8 glasses of water per day to prevent dehydration

Adopted from Calfee R, Fadale P: Pediatrics 2006;117:577-589.

CONCLUSION

The overweight epidemic is an enormous public health problem. Understanding the benefits of exercise, being aware of barriers to exercise, and actively overcoming these barriers with children and parents must be a high priority for every sports medicine provider. Increases in physical activity decrease all-cause mortality, reduce healthcare costs, and improve patient well being. A prescription for exercise is arguably the most valuable tool in the doctor's bag. Physicians should motivate all patients, both young and old, to increase physical activity levels and improve their health.

REFERENCES

1. Pollock M, Gaesser G, Butcher J, et al: ACSM position stand: the recommended quantity and quality of exercise for developing and maintaining cardiorespiratory and muscular fitness and flexibility in healthy adults. Med Sci Sports Exerc 1998;30(6):975-991.
2. Pate R, Pratt M, Blair S, et al: Physical activity and public health: a recommendation from the Centers for Disease Control and Prevention and the American College of Sports Medicine. JAMA 1995;273(5):402-407.
3. US Department of Health and Human Services: Healthy People 2010: Understanding and Improving Health. Washington, DC, US Department of Health and Human Services, US Government Printing Office, 2000.
4. US Department of Health and Human Services: The Surgeon General's Call to Action to Prevent and Decrease Overweight and Obesity. Washington, DC, US Department of Health and Human Services, Public Health Service, Office of the Surgeon General, 2001.
5. NIH Consensus Development Panel: Physical activity and cardiovascular health. JAMA 1996;276:241-246.
6. Biddle S, Gorely T, Stensel D, et al: Health-enhancing physical activity and sedentary behavior in children and adolescents. J Sports Sci 2004;22:679-701.
7. Penedo F, Dahn J: Exercise and well-being: a review of mental and physical health benefits associated with physical activity. Curr Opin Psychiatry 2005;18:189-193.
8. Gordon-Larsen P, Nelson M, Popkin B, et al: Longitudinal physical activity and sedentary behavior trends: adolescence to adulthood. Am J Prev Med 2004;27:277-283.
9. National Center for Health Statistics: Prevalence of Overweight Among Children and Adolescents: United States, 1999-2002 (Web site). Available at www.cdc.gov/nchs/products/pubs/pubd/hestats/overwght99.htm. Accessed July 28, 2007.
10. American Academy of Pediatrics: Active healthy living: prevention of childhood obesity through increased physical activity. Pediatrics 2006;117(5):1834-1842.
11. NIH Consensus Development Panel: Physical activity and cardiovascular health. JAMA 1996;276:241-246.
12. Yang X, Telama R, Viikari J, et al: Risk of obesity in relation to physical activity: tracking for youth to adulthood. Med Sci Sports Exerc 2006;38(5):919-925.
13. Council on Sports Medicine and Council on School Health: Active healthy living: prevention of childhood obesity through increased physical activity; American Academy of Pediatrics policy statement. Pediatrics 2006;117(5):1834-1842.
14. Lowry R, Wechster H, Kann L, et al: Recent trends in participation in physical education among US high school students. J Sch Health 2001;71(4):145-152.
15. Telama R, Yang X, Laakso L, et al: Physical activity in childhood and adolescence as predictor of physical activity in young adulthood. Am J Prev Med 1997;13(4):317-323.
16. Gordon-Larsen P, McMurray R, Popkin B: Determinants of adolescent physical activity and inactivity patterns. Pediatrics 2000;105(6):e83.
17. Tammelin T, Nayha S, Laitinen J, et al: Physical activity and social status in adolescence as predictors of physical inactivity in adulthood. Prev Med 2003;37:375-381.
18. Levin S, Lowry B, Brown D, et al: Physical activity and body mass index among US adolescents: youth risk behavior survey, 1999. Arch Pediatr Adolesc Med 2003;157:816-820.
19. Nelson M, Gordon-Larson P, Adair L, et al: Adolescent physical activity and sedentary behavior: patterning and long-term maintenance. Am J Prev Med 2005;28(3):259-266.
20. Anderson R, Crespo C, Bartlett S, et al: Relationship of physical activity and television watching with body weight and level of fatness among children: results from the Third National Health and Nutrition Examination Survey. JAMA 1998;279(12):938-942.
21. Patrick K, Sallis J, Prochaska J, et al: A multicomponent program for nutrition and physical activity change in primary care: PACE + for adolescents. Arch Pediatr Adolesc Med 2001;155:940-946.
22. Ortega-Sanchez R, Jimenez-Mena C, Cordoba-Garcia R, et al: The effect of office-based physician's advice on adolescent exercise behavior. Prev Med 2004;38:219-226.

23. Ma J, Wang Y, Stafford R: US adolescents receive suboptimal preventive counseling during ambulatory care. J Adolesc Health 2005;36:441.e1-441.e7.

24. Wang Y: Worldwide trends in childhood overweight and obesity. Int J Pediatr Obesity 2006;1(1):11-25.

25. O'Connor F: Sudden death in young athletes: screening for the needle in a haystack. Am Fam Physician 1998;57(11):2763-2770.

26. Centers for Disease Control and Prevention: NHANES CDC growth charts: United States (Web site). Available at www.cdc.gov/nchs/about/major/nhanes/growth charts/background.htm. Accessed July 28, 2007.

27. Daee A, Robinson P, Lawson M, et al: Psychologic and physiologic effects of dieting in adolescents. South Med J 2002;95(9):1032-1041.

28. Neumark-Sztainer D, Hannan P, Story M, et al: Weight-control behaviors among adolescent girls and boys: implications for dietary intake. J Am Diet Assoc 2004;104:913-920.

29. Payne G, Morrow J, Jonson L, et al: Resistance training in children and youth: a meta-analysis. Res Q Exerc Sport 1997;68:80-88.

30. Faigenbaum A: Strength training for children and adolescents. Clin Sports Med 2000;19(4)593-619.

31. Hobart J, Smucker D: The female athlete triad. Am Fam Physician 2000;61:3357-3364.

32. Brunet M: Female athlete triad. Clin Sports Med 2005;24:623-626.

33. Laos C, Metzl J: Performance-enhancing drug use in young athletes. Adolesc Med Clin 2006;17:719-731.

34. Congeni J, Miller S: Supplements and drugs used to enhance athletic performance. Pediatr Clin North Am 2002;49:435-461.

35. Calfee R, Fadale P: Popular ergogenic drugs and supplements in young athletes. Pediatrics 2006;117:577-589.

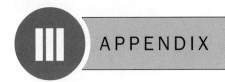

Exercise Prescription for Pregnant Patients

Pamela M. Williams, MD, and Michael Barron, MD

KEY POINTS

- With an uncomplicated pregnancy, women should be encouraged to perform at least 30 minutes of moderate exercise every day.
- Regular exercise during pregnancy appears to improve or maintain fitness.
- Available data about regular, moderate exercise is insufficient to infer any other important risk or benefit to the mother or infant.
- Women should choose activities that will minimize risk of a loss of balance and fetal trauma.
- Women should be advised that moderate exercise during lactation does not affect either the quantity or composition of breast milk or have an impact on infant growth.
- Pregnant competitive athletes may maintain a more strenuous training schedule under close physician supervision.

INTRODUCTION

Physical fitness is essential to the health of women across their life span, including during their childbearing years. Pregnancy is a normal health condition for the vast majority of women. Most women who participate in a regular exercise program will continue to exercise for at least a portion of their pregnancy. Fortunately, the majority of available evidence supports the safety of exercise as part of a normal pregnancy. In the absence of medical or obstetric complications, pregnant women should be encouraged by their prenatal care provider to begin or continue a program of regular, moderate-intensity exercise.[1,2] A basic knowledge of the physiologic changes of pregnancy and their impact on exercise, the benefits of exercise in pregnancy, and the recommended guidelines for exercise during pregnancy and the postpartum period allows a health-care provider to optimally counsel the pregnant woman about exercise.

PHYSIOLOGIC CHANGES OF PREGNANCY AND THEIR INTERACTIONS WITH EXERCISE

Multiple physiologic changes occur during the course of a normal pregnancy. The underlying concerns about exercise during pregnancy surround exercise-induced increases in maternal body temperature, circulating stress hormones, caloric expenditure, and biomechanical stress. Increases in these factors coupled with exercise-induced decreases in visceral blood flow could have adverse effects on the course and outcome of pregnancy. Potential adverse effects include spontaneous abortions, congenital malformations, growth retardation, preterm labor or birth, fetal trauma, premature rupture of membranes, uterine bleeding, and maternal musculoskeletal injury. However, available data does not infer any important risk for the mother or infant. Trials assessing the impact of exercise on the mother, the fetus, and the course of pregnancy are typically small and variable in quality.[3] Nonetheless, an understanding of these fundamental physiologic changes of pregnancy, the theoretic concerns superimposed by exercise, and the available data regarding exercise during pregnancy is invaluable for the clinician who cares for pregnant women.

PHYSIOLOGIC CHANGES OF PREGNANCY BY SYSTEM

Cardiovascular

During both pregnancy and exercise, the heart rate, cardiac output, and stroke volume increase. The pregnancy-induced increase in heart rate is thought to be the result of decreased vagal tone or increased sympathetic drive. Cardiac output increases largely as a result of increased venous return in combination with increased myocardial contractility. However, exercise and pregnancy have opposite effects on splanchnic blood flow. During exercise, splanchnic blood flow is diminished as perfusion is redistributed to skin and exercising muscle, whereas, during pregnancy, blood flow is shunted preferentially to the uterine, renal, and cutaneous circulations. These conflicting effects raise the theoretic concern of fetal hypoxemia during exercise. However, several factors appear to mitigate exercise-induced decreases in splanchnic blood flow during exercise. First, pregnancy causes increased plasma volume. Women who exercise when pregnant have blood volumes that are approximately 20% greater than the volumes of their sedentary controls.[4] Additionally, regular and sustained forms of weight-bearing exercise stimulate placental growth, thus leading to increased placental size and concomitant increases in villous vascular volume.[5] Repeated studies measuring the effect of exercise on fetal heart rate have shown insignificant, short-term fetal heart rate increases of 5 to 15 bpm. Transient episodes of fetal bradycardia were seen in a few studies of untrained women performing at near maximal capacity; pregnancy outcomes were not statistically significant from subjects in whom this finding was not seen.[6]

Maternal body position also affects cardiac output during pregnancy. In the supine position, uterine blood flow falls significantly as a result of the compression of the inferior vena cava by the pregnant uterus. This results in decreased venous return and cardiac output coupled with peripheral vasoconstriction and redistributed blood flow away from the splanchnic and uterine circulations. In physically active women, uterine blood flow decreases during both supine rest and supine exercise, but the decrease in the former is twice that seen in the latter.[7]

Pulmonary

During both exercise and pregnancy, minute ventilation and oxygen consumption increase. During pregnancy, the elevated minute ventilation is predominantly the result of small increases in tidal volume, and this results in increased arterial oxygen tension. However, the higher resting oxygen requirements of pregnancy coupled with the increased work of breathing required for any given workload raise the concern of decreased fetal oxygen availability during aerobic exercise. With mild exercise, pregnant women have a greater increase in respiratory frequency and oxygen consumption to meet their increased oxygen demand. As exercise intensifies to moderate or maximal levels, however, pregnant women demonstrate decreased respiratory frequency, lower tidal volume, and lower maximal oxygen consumption, which could overwhelm the adaptive changes that occur at lower levels of exertion. Most pregnant women will note a subjective increase in workload and a decline in maximal exercise performance throughout their pregnancies.[8]

Musculoskeletal

Significant musculoskeletal changes occur to a woman's body during the course of pregnancy. Growth of the breasts, the uterus, and the fetus accentuate the normal lumbar lordosis, shifting a woman's center of gravity and potentially leading to problems with balance. During weight-bearing exercises, the additional body weight of pregnancy increases ground reaction forces, further heightening the potential for injury. Increased ligamentous laxity, which is thought to be the result of higher levels of the hormones estrogen and relaxin, may raise the risk of sprains and strains during pregnancy. Finally, soft tissue swelling, which is a common symptom during the course of a normal pregnancy, can exacerbate compression-related disorders such as carpal tunnel syndrome. These compressive disorders may be further exacerbated by certain types of exercise.[9]

Most women will report greater physical discomfort during the later stages of pregnancy, with low back pain, abdominal and pelvic discomfort as a result of sacroiliac joint dysfunction, round ligament pain, increased uterine mobility, and pelvic instability being very common. However, studies of exercise during pregnancy have not documented increased injury rates among exercising pregnant patients. Indeed, regular exercise appears to reduce the frequency and severity of the musculoskeletal complaints associated with pregnancy.[4] Aquatic exercise programs, therapy to increase abdominal muscle strength and decrease lumbar lordosis,

and maternity support belts may help to alleviate exercise-associated symptoms in pregnant patients.

Thermoregulatory

Both pregnancy and exercise result in increased maternal heat production. During exercise, significant increases in core temperature can occur, although most excess heat is dissipated through increased skin blood flow and sweating. A normal fetal core temperature is approximately 0.5° C to 1° C higher than the maternal core temperature, with heat dissipation typically occurring through umbilical and uterine circulation. The theoretic concern is that an elevated core temperature (1.5° C to 2.5° C above the basal temperature) could be detrimental to fetal well being. In particular, animal studies linking hyperthermia to congenital malformations raised the concern that teratogenesis may occur as a result of increased thermal stress, especially among women participating in vigorous exercise during early pregnancy. However, no studies to date have produced an increase of more than 1.1° C in maternal core temperature in response to exercise, and no study has demonstrated an increased risk of teratogenesis.[10] By contrast, healthy, fit women appear to tolerate thermal stress better during pregnancy as a result of maternal adaptations that produce faster vasodilation and sweat initiation as compared with untrained subjects.[10]

Metabolic

Maternal metabolic changes oppose the normal physiologic response to exercise. The metabolic upregulation of pregnancy occurs to support the energy needs of the growing fetus and to store fat for later use during pregnancy and the postpartum period. Exercise also causes an increased demand for energy, and it increases the uptake of blood glucose by exercising muscles. These conflicting needs raise the theoretic concern for maternal hypoglycemia and a possible decrease in glucose availability for the fetus, which could lead to a lower birth weight. However, studies of women who exercise at moderate levels have demonstrated no decrease in fetal birth weight.[11] Blood glucose response to exercise depends on the duration and intensity of exercise, with glucose levels declining during moderate or prolonged exercise. Mild exercise results in no significant change.[11]

Neuroendocrine

Exercise is known to increase circulating levels of norepinephrine and epinephrine, which leads to theoretic concerns about premature labor among women who exercise during the third trimester of pregnancy. Norepinephrine increases both the strength and frequency of contractions, whereas epinephrine inhibits uterine activity. Pregnant runners often report uterine contractions during exercise, but studies do not consistently demonstrate changes in uterine activity. Meta-analyses of the effects of physical exercise on pregnancy outcome have not demonstrated significant differences in the risk of preterm labor or the length of gestation.[3,12]

EXERCISE AND THE COMPETITIVE ATHLETE

Competitive athletes will experience the same physiologic challenges of pregnancy and the accompanying theoretic risks of exercise. The pregnant athlete will typically decrease both cardiovascular and resistance training during pregnancy, but she will often maintain a more strenuous training level than the recreational athlete, and she will resume a high intensity of training sooner during the postpartum period. Studies indicate that athletes who continue to exercise may experience little decline in their aerobic fitness (as measured by their maximal oxygen consumption) over the course of pregnancy and during the postpartum period. This is theorized to be partly the result of the fact that pregnant athletes gain less fat than sedentary controls.[13] Data supporting the safety of athletic training during pregnancy, although limited in quantity, favors an athlete's ability to continue training with close monitoring by her health-care provider.[1,13]

BENEFITS OF EXERCISE

Regular aerobic exercise during pregnancy does appear to improve or maintain physical fitness.[3] However, similar to the risks of exercise during pregnancy, available data is insufficient to infer any additional definitive benefits for the mother or infant.[3] Nonetheless, some interesting findings are worthy of note and need to be further explored with larger, randomized trials. Regular exercise may have a favorable effect on the subjective experience of discomfort during pregnancy, enhance feelings of well-being, improve body image, and decrease maternal weight gain and fat deposition during late pregnancy.[4,14] Women who are exercising before pregnancy appear to feel better during the first trimester than those who did not engage in regular exercise.[4] Exercise during the first and second trimesters similarly correlates with an improved sense of well-being during the third trimester.[12] These benefits may translate into postpartum well-being, especially when regular exercise is continued. Although the length of labor does not appear to be altered in women who exercise, their perception of exertion during labor is decreased.[12] In addition, neither the quantity nor quality of breast milk appears to be significantly affected in breastfeeding mothers who continue a moderate exercise regimen.[13]

The role of exercise in the prevention of preeclampsia and in both preventing and treating gestational diabetes are areas of active research. Although there are currently no randomized trials confirming an association between an increase in regular physical activity and a reduction of preeclampsia risk,[15] case-control studies do demonstrate this association.[16] Additionally, prospective cohort studies have demonstrated that a preconception pattern of regular physical activity is associated with a lower risk of gestational diabetes,[17] but there is currently insufficient evidence to recommend for or against the prescription of exercise for the treatment of gestational diabetes.[18]

Limited research has explored the effects of exercise on neonatal well being. Repeated meta-analyses have failed to demonstrate significant differences in mean birth weights for infants of exercising mothers except for endurance athletes who participated in vigorous exercise programs during the third trimester. In the case of the latter, the fetuses were likely to weigh 200 to 400 g less than comparable controls; the significance of this weight difference is unclear.[19] No difference in birth Apgar scores was demonstrated among infants born to mothers who exercised.[12] However, one small study of early neonatal behavior indicates that infants born to exercising mothers have a different neurobehavioral profile as early as the fifth day after birth, with a higher ability to orient to environmental stimuli and to calm themselves after being exposed to stimuli.[20] Further preliminary neonatal and childhood benefits are suggested by additional research that needs to be confirmed in larger, randomized trials. Clapp[21] reported on morphometric and neurodevelopmental outcomes at birth and at the age of 5 years in the offspring of a small group of women exercisers and a control group. He found that, at both ages, head circumference and length were similar, but the offspring of exercising women had less body fat. Similar motor, integrative, and academic skills were found between the two groups. However, children of exercising mothers had higher scores on Wechsler intelligence scales and on oral language skill tests.[21]

GUIDELINES FOR EXERCISE DURING PREGNANCY

In 2002 and 2003, the American College of Obstetricians and Gynecologists followed by the Society of Obstetricians and Gynaecologists of Canada in conjunction with representation from the Canadian Society for Exercise Physiology released their most current opinions, which support moderate exercise as both safe and beneficial in uncomplicated pregnancies.[1,2] These statements continue a long, gradual trend away from treating pregnancy with inactivity and confinement. In the absence of medical or obstetric complications, both guidelines recommend that pregnant women should be encouraged to participate in regular aerobic exercise. Further, the American College of Obstetricians and Gynecologists recommends 30 minutes or more of moderate exercise on a daily basis in recognition of the recommendations of the Centers for Disease Control and Prevention and the American College of Sports Medicine recommendations, whereas the Society of Obstetricians and Gynaecologists of Canada includes a recommendation promoting strength and conditioning exercises as well.[1,2]

All pregnant women should undergo an evaluation early during pregnancy to assess for absolute and relative contraindications for initiating or continuing exercise during pregnancy. Although most women have uncomplicated pregnancies that proceed without significant interventions beyond routine screening, women with certain complications should be encouraged to limit their activities. **Box App-III.1** lists the absolute and relative contraindications to exercise during pregnancy.[1,2] A detailed history and physical examination (typically performed at the initial prenatal visit) in addition to the routine blood work done at that time are nearly always adequate for detecting contraindications. An ultrasound performed around 20 weeks with a Doppler study of umbilical cord flow may also yield valuable information concerning the location of the placenta, the cervical length, and fetuses who are at risk for intrauterine growth restriction. Even with a normal initial evaluation, some of the previously mentioned conditions may develop during pregnancy. **Box App-III.2** lists signs that should warn a woman to stop exercising and contact her physician.[1,2]

Participation in activities that increase the risk of fetal and maternal injury through abdominal trauma should be limited.[1,2] In addition, activities that require significant balance or range of motion should be avoided during later pregnancy. **Box App-III.3** provides a partial list of activities that should be avoided. Scuba diving should be avoided throughout pregnancy as a result of an increased risk for decompression sickness in the fetus, which is unable to filter bubble formation.[1,22] Pregnant women who are exercising above 6000 feet (≥ 1600 m) are believed to be at risk for decreased fetal oxygen delivery as a result of decreased arterial oxygen content coupled with decreased uterine artery blood flow from the combined effects of altitude and exercise. Women should be advised to limit their exercise at altitude, and they should be educated about signs of altitude sickness. It should be recommended to them that they immediately descend from altitude and seek medical attention should they experience symptoms.[1,23]

EXERCISE PRESCRIPTIONS DURING PREGNANCY

The overall goal of exercise during pregnancy should be to improve or maintain maternal fitness levels while minimizing risk to the developing fetus. A woman's prepregnancy level of fitness must be considered when individually tailoring a safe exercise program. The exercise program should allow flexibility

Box App-III.1: Contraindications to Exercise During Pregnancy[1,2]

Absolute

- Significant heart disease
- Restrictive lung disease
- Hypertensive disorders of pregnancy
  - Pregnancy-induced hypertension
  - Preeclampsia
- Ruptured membranes
- Premature labor during the current pregnancy
- Placenta previa during the third trimester
- Persistent second-trimester or third-trimester bleeding
- Incompetent cervix/cerclage
- Multiple gestation

Relative

- Severe anemia
- Cardiac arrhythmia
- Chronic bronchitis
- Poorly controlled type I diabetes
- Extremes of weight
  - Extreme morbid obesity
  - Excessively underweight (body mass index of < 12)
- Significant uncontrolled medical condition (e.g., poorly controlled hyperthyroidism, seizure disorder, or hypertension)
- Orthopedic limitations
- Intrauterine growth restriction (current pregnancy)
- Extremely sedentary lifestyle
- Heavy smoker
- Prior spontaneous abortion
- Prior preterm birth

Box App-III.2: Warning Signs to Stop Exercising[1,2]

- Leakage of amniotic fluid
- Vaginal bleeding
- Muscle weakness
- Chest pain
- Headache
- Dizziness or presyncope
- Preterm labor
- Decreased fetal movement
- Painful uterine contractions
- Dyspnea before exercise
- Excessive shortness of breath
- Calf pain or swelling

Box App-III.3: Contraindicated Sports during Normal Pregnancy

Contact Sports

- Boxing
- Basketball
- Football
- Hockey (ice and field)
- Martial arts
- Rugby
- Soccer
- Wrestling

Sports with Increased Risk for Falls or Abdominal Trauma

- Fencing
- Gymnastics
- Horseback riding
- Power weight lifting
- Racquet sports
- Rock climbing
- Scuba diving
- Skating
- Skiing (downhill snow and water)
- Skydiving/hang gliding
- Springboard diving

to accommodate anticipated changes that will occur across the course of pregnancy. When designing an exercise program, a woman's individual fitness goals (e.g., maintaining fitness, stress relief, competitive activities) as well as her daily activity levels and gestational age need to be considered. Pregnancy may be an opportunity to promote lasting behavioral change because iterative prenatal care allows for frequent feedback.

Understanding what constitutes moderate exercise is critical to a pregnant woman who is participating in an exercise program. The Borg rating of perceived exercise scale is a useful tool that is often used to monitor desired exercise intensity **(Box App-III.4).** One advantage of this scale is that it is equally appropriate for exercise during pregnancy or during the nonpregnant state. A perceived exertion rating in the range of 12 to 14 (somewhat hard) is appropriate for the majority of pregnant women. A brisk walk in which conversation would be periodically interrupted by breathing may be a good place to start for novices. Patients may be educated to use the "talk test" to monitor for overexertion. For example, a level of exercise at which talking would be comfortable but singing would not be is appropriate. Exercise intensity is excessive if a patient would be unable to carry on a verbal conversation while exercising. More experienced athletes will typically be able to identify moderate workouts that can be adjusted to their sense of well being as the pregnancy progresses. Those desiring more than moderate-intensity exercise should be closely monitored by an experienced health-care provider.

The mnemonic *FITT* is helpful to apply clinically when providing a woman with an exercise prescription during pregnancy; it stands for *frequency, intensity, time,* and *type.*[24] The recommended frequency of exercise is to start at three times per week and to progress to most days of the week. The intensity should be within the appropriate rating of perceived exercise range. The initial start time for the duration of exercise is 15 minutes, with

Box App-III.4: Borg Rating of Perceived Exertion

6 No exertion at all
7 Very, very light
8
9 Somewhat light
10
11 Fairly light
12
13 Somewhat hard
14
15 Hard
16
17 Very hard
18
19 Extremely hard
20 Maximal exertion

a goal of working up to 30 minutes. The type of exercise recommended for most should be no weight bearing or low-impact endurance exercise that makes use of large muscle groups (e.g., walking, stationary cycling, swimming, aquatic exercises, low-impact aerobics). As pregnancy progresses, physicians should provide anticipatory guidance to assist women with switching from a low-impact to a non–weight-bearing activity because this will allow more women to continue with a moderate-intensity program throughout pregnancy.

Women who exercise during pregnancy should be counseled to be aware of environmental conditions, and they should be warned about the potential impact of adverse conditions on maternal and fetal stress. They should be encouraged to exercise during the coolest hours of the day, to dress appropriately to minimize thermal stress, and to consume fluids before, during, and after exercise. Women should be made aware of the signals to stop exercising (see Box App-III.2), including they should be counseled about activities to avoid (see Box App-III.3), including the recommendation to avoid supine exercises, especially after the first trimester. Finally, periodic nutritional assessments should be performed. The most critical of these assessments is the careful monitoring of maternal weight gain to ensure that a patient's caloric intake is adequately meeting maternal energy expenditure as well as the developmental requirements of the growing fetus.

CONCLUSION

In summary, the American College of Obstetrics and Gynecology and its Canadian counterparts recommend that most pregnant women should engage in moderate exercise for 30 minutes each day. Although exercise and pregnancy often place competing demands on the maternal physiology, compensatory mechanisms safely allow for moderate exercise during an uncomplicated pregnancy. Understanding the basic physiology of exercise and pregnancy and having some familiarity with the sparse literature examining the risks and benefits of exercise during pregnancy will allow the sports medicine physician to provide the best possible support and counseling to female patients and athletes. Currently the available evidence is insufficient to show definitive benefits or risks of exercise in pregnancy. However, robust and irrefutable evidence supports regular exercise as an essential part of a healthy, long-term lifestyle. Because pregnancy is a natural, normal state of health for most women, the continuation or initiation of regular exercise should be encouraged.

REFERENCES

1. Exercise during pregnancy and the postpartum period. American College of Obstetricians and Gynecologists (ACOG) Committee Opinion No. 267. Obstet Gynecol 2002;99:171-173.
2. Davies GA, Wolfe LA, Mottola MF, MacKinnon C: Society of Obstetricians and Gynecologists of Canada; SGOC Clinical Practice Obstetrics Committee: Joint SOGC/CSEP clinical practice guideline: exercise in pregnancy and postpartum period. Can J Appl Physiol 2003;28:330-341.
3. Kramer MS, McDonald SW: Aerobic exercise for women during pregnancy. Cochrane Database Syst Rev 2006;3:CD000180.
4. Clapp JF 3rd: Exercise during pregnancy: a clinical update. Clin Sports Med 2000;19:273-286.
5. Bergmann A, Zygmunt M, Clapp JF 3rd: Running throughout pregnancy; effect on placental villous vascular volume and cell proliferation. Placenta 2004;25:694-698.
6. Artal R, Sherman C: Exercise during pregnancy: safe and beneficial for most. Phys Sportsmed 1999;27:51-52.
7. Jeffreys RM, Stepanchak W, Lobez B, et al: Uterine blood flow during supine rest and exercise after 28 weeks of gestation. BJOG 2006;113:1239-1247.
8. O'Toole M: Physiologic aspects of exercise in pregnancy. Clin Obstetric Gynecol 2003;46:379-389.
9. Ritchie JR: Orthopedic considerations during pregnancy. Clin Obstet Gynecol 2003;46:456-466.
10. Soultanakis-Aligianni H: Thermoregulation during exercise in pregnancy. Clin Obstet Gynecol 2003;46:442-455.
11. Bessinger RC, McMurray RG: Substrate utilization and hormonal response to exercise in pregnancy. Clin Obstet Gynecol 2003;46:467-478.
12. Wang T, Apgar B: Exercise during pregnancy. Am Fam Physician 1998;57:1846-1852.
13. Pivarnik JM, Perkins CD, Moyerbrailean T: Athletes and pregnancy. Clin Obstetric Gynecol 2003;46:403-414.
14. Goodwin A: Body image and psychological well-being in pregnancy: a comparison of exercises and non-exercises. Aust N Z J Obstet Gynaecol 2000;40:442-447.
15. Meher S, Duley L: Exercise or other physical activity for preventing pre-eclampsia and its complications. Cochrane Database Syst Rev 2006;19:CD005942.
16. Sorensen TK, Williams MA, Lee I, et al: Recreational physical activity during pregnancy and risk of preeclampsia. Hypertension 2004;41:1273-1280.
17. Zhang C, Solomon C, Manson J, Hu F: A prospective study of pregravid physical activity and sedentary behaviors in relation to risk of gestational diabetes mellitus. Arch Intern Med 2006;166:543-548.
18. Ceysens G, Rouiller D, Boulvain M: Exercise for diabetic pregnant women. Cochrane Database Syst Rev 2006;19:CD004225.
19. Leet T, Flick L: Effect of exercise on birth weight. Clin Obstet Gynecol 2003;46:423-431.
20. Clapp JF 3rd, Lopez B: Neonatal behavioral profile of the offspring of women who continued to exercise regularly throughout pregnancy. Am J Obstet Gynecol 1999;181:1038-1039.
21. Clapp JF 3rd: Morphometric and neurodevelopmental outcomes at age five years of the offspring of women who continued to exercise regularly throughout pregnancy. J Pediatr 1996;129:856-863.
22. St Leger Dowse M, Gunby A, Moncad R, et al: Scuba diving in pregnancy: can we determine safe limits? J Obstet Gynaecol 2006;26:509-513.
23. Entin PL, Coffin L: Physiological basis for recommendations regarding exercise during pregnancy at high altitude. High Alt Med Biol 2004;5:321-334.
24. Wolfe LA, Davies GA: Canadian guidelines for exercise in pregnancy. Clin Obstet Gynecol 2003;46:488-495.

Exercise Prescription for Geriatric Patients

Brian K. Unwin, MD

GERIATRIC CARE AS A DEMOGRAPHIC IMPERATIVE

A separate discussion of exercise prescription in the elderly is relevant for several reasons. This population is a high-risk, problem-prone population that often has multiple comorbidities that can affect the type and intensity of exercise performed. Exercise and an active lifestyle are instrumental to the prevention of disease and disability. It is also relevant to discuss this population subset because of the growing numbers of elderly patients in our country:

> In the United States, 20% of all Americans, or about 70 million people, will have passed their 65th birthday by 2030. The demographic tidal wave is coming. Aging in the 21st century, however, is more than just a matter of numbers. The average 75-year-old has three chronic conditions and uses five prescription drugs. Older adults also have unique challenges and different medical needs than younger adults. Consequently, it is not enough to be aware of the demographic imperative, we must be prepared for it.

—Patricia P. Barry, MD, MPH, Executive Director, Merck Institute of Aging and Health

In 2000, 40% of all deaths in Americans over the age of 65 years were linked to hyperlipidemia. Heart disease accounted for 32.4% of these deaths, and stroke accounted for 8%.[1] Coronary artery disease mortality and morbidity rates are highest among elderly men and women, with more than 80% of the deaths from coronary heart disease seen among individuals who are more than 65 years old.[2] Exercise can plan a significant role in reducing or mitigating the disability of individuals with these conditions, but it can also potentially play a role in reducing the impact of these conditions from a cultural and societal perspective. Only 43% of men and women over the age of 65 years report very good or excellent health.[3] By 2050, 20% of all elderly will be more than 80 years old, with this cohort being the fasting growing age group in the world. This cohort is also the population with the greatest disease burden and the need for long-term care services. The number of working individuals that financially support individuals who are 65 years of age and older will fall from 12 (in 1950) to 4 (by the year 2050). The financial cost

of these health problems results in increased direct health-care costs, especially Medicare costs, which are predicted to double to $500 million in 2010. Indirect costs borne by household caregivers who are caring for disabled elders is approaching almost 39 million households, and this was valued at $257 billion dollars in 2002.[4] These costs could be substantially mitigated if the tremendously beneficial effects of regular exercise were realized by a larger portion of senior society.

FUNCTIONAL AND PHYSIOLOGIC EFFECTS OF EXERCISE AND ACTIVITY

Although many seniors may exercise for competition, exercise for seniors takes on the more fundamental roles of preserving independence and the maintenance of function. Research has also demonstrated that an active lifestyle yields functional benefits that are comparable to exercise training. Aging research clearly shows that a loss of function and age-associated disease are not inherent parts of the aging process. Rather, wellness and function are determined by an interplay of genetic factors, disease, and disuse. Exercise and activity obviously have the greatest impact in this last domain. The succinct review by Schwartz and Kohrt[5] will primarily be used in this brief summary of how exercise affects elderly individuals.

Exercise and aerobic capacity

The age-associated change in aerobic muscle capacity as measured by maximal oxygen consumption appears to decline by 1% annually ($0.5 \text{ mL/min}^{-1}/\text{kg}^{-1}$ per year in longitudinal studies). A variety of studies demonstrate that patients with higher physical fitness levels seem to preserve higher aerobic capacity as compared with their sedentary counterparts, partly by slowing the rate of decline as well as by starting the aging process with greater aerobic capacity. Many studies demonstrate that changes in body composition develop with aging, including an increase in adipose tissue and a decrease in fat-free mass (or lean body mass). Hence, the attenuated decline in maximal oxygen consumption among elder athletes may also be related to preserved fat-free mass as a result of conditioning. In the absence of hypertension and coronary artery disease, resting cardiac output, heart rate, and heart size are normal in older individuals. Maximal heart rate has been consistently demonstrated to decline with aging, and this is likely related to changes in β-adrenergic sensitivity.

Research into the endurance capacity of older adults is confounded by the intensity and duration of the program, the baseline health and fitness of the individual, and the testing methodology. However, studies demonstrate that aerobic capacity can be improved by 10% to 30% with training, with comparable training effects seen between men and women and between older versus younger cohorts. Maximal cardiac output is greater among trained elderly athletes as compared with sedentary controls, and this is largely related to a larger stroke volume in the trained senior without a significant difference in the maximal heart rate. Healthy older individuals can train at relatively intense levels (85% of heart rate reserve), with most studies demonstrating that cardiovascular improvements can be obtained when training at 50% of heart rate reserve. Heart rate reserve is calculated as follows:

$$\text{Heart rate reserve} = 0.85 \: [(\text{Maximal heart rate} \\ - \text{Resting heart rate})]$$
$$\text{Target exercise heart rate} = \% \text{ of target intensity (Maximal} \\ \text{heart rate} - \text{Resting heart rate)} \\ + \text{Resting heart rate}$$

Benefits of exercise

The benefits of habitual exercise have been extensively studied and conclusively demonstrated in many populations, including the elderly. The following section summarizes the geriatric-specific benefits of regular physical activity.

Body composition

Longitudinal and cross-sectional studies show that body fat is consistently lower among active older adults and similar to that of active young adults. Fat mass can be reduced with exercise training with a preferential decrease in central adiposity, which is an important risk factor for diabetes and heart disease. However, the loss of weight or fat is greatest when it is coupled with caloric restriction. Unique to the elderly is a phenomenon in which increases in exercise may result in a concomitant decrease in non-exercise activity, thereby leading to no overall difference in energy expenditure over time.

Muscle strength and power

Cross-sectional studies likely underestimate the loss of muscle strength that occurs with aging (i.e., a 40% loss [cross-sectional] versus a 60% loss [longitudinal] in grip strength from young adulthood to the age of 80 years). Associated with this loss of strength is an equivalent loss of muscle mass and associated losses of muscle power. Muscle type, quality, and motor unit composition may also change with aging.

The positive effects of strength training in the elderly are well documented in a variety of studies, with the effect of the training varying as a result of the intensity of training, the baseline characteristics of the trainees, the measurement methodology, and the duration. In general, studies with longer durations and higher training intensities derive the greatest relative gains (50% to 200%) in strength.

Effect of exercise on functional status

In general, a variety of studies support the intuition that exercise and greater physical activity improve function in adults. The mixed results of some studies can be attributed to the type, duration, and intensity of exercise; the functional limitations of interest (e.g., walking distance versus falls); the methods of measurement; and the target population (e.g., community-dwelling versus frail elderly). Further complicating the assessment of functional

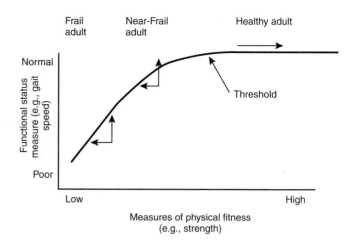

Figure App-IV.1 Nonlinear relationship between fitness and functional status.

improvements with exercise is the nonlinear relationship observed between physical fitness, functional status measures, and the target group[6] **(Figure App-IV.1).** Because each individual starts at a different point on the functional curve, a similar improvement in fitness measure may result in vastly different improvements in function, depending on the baseline function of the individual. This effect is particularly pronounced for functional, healthy adults. These individuals experience little measurable change in functional status with increased fitness because they are already functioning at a high level.[6]

Exercise and geriatric conditions

In addition to fitness and functional parameters, multiple medical conditions that are commonly seen among geriatric patients are improved with increased exercise and activity.

Insulin sensitivity and diabetes prevention

Endurance and strength training in older adults improves insulin sensitivity at a magnitude similar to that of younger adults. Insulin sensitivity improves as a result of the associated decline in insulin levels and improved glucose tolerance achieved with exercise. Through this and other mechanisms, exercise plays a critical role in the prevention of type II diabetes.

Cholesterol

Regular exercise has demonstrated benefits for atherogenic lipoprotein profiles by increasing high-density lipoprotein cholesterol concentrations. However, no studies quantify the effects of exercise on lipoprotein profiles and resultant morbidity and mortality in the elderly.

Blood pressure

Endurance training has demonstrated a consistent 3 to 4 mm Hg decline in both systolic and diastolic blood pressures, with an equivalent effect with low to moderate exercise as compared with more vigorous exercise. The evidence of the effect of strength training on lowering blood pressure is less robust as a result of fewer studies having been performed. Among younger populations, blood pressure reductions from resistance exercise appear to have a smaller but additive benefit.

Coronary and peripheral vascular disease

The benefit of exercise on atherosclerotic cardiovascular disease and overall mortality is well supported by prospective and retrospective population studies, with the effect of a sedentary lifestyle being equivalent to that of smoking. Improvement in symptomatic claudication is also demonstrated with endurance exercise training, and so is a 40% increase in overall physical activity. Patients with congestive heart failure and chronic obstructive pulmonary disease also demonstrate benefit with regard to exercise duration and physical endurance.

Osteoarthritis
Randomized trials of exercise therapy for arthritis demonstrate that patients with an exercise program show a functional status improvement of 10% to 25% that includes the benefits of lower subjective pain, improved gait speed, lower depression scores, and less use of pain medications.

Osteoporosis
Exercise during youth may predispose an individual to greater peak bone mass, and it may also mitigate the effects of osteoporosis. In general, well-designed studies demonstrate improvements in bone density, and they also show that either resistance or weight-bearing endurance exercise may have similar positive effects on bone density.

Cancer
Links between the beneficial effects of exercise/activity and cancer have long been postulated, with the greatest relationships being demonstrated in colon cancer (via cohort and case–control studies) and breast cancer. Seventeen out of 22 studies involving this topic suggest a benefit from exercise. Most importantly, no studies demonstrate an increase in cancer incidence as a result of exercise.

In summary, a multitude of well-designed studies consistently demonstrate the wide-ranging benefits of habitual exercise in the elderly population. These benefits range from improved body composition and function to improved risk profiles and outcomes for a multitude of common medical conditions.

Risks associated with exercise in the elderly
The risks associated with exercise are orthopedic injury and cardiovascular events. These risks are multifactorial, and they involve the interplay between the patient, the exercise performed, and environmental factors. The most common type of injury sustained is overuse musculoskeletal injury. For the elderly, injuries may be prevented by employing less-intense activities, moderating eccentric components of exercise, and emphasizing balance training. Common-sense measures also include appropriate footwear and foot care; monitoring, prevention, and treatment of exercise-associated hypoglycemia; safe exercise environments and equipment; and routine eye and hearing care. The risk of sudden death from exercise is largely associated with sudden vigorous exercise in previously sedentary individuals. The overall risk for sudden death in habitually active men is 30% of that seen in habitually sedentary men.

An excellent instructional patient guide (and video) called *Exercise: A Guide from the National Institute on Aging* (www.nih.gov/nia) provides an overview of the benefits of exercise, related safety concerns, motivational methods, nutrition, exercise techniques, and progress-monitoring tools.

Clearly the benefits of regular exercise far outweigh any associated risk, provided that the individual's risks are anticipated and addressed prospectively. How, then, can physicians encourage their older patients to adopt a lifestyle that incorporates habitual exercise?

PRINCIPLES OF BEHAVIORAL CHANGE

The first step in exercise advocacy or exercise prescription is to understand relevant patient exercise-related behaviors and patient knowledge and attitudes related to exercise. For many older Americans, beginning an exercise program will require significant behavioral changes. Their lack of habitual exercise may be the result of a lifetime of inactivity, illness, disability, or beliefs and attitudes that result in inactivity. The first step in developing an exercise prescription for seniors is to understand these issues before giving empiric advice about a course of action. An excellent introduction to health behavior change is provided by Rollnick, Mason, and Butler,[7] and a brief review of the principles will be described here. An exercise prescription, especially for a geriatric patient, is a futile effort unless the patient's exercise behaviors and attitudes are addressed.

The theoretic framework posed by Rollnick and colleagues is based on research reported by DiClemente and Prochaska[8] regarding the stages of change of behaviors. An individual that would benefit from an exercise might be in a state of precontemplation of exercise, and he or she may need assistance to progress to full contemplation of an exercise program. After the contemplation of the behavioral change (exercise), the individual will act only after adequate preparation has taken place. Behaviors will then need to be maintained to meet desired goals and prevent relapse **(Figure App-IV.2).**

Rollnick and colleagues state that the process of behavioral change begins with the patient and provider establishing a rapport and then setting an agenda. The agenda is established in collaboration between the provider and the patient. Often the agendas of the patient and the physician are the same; at times, however, there can be minor or major discrepancies between the agendas. In the context of an exercise prescription, a provider may be communicating an agenda of improving the patient's hypertension and diabetes control, whereas the patient's agenda may be narrowly focused on the treatment of erectile dysfunction. Clear communication of their respective agendas allows the provider and the patient to prioritize approaches and treatments to the satisfaction of both parties.

Developing an agenda allows the clinician to establish how a patient views the importance of a behavior change (in this case, how the patient will view exercise as a treatment of hypertension and diabetes) and assists the patient with developing confidence in his or her ability to perform physical activity and to realize the value of exercise as a treatment. The patient's confidence and sense of importance are intertwined and ultimately define patient readiness for change. If a patient is not confident that exercise will

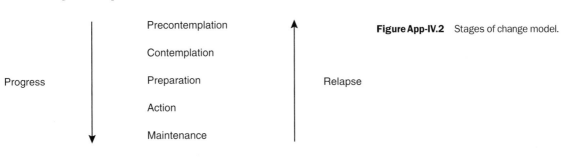

Figure App-IV.2 Stages of change model.

benefit his or her condition or if the patient is not confident he or she has the means or ability to exercise), then that patient will ascribe little importance to the activity. The patient is ready for change when the importance of and confidence in a behavioral change (exercise) are both developed; without this readiness, the exercise prescription will not work.

Patient resistance can have multifactorial causes, including interpersonal problems between the patient and the provider. Rollnick and colleagues emphasize that resistance to behavioral change can successfully be countered by physician strategies that focus on patient-centeredness. Patient-centeredness begins with carefully listening to the patient and developing an understanding of the patient's world of experiences related to the illness or condition. Included in this model is the integration of the patient's concepts of the disease or illness and the intervention. For example, a patient may have the view that the only form of exercise is jogging, whereas the provider is thinking of walking or swimming and stretching, strengthening, and mobility exercises. By collaboratively developing treatment goals, each clinical contact can help build a therapeutic relationship that encourages health promotion. Rollnick and colleagues define the patient role as one of being the ultimate decision maker. The physician's role is to respect the patient's autonomy and choices and to provide information to assist the patient with achieving mutually agreed-upon goals. By continuously monitoring the patient's views of what is important and the patient's confidence, the physician can propose new goals at the proper time **(Table App-IV.1)**. To continue with the previous patient example, the patient may experience significant improvements in readiness for an exercise program only after successful treatment of his erectile dysfunction.

BEFORE THE EXERCISE PRESCRIPTION

The exercise prescription begins with an assessment of physical limitations, cardiorespiratory risk factors, and signs and symptoms that could be worsened with physical activity. There are very few absolute or relative contraindications to mild to moderate physical activity. A routine history and physical examination can provide the information necessary to advise a patient about the initiation of a mild to moderate exercise program. High-risk conditions that may preclude the prescription of even mild to moderate exercise are listed in **Box App-IV.1.**

Medications requiring special patient education efforts include agents that might cause bradycardia or hypoglycemia. Patients receiving β-blockers or calcium-channel blockers may have exercise-limiting bradycardia, and they should use perceived exertion scales to guide the intensity of their workouts (described later). Oral hypoglycemics and insulin injections may need to be reduced in dose or changed with regard to timing to allow for the

Box App-IV.1: Conditions Precluding Prescription of Mild to Moderate Exercise

High-Risk Medical Conditions
- Recent electrocardiogram changes
- Recent myocardial infarction
- Unstable angina
- Complete (third-degree) heart block
- Decompensated heart failure
- Uncontrolled severe hypertension
- Uncontrolled metabolic disease
- Unstable arrhythmia
- Severe emphysema or chronic obstructive pulmonary disease causing dyspnea at rest
- Dissecting aneurysm
- Acute infection
- Severe cardiomyopathy
- Severe valvular heart disease

Common Geriatric Syndromes
- Cognitive impairment
- Falls
- Seizures
- Unstable anticoagulation
- Self-neglect
- Malnutrition

caloric burn than will occur with exercise. Diuretic use may cause electrolyte disturbances or exacerbate continence problems.

Before issuing an exercise prescription, the physician should always assess the patient's cardiovascular risk. As discussed previously, nearly all individuals can and should exercise at a mild or moderate intensity. However, an exercise treadmill test may be indicated to ensure adequate myocardial perfusion in individuals with high-risk medical conditions or in those who wish to begin a vigorous-intensity exercise program. The American College of Sports Medicine (ACSM) has issued consensus guidelines regarding which patients require exercise treadmill testing before beginning prescribed exercise **(Table App-IV.2).** The application of the American College of Sports Medicine guidelines requires characterizing the patient as being at low, moderate, or high risk for coronary artery disease (CAD) and understanding the difference between moderate-intensity and vigorous-intensity exercise. Categorizing patients as low, moderate, or high risk is done by examining their risk factors and determining if they currently exhibit signs or symptoms of CAD.

Low-risk individuals are asymptomatic men 45 years of age or younger and women 55 years of age or younger who have no more than one risk factor for CAD **(Box App-IV.2)**. Moderate-risk individuals are males who are more than 45 years of age and women more than 55 years of age who have two or more risk factors. High-risk patients include those patients with signs or symptoms of CAD **(Box App-IV.3)** or those with known cardiovascular (e.g., CAD), pulmonary (e.g., chronic obstructive pulmonary disease), or metabolic (e.g., diabetes) disease.

CAD risk factors and its signs and symptoms are listed in Boxes App-IV.2 and App-IV.3, respectively. These guidelines can be summarized by the observation that there is no indication for exercise stress testing in a generally healthy individual who plans to undertake a mild-intensity to moderate-intensity walking or cycling program.[9-11] If treadmill testing is indicated, the patient

Table App-IV.1   Questions of Importance, Confidence, and Readiness[7]

Importance	Confidence	Readiness
Is it worthwhile?	Can I?	Should I do it now?
Why should I?	How will I do it?	What about other priorities?
How will I benefit?	How will I cope with ____?	
What will change?		
At what cost?	How will I succeed if ____?	
Do I really want to?		
Will it make a difference?	What will change?	

Table App-IV.2 Does My Patient Need an Exercise Treadmill Test before Beginning an Exercise Program?

	Patient's Risk of Coronary Artery Disease		
	Low	*Moderate*	*High*
Moderate exercise	Not necessary	Not necessary	Recommended
Vigorous exercise	Not necessary	Recommended	Recommended

Box App-IV.2: Risk Factors for Coronary Artery Disease

- Family history of myocardial infarction in first-degree male relative before 55 years of age or in a female relative before 65 years of age
- Smoking currently or cessation within the previous 6 months
- Hypertension
- Hypercholesterolemia (any of the below values)
  - Total cholesterol > 200 mg/dL
  - High-density lipoprotein cholesterol < 35 mg/dL*
  - Low-density lipoprotein cholesterol > 130 mg/dL
- Impaired fasting glucose (> 110 mg/dL)
- Obesity (body mass index > 30)
- Sedentary lifestyle

*A high-density lipoprotein cholesterol value of greater than 60 mg/dL is considered a "negative risk factor". In other words, a 36-year-old obese male with hypertension and a high-density lipoprotein level of 65 mg/dL would be judged to have only one risk factor. Barring other diagnoses, this patient would therefore be categorized as low risk.

Box App-IV.3: Signs and Symptoms of Coronary Artery Disease

- Chest, neck, jaw, or arm pain that may be the result of ischemia
- Dyspnea with exertion or at rest
- Unexplained dizziness or syncope
- Orthopnea/paroxysmal nocturnal dyspnea (PND)
- Ankle edema
- Claudication
- Valvular heart disease
- Increasing fatigue with usual activities

Box App-IV.4: Contraindications to Exercise Treadmill Testing

Absolute

- Acute myocardial infarction (within 48 hours)
- Unstable angina
- Uncontrolled arrhythmias causing hemodynamic compromise
- Severe symptomatic aortic stenosis
- Acute pulmonary embolism
- Acute myocarditis/pericarditis
- Aortic dissection

Relative

- Left main coronary stenosis
- Moderate stenotic valvular heart disease
- Electrolyte abnormalities
- Severe hypertension (> 200/110 mm Hg)
- Tachy/bradyarrhythmias
- Hypertrophic cardiomyopathy
- Mental or physical impairment that impedes ability to exercise adequately
- High-degree atrioventricular block

for formal orthopedic care, as necessary) should be directed at problem areas.

The exercise prescription for older adults must also consider other impairments that may influence the individual's ability and safety to exercise. Vision should be assessed for age-related conditions such as cataracts, glaucoma, macular degeneration, or retinopathy. The assessment of hearing is important to ensure that the patient is receiving the aural information from the physician as well as for safety issues of participating in team sports or indoor or outdoor activities. Adequate vision and hearing are also important for promoting the socialization that comes with exercise.

Other impairments or limitations that may influence the exercise prescription include the assessment of appropriate adaptive equipment use such as canes, walkers, splints, and braces. Other equipment considerations depend on the medical condition of the patient and include blood sugar monitoring devices (as needed), a watch for monitoring the pulse, a quick-energy drink or food or glucagon for hypoglycemic episodes, a fast-acting β-agonist for bronchospasm, nitroglycerin for angina, pain relievers, a scale to monitor weight, a medical alert bracelet, a pocket list of medical conditions and medications, a cell phone, and access to transportation.

Exercise may also be challenged by seemingly unrelated conditions such as patient problems with urinary incontinence or bowel problems that require access to bathroom facilities. Vasomotor rhinitis may be a significant impediment to patient exercise, especially in cold weather. Patient phobias, anxiety, or depression may require treatment before or in conjunction with the exercise plan.

Additional time must also be spent to advise the patient about environmental precautions to take, such as proper clothing in cold or hot weather, hydration, and acclimatization. Heat-injury and cold-injury risk increases with such conditions as advancing age, hypertension, arteriosclerotic cardiovascular disease, diabetes, and neuropathies as well as medications such as diuretics, β-blockers, α-agonists, psychotropics, cholinesterase inhibitors, antidepressants, vasodilators, and alcohol. Travel to higher elevations may result in increased tachycardia, tachypnea, and an overall sense of "breathlessness."

should be assessed for absolute and relative contraindications to treadmill testing **(Box App-IV.4)** so that appropriate referral can be made, if indicated. More extensive discussion about the indications for and evaluation techniques of the exercise treadmill test are covered more extensively in the American College of Sports Medicine *Guidelines for Exercise Testing and Prescription*[9] and in Chapter 40 of this text. After determining the cardiopulmonary fitness of the patient, the second key assessment is the musculoskeletal examination. The focus of this examination is to identify limitations in range of motion, strength, or pain involving the neck, the spine, and the proximal and distal extremities. Stretching techniques and pain modality treatments (or referrals

THE EXERCISE PRESCRIPTION

The exercise prescription for the older adult begins with the consideration of five types of exercise (also called the *mode of exercise*). For the elderly, the five modes of exercise include general activities, cardiopulmonary (aerobic), resistance, flexibility and balance training. Each individual mode of exercise is then governed by the duration, the frequency, and the intensity of the exercise event, which should be followed by timely follow up. The useful mnemonic *MDFIT* (for *mode, duration, frequency, intensity,* and *follow-up*) can be used as an aid when writing the exercise prescription.[11] The American College of Sports Medicine's *Guidelines for Exercise Testing and Prescription,* seventh edition, is an excellent reference for and review of the process.

All exercise should begin with a warm up phase. The warm up should focus on promoting a full range of motion of the major joints of the upper and lower extremities, especially those joints and muscle groups that can be expected to be used during the activity or exercise period. Warming up before mundane activities such as mowing, gardening, and painting should also be encouraged, especially if the activity does not occur on a daily basis. The goal of the warm up is to do exactly that: to take the participant to near-exercise levels of aerobic activity, strength, and expected range of motion.

General activities

General (daily) exercise activities include walking the dog, walking greater distances when parking, taking the stairs, and walking instead of driving. Starting with daily activities could promote a positive attitude toward exercise, promote self-efficacy, reduce disability, and promote the habit of exercise. The ACSM guidelines recognize the importance of maintaining a generally active lifestyle. However, the guidelines also state that general activities are not sufficient for maintaining fitness in adults.[12] Additional cardiovascular, resistance, and flexibility exercises are required to maintain optimum health and fitness in older individuals.

Cardiovascular (aerobic) exercise

Cardiovascular (aerobic) exercise for the elderly should be designed around patient preferences and impairments. Walking is suitable for most individuals, with bicycling and swimming as other alternatives. The duration of exercise should progress to the point at which the patient is able to perform the activity for at least 30 minutes continuously or in accumulated bouts of at least 10 minutes of exercise over the day. The frequency of aerobic exercise should also be advanced gradually until moderate exercise occurs 5 days of the week. Alternatively, vigorous cardiovascular exercise can be performed for at least 20 minutes on 3 days of the week to meet this guideline. The intensity of the exercise can be governed by perceived exertion (12 to 14 for moderate exercise or 15 to 17 for vigorous exercise on the Borg scale) or on the basis of the heart rate. Perceived exertion scales are particularly effective for individuals who cannot obtain a target heart rate as a result of medications such as β-blockers, calcium-channel blockers, and clonidine. The intensity of the exercise can also be guided by providing a heart rate range for the patient to maintain during exercise. There are a number of methodologies involving the patient's pulse that can establish this exercise range with the patient. A key aspect of using the heart rate as a guide to exertion intensity is to recognize that, for any given individual, his or her true maximal heart rate can vary widely (± 15 bpm); this may require an upward or downward titration of the exercise range. Although this variation in individual heart rate response makes scales of perceived exertion even more attractive, there

are circumstances that warrant the formal determination of a patient's maximal heart rate, as outlined by the American College of Sports Medicine's recent guidance.[9]

Some recreational sports can provide significant cardiopulmonary activity and should be considered in the elderly individual who is capable of performing these activities. Activities such as cross-country skiing, basketball, racquetball, and tennis can be considered for those patients with the physical skills to perform them. Optimally, these should be played at a lower intensity to avoid injury; this may an adjustment of the individual's attitude from winning to just enjoying the game. Games themselves can be modified to allow more seniors to participate, such as playing water polo in shallow water, using smaller courts and fields, and adopting modified rules to promote participation and the enjoyment of a game. Involvement of the senior's family (intergenerational activities) may also promote exercise and sports among an entire family.

Resistance training

The incorporation of resistance training into an elder patient's exercise prescription is a necessity to promote function and independence. The loss of an individual's ability to perform the basic tasks of daily living (e.g., walking, transferring, toileting) predicts nursing home placement as well as increased morbidity and mortality. Upper-extremity strength is particularly critical during rehabilitation after a stroke, after lower-extremity joint replacement, or while recuperating from a lower-extremity fracture. The resistance training guidelines for a senior are similar to those of a younger adult, with some modifications. Initial sessions should be under supervision to ensure proper technique and further definition of the exercise plan. One potential method is by providing the patient with a referral to a physical therapist who is knowledgeable about the exercise needs of seniors; another is for the patient to use a reputable exercise trainer.

The first weeks of training should involve minimal resistance followed by slow increases in weight. The focus should be on 8-10 core muscle groups, such as the back, chest, shoulders, arms, hips, buttocks, knees, and ankles. Approximately 10 to 15 repetitions should be performed within each set of exercises for each muscle group. The frequency of strength training depends on the individual, but it should ideally occur on two to three nonconsecutive days a week to allow for adequate muscle rest between sessions. The level of intensity should be assessed as 12 to 13 on the Borg scale (i.e., somewhat hard). Increasing resistance (weight) should only occur after increasing the number of repetitions and after the perceived intensity has decreased. Multiple sets for each muscle group can be performed, but studies demonstrate that strength in seniors can be measurably benefited by performing only one set of each exercise.[5]

Technique must be emphasized to promote strength gains as well as to prevent injury. The Valsalva maneuver (straining) should be avoided. The patient should be able to move involved joints through a "pain-free arc" when performing the exercise. Often weight machines are preferred for seniors because they require less skill and provide more control for lifting and lowering weights, small incremental changes in resistance, and the promotion a full range of motion with a reduced fear of dropping weights. The patient should also be cautioned to perform slow transitions in posture (i.e., from supine to sitting or from sitting to standing) to avoid orthostasis. Resistance should be decreased by 50% if breaks in training of 3 weeks or more occur.

Flexibility exercises

The preservation of flexibility is linked with increased functional capacity and independence. Flexibility also intuitively reduces the chance for injury. For example, a frozen shoulder may impair an individual's ability to eat independently or to perform toileting activities, or a hip contracture can limit a senior's ability to enjoy recreational activities or to walk. The return of flexibility is perhaps the most important factor to emphasize to a senior patient after an injury. The flexibility of major joints is also crucial for the patient to conduct aerobic, resistance, and balance exercises. Neck and back flexion, extension, rotation, and side-bending exercises can be performed three or more times a day to preserve functions such as looking up and down when grasping objects or when operating a vehicle. Back and shoulder flexibility are critical for an individual to be able to dress. Back and lower-extremity flexibility are important for the donning of shoes, socks, and orthopedic appliances and for the inspection of the skin of the feet (if a patient has a peripheral neuropathy).

Flexibility exercises can and should be incorporated into day-to-day activities, and they should involve joints other than just the extremities. These exercises can be incorporated into daily activities (e.g., immediately before dressing, driving the car, or gardening and upon awakening or going to bed). Stretching should also be performed as part of warm up and cool-down activities after exercise sessions. Static stretching studies indicate that optimal benefit occurs within the first 15 seconds of stretching,[9] with two to four stretches per muscle group. Static stretching exercises are likely to be the most beneficial for most elders. Stretching should not cause pain, but it should be taken to a range of motion limit that is described as "tightness" by the patient. The ACSM recommends activities that maintain or increase flexibility for 10 minutes at least 2 days per week.

Dynamic stretching (using momentum by repetitive bouncing movements) is generally not recommended for seniors because of the possible resulting discomfort and injury. Proprioceptive neuromuscular facilitation typically requires the presence of a partner to perform it correctly, it is more time intensive, and it again may result in muscle soreness.

Balance exercises

Balance exercises are often rolled into flexibility exercises, but balance is dealt with here as a separate issue because of the critical role that balance plays in preventing falls and injury. It may be the most important exercise activity for those frail individuals who are at high risk for falls. Balance exercises should focus on the maintenance of an upright position with both stationary activities (static) and moving equilibrium (dynamic). Often these exercises can be worked into day-to-day activities that are functionally important to the patient.

This part of the exercise prescription is governed by findings from the history and physical examination. The history should focus on the history of not just falls but also of "near misses" (i.e., stumbles and trips), positional orthostasis, and avoidance behaviors (i.e., not walking on grass or uneven walkways). The history should also include any instances of central nervous system disorders such as stroke, syncope, or presyncope. The physical examination should include a detailed examination of the feet, the gait, the cardiovascular system, the orthostatic vital signs, the neurologic system, and the lower extremities. Additional predictive examination tools include the timed "up-and-go" test and the "standing reach" test. The timed up-and-go test evaluates dynamic balance **(Figure App-IV.3)**. Normal elders should be able to rise from a chair without using their arms to push off, walk 10 feet, turn around, and return to the chair and sit down within 10 seconds while walking at a normal pace. The standing reach test **(Figure App-IV.4** on page 640) addresses static balance, and it involves the individual standing with his or her side against a wall with the feet close together. The individual is then asked to raise the arm closest to the wall and to lean as far forward as possible without falling or shifting the feet. A horizontal distance covered of 6 inches or more is normal; less than 6 inches demonstrates that an individual at high risk for falls.

If an elder is falling at home or is deemed to be at high risk for falls, a home safety assessment by an occupational (or physical) therapist or by a visiting nurse or physician can be valuable for enhancing safety at home. Physical therapy consultation can also be valuable for addressing issues that involving the gait, neurologic issues, or adaptive equipment needs. These actions could then reformulate the exercise prescription. Recent ASCM guidance suggests that community-dwelling elders who are at risk for falls should perform exercises to maintain or improve balance.[12]

Yoga and tai chi are often mentioned as evidenced-based activities that improve patient balance and flexibility, but they may be difficult to implement on the basis of availability and the knowledge and preferences of the patient. Balance exercises should probably begin in a supervised environment to reduce the risk of falls and injury. Patients with greater balance needs should be encouraged to develop and maintain balance through repetitive static exercises such as standing on one leg while not touching other objects. This exercise can begin with raising one leg and maintaining contact with a steady object with one hand. The duration of this activity can be timed. With practice, balance time is increased and touch contact reduced. Dynamic balance can begin with chair exercises with the patient sitting and performing rotation, flexion, and extension movements as tolerated and then graduating to standing exercises, performing similar activities using support as needed. Dynamic balance can also be aided by supervised practice doing functional activities, such as getting in and out of the car and walking on uneven surfaces.

Timely follow-up

Timely follow-up is essential for the exercise prescription to be effective, for multiple reasons. First, it is a way to access and encourage compliance. Exercise may only become important for some patients if the physician emphasizes its importance. Compliance with the prescription should be assessed without judgment, and it should be approached in a fashion that allows the patient to discuss his or her limitations and confidence in the activities. The follow-up visit is also a means of accessing progress. One approach is to encourage the use of an exercise diary. Another simple process is to do a "timed walk" before the start of the exercise prescription and at intervals during follow-up care. For example, having nursing personnel complete a timed walk within or around the clinic may serve as an additional "vital sign" for the encounter. The visit also serves as a means of addressing any injuries and developing pain treatment and prevention plans. Finally, the visit could serve as a means for setting new goals within the exercise prescription or for promoting wellness in other domains, such as smoking cessation, mental health, hypertension, diabetes, or weight control.

CONCLUSION

Extensive literature supports the beneficial effect that exercise can have on senior patients' health and wellness. With the retirement of the baby boomer generation, more individuals can be expected to develop medical conditions and resultant disabilities that will directly benefit from a knowledgeable physician's application of the exercise prescription to treat these conditions. Additionally, the adoption and promotion of an active, healthy lifestyle has tremendous potential to prevent disease and maintain quality of life.

The exercise prescription begins with the physician promoting a patient's positive attitude toward exercise. This is done by developing the patient's awareness of the importance of exercise in his or

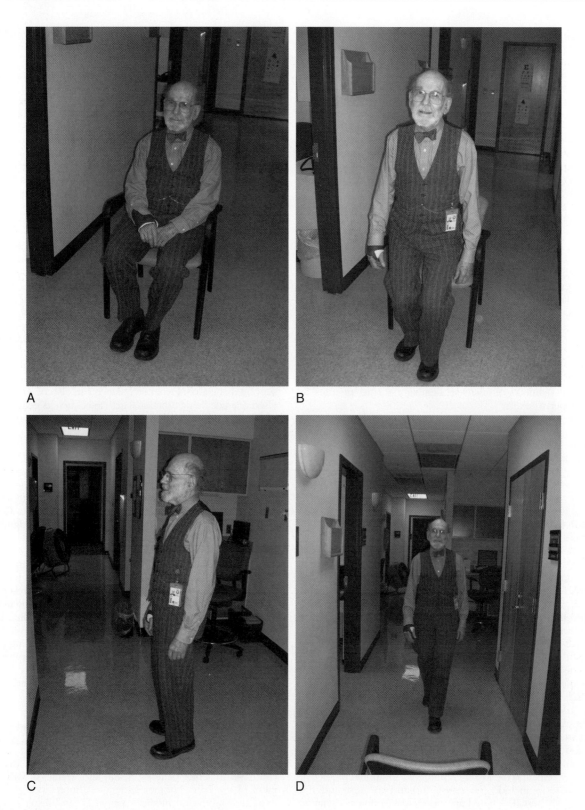

Figure App-IV.3 *A through D,* Timed up-and-go test. The doctor measures the time that it takes for the patient to rise from a chair, walk 10 feet, turn around, walk back, and sit down again. If this time is more than 15 seconds, the patient is at an increased risk for falls. This test is also an excellent tool for evaluating other aspects of geriatric physical function. Special attention should be paid to multiple versus single attempts to get out of the chair; the need to push up out of the chair with the arms; immediate balance on standing; gait (stance, path, swing, step width); turning balance; and controlled seating versus crashing into the seat.

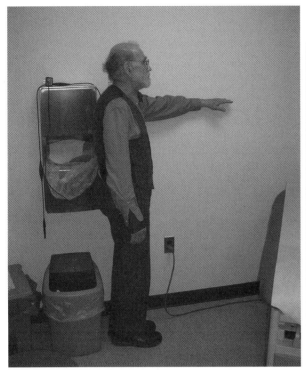

A

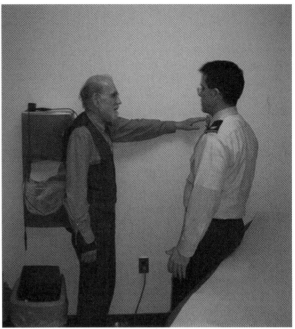

B

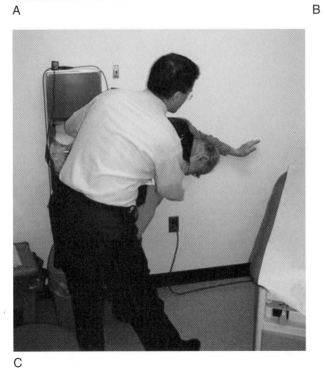

C

Figure App-IV.4 The standing reach test. *A,* The patient stands against the wall with an arm outstretched and the feet comfortably together. *B,* The physician stands close to the patient (in case of surprises) and marks on the wall the furthest extent of the patient's hand. *C,* The patient is instructed with a statement similar to the following: "Bend forward at the waist as far as you can without falling or shifting your feet. I will not let you fall." The patient bends forward and a second mark is made at the farthest reach of the fingers. The distance between the patient's standing reach mark and their bending-forward reach mark should be greater than 6 inches.

her life and the role that exercise can play in promoting wellness and independence. Confidence is built to initiate or maintain exercise by the therapeutic relationship, and the communication between the patient and the physician promotes progress and reduces barriers (friction) to exercise. The collaborative plan for exercise via the exercise prescription readies the patient for changes in exercise and activity.

There are few absolute contraindications to exercise and enhanced physical activity. However, a multitude of barriers and limitations to exercise and activity can come from a variety of intrinsic (i.e., patient) and extrinsic (e.g., environmental, social, financial) factors. Understanding these factors allows the physician to collaboratively tailor an exercise and lifestyle plan that is acceptable and attainable for the patient and that promotes health and wellness.

After assessing the patient's cardiorespiratory and musculoskeletal risks, the exercise prescription in the elderly patient involves the initiation of five different types (modes) of exercise: general activities, cardiopulmonary, strength, flexibility, and balance. The amount of exercise is quantified by advice regarding the duration, frequency, and intensity of the selected exercises and activities. Timely follow-up regarding the patient's compliance with the prescription along with the other ongoing medical issues allows the patient and the physician to chart progress and to make adjustments to continue the promotion of wellness and functionality in the elderly patient.

REFERENCES

1. Anderson RN, Smith BL: Deaths: Leading Causes for 2002. National Center for Health Statistics. Vital Health Statistics Series 2002:53(17).

2. Lerner D, Kannel WB: Patterns of coronary heart disease morbidity and mortality in the sexes: a 26-year follow-up of the Framingham population. Am Heart J 1986;111:383-390.

3. Moore MJ, Moir P, Patrick MM. The state of aging and health in America 2004. CDC. National Center for Health Statistics, National Health Interview Survey, 2001. Available at http://0-www.cdc.gov.mill1.sjlibrary.org/nchs/data/factsheets/aging-factsheet.pdf. Accessed September 9, 2007.

4. Arno PS: Well being of caregivers: The economic issues of caregivers. In McRae T (chair): New Caregiver Research. Symposium conducted at the annual meeting of the American Association of Geriatric Psychiatry. Orlando, FL, data from 1987/1988 National Survey of Families and Households (NSFH), 2002.

5. Schwartz RS, Kohrt WM: Exercise in elderly people: physiologic and functional effects. In Hazzard WR, Blass JP, Halter JB, et al (eds): Principles of Geriatric Medicine and Gerontology, 5th. New York, McGraw-Hill, 2003, pp 931-946.

6. Buchner DM, Larson EB, Wagner EH, et al: Evidence for a non-linear relationship between leg strength and gait speed. Age Ageing 1996;25(5):386-391.

7. Rollnick S, Mason P, Butler C. Health Behavior Change: A Guide for Practitioners. New York, Churchill Livingstone, 1999, pp 225.

8. DiClemente CC, Prochaska J: Toward a comprehensive, transtheoretical model of change: Stages of change and addictive behaviors. In Miller WR, Heather N (eds): Treating Addictive Behaviors, 2nd. New York, Plenum, 1998.

9. ACSM's Guidelines for Exercise Testing and Prescription, 7th ed. Philadelphia, Lippincott Williams & Wilkins, 2006.

10. Gill TM, DiPietro L, Krumholz HM: Role of exercise stress testing and safety monitoring for older persons starting an exercise program. JAMA 2000;284(3):342-349.

11. Brennan F: Exercise prescriptions for active seniors. Phys Sportsmed 2002;30(2):19-30.

12. Nelson ME, Rjeski WJ, Blair SN, et al: Physical activity and public health in older adults: Recommendation from the American College of Sports Medicine and the American Heart Association. Med Sci Sports Exerc 2007;39(8):1435.

Index

Page numbers followed by f refer to figures; those followed by t refer to tables; and those followed by b refer to boxed material.